Management of Hematologic Malignancies

Management of Hematologic Malignancies

Edited by

Susan M. O'Brien
The University of Texas MD Anderson Cancer Center, USA

Julie M. Vose
The University of Nebraska Medical Center, USA

Hagop M. Kantarjian
The University of Texas MD Anderson Cancer Center, USA

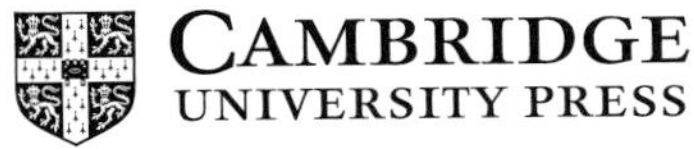

CAMBRIDGE UNIVERSITY PRESS
Cambridge, New York, Melbourne, Madrid, Cape Town, Singapore,
São Paulo, Delhi, Dubai, Tokyo, Mexico City

Cambridge University Press
The Edinburgh Building, Cambridge CB2 8RU, UK

Published in the United States of America by
Cambridge University Press, New York

www.cambridge.org
Information on this title: www.cambridge.org/9780521896405

First published 2011

Printed in the United Kingdom at the University Press, Cambridge

A catalog record for this publication is available from the British Library

Library of Congress Cataloging-in-Publication Data

Management of hematologic malignancies / edited by Susan O'Brien, Julie M. Vose,
Hagop M. Kantarjian.
p. ; cm.
Includes bibliographical references and index.
ISBN 978-0-521-89640-5 (hardback)
1. Lymphoproliferative disorders. 2. Lymphoproliferative disorders–
Treatment. I. O'Brien, Susan, 1954– II. Vose, Julie M. III. Kantarjian,
Hagop, 1952– IV. Title.
[DNLM: 1. Hematologic Neoplasms–diagnosis. 2. Hematologic Neoplasms–
therapy. WH 525 M2657 2010]
RC646.2.M35 2010
616.99′418–dc22

2010022725

ISBN 978-0-521-89640-5 Hardback

Contents

List of contributors vi

1. **Molecular pathology of leukemia** 1
Maher Albitar and Amber Donahue

2. **Management of acute myeloid leukemia** 26
Alan K. Burnett

3. **Treatment of acute lymphoblastic leukemia (ALL) in adults** 43
Ryan Mattison, Sarah Larson, and Wendy Stock

4. **Chronic myeloid leukemia** 68
Elias Jabbour, Hagop M. Kantarjian, and Jorge E. Cortés

5. **Chronic lymphocytic leukemia/small lymphocytic lymphoma** 81
Karen W. L. Yee and Susan M. O'Brien

6. **Myelodysplastic syndromes (MDS)** 103
Stefan H. Faderl, Guillermo Garcia-Manero, and Hagop M. Kantarjian

7. **Hairy cell leukemia** 116
Darren S. Sigal and Alan Saven

8. **Acute promyelocytic leukemia: pathophysiology and clinical results update** 131
Francesco Lo-Coco, Massimo Breccia, and Syed Khizer Hasan

9. **Myeloproliferative neoplasms** 141
Ayalew Tefferi

10. **Monoclonal gammopathy of undetermined significance, smoldering multiple myeloma, and multiple myeloma** 155
S. Vincent Rajkumar and Suzanne R. Hayman

11. **Amyloidosis and other rare plasma cell dyscrasias** 184
Angela Dispenzieri and Suzanne R. Hayman

12. **Waldenstrom's macroglobulinemia/ lymphoplasmacytic lymphoma** 207
Steven P. Treon and Giampaolo Merlini

13. **WHO classification of lymphomas** 228
William W. L. Choi and Wing C. Chan

14. **Molecular pathology of lymphoma** 257
David J. Good and Randy D. Gascoyne

15. **International staging and response criteria for lymphomas** 277
Bruce D. Cheson

16. **Treatment approach to diffuse large B-cell lymphomas** 286
Sonali M. Smith and Julie M. Vose

17. **Mantle cell lymphoma** 308
Andre Goy

18. **Follicular lymphomas** 338
Francisco J. Hernandez-Ilizaliturri and Myron S. Czuczman

19. **Hodgkin lymphoma: epidemiology, diagnosis, and treatment** 367
Andrew M. Evens and Sandra J. Horning

20. **Treatment approaches to MALT/marginal zone lymphoma** 404
Stephanie A. Gregory and Parameswaran Venugopal

21. **Peripheral T-cell lymphomas** 410
Matthew J. Matasar and Steven M. Horwitz

22. **Mycosis fungoides and Sézary syndrome** 432
Christiane Querfeld and Steven T. Rosen

23. **Central nervous system lymphoma** 449
Elizabeth R. Gerstner and Tracy T. Batchelor

24. **HIV-related lymphomas** 462
Caroline M. Behler and Lawrence D. Kaplan

25. **Lymphoblastic lymphoma** 487
Anuj Mahindra and John W. Sweetenham

26. **Burkitt lymphoma** 494
Julie M. Vose

Index 503

Contributors

Maher Albitar MD
Hematopathology and Oncology Department,
Quest Diagnostics Nichols Institute,
San Juan Capistrano, CA, USA

Tracy T. Batchelor MD
The Stephen E. and Catherine Pappas Center for Neuro-Oncology,
Massachusetts General Hospital Cancer Center,
Boston, MA, USA

Caroline M. Behler MD MS
San Francisco Veterans Affairs Medical Center, 4150 Clement Street, 111H1, San Francisco, CA, USA

Massimo Breccia MD
Department of Biotechnologies and Cellular Hematology,
Sapienza University, Rome, Italy

Alan K. Burnett MBChB MD
Department of Haematology, University of Wales College of Medicine, Cardiff, UK

Wing C. Chan MD
Center for Lymphoma and Leukemia Research, Department of Pathology, Nebraska Medical Center, Omaha, NE, USA

Bruce D. Cheson MD
Georgetown University Hospital, Lombardi Comprehensive Cancer Center, Washington DC, USA

William W. L. Choi MBBS MRCP DABPath
Department of Pathology, University of Hong Kong,
Queen Mary Hospital, Hong Kong

Jorge E. Cortés MD
Department of Leukemia, The University of Texas
MD Anderson Cancer Center, Houston, TX, USA

Myron S. Czuczman MD
Departments of Medicine and Immunology,
Roswell Park Institute, Buffalo, NY, USA

Angela Dispenzieri MD
Mayo Clinic College of Medicine, Division of Hematology,
Mayo Clinic, Rochester, MN, USA

Amber Donahue PhD
Hematopathology and Oncology Department,
Quest Diagnostics Nichols Institute,
San Juan Capistrano, CA, USA

Andrew M. Evens DO MSc
Division of Hematology/Oncology, Northwestern University Feinberg School of Medicine, Chicago, IL, USA

Stefan H. Faderl MD
Department of Leukemia, The University of Texas
MD Anderson Cancer Center, Houston, TX, USA

Guillermo Garcia-Manero MD
Department of Leukemia, The University of Texas
MD Anderson Cancer Center, Houston, TX, USA

Randy D. Gascoyne MD FRCPC
Department of Pathology and Laboratory Medicine, British Columbia Cancer Agency, Vancouver, BC, Canada

Elizabeth R. Gerstner MD
The Stephen E. and Catherine Pappas Center for
Neuro-Oncology, Massachusetts General Hospital Cancer Center,
Boston, MA, USA

David J. Good MD FRCPC
Department of Pathology and Laboratory Medicine, British Columbia Cancer Agency, Vancouver, BC, Canada

Andre Goy MD
The John Theurer Cancer Center, Hackensack University Medical Center, NJ, USA

Stephanie A. Gregory MD
Department of Hematology, Rush University Medical Center, Chicago, IL, USA

Suzanne R. Hayman MD
Mayo Clinic College of Medicine, Division of Hematology,
Mayo Clinic, Rochester, MN, USA

Francisco J. Hernandez-Ilizaliturri MD
Departments of Medicine and Immunology, Roswell Park Institute, Buffalo, NY, USA

Sandra J. Horning MD
Stanford University School of Medicine, Stanford, CA, USA

Steven M. Horwitz MD
Department of Medicine, Lymphoma Service, Memorial Sloan-Kettering Cancer Center, New York, NY, USA

Elias Jabbour MD
Department of Leukemia, The University of Texas MD Anderson Cancer Center, Houston, TX, USA

Hagop M. Kantarjian MD
Department of Leukemia, The University of Texas MD Anderson Cancer Center, Houston, TX, USA

Lawrence D. Kaplan MD
Division of Hematology/Oncology, University of California San Francisco, CA, USA

Syed Khizer Hasan MD
Department of Biopathology, University Tor Vergata, Rome, Italy

Sarah Larson MD
Section of Hematology-Oncology, Department of Medicine, University of Chicago Medical Center, Chicago, IL, USA

Francesco Lo-Coco MD
Department of Biopathology, University Tor Vergata, Rome, Italy

Anuj Mahindra MD
Hematology and Medical Oncology, Taussig Cancer Institute, Cleveland Clinic, Cleveland, OH, USA

Matthew J. Matasar MD
Department of Medicine, Lymphoma Service and Hematology Service, Memorial Sloan-Kettering Cancer Center, New York, NY, USA

Ryan Mattison MD
Division of Hematology/Oncology, School of Medicine and Public Health, University of Wisconsin, Madison, WI, USA

Giampaolo Merlini MD
Department of Biochemistry at the University of Pavia and Biotechnology Research Laboratories, University Hospital Policlinico San Matteo, Pavia, Italy

Susan M. O'Brien MD
Department of Leukemia, University of Texas MD Anderson Cancer Center, Houston, TX, USA

Christiane Querfeld MD PhD
Section of Dermatology, Department of Medicine, University of Chicago, Chicago, IL, USA

S. Vincent Rajkumar MD
Mayo Clinic College of Medicine, Division of Hematology, Mayo Clinic, Rochester, MN, USA

Steven T. Rosen MD FACP
Robert H. Lurie Comprehensive Cancer Center, Northwestern University, Chicago, IL, USA

Alan Saven MD
Division of Hematology/Oncology, and Ida M. and Cecil H. Green Cancer Center, Scripps Clinic, La Jolla, CA, USA

Darren S. Sigal MD
Division of Hematology/Oncology, Scripps Clinic, La Jolla, CA, USA

Sonali M. Smith MD
The University of Chicago, Chicago, IL, USA

Wendy Stock MD
Section of Hematology-Oncology, Department of Medicine, University of Chicago Medical Center, Chicago, IL, USA

John W. Sweetenham MD
Taussig Cancer Institute, Cleveland Clinic, Cleveland, OH, USA

Ayalew Tefferi MD
Division of Hematology, Department of Medicine, Mayo Clinic, Rochester, MN, USA

Steven P. Treon MD PhD
Bing Center for Waldenstrom's Macroglobulinemia, Dana-Farber Cancer Institute, Harvard Medical School, Boston, MA, USA

Parameswaran Venugopal MD
Department of Internal Medicine, Rush University Medical Center, Chicago, IL, USA

Julie M. Vose MD
Section of Hematology/Oncology, Nebraska Medical Center, Omaha, NE, USA

Karen W. L. Yee MD
Department of Medical Oncology and Hematology, Princess Margaret Hospital, Toronto, ON, Canada

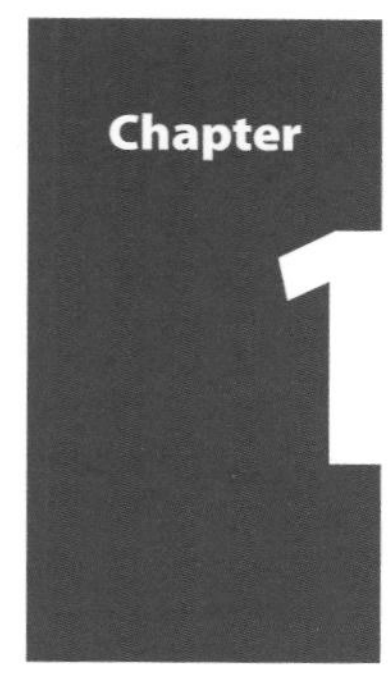

Molecular pathology of leukemia

Maher Albitar and Amber Donahue

Introduction

Most of the current knowledge of the molecular basis of leukemias indicates that leukemias are heterogeneous groups of neoplasms. Even when the clinical and phenotypic presentations are similar, biologically the leukemias may differ, and molecular characterization of the individual leukemia is therefore essential for predicting prognosis and determining therapeutic approaches. This observation is not only relevant to leukemias, but is true of the complexity of cancer in general.

With the recent advances in targeted therapy, and the ability to develop more specific inhibitors which target a specific pathway, precise understanding of the molecular abnormalities in a specific leukemia is becoming more crucial. It is widely accepted at this time that leukemia is a disease of hematopoietic cells, occurring when these cells become capable of independent self-renewal irrespective of physiologic needs. Most leukemic processes are believed to be initiated at the level of stem cells.[1] The definition of stem cells varies, however, dependent on the stage of differentiation. For example, it is believed that in some diseases, particularly chronic leukemias, the leukemic process is initiated at the stem cell level, but that the cells manage to differentiate to a certain extent, allowing the disease to manifest as a chronic leukemic process of the mature cells.[2] While some leukemias are characterized and defined by a specific molecular abnormality, considered the hallmark of the disease, most investigators believe that additional molecular abnormalities must accumulate for the disease to manifest itself, or progress to acute disease.[3] Therefore collaboration between two or more molecular abnormalities is likely to be common in leukemias.

Here we will review the basic molecular abnormalities detected in patients with leukemias, then discuss specifically the most common leukemias. It should be emphasized that most of the genes targeted in these malignancies could be altered through multiple mechanisms. The same gene could become abnormal through amplification and thus display increased expression in one patient, or become abnormal through a point mutation and exhibit increased activity in another patient. It is also possible for the gene to sustain a point mutation and be amplified in the same patient. For this reason, it is imperative to determine the molecular signature of each malignancy.

Chromosomal translocations

More chromosomal translocations have been reported in leukemia than in any other cancer. The reason for this is unknown. These translocations frequently lead to the expression of a fusion protein, although some translocations have been found to contribute to the deregulation of an oncogene without changing its protein product. Most of the translocations in a given disease involve a specific gene, but the partner gene may differ. In addition, some of the translocation can be on the same chromosome, manifesting as an inversion. The list of translocations reported in various types of leukemias is given in Table 1.1.

Gene mutations

Numerous pivotal mutations have been reported in various genes in specific diseases. Many mutations can be seen in the primary tumor, but certain others are seen as disease progresses, or as the tumor develops resistance to therapy. Most mutations lead to the constitutive activation of specific oncogenes, but it has recently been discovered that, following the use of targeted therapy, some mutations render tumor cells resistant to the targeting agent by altering the structure of the protein. This structural change prevents the binding of the targeting agent, and thus avoids the inactivation of the targeted protein.[4,5] Other recently described mutations include the expression of alternative splicing transcripts which may change the reading frame used for translation, and thus express a protein that is functionally different from the original protein. The list of genes found to be mutated in leukemias is shown in Table 1.2.

Management of Hematologic Malignancies, ed. Susan M. O'Brien, Julie M. Vose, and Hagop M. Kantarjian. Published by Cambridge University Press.

Table 1.1. Translocations reported in leukemias

Cytogenetic data	Chromosome band	Symbol	Names of genes
T-ALL			
t(1;3)(p32;p21)	1p32; 3p21[a]	TAL1-TCTA[b]	T-cell acute lymphocytic leukemia 1 (SCL, TCL5)[c]; T-cell leukemia translocation altered gene
t(1;5)(p32;q31)	1p32; 5q31	TAL1-??	T-cell acute lymphocytic leukemia 1 (SCL, TCL5); ??
t(1;7)(p32;q34)	1p32; 7q35[c]	TAL1-TRB	T-cell acute lymphocytic leukemia 1 (SCL, TCL5); T-cell receptor beta locus (TCRB)
t(1;7)(p34;q34)	1p35-p34.3; 7q35	LCK-TRB	lymphocyte-specific protein tyrosine kinase; T-cell receptor beta locus (TCRB)
t(1;14)(p32;q11)	1p32; 14q11.2	TAL1-TRA/TRD	T-cell acute lymphocytic leukemia 1 (SCL, TCL5); T-cell receptor alpha locus/T-cell receptor delta locus
t(1;19)(q23;p13)	1q23; 19p13	PBX1-TCF3	pre-B-cell leukemia transcription factor 1; transcription factor 3 (E2A immunoglobulin enhancer binding factors E12/E47)
t(2;14)(p13;q32)	2p13; 14q32.33	BCL11A-IGH	B-cell CLL/lymphoma 11A; immunoglobulin heavy locus
t(3;11)(q29;p15)	3q29; 11p15.5	IQCG-NUP98	IQ motif containing G; nucleoporin 98 kDa
t(4;11)(q21;p15)	4q21-q25; 11p15.5	RAP1GDS1-NUP98	RAP1, GTP-GDP dissociation stimulator 1; nucleoporin 98 kDa
t(4;11)(q21;q23)	4q21; 11q23	AFF1-MLL	AF4/FMR2 family, member 1 (AF4); myeloid/lymphoid or mixed-lineage leukemia (trithorax homolog, *Drosophila*)
t(4;21)(q31;q22)	4q31.1; 21q22.3	SH3D19-CBFA2	SH3 domain containing 19 (EBP, EVE1); runt-related transcription factor 1 (AML1, RUNX1)
t(5;14)(q35;q32)	5q35.1; 14q32.2	TLX3-BCL11B	T-cell leukemia, homeobox 3 (HOX11L2); B-cell CLL/lymphoma 11B
t(5;14)(q35;q32.2)	5q35.1; 14q32.2	TLX3-BCL11B	T-cell leukemia, homeobox 3 (HOX11L2); B-cell CLL/lymphoma 11B
t(5;14)(q35;q32.2)	5q35.2; 14q32.2	NKX2-5-BCL11B	NK2 transcription factor related, locus 5 (*Drosophila*); B-cell CLL/lymphoma 11B
t(5;17)(q13;q21)	5q13; 17q21	??	??
t(6;7)(q23;q34)	6q23.3; 7q35	MYB-TRB	v-myb myeloblastosis viral oncogene homolog (avian) (c-Myb); T-cell receptor beta locus (TCRB)
t(6;7)(q23;q34)	6q23.3; 7q35	AHI1-TRB	Abelson helper integration site 1 (AHI-1); T-cell receptor beta locus (TCRB)
t(6;11)(q27;q23)	6q27; 11q23	MLLT4-MLL	myeloid/lymphoid or mixed-lineage leukemia (trithorax homolog, *Drosophila*); translocated to, 4 (AF6); myeloid/lymphoid or mixed-lineage leukemia (trithorax homolog, *Drosophila*)
t(7;7)(p15;q34); inv(7)(p15q34)	7p15-p14; 7q35	HOXA10-TRB	homeobox A10 (HOX1, HOX1H); T-cell receptor beta locus (TCRB)
t(7;9)(q34;q32)	7q35; 9q32	TRB-TAL2	T-cell receptor beta locus (TCRB); T-cell acute lymphocytic leukemia 2
t(7;9)(q34;q34)	7q35; 9q34.3	TRB-NOTCH1	T-cell receptor beta locus (TCRB); Notch homolog 1, translocation-associated (*Drosophila*) (TAN1)
t(7;10)(q34;q24)	7q35; 10q24	TRB-TLX1	T-cell receptor beta locus (TCRB); T-cell leukemia, homeobox 1 (HOX11)
t(7;11)(q35;p13)	7q35; 11p13	TRB-LMO2	T-cell receptor beta locus (TCRB); LIM domain only 2 (rhombotin-like 1) (RBTN2)
t(7;12)(q34;p13)	7q35; 12p13	TRB-CCND2	T-cell receptor beta locus (TCRB); cyclin D2

Table 1.1. *(cont.)*

Cytogenetic data	Chromosome band	Symbol	Names of genes
t(7;14)(p15;q11-q11.2)	7p15-p14; 14q11.2	HOXA6/ HOXA7-TRD	homeobox A6/A7; T-cell receptor delta locus
t(7;14)(q35;q32.1)	7q34; 14q32.1	TBR-TCL1A	T-cell receptor beta locus (TCRB); T-cell leukemia/lymphoma 1A
t(7;19)(q34;p13)	7q34; 19p13.2	TBR-LYL1	T-cell receptor beta locus (TCRB); lymphoblastic leukemia derived sequence 1
t(8;9)(p22;p24)	8p22-p21.3; 9p24	PCM1-JAK2	pericentriolar material 1 (PTC4); Janus kinase 2
t(8;14)(q24;q11)	8q24.21; 14q11.2	C-MYC-TRA/TRD	v-myc myelocytomatosis viral oncogene homolog (avian) (c-Myc); T-cell receptor alpha locus/T-cell receptor delta locus
t(8;21)(q24;q22)	8q24.12; 21q22	TRPS1-CBFA2	trichorhinophalangeal syndrome I (LGCR); runt-related transcription factor 1 (AML1, RUNX1)
t(9;12)(p24;p13)	9p24; 12p13	JAK2-ETV6	Janus kinase 2; ets variant gene 6 (TEL oncogene)
dic(9;12)(p13;p13)	9p13; 12p13	PAX5-ETV6	paired box gene 5 (B-cell lineage-specific activator protein); ets variant gene 6 (TEL oncogene)
t(9;14)(q34;q32)	9q34.1; 14q32	ABL1-EML1	v-abl Abelson murine leukemia viral oncogene homolog 1; echinoderm microtubule associated protein like 1 (EMAP)
t(9;22)(q34;q11)	9q34.1; 22q11.21	ABL1-BCR1	v-abl Abelson murine leukemia viral oncogene homolog 1; breakpoint cluster region
t(10;11)(p13;q21)	10p12; 11q14-q21	MLLT10-PICALM	myeloid/lymphoid or mixed-lineage leukemia (trithorax homolog, *Drosophila*); translocated to, 10 (AF10); phosphatidylinositol binding clathrin assembly protein (CALM)
t(10;11)(q25;p15)	10q24.2-q24.3; 11p15.5	ADD3-NUP98	adducin 3 (gamma) (ADDL); nucleoporin 98 kDa
t(10;14)(q24;q11)	10q24; 14q11.2	TLX1-TRD	T-cell leukemia, homeobox 1 (HOX11); T-cell receptor delta locus
t(11;14)(p13;q11)	11p13; 14q11.2	LMO2-TRA/TRD	LIM domain only 2 (rhombotin-like 1) (RBTN2); T-cell receptor alpha locus/T-cell receptor delta locus
t(11;14)(p15;q11)	11p15.5; 14q11.2	LMO1-TRA/TRD	LIM domain only 1 (rhombotin 1); T-cell receptor alpha locus/T-cell receptor delta locus
t(11;19)(q23;p13.3)	11q23; 19p13.3	MLL-MLLT1	myeloid/lymphoid or mixed-lineage leukemia (trithorax homolog, *Drosophila*); myeloid/lymphoid or mixed-lineage leukemia (trithorax homolog, *Drosophila*); translocated to, 1 (ENL)
t(12;13)(p12;q12-q14)	12p13; 13q12.3	ETV6-CDX2	ets variant gene 6 (TEL oncogene); caudal type homeobox transcription factor 2 (CDX3)
t(12;14)(p13;q11)	12p13; 14q11.2	CCND2-TRA/TRD	cyclin D2; T-cell receptor alpha locus/T-cell receptor delta locus
t(14;14)(q11;q32.1)	14q11.2; 14q32.1	TRA/TRD-TCL1A	T-cell receptor alpha locus/T-cell receptor delta locus; T-cell leukemia/lymphoma 1A
t(14;21)(q11;q22)	14q11.2; 21q22.11	TRA-OLIG2	T-cell receptor alpha locus; oligodendrocyte lineage transcription factor 2 (BHLHB1)
t(X;11)(q13;q23)	Xq13.1; 11q23	MLLT7-MLL	myeloid/lymphoid or mixed-lineage leukemia (trithorax homolog, *Drosophila*); translocated to, 7 (AFX1); myeloid/ lymphoid or mixed-lineage leukemia (trithorax homolog, *Drosophila*)
B-ALL			
t(1;2)(q12;q37)	1q12; 2q37	??	??
t(1;3)(p36;p21)	1p36.23-p33	??	??

Table 1.1. *(cont.)*

Cytogenetic data	Chromosome band	Symbol	Names of genes
t(1;5)(q22;q33)	1q12; 5q31-q32	PDE4DIP-PDGFRB	phosphodiesterase 4D interacting protein (myomegalin); platelet-derived growth factor receptor, beta polypeptide
t(1;9)(q24;q34)	1q22-q24; 9q34.1	RCSD1-ABL1	RCSD domain containing 1 (MK2S4, CAPZIP); v-abl Abelson murine leukemia viral oncogene homolog 1
t(1;14)(q21;q32)	1q21; 14q32.33	BCL9-IGH	B-cell CLL/lymphoma 9; immunoglobulin heavy locus
t(1;14)(q25;q32)	1q25.2; 14q32.33	LHX4-IGH	LIM homeobox 4 (Gsh4); immunoglobulin heavy locus
t(1;18)(q25;q23)	1q25; 18q23	??	??
t(1;19)(q23;p13)	1q23; 19p13	PBX1-TCF3	pre-B-cell leukemia transcription factor 1; transcription factor 3 (E2A immunoglobulin enhancer binding factors E12/E47)
t(1;22)(q21;q11)	1q21; 22q11.1-q11.2	BCL9-IGL	B-cell CLL/lymphoma 9; immunoglobulin lambda locus
t(2;8)(p12;q24)	2p12; 8q24.21	MYC-IGK	v-myc myelocytomatosis viral oncogene homolog (avian) (c-Myc); immunoglobulin kappa locus
t(2;9)(p11;p13)	2p11; 9p13	??-PAX5	??; paired box gene 5 (B-cell lineage-specific activator protein)
t(2;11)(p21;q23)	2p21; 11q23	??-MLL	??; myeloid/lymphoid or mixed-lineage leukemia (trithorax homolog, *Drosophila*)
AML			
t(1;2)(q12;q37)	1q12; 2q37	??	??
t(1;3)(p36;p21)	1p36; 3p21	??	??
t(1;3)(p36;q21)	1p36.23-p33; 3q21.3	PRDM16-RPN1	PR domain containing 16; ribophorin I (RBPH1)
t(1;7)(p36;q34)	1p36; 7q34	??	??
t(1;7)(q10;p10)	1q10; 7p10	??	??
t(1;8)(p22-p32;q22-q23)	1p22-p32; 8q22-q23	??	??
t(1;11)(q21;q23)	1q21; 11q23	AF1Q-MLL	ALL1-fused gene from chromosome 1q; myeloid/lymphoid or mixed-lineage leukemia (trithorax homolog, *Drosophila*)
t(1;12)(q21;q24)	1q21; 12q24	??	??
t(1;12)(q25;p13)	1q24-q25; 12p13	ABL2-ETV6	v-abl Abelson murine leukemia viral oncogene homolog 2; ets variant gene 6 (TEL oncogene)
t(1;14)(q25;q32)	1q25.2; 14q32.33	LHX4-IGH	LIM homeobox 4 (Gsh4); immunoglobulin heavy locus
dic(1;15)(p11;p11)	1p11; 15p11	??	??
t(1;16)(q12;q24)	1q12; 16q24	??	??
t(1;18)(q25;q23)	1q25; 18q23	??	??
t(1;19)(p13;p13.1)	1p13; 19p13.1	??	??
t(1;19)(q23;p13)	1q23; 19p13	PBX1-TCF3	pre-B-cell leukemia transcription factor 1; transcription factor 3 (E2A immunoglobulin enhancer binding factors E12/E47)
t(1;21)(p32;q22)	1p32; 21q22.3	??-CBFA2	??; runt-related transcription factor 1 (AML1, RUNX1)
t(1;21)(p35;q22)	1p35; 21q22.3	YTHDF2-CBFA2	YTH domain family member 2; runt-related transcription factor 1 (AML1, RUNX1)
t(1;21)(p36;q22)	1p36.23-p33; 21q22.3	PRDM16-CBFA2	PR domain containing 16; ribophorin I (RBPH1); runt-related transcription factor 1 (AML1, RUNX1)
t(1;21)(q21;q22)	1q21; 21q22.3	ZNF687-CBFA2	zinc finger protein 687; runt-related transcription factor 1 (AML1, RUNX1)
t(1;22)(p13;q13)	1p13; 22q13	RBM15-MKL1	RNA binding motif protein 15 (OTT); megakaryoblastic leukemia (translocation) 1 (MAL)

Table 1.1. *(cont.)*

Cytogenetic data	Chromosome band	Symbol	Names of genes
t(2;3)(p15-p23;q26-q27)	2p15-p23; 3q24-q28	??-EVI1	??; ecotropic viral integration site 1
t(2;4)(p23;q25-q35)	2p23; 4q25-q35	??	??
t(2;11)(p21;q23)	2p21; 11q23	??-MLL	??; myeloid/lymphoid or mixed-lineage leukemia (trithorax homolog, *Drosophila*)
t(2;11)(q37;q23) in AML	2q37; 11q23	SEPT2-MLL	septin 2 (DIFF6, NEDD5, Pnutl3); myeloid/lymphoid or mixed-lineage leukemia (trithorax homolog, *Drosophila*)
t(2;19)(p11;p13)	2p11; 19p13	??	??
t(2;21)(p11;q22)	2p11; 21q22	??-CBFA2	??; runt-related transcription factor 1 (AML1, RUNX1)
ins(3;3)(q26;q21-q26); inv(3)(q21q26); t(3;3)(q21;q26)	3q21; 3q24-q28	RPN1-EVI1	ribophorin 1; ecotropic viral integration site 1
t(3;4)(p21;q34)	3p21; 4q34	??	??
t(3;5)(q25;q34)	3q25.1; 5q35	MLF1-NPM1	myeloid leukemia factor 1; nucleophosmin (nucleolar phosphoprotein B23, numatrin)
t(3;5)(q26;q34)	3q24-q28; 5q34	EVI1-??	ecotropic viral integration site 1; ??
t(3;6)(q25;q26)	3q24-q28; 6q26	EVI1-??	ecotropic viral integration site 1; ??
t(3;7)(q26;q21)	3q24-q28; 7q21-q22	EVI1-CDK6	ecotropic viral integration site 1; cyclin-dependent kinase 6
t(3;8)(q26;q24)	3q26; 8q24	EVI1/MDS1-PVT1/C-MYC	ecotropic viral integration site 1 OR myelodysplastic syndrome 1; Pvt1 oncogene OR MYC activator
t(3;12)(q26;p13)	3q26; 12p13	EVI1/MDS1-PVT1/C-MYC-ETV6	ecotropic viral integration site 1 OR myelodysplastic syndrome 1; ets variant gene 6 (TEL oncogene)
t(3;16)(q21;q22)	3q21; 16q22	??-CBFB	??; core binding factor, beta subunit
t(3;17)(q26;q22)	3q24-q28; 17q22	EVI1-??	ecotropic viral integration site 1; ??
t(3;21)(q26;q22)	3q24-q28; 21q22.3	EVI1-CBFA2	ecotropic viral integration site 1; runt-related transcription factor 1 (AML1, RUNX1)
t(4;5)(q31;q31)	4q31; 5q31	??	??
t(4;11)(q21;q23)	4q21; 11q23	AFF1-MLL	AF4/FMR2 family, member 1 (AF4); myeloid/lymphoid or mixed-lineage leukemia (trithorax homolog, *Drosophila*)
t(4;11)(q35;q23)	4q35.1; 11q23	SORBS2-MLL	sorbin and SH3 domain containing 2 (ARGBP2); myeloid/lymphoid or mixed-lineage leukemia (trithorax homolog, *Drosophila*)
t(4;12)(q11-q21;p13)	4q11-q12; 12p13	CHIC2-ETV6	cysteine-rich hydrophobic domain 2; ets variant gene 6 (TEL oncogene)
t(4;21)(q31;q22)	4q31.1; 21q22.3	SH3D19-CBFA2	SH3 domain containing 19 (EBP, EVE1); runt-related transcription factor 1 (AML1, RUNX1)
t(5;11)(q31;q23)	5q31; 11q23	GRAF-MLL	GTPase regulator associated with focal adhesion kinase pp125 (FAK); (ARHGAP26; Rho GTPase activating protein 26); myeloid/lymphoid or mixed-lineage leukemia (trithorax homolog, *Drosophila*)
t(5;11)(q35;p15.5)	5q35; 11p15.5	NSD1-NUP98	nuclear receptor binding SET domain protein 1; nucleoporin 98 kDa
t(5;12)(q31;p13) in MDS, AML and AEL	5q31; 12p13	FACL6-ETV6	fatty-acid-coenzyme A ligase, long-chain 6 (ACSL6); ets variant gene 6 (TEL oncogene)

Table 1.1. *(cont.)*

Cytogenetic data	Chromosome band	Symbol	Names of genes
t(5;14)(q33;q32) PDGFRB/TRIP11	5q31-q32; 14q31-q32	PDGFRB-TRIP11	platelet-derived growth factor receptor, beta polypeptide; thyroid hormone interactor receptor 11 (CEV14)
t(5;17)(q35;q21)	5q35; 17q21	NPM1-RARA	nucleophosmin (nucleolar phosphoprotein B23, numatrin); retinoic acid receptor, alpha
t(5;21)(q13;q22)	5q13; 21q22	??-CBFA2	??; runt-related transcription factor 1 (AML1, RUNX1)
t(6;9)(p23;q34)	6p23; 9q34	DEK-NUP214	DEK oncogene (DNA binding); nucleoporin 214 kDa (CAN)
t(6;11)(q13;q23)	6q13; 11q23	SMAP1-MLL	small ArfGAP1; myeloid/lymphoid or mixed-lineage leukemia (trithorax homolog, *Drosophila*)
t(6;11)(q15;q23)	6q15; 11q23	??-MLL	??; myeloid/lymphoid or mixed-lineage leukemia (trithorax homolog, *Drosophila*)
t(6;11)(q27;q23)	6q27; 11q23	MLLT4-MLL	myeloid/lymphoid or mixed-lineage leukemia (trithorax homolog, *Drosophila*); translocated to, 4 (AF6); myeloid/lymphoid or mixed-lineage leukemia (trithorax homolog, *Drosophila*)
t(6;14)(q25-27;q32)	6q25-q27; 14q32	??-BCL11B	??; B-cell CLL/lymphoma 11B (CTIP2)
t(7;8)(q34;p11)	7q32-q34; 8p11.2-p11.1	TIF1-FGFR1	transcriptional intermediary factor 1 (PTC6, TIF1A, TRIM24); fibroblast growth factor receptor 1
t(7;11)(p15;p15)	7p15-p14.2; 11p15	HOXA9-NUP98	homeobox A9; nucleoporin 98 kDa
t(7;12)(q36;p13)	7q36; 12p13	HLXB9-ETV6	homeobox HB9; ets variant gene 6 (TEL oncogene)
t(7;14)(q21;q13)	7q21; 14q13	??	??
t(7;14)(q22;q11)	7q22; 14q11	??	??
t(7;14)(q35;q32.1)	7q34; 14q32.1	TBR-TCL1A	T-cell receptor beta locus (TCRB); T-cell leukemia/lymphoma 1A
t(7;21)(p22;q22)	7p22.1; 21q22	USP42-CBFA2	ubiquitin-specific peptidase 42; runt-related transcription factor 1 (AML1, RUNX1)
inv(8)(p11q13)	8p11; 8q13.3	MYST3-NCOA2	MYST histone acetyltransferase (monocytic leukemia) 3 (MOZ); nuclear receptor coactivator 2
i(8)(q10)	i(8)(q10)	??	??
t(8;9)(p22;p24)	8p22-p21.3; 9p24	PCM1-JAK2	pericentriolar material 1 (PTC4); Janus kinase 2
t(8;11)(p11;p15)	8p11.2; 11p15.5	WHSC1L1-NUP98	Wolf-Hirschhorn syndrome candidate 1-like 1 (NSD3); nucleoporin 98 kDa
t(8;11)(p12;p15)	8p12; 11p15	??	??
t(8;12)(q12;p13)	8q12; 12p13	??	??
t(8;16)(p11;p13)	8p11; 16p3.3	MYST3-CREBBP	MYST histone acetyltransferase (monocytic leukemia) 3 (MOZ); CREB binding protein (CBP)
t(8;19)(p11;q13)	8p11; 19q13	MYST3-??	MYST histone acetyltransferase (monocytic leukemia) 3 (MOZ); ??
t(8;19)(p12;q13)	8p11.2-p11.1; 19q13	FGFR1-ERVK3	fibroblast growth factor receptor 1; endogenous retroviral sequence K(C4), 3 (HERV-K)
t(8;21)(q22;q22)	8q22; 21q22	CBFA2T1-CBFA2	core-binding factor, runt domain, alpha subunit 2; translocated to, 1 (ETO); runt-related transcription factor 1 (AML1, RUNX1)
t(8;21)(q24;q22)	8q24.12; 21q22	TRPS1-CBFA2	trichorhinophalangeal syndrome I (LGCR); runt-related transcription factor 1 (AML1, RUNX1)

Table 1.1. *(cont.)*

Cytogenetic data	Chromosome band	Symbol	Names of genes
t(8;22)(p11;q13)	8p11; 22q13.2	MYST3-EP300	MYST histone acetyltransferase (monocytic leukemia) 3 (MOZ); 300 kDa E1A-Binding protein gene (p300)
t(9;9)(q34;q34)	9q34; 9q34	SET-NUP214	SET translocation; nucleoporin 214 kDa (CAN)
t(9;11)(p22;p15)	9p22.3; 11p15	PSIP2-NUP98	PC4 and SFRS1 interacting protein 2 (LEDGF, PSIP1); nucleoporin 98 kDa
t(9;11)(p22;q23)	9p22; 11q23	MLLT3-MLL	myeloid/lymphoid or mixed-lineage leukemia (trithorax homolog, *Drosophila*); translocated to, 3 (AF9); myeloid/ lymphoid or mixed-lineage leukemia (trithorax homolog, *Drosophila*)
t(9;11)(q34;p15)	9q34.1; 11p15	PRRX2-NUP98	paired related homeobox 2 (PMX2, PRX2); nucleoporin 98 kDa
t(9;11)(q34;q23)	9q33.3; 11q23	AF9Q34-MLL	nGAP-like protein; myeloid/lymphoid or mixed-lineage leukemia (trithorax homolog, *Drosophila*)
t(9;11)(q34;q23)	9q34; 11q23	FNBP1-MLL	formin binding protein 1 (FBP17); myeloid/lymphoid or mixed-lineage leukemia (trithorax homolog, *Drosophila*)
t(9;12)(q34;p13)	9q34.1; 12p13	ABL1-ETV6	v-abl Abelson murine leukemia viral oncogene homolog 1; ets variant gene 6 (TEL oncogene)
t(9;21)(q34;q22)	9q34; 21q22	??-CBFA2	??; runt-related transcription factor 1 (AML1, RUNX1)
t(9;22)(q34;q11)	9q34.1; 22q11.21	ABL1-BCR	v-abl Abelson murine leukemia viral oncogene homolog 1; breakpoint cluster region
t(10;11)(p11.2;q23)	10p11.2; 11q23	ABI1-MLL	abl-interactor 1 (E3B1); myeloid/lymphoid or mixed-lineage leukemia (trithorax homolog, *Drosophila*)
t(10;11)(p12;q23)	10p12; 11q23	MLLT10; MLL	myeloid/lymphoid or mixed-lineage leukemia (trithorax homolog, *Drosophila*); translocated to, 10 (AF10); myeloid/ lymphoid or mixed-lineage leukemia (trithorax homolog, *Drosophila*)
t(10;11)(p13;q21)	10p12; 11q14-21	MLLT10-PICALM	myeloid/lymphoid or mixed-lineage leukemia (trithorax homolog, *Drosophila*); translocated to, 10 (AF10); phosphatidylinositol binding clathrin assembly protein (CALM)
t(10;11)(q22;q23)	10q21; 11q23	TET1-MLL	tet oncogene 1 (CXXC6); myeloid/lymphoid or mixed-lineage leukemia (trithorax homolog, *Drosophila*)
t(10;16)(q22;p13)	10q22; 16p13.3	MYST4-CREBBP	MYST histone acetyltransferase (monocytic leukemia) 4 (MORF); CREB binding protein (CBP)
inv(11)(p15q22); t(11;11)(p15;q22)	11p15.5; 11q22	NUP98-DDX10	nucleoporin 98 kDa; DEAD (Asp-Glu-Ala-Asp) box polypeptide 10
t(11;12)(p15;p13)	11p15.5; 12p11	NUP98-KDM5A	nucleoporin 98 kDa; lysine (K)-specific demethylase 5A (RBP2, RBBP2, JARID1A)
t(11;12)(q23;q13) (MLL/CIP29)	11q23; 12q13.2	MLL-SARNP	myeloid/lymphoid or mixed-lineage leukemia (trithorax homolog, *Drosophila*); SAP domain containing ribonucleoprotein (CIP29)
t(11;16)(q23;p13.3)	11q23; 16p13.3	MLL-CREBBP	myeloid/lymphoid or mixed-lineage leukemia (trithorax homolog, *Drosophila*); CREB binding protein (CBP)
t(11;17)(p15;p13)	11p15.5; 17p13.1	NUP98-PHF23	nucleoporin 98 kDa; PHD finger protein 23 (hJUNE-1b)
t(11;17)(q13;q21)	11q13; 17q21	NUMA1-RARA	nuclear mitotic apparatus protein 1; retinoic acid receptor, alpha
t(11;17)(q23;p13)	11q23; 17p13.1	MLL-GAS7	myeloid/lymphoid or mixed-lineage leukemia (trithorax homolog, *Drosophila*); growth arrest-specific 7

Table 1.1. *(cont.)*

Cytogenetic data	Chromosome band	Symbol	Names of genes
t(11;17)(q23;q12) MLL/RARα	11q23; 17q21	MLL-RARA	myeloid/lymphoid or mixed-lineage leukemia (trithorax homolog, *Drosophila*); retinoic acid receptor, alpha
t(11;17)(q23;q12-q21) MLL/AF17	11q23; 17q21	MLL-MLLT6	myeloid/lymphoid or mixed-lineage leukemia (trithorax homolog, *Drosophila*); myeloid/lymphoid or mixed-lineage leukemia (trithorax homolog, *Drosophila*); translocated to, 6 (AF17)
t(11;17)(q23;q12-q21) MLL/LASP1	11q23; 17q11-q21.3	MLL-LASP1	myeloid/lymphoid or mixed-lineage leukemia (trithorax homolog, *Drosophila*); LIM and SH3 protein 1
t(11;17)(q23;q21)	11q23.1; 17q21	ZNF145-RARA	zinc finger protein 145 (PLZF); retinoic acid receptor, alpha
t(11;17)(q23;q25)	11q23; 17q25	MLL-MSF	myeloid/lymphoid or mixed-lineage leukemia (trithorax homolog, *Drosophila*); MLL septin-like fusion
t(11;19)(q23;p13.1)	11q23; 19p13.1	MLL-ELL	myeloid/lymphoid or mixed-lineage leukemia (trithorax homolog, *Drosophila*); ELL gene (11-19 lysine-rich leukemia gene)
t(11;19)(q23;p13.3)	11q23; 19p13.3	MLL-MLLT1	myeloid/lymphoid or mixed-lineage leukemia (trithorax homolog, *Drosophila*); myeloid/lymphoid or mixed-lineage leukemia (trithorax homolog, *Drosophila*); translocated to, 1 (ENL)
t(11;20)(p15;q11)	11p15.5; 20q12-q13.1	NUP98-TOP1	nucleoporin 98 kDa; topoisomerase (DNA) I
t(11;22)(q23;q11.2)	11q23; 17q22-q23	MLL-SEPT4	myeloid/lymphoid or mixed-lineage leukemia (trithorax homolog, *Drosophila*); septin 4 (hCDCREL-2, SEP4)
t(12;13)(p12;q12-q14)	12p13; 13q12.3	ETV6-CDX2	ets variant gene 6 (TEL oncogene); caudal type homeobox transcription factor 2 (CDX3)
t(12;13)(p13;q12) ETV6/FLT3	12p13; 13q12	ETV6-FLT3	ets variant gene 6 (TEL oncogene); fms-related tyrosine kinase 3
t(12;13)(p13;q14)	12p13; 13q14.11	ETV6-TTL	ets variant gene 6 (TEL oncogene); twelve-thirteen translocation leukemia gene (LOC646982; FLJ21437)
t(12;15)(p13;q25)	12p13; 15q25	ETV6-NTRK3	ets variant gene 6 (TEL oncogene); neurotrophic tyrosine kinase receptor, type 3
t(12;17)(p11;q11)	12p11; 17q11	??	??
t(12;17)(p13;q11)	12p12; 17q11.1-q11.2	ZNF384-TAF15	zinc finger protein 384 (CIZ/NMP4); TAF15 RNA polymerase II
t(12;19)(q13;q13)	12q13; 19q13	??	??
t(12;21)(q12;q22)	12q12; 21q22	CPNE8-CBFA2	copine VIII; runt-related transcription factor 1 (AML1, RUNX1)
t(12;22)(p13;q11-q12)	12p13; 22q11	ETV6-MN1	ets variant gene 6 (TEL oncogene); meningioma (disrupted in balanced translocation) 1
t(12;22)(p13;q12)	12p12; 22q12	ZNF384-EWSR1	zinc finger protein 384 (CIZ/NMP4); Ewing sarcoma breakpoint region 1 (EWS)
inv(14)(q11q32.1); t(14;14)(q11;q32.1)	14q11.2; 14q32.1	TRA/TRD-TCL1A	T-cell receptor alpha locus/T-cell receptor delta locus; T-cell leukemia/lymphoma 1A
t(14;22)(q32;q11)	14q32.33; 22q11.1-q11.2	IGH-IGL	immunoglobulin heavy locus; immunoglobulin lambda locus
t(15;17)(q22;q21)	15q22; 17q21	PML-RARA	promyelocytic leukemia; retinoic acid receptor, alpha
inv(16)(p13q22); t(16;16)(p13;q22)	16p13; 16q22	MYH11-CBFB	myosin, heavy polypeptide 11, smooth muscle; core-binding factor, beta subunit
t(16;21)(p11;q22)	16p11.2; 21q22.3	FUS-ERG	fusion, derived from t(12;16) malignant liposarcoma; v-ets erythroblastosis virus E26 oncogene like (avian)

Table 1.1. *(cont.)*

Cytogenetic data	Chromosome band	Symbol	Names of genes
t(16;21)(q24;q22)	16q24; 21q22	CBFA2T3-CBFA2	core-binding factor, runt domain, alpha subunit 2; translocated to, 3 (MTG-16); runt-related transcription factor 1 (AML1, RUNX1)
dic(17;20)(p11.2;q11.2)	17p13; 20q11.2	TP53-??	tumor protein p53-??
t(17;17)(q21;q21)	17q11.2-17q21	STAT5B-RARA	signal transducer and activator of transcription 5B; retinoic acid receptor, alpha
t(17;21)(q11.2;q22)	17q11; 21q22	??-CBFA2	??-runt-related transcription factor 1 (AML1, RUNX1)
t(20;21)(q11;q22)	20q11; 21q22	??-CBFA2	??-runt-related transcription factor 1 (AML1, RUNX1)
t(20;21)(q13;q22)	20q13; 21q22	??-CBFA2	??-runt-related transcription factor 1 (AML1, RUNX1)
t(X;6)(p11;q23)	Xp10; 6q23	??	??
t(X;10)(p10;p10)	Xp10; 10p10	??	??
t(X;11)(q13;q23)	Xq13.1; 11q23	MLLT7-MLL	myeloid/lymphoid or mixed-lineage leukemia (trithorax homolog, *Drosophila*); translocated to, 7 (AFX1); myeloid/ lymphoid or mixed-lineage leukemia (trithorax homolog, *Drosophila*)
t(X;21)(p22;q22)	Xp22.11; 21q22	PRDX4-CBFA2	peroxiredoxin 4 (PRX-4); runt-related transcription factor 1 (AML1, RUNX1)
t(X;21)(q26;q22)	Xq26; 21q22.3	ELF4-ERG	E74-like factor 4 (ets domain transcription factor); v-ets erythroblastosis virus E26 oncogene like (avian)
t(Y;1)(q12;q12)	Yq12; 1q12	??	??
MDS			
t(1;3)(p36;q21)	1p36.23-p33; 3q21.3	PRDM16-RPN1	PR domain containing 16; ribophorin I (RBPH1)
t(1;3)(p36;p21)	1p36.23-p33; 3p21	??	??
t(1;6)(p36;p21)	1p36; 3p21	??	??
t(1;7)(q10;p10)	1q10; 7p10	??	??
t(1;12)(p36;p13)	1p36; 12p13	MDS2-ETV6	myelodysplastic syndrome 2; ets variant gene 6 (TEL oncogene)
dic(1;15)(p11;p11)	1p11; 15p11	??	??
t(1;16)(q11;q11)	1q11; 16q11	??	??
t(1;18)(q10;q10)	1q10; 18q10	??	??
t(1;19)(p13;p13.1)	1p13; 19p13.1	??	??
t(1;21)(p36;q22)	1p36.23-p33; 21q22.3	PRDM16-CBFA2	PR domain containing 16; ribophorin I (RBPH1); runt-related transcription factor 1 (AML1, RUNX1)
t(2;3)(p15-p23;q26-q27)	2p15-p23; 3q24-q28	??-EVI1	??; ecotropic viral integration site 1
t(2;4)(p23;q25-q35)	2p23; 4q25-q35	??	??
t(2;11)(p21;q23)	2p21; 11q23	??-MLL	??; myeloid/lymphoid or mixed-lineage leukemia (trithorax homolog, *Drosophila*)
t(2;12)(q31;p13)	2q31; 12p13	??-ETV6	??-ets variant gene 6 (TEL oncogene)
t(3;3)(p24;q26)	3p24; 3q24-q28	??-EVI1	??-ecotropic viral integration site 1
ins(3;3)(q26;q21q26); inv(3)(q21q26); t(3;3)(q21;q26)	3q21; 3q24-q28	RPN1-EVI1	ribophorin 1 (RBPH1); ecotropic viral integration site 1
t(3;4)(p21;q34)	3p21; 4q34	??	??

Table 1.1. *(cont.)*

Cytogenetic data	Chromosome band	Symbol	Names of genes
t(3;5)(q25;q34)	3q25.1; 5q35	MLF1-NPM1	myeloid leukemia factor 1; nucleophosmin (nucleolar phosphoprotein B23, numatrin)
t(3;8)(q26;q24)	3q26; 8q24	EVI1/MDS1-PVT1/C-MYC	ecotropic viral integration site 1 OR myelodysplastic syndrome 1; Pvt1 oncogene OR MYC activator
t(3;12)(q26;p13)	3q26; 12p13	EVI1/MDS1-PVT1/C-MYC-ETV6	ecotropic viral integration site 1 OR myelodysplastic syndrome 1; ets variant gene 6 (TEL oncogene)
t(3;16)(q21;q22)	3q21; 16q22	??-CBFB	??; core binding factor, beta subunit
t(3;18)(q26;q11)	3q24-q28; 18q11	EVI1-??	ecotropic viral integration site 1; ??
t(3;21)(q26;q22)	3q24-q28; 21q22.3	EVI1-CBFA2	ecotropic viral integration site 1; runt-related transcription factor 1 (AML1, RUNX1)
t(4;5)(q31;q31)	4q31; 5q31	??	??
t(4;11)(p12;q23)	4p12; 11q23	FRYL-MLL	FRY-like (KIAA0826, FLJ16177, furry homolog, *Drosophila*); myeloid/lymphoid or mixed-lineage leukemia (trithorax homolog, *Drosophila*)
t(4;17)(q12;q21)	4q12; 17q21	FIP1L1; RARA	FIP1 like 1 (*Saccharomyces cerevisiae*); retinoic acid receptor, alpha
t(5;7)(q33;q11)	5q31-q32; 7q11	PDGFRB-HIP1	platelet-derived growth factor receptor, beta polypeptide; huntingtin interacting protein 1
t(5;11)(q31;q23)	5q31; 11q23	GRAF-MLL	GTPase regulator associated with focal adhesion kinase pp125 (FAK); (ARHGAP26; Rho GTPase activating protein 26); myeloid/lymphoid or mixed-lineage leukemia (trithorax homolog, *Drosophila*)
t(5;12)(q31;p13) in MDS, AML and AEL	5q31; 12p13	FACL6-ETV6	fatty-acid-coenzyme A ligase, long-chain 6 (ACSL6); ets variant gene 6 (TEL oncogene)
t(5;12)(q33;p13)	5q31-q32; 12p13	PDGFRB-ETV6	platelet-derived growth factor receptor; ets variant gene 6 (TEL oncogene)
t(5;17)(q33;p11.2)	5q31-q32; 17p11.2	PDGFRB-HCMOGT-1	platelet-derived growth factor receptor, beta polypeptide; sperm antigen HCMOGT-1
t(5;17)(q33;p13)	5q31-q32; 17p13	PDGFRB-RAB5EP	platelet-derived growth factor receptor, beta polypeptide; rabaptin, RAB GTPase binding effector protein 1 (RABPT5)
t(5;21)(q13;q22)	5q13; 21q22	??-CBFA2	??; runt-related transcription factor 1 (AML1, RUNX1)
inv(6)(p15q13)	6p15; 6q13	??	??
inv(6)(p25q13)	6p25; 6q13	??	??
t(6;8)(q27;p12)	6q27; 8p11.2-p11.1	FGFR1OP-FGFR1	FGFR1 oncogene partner (FOP); fibroblast growth factor receptor 1
t(6;9)(p23;q34)	6p23; 9q34	DEK-NUP214	DEK oncogene (DNA binding); nucleoporin 214 kDa (CAN)
t(6;12)(p21;p13)	6p21; 12p13	CCND3-ETV6	cyclin D3; ets variant gene 6 (TEL oncogene)
t(6;21)(p22;q22)	6p22; 21q22	??-CBFA2	??; runt-related transcription factor 1 (AML1, RUNX1)
t(7;12)(p12;q13)	7p12; 12q15	??-HMGA2	??; high mobility group AT-hook 2 (HMGIC)
t(7;12)(q36;p13)	7q36; 12p13	HLXB9-ETV6	homeobox HB9; ets variant gene 6 (TEL oncogene)
t(8;9)(p22;p24)	8p22-p21.3; 9p24	PCM1-JAK2	pericentriolar material 1 (PTC4); Janus kinase 2
t(8;12)(q12;p13)	8q12; 12p13	??	??
t(8;12)(q22;q13)	8q22; 12q15	??-HMGA2	??; high mobility group AT-hook 2 (HMGIC)

Table 1.1. *(cont.)*

Cytogenetic data	Chromosome band	Symbol	Names of genes
t(8;13)(p12;q12)	8p11.2-p11.1; 13q11-q12	FGFR1-ZNF198	fibroblast growth factor receptor 1; zinc finger protein 198
t(8;21)(q23;q22)	8q23; 21q22	ZFPM2-CBFA2	zinc finger protein, multitype 2 (FOG2); runt-related transcription factor 1 (AML1, RUNX1)
t(9;12)(q22;p12)	9q22; 12p13	SYK-ETV6	spleen tyrosine kinase; ets variant gene 6 (TEL oncogene)
t(10;12)(q24;p13)	10q24.1-q25.1; 12p13	GOT1-ETV6	glutamic-oxaloacetic transaminase 1 (GIG18); ets variant gene 6 (TEL oncogene)
t(10;16)(q22;p13)	10q22; 16p13.3	MYST4-CREBBP	MYST histone acetyltransferase (monocytic leukemia) 4 (MORF); CREB binding protein (CBP)
t(11;11)(p15;q22)	11p15.5	NUP98	nucleoporin 98 kDa
inv(11)(p15q22)	11p15.5; 11q22	NUP98-DDX10	nucleoporin 98 kDa; DEAD (Asp-Glu-Ala-Asp) box polypeptide 10
t(11;16)(q23;p13.3)	11q23; 16p13.3	MLL-CREBBP	myeloid/lymphoid or mixed-lineage leukemia (trithorax homolog, *Drosophila*); CREB binding protein (CBP)
t(11;17)(q23;q25)	11q23; 17q25	MLL-MSF	myeloid/lymphoid or mixed-lineage leukemia (trithorax homolog, *Drosophila*); MLL septin-like fusion
t(11;20)(p15;q11)	11p15.5; 20q12-q13.1	NUP98-TOP1	nucleoporin 98 kDa; topoisomerase (DNA) I
t(12;12)(p13;q13)	12p13; 12q15	??-HMGA2	??-high mobility group AT-hook 2 (HMGIC)
t(12;13)(p12;q12-q14)	12p13; 13q12.3	ETV6-CDX2	ets variant gene 6 (TEL oncogene); caudal type homeobox transcription factor 2 (CDX3)
t(12;13)(p13;q12) ETV6/FLT3	12p13; 13q12	ETV6-FLT3	ets variant gene 6 (TEL oncogene); fms-related tyrosine kinase 3
t(12;13)(p13;q14)	12p13; 13q14.11	ETV6-TTL	ets variant gene 6 (TEL oncogene); twelve-thirteen translocation leukemia gene (LOC646982; FLJ21437)
t(12;14)(q13;q31)	12q15; 14q31	HMGA2-??	high mobility group AT-hook 2 (HMGIC); ??
t(12;17)(p13;p13)	12p13; 17p13.1-p12	ETV6-PER1	ets variant gene 6 (TEL oncogene); period homolog 1 (*Drosophila*)
t(12;20) (q15;q11.2)	12q15; 20q11.2	HMGA2-??	high mobility group AT-hook 2 (HMGIC); ??
t(12;22) (p13;q11-q12)	12p13; 22q11	ETV6-MN1	ets variant gene 6 (TEL oncogene); meningioma (disrupted in balanced translocation) 1
t(14;21)(q22;q22)	14q22; 21q22	??-CBFA2	??; runt-related transcription factor 1 (AML1, RUNX1)
t(15;21)(q22;q22)	15q22; 21q22	??-CBFA2	??; runt-related transcription factor 1 (AML1, RUNX1)
inv(16)(p13q22); t(16;16)(p13;q22)	16p13; 16q22	MYH11-CBFB	myosin, heavy polypeptide 11, smooth muscle; core-binding factor, beta subunit
t(16;21)(q24;q22)	16q24; 21q22	CBFA2T3-CBFA2	core-binding factor, runt domain, alpha subunit 2; translocated to, 3 (MTG-16); runt-related transcription factor 1 (AML1, RUNX1)
dic(17;20)(p11.2;q11.2)	17p13; 20q11.2	TP53-??	tumor protein p53-??
t(20;21)(q13;q22)	20q13; 21q22	??-CBFA2	??-runt-related transcription factor 1 (AML1, RUNX1)
t(X;20)(q13;q13.3)	Xq13.1; 20q13.3	??	??
t(Y;1)(q12;q12)	Yq12; 1q12	??	??
MPD			
t(1;3)(p36;p21)	1p36.23-p33; 3p21	??	??

Table 1.1. *(cont.)*

Cytogenetic data	Chromosome band	Symbol	Names of genes
t(1;5)(q22;q33)	1q22; 5q31-q32	PDE4DIP-PDGFRB	phosphodiesterase 4D interacting protein (myomegalin); platelet-derived growth factor receptor, beta polypeptide
t(1;7)(q10;p10)	1q10; 7p10	??	??
t(1;12)(p36;p13)	1p36; 12p13	MDS2-ETV6	myelodysplastic syndrome 2; ets variant gene 6 (TEL oncogene)
dic(1;15)(p11;p11)	1p11; 15p11	??	??
t(1;18)(q10;q10)	1q10; 18q10	??	??
t(2;3)(p15-p23;q26-q27)	2p15-p23; 3q24-q28	??-EVI1	??; ecotropic viral integration site 1
t(2;4)(p23;q25-q35)	2p23; 4q25-q35	??	??
t(2;13)(p16;q12)	2p21; 13q12	SPTBN1; FLT3	pectrin, beta, non-erythrocytic 1; fms-related tyrosine kinase 3
inv(3)(p12q26)	3q24-q28; 3p12	EVI1-??	ecotropic viral integration site 1; ??
inv(3)(q21q26)	3q21; 3q24-q28	RPN1-EVI1	ribophorin 1; ecotropic viral integration site 1
inv(3)(q23q26)	3q24-q28; 3q23	EVI1-??	ecotropic viral integration site 1; ??
ins(3;3)(q26;q21q26); t(3;3)(q21;q26)	3q21.3-q25.2	RPN1-EVI1	ribophorin 1
t(3;5)(q25;q34)	3q25.1; 5q35	MLF1-NPM1	myeloid leukemia factor 1; nucleophosmin (nucleolar phosphoprotein B23, numatrin)
t(3;7)(q26;q21)	3q24-q28; 7q21-q22	EVI1-CDK6	ecotropic viral integration site 1; cyclin-dependent kinase 6
t(3;11)(q26;p15)	3q24-q28; 11p15	EVI1-??	ecotropic viral integration site 1; ??
t(3;17)(q26;q22)	3q24-q28; 17q22	EVI1-??	ecotropic viral integration site 1; ??
t(4;10)(q12;p11)	4q11-q13; 10p11	PDGFRA-KIF5B	platelet-derived growth factor, alpha-receptor; kinesin family member 5B
t(4;12)(q12;p13) PDGFRA/ETV6	4q11-q13; 12p13	PDGFRA-ETV6	platelet-derived growth factor, ets variant gene 6 (TEL oncogene)
t(4;22)(q12;q11.2)	4q11-q13; 22q11.21	PDGFRA-BCR	platelet-derived growth factor, alpha-receptor; breakpoint cluster region
t(5;10)(q33;q21)	5q31-q32; 10q21	PDGFRB-D10S170	platelet-derived growth factor receptor, beta polypeptide; DNA segment on chromosome 10 (unique) 170, H4 gene (PTC1; CCDC6)
t(5;11)(q31;q23)	5q31; 11q23	GRAF-MLL	GTPase regulator associated with focal adhesion kinase pp125 (FAK); (ARHGAP26; Rho GTPase activating protein 26); myeloid/lymphoid or mixed-lineage leukemia (trithorax homolog, *Drosophila*)
t(5;12)(q31;p13)	5q31; 12p13	FACL6-ETV6	fatty-acid-coenzyme A ligase, long-chain 6 (ACSL6); ets variant gene 6 (TEL oncogene)
t(5;12)(q33;p13)	5q31-q32; 12p13	PDGFRB-ETV6	platelet-derived growth factor receptor; ets variant gene 6 (TEL oncogene)
t(5;14)(q33;q32) PDGFRB/KIAA1509	5q31-q32; 14q32.12	PDGFRB-KIAA1509	platelet-derived growth factor receptor, beta polypeptide; now known as CCDC88C (coiled-coil domain containing 88C)
t(5;15)(q33;q22)	5q31-q32; 15q22	PDGFRB-TP53BP1	platelet-derived growth factor receptor, beta polypeptide; tumor protein p53 binding protein 1 (53BP1)
t(7;8)(q34;p11)	7q32-q34; 8p11.2-p11.1	TIF1-FGFR1	transcriptional intermediary factor 1 (PTC6, TIF1A, TRIM24); fibroblast growth factor receptor 1
t(7;11)(p15;p15)	7p15-p14.2; 11p15	HOXA9-NUP98	homeobox A9; nucleoporin 98 kDa

Table 1.1. *(cont.)*

Cytogenetic data	Chromosome band	Symbol	Names of genes
t(7;14)(q21;q13)	7q21; 14q13	??	??
t(7;17)(p15;q23)	7p15-p14.2; 17q23	HOXA9-MSI2	homeobox A9; musashi homolog 2 (*Drosophila*)
t(7;17)(q32-34;q23)	7q32-q34; 17q23.3	??-MSI2	??; musashi homolog 2 (*Drosophila*)
t(8;9)(p12;q33)	8p11.2-p11.1; 9q33	FGFR1-CEP1	fibroblast growth factor receptor 1; centrosomal protein 1 (CEP110)
t(8;12)(p12;p11)	8p11.2-p11.1; 12p11.23	FGFR1-FGFR1OP2	fibroblast growth factor receptor 1; FGFR1 oncogene partner 2
t(8;12)(p12;q15)	8p11.2-p11.1; 12q15	FGFR1-CPSF6	fibroblast growth factor receptor 1; cleavage and polyadenylation specific factor 6
t(8;12)(q22;q13)	8q22; 12q15	??-HMGA2	??; high mobility group AT-hook 2 (HMGIC)
t(8;14)(q11;q32)	8q11; 14q32.33	CEBPD-IGH	CCAAT/enhancer binding protein (C/EBP), delta; immunoglobulin heavy locus
t(8;17)(p12;q23)	8p11.2-p11.1; 17q11.2	FGFR1	fibroblast growth factor receptor 1; myosin XVIIIA
t(8;17)(p12;q25)	8p11.2-p11.1; 17q25.3	FGFR1-??	fibroblast growth factor receptor 1; ??
t(8;22)(p11;q11)	8p11.2-p11.1; 22q11.21	FGFR1-BCR	fibroblast growth factor receptor 1; breakpoint cluster region
t(9;11)(p22;p15)	9p22.3; 11p15	PSIP2-NUP98	PC4 and SFRS1 interacting protein 2 (LEDGF, PSIP1); nucleoporin 98 kDa
t(9;12)(p24;p13)	9p24; 12p13	JAK2-ETV6	Janus kinase 2; ets variant gene 6 (TEL oncogene)
t(9;12)(q34;p13)	9q34.1; 12p13	ABL1-ETV6	v-abl Abelson murine leukemia viral oncogene homolog 1; ets variant gene 6 (TEL oncogene)
der(9;18)(p10;q10)	9p10; 18q10	??	??
t(9;22)(p24;q11.2)	9p24; 22q11.21	JAK2-BCR	Janus kinase 2; breakpoint cluster region
t(9;22)(q34;q11) in CML	9q34.1; 22q11.21	ABL1-BCR	v-abl Abelson murine leukemia viral oncogene homolog 1; breakpoint cluster region
t(10;12)(q24;p13)	10q24.1-q25.1; 12p13	GOT1-ETV6	glutamic-oxaloacetic transaminase 1 (GIG18); ets variant gene 6 (TEL oncogene)
inv(11)(p15q22); t(11;11) (p15;q22)	11p15.5; 11q22	NUP98-DDX10	nucleoporin 98 kDa; DEAD (Asp-Glu-Ala-Asp) box polypeptide 10
ins(12;8)(p11;p12p22)	12p11.23; 8p12	FGFR1OP2-FGFR	FGFR1 oncogene partner 2; fibroblast growth factor receptor 1
t(12;13)(p12;q12-q14)	12p13; 13q12.3	ETV6-CDX2	ets variant gene 6 (TEL oncogene); caudal type homeobox transcription factor 2 (CDX3)
t(12;13)(p13;q12) ETV6/FLT3	12p13; 13q12	ETV6-FLT3	ets variant gene 6 (TEL oncogene); fms-related tyrosine kinase 3
t(12;13)(p13;q14)	12p13; 13q14.11	ETV6-TTL	ets variant gene 6 (TEL oncogene); twelve-thirteen translocation leukemia gene (LOC646982; FLJ21437)
t(12;22)(p13;q11-q12)	12p13; 22q11	ETV6-MN1	ets variant gene 6 (TEL oncogene); meningioma (disrupted in balanced translocation) 1
inv(16)(p13q22); t(16;16) (p13;q22)	16p13; 16q22	MYH11-CBFB	myosin, heavy polypeptide 11, smooth muscle; core binding factor, beta subunit
t(X;20)(q13;q13.3)	Xq13.1; 20q13.3	??	??
t(Y;1)(q12;q12)	Yq12; 1q12	??	??
CLPD			
t(1;3)(p36;q21)	1p36.23-p33; 3q21.3	PRDM16-RPN1	PR domain containing 16; ribophorin I (RBPH1)

Table 1.1. *(cont.)*

Cytogenetic data	Chromosome band	Symbol	Names of genes
t(1;6)(p35;p25)	1p35; 6p25-p23	??-IRF4	??; interferon regulatory factor 4
t(1;14)(q21;q32) IRTA1/IGH	1q21; 14q32.33	FCRL4-IGH	Fc receptor-like 4 (IRTA1); immunoglobulin heavy locus
t(2;14)(p13;q32)	2p13; 14q32.33	BCL11A-IGH	B-cell CLL/lymphoma 11A; immunoglobulin heavy locus
t(2;18)(p11;q21)	2p11; 18q21.3	??-BCL2	??; B-cell CLL/lymphoma 2
t(2;19)(p12;q13) IGK/BCL3	2p12; 19q13	IGK-BCL3	immunoglobulin kappa locus; B-cell CLL/lymphoma 3
t(6;12)(p21;p13)	6p21; 12p13	CCND3-ETV6	cyclin D3; ets variant gene 6 (TEL oncogene)
t(6;14)(p21;q32)	6p21; 14q32.33	CCND3-IGH	cyclin D3; immunoglobulin heavy locus
t(6;14)(q25-q27;q32)	6q25-q27; 14q32	??-BCL11B	??; B-cell CLL/lymphoma 11B (CTIP2)
t(7;14)(q35;q32.1)	7q34; 14q32.1	TBR-TCL1A	T-cell receptor beta locus (TCRB); T-cell leukemia/lymphoma 1A
t(8;12)(q24;q22)	8q24.21; 12q22	MYC-BTG1	v-myc myelocytomatosis viral oncogene homolog (avian) (c-Myc); B-cell translocation gene 1
t(9;14)(p13;q32)	9p13; 14q32.33	PAX5-IGH	paired box gene 5 (B-cell lineage-specific activator protein); immunoglobulin heavy locus
t(11;14)(p11;q32)	11p11; 14q32	??-IGH	??; immunoglobulin heavy locus
t(11;14)(q13;q32)	11q13; 14q32.33	CCND1-IGH	cyclin D1; immunoglobulin heavy locus
t(14;14)(q11;q32.1); inv(14)(q11q32.1)	14q11.2; 14q32.1	TRA/TRD-TCL1A	T-cell receptor alpha locus/T-cell receptor delta locus; T-cell leukemia/lymphoma 1A
t(14;18)(q32;q21)	14q32.33; 18q21.3	IGH-BCL2	immunoglobulin heavy locus; B-cell CLL/lymphoma 2
t(14;19)(q32;q13)	14q32.33; 19q13	IGH-BCL3	immunoglobulin heavy locus; B-cell CLL/lymphoma 3
t(14;22)(q32;q11)	14q32.33; 22q11.1-q11.2	IGH-IGL	immunoglobulin heavy locus; immunoglobulin lambda locus
t(18;22)(q21;q11)	18q21.3; 22q11	BCL2-??	B-cell CLL/lymphoma 2; ??
t(19;19)(p13;q13); inv(19)(p13q13)	19p13.3; 19q13	TCF3-TFPT	transcription factor 3 (E2A immunoglobulin enhancer binding factors E12/E47); TCF3 (E2A) fusion partner (in childhood leukemia)
t(19;22)(q13;q11)	19q13; 22q11.1-q11.2	BCL3-IGL	B-cell CLL/lymphoma 3; immunoglobulin lambda locus
t(X;11)(q21;q23)	Xq21.1; 11q22.3-q23.1	BRWD3-ARHGAP20	bromodomain and WD repeat domain containing 3 (BRODL); Rho GTPase activating protein 20 (RARHOGAP)

Notes:
[a]Chromosome bands listed are those given in EntrezGene for the genes demonstrated to be involved in the translocation.
[b]Genes involved in the translocation are listed in the order given in the Chromosome band column.
[c]Gene names given in parentheses are synonyms; genes are listed in the order given in the Chromosome band column.
T-ALL: T-cell acute lymphoblastic leukemia; B-ALL: B-cell acute lymphoblastic leukemia; AML: acute myeloid leukemia; MDS: myelodysplastic syndrome; AEL: acute erythroleukemia; MPD: myeloproliferative disease; CML: chronic myeloid leukemia; CLPD: chronic lymphoproliferative disorders.

Gene deletions and amplifications

The deletion of tumor suppressor genes is another mechanism for leukemogenesis. Some of the deletions most recently described involve the loss of microRNAs (miRNAs) that function as suppressors. Amplifications are rare in leukemias, but have been documented. Table 1.3 gives a list of genes found to be deleted or amplified in leukemias.

Changes in expression

Deregulation of gene expression, such as the downregulation of tumor suppressors or the overexpression of oncogenes, is a common abnormality seen in leukemias. Most instances of downregulation are caused by deletion of the gene, or by hypermethylation as explained below. However, some deregulation and downregulation can be caused by other mechanisms

Table 1.2. Genes mutated in leukemias

Symbol	Name	Chromosome band
IKZF1	IKAROS family zinc finger 1	7p12.2
MAP2K4	mitogen-activated protein kinase kinase 4	17p11.2
FANCD2	Fanconi anemia, complementation group D2	3p26
ATM	ataxia telangiectasia mutated	11q22.3
CDKN2A-p16 (INK4a)	cyclin-dependent kinase inhibitor 2A (p16(INK4a)) gene	9p21
FANCA	Fanconi anemia, complementation group A	16q24.3
FANCC	Fanconi anemia, complementation group C	9q22.3
PTEN	phosphatase and tensin homolog gene	10q23.3
RB1	retinoblastoma gene	13q14
WT1	Wilms tumor 1 gene	11p13
NF1	neurofibromatosis type 1 gene	17q12
NF2	neurofibromatosis type 2 gene	22q12.2
CDKN2A-p14ARF	cyclin-dependent kinase inhibitor 2A-p14ARF protein	9p21
CHEK2	CHK2 checkpoint homolog (*Schizosaccharomyces pombe*)	22q12.1
CTNNB1	catenin (cadherin-associated protein), beta 1	3p22-p21.3
AKT1	v-akt murine thymoma viral oncogene homolog 1	14q32.32
CARD11	caspase recruitment domain family, member 11	7p22
CDK4	cyclin-dependent kinase 4	12q14
FGFR2	fibroblast growth factor receptor 2	10q26
GATA2	GATA binding protein 2	3q21.3
HRAS	v-Ha-ras Harvey rat sarcoma viral oncogene homolog	11p15.5
JAK3	Janus kinase 3	19p13.1
KRAS	v-Ki-ras2 Kirsten rat sarcoma 2 viral oncogene homolog	12p12.1
MET	met proto-oncogene (hepatocyte growth factor receptor)	7q31
MPL	myeloproliferative leukemia virus oncogene, thrombopoietin receptor	p34
MUTYH	mutY homolog (*Escherichia coli*)	1p34.3-1p32.1
NRAS	neuroblastoma RAS viral (v-ras) oncogene homolog	1p13.2
PIK3CA	phosphoinositide-3-kinase, catalytic, alpha polypeptide	3q26.3
PTPN11	protein tyrosine phosphatase, non-receptor type 11	12q24.1
TNFRSF6	tumor necrosis factor receptor superfamily, member 6 (FAS)	10q24.1
GATA1	GATA binding protein 1 (globin transcription factor 1)	Xp11.23
PHOX2B	paired-like homeobox 2b	4p12
TCF1	transcription factor 1, hepatic (HNF1)	12q24.2
PIK3R1	phosphoinositide-3-kinase, regulatory subunit 1 (alpha)	5q13.1
BLM	Bloom syndrome	15q26.1
CEBPA	CCAAT/enhancer binding protein (C/EBP), alpha	11p15.5
TP53	tumor protein p53	17p13
ERCC2	excision repair cross-complementing rodent repair deficiency, complementation group 2 (xeroderma pigmentosum D)	19q13.2-q13.3
FANCG	Fanconi anemia, complementation group G	9p13
FLT3	fms-related tyrosine kinase 3	13q12
KIT	v-kit Hardy-Zuckerman 4 feline sarcoma viral oncogene homolog	4q12
ERCC3	excision repair cross-complementing rodent repair deficiency, complementation group 3 (xeroderma pigmentosum group B complementing)	2q21
BRAF	v-raf murine sarcoma viral oncogene homolog B1	7q34
FANCF	Fanconi anemia, complementation group F	11p15
FANCE	Fanconi anemia, complementation group E	6p21-p22
IL6ST	interleukin 6 signal transducer (gp130, oncostatin M receptor)	5q11
NPM1	nucleophosmin (nucleolar phosphoprotein B23, numatrin)	5q35
GRAF	GTPase regulator associated with focal adhesion kinase pp125(FAK)	5q31

Table 1.2. *(cont.)*

Symbol	Name	Chromosome band
BCL6	B-cell CLL/lymphoma 6	3q27
JAK2	Janus kinase 2	9p24
PRKAR1A	protein kinase, cAMP-dependent, regulatory, type I, alpha (tissue-specific extinguisher 1)	17q23-q24
PDGFRA	platelet-derived growth factor, alpha-receptor	4q11-q13
MLL	myeloid/lymphoid or mixed-lineage leukemia (trithorax homolog, *Drosophila*)	11q23

regulate the expression of genes, and they themselves can be deregulated. Post-transcriptional regulation is also well documented.

Methylation

Methylation as a mechanism for the regulation of gene expression has been extensively studied in cancer, and every indication suggests that this phenomenon plays a major role in leukemogenesis. This is particularly important in light of the many methylation inhibitors that are currently being used in treating patients with various types of leukemias.[6,7]

Acute myeloid leukemia (AML)

Numerous genomic abnormalities have been described in AML, and most have been demonstrated to confer high proliferation rate and uncontrolled growth of cells. Chromosomal translocations are common in AML, but more common are large deletions (Table 1.3). Here we will discuss the molecular abnormalities that appear to dictate a particular clinical behavior, and which may indicate a specific therapeutic approach.

Core binding factor (CBF) abnormalities

Core binding factors (CBFs) are transcription factors, or coactivators of transcription factors, and play a major role in hematopoietic cell development.[8] They exist in cells as heterodimers that bind to DNA to activate transcription. Three genes (*CBFA1, CBFA2, CBFA3*) encode alpha subunits, which bind DNA, and one gene, *CBFB*, encodes the non-DNA-binding beta subunit.[9] The t(8;21)(q22;q22) translocation fuses *CBFA2* (also called *AML1* and *RUNX1*) to *ETO* (also called *RUNXIT1* and *CBFA2T1*), and inv(16)(p13q22)/t(16;16)(p13;q22) similarly disrupts *CBFB* by fusing the N-terminal portion of the CBF beta subunit to the carboxy terminal of the MYH11 protein (also called SMMHC). These abnormalities are associated with good outcomes in AML, but other translocations involving *CBFA2* and additional genes have been reported to be associated with poor outcome.[10–12] For example, t(3;21)(q26;q22) results in fusion of *CBFA2* to *EAP, MDS1*, or *EVI1* and is associated with poor outcome.[13,14] In addition, mutations in the *CBFA2* gene have been reported in rare cases of AML, and germline *CBFA2* mutations have been reported in rare autosomal dominant familial platelet disorders with predisposition to AML.[15] Translocation of the *CBFA2* gene to the *TEL* gene in t(12;21)(p13;q22) leads to acute lymphoblastic leukemia (ALL), rather than AML, and represents the most common abnormality in pediatric ALL.[16]

Table 1.3. Deletions and amplifications in leukemias

Symbol	Name	Chromosomal band
AKT2	v-akt murine thymoma viral oncogene homolog 2	19q13.1-q13.2
MDM2	Mdm2 p53 binding protein homolog	12q15
MYC	v-myc myelocytomatosis viral oncogene homolog (avian)	8q24.12-q24.13
IKZF1	IKAROS family zinc finger 1	7p12.2
MAP2K4	mitogen-activated protein kinase kinase 4	17p11.2
FANCD2	Fanconi anemia, complementation group D2	3p26
ATM	ataxia telangiectasia mutated	11q22.3
CDKN2A-p16 (INK4a)	cyclin-dependent kinase inhibitor 2A (p16(INK4a)) gene	9p21
FANCA	Fanconi anemia, complementation group A	16q24.3
FANCC	Fanconi anemia, complementation group C	9q22.3
PTEN	phosphatase and tensin homolog gene	10q23.3
RB1	retinoblastoma gene	13q14
STK11	serine/threonine kinase 11 gene (LKB1)	19p13.3
CDKN2A-p14ARF	cyclin-dependent kinase inhibitor 2A–p14ARF protein	9p21

Abnormalities involving CBF alpha/beta are thought to require additional, complementary molecular abnormalities to cause a leukemic phenotype. Mutations in exon 8 of *c-Kit* have been reported at a relatively high frequency (approximately 22%) in leukemias with *AML1* translocation, and (varied from 9% to 29%) in leukemias with CBF beta translocations.[17] Patients with CBF beta abnormalities have a relatively high rate of mutations in the *RAS* oncogene, similar to that reported in acute monocytic leukemias. Mutations in the fms-like tyrosine kinase 3 (FLT3) also have been reported in cases with CBF beta abnormality.[17] The presence of these mutations in this group of patients is also associated with adverse outcome.

Retinoic acid receptor alpha (RARA) abnormalities

Deregulation of the *RARA* gene is believed to cause maturation arrest of myeloid cells at the promyelocyte state, leading to acute promyelocytic leukemia (APL). The most common fusion partner gene (90–95%) is promyelocytic leukemia gene (*PML*), located on chromosome 15, which is fused to *RARA* as a result of t(15;17)(q21;q22).[18–20] In 5% to 10% of APL cases, however, the partner gene is not *PML*. APL cases with t(11;17)(q23;q21), t(5;17)(q35;q21), and t(11;17)(q13;q21) have been reported in which the *RARA* is fused to the *PLZF* (promyelocytic leukemia zinc finger), *NPM* (nucleophosmin), and *NuMA* (nuclear mitotic apparatus) genes, respectively.[18,21–24] Translocations of *RARA* to the *STAT5b* gene on 17q21 and the *PRKAR1A* gene on 17q22-q24 have also been reported.[25,26] *PRKAR1A* encodes the regulatory subunit type I-α (RIα) of cyclic adenosine monophosphate (cAMP)-dependent protein kinase (PKA). It is important to distinguish these cases due to the fact that combination therapy for APL with all-*trans* retinoic acid (ATRA) and arsenic trioxide (ATO) is successful except in the presence of *PLZF/RARA* or *STAT5b* fusion gene.[27] Mutations in *FLT3* have also been reported to be more frequent in APL and to be associated with a higher white blood cell count.[28]

11q23 (*MLL*) abnormalities

The *MLL* gene has been reported to translocate into almost any chromosome, and a number of these abnormalities can be seen in ALL as well as AML (Table 1.1). Some of these translocations cannot be detected by routine karyotyping, and it is therefore necessary to perform fluorescence *in situ* hybridization (FISH) or molecular studies. In addition, about 10% of AML patients with normal karyotype may have partial internal tandem duplications in the *MLL* gene, which can be detected by molecular testing only.[29,30] *MLL* abnormalities are associated with more aggressive disease, frequently with monocytic differentiation.[31,32] This abnormality is also more frequent in therapy-related leukemia.

Trisomy 8

AML cases with trisomy 8 are fairly common (5%), either as the sole abnormality or in combination with other abnormalities. Trisomy 8 is considered of intermediate prognosis.[33] However, some studies suggest that trisomy 8 should be included as an unfavorable cytogenetic abnormality. Multiple important genes have been described on chromosome 8, with the *c-MYC* oncogene as a leading candidate, but the exact molecular abnormalities in +8 are not defined at present. Most likely this abnormality is associated with additional genomic abnormalites in the leukemic cells that are as yet undiscovered.

Monosomy 5 and del(5q) abnormalities

Monosomy 5 is common in AML (5%), and is frequently associated with -7, del(7q) or del(17p).[34] In contrast, del(5q) is more common (10%) and more frequently present with additional chromosomal abnormalities in AML.[35] This abnormality is more frequent in older patients, and is usually associated with resistance to chemotherapy and short survival.[36] The pathogenic abnormalities resulting from -5 or 5q- are not known, despite significant work and research in this field. Several studies have demonstrated that in -5, there are chromosome 5 species integrated in other chromosomes, raising the possibility that most -5 are, in reality, 5q-. The important region is believed to be in the vicinity of 5q31, where the genes for interleukin 3 (IL-3), colony-stimulating factor 1 receptor (CSF1R), and granulocyte-macrophage colony-stimulating factor (GMCSF) are located, but extensive studies have not confirmed that these genes are the target of this abnormality. New genes have recently been described in this region, but these potential targets require confirmation.

Monosomy 7 and del(7q) abnormalities

This abnormality is similar to that described for chromosome 5, and is frequently associated with 5q abnormalities. Monosomy 7 has been reported in 50% of AML cases with inv(3)(q21;q26)/t(3;3)(q21;q26), and is frequently seen at high rates in any abnormality involving 3q21.[37] This abnormality is associated with resistance to therapy and poor survival and is seen more frequently in older patients. Furthermore, this abnormality is more frequent in therapy-related AML, especially after alkylating therapy or radiotherapy.[38] The pathogenic abnormality resulting from this chromosomal abnormality is not known.

fms-related tyrosine kinase 3 (*FLT3*)

Mutations in the *FLT3* gene are the most common molecular abnormalities in AML, appearing at a frequency of 30% to 35% of cases. Most *FLT3* mutations are internal tandem duplications (ITD) in the juxtamembrane domain of *FLT3*, leading to the addition of amino acids, from just a few to more than 50 new residues. The reading frame is always maintained in these mutations, and these additional amino acids are believed to lead to loss of function and inhibition of protein kinase activity. Mutations in the activation loop, especially at aspartic acid 835 (D835), have also been reported. Most studies suggest that *FLT3* mutations lead to poor outcome in patients younger than 65, while patients with *FLT3* mutations in both alleles have significantly more aggressive disease.[39]

Nucleophosmin (*NPM1*)

NPM1 is a nucleo-cytoplasmic shuttling protein predominantly found in the nucleus, whose functions include binding of nucleic acids, regulation of centrosome duplication, and ribosomal function.[40] The *NPM1* gene is located on chromosome

5q35. Mutations in exon 12 of the *NPM1* gene have been described in 25% of AML cases.[41] These mutations lead to frame shifts, generating an elongated protein which is retained in the cytoplasm. Using immunohistochemical methods, Falini and colleagues detected aberrant cytoplasmic localization of the NPM1 protein in 35% of patients with AML, and in 60% of those patients with a diploid karyotype. These patients also display an increased incidence of *FLT3* mutation, most of the mutations involving the insertion of four nucleotides.[41] The presence of these mutations has been shown to be associated with a higher likelihood of achieving complete response to standard induction chemotherapy and longer event-free survival.[42]

Wilms tumor (*WT1*)

The *WT1* gene is located on 11p13 and encodes a transcription factor that is now demonstrated to act both as a tumor suppressor gene and as an oncogene. The gene is mutated in 5% of cases of Wilms tumor. However, it was recently reported to be mutated in 5–10% of cases of AML as well.[43] Most *WT1* mutations fall in exons 7 and 9, and include both point mutations and insertions.[44] The presence of *WT1* mutations is associated with shorter survival and progression-free survival in patients with AML who are younger than 60.[45] These mutations are more common in patients with diploid karyotype.

CCAAT/enhancer binding protein alpha (*CEBPA*)

The *CEBPA* gene is a member of the leucine zipper transcription factor family that is crucial for the proliferation and terminal differentiation of granulocytes. The wild-type CEBPA protein exists as two isoforms, p42 and p30. CEBPA inhibits the E2F pathway and downregulates c-Myc expression, thus allowing myeloid cells to enter terminal differentiation.[46] Most of the described mutations of CEBPA involve insertion/deletion and termination of transcription. Mutations in CEBPA have been reported in 5% to 15% of cases of AML.[47] The presence of this mutation has been reported to be associated with favorable outcome, especially in patients with normal cytogenetics who lack *FLT3* mutation.[45]

Acute lymphoblastic leukemia (ALL)

ALL is a disease more common in the pediatric group than in adults. Despite some overlap in biology between pediatric and adult ALL, the clinical behavior and outcome differ significantly between the two groups. Even within the pediatric group, children aged 1 to 9 years have significantly better outcome than children aged 10 years or older; and older children in turn have better outcome than adults. The clinical differences between pediatric ALL and adult ALL reflect differences not only in the host, but also in the disease. The following subcategories of ALL should be distinguished based on their specific therapeutic approach and clinical outcome.

Ploidy groups

Ploidy grouping is well established in ALL, and different groups have different clinical and biologic behavior. Hyperdiploidy (51–65 chromosomes) is more common in pediatric patients with B-cell ALL, and this abnormality is associated with better outcome.[48] *PAX5* mutation and deletion is infrequently seen in pediatric patients with hyperdiploidy.[49] In contrast, hypodiploidy (< 44 chromosomes), which is seen in both adult and pediatric ALL, is associated with poor outcome. These patients have higher incidence of complex abnormalities and preferential involvement of chromosomes 7, 9, and 12.[50,51]

Philadelphia-positive ALL

Translocation (9;22), or the Philadelphia chromosome, is the most frequent primary abnormality in ALL, and expression of the resulting Bcr-Abl fusion protein is associated with more aggressive disease.[52] Therapy with kinase inhibitors (imatinib, nilotinib, or dasatinib) in patients with *BCR-ABL* translocation may lead to the development of Abl kinase mutations associated with drug resistance. Testing for Abl kinase mutations is thus a key consideration when treating patients with kinase inhibitors. However, most laboratories design the Abl kinase domain mutation analysis around the expression of the P210 protein, which is expressed in chronic myeloid leukemia (CML), and some of these procedures may not adequately amplify the P190 fusion transcript, which is expressed in ALL.[53] Therefore, the assay should be designed specifically to encompass the P190 transcript, in order to most accurately characterize the molecular basis of each patient's disease.

t(12;21)(p13;q22)

This is a common translocation in childhood ALL, detected in 25–30% of precursor B-cell ALL, and is extremely rare in adult ALL. The genes involved in this translocation are *CBFA2* (also known as *AML1* and *RUNX1*) and *ETV6* (ETS-type variant 6), also known as *TEL*. The two genes form a fusion gene that has been shown to occur as a prenatal event in some patients. This abnormality is usually associated with good outcome.[54]

IKZF1 abnormalities

A recent report suggested that the *IKZF1* gene, which codes for the lymphoid transcription factor IKAROS, is abnormal (deleted or mutated) in 28.6% of pediatric patients with ALL, and that patients with this abnormality have higher rates of failure and relapse.[55] While these data need further confirmation, this abnormality should be considered in ALL patients.

Burkitt-type ALL

ALL with B-cell immunophenotype is usually associated with t(8;14)(q24.1;q32) or t(8;22)(q24.1;q11.2). Patients with Burkitt-type lymphoma typically have a very aggressive disease course and short survival. CD20 expression is more common in these patients, and the addition of rituximab to chemotherapy has been shown to improve outcome.[56,57]

IL3-IGH translocation [t(5;14)(q31;q32)]

Patients with this abnormality should be distinguished because they may present with eosinophilia and a slight increase in blasts.[58–59] Therefore, the diagnosis can be confusing or missed. High levels of IL-3 are detected in these patients and are considered the cause of the eosinophilia.

Translocations in ALL

Numerous translocations have been reported in ALL as shown in Table 1.1. Some of these translocations are associated with good outcome as in t(12;21)/*TEL-AML1*, but other cytogenetic abnormalities are associated with unfavorable outcome, including t(4;11)/*MLL-AF4* and t(1;19)/*E2A-PBX1*.[54,61]

HOX gene family

There are four clusters of highly conserved homeobox (*HOX*) genes, each encoding 61 amino acids: the *HOXA* cluster on chromosome 7, *HOXB* on chromosome 17, *HOXC* on chromosome 12, and *HOXD* on chromosome 2. These *HOX* genes constitute a highly conserved family of DNA-binding genes that play a significant role in hematopoiesis. In addition, deregulation of *HOX* genes and the more divergent homeobox genes scattered throughout the genome are involved in leukemogenesis in myeloid and lymphoid cells.[62–64] For example, the homeobox gene *PBX1* mentioned above is translocated to the *E2A* gene in precursor B-cell ALL with t(1;19), and the *HOX11* gene is involved in the translocation t(10;14) in precursor T-cell ALL.[65–66] ALL with t(1;19) rarely expresses CD34 and is, in general, considered more aggressive.[67–69]

NOTCH gene and precursor ALL

The Notch signaling pathway is important for cell–cell interaction and is involved in the control of cell differentiation and survival.[70,71] Notch receptors are transmembrane glycoproteins that heterodimerize in order to be stabilized on the surface. When activated by ligands, the intracellular domain of Notch is cleaved and shuttled into the nucleus where it activates the transcription of target genes. *NOTCH1*, a member of the *NOTCH* gene family, contains activating mutations in 50% to 70% of precursor T-cell ALL.[72,73] Most of the *NOTCH1* mutations in ALL involve the heterodimerization domain. Available data suggest that *NOTCH1* gain-of-function mutations correlate with good outcome in children and in adult T-ALL.[74–76] The *NOTCH* gene pathway is also affected by abnormalities in the IKAROS gene *IKZF1*; the IKAROS protein is a direct repressor of Notch target genes.[77] However, additional data are necessary before implementing testing of these genes in the diagnosis and classification of ALL.

Chronic lymphoproliferative diseases

Chronic lymphoproliferative diseases include multiple B- and T-cell diseases that usually involve mature cells and demonstrate chronic clinical course. Most of these are B cell in origin and include chronic lymphocytic leukemia (CLL), marginal zone lymphoma, splenic marginal zone lymphoma, hairy cell leukemia, and follicular lymphoma. Rare T-cell diseases act in chronic fashion. The most appropriate disease is large granular lymphocytic lymphoma including the T-cell and natural killer (NK) subtypes. The major molecular changes in this group of diseases are described in Tables 1.1 to 1.3.

Chronic lymphocytic leukemia (CLL)

The diagnosis of CLL requires the presence of greater than 5000 clonal B lymphocytes/μL in the peripheral blood; otherwise the disease should be considered "monoclonal B-cell lymphocytosis" (MBL). MBL is defined by the presence of clonal B cells, but less than 5000 B lymphocytes/μL blood in the absence of lymphadenopathy or organomegaly.[78] MBL is considered analogous to monoclonal gammopathy of undetermined significance (MGUS) and is believed to progress to frank CLL at a rate of 1–2% per year.[79,80] CLL should be also distinguished from the more aggressive form prolymphocytic leukemia, a morphologic distinction based on the presence of prolymphocytes comprising at least 55% of the blood lymphocytes.

IGHV mutation status

Patients with CLL expressing unmutated ($<$ 3% mutation rate) *IgHV* show aggressive disease and should be distinguished from those expressing a mutated *IgHV* gene.[81–82] The *IGHV* mutation status is not relevant to the oncogenic process, however, and is most likely a marker for the stage of differentiation of the initiating leukemic cells.

Del(11q)

The 11q22 deletion is seen in 10% of CLL cases and the targeted gene is most likely the *ATM* gene. This abnormality is always associated with more aggressive disease, irrespective of the mutation status.[83]

Del(13q)

Deletion of 13q14 leads to abnormalities in miRNAs, which have been shown to repress translation and regulate the degradation of transcripts of a variety of genes. Both miR15a and miR16–1 are deleted with 13q14.[84] Data show that these two miRNAs act as tumor suppressors by downregulating the translation of AU-rich elements found in oncogenes such as *MCL1, BCL2, ETS1*, and *JUN*, which are involved in apoptosis and cell cycle regulation.[85]

Del(17p)

This deletion is detected in $<$ 5% of patients with CLL and the target gene is believed to be the *TP53* gene. Detecting this abnormality is important, because it implies more aggressive disease and resistance to therapy irrespective of the mutation status. Most frequently this abnormality is detected as a late event in the course of the disease.[86]

Follicular lymphoma/leukemia

The hallmark of this disease is the presence of t(14;18)(q32; q21) involving the *IGH* and *BCL2* gene, and overexpression of BCL2, which make the mature follicular cells resistant to apoptosis. This abnormality is detected in 80–90% of cases.[87]

Other chronic lymphoproliferative diseases

Less common B- and T-cell diseases can be classified under this category, including hairy cell leukemia, marginal zone lymphoma, T-cell prolymphocytic leukemia, and T-cell large granular lymphocytes. Multiple genomic abnormalities have been reported in these diseases including deletions and rare translocations, but no specific genomic abnormality. The extranodal marginal zone lymphoma, which is not discussed here, is unusual and despite its similarity to nodal marginal zone has specific chromosomal abnormalities.

Chronic myeloproliferative diseases

Chronic myeloid leukemia (CML)

CML is characterized by the proliferation of maturing myeloid cells and the presence of the t(9;22)(q34;q11) chromosomal translocation, resulting in a shortened chromosome 22 (the Philadelphia chromosome). This translocation fuses the *BCR* gene with the *ABL1* gene, leading to the expression of a fusion mRNA and protein. Although rare, translocations fusing *ABL1* to a gene other than *BCR* have been described, and t(9;12)(q34; p13) resulting in an *ETV6-ABL1* gene rearrangement/fusion has been reported in patients with a disease similar to CML.[88] In addition, cases with *BCR/JAK2* fusion with t(9;22)(p24;q11) have been reported.[89–91] Unusual t(8;9)(p22;p24) translocations with a molecular abnormality involving the *PCM1* and *JAK2* genes were reported in patients presenting with chronic myeloproliferative neoplasia (MPN). However, this disease did not respond to standard kinase inhibitor therapy, which suggests a different clinical entity.[92,93] The most common fusion transcripts resulting from the Philadelphia chromosome are b2a2 and b3a2, resulting from two different breakpoints on chromosome 22 at the *BCR* gene. Rare transcript e19a2 has also been reported in some patients. The first two transcripts result in the expression of a 210 kilodalton (kDa) protein, while the protein resulting from the third transcript is 230 kDa.[94,95]

The development of imatinib and next-generation kinase inhibitors has changed the course of CML disease. Five-year survival is now greater than 80%. However, some patients demonstrate primary or secondary resistance, and some progress to accelerated or blast phase. While determination of imatinib resistance should be based on lack or loss of hematologic, cytogenetic, or molecular responses rather than on the detection of mutation alone, in general the presence of *ABL1* mutation in a CML patient being treated with imatinib will indicate resistance. For instance, mutations such as Y253H, E255K/V, and T315I, when detected using direct sequencing, are usually indicative of resistance.[96–98] *ABL1* mutations are detected in 30% to 40% of resistant patients.[99–102] However, Abl1-kinase domain mutations can be detected transiently during therapy and on occasion may disappear with continued therapy.[103] Early detection of resistance is important. Switching to one of the newly available kinase inhibitors at early signs of resistance, or even increasing the dosage of imatinib, may prevent overt resistance.[104–107] Recent findings indicate that an alternatively spliced *BCR-ABL1* mRNA, causing the insertion of 35 nucleotides between exons 8 and 9, leads to the expression of a truncated but highly resistant species of Bcr-Abl1 protein.[5] Low-level expression of this alternatively spliced *BCR-ABL1* could allow some cells to evade kinase inhibitor therapy, providing more opportunity to develop additional mutations and overtly resistant disease. One method for detecting Abl kinase mutations at early stages without compromising specificity is to test plasma rather than cells from bone marrow or peripheral blood.[108] Transformation from chronic phase into accelerated or blast crisis is frequently associated with secondary genomic abnormalities. The most common lesions are +8, i(17q), and a second Philadelphia chromosome.

Non-CML chronic myeloproliferative diseases

Because of the specific molecular abnormality in CML (i.e., the Philadelphia chromosome), the term chronic myeloproliferative disease or neoplasia (MPD or MPN) frequently refers to chronic myeloproliferative diseases excluding CML. MPNs include polycythemia vera (PV); primary myelofibrosis (PMF); essential thrombocytemia (ET); hypereosinophilic syndrome (HES); and chronic eosinophilic leukemia, mastocytosis, and chronic neutrophilic leukemia (CNL). The various MPNs exhibit significant similarity at the clinical, morphologic, and molecular levels. CNL remains a distinct entity with an aggressive course, but without a specific defined molecular abnormality. However, diagnosis is relatively straightforward based on morphology and clinical presentation. PV, ET, and PMF show significant overlap, and most affected patients develop marrow fibrosis. Translocations have been reported in this group of diseases (Table 1.1), but the most common abnormalities are discussed below.

JAK2 mutation status

JAK2 mutations in exons 12, 13, 14, and 15 are the most common mutations in this group of diseases. All reported mutations are in the pseudokinase domain, and are expected to relieve the auto-inhibitory function of this domain on JAK2 kinase activity.[109] When screening for *JAK2* mutations, the use of plasma rather than cells for RNA extraction may allow more timely detection of disease. Early disease, in which platelets are the main neoplastic cell type, can be missed if cells rather than plasma are used for testing.[110]

Among *JAK2* mutations, V617F represents the most common abnormality and is present in 80% to 90% of patients with PV,

35% to 45% of those with ET, and 35% to 45% of those with PMF. *JAK2* mutations other than V617F are rare, accounting for only about 1% to 2% of *JAK2* mutations. Most of the other *JAK2* reported mutations are in exon 12, but rare mutations in exons 13, 14, and 15 have also been described.[109,111]

MPL mutations

It has been estimated that 5% of patients with PV, ET, or PMF without *JAK2* mutation may have a mutation in the thrombopoietin receptor MPL (myeloproliferative leukemia virus oncogene).[112,113] The W515L/K mutation has been reported in sporadic cases and the S505N as well as P106L have been reported in familial forms of MPD.[114,115] These mutations typically occur in the absence of *JAK2* V617F mutation, and should be tested for after *JAK2* mutations have been ruled out in patients whose clinical presentation suggests MPD.[116,117] Recent studies, however, have demonstrated concurrence of *MPL* and *JAK2* V617F mutations in some cases.[118,119] Our data suggest that *MPL* mutations are twice as common as *JAK2* exon 12 and 13 mutations in patients with *JAK2* V617F-negative non-CML MPNs.

FGFR1 abnormalities

Translocations affecting the *FGFR1* gene are associated with the 8p11 myeloproliferative syndrome, a specific disease that usually presents with eosinophilia and myeloproliferative features but may also progress to AML or ALL.[120] Multiple *FGFR1* fusion partners have been reported, and the most common translocations are: t(8;13)(p11;q12), t(8;9)(p11;q33), t(6;8)(q27;p11), t(8;22)(p11;q11), t(8;17)(p11;q23), t(8;19)(p11;q13), and t(7;8)(q34;p11). Frequently these abnormalities are detected by routine karyotype analysis.

FIP1L1-PDGFRA fusion

Patients with eosinophilia and increased mast cells have a specific class of MPN that is frequently associated with the *FIP1L1-PDGFRA* (FIP1-like-1–platelet-derived growth factor receptor-α) fusion, formed by a cryptic deletion at 4q12. These patients should be distinguished because they respond to imatinib therapy.[121] However, some of the patients with this abnormality may also present with AML and ALL.[122] This abnormality cannot be seen by routine karyotyping, but can be detected by FISH as well as real time-polymerase chain reaction (PCR)-based molecular testing.

PDGFRB rearrangement

The *PDGFRB* gene is located on 5q31~33 and can be translocated and fused with one of multiple genes. The most common translocation is t(5;12)(q32;p12), resulting in fusion with the *ETV6* gene.[123–125] Some patients with MPN and eosinophilia may present with this abnormality, but *PDGFRB* rearrangement can also be seen in acute leukemia, myelodysplasia, and chronic myelomonocytic leukemia (CMML). Given the possibility of multiple fusion partners when the *PDGFRB* is involved, break-apart FISH testing is recommended when *PDGFRB* rearrangement is suspected and conventional karyotyping is negative.

Conclusions

We have provided a brief overview of some of the most common genetic alterations seen in leukemia. The contents of Tables 1.1–1.3 and the wealth of literature dealing with hematologic malignancies are excellent indicators of the remarkable complexity of these diseases. Each year, the efforts of researchers and clinicians around the world further elucidate the etiology and intricate interactions in each of these leukemias. As we learn more about these diseases, it becomes increasingly clear that as much information as possible must be gathered about each patient's disease. With a detailed picture of the malignancy, treatment can be tailored more efficiently and more specifically to the individual patient.

References

1. Jones RJ, Armstrong SA. Cancer stem cells in hematopoietic malignancies. *Biol Blood Marrow Transplant* 2008;**14**:12–16.
2. Passegue E, Jamieson CH, Ailles LE, *et al.* Normal and leukemic hematopoiesis: are leukemias a stem cell disorder or a reacquisition of stem cell characteristics? *Proc Natl Acad Sci U S A* 2003;**100** Suppl 1:11 842–9.
3. Moore MA. Converging pathways in leukemogenesis and stem cell self-renewal. *Exp Hematol* 2005;**33**:719–37.
4. Hochhaus A, Erben P, Ernst T, *et al.* Resistance to targeted therapy in chronic myelogenous leukemia. *Semin Hematol* 2007;**44**:S15–24.
5. Lee TS, Ma W, Zhang X, *et al.* BCR-ABL alternative splicing as a common mechanism for imatinib resistance: evidence from molecular dynamics simulations. *Mol Cancer Ther* 2008;**7**:3834–41.
6. Ghoshal K, Bai S. DNA methyltransferases as targets for cancer therapy. *Drugs Today (Barc)* 2007;**43**:395–422.
7. Plimack ER, Kantarjian HM, Issa JP. Decitabine and its role in the treatment of hematopoietic malignancies. *Leuk Lymphoma* 2007;**48**:1472–81.
8. Friedman AD. Cell cycle and developmental control of hematopoiesis by Runx1. *J Cell Physiol* 2009; **219**:520–4.
9. Levanon D, Groner Y. Structure and regulated expression of mammalian RUNX genes. *Oncogene* 2004;**23**:4211–19.
10. Byrd JC, Mrozek K, Dodge RK, *et al.* Pretreatment cytogenetic abnormalities are predictive of induction success, cumulative incidence of relapse, and overall survival in adult patients with de novo acute myeloid leukemia: results from Cancer and Leukemia Group B (CALGB 8461). *Blood* 2002;**100**:4325–36.
11. Grimwade D, Walker H, Harrison G, *et al.* The predictive value of hierarchical cytogenetic classification in older adults with acute myeloid leukemia (AML): analysis of 1065 patients entered into the United Kingdom Medical Research Council AML11 trial. *Blood* 2001;**98**:1312–20.

12. Marcucci G, Mrozek K, Ruppert AS, *et al.* Prognostic factors and outcome of core binding factor acute myeloid leukemia patients with t(8;21) differ from those of patients with inv(16): a Cancer and Leukemia Group B study. *J Clin Oncol* 2005;**23**:5705–17.
13. Nucifora G, Begy CR, Kobayashi H, *et al.* Consistent intergenic splicing and production of multiple transcripts between AML1 at 21q22 and unrelated genes at 3q26 in (3;21)(q26;q22) translocations. *Proc Natl Acad Sci U S A* 1994;**91**:4004–8.
14. Zent C, Kim N, Hiebert S, *et al.* Rearrangement of the AML1/CBFA2 gene in myeloid leukemia with the 3;21 translocation: expression of co-existing multiple chimeric genes with similar functions as transcriptional repressors, but with opposite tumorigenic properties. *Curr Top Microbiol Immunol* 1996;**211**:243–52.
15. Michaud J, Wu F, Osato M, *et al.* In vitro analyses of known and novel RUNX1/AML1 mutations in dominant familial platelet disorder with predisposition to acute myelogenous leukemia: implications for mechanisms of pathogenesis. *Blood* 2002; **99**:1364–72.
16. Zelent A, Greaves M, Enver T. Role of the TEL-AML1 fusion gene in the molecular pathogenesis of childhood acute lymphoblastic leukaemia. *Oncogene* 2004;**23**:4275–83.
17. Boissel N, Leroy H, Brethon B, *et al.* Incidence and prognostic impact of c-Kit, FLT3, and Ras gene mutations in core binding factor acute myeloid leukemia (CBF-AML). *Leukemia* 2006;**20**:965–70.
18. Grimwade D, Biondi A, Mozziconacci MJ, *et al.* Characterization of acute promyelocytic leukemia cases lacking the classic t(15;17): results of the European Working Party. Groupe Francais de Cytogenetique Hematologique, Groupe de Francais d'Hematologie Cellulaire, UK Cancer Cytogenetics Group and BIOMED 1 European Community-Concerted Action "Molecular Cytogenetic Diagnosis in Haematological Malignancies." *Blood* 2000;**96**:1297–308.
19. Larson RA, Kondo K, Vardiman JW, *et al.* Evidence for a 15;17 translocation in every patient with acute promyelocytic leukemia. *Am J Med* 1984;**76**:827–41.
20. Rowley JD, Golomb HM, Dougherty C. 15/17 translocation, a consistent chromosomal change in acute promyelocytic leukaemia. *Lancet* 1977;**1**:549–50.
21. Chen SJ, Zelent A, Tong JH, *et al.* Rearrangements of the retinoic acid receptor alpha and promyelocytic leukemia zinc finger genes resulting from t(11;17)(q23;q21) in a patient with acute promyelocytic leukemia. *J Clin Invest* 1993;**91**:2260–7.
22. Redner RL. Variations on a theme: the alternate translocations in APL. *Leukemia* 2002;**16**:1927–32.
23. Redner RL, Rush EA, Faas S, *et al.* The t (5;17) variant of acute promyelocytic leukemia expresses a nucleophosmin-retinoic acid receptor fusion. *Blood* 1996;**87**:882–6.
24. Wells RA, Catzavelos C, Kamel-Reid S. Fusion of retinoic acid receptor alpha to NuMA, the nuclear mitotic apparatus protein, by a variant translocation in acute promyelocytic leukaemia. *Nat Genet* 1997;**17**:109–13.
25. Arnould C, Philippe C, Bourdon V, *et al.* The signal transducer and activator of transcription STAT5b gene is a new partner of retinoic acid receptor alpha in acute promyelocytic-like leukaemia. *Hum Mol Genet* 1999;**8**:1741–9.
26. Catalano A, Dawson MA, Somana K, *et al.* The PRKAR1A gene is fused to RARA in a new variant acute promyelocytic leukemia. *Blood* 2007;**110**:4073–6.
27. Guidez F, Ivins S, Zhu J, *et al.* Reduced retinoic acid-sensitivities of nuclear receptor corepressor binding to PML- and PLZF-RARalpha underlie molecular pathogenesis and treatment of acute promyelocytic leukemia. *Blood* 1998;**91**:2634–42.
28. Gale RE, Hills R, Pizzey AR, *et al.* Relationship between FLT3 mutation status, biologic characteristics, and response to targeted therapy in acute promyelocytic leukemia. *Blood* 2005;**106**:3768–76.
29. Caligiuri MA, Strout MP, Lawrence D, *et al.* Rearrangement of ALL1 (MLL) in acute myeloid leukemia with normal cytogenetics. *Cancer Res* 1998;**58**:55–9.
30. Dohner K, Tobis K, Ulrich R, *et al.* Prognostic significance of partial tandem duplications of the MLL gene in adult patients 16 to 60 years old with acute myeloid leukemia and normal cytogenetics: a study of the Acute Myeloid Leukemia Study Group Ulm. *J Clin Oncol* 2002;**20**:3254–61.
31. Munoz L, Nomdedeu JF, Villamor N, *et al.* Acute myeloid leukemia with MLL rearrangements: clinicobiological features, prognostic impact and value of flow cytometry in the detection of residual leukemic cells. *Leukemia* 2003;**17**:76–82.
32. Shiah HS, Kuo YY, Tang JL, *et al.* Clinical and biologic implications of partial tandem duplication of the MLL gene in acute myeloid leukemia without chromosomal abnormalities at 11q23. *Leukemia* 2002;**16**:196–202.
33. Wolman SR, Gundacker H, Appelbaum FR, *et al.* Impact of trisomy 8 (+8) on clinical presentation, treatment response, and survival in acute myeloid leukemia: a Southwest Oncology Group study. *Blood* 2002;**100**:29–35.
34. Johansson B, Mertens F, Heim S, *et al.* Cytogenetics of secondary myelodysplasia (sMDS) and acute nonlymphocytic leukemia (sANLL). *Eur J Haematol* 1991;**47**:17–27.
35. Van den Berghe H, Michaux L. 5q-, twenty-five years later: a synopsis. *Cancer Genet Cytogenet* 1997;**94**:1–7.
36. Herry A, Douet-Guilbert N, Gueganic N, *et al.* Del(5q) and MLL amplification in homogeneously staining region in acute myeloblastic leukemia: a recurrent cytogenetic association. *Ann Hematol* 2006;**85**:244–9.
37. Horsman DE, Gascoyne RD, Barnett MJ. Acute leukemia with structural rearrangements of chromosome 3. *Leuk Lymphoma* 1995;**16**:369–77.
38. Larson RA. Is secondary leukemia an independent poor prognostic factor in acute myeloid leukemia? *Best Pract Res Clin Haematol* 2007;**20**:29–37.
39. Kiyoi H, Naoe T. Biology, clinical relevance, and molecularly targeted therapy in acute leukemia with FLT3 mutation. *Int J Hematol* 2006;**83**:301–8.
40. Okuwaki M. The structure and functions of NPM1/Nucleophosmin/B23, a multifunctional nucleolar acidic protein. *J Biochem* 2008;**143**:441–8.
41. Falini B, Mecucci C, Tiacci E, *et al.* Cytoplasmic nucleophosmin in acute myelogenous leukemia with a normal karyotype. *N Engl J Med* 2005;**352**:254–66.

42. Dohner K, Schlenk RF, Habdank M, *et al.* Mutant nucleophosmin (NPM1) predicts favorable prognosis in younger adults with acute myeloid leukemia and normal cytogenetics: interaction with other gene mutations. *Blood* 2005; **106**:3740–6.

43. Yang L, Han Y, Suarez Saiz F, *et al.* A tumor suppressor and oncogene: the WT1 story. *Leukemia* 2007;**21**:868–76.

44. Gaidzik VI, Schlenk RF, Moschny S, *et al.* Prognostic impact of WT1 mutations in cytogenetically normal acute myeloid leukemia: a study of the German-Austrian AML Study Group. *Blood* 2009;**113**:4505–11.

45. Renneville A, Boissel N, Zurawski V, *et al.* Wilms tumor 1 gene mutations are associated with a higher risk of recurrence in young adults with acute myeloid leukemia: a study from the Acute Leukemia French Association. *Cancer* 2009;**115**:3719–27.

46. Koschmieder S, Halmos B, Levantini E, *et al.* Dysregulation of the C/EBPalpha differentiation pathway in human cancer. *J Clin Oncol* 2009;**27**:619–28.

47. Fuchs O, Provaznikova D, Kocova M, *et al.* CEBPA polymorphisms and mutations in patients with acute myeloid leukemia, myelodysplastic syndrome, multiple myeloma and non-Hodgkin's lymphoma. *Blood Cells Mol Dis* 2008;**40**:401–5.

48. Harrison CJ, Foroni L. Cytogenetics and molecular genetics of acute lymphoblastic leukemia. *Rev Clin Exp Hematol* 2002;**6**:91–113; discussion 200–2.

49. Mullighan CG, Goorha S, Radtke I, *et al.* Genome-wide analysis of genetic alterations in acute lymphoblastic leukaemia. *Nature* 2007;**446**:758–64.

50. Charrin C, Thomas X, Ffrench M, *et al.* A report from the LALA-94 and LALA-SA groups on hypodiploidy with 30 to 39 chromosomes and near-triploidy: 2 possible expressions of a sole entity conferring poor prognosis in adult acute lymphoblastic leukemia (ALL). *Blood* 2004;**104**:2444–51.

51. Heerema NA, Nachman JB, Sather HN, *et al.* Hypodiploidy with less than 45 chromosomes confers adverse risk in childhood acute lymphoblastic leukemia: a report from the children's cancer group. *Blood* 1999;**94**:4036–45.

52. Radich JP. Philadelphia chromosome-positive acute lymphocytic leukemia. *Hematol Oncol Clin North Am* 2001;**15**:21–36.

53. Jones CD, Yeung C, Zehnder JL. Comprehensive validation of a real-time quantitative bcr-abl assay for clinical laboratory use. *Am J Clin Pathol* 2003;**120**:42–8.

54. Mosad E, Hamed HB, Bakry RM, *et al.* Persistence of TEL-AML1 fusion gene as minimal residual disease has no additive prognostic value in CD 10 positive B-acute lymphoblastic leukemia: a FISH study. *J Hematol Oncol* 2008;**1**:17.

55. Mullighan CG, Su X, Zhang J, *et al.* Deletion of IKZF1 and prognosis in acute lymphoblastic leukemia. *N Engl J Med* 2009;**360**:470–80.

56. Thomas DA, Faderl S, O'Brien S, *et al.* Chemoimmunotherapy with hyper-CVAD plus rituximab for the treatment of adult Burkitt and Burkitt-type lymphoma or acute lymphoblastic leukemia. *Cancer* 2006;**106**:1569–80.

57. Grimaldi JC, Meeker TC. The t(5;14) chromosomal translocation in a case of acute lymphocytic leukemia joins the interleukin-3 gene to the immunoglobulin heavy chain gene. *Blood* 1989;**73**:2081–5.

58. Hogan TF, Koss W, Murgo AJ, *et al.* Acute lymphoblastic leukemia with chromosomal 5;14 translocation and hypereosinophilia: case report and literature review. *J Clin Oncol* 1987;**5**:382–90.

59. Tono-oka T, Sato Y, Matsumoto T, *et al.* Hypereosinophilic syndrome in acute lymphoblastic leukemia with a chromosome translocation [t(5q;14q)]. *Med Pediatr Oncol* 1984;**12**:33–7.

60. Mancini M, Scappaticci D, Cimino G, *et al.* A comprehensive genetic classification of adult acute lymphoblastic leukemia (ALL): analysis of the GIMEMA 0496 protocol. *Blood* 2005;**105**:3434–41.

61. Argiropoulos B, Humphries RK. Hox genes in hematopoiesis and leukemogenesis. *Oncogene* 2007;**26**:6766–76.

62. Chiba S. Homeobox genes in normal hematopoiesis and leukemogenesis. *Int J Hematol* 1998;**68**:343–53.

63. Owens BM, Hawley RG. HOX and non-HOX homeobox genes in leukemic hematopoiesis. *Stem Cells* 2002; **20**:364–79.

64. Hatano M, Roberts CW, Minden M, *et al.* Deregulation of a homeobox gene, HOX11, by the t(10;14) in T cell leukemia. *Science* 1991;**253**:79–82.

65. Hunger SP, Galili N, Carroll AJ, *et al.* The t(1;19)(q23;p13) results in consistent fusion of E2A and PBX1 coding sequences in acute lymphoblastic leukemias. *Blood* 1991;**77**:687–93.

66. Kennedy MA, Gonzalez-Sarmiento R, Kees UR, *et al.* HOX11, a homeobox-containing T-cell oncogene on human chromosome 10q24. *Proc Natl Acad Sci U S A* 1991;**88**:8900–4.

67. Borowitz MJ, Hunger SP, Carroll AJ, *et al.* Predictability of the t(1;19)(q23; p13) from surface antigen phenotype: implications for screening cases of childhood acute lymphoblastic leukemia for molecular analysis: a Pediatric Oncology Group study. *Blood* 1993;**82**:1086–91.

68. Foa R, Vitale A, Mancini M, *et al.* E2A-PBX1 fusion in adult acute lymphoblastic leukaemia: biologic and clinical features. *Br J Haematol* 2003;**120**:484–7.

69. Privitera E, Kamps MP, Hayashi Y, *et al.* Different molecular consequences of the 1;19 chromosomal translocation in childhood B-cell precursor acute lymphoblastic leukemia. *Blood* 1992;**79**:1781–8.

70. Fortini ME. Notch signaling: the core pathway and its posttranslational regulation. *Dev Cell* 2009;**16**:633–47.

71. Joshi I, Minter LM, Telfer J, *et al.* Notch signaling mediates G1/S cell-cycle progression in T cells via cyclin D3 and its dependent kinases. *Blood* 2009;**113**:1689–98.

72. Mansour MR, Linch DC, Foroni L, *et al.* High incidence of Notch-1 mutations in adult patients with T-cell acute lymphoblastic leukemia. *Leukemia* 2006;**20**:537–9.

73. Weng AP, Ferrando AA, Lee W, *et al.* Activating mutations of NOTCH1 in human T cell acute lymphoblastic leukemia. *Science* 2004;**306**:269–71.

74. Breit S, Stanulla M, Flohr T, *et al.* Activating NOTCH1 mutations predict favorable early treatment response and long-term outcome in childhood precursor T-cell lymphoblastic leukemia. *Blood* 2006;**108**:1151–7.

75. Park MJ, Taki T, Oda M, *et al.* FBXW7 and NOTCH1 mutations in childhood

T cell acute lymphoblastic leukaemia and T cell non-Hodgkin lymphoma. *Br J Haematol* 2009;**145**:198–206.

76. van Grotel M, Meijerink JP, van Wering ER, *et al.* Prognostic significance of molecular-cytogenetic abnormalities in pediatric T-ALL is not explained by immunophenotypic differences. *Leukemia* 2008;**22**:124–31.

77. Kathrein KL, Chari S, Winandy S. Ikaros directly represses the notch target gene Hes1 in a leukemia T cell line: implications for CD4 regulation. *J Biol Chem* 2008;**283**:10 476–84.

78. Marti GE, Rawstron AC, Ghia P, *et al.* Diagnostic criteria for monoclonal B-cell lymphocytosis. *Br J Haematol* 2005;**130**:325–32.

79. Rawstron AC, Bennett FL, O'Connor SJ, *et al.* Monoclonal B-cell lymphocytosis and chronic lymphocytic leukemia. *N Engl J Med* 2008;**359**:575–83.

80. Damle RN, Wasil T, Fais F, *et al.* Ig V gene mutation status and CD38 expression as novel prognostic indicators in chronic lymphocytic leukemia. *Blood* 1999;**94**:1840–7.

81. Hamblin TJ, Davis Z, Gardiner A, *et al.* Unmutated Ig V(H) genes are associated with a more aggressive form of chronic lymphocytic leukemia. *Blood* 1999;**94**:1848–54.

82. Kharfan-Dabaja MA, Chavez JC, Khorfan KA, *et al.* Clinical and therapeutic implications of the mutational status of *IGHV* in patients with chronic lymphocytic leukemia. *Cancer* 2008;**113**:897–906.

83. Gumy-Pause F, Wacker P, Sappino AP. ATM gene and lymphoid malignancies. *Leukemia* 2004;**18**:238–42.

84. Calin GA, Cimmino A, Fabbri M, *et al.* MiR-15a and miR-16-1 cluster functions in human leukemia. *Proc Natl Acad Sci U S A* 2008;**105**:5166–71.

85. Calin GA, Dumitru CD, Shimizu M, *et al.* Frequent deletions and down-regulation of micro-RNA genes miR15 and miR16 at 13q14 in chronic lymphocytic leukemia. *Proc Natl Acad Sci U S A* 2002;**99**:15 524–9.

86. Montserrat E. New prognostic markers in CLL. *Hematology Am Soc Hematol Educ Program* 2006;279–84.

87. Rabkin CS, Hirt C, Janz S, *et al.* t(14;18) translocations and risk of follicular lymphoma. *J Natl Cancer Inst Monogr* 2008;(39):48–51.

88. Andreasson P, Johansson B, Carlsson M, *et al.* BCR/ABL-negative chronic myeloid leukemia with ETV6/ABL fusion. *Genes Chromosomes Cancer* 1997;**20**:299–304.

89. Cirmena G, Aliano S, Fugazza G, *et al.* A BCR-JAK2 fusion gene as the result of a t(9;22)(p24;q11) in a patient with acute myeloid leukemia. *Cancer Genet Cytogenet* 2008;**183**:105–8.

90. Griesinger F, Hennig H, Hillmer F, *et al.* A BCR-JAK2 fusion gene as the result of a t(9;22)(p24;q11.2) translocation in a patient with a clinically typical chronic myeloid leukemia. *Genes Chromosomes Cancer* 2005;**44**:329–33.

91. Lane SW, Fairbairn DJ, McCarthy C, *et al.* Leukaemia cutis in atypical chronic myeloid leukaemia with a t (9;22) (p24;q11.2) leading to BCR-JAK2 fusion. *Br J Haematol* 2008;**142**:503.

92. Bousquet M, Quelen C, De Mas V, *et al.* The t(8;9)(p22;p24) translocation in atypical chronic myeloid leukaemia yields a new PCM1-JAK2 fusion gene. *Oncogene* 2005;**24**:7248–52.

93. Reiter A, Walz C, Watmore A, *et al.* The t(8;9)(p22;p24) is a recurrent abnormality in chronic and acute leukemia that fuses PCM1 to JAK2. *Cancer Res* 2005;**65**:2662–7.

94. Bernasconi P, Calatroni S, Boni M, *et al.* p230 does not always predict a mild clinical course in myeloid malignancies: e19a2 bcr/abl fusion transcript with additional chromosome abnormalities in a patient with acute monoblastic leukemia (M5a). *Haematologica* 2001;**86**:320–1.

95. Wang L, Seale J, Woodcock BE, *et al.* e19a2-positive chronic myeloid leukaemia with BCR exon e16-deleted transcripts. *Leukemia* 2002;**16**:1562–3.

96. Branford S, Rudzki Z, Walsh S, *et al.* Detection of BCR-ABL mutations in patients with CML treated with imatinib is virtually always accompanied by clinical resistance, and mutations in the ATP phosphate-binding loop (P-loop) are associated with a poor prognosis. *Blood* 2003;**102**:276–83.

97. Corbin AS, Buchdunger E, Pascal F, *et al.* Analysis of the structural basis of specificity of inhibition of the Abl kinase by STI571. *J Biol Chem* 2002;**277**:32 214–19.

98. Hochhaus A, Kreil S, Corbin AS, *et al.* Molecular and chromosomal mechanisms of resistance to imatinib (STI571) therapy. *Leukemia* 2002;**16**:2190–6.

99. Jabbour E, Kantarjian H, Jones D, *et al.* Frequency and clinical significance of BCR-ABL mutations in patients with chronic myeloid leukemia treated with imatinib mesylate. *Leukemia* 2006;**20**:1767–73.

100. Shah NP, Nicoll JM, Nagar B, *et al.* Multiple BCR-ABL kinase domain mutations confer polyclonal resistance to the tyrosine kinase inhibitor imatinib (STI571) in chronic phase and blast crisis chronic myeloid leukemia. *Cancer Cell* 2002;**2**:117–25.

101. Soverini S, Colarossi S, Gnani A, *et al.* Contribution of ABL kinase domain mutations to imatinib resistance in different subsets of Philadelphia-positive patients: by the GIMEMA Working Party on Chronic Myeloid Leukemia. *Clin Cancer Res* 2006;**12**:7374–9.

102. Talpaz M, Shah NP, Kantarjian H, *et al.* Dasatinib in imatinib-resistant Philadelphia chromosome-positive leukemias. *N Engl J Med* 2006;**354**:2531–41.

103. Apperley JF. Part I: mechanisms of resistance to imatinib in chronic myeloid leukaemia. *Lancet Oncol* 2007;**8**:1018–29.

104. Gruber FX, Lamark T, Anonli A, *et al.* Selecting and deselecting imatinib-resistant clones: observations made by longitudinal, quantitative monitoring of mutated BCR-ABL. *Leukemia* 2005;**19**:2159–65.

105. Martinelli G, Iacobucci I, Soverini S, *et al.* Monitoring minimal residual disease and controlling drug resistance in chronic myeloid leukaemia patients in treatment with imatinib as a guide to clinical management. *Hematol Oncol* 2006;**24**:196–204.

106. O'Hare T, Walters DK, Stoffregen EP, *et al.* Combined Abl inhibitor therapy for minimizing drug resistance in chronic myeloid leukemia: Src/Abl inhibitors are compatible with imatinib. *Clin Cancer Res* 2005;**11**:6987–93.

107. Weisberg E, Manley PW, Cowan-Jacob SW, *et al.* Second generation inhibitors of BCR-ABL for the treatment of imatinib-resistant chronic myeloid leukaemia. *Nat Rev Cancer* 2007;**7**:345–56.

108. Ma W, Tseng R, Gorre M, *et al.* Plasma RNA as an alternative to cells for

monitoring molecular response in patients with chronic myeloid leukemia. *Haematologica* 2007; **92**:170–5.

109. Ma W, Kantarjian H, Zhang X, *et al.* Mutation profile of JAK2 transcripts in patients with chronic myeloproliferative neoplasias. *J Mol Diagn* 2009;**11**:49–53.

110. Ma W, Kantarjian H, Verstovsek S, *et al.* Hemizygous/homozygous and heterozygous JAK2 mutation detected in plasma of patients with myeloproliferative diseases: correlation with clinical behaviour. *Br J Haematol* 2006;**134**:341–3.

111. Pardanani A, Lasho TL, Finke C, *et al.* Prevalence and clinicopathologic correlates of JAK2 exon 12 mutations in JAK2V617F-negative polycythemia vera. *Leukemia* 2007;**21**:1960–3.

112. Pancrazzi A, Guglielmelli P, Ponziani V, *et al.* A sensitive detection method for MPLW515L or MPLW515K mutation in chronic myeloproliferative disorders with locked nucleic acid-modified probes and real-time polymerase chain reaction. *J Mol Diagn* 2008;**10**:435–41.

113. Pikman Y, Lee BH, Mercher T, *et al.* MPLW515L is a novel somatic activating mutation in myelofibrosis with myeloid metaplasia. *PLoS Med* 2006;**3**:e270.

114. Ding J, Komatsu H, Wakita A, *et al.* Familial essential thrombocythemia associated with a dominant-positive activating mutation of the c-MPL gene, which encodes for the receptor for thrombopoietin. *Blood* 2004;**103**:4198–200.

115. El-Harith el-HA, Roesl C, Ballmaier M, *et al.* Familial thrombocytosis caused by the novel germ-line mutation p. Pro106Leu in the MPL gene. *Br J Haematol* 2009;**144**:185–94.

116. Beer PA, Campbell PJ, Scott LM, *et al.* MPL mutations in myeloproliferative disorders: analysis of the PT-1 cohort. *Blood* 2008;**112**:141–9.

117. Schnittger S, Bacher U, Haferlach C, *et al.* Characterization of 35 new cases with four different MPLW515 mutations and essential thrombocytosis or primary myelofibrosis. *Haematologica* 2009;**94**:141–4.

118. Lasho TL, Pardanani A, McClure RF, *et al.* Concurrent MPL515 and JAK2V617F mutations in myelofibrosis: chronology of clonal emergence and changes in mutant allele burden over time. *Br J Haematol* 2006;**135**:683–7.

119. Vannucchi AM, Antonioli E, Guglielmelli P, *et al.* Characteristics and clinical correlates of MPL 515W>L/K mutation in essential thrombocythemia. *Blood* 2008;**112**:844–7.

120. Cross NC, Reiter A. Fibroblast growth factor receptor and platelet-derived growth factor receptor abnormalities in eosinophilic myeloproliferative disorders. *Acta Haematol* 2008;**119**:199–206.

121. Cools J, DeAngelo DJ, Gotlib J, *et al.* A tyrosine kinase created by fusion of the PDGFRA and FIP1L1 genes as a therapeutic target of imatinib in idiopathic hypereosinophilic syndrome. *N Engl J Med* 2003;**348**:1201–14.

122. Metzgeroth G, Walz C, Score J, *et al.* Recurrent finding of the FIP1L1-PDGFRA fusion gene in eosinophilia-associated acute myeloid leukemia and lymphoblastic T-cell lymphoma. *Leukemia* 2007;**21**:1183–8.

123. Bain BJ, Fletcher SH. Chronic eosinophilic leukemias and the myeloproliferative variant of the hypereosinophilic syndrome. *Immunol Allergy Clin North Am* 2007;**27**:377–88.

124. Golub TR, Barker GF, Lovett M, *et al.* Fusion of PDGF receptor beta to a novel ets-like gene, tel, in chronic myelomonocytic leukemia with t(5;12) chromosomal translocation. *Cell* 1994;**77**:307–16.

125. Steer EJ, Cross NC. Myeloproliferative disorders with translocations of chromosome 5q31–35: role of the platelet-derived growth factor receptor Beta. *Acta Haematol* 2002;**107**:113–22.

Chapter 2

Management of acute myeloid leukemia

Alan K. Burnett

Introduction

In light of the age distribution of acute myeloid leukemia (AML) decisions on the approach to treatment are primarily determined by patient age. Unless there are compelling reasons to the contrary, patients up to 60 years or so will be offered intensive induction and consolidation treatment.[1,2] Population-based studies in Europe and the United States indicate that patients above this age are less likely (i.e., 30%) to receive conventional chemotherapy.[3,4] One of the current treatment dilemmas is who in the older population should be offered conventional chemotherapy and who should not. This is usually decided by patient-related factors such as age, performance score, and presence of comorbidities, but frequently other factors are influential such as social circumstances and the wishes of the patient. Less frequently disease-related factors, such as the presence of high-risk cytogenetics, might suggest that there is little to be gained from conventional treatment.

Although by no means definitive this dilemma has stimulated the development of a number of prognostic scoring systems in the older patient.[5–7] These can provide a more realistic estimate of outcome to inform patient decisions and, if appropriate, can define patients where an experimental approach is justifiable.

Induction chemotherapy

Conventional treatment is a combination of an anthracycline and cytarabine (cytosine arabinoside [Ara-C]). The anthracycline is usually daunorubicin, mitoxantrone, or idarubicin. Ara-C may be given as a 12-hourly bolus or by continuous infusion over 7 to 10 days. Which anthracycline? In terms of overall benefit there are few consistent data to suggest a best choice. In some studies mitoxantrone or idarubicin tended to have a modest advantage, but are associated with more myelosuppression. In an extensive formal meta-analysis of seven comparative trials the conclusion confirmed this perception.[8] Recently published studies suggest that 90 mg/m^2 of daunorubicin is superior to 45 mg/m^2 suggesting that higher doses may provide benefit.[9,10] However, the outcome in these reports is matched by several other studies in which conventional doses were used. Since there is a dose response to Ara-C in AML, three major studies have assessed the value of dose escalation of high- or intermediate-dose Ara-C during induction.[11–13] The observations were that there was no convincing overall survival benefit.

A large study conducted by the Australian Leukemia Study Group suggested that the addition of etoposide as a third drug improved outcome.[14] Older trials assessed the addition of thioguanine as the third drug but did not find a clear benefit; however, it has been traditionally used in the UK Medical Research Council (MRC) trials. In a major randomized comparison of daunorubicin plus Ara-C combined with either etoposide or thioguanine as the third drug, no significant differences were observed with respect to remission rate or survival overall or in any patient subgroup.[2] The conclusion for standard practice at the present time is that a combination of anthracycline 3 days and Ara-C by continuous infusion over 7 days, or 12-hourly bolus over 10 days, is standard care.

Results of induction chemotherapy

As a general estimate, combination chemotherapy will achieve complete disease remission (CR) in 75–80% of patients under 60 years and is age related. For patients over 60, 45–60% will enter CR (Table 2.1). It should be borne in mind that older patients who receive a conventional induction schedule are a selected group. So the relatively encouraging results seen in older patients ignores contemporary patients not subjected to, or thought fit for treatment. As can be seen from Table 2.1 there has been improvement in the remission rate over the last 20 years in all ages. Since the basic anthracycline–Ara-C approach has changed little, these improvements can probably be accounted for by improved supportive care – which is a crucial component of effective development of more intensive treatments.

Definition of response

Particularly in relation to novel agents, the category of CRp or CRi has emerged. This defines patients who fulfill the

Management of Hematologic Malignancies, ed. Susan M. O'Brien, Julie M. Vose, and Hagop M. Kantarjian. Published by Cambridge University Press.

Table 2.1. Remission rates for AML in UK Medical Research Council trials

Changes in outcome with time						
	Pre-1980	1980–4	1985–9	1990–4	1995–9	2000–5
Age < 15	39%	82%	90%	92%	92%	93%
Age 15–59	40%	73%	76%	79%	83%	85%
Age 60–69	25%	52%	47%	58%	60%	65%
Age 70+	18%	36%	40%	48%	47%	62%
Overall	34%	66%	70%	74%	77%	79%

conventional definition of bone marrow response, but have not recovered platelets (CRp) or neutrophils. CRi therefore has been developed as a category of response to induction therapy. In the UK MRC studies illustrated in Table 2.1, peripheral blood criteria were not required; however, by current definition[15] about 6% of younger patients and 8–10% of older patients would now be in the CRi category of response. In terms of survival it has been less clear whether CR and CRi were equivalent. In a recent retrospective comparison of two large databases CRp had an inferior overall survival compared with CR by Cheson Criteria.[15] In some studies an early marrow assessment on day 14 or 16 has been used as an indicator for immediate additional therapy and poorer outcome.[17]

Most patients who enter CR do so with the first induction course. Patients who do not achieve CR or CRi can be classed as partial (PR) or non-response. About half of PR patients will enter CR with a second induction course involving the same drugs. Patients who achieve less than a PR are refractory, and although there is little direct evidence to support it, it is normal practice to use an alternative treatment. In the UK MRC experience, the response to course 1, whether CR, CRi, PR, or refractory disease, is highly predictive for subsequent survival even though they achieve CR with the next or subsequent treatments.[18] Interestingly, there is little survival difference between CR and PR patients who enter CR; however, both are better than patients who enter CR and have achieved less than a PR to course 1.

Alternative schedules

Even in younger patients where the remission rate is high, there is justification to try to improve both the rate and quality of CR. There are several examples of treatment which do not appear to improve the rate of CR but lead to a reduction in relapse risk and thereby improve survival.

Growth factors

Several randomized trials have evaluated what contribution growth factors (granulocyte colony-stimulating factor [G-CSF] or granulocyte–macrophage colony-stimulating factor [GM-CSF]) can make.[19] In general these have been used to curtail the duration of post-induction neutropenia. Some studies have intended to "prime" leukemic cells by exploiting the fact that they have growth factor receptors which can stimulate cells into cycle and thereby make the cells more sensitive to chemotherapy.[20] On the whole these studies have been disappointing in that they have usually not improved survival.[21,22] Concerns that they may stimulate leukemic proliferation have not been realized. The duration of neutropenia has been reduced usually by 2 to 4 days but this has not necessarily resulted in reduction in days on antibiotics or in hospital. Most, but not all, studies have not shown a difference in response rate or subsequent relapse risk. Fewer studies have attempted the priming strategy of which most have been negative. The most recent trial conducted by the HOVON group in Europe was able to demonstrate a small survival benefit in standard-risk patients due to a reduction in relapse risk.[23] This, however, is a subgroup analysis of a trial which has not been corroborated in other studies. The duration of neutropenia is more prolonged following consolidation therapy. Growth factor studies in this setting have a more pronounced benefit in reduction of neutropenia and duration of hospitalization.

Overall there is no consistent evidence that routine use of growth factors, although safe, improves survival. It may be that for socioeconomic reasons and in certain healthcare systems curtailment of neutropenia – particularly in consolidation – is reasonable. Current guidelines from the British Committee for Standards in Haematology and American Society of Clinical Oncology (ASCO) concur that routine use can be recommended only in consolidation.[24,25]

Resistance modulation

A number of biochemical mechanisms can make cells resistant to the frequently used agents such as daunorubicin or etoposide. These include P-glycoprotein (Pgp), which is a product of the *MDR1* gene, MRP (multidrug resistance-associated protein), LRP (lung resistance protein), and BCL2. P-glycoprotein overexpression is frequently seen in AML, particularly in older patients where more than 70% have this feature, which is assumed to, at least in part, explain why older patients are less responsive to treatment.[26,27] As well as being a prognostic factor for induction, response, and survival, Pgp has been a therapeutic target because drugs like ciclosporin or its

Table 2.2. Randomized trials of gemtuzumab ozogamicin

Trial	Age	Intervention	Status
MRC AML 15	<60	GO (3 mg/m^2) Course 1 and/or 3	Closed
SWOG 106	<60	D (45 mg/m^2), A + GO (6 mg/m^2) vs. D (60 mg/m^2), A ± GO maintenance	Closed
HOVON–SAKK 43	>60	±GO maintenance 6 mg/m^2 4 weekly × 3	Closed
EORTC–GIMEMA AML 17	<60	GO (6 + 6 mg/m^2) + MICE vs. MICE induction ± GO + mini-ICE in consolidation	Open
EORTC–GIMEMA AML 19	>60 (unfit)	GO monotherapy 6 mg/m^2 day 1, 3 mg/m^2 day 8 vs. best supportive care	Open
ECOG E1900		±GO 6 mg/m^2 pre-autograft consolidation	Closed
NCRI AML 17	<60	Induction chemotherapy + GO 3 mg/m^2 vs. 6 mg/m^2	Open
NCRI AML 16	>60 (unfit)	Low dose Ara-C ± GO 5 mg on day 1	Closed
NCRI AML 16	>60	Induction chemotherapy ± GO 3 mg/m^2	Closed

Notes: MRC: Medical Research Council; SWOG: Southwest Oncology Group;
HOVON–SAKK: Haemato-oncologie voor volwassenen Nederland-schweizerische Arbeitsgemeinschaft fur Klinische Krebsforschung;
EORTC–GIMEMA: European Organization for Research and Treatment of Cancer–Gruppo Italiano Malattie Ematologiche dell'Adulto;
ECOG: Eastern Cooperative Oncology Group; NCRI: National Cancer Research Institute; GO: gemtuzumab ozogamicin; D: daunorubicin; A: cytarabine;
MICE: mitoxantrone, cytarabine, and etoposide; ICE: idarubicin, cytarabine, and etaposide.

derivative PSC-833, and next-generation agents such as zosiquidar, are very effective Pgp reversal agents in preclinical studies. In spite of the clear preclinical effect, clinical trials of reversal agents have disappointed. The strategy was given early encouragement by a study in relapsed disease reported by the Southwest Oncology Group in which patients were treated with ciclosporin combined with daunorubicin – given by continuous infusion – and Ara-C versus daunorubicin-Ara-C alone.[28] Survival was superior in the ciclosporin arm. An MRC trial also tested ciclosporin in relapsed disease but was unable to show benefit; however, the ciclosporin dose was probably inadequate, and infusional daunorubicin was not used.[29] PSC-833 was perceived to have advantages over ciclosporin in that it is less immunosuppressive with less potential renal toxicity. Because both ciclosporin and PSC-833 increase the area under the curve (AUC) of target drugs, trials required the standard dose of daunorubicin and etoposide to be reduced. In the trials reported in untreated patients no benefit has been observed.[30–32] Preliminary reports of the next-generation agent, zosiquidar, do not suggest a likely benefit.[33]

The fact that reversal of resistance, while impressive in vitro, has not shown clinical benefit might be explained by the coexistence of other resistance mechanisms that are not susceptible to the agents developed so far.[34]

Antibody-directed chemotherapy

Initial studies using a naked anti-CD33 humanized monoclonal antibody showed some activity in acute promyelocytic leukemia (APL) by converting patients who were in remission, but molecularly positive, to molecular negativity.[35] However, in a randomized trial in relapsed AML, when added or not to conventional chemotherapy there was no improvement in remission rate or survival.[36] Recently, new studies have been initiated using this unconjugated antibody as monotherapy in older patients who are not suitable for standard chemotherapy.[37]

A more recent strategy is to deliver chemotherapy as an immunoconjugate. Gemtuzumab ozogamicin (GO; Mylotarg) was developed for this purpose. It is an IgG_3 humanized anti-CD33 monoclonal antibody which is attached by a unique chemical linker to the powerful intercalator, calicheamicin. On the basis of unrandomized phase II trials[38] in older patients in relapsed disease it gained regulatory approval in the USA, but not in Europe. In this context reinduction rates (CR and CRi) of approximately 1 in 3 were observed. When given at full dose, i.e., 9 mg/m^2, in patients who have had or will have a stem cell transplant, extra liver toxicity in the form of veno-occlusive disease (VOD) – otherwise described as sinusoidal obstructive syndrome – was observed.[39] This was also observed when added in full dose to chemotherapy.[40] Because of the unique mechanism of action there has been considerable interest – particularly in Europe – in assessing its role in various settings of AML.

In induction GO is seen as a way of either improving the quality of remission by simultaneously combining it with chemotherapy, or improving overall response by pretreating patients with GO as monotherapy before standard chemotherapy (Table 2.2).[41] Preliminary phase II studies established that doses of 6 mg/m^2 or 3 mg/m^2 given simultaneously with chemotherapy were safe.[42,43] Randomized trials have yet to be fully completed or reported. However, a preliminary analysis of the UK MRC AML15 trial demonstrated no improvement in remission rate, but a reduction in relapse risk and improved disease free survival. However, there was no significant improvement in overall survival.[44] It appears that the benefit is limited to the more favorable risk patients defined by age and cytogenetics. This and other studies will need analysis on mature data.

All-*trans* retinoic acid (ATRA)

The inclusion of ATRA treatment in APL has revolutionized the survival in that disease. APL cells are amenable to the proapoptotic effects of ATRA. Preclinical studies conducted by Lishner and colleagues demonstrated that pretreatment of non-APL AML cells with ATRA increased sensitivity to Ara-C, probably by reducing the expression of BCL2.[45] This provided the rationale for testing the combination of ATRA with chemotherapy in non-APL patients. The first study was initially encouraging but in final analysis showed no benefit.[46] The UK MRC Group was unable to show any benefit when added to low-dose Ara-C in frontline treatment of older patients[47] or when combined with fludarabine-Ara-C in relapsed patients,[48] or in a large trial of first-line treatment in younger patients.[13] A similar study conducted by the Ulm group, however, has shown a survival benefit in older patients.[49] They also suggested that response was associated with the presence of a mutation of the nucleophosmin 1 (*NPM1*) gene or the expression of the meningioma 1 gene (*MN1*).[50] These findings have not been confirmed in the large MRC study.[51,52]

Fludarabine-based induction combinations

Fludarabine as a single agent is active in AML but only at doses associated with unacceptable neurotoxicity. The biochemical rationale for combining with Ara-C resulted in several similar schedules of fludarabine/Ara-C/idarubicin usually with additional G-CSF being developed and tested in the phase II settings. The issue of whether G-CSF or even idarubicin are important contributions has received modest attention. The MRC AMLHR trial compared fludarabine/Ara-C (FA) ± G-CSF against Ara-C/daunorubicin/etoposide (ADE ± G-CSF) in patients with high-risk disease or relapse and found that FA was not superior and the addition of G-CSF did not improve results.[48] In the MRC AML15 trial FLAG-Ida (fludarabine, Ara-C, G-CSF, idarubicin) was compared to DA and ADE. It appeared to have more antileukemic effect but this advantage was neutralized by significantly more myelosuppression and difficulty in complying with subsequent consolidation. Of interest was that it was possible to add GO to FLAG-Ida to enhance the antileukemic effect without additional myelosuppression.[42]

Consolidation treatment

Consolidation chemotherapy

Historically post-induction treatment was delivered with the same drugs but in a less intensive fashion, which may or may not have been followed by maintenance. In the modern era intensive consolidation is given. The landmark Cancer and Leukemia Group B (CALGB) trial[53] established the evidence of an Ara-C dose response. The aim of the trial was to compare three doses in consolidation, 100 mg/m^2 versus 400 mg/m^2 versus 3.0 g/m^2. This established 3 g/m^2 as a standard of care for consolidation, which might be particularly suitable for patients with favorable cytogenetics.[54] While high-dose Ara-C is a standard of care for consolidation but its use in induction has not been found to be of value in all studies, the option to use it in both induction and consolidation has been prospectively tested in one Australasian trial. There was no advantage in deploying it in both phases.[55]

Treatment outcomes

In younger patients treatment results have improved, particularly in children and to some extent in younger adults up to 60 years of age. However, results from the experience of major collaborative groups do not suggest that similar benefits have been delivered to older patients (Figure 2.1). It should also be borne in mind that the median age of AML patients is 68 years and these outcomes in older patients only apply to those given conventional therapy and do not represent the patients given only palliation with best supportive care.

Stem cell transplantation

There are now a variety of techniques being undertaken to establish a full chimera of donor hemopoiesis. The purpose of autologous transplantation was to permit the marrow to be exposed to sublethal irradiation and rescue hemopoiesis with harvested peripheral blood or bone marrow which had been collected in remission. This approach is relatively safe in patients up to 60 years and has a powerful antileukemic effect, but the main reason for failure is disease recurrence which is likely to develop from residual disease in the patient or possibly the regrafted marrow. Using a donor as a source of stem cells has the additional benefits of ensuring that the new marrow is not a source of disease, but more importantly provides a graft-versus-leukemia (GVL) reaction. There is a growing belief that it is the GVL effect that mediates the major component of the antileukemic mechanism.

Major collaborative group trials have evaluated the role of a standard transplant incorporating myeloablative conditioning with a match sibling donor. The EORTC,[56] HOVON,[57] GOELAM,[58] and US Intergroup[59] studies set out to compare transplant with consolidation chemotherapy – usually high-dose Ara-C. The UK MRC AML10 trial evaluated consolidation chemotherapy with or without an additional transplant.[60] The overall results (Figure 2.2) were generally similar, and have influenced current practice. None of these comparisons were truly randomized except the subsequent MRC AML12 trial[13] and a "genetic" randomization was undertaken, i.e., "donor versus no donor." This is not an ideal comparison, particularly since not every patient who had a donor received a transplant. With these reservations in mind a number of general conclusions can be made. There is a consistent picture that transplant reduces the risk of relapse in most risk groups and age strata; this in some, but not all, studies results in a significantly better disease-free survival, but not overall survival. This discrepancy is explained by the fact that there

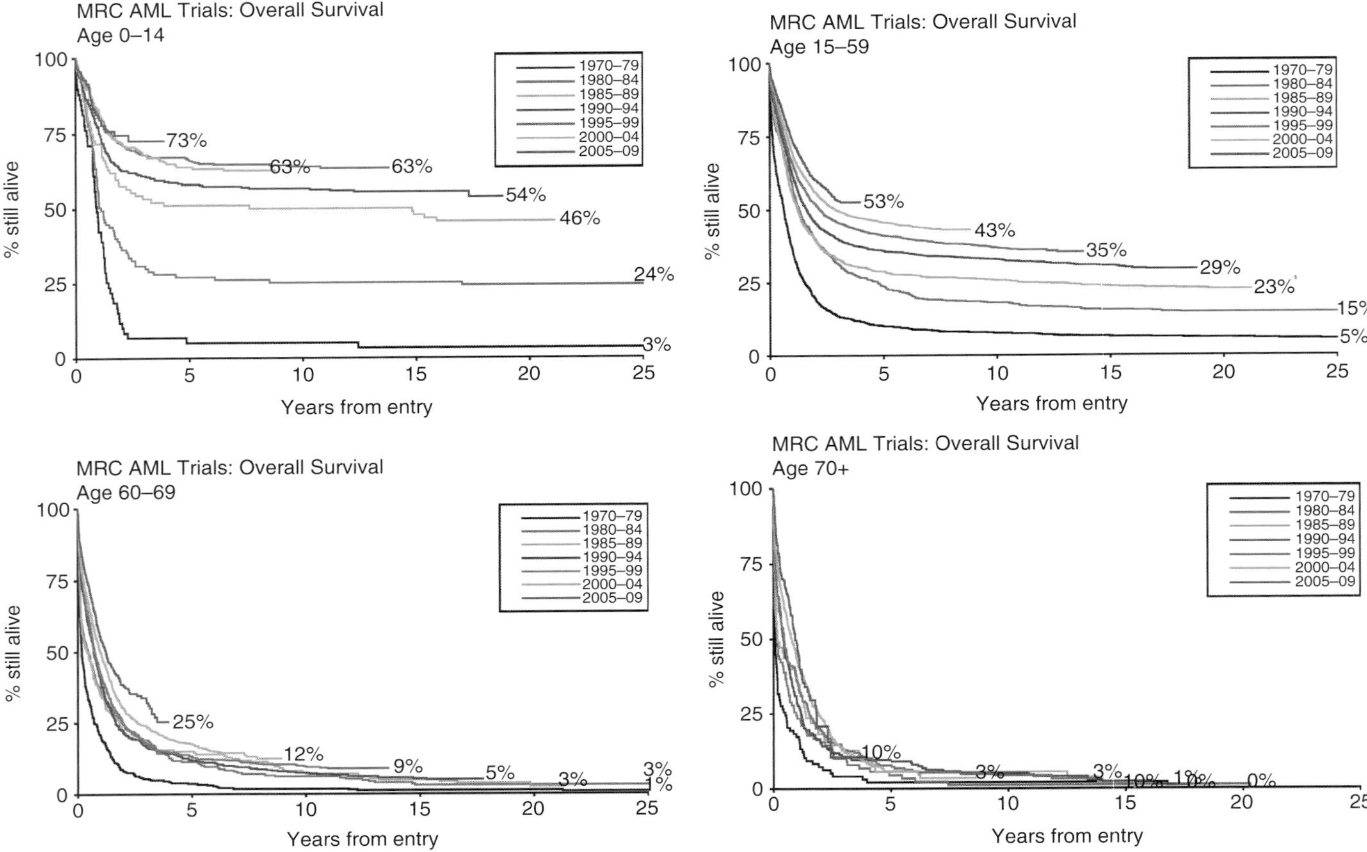

Figure 2.1 Survival changes with time in major age groups.

remains an important procedure-related mortality, and that a higher proportion of patients who received chemotherapy alone could be salvaged when they relapsed, compared with those who were transplanted. As will be discussed below, patients who enter remission have significant differences in their individual relapse risk. This is predominantly defined by cytogenetics at diagnosis. Most studies are consistent in that patients who are at low risk do not have a better survival with a transplant in CR1. The data are variable in patients with high-risk disease, where there is also the issue of early relapse occurring before a transplant can be delivered, which in turn weakens the donor vs. no donor analysis. Of the five major studies a clear survival benefit in poor-risk disease was only seen in the US Intergroup trial. The patient numbers in the individual studies are small so it is still accepted practice to offer high-risk patients this treatment approach with the recommendation that patients should be identified early and move to transplant promptly. This is also justified by the poor chance of salvaging poor-risk patients if they relapse.

The remaining difficulty remains with patients who are neither good nor poor risk, who comprise 60% of patients in the transplantable age range. None of the studies showed an overall survival benefit in these standard-risk patients. These trials were primarily designed to assess autologous transplantation. In this respect the results generate similar conclusions as just summarized, although the main reason for failure was disease relapse. These studies have been useful and have demonstrated the importance of using relapse risk in decision making with respect to transplantation. They are however out of date and several new issues have to be taken into account.

Cytogenetics is not the only determinant of relapse risk as discussed below. Other features such as presenting white count, age, de novo or secondary disease, sex, and marrow response to first treatment course are all readily available factors, each of which is an independent predictor. All or any of these factors may cause concern in patients who are of standard cytogenetic risk. On retrospectively reviewing a composite score derived from a Cox regression model, which was prospectively validated, approximately 20% of standard-risk patients can be redefined as high risk.[61] Whereas no overall survival benefit was seen in the cytogenetically defined high-risk patients, the transfer of the redefined intermediate risk to the high-risk category results in a clear trend for benefit in the

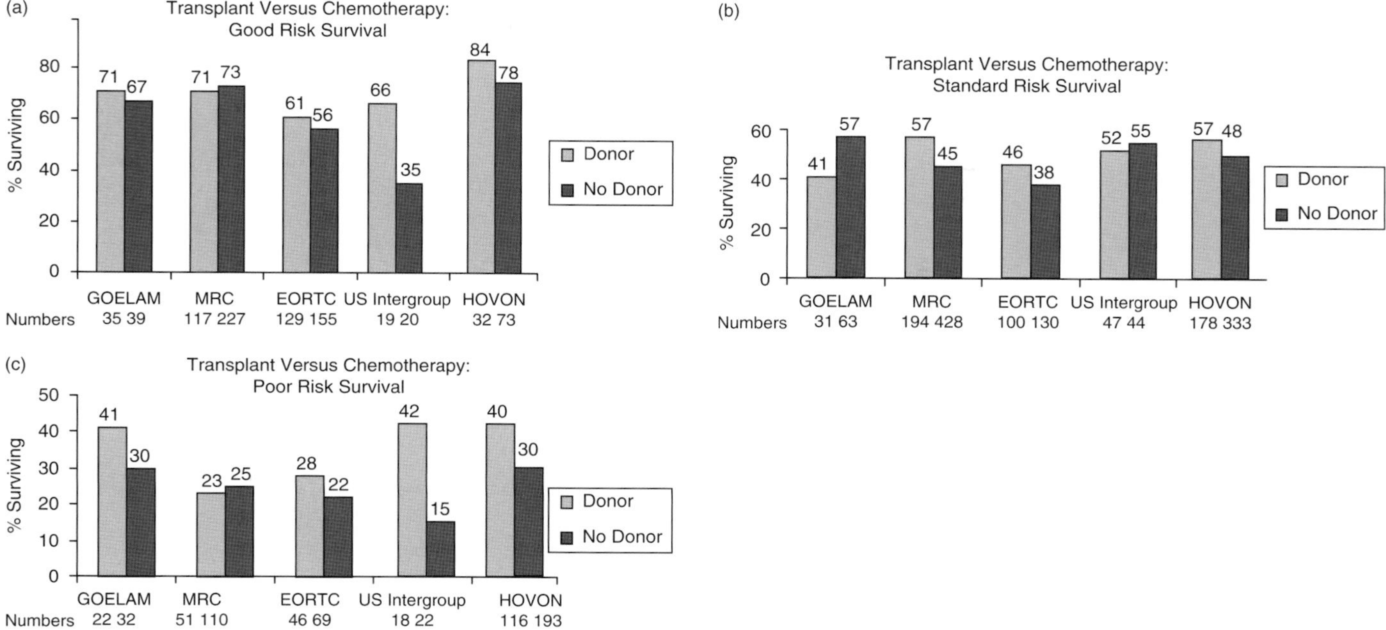

Figure 2.2 Overall survival by risk group in collaborative group trials. (a) Good risk, (b) intermediate risk, and (c) poor risk.

new high-risk group in this study. This illustrates that there are subgroups of patients who can be identified where there is evidence of survival benefit and the priority must be to improve the proportion of such patients who actually receive the transplant.

The molecular heterogeneity of AML has delineated mutations which have prognostic implications, for example mutations of *NPM1* and *CEBPα* tend to be favorable whereas *FLT3, EVI1*, and *WT1* mutations predict for a higher relapse risk. Setting these additional factors in the context of existing factors and using them to direct therapy is a major challenge which is now beginning.

While defining which patients will have their survival improved by a standard myeloablative transplant is very complicated, it has also been limited in its applicability by the need to find a matched donor and by age. In the studies mentioned above there was no evidence of a survival benefit for patients > 35–40 years of age. New transplant techniques have now opened up opportunities for a substantially greater proportion of cases. Expansion of volunteer donor panels and improved tissue typing techniques now mean that unrelated transplant is safe and the emerging results suggest can produce survival that is similar to that delivered by a standard matched sibling allograft. The recognition that myeloablative treatment was not a prerequisite for establishing a full chimera has raised the prospect in AML that a reduced intensity conditioned (RIC) allograft could confer the same GVL effect. The emerging evidence suggests that this is a feasible option for older patients with encouraging survival (Table 2.3). This approach has, as yet, not been proven to be superior to chemotherapy and should therefore be undertaken in the context of a clinical trial. While it does offer the transplant prospect to older patients, current evidence suggests that the actual proportion of older patients receiving it is small.[80]

Transplantation in second remission

Overall transplantation in second remission improves survival from 20% to 40%. The most powerful predictors of outcome if a patient relapses and enters a second remission are age, duration of CR1, and the original cytogenetic risk group.[81,82] Of those receiving a transplant and using a donor versus no donor assessment, good- and intermediate-risk but not poor-risk patients had a survival benefit.[83] Similarly patients with CR1 of < 6 months did not benefit. The hurdles for patients are the achievement of second remission, receiving a transplant, and surviving post transplant. With respect to understanding how many patients who relapse can be salvaged the MRC group reported the 20-year experience in 730 patients who avoided a transplant in CR1 (Figure 2.3).[84] The respective rates of CR2 were 72%, 43%, and 25% respectively in the good-, intermediate- and poor-risk groups. Of those who gained remission, 73%, 62%, and 63% respectively received a transplant of some sort. So 53%, 27%, and 16% of each respective group who relapsed received a transplant. When the outcome of transplant is taken into account, 32%, 11%, and 4% of good-, intermediate- and poor-risk patients are salvaged.

Immunologic approaches

Since it is possible to expand an autoreactive T-cell population which could mount immunologic control over residual disease, there has been interest in augmenting this effect with maintenance interleukin 2 (IL-2). At least two randomized

Table 2.3. Reduced intensity conditioning hematopoietic stem cell transplantation in AML: summary of trials including at least 20 patients

Reference	No. patients AML (total)	Median age (range)	Conditioning regimen	Donor type (related/unrelated)	Graft failure	TRM/NRM	Acute GVHD (II–IV)/Chronic GVHD	Relapse	LFS/PFS	OS
Giralt *et al.*, 2001[62]	43 (86)	52 (22–70)	Flu/Mel or 2-CdA/Mel	46/40	NA	37% (100-day)	49%/68%	27%	23% (2-yr)	28% (2-yr)
Sayer *et al.*, 2003[63]	113	51 (16–67)	Flu/Cy/Bu or TBI (4–8 Gy)/Flu	51/62	5%	53% (2-yr)	42%/33%	NA	29% (2-yr)	32% (2-yr)
Hamaki *et al.*, 2004[64]	24 (36)	55 (27–67)	2-CdA or Flu/Bu ± ATG	24/0	3%	3% (100-day)	48%/82%	22%	85% (1-yr) low-risk, 64% (1-yr) high-risk	NA
Ho *et al.*, 2004[65]	23 (62)	53 (22–70)	Flu/Bu/Campath	7/16	3%	15% (1-yr)	NA	NA	62% (1-yr)	74% (1-yr)
Gomez-Nunez *et al.*, 2004[66]	20 (145)	54 (19–67)	Flu/Mel or Flu/Bu	20/0	NA	20% (1-yr)	34%/41% (1-yr)	NA	52% (1-yr)	60% (1-yr)
de Lima *et al.*, 2004[67]	68 (94)	54 (22–75) FM 61 (27–74) FAI	Flu/Mel (FM) or Flu/Ara-C/Ida (FAI)	65/29	3% FM 19% FAI	26% (100-day) FM 13% (100-day) FAI	39%/39% FM 25%/27% FAI	30% FM 61% FAI	32% (3-yr) FM 19% (3-yr) FAI	35% (3-yr) FM 30% (3-yr) FAI
Hallemeier *et al.*, 2004[68]	32	47 (32–60)	Cy/TBI (5.5 Gy)	29/3	0%	28%	3%[a]/54%	22%	57% (3-yr) CR1, 39% (3-yr) CR2+	55% (3-yr) CR1, 39% (3-yr) CR2+
Aoudjhane *et al.*, 2005[69]	315	57 (50–73)	Flu/Bu or Flu/TBI (< 3 Gy)	315/0	NA	18% (1-yr)	22%/48% (2-yr)	41%	40% (2-yr)	47% (2-yr)
Baron *et al.*, 2005[70]	46 (322)	54 (5–72)	TBI (2 Gy) ± Flu	192/130	7%	NA	58%/56%	34%	39% (3-yr)	50% (3-yr)
van Besien *et al.*, 2005[71]	41 (52)	52 (17–71)	Flu/Mel/Campath	27/25	4%	33% (2-yr)	33%/18% (1-yr)	40% (2-yr)	31% (2-yr)	39% (2-yr)
Tauro *et al.*, 2005[72]	56 (76)	52 (18–71)	Flu/Mel/Campath	35/41	3%	19% (1-yr)	28%/11%	36%	37% (3-yr)	41% (3-yr)
Schmid *et al.*, 2005[73]	75	52 (19–66)	Sequential Flu/Ara-C/Amsa then Cy/TBI (4 Gy)/ATG	31/44	7%	33% (1-yr)	49%/35%	17%	40% (2-yr)	42% (2-yr)
Claxton *et al.*, 2005[74]	23	59 (28–72)	Flu/Cy/Sirolimus ± ATG	6/17	0%	8%	43%/77%	NA	NA	50% (2-yr)

Mohty *et al.*, 2005[75]	25 (35)	52 (26–55)	Flu/Bu/ATG	25/0	NA	12%	NA	12% (4-yr)	62% (4-yr)	NA
Hegenbart *et al.*, 2006[76]	122	57 (17–74)	TBI (2 Gy) ± Flu	58/64	5%	16% (2-yr)	40%/36%	39% (2-yr)	44% (2-yr)	48% (2-yr)
Platzbecker *et al.*, 2006[77]	26	49 (17–68)	Flu/Mel or Flu/Bu	11/15	NA	15% (2-yr)	54%/64%	11%	63% (3-yr)	63% (3-yr)
Scott *et al.*, 2006[78]	20 (38)	62 (40–72)	TBI (2 Gy) ± Flu	26/12	12%	39% (3-yr)	54%/55% (2-yr)	31% (3-yr)	27% (3-yr)	28% (3-yr)
Shimoni *et al.*, 2006[79]	56 (67)	50 (17–70)	Flu/Bu (either FB2: Bu 6.4 mg/kg or FB4: Bu 12.8 mg/kg)	29/38	7% FB2 4% FB4	8% (2-yr) FB2 & FB4	8%[a]/31% FB2 8%[a]/59% FB4	49% FB2 43% FB4	43% (2-yr) FB2 49% (2-yr) FB4	47% (2-yr) FB2 49% (2-yr) FB4

Notes: [a]Grade III–IV acute graft-versus-host disease Ara-C: cytosine arabinoside; ATG: anti-thymocyte globulin; Bu: busulfan; CR1: first complete remission; CR2+: second or subsequent complete remission; Cy: cyclophosphamide; Flu: fludarabine; GVHD: graft-versus-host disease; Gy: gray; Ida: idarubicin; LFS: leukemia-free survival; Mel: melphalan; NA, not available; NRM: non-relapse mortality; OS: overall survival; PFS: progression-free survival; 2-CdA: cladribine; Amsa: amsacrine; TBI: total body irradiation; TRM: transplant-related mortality; yr: year.

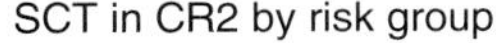

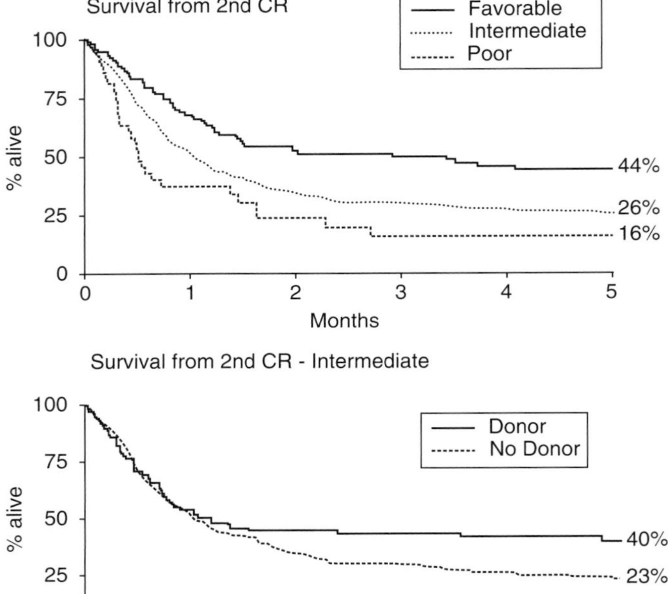

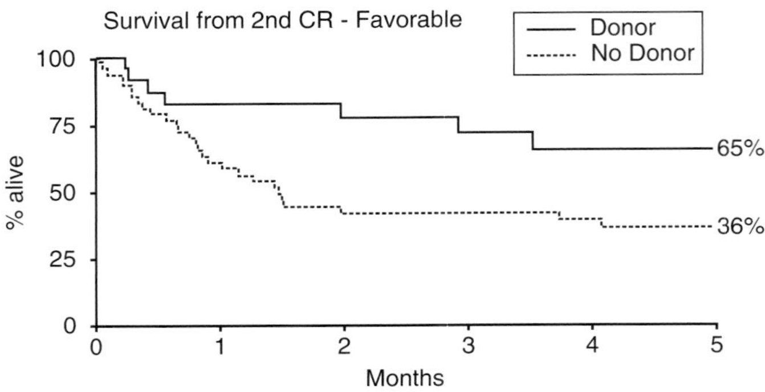

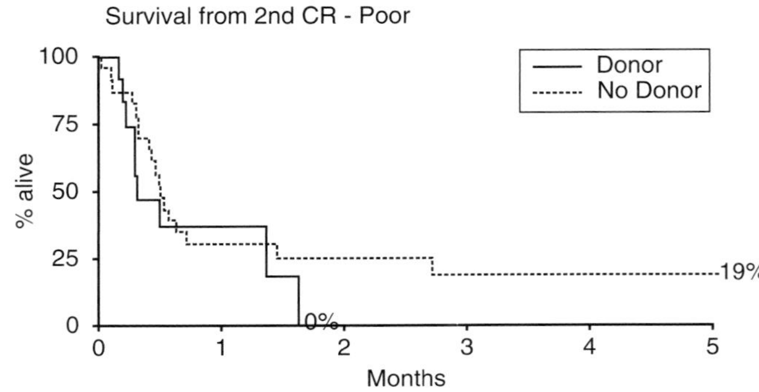

Figure 2.3 Transplantation in second remission.

trials have been disappointing.[85,86] Recently a new approach of combining lower doses of IL-2 with histamine has been developed based on preclinical observations that the combination is more efficient than either alone. Patients randomized after consolidation in CR1 had a significantly improved leukemia-free survival with this combination, although the overall survival was not statistically significant.[87] This is of interest, but probably needs to be confirmed.

Prognostic factors

The literature is replete with reports of factors which appear capable of predicting which patients will respond to treatment and who are at differing risk of relapse. It is of critical importance that such factors are prospectively validated on a separate dataset which is of adequate size to make the prediction statistically robust and independent in multivariate analysis. The most reliable tend to override treatment effects. The clinical interest in prognostic factors is either to provide information about disease biology, to delineate potential targets for therapy, or to make treatment decisions. While several factors are prognostic, far fewer are predictive, i.e., provide a validated basis to adopt a particular treatment approach. It is easy to omit the validation step and also to make the assumption that a prognostic factor is in fact predictive. Stem cell transplantation is often felt to be appropriate for a patient who is at an increased risk without evidence that such an approach is validated. What is poor prognosis for chemotherapy is usually also poor prognosis for transplantation. However, there are emerging situations where relevant new therapeutic possibilities are available, e.g., FLT3 inhibitors for FLT3 mutated patients.

Table 2.4. Prognostic factors in remission

Cytogenetics	Mutations	Impact
Age	*FLT3* ITD (25%)[a]	−ve
Presenting white count	*FLT3* TK (7%)	−ve
Marrow response to course 1	*RAS* (12%)	nil
Persistence of minimal residual disease	*CEBPa* (5–10%)	+ve
Sex	*NPM1* (40%)	+ve
	EVI1 (8%)	−ve
	WT1 (8%)	−ve
	MLL (7%)	−ve

Note: [a]Incidence.

Validated prognostic factors

Age, cytogenetic risk group, response to course 1 of treatment, presenting white count, and de novo, secondary, or treatment-related disease are among the most widely recognized, and are used to make treatment decisions (Table 2.4). The subtlety of

Table 2.5. Collaborative group cytogenetic risk classification

	Variation in cytogenetic risk group classification in AML				
	MRC	SWOG/ECOG	CALGB	GIMEMA/ AML10	German AMLCG
Favorable	t(15;17) t(8;21) inv(16)/ t(16;16)	t(15;17) t(8;21) (lacking del (9q), complex i.e. > 3 unrel abn) inv(16)/t(16;16)/del (16q)	t(15;17) t(8;21) inv(16)/t(16;16)	t(15;17) t(8;21) inv (16)/ t(16;16)	t(15;17) t(8;21) inv(16)/t(16;16)
Intermediate	Normal Other non-complex	Normal +6, +8, -Y, del (12p)	Normal Other non-complex	Normal -Y	Normal Other non-complex
Adverse	abn(3q) -5/del(5q) -7 complex (> 5 unrel abn) (excluding those with favorable changes)	abn(3q), (9q), (11q), (21q), abn(17p) -5/del(5q) -7/del (7q) t(6;9) t(9;22) complex (> 3 unrel abn)	inv(3)/t(3;3) -7 t(6;9) t(6;11) t(11;19) +8 complex (> 3 unrel abn) (excluding those with favorable changes)	Other	inv(3)/t(3;3) -5/ del(5q) -7/del (7q) abn(11q23) del(12p) abn (17p)

Note: AMLCG: AML Cooperative Group.

cytogenetic risk groups and prognosis continues to evolve and enter new classifications (Table 2.5). In general age is the first discriminant in management. While this is a continuous variable, age becomes important in that there are limitations to the intensity of treatment that can be given to older patients, which would be routine in younger patients. The independence of cytogenetics is well validated. Although there are some differences between collaborative groups in relation to the definition of cytogenetic risk groups and new subcategories continue to be developed, chromosome changes have a dominant effect on treatment outcome. Patients who are under 60 years with favorable characteristics have a survival expectation of 65% on current chemotherapy and are generally not advised to undergo stem cell transplant. There has been little evidence of improved outcome in poor-risk young patients over the years leading some to question the value of persisting with a conventional chemotherapy approach. Most investigators would support the use of stem cell transplantation from a sibling or unrelated donor in this group even though the prospective trials carried out by the collaborative groups did not consistently show a survival benefit for this approach.

The intermediate cytogenetic risk group comprises 60% of all patients under 60 years. Once again the transplant trials have not consistently shown a survival benefit in this group although a significant reduction in relapse risk and disease-free survival is apparent. This discrepancy is due to the negative effect of greater treatment-related mortality in transplant recipients, and an increased ability to salvage patients who relapse from chemotherapy. It is primarily in this intermediate-risk group that the new molecular information has emerged – much of which appears to lack prognostic implications – some of which has been prognostically validated. In older patients prognostic factors are more difficult to find, and less useful, because treatment outcome remains poor. However, the same factors apply, but with less discrimination than in younger patients. In general older patients tend to have a preponderance of unfavorable factors and a higher proportion of cases with a chemotherapy "resistant" phenotype.

Molecular information

Information concerning mutations and genes that are overexpressed and have prognostic implication is rapidly emerging, and is further dissecting those established major risk groupings. Several publications have indicated that 25–30% of patients will have a mutation of the growth factor receptor FLT3.[88] This mutation has little effect on induction treatment outcome, but is highly predictive of patients likely to relapse, particularly in the intermediate cytogenetic risk group. Whether this automatically identifies patients who should be transplanted is not yet clear. The situation is further complicated by the observation that the relapse risk is not the same for all allelic ratios with high mutant:wild type presenting a higher risk. Increasing complexity has been introduced by the discovery that the cytoplasmic shuttling protein NPM1 is mutated in a high proportion (50%) of patients with a normal karyotype and consistently appears in 60% of patients with an *FLT3* mutation. In general *NPM1* predicts for a better response to induction and a reduced risk of relapse, and is therefore a favorable factor when it occurs on its own. It also appears to counteract the negative impact of *FLT3*.[89–92] So the poorest outcome occurs in *FLT3* mutants who do not have an NPM1 mutation. Patients who have an *NPM1* mutation without mutant *FLT3* have a survival similar to that of favorable (core binding factor) leukemias. It also appears that a double mutant of CEBPα confers a favorable outcome[93] while *EVI1* and *BAALC* overexpression have a negative impact.[94,95] Information will continue to accumulate as advancing technology is exploited. There are still issues with respect to standardization of assay, prospective validation, and inter-reaction between factors that remain to be settled. A major challenge is to integrate them into patient management. Some will emerge as therapeutic targets such as FLT3 or cKIT within the core binding factor leukemias.

Most guidance recommends that patients with high-risk cytogenetics should proceed to transplant as soon as possible, but even then the overall survival benefit is not unanimous between all studies when subjected to a donor versus no donor analysis. Opinion generally accepts that survival is not improved by transplant in favorable-risk patients (t(8;21), inv(16), or intermediate risk with *NPM1* mutation). It is now recognized that 20–30% of core binding factor leukemias have a cKIT mutation,[93–95] and that this confers a higher risk of relapse. There is so far no information as to whether this makes these patients candidates for transplant or indeed whether one of the tyrosine kinase inhibitors, such as Glivec, disatinib, or PKC416 (Staurosporin), may be beneficial. Of interest, the addition of GO to induction therapy of core binding factor leukemia in the UK MRC AML15 trial was particularly beneficial with a survival at 4 years of 84%. However, the effect on the cKIT subgroup is not yet known. Several molecules with anti-FLT3 activity have emerged and large randomized trials have been initiated which incorporate an inhibitor into standard chemotherapy. While the presence or overexpression of other molecular markers have emerged which have favorable (CEBPα, NPM1) or unfavorable (EVI1, FLT3+/NPM1$^-$) implications, they are not predictive with respect to what action to take.

Minimal residual disease

The emerging molecular knowledge and improved fluorescence activated cell sorting (FACS) technology have provided opportunities to monitor disease response at a level of detection well beyond conventional microscopy. There are several studies which provide clear evidence that patients at higher risk of relapse can be identified 3–6 months before clinical relapse (Table 2.6). It is important to be aware that the detection of minimal residual disease (MRD) does not always predict relapse. Most information available so far derives a threshold of detection that best correlated with relapse risk on a retrospective analysis; fewer have been prospectively validated and could be treatment dependent. Some approaches appear to be more useful as a single point analysis, e.g., a log reduction after induction or on completion of treatment, while others may be more useful as a disease monitor based on a particular sensitivity level.

The paradigm for this approach is APL where detection at a transcript level of 1×10^4 at the end of treatment predicts a high – almost inevitable – risk of relapse.[103,104]

However, since most cases are PCR negative at this point, more relapses come from the patients who are PCR negative at this time. So although the risk is lower, this group is bigger so a larger number of patients who relapse come from that group. The substitution of real-time quantitative (RQ)-PCR which has value in assessing the quality of the RNA does not add much if used as a single point assay; however, careful sequential monitoring of bone marrow at 3-monthly intervals is more successful.

Table 2.6. Studies of minimal residual disease detection by immunophenotyping

Venditti *et al.*[96]	56	3.5×10^4 cells after consolidation predicts relapse 77% vs. 17%
San Miguel *et al.*[97]	126	Increased risk of relapse 14% vs. 50%
Sievers *et al.*[98]	252	Relapse risk 69% vs. 41% (p = 0.0058)
Kern W *et al.*[99]	60	Log reduction after induction and consolidation -> DFS; after consolidation to OS 88% vs. 51% at 2 years
Coustan-Smith *et al.*[100]	46	72% vs. 33% relapse prediction
Feller *et al.*[101]	72	Predictive of relapse after course 1 and 3
Langebrake *et al.*[102]	542	Predicts relapse 71% vs. 48% and 70% vs. 50%. Does not provide additional predictive information

Note: DFS: disease-free survival; OS: overall survival.

The implication of MRD detection is that therapeutic intervention at the time of MRD positivity improves survival, compared to treating at the time of hematologic relapse. This is far from being established because in most cases a therapeutic option has not been validated. The exception to this is APL where intervention with arsenic trioxide is very effective. Ironically the relapse risk of APL treated with modern therapy is so low that the cost of regular RQ-PCR monitoring when less than 10% of patients relapse could be questioned.

The question of reliability of the chosen end point needs to be established for each method, and it requires to be prospectively validated. MRD is clearly an additional prognostic factor, but what additional information it provides beyond those which are currently available requires more careful study.

Novel agents

There are several challenges remaining in the treatment of AML and standard treatment has probably reached its potential. Several novel treatments are currently under evaluation but are not yet approved.

Gemtuzumab ozogamicin (Mylotarg)

Although approved for the treatment of older patients who relapse, several prospective trials are underway in first line – in induction, consolidation, or as maintenance, or in more than one phase. The MRC AML15 trial combines a single dose given simultaneously with induction and/or consolidation in a 2×2 design in younger patients. The SWOG-106 trial also combines with standard $7 + 3$ and also randomizes as maintenance. The ECOG trial randomly gives GO before autologous transplant in consolidation.

The GIMEMA-EORTC trials AML17 and 19 give single-agent GO or not followed by conventional induction chemotherapy followed by consolidation with or without GO. In unfit patients (AML18 trial) monotherapy with GO is compared with best supportive care. The HOVON 43 trial in older patients randomizes patients to GO maintenance after they have received standard induction and consolidation treatment. These are major trials which are either closed to recruitment or well advanced so results are awaited. The UK MRC group have initiated a comparison (AML16 trial) of low-dose Ara-C with or without GO in older patients who are not candidates for standard therapy. In older patients who are fit the combination of daunorubicin/Ara-C is being compared with daunorubicin/clofarabine each with or without GO as induction. In younger patients two doses (3 mg/m^2 versus 6 mg/m^2) are being compared in induction (AML17 trial).

In the early unrandomized studies of GO the licenced dose of 9 mg/m^2 was used as monotherapy.[38] When used at this dose in association with allogeneic transplant there was increased liver toxicity in the form of renal-occlusive disease.[39] In preliminary combinations of 9 mg/m^2 with chemotherapy similar liver toxicity was observed.[40] Based on dose-finding studies the prospective trials have found that doses of 3 mg/m^2 or 6 mg/m^2 are safe when used in combination.

Clofarabine

Clofarabine is a new-generation purine analog that was engineered to capture the advantageous properties of fludarabine and cladribine, giving it the potential benefits of resistance to decontamination and direct mitochondrial-mediated apoptosis with reduced neurotoxicity due to substitution by a C-2' fluorine, which resulted in the innocuous 2-chloroadenine rather than the neurotoxic 2-fluoroadenine. The latter characteristic also has the additional advantage of a potential for oral dosing. Preliminary studies by the MD Anderson group established efficacy in relapsed acute leukemia. In phase II evaluation in relapsed AML in a schedule of 40 mg/m^2 on day 1–5 over 40% of patients achieved a CR which is encouraging for a single agent.[105] Its efficacy and future potential for oral administration encouraged its evaluation as a single agent in older patients who would not normally be offered standard chemotherapy predominantly on age criteria. Although separate and with slightly different entry criteria, three unrandomized phase II trials have delivered similar and encouraging results.[106–108] Between 40% and 50% achieved CR or CRi, usually with a course of treatment, responses occurred at a similar level in patients $>$ 70 years, and a response rate of around 43% was observed in patients with high-risk cytogenetics. While intended to be a non-intensive approach for older patients, even the reduced dose (30 mg/m^2 per day and days 1–5) used in these trials was associated with myelosuppression and its consequences. Care is required with respect to renal function. In the absence of a control arm the question arises as to what the standard of care would be for the patients involved. The investigators believe that it would have been best supportive care or low-dose Ara-C rather than standard chemotherapy, in which case the results give grounds for optimism, particularly with respect to the response to patients with poor-risk cytogenetics. There is a biochemical rationale for combining clofarabine with Ara-C. One completed randomized study using the unconventional "adaptive" randomization design suggested that clofarabine combined with low-dose Ara-C was superior to clofarabine alone.[109] Several prospective studies are underway or being established to evaluate this agent in a phase II setting. Although in receipt of regulatory approval in advanced ALL in young patients, it is not yet approved in AML.

Farnesyl transferase inhibition

Although only mutated in 12–15% of cases, and not being of prognostic significance, inhibition of RAS is a strategy of interest. Farnesyl transferase is required in the essential process of prenylation of cytoplasmic proteins to enable attachment to the inner aspect of the cell membrane to enable signaling. Target proteins include RhoB, RAC, and transforming growth factor beta (TGF-β) as well as RAS. If leukemic cells are dependent on the relevant pathway activation then farnesyl transferase inhibition may be an effective treatment. Farnesyl transferase inhibitors divide into four classes: bisubstrate analogs, peptidomitres, non-peptidomimetion, and farnesyl diphosphate analogs. In AML the lead compound has been tipifarnib (R115777, Zarnestra) which is a member of the non-peptidomimetic class of inhibitors. A large phase II study in relapse showed a modest response with a CR rate of 6%.[110] A similarly large study in older unfit patients produced a remission rate of around 15–18%, and of interest, potential durable benefit in patients who achieved only a partial response.[111] It was noted that responses were not dependent on the presence of a RAS mutation. However, when assessed in older patients randomized against best supportive care no survival benefit was observed and the remission rate was less than 10%.[112] While disappointing, prospective studies in combination with chemotherapy are now in progress.

Cloretazine

Cloretazine is a novel alkylator of the sulfonyl hydrazine class which was initially shown to be effective in relapsed disease. In a first-line study in older patients ($>$ 60 years) a 41% CR rate following a single infusion of 600 mg/m^2 was seen.[113] The responses seen included patients with poor-risk cytogenetics, poor performance score, and aged over 70 years. The survival in responders at 12 months was approximately 30%. This encouraged an ongoing randomized trial in patients in first relapse in combination with Ara-C 1.5 g/m^2 versus Ara-C alone. This important trial has still to complete recruitment.

Cloretazine clearly an effective agent, but associated with significant myelosuppression and possible pulmonary toxicity that implies that testing of different doses and in combinations is justified in order to assess its potential.

Future approaches

Important progress has been made in younger patients with various schedules of conventional chemotherapy and appropriate use of stem cell transplantation. As results have improved, so it has been possible to dissect out many factors which are prognostic and to some extent they can be used to direct therapy, but for the most part they are not predictive, i.e., there is no proven treatment to apply. Molecular targets are now defined which are amenable to therapy based on preclinical data. Of particular interest is FLT3 inhibitors. As single agents these have not lived up to the preclinical promise, but there is considerable momentum to examine them in combination with chemotherapy. This will probably be the pattern of their development. Among such strategies are agents which are antiapoptotic, anti-VEGF (vascular endothelial growth factor), anti-KIT, etc. Epigenetic mechanisms may well be relevant and clinical data from studies in myelodysplastic syndromes have shown efficacy which may be applicable to older patients in particular. This concept is being tested in ongoing randomized trials.

Since there is no shortage of new therapeutic agents to test, the issue becomes how to do so in the most efficient manner. Traditional trials consume large numbers of patients, and are of course required for definitive proof, but in a rare disease like AML this is problematic with so many emerging agents to be tested in defined subgroups. Perhaps the time is right for some statistical compromise in order to find winning agents or combinations. This is attractive if progress is to be rapid enough and since new agents in rarer subgroups of patients are very likely to be expensive, larger benefits will be required.

References

1. Lowenberg B, Downing JR, Burnett A. Acute myeloid leukemia. *N Engl J Med* 1999;**341**(14):1051–62.
2. Hann IM, Stevens RF, Goldstone AH, *et al.* Randomized comparison of DAT versus ADE as induction chemotherapy in children and younger adults with acute myeloid leukemia. Results of the Medical Research Council's 10th AML Trial (MRC AML 10). *Blood* 1997;**89**:2311–18.
3. Juliusson G, Billstrom R, Gruber A, *et al.* Attitude towards remission induction for elderly patients with acute myeloid leukemia influences survival. *Leukemia* 2006;**20**(1):42–7.
4. Menzin J, Lang K, Earle C, *et al.* The outcomes and costs of acute myeloid leukemia among the elderly. *Arch Intern Med* 2002;**162**:1597–603.
5. Giles FJ, Borthakur G, Ravandi F, *et al.* The haematopoietic cell transplantation comorbidity index score is predictive of early death and survival in patients over 60 years of age receiving induction therapy for acute myeloid leukemia. *Br J Haematol* 2007;**136**(4):624–7.
6. Kantarjian H, O'Brien S, Cortes J, *et al.* Results of intensive chemotherapy in 998 patients age 65 years or older with acute myeloid leukemia or high-risk myelodysplastic syndrome. *Cancer* 2006;**106**(5):1090–8.
7. Wheatley K, Brookes CL, Hills RK, *et al.* Prognostic factors in older AML patients receiving intensive and non-intensive therapy: analysis of the UK AML11 and AML14 Trials. *Blood* 2005;**106**(11):199a.
8. Wheatley K. A systemic collaborative overview of randomized trials comparing idarubicin with daunorubicin (or other anthracyclines) as induction therapy for acute myeloid leukemia. *Br J Haematol* 1998;**103**:100–9.
9. Fernandez HF, Sun Z, Yao X, *et al.* Anthracycline dose intensification in acute myeloid leukemia. *N Engl J Med* 2009;**361**(13):1249–59.
10. Löwenberg B, Ossenkoppele GJ, Van Putten W, *et al.* High-dose daunorubicin in older patients with acute myeloid leukemia. *N Engl J Med* 2009;**361**(13):1235–48.
11. Bishop JF, Matthews JP, Young GA, *et al.* A randomized study of high-dose cytarabine in induction in acute myeloid leukemia. *Blood* 1996;**87**: 1710–17.
12. Weick JK, Kopecky KJ, Appelbaum FR, *et al.* A randomized investigation of high-dose versus standard dose cytosine arabinoside with daunorubicin in patients with previously untreated acute myeloid leukemia: a Southwest Oncology Group Study. *Blood* 1996;**88** (8):2841–51.
13. Burnett AK, Wheatley K, Goldstone AH, *et al.* MRC AML12: a comparison of ADE vs. MAE and S-DAT vs. H-DAT ± retinoic acid for induction and four vs. five total courses using chemotherapy or stem cell transplant in consolidation in 3459 patients under 60 years with AML. *Blood* 2002; **100**(11):155a.
14. Bishop JF, Lowenthal PM, Joshua D, *et al.* Etoposide in acute non-lymphoblastic leukemia. *Blood* 1990;**75**:27–32.
15. Cheson BD, Bennett JM, Kopecky KJ, *et al.* Revised recommendations of the International Working Group for Diagnosis, Standardization of Response Criteria Treatment Outcomes, and Reporting Standards for Therapeutic Trials in Acute Myeloid Leukemia. *J Clin Oncol* 2003; **21**(24):4642–9.
16. Estey E, Sun Z, Rowe J, *et al.* A 3,239-patient combined Eastern Cooperative Oncology Group (ECOG), MD Anderson Cancer Center (MDA) analysis of the effect of CR vs. responses < CR on long-term survival in newly diagnosed AML treated with Ara-C-containing regimens: implications for targeted drug development. *Blood* 2007;**110**(11):94a.
17. Kern W, Haferlach T, Schoch C, *et al.* Early blast clearance by remission induction therapy is a major independent prognostic factor for both achievement of complete remission and long-term outcome in acute myeloid leukemia: data from the German AML Cooperative Group (AMLCF) 1992 Trial. *Blood* 2002;**101**(1):64–70.
18. Wheatley K, Burnett AK, Goldstone AH, *et al.* A simple, robust, validated and highly predictive index for the determination of risk-directed therapy in acute myeloid leukemia derived from the MRC AML 10 trial. United Kingdom Medical Research Council's Adult and Childhood Leukemia Working Parties. *Br J Haematol* 1999;**107**(1):69–79.
19. Estey EH. Growth factors in acute myeloid leukemia. In: Burnett AK, ed. *Clinical Haematology*. London, Bailliere Tindall. 2001; 175–87.

20. Buchner T, Hiddemann W, Rottmann R, *et al.* Multiple course chemotherapy with or without GM-CSF priming and long term administration for newly diagnosed AML. *Proc Am Soc Clin Oncol* 1993;**12**:301.

21. Thomas X, Raffoux E, Botton S, *et al.* Effect of priming with granulocyte-macrophage colony-stimulating factor in younger adults with newly diagnosed acute myeloid leukemia: a trial by the Acute Leukemia French Association (ALFA) Group. *Leukemia* 2007;**21** (3):453–61.

22. Rowe JM, Neuberg D, Friedenberg W, *et al.* & Eastern Cooperative Oncology. A phase 3 study of three induction regimens and of priming with GM-CSF in older adults with acute myeloid leukemia: a trial by the Eastern Cooperative Oncology Group. *Blood* 2004;**103**:479–85.

23. Lowenberg B, van Putten W, Theobald M, *et al.* Effect of priming with granulocyte colony-stimulating factor on the outcome of chemotherapy for acute myeloid leukemia. *N Engl J Med* 2003;**349**(8):743–52.

24. Pagliuca A, Carrington P, Pettengell R, *et al.* Guidelines on the use of colony-stimulating factors in haematological malignancies. *Br J Haematol* 2003;**123**:22–33.

25. Smith TJ, Khatcheressian J, Lyman GH, *et al.* 2006 Update of recommendations for the use of white blood cell growth factors: an evidence-based clinical practice guideline. *J Clin Oncol* 2006;**24**:3187–205.

26. Leith CP, Chen IM, Kopecky KJ, *et al.* Correlation of multidrug resistance (MDR1) protein expression with functional dye/drug efflux in acute myeloid leukemia by multiparameter flow cytometry: identification of discordant MDR-/Efflux+ and MDR1+/Efflux- cases. *Blood* 1995;**86** (6):2329–42.

27. Leith CP, Kopecky K, Godwin JE, *et al.* Acute myeloid leukemia in the elderly: assessment of multidrug resistance (MDR1) and cytogenetics distinguishes biologic subgroups with remarkably distinct responses to standard chemotherapy. A Southwest Oncology Group Study. *Blood* 1997;**89**(9):3323–9.

28. List AF, Kopecky KJ, Willman C, *et al.* Benefit of cyclosporin modulation of drug resistance in patients with poor-risk acute myeloid leukemia: a Southwest Oncology Group study. *Blood* 2001;**98**:3212–20.

29. Yin JA, Wheatley K, Rees JK, *et al.* Comparison of 'sequential' versus 'standard' chemotherapy as re-induction treatment, with or without cyclosporine, in refractory/relapsed acute myeloid leukemia (AML): results of the UK Medical Research Council AML-R trial. *Br J Haematol* 2001;**122**:164–5.

30. Holt B, van der Lowenberg B, Burnett AK, *et al.* The value of the MDR1 reversal agent PSC-833 in addition to daunorubicin and cytarabine in the treatment of elderly patients with previously untreated acute myeloid leukemia (AML), in relation to MDR1 status at diagnosis. *Blood* 2005;**106** (8):2646–54.

31. Baer MR, George SL, Dodge RK, *et al.* Phase 3 study of the multidrug resistance modulator PSC-833 in previously untreated patients 60 years of age and older with acute myeloid leukemia: Cancer and Leukemia Group B Study 9720. *Blood* 2002;**100**(4): 1224–32.

32. Burnett AK, Hills RK, Goldstone AH, *et al.* Attempts to modulate chemoresistance in older patients with AML using PSC-833 – results of LRF AML14 Trial. *Blood* 2003;**102**:614a.

33. Lancet JE, Gotlib J, Wetzler M, *et al.* Phase I/II study of the P-glycoprotein (Pgp) inhibitor zosuquidar administered by continuous infusion (CIV) with daunorubicin (DNR) and cytarabine (ARA-C) as primary therapy in older patients with Pgp-positive acute myeloid leukemia (AML). *Blood* 2007;**110**(11):94a–5a.

34. Schaich M, Soucek S, Thiede C, *et al.* MDR1 and MRP1 gene expression are independent predictors for treatment outcome in adult acute myeloid leukemia. *Br J Haematol* 2005;**128** (3):324–32.

35. Jurcic JG, DeBlasio T, Dumont L, *et al.* Molecular remission induction with retinoic acid and anti-CD33 monoclonal antibody HuM195 in acute promyelocytic leukemia. *Clin Cancer Res* 2000;**6**:372–80.

36. Feldman EJ, Brandwein J, Stone R, *et al.* Phase III randomized multicenter study of a humanized anti-CD33 monoclonal antibody, lintuzumab, in combination with chemotherapy, versus chemotherapy alone in patients with refractory or first-relapsed acute myeloid leukemia. *J Clin Oncol* 2005; **23**(28):4110–16.

37. Raza A, Jurcic JG, Roboz GJ, *et al.* Complete remissions observed in acute myeloid leukemia following prolonged exposure to SGN-33 (lintuzumab), a humanized monoclonal antibody targeting CD33. *Blood* 2007;**110**(11):54a.

38. Larson RA, Boogaerts MA, Estey E, *et al.* Antibody-targeted chemotherapy of older patients with acute myeloid leukemia in first relapse using Mylotarg (gemtuzumab ozogamicin). *Leukemia* 2002;**16**:1627–36.

39. Wadleigh M, Richardson PG, Zahrieh D, *et al.* Prior gemtuzumab ozogamicin exposure significantly increases the risk of veno-occlusive disease in patients who undergo myeloablative allogeneic stem cell transplantation. *Blood* 2003;**102**(5):1578–82.

40. Giles FJ, Kantarjian HM, Kornblau SM, *et al.* Mylotarg (gemtuzumab ozogamicin) therapy is associated with hepatic venoocclusive disease in patients who have not received stem cell transplantation. *Cancer* 2001;**92** (2):406–13.

41. Amadori S, Suciu S, Willemze R, *et al.* Sequential administration of gemtuzumab ozogamicin and conventional chemotherapy as first line therapy in elderly patients with acute myeloid leukemia: a phase II study (AML-15) of the EORTC and GIMEMA leukemia groups. *Haematologica* 2004;**89**(8):950–6.

42. Kell WJ, Burnett AK, Chopra R, *et al.* A feasibility study of simultaneous administration of gemtuzumab ozogamicin with intensive chemotherapy in induction and consolidation in younger patients with acute myeloid leukemia. *Blood* 2003; **102**(13):4277–83.

43. Deangelo DJ, Liu D, Stone R, *et al.* Preliminary report of a phase 2 study of gemtuzumab ozogamicin in combination with cytarabine and daunorubicin in patients <60 years of age with de novo acute myeloid leukemia. *J Clin Oncol* 2003;**22**:578a.

44. Burnett AK, Kell WJ, Goldstone AH, *et al.* The addition of gemtuzumab ozogamicin to induction chemotherapy for AML improves disease free survival without extra toxicity: preliminary analysis of 1115 patients in the MRC AML15 trial. *Blood* 2006;**108**(11):8a.

45. Lishner M, Curtis JE, Minkin S, *et al.* Interaction between retinoic acid and cytosine arabinoside affecting the blast cells of acute myeloblastic leukemia. *Leukemia* 1989;**3**(11):784–8.

46. Estey EH, Thall PF, Pierce S, *et al.* Randomized phase II study of fludarabine + cytosine arabinoside + idarubicin +/- all-*trans* retinoic acid +/- granulocyte colony-stimulating factor in poor prognosis newly diagnosed acute myeloid leukemia and myelodysplastic syndrome. *Blood* 1999;**93**(8):2478–84.

47. Burnett AK, Milligan D, Prentice AG, *et al.* A comparison of low-dose cytarabine and hydroxyurea with or without all-*trans* retinoic acid for acute myeloid leukemia and high-risk myelodysplastic syndrome in patients not considered fit for intensive treatment. *Cancer* 2007;**109**(6):1114–24.

48. Milligan D, Wheatley K, Littlewood TJ, *et al.* for the NCRI Haematological Oncology Clinical Studies Group. Fludarabine and cytosine are less effective than standard ADE chemotherapy in high-risk acute myeloid leukemia, and addition of G-CSF and ATRA are not beneficial: results of the MRC AML-HR randomized trial. *Blood* 2006; **107**:4614–22.

49. Schlenk RF, Frohling S, Hartmann F, *et al.* Phase III study of all-*trans* retinoic acid in previously untreated patients 61 years or older with acute myeloid leukemia. *Leukemia* 2004;**18**(11):1798–803.

50. Heuser M, Argiropoulos B, Kuchenbauer F, *et al.* MNI overexpression induces acute myeloid leukemia in mice and predicts ATRA resistance in patients with AML. *Blood* 2007;**110**(5):1639–47.

51. Hills R, Green C, Patel Y, *et al.* The impact of FLT3-ITD and NPM1 mutational status on the outcome of ATRA therapy in patients with non-APL AML: results of the UK MRC AML12 trial. *Blood* 2008;**112**(11):554a.

52. Guy C, Gilkes A, Gale R, *et al.* The impact of MN1 overexpression on the outcome of younger patients with AML treated with intensive chemotherapy with or without ATRA therapy. *Blood* 2008;**112**(11):2978a.

53. Mayer RJ, Davis RB, Schiffer CA, *et al.* Intensive postremission chemotherapy in adults with acute myeloid leukemia. Cancer and Leukemia Group B. *N Engl J Med* 1994;**331**(14):896–903.

54. Byrd JC, Dodge RK, Carroll A, *et al.* Patients with t(8;21)(q22;q22) and acute myeloid leukemia have superior failure-free and overall survival when repetitive cycles of high-dose cytarabine are administered. *J Clin Oncol* 1999; **17**:3767–75.

55. Bradstock KF, Matthews JP, Lowenthal RM, *et al.* A randomized trial of high-versus conventional-dose cytarabine in consolidation chemotherapy for adult de novo acute myeloid leukemia in first remission after induction therapy containing high-dose cytarabine. *Blood* 2005;**105**(2):481–8.

56. Zittoun RA, Mandelli F, Willemze R, *et al.* Autologous or allogeneic bone marrow transplantation compared with intensive chemotherapy in acute myelogenous leukemia. European Organization for Research and Treatment of Cancer (EORTC) and the Gruppo Italiano Malattie Ematologiche Maligne dell'Adulto (GIMEMA) Leukemia Cooperative Groups. *N Engl J Med* 1995;**332**(4):217–23.

57. Cornelissen JJ, van Putten WL, Verdonck LF, *et al.* Results of a HOVON/SAKK donor versus no-donor analysis of myeloablative HLA-identical sibling stem cell transplantation in first remission acute myeloid leukemia in young and middle-aged adults: benefits for whom? *Blood* 2007;**109**(9):3658–66.

58. Harousseau JL, Cahn JY, Pignon B, *et al.* Comparison of autologous bone marrow transplantation and intensive chemotherapy as postremission therapy in adult acute myeloid leukemia. *Blood* 1997;**90**:2978–86.

59. Cassileth PA, Harrington DP, Appelbaum F, *et al.* Chemotherapy compared with autologous or allogeneic bone marrow transplantation in the management of acute myeloid leukemia in first remission. *N Engl J Med* 1998;**339**(23):1649–56.

60. Burnett AK, Wheatley K, Goldstone AH, *et al.* The value of allogeneic bone marrow transplant in patients with acute myeloid leukemia at differing risk of relapse: results of the UK MRC AML10 trial. *Br J Haematol* 2002;**118**:385–400.

61. Burnett AK, Hills RK, Wheatley K, *et al.* A sensitive risk score for directing treatment in younger patients with AML. *Blood* 2006;**108**(11):10a.

62. Giralt S, Thall PF, Khouri I, *et al.* Melphalan and purine analog-containing preparative regimens: reduced-intensity conditioning for patients with hematologic malignancies undergoing allogeneic progenitor cell transplantation. *Blood* 2001; **97**(3):631–7.

63. Sayer HG, Kroger M, Geyer J, *et al.* Reduced intensity conditioning for allogeneic hematopoietic stem cell transplantation in patients with acute myeloid leukemia: disease status by marrow blasts is the strongest prognostic factor. *Bone Marrow Transplant* 2003; **31**:1089–95.

64. Hamaki T, Kami M, Kim SW, *et al.* Reduced-intensity stem cell transplantation from an HLA-identical sibling donor in patients with myeloid malignancies. *Bone Marrow Transplant* 2004;**33**(9):891–900.

65. Ho AY, Pagliuca A, Kenyon M, *et al.* Reduced-intensity allogeneic hematopoietic stem cell transplantation for myelodysplastic syndrome and acute myeloid leukemia with multilineage dysplasia using fludarabine, busulfan, and alemtuzumab (FBC) conditioning. *Blood* 2004;**104**(6):1616–23.

66. Gomez-Nunez M, Martino R, Caballero MD, *et al.* Elderly age and prior autologous transplantation have a deleterious effect on survival following allogeneic peripheral blood stem cell transplantation with reduced-intensity conditioning: results from the Spanish multicenter prospective trial. *Bone Marrow Transplant* 2004;**33**(5):477–82.

67. de Lima M, Anagnostopoulos A, Munsell M, *et al.* Nonablative versus reduced-intensity conditioning regimens in the treatment of acute myeloid leukemia and high-risk myelodysplastic syndrome: dose is relevant for long-term disease control after allogeneic hematopoietic stem cell transplantation. *Blood* 2004; **104**(3):865–72.

68. Hallemeier C, Girgis M, Blum W, *et al.* Outcomes of adults with acute myelogenous leukemia in remission given 550 cGy of single-exposure total body irradiation, cyclophosphamide, and unrelated donor bone marrow transplants. *Biol Blood Marrow Transplant* 2004;**10**(5):310–19.

69. Aoudjhane M, Labopin M, Gorin NC, *et al.* Comparative outcome of reduced

intensity and myeloablative conditioning regimen in HLA identical sibling allogeneic haematopoietic stem cell transplantation for patients older than 50 years of age with acute myeloblastic leukemia: a retrospective survey from the Acute Leukemia Working Party (ALWP) of the European group for Blood and Marrow Transplantation (EBMT). *Leukemia* 2005;**19**(12):2304–12.

70. Baron F, Maris MB, Sandmaier BM, *et al.* Graft-versus-tumor effects after allogeneic hematopoietic cell transplantation with nonmyeloablative conditioning. *J Clin Oncol* 2005; **23**(9):1993–2003.

71. van Besien K, Artz A, Smith S, *et al.* Fludarabine, melphalan, and alemtuzumab conditioning in adults with standard-risk advanced acute myeloid leukemia and myelodysplastic syndrome. *J Clin Oncol* 2005;**23**(24): 5728–38.

72. Tauro S, Craddock C, Peggs K, *et al.* Allogeneic stem-cell transplantation using a reduced-intensity conditioning regimen has the capacity to produce durable remissions and long-term disease-free survival in patients with high-risk acute myeloid leukemia and myelodysplasia. *J Clin Oncol* 2005; **23**(36):9387–93.

73. Schmid C, Schleuning M, Ledderose G, *et al.* Sequential regimen of chemotherapy, reduced-intensity conditioning for allogeneic stem-cell transplantation, and prophylactic donor lymphocyte transfusion in high-risk acute myeloid leukemia and myelodysplastic syndrome. *J Clin Oncol* 2005;**23**(24):5675–87.

74. Claxton DF, Ehmann C, Rybka W. Control of advanced and refractory acute myelogenous leukemia with sirolimus-based non-myeloablative allogeneic stem cell transplantation. *Br J Haematol* 2005;**130**(2):256–64.

75. Mohty M, de Lavallade H, Ladaique P, *et al.* The role of reduced intensity conditioning allogeneic stem cell transplantation in patients with acute myeloid leukemia: a donor vs. no donor comparison. *Leukemia* 2005;**19**(6): 916–20.

76. Hegenbart U, Niederwieser D, Sandmaier BM, *et al.* Treatment for acute myelogenous leukemia by low-dose, total-body, irradiation-based conditioning and hematopoietic cell transplantation from related and unrelated donors. *J Clin Oncol* 2006; **24**(3):444–53.

77. Platzbecker U, Thiede C, Fussel M, *et al.* Reduced intensity conditioning allows for up-front allogeneic hematopoietic stem cell transplantation after cytoreductive induction therapy in newly-diagnosed high-risk acute myeloid leukemia. *Leukemia* 2006; **20**(4):707–14.

78. Scott BL, Sandmaier BM, Storer B, *et al.* Myeloablative vs. nonmyeloablative allogeneic transplantation for patients with myelodysplastic syndrome or acute myelogenous leukemia with multilineage dysplasia: a retrospective analysis. *Leukemia* 2006;**20**(1):128–35.

79. Shimoni A, Hardan I, Shem-Tov N, *et al.* Allogeneic hematopoietic stem-cell transplantation in AML and MDS using myeloablative versus reduced-intensity conditioning: the role of dose intensity. *Leukemia* 2006;**20**(2):322–8.

80. Estey E, de Lima M, Tibes R, *et al.* Prospective feasibility analysis of reduced-intensity conditioning (RIC) regimens for hematopoietic stem cell transplantation (HSCT) in elderly patients with acute myeloid leukemia (AML) and high-risk myelodysplastic syndrome (MDS). *Blood* 2007; **109**(4):1395–400.

81. Rees JKH, Gray RG, Swirsky D, *et al.* Principal results of the Medical Research Council's 8th acute myeloid leukemia trial. *Lancet* 1986; **2**:1236–41.

82. Breems DA, van Putten WL, Huijgens PC, *et al.* Prognostic index for adult patients with acute myeloid leukemia in first relapse. *J Clin Oncol* 2005; **23**(9):1969–78.

83. Burnett AK, Hills R, Goldstone AH, *et al.* The impact of transplant in AML in 2nd CR: a prospective study of 741 in the MRC AML10 and 12 trials. *Blood* 2004;**104**(11):179a.

84. Blaise D, Attal M, Reiffers J, *et al.* Randomized study of recombinant interleukin-2 after autologous bone marrow transplantation for acute leukemia in first complete remission. *Eur Cytokine Netw* 2000;**11**:91–8.

85. Blaise D, Olive D, Michallet M, *et al.* Impairment of leukemia-free survival by addition of interleukin-2-receptor antibody to standard graft-versus-host prophylaxis. *Lancet* 1995;**345** (8958):1144–6.

86. Cortes JE, Kantarjian HM, O'Brien S, *et al.* A pilot study of interleukin-2 for adult patients with acute myelogenous leukemia in first complete remission. *Cancer* 1999;**85**(7):1506–13.

87. Brune M, Castaigne S, Catalano J, *et al.* Improved leukemia-free survival after postconsolidation immunotherapy with histamine dihydrochloride and interleukin-2 in acute myeloid leukemia: results of a randomized phase 3 trial. *Blood* 2006;**108**(1):88–96.

88. Knapper S. FLT3 inhibition in acute myeloid leukemia. *Br J Haematol* 2007;**138**(6):687–99.

89. Abu-Duhier FM, Goodeve AC, Wilson GA, *et al.* FLT3 internal tandem duplication mutations in adult acute myeloid leukemia define a high-risk group. *Br J Haematol* 2000;**111**:190–5.

90. Kottaridis PD, Gale RE, Frew ME, *et al.* The presence of a FLT3 internal tandem duplication in patients with acute myeloid leukemia (AML) adds important prognostic information to cytogenetic risk group and response to the first cycle of chemotherapy: analysis of 854 patients from the United Kingdom Medical Research Council AML 10 and 12 trials. *Blood* 2001;**98**:1752–9.

91. Levis M, Small D. ITD does matter in leukemia. *Leukemia* 2003;**17**:1738–52.

92. Frohling S, Schlenk RF, Breitruck J, *et al.* Prognostic significance of activating FLT3 mutations in younger adults (16 to 60 years) with acute myeloid leukemia and normal cytogenetics: a study of the AML Study Group Ulm. *Blood* 2002;**100**:4372–80.

93. Cairoli R, Beghini A, Grillo G, *et al.* Prognostic impact of c-KIT mutations in core binding factor leukemias: an Italian retrospective study. *Blood* 2006;**107**(9):3463–8.

94. Paschka P, Marcucci G, Ruppert AS, *et al.* Adverse prognostic significance of KIT mutations in adult acute myeloid leukemia with inv(16) and t(8;21): a Cancer and Leukemia Group B Study. *J Clin Oncol* 2006;**24**(24):3904–11.

95. Care RS, Valk PJ, Goodeve AC, *et al.* Incidence and prognosis of c-KIT and FLT3 mutations in core binding factor (CBF) acute myeloid leukemias. *Br J Haematol* 2003;**121**:775–7.

96. Venditti A, Buccisano F, Del Poeta C, *et al.* Level of minimal residual disease after consolidation therapy predicts

outcome in acute myeloid leukemia. *Blood* 2000;**96**:3948–52.

97. San Miguel JF, Martinez A, Macedo A, *et al.* Immunophenotyping investigation of minimal residual disease is a useful approach for predicting relapse in acute myeloid leukemia patients. *Blood* 1997;**90**:2465–70.
98. Sievers EL, Lange BJ, Alonzo TA, *et al.* Immunophenotypic evidence of leukemia after induction therapy predicts relapse, results from a prospective Children's Cancer Group study of 252 patients with acute myeloid leukemia. *Blood* 2003;**101**:3398–406.
99. Kern W, Voskova D, Schoch C, *et al.* Determination of relapse risk based on assessment of minimal residual disease during complete remission by multiparameter flow cytometry in unselected patients with acute myeloid leukemia. *Blood* 2004;**104**(10):3078–85.
100. Coustan-Smith E, Ribeiro RC, Rubnitz JE, *et al.* Clinical significance of residual disease during treatment in childhood acute myeloid leukemia. *Br J Haematol* 2003;**123**:243–52.
101. Feller N, van der Pol MA, van Stijn A, *et al.* MRD parameters using immunophenotypic detection methods are highly reliable in predicting survival in acute myeloid leukemia. *Leukemia* 2004;**18**(8):1380–90.
102. Langebrake C, Creutzig U, Dworzak M, *et al.* Residual disease monitoring in childhood acute myeloid leukemia by multiparameter flow cytometry: the MRD-AML-BFM Study Group. *J Clin Oncol* 2006;**24**(22):3686–92.
103. Freeman SD, Jovanovic JV, Grimwade D. Development of minimal residual disease-directed therapy in acute myeloid leukemia. *Semin Oncol* 2008;**35**(4):388–400.
104. Grimwade DJ, Jovanovic J, Hills R, *et al.* Evaluation of prospective detection of PML-RARA and RARA-PML fusion transcripts by real-time quantitative PCR (RQ-PCR) to direct pre-emptive therapy with arsenic trioxide (ATO) in acute promyelocytic leukemia (APL) patients treated in the UK MRC AML15 trial. *Blood* 2007;**110**(11):166A–7A.
105. Kantarjian H, Gandhi V, Cortes J, *et al.* Phase 2 clinical and pharmacologic study of clofarabine in patients with refractory or relapsed acute leukemia. *Blood* 2003;**102**(7):2379–86.
106. Burnett AK, Russell N, Kell WJ, *et al.* A phase 2 evaluation of single agent clofarabine as first line treatment for older patients with AML who are not considered fit for intensive chemotherapy. *Blood* 2004;**104**:248a.
107. Burnett AK, Russell NH, Kell J, *et al.* European development of clofarabine as treatment for older patients with acute myeloid leukemia considered unsuitable for intensive chemotherapy. *J Clin Oncol* published online April 12, 2010, DOI: 10.1200/JCO. 2009.26.4242.
108. Kantarjian HM, Erba HP, Claxton D, *et al.* Phase II study of clofarabine monotherapy in previously untreated older adults with acute myeloid leukemia and unfavorable prognostic factors. *J Clin Oncol* 2010; **28**(4):549–55.
109. Faderl S, Ravandi F, Huang X, *et al.* A randomized study of clofarabine versus clofarabine plus low-dose cytarabine as front-line therapy for patients aged 60 years and older with acute myeloid leukemia and high-risk myelodysplastic syndrome *Blood* 2008;**112**:1638–45.
110. Harousseau JL, Lancet JE, Reiffers J, *et al.* A phase 2 study of the oral farnesyltransferase inhibitor tipifarnib in patients with refractory or relapsed acute myeloid leukemia. *Blood* 2007; **109**(12):5151–6.
111. Lancet JE, Gojo I, Gotlib J, *et al.* A phase 2 study of the farnesyltransferase inhibitor tipifarnib in poor-risk and elderly patients with previously untreated acute myelogenous leukemia. *Blood* 2007;**109**(4):1387–94.
112. Harousseau JL, Martinelli G, Jedrlejczak WW, *et al.* A randomized phase 3 study of tipifarnib compared to best supportive care (including hydroxyurea) in the treatment of newly diagnosed acute myeloid leukemia (AML) in patients 70 years or older. *Blood* 2007;**110**(11):135A–6A.
113. Giles F, Rizzieri D, Karp J, *et al.* Cloretazine (VNP40101M), a novel sulfonylhydrazine alkylating agent, in patients age 60 years or older with previously untreated acute myeloid leukemia. *J Clin Oncol* 2007;**25**(1): 25–31.

Chapter 3

Treatment of acute lymphoblastic leukemia (ALL) in adults

Ryan Mattison, Sarah Larson, and Wendy Stock

Introduction

Acute lymphoblastic leukemia (ALL) is a neoplastic clonal disorder resulting from the maturation arrest of lymphoid progenitors. While both T-cell precursors and B-cell precursors can be transformed, greater than 85% of cases are derived from precursor B cells. Accumulation of lymphoblasts within the bone marrow can result in anemia, thrombocytopenia, and neutropenia. Symptoms of fatigue, bleeding, bruising, and infection are frequent initial manifestations of the disease. There are a number of ALL subtypes that are characterized by particular morphologic, immunophenotypic, cytogenetics, and molecular findings. Treatment of ALL in the pediatric population has been a success story in hematology/oncology, with cure rates approaching 80%. Unfortunately, a majority of adult patients, approximately 65%, succumb to their disease. The use of novel agents and the introduction of risk-adapted therapies, including stem cell transplantation (SCT), the identification of new molecular targets, and the application of pediatric treatment approaches to adult patients are promising strategies that offer hope to improve treatment outcomes for adults with this heterogeneous group of diseases.

Epidemiology/etiology

Incidence

ALL comprises 20% of newly diagnosed acute leukemias in adults. Approximately 5200 new cases were diagnosed in the United States in 2007, and 1420 patients died from the disease that year.[1] Most cases occur de novo, though prior exposure to chemotherapy, especially topoisomerase II inhibitors[2] and alkylating agents,[3] is a risk factor for both ALL and acute myeloid leukemia (AML). Therapy-related leukemias are strongly associated with rearrangements of the *MLL* (mixed-lineage leukemia) gene located on chromosome 11q23.[2]

Etiology, risk factors, and inherited cancer syndromes

In the majority of cases, ALL is an acquired disease without a clearly defined initiating event. Though viruses, ionizing radiation, and hereditary disposition have been implicated in the etiology of ALL, no single factor has been definitively identified as a cause.

Approximately 5% of myeloid and lymphoid leukemia cases are linked to inherited genetic syndromes that involve genes that relate to DNA repair and genomic stability. A well-known example is trisomy 21 (Down syndrome), which confers a 10- to 20-fold higher risk of acute leukemia than in children without Down syndrome. Mechanisms that may link Down syndrome with acute leukemia include altered folate metabolism, mutations of the transcription factor GATA1 and other genes, or disomy of a leukemia predisposition gene on chromosome 21.[4,5] Inherited syndromes such as Fanconi's anemia, Bloom's syndrome, and ataxia-telangectasia that lead to excessive chromosomal fragility are associated with an excess risk of ALL.[6–8]

There have been elegant clinical studies performed that shed light on the prenatal origin of some pediatric leukemia cases. When observing the incidence of acute leukemia in monozygotic twin pairs, investigators have observed a concordance rate ranging from 5% to 25% in patients between the ages of 0 and 15 years. However, in infants younger than one year of age, the concordance rate reaches nearly 100%. Through the analysis of blood samples collected for routine neonatal screening purposes, investigators have determined that the identical clonal origin of acute leukemia in monozygotic twin pairs is strong evidence of in utero origin of leukemogenesis.[9] Furthermore, the presence of detectable *TEL-AML1* (*ETV6-RUNX1*) fusion gene or clonal rearrangements of the *IGH* sequence in archived neonatal blood samples in children who later develop ALL is evidence that many cases of leukemia had initiation steps that developed in utero.[10,11]

ALL occurring in twin children older than one year often involves the *TEL-AML1* fusion gene and requires a longer period of postnatal development, suggesting that other genetic changes are required for the development of leukemia.[9] In addition, another study observed an incidence

Management of Hematologic Malignancies, ed. Susan M. O'Brien, Julie M. Vose, and Hagop M. Kantarjian. Published by Cambridge University Press.

of 1% of the *TEL-AML1* fusion gene in neonatal blood samples, though the observed incidence of ALL involving that genetic abnormality was 100-fold less, suggesting that other molecular changes are necessary for leukemogenesis.[12]

Some environmental factors have also been linked to the development of ALL. A prominent example includes the exposure to high doses of ionizing radiation in the atomic bomb survivors of Hiroshima and Nagasaki and the subsequent development of acute leukemia.[13] The link between cigarette smoking and the development of ALL was seen in a Cancer and Leukemia Group B (CALGB) study that observed an increased risk of ALL in smokers older than 60 years. That case–control study showed a greater than threefold risk of ALL development in those who smoked compared to those who did not smoke (odds ratio = 3.40; 95% confidence interval = 0.97–11.9).[14] In contrast, while chronic exposure to the non-ionizing radiation associated with high-voltage power lines had been associated with the development of ALL, a more recent study has excluded this exposure as a causative factor.[15]

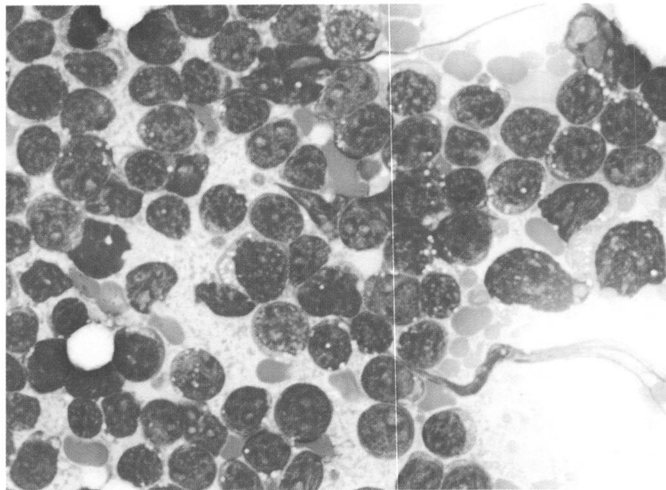

Figure 3.1 Burkitt lymphoma: bone marrow aspirate smear from a patient diagnosed with Burkitt lymphoma involving the bone marrow. The cells are uniformly intermediate in size with deeply basophilic cytoplasm and prominent lipid vacuoles. The nuclear chromatin is clumped and cells contain two to three small, centrally placed nucleoli. Photo courtesy of Sandeep Gurbuxani MBBS, PhD Instructor, Department of Pathology, University of Chicago.

Pathology

Clinical and laboratory features

When ALL is suspected, basic laboratory studies must be performed including a complete blood count with differential and smear, a complete electrolyte panel with liver function tests, and tumor lysis labs including lactate dehydrogenase (LDH), calcium, phosphorus, and uric acid. A chest radiograph should also be included. Bone marrow aspirate and biopsy are required, and the sample must be evaluated for morphology, cytogenetics, immunohistochemical and immunophenotypic studies, as well as molecular studies. As discussed later, these studies are needed to assign risk and to tailor therapy accordingly.

Morphology and immunophenotyping

The current WHO (World Health Organization) classification incorporates immunophenotypic and cytogenetics information into the classification schema with the goal of making disease categories more clinically relevant.[16] The WHO classification includes precursor B-cell, precursor T-cell, and Burkitt (mature B-cell) lymphoma/leukemia. Flow cytometry is key to defining immunophenotype.[16] Precursor B-cell ALL is terminal deoxynucleotidyl transferase (TdT) positive and often expresses CD34. The B-cell markers CD19, CD22, and CD79a are also present, and surface immunoglobulin is negative. CD20 is expressed, usually weakly, in 40% to 50% of cases.[17] Precursor T-cell ALL is also TdT positive, but lacks the B-cell markers mentioned. Precursor T-cell ALL is CD3+, and many cases coexpress the T-cell markers CD2, CD4, and CD8. Burkitt lymphoma/leukemia is notable for the expression of B-cell markers CD19 and CD22, and is positive for surface immunoglobulin. In addition, Burkitt lymphoma/leukemia is kappa or lambda light chain restricted. In contrast to precursor B-cell ALL, Burkitt lymphoma/leukemia is strongly CD20+, but is TdT and CD34 negative. The vast majority of ALL cases are myeloperoxidase (MPO) and non-specific esterase negative. The presence of these cytochemical markers is more consistent with AML. However, there are rare cases of ALL that are MPO positive but that have the typical pattern of lymphoid surface markers present that help to define ALL lymphoblasts.

Before the WHO classification, ALL classification had been categorized by morphology according to the French–American–British (FAB) classification that relied on morphologic appearance (Figures 3.1 and 3.2). Under the FAB system, L1 blasts appear smaller with finer chromatin and fewer nucleoli. L1 subtype was present in 74% of pediatric cases (children younger than 15 years), and the prognosis was generally better than the L2 subtype. L2 lymphoblasts appear larger with more prominent nucleoli. This type was seen in 66% of adult patients, with a generally poorer outcome than L1 subtype. L3 subtype (Burkitt) is mature B-cell leukemia and is retained in the WHO classification system. L3 blasts have prominent vacuoles and a classic "starry sky" appearance from the tingible body macrophages due to the extremely high proliferation rate seen in this disease.

Cytogenetics

Recurring abnormalities in the number of chromosomes, translocations, and partial deletions are seen in 60–70% of ALL cases.[18] Cytogenetic analysis is important both for prognostic assessment in an individual patient and as a tool for investigators to gain insight into the molecular pathogenesis of

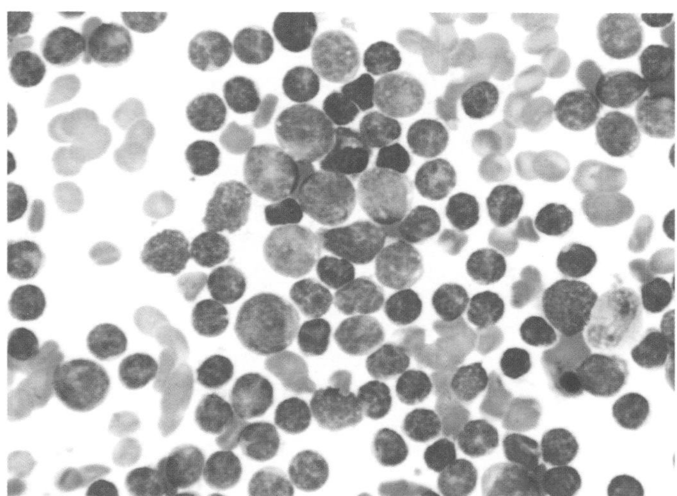

Figure 3.2 Precursor B-cell ALL: bone marrow aspirate smear from a patient diagnosed with precursor B-lymphoblastic leukemia. The bone marrow is almost entirely replaced by small- to intermediate-sized blasts with high nuclear cytoplasmic ratio, variably condensed nuclear chromatin, and small to absent nucleoli. Photo courtesy of Sandeep Gurbuxani MBBS, PhD Instructor, Department of Pathology, University of Chicago.

ALL. The incidence and clinical impact of common cytogenetics findings are listed in Table 3.1.

Hyperdiploidy is the addition of whole chromosomes resulting in a number greater than the 46 chromosomes seen in normal human cells. Hyperdiploidy is seen in pediatric ALL more commonly than in adult ALL, and the presence of more than 50 chromosomes in pediatric patients is associated with a favorable prognosis. Adults with hyperdiploid karyotype typically have a less favorable prognosis than in children, a phenomenon that may be explained by the presence of poor-prognosis features such as the Philadelphia chromosome.[19] Hypodiploidy occurs in approximately 5% of adult ALL patients, and confers a poor prognosis.[18]

Chromosomal translocations occur when material between two or more chromosomes is exchanged, resulting in either novel fusion genes or dysregulation of normal gene expression. Fusion gene products may involve transcription factors that are normally involved in cellular differentiation and proliferation. When translocations occur, differentiation can be blocked, leading to the accumulation of immature lymphocyte precursors. Abnormal proliferation can occur due to aberrant growth factor signaling. The most common translocation in adults is the Philadelphia chromosome (Ph+) t(9;22)(q34;q11), present in 25–30% of ALL patients.[20] The fusion protein, also seen as the hallmark finding in chronic myeloid leukemia (CML), leads to continuous activation of the Abl tyrosine kinase and lack of control over the normally well-regulated RAS and phosphatidyl inositol 3 kinase (PI 3K)/AKT pathways, resulting in abnormal proliferation and a block in apoptosis.[21] Ph+ ALL (*BCR-ABL+*) has a poor prognosis, though apparently dramatic improvements in clinical outcomes have been seen with the introduction of imatinib and other tyrosine kinase inhibitors as will be discussed in later sections. Another common translocation partner is the *MLL* gene located on 11q23. *MLL* is known to fuse with more than 50 partner genes, the most common of which is *AF4* located on 4q21. The t(4;11)(q21;q23) translocation is involved in 60% of infant ALL cases and is seen in 10% of adult ALL patients.[22] *MLL* is also implicated in many cases of AML and myelodysplastic syndrome, and its involvement is often seen in patients who had previously been treated with topoisomerase II inhibitors for other malignancies. *MLL*-related leukemias often are resistant to treatment and have a poor prognosis.

The t(12;21)(p13;q22) translocation results in the *TEL-AML1* fusion gene that is the most common rearrangement seen in pediatric ALL.[23] This cryptic translocation is not readily apparent when standard cytogenetic analysis is performed, but the fusion transcript can be detected using reverse

Table 3.1. Cytogenetics in ALL

Karyotype	Frequency %	% DFS/EFS (5 year)	% OS (5 year)
Good			
t(14q11-q13)	4.7–6	78	78
del(12p) or t(12p)	4–5.5	34–76	41–82
Intermediate			
Normal	25–30	38–43	37–48
t(10;14)(q24; q11.2)	2–8	34	41
t(1;19)(q21; p13.3)	0.8–3	29	32
del(9p) or t(9p)	0.5–15	44–49	38–58
Hyperdiploid	6.6–35	50	53
+21	13.7	29	26
Poor			
del 7	2–6	25–36	14–36
+8	3–10	15–22	12–22
Low hypodiploidy/ near triploidy	9	18	22
t(8;14)	2–5	60–88 (3 year)	50–79 (3 year)
t(4;11) (q21;q23)	1–7	15–25	18–24
t(9;22) (q34;q11)	17–29	5–10 pre-imatinib	5–11 pre-imatinib
	Up to 50% in elderly patients	51–60 (1 year) with imatinib	65–76 (1 year) with imatinib

Notes: DFS: disease-free survival; EFS: event-free survival; OS: overall survival.

transcriptase-polymerase chain reaction (RT-PCR) analysis. Its presence is associated with a good prognosis in children, and it is very rarely detected in adult ALL.[24]

The translocations involving 8q24 and *c-MYC*, seen commonly in Burkitt lymphoma/leukemia, are examples of normal genes that have unregulated expression due to promoter substitution and subsequent overactivity. The common t(8;14)(q24;q32) as well as the less prevalent t(2;8)(p12;q24) and t(8;22)(q24;q11) are involved in almost all cases of Burkitt lymphoma/leukemia. The mechanism of disease involves bringing *c-MYC* under the control of the immunoglobulin gene regulatory elements that are located on chromosome bands 14q32 (*IgH*), 2p12 (*IGL*), and 22q11 (*IGK*).[25,26] However, the mechanisms for *c-MYC*-controlled malignant progression are not yet completely understood. Similarly, in T-lineage ALL, there are recurrent translocations that join together the enhancer elements of the T-cell receptor genes leading to aberrant expression of the partner fusion genes. The T-cell receptor alpha (*TCR-α*) and delta (*TCR-δ*) located on 14q11, the T-cell receptor beta (*TCR-β*) on 7q32-q36, and the T-cell receptor gamma (*TCR-γ*) on 7p15 have been shown to fuse with a number of partner genes, including the transcription factors *c-MYC* (8q24), *TAL1/SCL* (1p32), *TAL2* (9q32), *LYL1* (19p13), *LMP1/RBTN1* (11p15), *LMO2/RBTN2* (11p13), and *HOX11* (10q24). Finally, the *NOTCH1* gene that encodes a transmembrane receptor has been implicated in precursor T-cell ALL as discussed below.

Molecular genetics

While karyotypic analysis currently remains the most important clinical prognosticator in ALL and provides critical information about disease pathogenesis, genome-wide expression analyses and identification of genes and pathways that are aberrantly expressed and regulated in ALL are providing new insights that may direct future targeted drug development. Inactivation of the tumor suppressor genes p16 (*CDKN2A, INK4A*) and p15 (*CDKN2B, INK4B*) occur frequently in ALL, usually as a result of chromosomal deletion involving the 9p21 locus. The reported frequency of both heterozygous and homozygous deletions of p16 varies from 6% to 33% in precursor B-cell ALL and from 30% to 83% in precursor T-cell ALL.[27] Both p15 and p16 specifically inhibit cyclin/CDK4/6 complexes that block cell division during the G1/S phase of the cell cycle and their loss results in loss of control of cell proliferation and tumor progression.[28] Loss of cell cycle regulatory control may also occur via mutations of the p53 tumor suppressor gene in up to 25% of adults with ALL and/or loss of the Rb tumor suppressor gene in as many as 50% of cases. Retrospective analysis demonstrated that adult ALL cases with aberrant expression of at least two of these tumor suppressor genes (p16, Rb, or p53) had a significantly worse disease-free survival than patients with only one or none of these abnormalities.[29]

Recent discoveries indicate that gain-of-function mutations in the *NOTCH1* gene are found in 50% to 70% of cases of precursor T-cell ALL in both children and adults making these mutations the most common acquired genetic lesion identified to date for this ALL subset (for review, see Aster *et al.*[30]). Interestingly, major downstream targets of *NOTCH1* activation include c-Myc, mTOR, and activation of the PI3K/AKT pathway. These effects are important in supporting the growth of precursor T-cell lymphoblasts.[31–35] While the interplay of NOTCH with other developmental pathways that contribute to the pathogenesis of precursor T-cell ALL remains to be clearly defined, these insights are already providing the impetus for the development of therapeutic strategies that might block these aberrantly regulated pathways (see *Emerging therapeutic options* section, p. 59).

Genome-wide analysis to identify cooperating mutations that may be important in the pathogenesis of precursor B-cell ALL has recently resulted in the identification of new molecular lesions in this disease subset in pediatric ALL.[36] Using high-resolution single-nucleotide polymorphism arrays with DNA sequencing, deletions, amplification, point mutations, and structural rearrangements in genes encoding key regulators of normal B-lymphocyte development and differentiation were identified in 40% of precursor B-cell ALL cases in children. The most frequent target of somatic mutation was the *PAX5* gene and these mutations resulted in reduced levels of the PAX5 protein. Deletions were also detected in the *TCF3, EBF1, LEF1, IKZF1* (*IKAROS*), and *IKZF3* (*AIOLOS*) genes. The mutations result in disruption of pathways controlling normal B-cell development and differentiation and may lead to development of ALL. The same investigators have also shown that deletion of the *IKAROS* gene occurs very commonly (84% of cases) in Ph+ ALL but not in chronic phase CML.[37] This suggests that the loss of IKAROS function is an important event in the development of ph+ ALL. Another layer of complexity in ALL pathogenesis that is being actively investigated is the epigenetic regulation of gene expression through modulation of target mRNAs by microRNAs (miRs).[38] Hyper-methylation of a specific miR, miR 203, resulted in decreased miR 203 expression and enhanced *BCR-ABL* gene expression in Ph+ ALL, suggesting that miR203 may function as a tumor suppressor and implicates that its re-expression might have therapeutic benefit. Further elucidation of the cooperating mutations and epigenetic modifications that result in ALL pathogenesis will help to identify new "druggable" targets and guide the direction of future experimental therapeutic development in ALL.

Differential diagnosis

Typical symptoms of ALL include fatigue, shortness of breath, pallor, bone pain, and anorexia. Hepatomegaly and splenomegaly are present in approximately 50% of patients and can result in abdominal fullness. Lymphadenopathy occurs in ALL more often than AML, but lymph node enlargement does not usually occur prior to bone marrow or peripheral blood involvement. Other diseases that have overlapping symptoms with ALL include AML, blast crisis CML, and high grade lymphomas. Non-neoplastic lymphoproliferative disorders including Epstein–Barr (EBV) or cytomegalovirus (CMV) infection should also be considered since the morphology of reactive lymphocytes can be similar to lymphoblasts.

Precursor T-cell ALL typically presents with a large mediastinal mass and higher white blood cell (WBC) count, and occurs more frequently in young men than in women. Burkitt lymphoma/leukemia is commonly accompanied by an elevated LDH, central nervous system (CNS) involvement, and bulky adenopathy.

Prognostic factors

There are a number of clinical features in ALL that have a known impact on prognosis, including age, WBC count at diagnosis, time to achievement of complete remission (CR), immunophenotype, cytogenetics, and the presence of minimal residual disease (MRD).

A number of trials have shown that patient age influences both CR rate and disease-free survival (DFS) in ALL.[39–42] Patients between the ages of 30 and 60 years are considered to be at standard risk, with those younger than 30 having a better outcome. Patients older than 60 years have an adverse prognosis, an observation that is due in large part to the increasing percentage of high-risk cytogenetics with increasing age. In an analysis of the British Medical Research Council (MRC) ALL trials, there was a decline in CR and remission-free survival as age increased.[43] Children aged 2–10 years have the best prognosis of all patients with ALL as they have a higher incidence of both the favorable *TEL-AML1* fusion gene resulting from a cryptic t(12;21) and hyperdiploid karyotype. Older adolescents and young adults have less favorable outcomes than younger children. Survival continues to decrease as the disease presents in older age, to the point where adults older than 60 years can expect to have less than a 20% chance of cure. Explanations include comorbid illnesses that make remission induction therapy more difficult to tolerate and more aggressive biology, particularly the presence of the t (9;22) Philadelphia chromosome, seen in up to 50% of adults older than 50 years.[44]

Leukocyte count at diagnosis is a risk factor as shown by a number of studies.[39,45–47] WBC counts of 15 000/μL to 30 000/μL lead to shorter remission duration in patients with precursor B-cell ALL, with those who have a WBC of 100 000/μL or greater at particularly high risk of short remissions.[48] Patients with precursor T-cell ALL often present with much higher WBC counts without associated poor outcomes until the WBC count is greater than 100 000/μL.[39]

Coexpression of myeloid antigens, especially CD13 and CD33, occurs in approximately 20–30% of ALL cases.[16,49] However, ALL cases are characteristically MPO negative. The presence of myeloid antigens does not necessarily define bilineage involvement, and the use of uniform grading systems helps to define biphenotypic disease.[50] In some studies, the presence of myeloid markers confers a worse prognosis than in conventional ALL.[49,51] However, other studies show that clinical outcomes are no worse in patients with myeloid marker expression.[52,53]

The presence of the CD20 antigen on precursor B-cell ALL blasts has been shown to be an independent poor prognostic factor. In a study by the MD Anderson investigators of 253 patients treated before rituximab became widely available, it was found that the expression of CD20 on more than 20% of blasts was associated with decreased 3-year overall survival (OS) (27% vs. 40%, $p = 0.03$).[17]

In the treatment of pediatric ALL, early clearance of blasts (within 7 days) has been shown to be an important predictor of survival. In adult ALL, attaining CR within 2–4 weeks is associated with improved survival while requiring more than 4 weeks of therapy before CR is achieved portends a worse outcome.[42,54]

Minimal residual disease

The use of qualitative and, more recently, quantitative Q-PCR and flow cytometry have been established as valid techniques to monitor for the presence of MRD during the treatment of patients with ALL. The presence of the *BCR-ABL* fusion gene in Ph+ ALL or a specific rearrangement of the immunoglobulin heavy chain (*IGH*) or T-cell receptor (*TCR*) gene are well-suited for amplification by real-time quantitative PCR (RQ-PCR) using specific primer pairs and probes for a patient's leukemia clone. Eighty percent to 95% of patients can have rearrangements detected at diagnosis.[55] This technique can detect 1 leukemia cell in the background of 10^4 to 10^6 normal cells. While it is a highly sensitive test, there is a significant problem with false positive results. In addition, the creation of patient-specific primers and probes when targeting rearranged *IGH* and *TCR* genes is a time-consuming and relatively expensive process. There is also substantial inter-laboratory variability that makes this technique difficult to standardize, though progress has been made in reducing variation.[56] A key adult study using semi-quantitative PCR showed that 9/13 (69%) of patients who were MRD positive at 1 month later had relapsed ALL compared to 3/10 (30%) who were MRD negative.[57] In the same study, 2/2 (100%) of patients who were MRD positive at 5 months eventually relapsed compared to 3/8 (37%) of patients who were MRD negative. Finally, 0/4 (0%) of patients who were MRD negative at 9 months relapsed. More recently, a German study showed that 196 adult ALL patients who had standard-risk disease could be divided into three prognostic groups based on the time point at which MRD declined to fewer than 1 leukemia cell in 10^4 cells. Patients who had such a decline at day +11 and day +24 after induction therapy were considered to be low risk and had a relapse rate of 0% at 3 years. Patients who had MRD present at a level higher than 1 cell in 10^4 cells at week 16 after induction were high risk and had a 3-year relapse rate of 94%. The remaining patients were at intermediate risk of relapse and had a 3-year relapse rate of 47%.[58]

Flow cytometry techniques utilize the presence of aberrant immunophenotypes expressed on the lymphoblast surface, such as the presence of myeloid antigens or coexpression of two or more antigens not usually present at the same stage of differentiation. Up to 95% of ALL patients have disease features that can be detected and followed by flow cytometry. One leukemia cell can be detected in the background of 10^3 to 10^4 normal cells.[59] In adult patients, detection of MRD by flow cytometry has shown that patients with precursor T-cell ALL are at increased risk of relapse when MRD is present prior to consolidation (83% vs. 51%), prior to the third post-remission module (72% vs. 33%), and prior to the sixth cycle of post-remission therapy (75% vs. 30%).[60]

While MRD detection has predictive power as an early marker for relapse, its real value is the potential to guide therapy. Patients who are at higher risk of relapse may benefit from more intense post-remission therapy through the use of early allogeneic SCT. This is a question that is currently under investigation by the German Multicenter Study Group for adult ALL (GMALL).[61]

Therapy

Chemotherapy regimens

Therapy for ALL consists of a series of complex chemotherapy combinations and treatment schedules. Treatment is divided into three distinct phases: (1) remission induction; (2) one or more phases of consolidation (intensification); and (3) long-term maintenance therapy for 2–3 years (except for Burkitt lymphoma/leukemia). Because of the high incidence of CNS involvement or relapse, all protocols utilize either intrathecal chemotherapy or a combination of intrathecal therapy with cranial irradiation. Systemic administration of drugs that penetrate the CNS is also a key component of the chemotherapy armamentarium. These regimens utilize many drugs with differing mechanisms of action, and they have evolved from successful treatment programs in pediatric ALL. The following section reviews the basic treatment components that have been employed in adult ALL during the last decade, focusing on outcomes of large single institution and cooperative group trials. The results of these trials are summarized in Table 3.2.

Induction

The purpose of induction therapy is to reduce quickly the leukemia cell burden and to restore normal hematopoiesis. Commonly used induction regimens initially contained a combination of drugs first shown to be successful in pediatric ALL, and included a corticosteroid, vincristine, and L-asparaginase. CR rates were only 40–65%, and the remission duration was short, 6 months or less. The addition of an anthracycline, either daunorubicin or doxorubicin, improved the CR rate to 72–92%.[40,68–71] A CALGB trial compared two different anthracyclines, daunorubicin and mitoxantrone, during induction, and found that CR rates using each agent were similar.[72] In a different strategy, investigators at Memorial Sloan-Kettering Cancer Center evaluated an induction regimen that avoided vincristine and corticosteroids, and instead used high-dose cytarabine (3 g/m^2 per day for 5 days) along with mitoxantrone (80 mg/m^2 for one dose on day 3) and granulocyte colony-stimulating factor (G-CSF) support. Their results in 37 patients showed an 84% CR rate with a median time to CR of 34 days.[73]

Cyclophosphamide has also been added to induction chemotherapy [39,64] with mixed results. The CALGB investigators showed an overall CR rate of 85% and improved DFS in their single-arm phase II trial compared with historical controls.[39] In contrast, the Italian study, which randomized nearly half of its 769 patients to receive cyclophosphamide at induction, showed no significant difference between those patients who did or did not receive cyclophosphamide.[64] The use of lower-dose cyclophosphamide has also been incorporated along with prednisone into a 5- to 7-day-long "pro-phase" therapy that precedes induction chemotherapy as a strategy to begin cytoreduction while minimizing the risk of tumor lysis syndrome.[74]

The use of G-CSF during induction was studied in the randomized trial CALGB 9111.[62] While the use of growth factor reduced the time of neutrophil recovery (16 days vs. 22 days, $p < 0.001$) and had a trend toward improved CR rates (87% vs. 77%, $p = 0.07$) there was no difference in DFS or OS between patients who did and did not receive G-CSF.

Thus, most regimens currently utilize a four or five drug combination consisting of vincristine, a corticosteroid, an anthracycline, and the use of either L-asparaginase, cyclophosphamide, or both.

Consolidation

While induction chemotherapy leads to CR rates that are greater than 90% in many series, the relapse rate in adult ALL patients is 50–75%, leading to many variations of post-remission consolidation treatment in an attempt to eradicate MRD and improve DFS. Adult consolidation regimens have evolved from pediatric schedules that have shown to be successful.[75] Post-remission therapy in ALL can include a wide range of drugs, including cytarabine, etoposide, VM26, methotrexate, 6-mercaptopurine (6-MP), and 6-thioguanine (6-TG). In addition, the use of autologous and allogeneic SCT has been incorporated into ALL treatment as will be discussed in a separate section.

The MD Anderson group used extended consolidation within its HyperCVAD regimen by alternating hyperfractionated cyclophosphamide, vincristine, doxorubicin, and dexamethasone (cycles 1, 3, 5, and 7) with high doses of methotrexate and cytarabine (cycles 2, 4, 6, and 8) in a single-arm trial. [76] In this study of 204 patients treated between 1992 and 1998, median survival was 35 months and the 5-year

Table 3.2. Trial results of chemotherapy regimens for adult ALL

Trial	Design	Number of patients	Median age (range)	CR (%)	DFS (%)	OS (%)	Comments
CALGB 9111[62]	Patients randomized to receive G-CSF or placebo with induction	Total 198	35 (16–83)	82	23 months[a]	23 months[a]	G-CSF shortened time to neutrophil recovery and increased CR, but did not affect toxicity, DFS, or OS
		G-CSF 102		87	2.3 years	2.4 years	
		Placebo 96		77	1.7 years	1.8 years	
JALSG ALL-93[63]	Increased doxorubicin during induction and randomized patients to sequential or intermittent intensification	263	31 (15–59)	78	30 63 months	33 63 months	No benefit from doxorubicin and no difference between intensification schedules
GIMEMA 0288[64]	Patients randomized to receive Cy during induction then randomized to post-CR intensification	Cy 387	27.5 (12–60)	81	31 8 year	28 8 year	Neither randomization had significant impact on CR, DFS, or OS
		No Cy 382		83	28 8 year	27 8 year	
MDACC[65]	Follow-up results of patients treated with HyperCVAD	288	40 (15–92)	92	38 5 year	38 5 year	No asparaginase improved outcome compared to VAD regimen
LALA-94[66]	Standard-risk[b] patients received induction course then randomized to receive intense consolidation	Total 307	33	83	35	44 5 year	Intensified consolidation regimen did not affect overall survival
		Intense consolidation Arm A 158				Arm A 45	
		Standard consolidation Arm B 154				Arm B 43	
UKALLXII/ ECOG 2993[67]	All patients received 2 phases of induction chemo regardless of disease risk factors	1153 Ph– patients	(15–59)	93	NR	41	Favorable CR rate
GMALL 07/03 [61]	Short, intense chemo and risk stratification including MRD	713	34 (15–55)	89	NR	54 5 year	Favorable outcomes: high survival and relapse rate in young standard-risk patients

Notes: [a]Median DFS and OS.
[b]Standard risk defined as lack of t(4;11), t(1;19), 11q23 rearrangement, WBC $< 30 \times 10^9$, no myeloid markers, and first CR achieved after one course of induction therapy.
G-CSF: granulocyte colony-stimulating factor; Cy: cyclophosphamide; HyperCVAD: hyperfractionated cyclophosphamide, vincistine, doxarubicin, and dexamethasone alternating with high-dose methotrexate and cytarabine; NR: not reported.

survival was 39%. The Italian GIMEMA group conducted a study that included randomization of 388 patients to post-remission intensification followed by maintenance chemotherapy versus early maintenance therapy without intensification.[64] The results showed no significant difference between the two groups at 8 years, with 36% DFS in patients treated with consolidation versus 37% in patients who went directly to maintenance therapy. However, only 35% of patients who were randomized to the consolidation/maintenance arm completed treatment as prescribed due to compliance problems and treatment-related toxicity.

The French LALA-94 trial investigated the use of intensive versus less-intense consolidation treatment in patients with standard-risk ALL.[66] In this trial, patients were considered to be at standard risk if they had (1) precursor B-cell ALL without CNS involvement; (2) the absence of the Ph chromosome, t(4;11), t(1;19), or other abnormalities involving 11q23 rearrangements; (3) WBC count less than 30×10^9/L; (4) an immunophenotype characterized by CD10+/CD19+, or CD20+/CD19+; (5) the absence of myeloid markers; (6) the achievement of CR after one course of chemotherapy. Intensive consolidation included the use of high-dose cytarabine and mitoxantrone, while standard consolidation included cyclophosphamide, lower-dose cytarabine, and 6-MP. Of 307 patients who had standard risk disease in this trial, there was no significant difference in OS between the more intense versus less intense consolidation arms (45% vs. 43%, $p = 0.73$).

Pioneered in the treatment of pediatric ALL, the contribution of L-asparaginase to response rates and duration of response in adults is not clear. Its toxicities in adults include pancreatitis, hepatotoxicity, and coagulopathy. An analysis of the CALGB 8811 study showed a marginal benefit in DFS at 3 years for patients who received all prescribed doses of L-asparaginase (55% vs. 48%, with overlapping 95% confidence intervals).[77] Eighty-five percent of the 197 patients in that trial achieved CR after induction.[39] In contrast, the well-established HyperCVAD regimen used by the MD Anderson group does not include L-asparaginase. In their trial of 204 patients, 91% achieved CR with 3- and 5-year DFS rates of 50% and 38%, respectively.[76]

Maintenance

Maintenance therapy also made its debut in the treatment of pediatric ALL and has been shown to be an important component of treatment. Despite the lack of randomized trials investigating the importance of maintenance treatment in adults with ALL, trials show inferior results compared to historical controls when maintenance therapy is not included. In a CALGB study designed to compare daunorubicin versus mitoxantrone during induction, all patients received vincristine, methotrexate, and prednisone during induction, followed by four cycles of intensification treatment along with CNS prophylaxis.[72] None of the patients received maintenance therapy. Though there was no difference between daunorubicin and mitoxantrone arms, the median duration remission times (10.2 months vs. 12.3 months, $p = 0.56$) were shorter than those of a previous trial, so the study was stopped earlier than planned.[72] In a Dutch study, investigators conducted a multicenter phase II trial that included standard induction chemotherapy followed by consolidation treatment with high-dose cytarabine along with amsacrine, mitoxantrone, and etoposide as well as intrathecal (IT) methotrexate for CNS prophylaxis. The patients did not receive maintenance therapy. Though CNS relapse rates were relatively low (3%), the 5-year OS rate of 22% was inferior to protocols that included long-term maintenance chemotherapy.[78]

The rationale behind the use of maintenance treatment is the elimination of slowly growing subclones that persist after induction and consolidation treatments by exposing them to antimetabolite drugs over long periods of time, ranging from 18 months up through 3 years after initial diagnosis. Commonly used components of maintenance therapy include daily 6-MP and oral weekly methotrexate, supplemented by monthly pulses of vincristine, corticosteroids, and periodic IT methotrexate. While the use of maintenance treatment is standard in precursor B-cell and precursor T-cell ALL, its use can be omitted in Burkitt lymphoma/leukemia since relapse rates after the first year of treatment are low.

CNS prophylaxis and treatment

While fewer than 10% of adults with ALL present with CNS involvement,[79,80] CNS relapse will occur in 35–75% of patients at one year if prophylactic CNS-directed therapy is not incorporated into treatment.[81,82] A lumbar puncture at the time of ALL diagnosis is essential. CNS disease is present when more than five leukocytes per microliter of cerebrospinal fluid are seen along with the presence of lymphoblasts in the cerebrospinal fluid.[83] Symptoms may include headache, meningismus, fever, or cranial nerve palsies. However, some patients have no symptoms. Risk factors for CNS involvement in adults include Burkitt lymphoma/leukemia, high serum LDH levels (> 600 units/liter), and the presence of a high proliferative index at diagnosis (greater than 14% of lymphoblasts in the S and G_2M phase of the cell cycle).[84]

Initially, CNS-directed therapy included the use of IT methotrexate and 2400 cGy cranial radiation in the pediatric population. This strategy was incorporated into an early adult trial that compared CNS prophylaxis with no CNS treatment, resulting in an improved CNS relapse rate of 19% versus 42% at 24 months.[82] While in children it is known that combination treatment can result in toxicities that include seizures, early dementia, cognitive dysfunction, and slow growth, the long-term effects on adults are less clear.[85] It is known that combined radiation and IT chemotherapy in adults can cause substantial acute toxicities that may delay post-remission consolidation treatment. Simultaneous use of cranial irradiation and systemic high-dose cytarabine or methotrexate leads to unacceptable neurologic toxicities and is not used. An alternative strategy that uses IT chemotherapy without radiation has been investigated. This treatment regimen includes "triple therapy" that combines IT methotrexate, cytarabine, and corticosteroids without radiation.[86]

CNS relapse rates as low as 5% have been achieved without radiation by using combination IT treatment in conjunction with high-dose systemic treatment that can penetrate the cerebrospinal fluid.[76,87] However, the GMALL investigators have reported higher CNS relapse rates of 9% versus 5% when CNS-directed radiation was postponed.[74] Similarly, investigators observed that the omission of cranial radiation therapy in pediatric patients with T-lineage ALL correlated with a higher 3-year CNS relapse rate (18% versus 7% in the irradiated group, $p = 0.012$).[88] Thus, pediatric oncologists routinely use prophylactic CNS radiation therapy for patients with precursor T-cell ALL.

If symptomatic CNS disease is present at diagnosis, IT chemotherapy using cytarabine, methotrexate, and methylprednisolone is given concurrently with 15–20 Gy radiation therapy.[79]

The role of stem cell transplant in Ph− ALL in first complete remission (CR1)

The efficacy of allogeneic SCT in ALL was first reported in 1973,[89] and the "graft-versus-leukemia effect" was described as early as 1979.[90] The role of allogeneic transplant has been established in patients with well-known risk factors such as t(9;22) and t(4;11) cytogenetics and may represent the optimal approach to curing these patients. Determining if other patients may also benefit from allogeneic SCT in CR1 has been an area of intense study. Results from recent trials suggest that specific disease subsets may benefit from an allogeneic SCT in first remission (Table 3.3).

In an earlier Dutch trial, 54 patients (age 15–51 years) with ALL and 15 patients with lymphoblastic lymphoma were treated with induction and consolidation chemotherapy. Thirty patients had an HLA-matched sibling, and 22 of those patients were scheduled to undergo allogeneic SCT.[96] The DFS of these patients was 58% (± 11%) at 5 years, a result not significantly different from the outcomes in the other patients on study who did not receive a transplant as part of their regimens.

The French LALA-87 trial was designed to evaluate the best post-remission strategy in ALL, comparing consolidation chemotherapy versus autologous SCT (ASCT) versus allogeneic transplant.[97] The results of this trial analyzing 572 patients with 10 years of follow-up data showed that survival was 46% for patients who received an allogeneic transplant versus 31% for those who received chemotherapy ($p = 0.04$). When broken into high-risk and standard-risk groups (with high risk including Ph+ status, age > 35 years, WBC $> 30 \times 10^6/\mu L$, and time to CR > 4 weeks), OS at 10 years was 44% in the allogeneic transplant group versus 11% for the chemotherapy group ($p = 0.009$). In the standard-risk group, survival rates in the allogeneic transplant group (49%) and the chemotherapy group (39%) were similar ($p = 0.6$). Thus, this study demonstrated a survival benefit for allogeneic transplant in high-risk patients.

Similarly, the LALA-94 trial re-evaluated the benefit of allogeneic transplant in high-risk patients.[66] In this study, 922 adult patients were divided into four risk groups consisting of (1) standard-risk ALL, (2) high-risk ALL, (3) Ph+ ALL, and (4) ALL with CNS involvement.[66] Patients in all but the standard-risk group were assigned to receive allogeneic transplant if they had an HLA-matched sibling. Those in groups 3 and 4 were assigned to ASCT if no family donor were available while those in group 2 were randomized to either ASCT or further chemotherapy. The results of this intent-to-treat analysis showed that patients with high-risk ALL and those with CNS involvement had a better outcome if a donor was available for transplant. Among high-risk patients, those allocated to the allogeneic transplant arm had a better median DFS of 20.8 months compared to a median DFS of 15.2 months in the ASCT arm and a median DFS of only 11 months in the chemotherapy arm ($p = 0.007$). These results confirm the findings of the LALA-87 trial showing benefit of allogeneic transplant in high-risk patients if a sibling donor is available.

The MRC UKALL XII/ECOG 2993 study is the largest prospective, randomized trial comparing allogeneic SCT with chemotherapy as a post-remission treatment strategy.[94] One thousand nine hundred and thirteen patients aged 15 years to 59 years were enrolled between 1993 and 2006, with the upper age limit extended to 64 years in 2003. The study schema allocated all patients younger than 50 years (later amended to 55 years) having an HLA-matched sibling to receive a transplant. All Ph+ patients were assigned to transplantation, using a matched unrelated donor if necessary. Younger patients without a family member donor and patients older than 50 years old (or 55 years old later in the study) were randomized to either ASCT or further chemotherapy for consolidation treatment. High-risk patients throughout the study period were defined by the following factors: (1) age greater than 35 years; (2) WBC count greater than 30 000/μL in B-lineage disease or greater than 100 000/μL in T-lineage disease; (3) all Ph+ patients. The median follow-up period was 4 years, 11 months (range, 1 month to 13 years, 11 months). Ph− patients with a matched sibling donor had a 5-year OS rate of 53% versus 45% for those without a donor ($p = 0.01$) in the intent-to-treat analysis. Standard-risk patients had the most benefit from transplant, with 5-year OS of 62% versus 52% ($p = 0.02$) in those who had a sibling donor compared to those who did not. The benefit from a transplant in high-risk patients was not statistically significant ($p = 0.2$), with OS of 41% and 35% in the donor group and no-donor group, respectively. The trial also showed that in all groups, autologous transplant offered no more benefit than chemotherapy alone. In contrast to the LALA trials, the joint Medical Research Council/Eastern Cooperative Oncology Group (MRC/ECOG) trial showed that transplant was most beneficial to standard-risk patients as defined rather than high-risk patients. However, in their study, it is important to be mindful of the fact that risk groups were defined differently compared to other transplant studies. Thus, allogeneic transplant in CR1 was not significantly better for patients over age 35 years (high risk) due to high transplant-related mortality.

ASCT has been studied as a treatment option for patients who do not have an HLA-matched sibling donor. In a review

Table 3.3. Trials evaluating the role of stem cell transplant in adult ALL

Trial	Design	Number of patients	Outcome measure	Chemotherapy (%)	Autologous transplant (%)	Allogeneic transplant (%)	Comments
JALSG/ IBMTR[91]	Compared outcome of chemotherapy on JALSG ALL87 to outcome of transplant from IBMTR database	Allo 214	DFS at 5 yrs	30 (≤ 30 yr)	–	53 (≤ 30 yrs)	Allogeneic transplant improved DFS, but had high TRM for patients > 30 years old
		Chemo 76		26 (> 30 yrs)	–	30 (> 30 yrs)	
GOELAMS[92]	Patients received allo-SCT if donor available. Patients without a donor received auto-SCT	Allo 41	DFS at 6 yrs	–	33	72	Improved DFS with allo-SCT compared to auto-SCT
		Auto 115		–	–	–	
LALA-94[73]	Risk stratification into 4 groups						Allogeneic SCT improved DFS in high-risk ALL in CR1. Auto-SCT did not confer benefit over chemotherapy
	1 = Standard risk[a]	307 standard risk	OS at 5 yrs	44	–	–	
	2 = High risk	211 high risk	OS at 5 yrs	21	32	51	
	3 = Ph+	140 Ph+	OS at 3 yrs	–	17	36	
	4 = CNS disease	48 CNS+	OS at 3 yrs	–	46	40	
PETHEMA ALL-93[93]	Standard risk treated with chemotherapy, remaining groups allocated to SCT. High risk[b] patients received sibling allo-SCT if available or randomized to auto-SCT vs. chemotherapy	Allo 57		–	–	–	Matched sibling allo-SCT did not show a survival benefit for patients with high-risk ALL
		Auto 34	OS at 5 yrs	45	54	44	
		Chemo 48		–	–	–	
MRC-UKALLXII/ ECOG 2993[94]	Matched sibling allo-SCT in CR1 if available (donor) or randomized to auto-SCT vs. chemotherapy (no donor)	1913	OS at 5 yrs	46	37	53	Allo-SCT in CR1 has survival benefit for standard risk, but not high risk patients[c]; auto-SCT not effective

Table 3.3. *(cont.)*

Trial	Design	Number of patients	Outcome measure	Chemotherapy (%)	Autologous transplant (%)	Allogeneic transplant (%)	Comments
Stanford University/ City of Hope[95]	Long-term follow-up of patients with Ph+ ALL treated with matched sibling allo-SCT	CR1 48		–	–	54	Improved survival in patients transplanted during CR1. Did not evaluate effect of imatinib on transplant outcome
		CR2 26	OS at 10 yrs	–	–	29	

Notes: [a]Standard risk defined as lack of t(4;11), t(1;19), 11q23 rearrangement, WBC < 30 × 10^9, no myeloid markers, and CR1 achieved after one course induction therapy.
[b]High risk defined by age 30–50 years, WBC greater than or equal to 25 × 10^9, t(9;22), t(4;11) or other 11q23 rearrangement and t(1;19).
[c]High risk defined by age > 35 years, WBC > 100 × 10^9 for B-cell lineage or > 30 × 10^9 for T-cell lineage, and t(9;22).

of the French LALA-85, -87, and -94 trials, investigators studied 175 patients who received ASCT and 174 patients who were treated with chemotherapy. Their results showed that receiving ASCT was associated with lower incidence of relapse than treatment with chemotherapy was (66% vs. 78% at 10 years, p = 0.05). However, DFS and OS were not significantly different between the groups.[98] Similarly, Yanada and colleagues performed a meta-analysis of seven trials conducted by Japanese and European cooperative groups that included 1274 patients. No benefit was seen when autologous transplant was compared to chemotherapy in those patients who lacked an HLA-matched sibling donor.[99]

Special considerations (mature B-cell ALL, Ph+ ALL, adolescent/young adults, elderly)

Burkitt lymphoma/leukemia (FAB L3) is an aggressive, rapidly proliferating disease that is relatively rare, comprising 2–4% of adult ALL cases and 1–2% of pediatric cases.[100] Clinical features include a high cell proliferation rate, bulky lymphadenopathy, and frequent CNS involvement. Characteristic immunophenotypic findings include CD10+/−, CD19+, CD20+, and CD34−. Surface immunoglobulin is present, unlike in precursor B-cell and precursor T-cell leukemia. Its pathogenesis involves overexpression of the *c-MYC* oncogene on chromosome 8q24 as a result of chromosomal translocations involving the immunoglobulin heavy or light chains. The most common translocation is the t(8;14)(q24;q32) seen in up to 85% of cases, while t(8;22)(q24;q11) and t(2;8)(p12;q24) rearrangements occur in a minority of cases.[101] The c-Myc protein is a transcription factor that plays a role in the regulation of hundreds of genes that are important to vital processes such as cell cycle regulation, signal transduction, and metabolism.[102] Gene expression profiling techniques have been a useful method of distinguishing Burkitt lymphoma/leukemia from other B-cell lymphomas.[103,104]

Prognosis for adults in the past has been very poor. During the last two decades, outcomes for patients with Burkitt lymphoma/leukemia have improved markedly following the development of intensive chemotherapy strategies. The group at St. Jude Children's Hospital pioneered the use of fractionated dosing schedules and alternating drug schedules in children to take advantage of rapid cell proliferation and to prevent drug resistance.[105] Their treatment schedule used high-dose cyclophosphamide, then doxorubicin, vincristine, and CNS-targeting therapy including IT methotrexate and cytarabine, high-dose intravenous (IV) methotrexate with leucovorin rescue, and IV cytarabine. Maintenance therapy was not a component of treatment. Using this strategy, 27 of 29 patients (93%) achieved CR.[105]

Due to the success of this pediatric regimen, French[106] and German [73] investigators applied a similar treatment schedule in adult patients. However, they added a "prophase" regimen of corticosteroids and pulsed cyclophosphamide prior to induction in order to reduce the risk of tumor lysis syndrome. As in the pediatric regimens, and in contrast to most other ALL treatment schedules, reinduction and maintenance phases were not used since relapses after 1 year are uncommon. Compared to historical controls, these studies yielded improved CR rates (63% and 74% versus 44%) and higher OS rates (49% and 51% versus 0%), thus setting a new standard in the treatment of adult Burkitt lymphoma/leukemia. Study results for Burkitt lymphoma/leukemia are summarized in Table 3.4.

Investigators at the MD Anderson Cancer Center developed the HyperCVAD regimen consisting of eight total

Table 3.4. Burkitt lymphoma/leukemia trials

Trial	Regimen	Number of patients	CR (%)	DFS (%)	OS (%)	Comments
Societe Francaise d'Oncologie Pediatrique (SFOP)[106]	Cytoreductive phase with COP followed by therapy using pediatric regimens	65	89	71	74	Young patient population with median age 26
				EFS 3 years	3 years	
MD Anderson Cancer Center	HyperCVAD alone	48	85	60	53	Adding rituximab to hyperCVAD appears to improve survival based on comparison to historical controls
(MDACC)[100,107]	HyperCVAD with rituximab	28	86	88	89	
				3 years estimated	3 years estimated	
CODOX-M/ IVAC/UKLG LY06[108]	Low-risk patients received 3 cycles CODOX-M, high-risk patients received 4 cycles alternating CODOX-M and IVAC	52	76	65 2 years	73 2 years	High-intensity regimen can be curative, but has significant toxicity
Cancer and Leukemia Group B (CALGB9251)[109]	Cytoreduction phase followed by 6 alternating cycles with cytarabine, doxorubicin, vincristine, high-dose MTX, cyclophosphamide, and decadron and 6 cycles intrathecal therapy	92				Eliminating intracranial radiation decreases neurotoxicity, but does not decrease efficacy
		Cohort 1 52	Cohort 1 71	Cohort 1 66	Cohort 1 54	
		Cohort 2 40	Cohort 2 68	Cohort 2 67	Cohort 2 50	
				3 years	3 years	
	Cohort 1 received intracranial radiotherapy					
Societe Francaise d'Oncologie Pediatrique	High intensity short duration with regimen intensification based upon disease burden	72	72	65	70	Consistent with previous SFOP results in an older patient population
				EFS 2 years	2 years	
GOELAMS[110]						
German Multicenter Study Group for the Treatment of ALL	6 short intense cycles with high-dose MTX and cytarabine, fractionated alkylating agents and rituximab. Two doses maintenance rituximab	70	90	NR	79 3 years	The addition of rituximab appears to improve survival
GMALL[111]						

Notes: COP: cyclophosphamide, vincristine, prednisone; CODOX-M: cyclophosphamide, vincristine, duxorubicin, and methotrexate; IVAC: ifosfamide, etoposide and high-dose methotrexate; MTX: methotrexate; EFS: event-free survival.

cycles of therapy using hyperfractionated cyclophosphamide, vincristine, doxorubicin, and dexamethasone alternating with high-dose IV methotrexate and cytarabine. CNS therapy was given with IT methotrexate and cytarabine.[100] Their patient population included 26 patients, with a mean age of 58 years, significantly older than in previously published trials. This regimen resulted in a CR rate of 81%, a 3-year OS rate of 49%, and a 3-year DFS rate of 61%.[100] There was a sharp decrease in survival for patients older than 60 years: 77% versus 17% ($p < 0.01$). Other risk factors for poor prognosis included female gender, decreased performance status, albumin < 3 g/dL, and hepatosplenomegaly.

Since CNS involvement is a significant concern in Burkitt lymphoma/leukemia, cranial-directed therapy is a critical component of treatment. However, the combination of IT chemotherapy and CNS-directed radiation therapy leads to significant neurotoxicity. The CALGB 9251 study was designed to test the hypothesis that CNS therapy could be reduced and still control disease while improving the toxicity profile.[109] Ninety-two patients were enrolled and treated with a cyclophosphamide/prednisone prophase followed by six alternating cycles of chemotherapy. Cycles 2, 4, and 6 included ifosfamide, methotrexate, vincristine, cytarabine, etoposide, and dexamethasone while cycles 3, 5, and 7 included cyclophosphamide, methotrexate, vincristine, doxorubicin, and dexamethasone. The first cohort of 52 patients received CNS-directed treatment that included 12 doses of IT methotrexate, cytarabine, hydrocortisone, and 2400 cGy of cranial irradiation with radiation administered in 12 fractions between cycles 3 and 4. The second cohort of 40 patients received fewer doses of IT chemotherapy (6 doses) and received 2400 cGy of cranial radiation after cycle 7 only if there were prior bone marrow involvement (27/40 patients). After median follow-up of 6.8 years in Cohort 1 and 4.1 years in Cohort 2, the first group of patients had nine serious incidents of neurotoxicity while no patients in the second group experienced such side effects. The serious neurologic events included transverse myelitis, aphasia, neuropathy, and blindness. Less severe neurologic side effects were also more common in Cohort 1 than in Cohort 2 (61% versus 26%, $p = 0.001$). Treatment responses were similar, with a 3-year event-free survival (EFS) of 52% in patients in Cohort 1 and 45% in patients in Cohort 2, with no statistically significant difference between the two groups. The authors concluded that omission of cranial irradiation in patients without CNS involvement adequately controlled disease while sparing patients the increased risk of neurologic toxicities.[109]

Because mature B-cell leukemia expresses CD20, it can be targeted by rituximab, a monoclonal antibody against the CD20 antigen. In preliminary reports, the addition of rituximab appears to improve CR rates and may improve survival. The addition of rituximab to the HyperCVAD regimen improved 3-year OS from 53% to 89% ($p < 0.01$) and 3-year DFS from 60% to 88% ($p = 0.03$) as demonstrated in a phase II study compared to historical controls.[107] Similarly, a study by the GMALL group showed that the addition of rituximab to aggressive chemotherapy led to a 3-year OS rate of 91% for patients younger than 55 years old and 84% for patients older than 55 years.[111] These data suggest that the use of rituximab may become a standard component of Burkitt lymphoma/leukemia therapy.

Philadelphia chromosome positive (Ph+) ALL

The presence of the t(9;22)(q34;q11) translocation (Ph+) and the resultant *BCR-ABL* fusion gene is the most common cytogenetic abnormality in adult ALL, and its presence has a significant adverse prognostic impact.[112,113] Median survival of Ph+ patients treated with standard ALL protocols was 9 months, with allogeneic stem cell transplant being the only curative treatment.[66,99,114] Fifty percent of patients with precursor B-cell ALL who are older than 60 years have t(9;22) involvement, and allogeneic transplant is particularly difficult in this older patient population.

The outcomes for patients with Ph+ ALL have begun to improve with the addition of targeted Bcr-Abl tyrosine kinase inhibitors (TKI) to frontline therapy (see Table 3.5). The MD Anderson group was the first to show that incorporating imatinib into induction chemotherapy with their standard HyperCVAD regimen improved CR rates to 90% and did so without increasing toxicity.[115] Another trial that confirmed the value of imatinib was conducted by the Group for Research on Adult Acute Lymphoblastic Leukemia (GRAAPH)-2003 study, in which 45 patients with Ph+ ALL were treated with imatinib during the consolidation or the induction phase of chemotherapy and continued until the time of allogeneic SCT. All 22 patients who had a CR and an HLA-matched donor went on to receive an allogeneic SCT in first remission. The overall CR rate was 96%, and DFS and OS were 51% and 65%, respectively, at a median of 18 months. These results were significantly better than the outcome for patients enrolled on the pre-imatinib LALA-94 trial who served as historical controls.[117] A Korean group demonstrated the feasibility of adding imatinib to post-induction treatment that was then followed by allogeneic transplant as consolidation therapy.[120] In their study of 29 patients with Ph+ ALL, the relapse rate during post-remission treatment with imatinib before SCT was 4.3% compared to 40.7% in a previous study that served as a historic control ($p = 0.003$).[120]

In a separate study by the Japan Adult Leukemia Study Group (JALSG), imatinib was added to standard chemotherapy. The one-year EFS and OS were estimated to be 60% and 76.1%, significantly improved over a previous study used as a historical comparison.[116] In this phase II trial, early and prolonged exposure to imatinib was key to success, and with very early, limited follow-up, the outcomes were significantly better than historical controls and were identical whether or not patients underwent SCT. Similar results come from a Children's Oncology Group (COG) study using escalating doses of imatinib in children with Ph+ ALL.[121] With short follow-up,

Table 3.5. Ph+ ALL

Trial	Regimen	Number of patients	CR (%)	DFS (%)	OS (%)
French Groupe d'Etude et de Traitement de la Leucemie Aigue Lymphoblastique de l'Adulte (LALA-94)[114]	Induction, consolidation, and pretransplant cycles followed by sibling, MUD, or autologous SCT based on donor availability	154	53	NR	19 3 year
MD Anderson Cancer Center (MDACC)[115]	HyperCVAD	48	92	14 5 year	12 5 year
	HyperCVAD with concurrent imatinib	20	93	75 20 month	75 20 month
United Kingdom Medical Research Council Adult Leukemia Working Party and Eastern Cooperative Oncology Group (UKALL XII/ECOG 2993)[67]	Two phases induction, intensification followed by consolidation/maintenance or SCT	293	83	NR	25 5 year
Japan Adult Leukemia Study Group (JALSG)[116]	Standard induction plus imatinib followed by consolidation with alternating courses of imatinib and high doses of MTX and Ara-C. SCT if donor available	80	96	60 1 year estimated	76 1 year estimated
Group for Research on Adult Lymphoblastic Leukemia (GRAAPH-2003)[117]	Imatinib incorporated into induction or consolidation based upon initial disease response. SCT for patients with available donor	45	96	51 18 months	65 18 months
German Multicenter Study Group for Adult Acute Lymphoblastic Leukemia (GMALL)[118]	Elderly patients randomized to standard induction or imatinib	Imatinib 28	96	30 18 months estimated	57 18 months estimated
		Chemotherapy 27	50	35 18 months estimated	41 18 months estimated
Italian Gruppo Italiano Malattie Ematologiche dell'Adulto (GIMEMA)[119]	Elderly patients treated with prednisone and imatinib	29	100	74 1 year estimated	48 1 year estimated

Notes: MUD: matched unrelated donor; Ara-c: cytarabine (cytosine arabinoside); MTX: methotrexate; NR: not reported.

Schultz and colleagues showed that DFS and OS were similar for children who underwent allogeneic stem cell transplant in CR1 compared to those who received consolidation chemotherapy and imatinib but who were not transplanted. Longer follow-up will be required to see if these early results apply to longer-term EFS.

The optimal timing and duration of imatinib has not yet been determined, although there is evidence that early administration along with chemotherapy rather than after induction and consolidation chemotherapy gives better results. Wassmann and colleagues conducted a study of 92 patients with 47 patients who received imatinib on an alternating schedule and 45 patients who received imatinib concurrent with chemotherapy.[122] Ninety-five percent of patients receiving concurrent chemotherapy and imatinib achieved CR. Importantly, 52% of patients receiving concurrent treatment were MRD negative by PCR, while only 19% were PCR negative among patients receiving alternating chemotherapy and imatinib ($p = 0.01$).

Imatinib is a particularly attractive treatment option for older adults with Ph+ ALL. As mentioned earlier, Ph+ ALL is more prevalent in older patients. The presence of comorbidities in older patients makes chemotherapy, and especially allogeneic transplant, more poorly tolerated than in younger patients. There have been several recent clinical investigations that assess the use of imatinib as frontline treatment in older adults with Ph+ ALL.[118,119] Vignetti and colleagues used imatinib and corticosteroids, without chemotherapy, as induction treatment in 30 patients between ages 61 and 83 years.[119] They reported no major toxicities and a median survival of 20 months without the need for hospitalization, an excellent outcome for a treatment with palliative intent. All of the patients reached CR and survival was significantly better than pre-imatinib regimens for older adults where the median survival was only seven to nine months.[123–126] Similarly, Delannoy *et al.* used imatinib in consolidation and maintenance for older adults with Ph+ ALL[127] and demonstrated significantly improved DFS and OS at one year compared to historical controls. Ottmann and colleagues randomized 55 patients with a median age of 68 years to induction therapy with imatinib alone versus age-adapted induction chemotherapy without imatinib, though all patients received imatinib during consolidation treatment.[118] Despite an improved CR rate in the imatinib group (96% vs. 50%, $p = 0.0001$), OS was the same in both cohorts, estimated to be 42% at 24 months. Thus, the use of imatinib in frontline therapies for older adults has resulted in significant improvements in both remission rates and improvements in survival.

Despite these significant improvements in response rates, the emergence of imatinib-resistant clones may result in relapse. Mutations in the kinase domain of the Bcr-Abl fusion protein lead to less avid imatinib binding and subsequent resistance to the drug.[128] Mutations generally involve one of four regions of the kinase domain. These are the ATP binding loop (P-loop), contact site (including the T315 and F317 amino acids), the SH2 binding site, and the A-loop.[129] The P-loop and T315I mutations are associated with very poor prognosis in CML and in Ph+ ALL.[130–132] In addition, the T315I mutation leads to resistance to second-generation TKIs, including dasatinib and nilotinib. While mutations often emerge after an initial response to therapy, there is evidence that *BCR-ABL* mutations are present in some patients who are refractory to upfront TKI therapy in CML.[131] Likewise, TKI resistance mutations in ALL were seen in a subpopulation of cells in 40% of patients enrolled on the GMALL ADE10 trial.[133] At the time of relapse, 90% of the dominant cell clone exhibited the same kinase domain mutation in that study.

The problem of relapsed/refractory ALL and patient intolerance to imatinib may be partially overcome by the introduction of the second-generation TKI dasatinib.[118,134,135] In an interim analysis of a phase II trial of Ph+ ALL patients who were resistant or intolerant to imatinib, a combination of dasatinib and prednisone induced a complete hematologic remission in 100% of 23 patients within 3 weeks of treatment initiation.[135] There was little toxicity reported in conjunction with these promising data, though median follow-up was limited to 4.5 months at the time of study presentation. In addition, dasatinib may effectively cross the blood–brain barrier and is efficacious against CNS disease.[136] Early promising results of combining dasatinib with combination chemotherapy have recently been reported.[137]

Nilotinib is another second-generation TKI with greater (20-fold) potency against BCR-ABL than imatinib,[138] though it is also ineffective against the T315I point mutation.[139] In a phase II study of patients with blast crisis CML or relapsed/refractory Ph+ ALL, 20 patients (24%) achieved a complete response, and no Ph+ ALL patient developed CNS disease with short follow-up.[140]

Adolescent/young adults and late complications of therapy

The adolescent and young adult (AYA) population of ALL patients is generally considered to encompass those between the ages of 15 and 30 years. This is a unique population in whom the observation was made that clinical outcome often depends heavily on whether a person is treated on a pediatric or an adult protocol. Because of community referral patterns, such patients may be treated by pediatric or adult oncologists who choose a regimen most appropriate for the population with which that physician is most familiar. Pediatric treatment protocols are often based on the Berlin–Frankfurt–Munster (BFM) regimens initially developed in the late 1970s.[141] Treatment consists of (1) an induction regimen including oral corticosteroids, IV vincristine and daunorubicin, intramuscular L-asparaginase, and IT cytarabine and methotrexate; (2) a consolidation regimen of 6-MP and IV and IT methotrexate; (3) a reintensification step including dexamethasone, vincristine, doxorubicin, and L-asparaginase alternating with cyclophosphamide, cytarabine, 6-TG, and IT methotrexate; and (4) maintenance therapy containing oral methotrexate and 6-MP for 2–3 years.[142] Pediatric regimens typically use higher doses of vincristine, corticosteroids, methotrexate, and L-asparaginase than adult protocols. Adult therapy contains higher doses of the myelosuppressive drugs daunorubicin, cytarabine, and cyclophosphamide.

In observations by CALGB and Children's Cancer Group (CCG) investigators,[143] AYA patients (aged 16 years to 21 years) who were treated on pediatric protocols had significantly better EFS than those treated on adult protocols. Their retrospective observations of separate CCG and CALGB trials showed that AYA patients with similar risk factors had 7-year EFS of 63% in those patients treated with pediatric regimens compared to 7-year EFS of 34% in patients treated with adult regimens. Similar results were seen in comparative trials in France,[144] the Netherlands,[145] Italy,[146] and the United Kingdom.[147] In all five studies, the ages and risk stratification criteria were well matched among patients treated on pediatric versus adult protocols. Thus, underlying biology alone is unlikely to explain superior outcomes for those patients treated on pediatric protocols. As mentioned previously, pediatric regimens contain significantly more corticosteroids, vincristine, methotrexate, and L-asparaginase than the drug combinations used in adult trials.

Because these agents have been considered too toxic to give to adults when dosed in a range for pediatric patients, it could be that AYA patients are relatively underdosed with these critical drugs. A recent study by Spanish investigators confirmed that the ALL-96 regimen, designed for pediatric patients, was equally effective in adolescents aged 15–18 years as it was in young adults aged 16–30 years, with a CR rate of 98% and an OS rate of 69% with median follow-up of over 4 years.[148] While there was a slightly higher incidence of hematologic toxicity in the young adults compared to the adolescent patients, overall outcomes were not affected. Pediatric regimens also contain more CNS-directed therapy and a prolonged maintenance phase. There has also been much written about how ALL is commonly seen and treated by pediatric oncologists and rarely encountered by adult oncologists.[149–151] Pediatric oncologists and supporting staff may be more inclined to avoid dose reductions, less likely to change treatment schedules based on non-medical factors, and more familiar with treatment side effects and supportive care strategies. Patients under the care of a pediatric oncologist may also be more likely to have a parent involved with their treatment and appointments, making adherence to therapy more likely, though no prospective comparative data are available to answer this question.

Given the better outcomes seen in AYA patients treated with pediatric protocols, much can be learned through this phenomenon to improve the treatment of all patients with ALL. There are major clinical trials under way that explore the feasibility and test the effectiveness of extending the pediatric approach to ALL to adults. An intergroup study, C-10403, jointly designed by the CALGB, the Southwest Oncology Group (SWOG), and the ECOG has been open since November 2007. The trial is enrolling patients aged 16–30 years old with newly diagnosed precursor B-cell or precursor T-cell ALL. The treatment schedule is the same as one arm of the COG AALL0232 regimen, a BFM-based schedule that resulted in improved 3-year DFS of 75% for patients 16–20 years old. The investigators have an enrollment goal of 300 patients over 5 years, and there is a plan to compare patient outcomes with historical controls. In another study, investigators at the Dana-Farber Cancer Institute are enrolling patients aged 18 to 50 years old on a pediatric-inspired protocol that showed excellent outcomes in an AYA patient population.[152] In the published results, 5-year EFS rates were 78% for patients aged 15–18 years old, with EFS rates of 77% for historical controls aged 10–15 years ($p = 0.09$). In addition, there was no increase in treatment-related complications in the older adolescents. These results inspired the current trial for patients up to age 50 years old, with preliminary results showing an estimated EFS rate of 75% and OS at 79% with a median patient age of 28 years and median follow-up of 18 months.[153]

Older adults

Older patients with ALL represent a challenging patient subset given their higher likelihood of comorbidities, sensitivity to drug toxicity, and unfavorable disease characteristics including a high prevalence of the Philadelphia chromosome. Further, response rates and outcomes of these patients are not well studied because they are not frequently enrolled on clinical trials. The limited number of patients enrolled on previous trials demonstrate worse CR, DFS, and OS compared to younger patients.[124–126,154–157] More recently the PETHEMA-ALL 96 trial enrolled 33 patients aged 56–77 without the Philadelphia chromosome.[158] Initially the induction chemotherapy regimen included vincristine, daunorubicin, prednisone, L-asparaginase, and cyclophosphamide and resulted in a CR rate of 30% and early death during induction of 70%. Removal of L-asparaginase and cyclophosphamide from the regimen increased the CR rate to 70% and reduced early death during induction to 22%, but did not affect DFS or OS. These results are consistent with previous studies showing that age-adjusted therapies are not sufficient alternatives for effective disease treatment.[125,156,159]

The high incidence of unfavorable karyotypes in elderly patients, specifically the Philadelphia chromosome, contributes to disease resistance and difficulty with drug toxicity.[20,64,112,160] Recent trials have explored the efficacy of imatinib as an alternative to, or in combination with, reduced intensity multidrug induction regimens for older adults with Ph+ ALL. The results of these investigations are described above in the section on Ph+ ALL and demonstrate improved responses and prolongation of survival for imatinib-treated older adults. These studies suggest that age-adjusted therapy with concomitant use of targeted therapy clearly benefit older patients with Ph+ ALL. The challenge for the future will be to define new regimens that continue to minimize toxicity and can overcome the emergence of drug resistance.

Supportive care

Effective treatment of adult ALL requires supportive management of complications associated with chemotherapy and frequently has a significant impact on outcome. Optimal infectious disease management during periods of neutropenia and management of tumor lysis syndrome are crucial areas of supportive care. Neutropenic fever necessitates immediate evaluation of the patient and initiation of therapy with antibiotics. The antibiotic coverage should be broad and chosen based upon the frequency and resistance of bacterial isolates within the specific hospital.[161] Additionally, afebrile neutropenic patients should receive antibiotic prophylaxis with evidence supporting the use of a fluoroquinolone, but ultimate decision based upon individual patient comorbidities and allergies.[162] Antifungal and antiviral prophylaxis should also be strongly considered as neutropenic patients are very susceptible to severe and invasive fungal infections and reactivation of latent viruses.[163,164] Due to the significant immunosuppression rendered by the agents used to treat ALL, patients should also receive prophylaxis for *Pneumocystis carinii* during the entire course of consolidation and maintenance therapy.

Shortening the period of neutropenia to prevent possibly fatal infections is the goal of using G-CSF, and previous studies demonstrate the utility of this drug with induction regimens for ALL.[62,165–167] Thomas *et al.* randomized patients on the

LALA-94 trial to receive G-CSF, granulocyte–macrophage colony-stimulating factor (GM-CSF), or no CSF.[167] When given on day four of induction until return of absolute neutrophil count (ANC) > 1000, patients receiving G-CSF had significantly shorter hospital stays, less time to neutrophil recovery, and fewer severe infections compared with patients that did not receive CSF. The previously discussed CALGB 9111 trial highlighted the benefit of using this drug in patients prone to difficulty with hematologic recovery, specifically older patients.[62] The study observed a trend towards increased CR rates in patients 60 years of age or older in the G-CSF arm compared with the placebo arm. Although G-CSF does not affect DFS or OS, it appears to be safe and assists patients to proceed with post-remission therapy.

Tumor lysis syndrome presents another cause of morbidity and possible mortality in adult ALL. Recent guidelines stress identification of patients at high risk for tumor lysis syndrome, which include ALL patients with an elevated WBC count at baseline, elevated LDH, and baseline renal dysfunction.[168] All patients should be treated aggressively with fluid hydration, allopurinol, and possibly rasburicase depending upon serum uric acid level.

Relapsed disease

Although the majority of adults with ALL reach CR, most of them will eventually relapse and subsequently be much less responsive to salvage therapy. First relapse typically occurs within the first two years after induction and remissions lasting longer than 18 months are associated with improved response to salvage regimens.[169–171] CR rates for salvage regimens range from 31% to 78% and survival for these patients remains poor.[170,172–175] The more effective salvage regimens are multidrug and usually contain intermediate to high-dose cytarabine.[169] For patients with relapsed or refractory precursor T-cell ALL, nelarabine, a deoxyguanosine analog prodrug, is a single-agent therapy with proven favorable results. DeAngelo *et al.* used nelarbine to treat relapsed and refractory patients and demonstrated a CR rate of 41% and OS of 28% at one year.[176] Despite this difficult patient population, nelarabine allowed patients to proceed to transplant and increased survival.

In order to evaluate the role of SCT in relapsed disease, the large MRC UKALL XII/ECOG 2993 trial evaluated the outcome of 609 relapsed patients treated with chemotherapy, ASCT or allogeneic SCT.[171] The 5-year OS rates for the chemotherapy, ASCT, matched unrelated donor (MUD) SCT, and sibling SCT arms were 4%, 15%, 16%, and 23% respectively with a significant survival difference between the chemotherapy and transplant groups. The LALA-94 trial observed similar results in relapsed patients with active disease or in CR2 with SCT producing improved DFS and OS with a 5-year OS of 25%. In these trials initial post-remission therapy and risk stratification group did not affect relapse rate; however, achieving CR2 prior to SCT did improve outcome. These, as well as previous studies,[170,172,177] show that allogeneic SCT is the only potentially curative therapy in relapsed or refractory ALL. However, even in patients able to tolerate SCT with an available donor the maximum 5-year OS reported is 25%, which highlights the importance of developing improved post-remission strategies to avoid disease recurrence.

Emerging therapeutic options

New purine analogs have shown activity in relapsed disease and are being considered for frontline therapies. As mentioned previously, nelarabine, a prodrug that when demethylated forms a deoxyguanosine analog toxic to immature T cells, has been approved for treatment of relapsed precursor T-cell ALL, and has been incorporated into a frontline COG regimen for this patient subset. A preliminary result of this study reported that the addition of nelarabine treatment modules does not appear to result in any additional toxicities and appears to improve survival. Compared with historical controls where survival was less than 50%, the 3-year EFS for high-risk children (defined as a slow response to prednisone pre-phase induction and/or high levels of MRD defined by flow cytometric analysis following induction chemotherapy) is over 70% with the addition of nelarabine.[178] Clofarabine, another novel purine nucleoside, has been recently approved for treatment of relapsed ALL in children. In a phase II trial of single-agent clofarabine in 61 children with relapsed/refractory ALL, the overall response rate was 30%.[179] Remissions were sufficiently durable to allow patients to proceed to hematopoietic stem cell transplantation. Limited activity of single-agent clofarabine has been reported in adults with relapsed ALL; however, this may be worthy of further exploration. In a phase I study of adults with refractory acute leukemias, clofarabine was combined with cyclophosphamide based on drug synergy that was demonstrated in vitro in primary leukemia cells.[180] In this study, the dose-limiting toxicity was prolonged marrow aplasia; nevertheless, significant clinical responses were noted in four of six patients with refractory ALL.

A new preparation of vincristine, sphingosomal vincristine (vincristine encapsulated in sphingomyelin liposomes or "sphingosomes" for IV injection) results in prolonged exposure to vincristine. Sphingosomal vincristine resulted in significantly greater antitumor activity in vitro and in animal models when compared with conventional vincristine.[181] In a phase II trial of single-agent sphingosomal vincristine given to adults with relapsed or refractory ALL, the overall response rate was 14%[182] and has prompted the further development of this drug in relapsed ALL.

New preparations of active drugs are also being incorporated into frontline therapies. A single IV infusion of the long-acting form of L-asparaginase, PEG-asparaginase, has been tested as part of a frontline standard induction regimen in adults with ALL. IV PEG-asparaginase was well tolerated and resulted in a long duration of asparagine depletion which, in earlier studies, correlated with improved DFS.[183] In a randomized study of native L-asparaginase versus PEG-asparaginase as part of induction and post-remission therapy performed by the CCG, there was no difference in EFS between the two arms. However, more effective asparagine depletion and the lower rate of antibody development in the PEG-asparaginase arm led these investigators to recommend PEG-asparaginase over native asparaginase for frontline therapy of ALL in children.[184]

From bench to bedside: evolution of targeted therapies

Better definition of the molecular pathogenesis of ALL will undoubtedly direct development of future subset-specific targeted therapies. As described previously, the most promising example of current targeted therapeutic development in ALL is the addition of the Abl TKI to the treatment of Ph+ ALL. New targeted inhibitors in development that may improve response rates and prevent the emergence of drug resistance are being evaluated in clinical trials. They include the dual SRC/Bcr-Abl inhibitors SKI-606 and INNO-406 (formerly NS-187),[185–187] both of which are active in most *BCR-ABL* mutations that confer resistance to imatinib, except for the T315I mutation. There was early success against the T315I mutation using the aurora kinase inhibitor MK-0457;[188] however, further testing of this agent was discontinued early due to unreasonable toxicities. Further phase I testing of this agent to determine an acceptable phase II dose may be required.

Another promising strategy, monoclonal antibody targeting of antigens specific to certain disease subsets, is being explored to enhance chemotherapeutic efficacy. The incorporation of rituximab into frontline therapies for Burkitt lymphoma/leukemia (described earlier) may also be effective for the 20–50% of precursor B-cell cases that express CD20. Preliminary data from a clinical trial combining rituximab with the HyperCVAD regimen in adults with precursor B-cell ALL with CD20 expression suggest that the addition of rituximab resulted in improvement in DFS to 56% compared with a historical control DFS of 35% for this patient subset.[189] Of note, the addition of rituximab appeared to improve DFS only for adults < 60 years old. Longer follow-up of these preliminary data is required to substantiate a beneficial role for direct targeting of CD20 in adult ALL. Epratuzumab, a humanized monoclonal antibody against CD22 located in the cytoplasm of precursor B cells and the surface of more mature B cells, may also have activity for this subset of patients and has already shown some activity in relapsed ALL. In a study for children with relapsed ALL, epratuzumab was combined with standard reinduction therapy.[190] Flow cytometric evaluation demonstrated the rapid eradication of surface CD22 within 24 hours of drug administration, indicating effective targeting of leukemic cells. Complete remissions were observed in 9 of 15 patients. CD52 is expressed in over 70% of all adult ALL cases and represents an attractive target. Alemtuzumab, an anti-CD52 antibody, has been explored in a recently completed CALGB phase I/II trial as an adjunct to standard chemotherapy to determine whether it has a role in the eradication of MRD.[191] This study demonstrated that it was possible to add alemtuzumab to frontline therapy without significant additional toxicity; however, clinical outcome data have not yet been reported.

New insights into ALL pathogenesis are leading to the development of preclinical therapeutic models and early-phase molecularly targeted clinical trials. As described above in the section on *Molecular genetics*, aberrant *NOTCH1* activation occurs in the majority of patients with precursor T-cell ALL. This observation led investigators to explore targeted inhibition of Notch1 protein activation. Gamma secretase is required for Notch1 cleavage and subsequent activation; thus, preclinical testing of compounds that inhibit gamma secretase have demonstrated decreased proliferation and subsequent differentiation of some T-cell ALL cell lines. Prolonged exposure resulted in apoptotic cell death.[192] An early phase I clinical trial of a gamma secretase inhibitor for patients with relapsed/refractory precursor T-cell ALL demonstrated pharmacodynamic evidence of Notch1 inhibition and resulted in one transient clinical response; further dose escalation was limited due to severe diarrhea.[193] Additional preclinical data suggest that Notch1 positively regulates the mTOR pathway in precursor T-cell ALL and that the combined inhibition of mTOR using rapamycin with a gamma secretase inhibitor could be a rational approach to treatment of these leukemias.[33]

Targeting the mTOR pathway may also be useful for other subsets of ALL. A recent gene expression-based chemical genomic study screening for agents whose expression profile overlapped with the gene expression signature of corticosteroid sensitivity or resistance in ALL cell lines identified that the mTOR inhibitor rapamycin induced corticosteroid sensitivity and apoptosis via modulation of the antiapoptotic MCL1 protein.[194] Targeting mTOR has also been tested in a preclinical NOD/SCID mouse xenograft ALL model. When mice with established ALL were treated with a second-generation mTOR inhibitor, CCI-779, they had a dramatic decrease in peripheral blood blasts and in splenomegaly.[195] Rapamycin has been shown to induce apoptosis of primary ALL cells by inhibiting signaling through the PI3K/*AKT* survival pathway.[196] Recent preclinical data also demonstrate a rationale for targeting PI3K in Ph+ ALL using a specific PI3K inhibitor in combination with rapamycin.[197]

Aberrant expression of cell cycle regulatory genes, as described above, occurs frequently in both precursor B- and T-cell ALL and represents potential therapeutic targets.[29] Flavopiridol, a serine/threonine kinase inhibitor that targets multiple cyclin-dependent kinases, induces cell cycle checkpoint arrest and may be an attractive targeted agent. In preclinical studies of ALL cell lines, flavopiridol induced cell cycle arrest with evidence of reduced cyclin-dependent kinase activity and induction of cell death.[198] In a phase I trial in relapsed ALL, flavopiridol was administered for three days, followed by cytarabine and mitoxantrone.[199] While it is difficult to ascertain the clinical benefit of the addition of flavopiridol to known active agents in relapsed ALL, pharmacodynamic studies suggested that flavopiridol induced significant cell cytotoxicity as a single agent.

Conclusions

Contemporary treatment strategies for adults with ALL are increasingly dependent on improved risk stratification with a focus on biologically based therapies. Significant progress using biologically risk-adapted strategies has already been demonstrated for adults with Ph+ ALL and those with Burkitt lymphoma/leukemia. Undoubtedly, the rapid evolution of insights into the molecular pathogenesis of ALL will prompt the development of targeted experimental therapeutic approaches. However, due to the relative rarity and tremendous biologic heterogeneity of ALL, future treatment progress will rely upon carefully designed prospective subset-specific studies that require the participation of large national and international cooperative groups to achieve the ultimate goal of improving cure rates for this challenging disease.

References

1. Jemal A, Siegel R, Ward E, *et al.* Cancer statistics, 2007. *CA Cancer J Clin* 2007;**57**:43–66.
2. Andersen MK, Christiansen DH, Jensen BA, *et al.* Therapy-related acute lymphoblastic leukaemia with MLL rearrangements following DNA topoisomerase II inhibitors, an increasing problem: report on two new cases and review of the literature since 1992. *Br J Haematol* 2001;**114**:539–43.
3. Leone G, Voso MT, Sica S, *et al.* Therapy related leukemias: susceptibility, prevention and treatment. *Leuk Lymphoma* 2001;**41**:255–76.
4. Zipursky A, Poon A, Doyle J. Leukemia in Down syndrome: a review. *Pediatr Hematol Oncol* 1992;**9**:139–49.
5. Gurbuxani S, Vyas P, Crispino JD. Recent insights into the mechanisms of myeloid leukemogenesis in Down syndrome. *Blood* 2004;**103**:399–406.
6. Shaw MP, Eden OB, Grace E, *et al.* Acute lymphoblastic leukemia and Klinefelter's syndrome. *Pediatr Hematol Oncol* 1992;**9**:81–5.
7. German J, Bloom D, Passarge E, *et al.* Bloom's syndrome. VI. The disorder in Israel and an estimation of the gene frequency in the Ashkenazim. *Am J Hum Genet* 1977;**29**:553–62.
8. Toledano SR, Lange BJ. Ataxia-telangiectasia and acute lymphoblastic leukemia. *Cancer* 1980;**45**:1675–8.
9. Greaves MF, Maia AT, Wiemels JL, *et al.* Leukemia in twins: lessons in natural history. *Blood* 2003;**102**:2321–33.
10. Wiemels JL, Cazzaniga G, Daniotti M, *et al.* Prenatal origin of acute lymphoblastic leukaemia in children. *Lancet* 1999;**354**:1499–503.
11. Fasching K, Panzer S, Haas OA, *et al.* Presence of clone-specific antigen receptor gene rearrangements at birth indicates an in utero origin of diverse types of early childhood acute lymphoblastic leukemia. *Blood* 2000;**95**:2722–4.
12. Mori H, Colman SM, Xiao Z, *et al.* Chromosome translocations and covert leukemic clones are generated during normal fetal development. *Proc Natl Acad Sci U S A* 2002;**99**:8242–7.
13. Preston DL, Kusumi S, Tomonaga M, *et al.* Cancer incidence in atomic bomb survivors. Part III. Leukemia, lymphoma and multiple myeloma, 1950–1987. *Radiat Res* 1994;**137**:S68–97.
14. Sandler DP, Shore DL, Anderson JR, *et al.* Cigarette smoking and risk of acute leukemia: associations with morphology and cytogenetic abnormalities in bone marrow. *J Natl Cancer Inst* 1993;**85**:1994–2003.
15. UK Childhood Cancer Study Investigators. Childhood cancer and residential proximity to power lines. *Br J Cancer* 2000;**83**:1573–80.
16. Jaffe E, Harris N, Stein H, *et al.* (eds.) *World Health Organization Classification of Tumours: Pathology and Genetics of Tumours of Haematopoietic and Lymphoid Tissues.* Lyon, IARC Press. 2001; 111–87.
17. Thomas DA, O'Brien S, Jorgensen JL, *et al.* Prognostic significance of CD20 expression in adults with de novo precursor B-lineage acute lymphoblastic leukemia. *Blood* 2009;**113**:6330–7.
18. Faderl S, Kantarjian HM, Talpaz M, *et al.* Clinical significance of cytogenetic abnormalities in adult acute lymphoblastic leukemia. *Blood* 1998;**91**:3995–4019.
19. Secker-Walker LM, Prentice HG, Durrant J, *et al.* Cytogenetics adds independent prognostic information in adults with acute lymphoblastic leukaemia on MRC trial UKALL XA. MRC Adult Leukaemia Working Party. *Br J Haematol* 1997; **96**:601–10.
20. Wetzler M, Dodge RK, Mrozek K, *et al.* Prospective karyotype analysis in adult acute lymphoblastic leukemia: the cancer and leukemia Group B experience. *Blood* 1999;**93**:3983–93.
21. Skorski T, Kanakaraj P, Nieborowska-Skorska M, *et al.* Phosphatidylinositol-3 kinase activity is regulated by BCR/ABL and is required for the growth of Philadelphia chromosome-positive cells. *Blood* 1995;**86**:726–36.
22. Ferrando AA, Look AT. Clinical implications of recurring chromosomal and associated molecular abnormalities in acute lymphoblastic leukemia. *Semin Hematol* 2000;**37**:381–95.
23. Golub TR, Barker GF, Bohlander SK, *et al.* Fusion of the TEL gene on 12p13 to the AML1 gene on 21q22 in acute lymphoblastic leukemia. *Proc Natl Acad Sci U S A* 1995;**92**:4917–21.
24. Shurtleff SA, Buijs A, Behm FG, *et al.* TEL/AML1 fusion resulting from a cryptic t(12;21) is the most common genetic lesion in pediatric ALL and defines a subgroup of patients with an excellent prognosis. *Leukemia* 1995;**9**:1985–9.
25. Dalla-Favera R, Bregni M, Erikson J, *et al.* Human c-myc onc gene is located on the region of chromosome 8 that is translocated in Burkitt lymphoma cells. *Proc Natl Acad Sci U S A* 1982;**79**:7824–7.
26. Taub R, Kirsch I, Morton C, *et al.* Translocation of the c-myc gene into the immunoglobulin heavy chain locus in human Burkitt lymphoma and murine plasmacytoma cells. *Proc Natl Acad Sci U S A* 1982;**79**:7837–41.
27. Bertin R, Acquaviva C, Mirebeau D, *et al.* CDKN2A, CDKN2B, and MTAP gene dosage permits precise

characterization of mono- and bi-allelic 9p21 deletions in childhood acute lymphoblastic leukemia. *Genes Chromosomes Cancer* 2003;**37**:44–57.

28. Sherr CJ, Roberts JM. CDK inhibitors: positive and negative regulators of G1-phase progression. *Genes Dev* 1999;**13**:1501–12.
29. Stock W, Tsai T, Golden C, *et al.* Cell cycle regulatory gene abnormalities are important determinants of leukemogenesis and disease biology in adult acute lymphoblastic leukemia. *Blood* 2000;**95**:2364–71.
30. Aster JC, Pear WS, Blacklow SC. Notch signaling in leukemia. *Annu Rev Pathol* 2008;**3**:587–613.
31. Weng AP, Millholland JM, Yashiro-Ohtani Y, *et al.* c-Myc is an important direct target of Notch1 in T-cell acute lymphoblastic leukemia/lymphoma. *Genes Dev* 2006;**20**:2096–109.
32. Palomero T, Lim WK, Odom DT, *et al.* NOTCH1 directly regulates c-MYC and activates a feed-forward-loop transcriptional network promoting leukemic cell growth. *Proc Natl Acad Sci U S A* 2006;**103**:18 261–6.
33. Chan SM, Weng AP, Tibshirani R, *et al.* Notch signals positively regulate activity of the mTOR pathway in T-cell acute lymphoblastic leukemia. *Blood* 2007;**110**:278–86.
34. Palomero T, Sulis ML, Cortina M, *et al.* Mutational loss of PTEN induces resistance to NOTCH1 inhibition in T-cell leukemia. *Nat Med* 2007;**13**:1203–10.
35. Palomero T, Dominguez M, Ferrando AA. The role of the PTEN/AKT pathway in NOTCH1-induced leukemia. *Cell Cycle* 2008;**7**:965–70.
36. Mullighan CG, Goorha S, Radtke I, *et al.* Genome-wide analysis of genetic alterations in acute lymphoblastic leukaemia. *Nature* 2007; **446**:758–64.
37. Mullighan CG, Miller CB, Radtke I, *et al.* BCR-ABL1 lymphoblastic leukaemia is characterized by the deletion of Ikaros. *Nature* 2008;**453**:110–14.
38. Mi S, Lu J, Sun M, *et al.* MicroRNA expression signatures accurately discriminate acute lymphoblastic leukemia from acute myeloid leukemia. *Proc Natl Acad Sci U S A* 2007;**104**:19 971–6.
39. Larson RA, Dodge RK, Burns CP, *et al.* A five-drug remission induction regimen with intensive consolidation for adults with acute lymphoblastic leukemia: cancer and leukemia group B study 8811. *Blood* 1995;**85**:2025–37.
40. Kantarjian HM, Walters RS, Keating MJ, *et al.* Results of the vincristine, doxorubicin, and dexamethasone regimen in adults with standard- and high-risk acute lymphocytic leukemia. *J Clin Oncol* 1990;**8**:994–1004.
41. Lazzarino M, Morra E, Alessandrino EP, *et al.* Adult acute lymphoblastic leukemia. Response to therapy according to presenting features in 62 patients. *Eur J Cancer Clin Oncol* 1982;**18**:813–19.
42. Hoelzer D, Thiel E, Loffler H, *et al.* Prognostic factors in a multicenter study for treatment of acute lymphoblastic leukemia in adults. *Blood* 1988;**71**:123–31.
43. Chessells JM, Hall E, Prentice HG, *et al.* The impact of age on outcome in lymphoblastic leukaemia; MRC UKALL X and XA compared: a report from the MRC Paediatric and Adult Working Parties. *Leukemia* 1998;**12**:463–73.
44. Secker-Walker LM, Craig JM, Hawkins JM, *et al.* Philadelphia positive acute lymphoblastic leukemia in adults: age distribution, BCR breakpoint and prognostic significance. *Leukemia* 1991;**5**:196–9.
45. Linker CA, Levitt LJ, O'Donnell M, *et al.* Treatment of adult acute lymphoblastic leukemia with intensive cyclical chemotherapy: a follow-up report. *Blood* 1991;**78**:2814–22.
46. Hoelzer D, Thiel E, Ludwig WD, *et al.* The German multicentre trials for treatment of acute lymphoblastic leukemia in adults. The German Adult ALL Study Group. *Leukemia* 1992;**6** Suppl 2:175–7.
47. Faderl S, Albitar M. Insights into the biologic and molecular abnormalities in adult acute lymphocytic leukemia. *Hematol Oncol Clin North Am* 2000;**14**:1267–88.
48. Mandelli F, Annino L, Rotoli B. The GIMEMA ALL 0183 trial: analysis of 10-year follow-up. GIMEMA Cooperative Group, Italy. *Br J Haematol* 1996;**92**:665–72.
49. Suggs JL, Cruse JM, Lewis RE. Aberrant myeloid marker expression in precursor B-cell and T-cell leukemias. *Exp Mol Pathol* 2007;**83**:471–3.
50. Matutes E, Morilla R, Farahat N, *et al.* Definition of acute biphenotypic leukemia. *Haematologica* 1997;**82**:64–6.
51. Boldt DH, Kopecky KJ, Head D, *et al.* Expression of myeloid antigens by blast cells in acute lymphoblastic leukemia of adults. The Southwest Oncology Group experience. *Leukemia* 1994;**8**:2118–26.
52. Pui CH, Behm FG, Singh B, *et al.* Myeloid-associated antigen expression lacks prognostic value in childhood acute lymphoblastic leukemia treated with intensive multiagent chemotherapy. *Blood* 1990;**75**:198–202.
53. Preti HA, Huh YO, O'Brien SM, *et al.* Myeloid markers in adult acute lymphocytic leukemia. Correlations with patient and disease characteristics and with prognosis. *Cancer* 1995;**76**:1564–70.
54. Gaynor J, Chapman D, Little C, *et al.* A cause-specific hazard rate analysis of prognostic factors among 199 adults with acute lymphoblastic leukemia: the Memorial Hospital experience since 1969. *J Clin Oncol* 1988;**6**:1014–30.
55. Pongers-Willemse MJ, Seriu T, Stolz F, *et al.* Primers and protocols for standardized detection of minimal residual disease in acute lymphoblastic leukemia using immunoglobulin and T cell receptor gene rearrangements and TAL1 deletions as PCR targets: report of the BIOMED-1 CONCERTED ACTION: investigation of minimal residual disease in acute leukemia. *Leukemia* 1999;**13**:110–18.
56. Gabert J, Beillard E, van der Velden VH, *et al.* Standardization and quality control studies of 'real-time' quantitative reverse transcriptase polymerase chain reaction of fusion gene transcripts for residual disease detection in leukemia – a Europe Against Cancer program. *Leukemia* 2003;**17**:2318–57.
57. Mortuza FY, Papaioannou M, Moreira IM, *et al.* Minimal residual disease tests provide an independent predictor of clinical outcome in adult acute lymphoblastic leukemia. *J Clin Oncol* 2002;**20**:1094–104.
58. Bruggemann M, Raff T, Flohr T, *et al.* Clinical significance of minimal residual disease quantification in adult patients with standard-risk acute

lymphoblastic leukemia. *Blood* 2006;**107**:1116–23.

59. Vidriales MB, San-Miguel JF, Orfao A, *et al.* Minimal residual disease monitoring by flow cytometry. *Best Pract Res Clin Haematol* 2003; **16**:599–612.

60. Krampera M, Vitale A, Vincenzi C, *et al.* Outcome prediction by immunophenotypic minimal residual disease detection in adult T-cell acute lymphoblastic leukaemia. *Br J Haematol* 2003;**120**:74–9.

61. Gokbuget N, Arnold R, Bohme A, *et al.* Improved outcome in high risk and very high risk ALL by risk adapted SCT and in standard risk ALL by intensive chemotherapy in 713 adult ALL patients treated according to the prospective GMALL study 07/2003. *ASH Annual Meeting Abstracts* 2007;**110**:12.

62. Larson RA, Dodge RK, Linker CA, *et al.* A randomized controlled trial of filgrastim during remission induction and consolidation chemotherapy for adults with acute lymphoblastic leukemia: CALGB study 9111. *Blood* 1998;**92**:1556–64.

63. Takeuchi J, Kyo T, Naito K, *et al.* Induction therapy by frequent administration of doxorubicin with four other drugs, followed by intensive consolidation and maintenance therapy for adult acute lymphoblastic leukemia: the JALSG-ALL93 study. *Leukemia* 2002;**16**:1259–66.

64. Annino L, Vegna ML, Camera A, *et al.* Treatment of adult acute lymphoblastic leukemia (ALL): long-term follow-up of the GIMEMA ALL 0288 randomized study. *Blood* 2002; **99**:863–71.

65. Kantarjian H, Thomas D, O'Brien S, *et al.* Long-term follow-up results of hyperfractionated cyclophosphamide, vincristine, doxorubicin, and dexamethasone (HyperCVAD), a dose-intensive regimen, in adult acute lymphocytic leukemia. *Cancer* 2004;**101**:2788–801.

66. Thomas X, Boiron JM, Huguet F, *et al.* Outcome of treatment in adults with acute lymphoblastic leukemia: analysis of the LALA-94 trial. *J Clin Oncol* 2004; **22**:4075–86.

67. Rowe JM, Buck G, Burnett AK, *et al.* Induction therapy for adults with acute lymphoblastic leukemia: results of more than 1500 patients from the international ALL trial: MRC UKALL XII/ECOG E2993. *Blood* 2005;**106**:3760–7.

68. Hussein KK, Dahlberg S, Head D, *et al.* Treatment of acute lymphoblastic leukemia in adults with intensive induction, consolidation, and maintenance chemotherapy. *Blood* 1989;**73**:57–63.

69. Schauer P, Arlin ZA, Mertelsmann R, *et al.* Treatment of acute lymphoblastic leukemia in adults: results of the L-10 and L-10M protocols. *J Clin Oncol* 1983;**1**:462–70.

70. Gottlieb AJ, Weinberg V, Ellison RR, *et al.* Efficacy of daunorubicin in the therapy of adult acute lymphocytic leukemia: a prospective randomized trial by cancer and leukemia group B. *Blood* 1984;**64**:267–74.

71. Radford JE Jr, Burns CP, Jones MP, *et al.* Adult acute lymphoblastic leukemia: results of the Iowa HOP-L protocol. *J Clin Oncol* 1989;**7**:58–66.

72. Cuttner J, Mick R, Budman DR, *et al.* Phase III trial of brief intensive treatment of adult acute lymphocytic leukemia comparing daunorubicin and mitoxantrone: a CALGB Study. *Leukemia* 1991;**5**:425–31.

73. Hoelzer D, Ludwig WD, Thiel E, *et al.* Improved outcome in adult B-cell acute lymphoblastic leukemia. *Blood* 1996;**87**:495–508.

74. Gokbuget N, Hoelzer D, Arnold R, *et al.* Treatment of adult ALL according to protocols of the German Multicenter Study Group for Adult ALL (GMALL). *Hematol Oncol Clin North Am* 2000;**14**:1307–25.

75. Nachman JB, Sather HN, Sensel MG, *et al.* Augmented post-induction therapy for children with high-risk acute lymphoblastic leukemia and a slow response to initial therapy. *N Engl J Med* 1998;**338**:1663–71.

76. Kantarjian HM, O'Brien S, Smith TL, *et al.* Results of treatment with HyperCVAD, a dose-intensive regimen, in adult acute lymphocytic leukemia. *J Clin Oncol* 2000;**18**:547–61.

77. Larson RA, Fretzin MH, Dodge RK, *et al.* Hypersensitivity reactions to L-asparaginase do not impact on the remission duration of adults with acute lymphoblastic leukemia. *Leukemia* 1998;**12**:660–5.

78. Dekker AW, van't Veer MB, Sizoo W, *et al.* Intensive postremission chemotherapy without maintenance therapy in adults with acute lymphoblastic leukemia. Dutch Hemato-Oncology Research Group. *J Clin Oncol* 1997;**15**:476–82.

79. Reman O, Pigneux A, Huguet F, *et al.* Central nervous system involvement in adult acute lymphoblastic leukemia at diagnosis and/or at first relapse: results from the GET-LALA group. *Leuk Res* 2008;**32**:1741–50.

80. Cortes J, O'Brien SM, Pierce S, *et al.* The value of high-dose systemic chemotherapy and intrathecal therapy for central nervous system prophylaxis in different risk groups of adult acute lymphoblastic leukemia. *Blood* 1995;**86**:2091–7.

81. Law IP, Blom J. Adult acute leukemia: frequency of central system involvement in long term survivors. *Cancer* 1977;**40**:1304–6.

82. Omura GA, Moffitt S, Vogler WR, *et al.* Combination chemotherapy of adult acute lymphoblastic leukemia with randomized central nervous system prophylaxis. *Blood* 1980;**55**:199–204.

83. Mastrangelo R. The problem of "staging" in childhood acute lymphoblastic leukemia: a review. *Med Pediatr Oncol* 1986;**14**:121–3.

84. Kantarjian HM, Walters RS, Smith TL, *et al.* Identification of risk groups for development of central nervous system leukemia in adults with acute lymphocytic leukemia. *Blood* 1988;**72**:1784–9.

85. Tucker J, Prior PF, Green CR, *et al.* Minimal neuropsychological sequelae following prophylactic treatment of the central nervous system in adult leukaemia and lymphoma. *Br J Cancer* 1989;**60**:775–80.

86. Pullen J, Boyett J, Shuster J, *et al.* Extended triple intrathecal chemotherapy trial for prevention of CNS relapse in good-risk and poor-risk patients with B-progenitor acute lymphoblastic leukemia: a Pediatric Oncology Group study. *J Clin Oncol* 1993;**11**:839–49.

87. Mandelli F, Annino L, Vegna ML, *et al.* GIMEMA ALL 0288: a multicentric study on adult acute lymphoblastic leukemia. Preliminary results. *Leukemia* 1992;**6** Suppl 2:182–5.

88. Laver JH, Barredo JC, Amylon M, *et al.* Effects of cranial radiation in children with high risk T cell acute lymphoblastic leukemia: a Pediatric

Oncology Group report. *Leukemia* 2000;**14**:369–73.

89. Storb R, Bryant JI, Buckner CD, *et al.* Allogeneic marrow grafting for acute lymphoblastic leukemia: leukemic relapse. *Transplant Proc* 1973;**5**:923–6.
90. Weiden PL, Flournoy N, Thomas ED, *et al.* Antileukemic effect of graft-versus-host disease in human recipients of allogeneic-marrow grafts. *N Engl J Med* 1979;**300**:1068–73.
91. Oh H, Gale RP, Zhang MJ, *et al.* Chemotherapy vs HLA-identical sibling bone marrow transplants for adults with acute lymphoblastic leukemia in first remission. *Bone Marrow Transplant* 1998;**22**:253–7.
92. Hunault M, Harousseau JL, Delain M, *et al.* Better outcome of adult acute lymphoblastic leukemia after early genoidentical allogeneic bone marrow transplantation (BMT) than after late high-dose therapy and autologous BMT: a GOELAMS trial. *Blood* 2004;**104**:3028–37.
93. Ribera JM, Oriol A, Bethencourt C, *et al.* Comparison of intensive chemotherapy, allogeneic or autologous stem cell transplantation as post-remission treatment for adult patients with high-risk acute lymphoblastic leukemia. Results of the PETHEMA ALL-93 trial. *Haematologica* 2005;**90**:1346–56.
94. Goldstone AH, Richards SM, Lazarus HM, *et al.* In adults with standard-risk acute lymphoblastic leukemia, the greatest benefit is achieved from a matched sibling allogeneic transplantation in first complete remission, and an autologous transplantation is less effective than conventional consolidation/maintenance chemotherapy in all patients: final results of the International ALL Trial (MRC UKALL XII/ECOG E2993). *Blood* 2008;**111**:1827–33.
95. Laport GG, Alvarnas JC, Palmer JM, *et al.* Long-term remission of Philadelphia chromosome-positive acute lymphoblastic leukemia after allogeneic hematopoietic cell transplantation from matched sibling donors: a 20-year experience with the fractionated total body irradiation-etoposide regimen. *Blood* 2008;**112**:903–9.
96. De Witte T, Awwad B, Boezeman J, *et al.* Role of allogenic bone marrow transplantation in adolescent or adult patients with acute lymphoblastic leukaemia or lymphoblastic lymphoma in first remission. *Bone Marrow Transplant* 1994; **14**:767–74.
97. Thiebaut A, Vernant JP, Degos L, *et al.* Adult acute lymphocytic leukemia study testing chemotherapy and autologous and allogeneic transplantation. A follow-up report of the French protocol LALA 87. *Hematol Oncol Clin North Am* 2000; **14**:1353–66.
98. Dhedin N, Dombret H, Thomas X, *et al.* Autologous stem cell transplantation in adults with acute lymphoblastic leukemia in first complete remission: analysis of the LALA-85, -87 and -94 trials. *Leukemia* 2006;**20**:336–44.
99. Yanada M, Matsuo K, Suzuki T, *et al.* Allogeneic hematopoietic stem cell transplantation as part of postremission therapy improves survival for adult patients with high-risk acute lymphoblastic leukemia: a metaanalysis. *Cancer* 2006;**106**:2657–63.
100. Thomas DA, Cortes J, O'Brien S, *et al.* HyperCVAD program in Burkitt's-type adult acute lymphoblastic leukemia. *J Clin Oncol* 1999;**17**:2461–70.
101. Yustein JT, Dang CV. Biology and treatment of Burkitt's lymphoma. *Curr Opin Hematol* 2007;**14**:375–81.
102. Zeller KI, Zhao X, Lee CW, *et al.* Global mapping of c-Myc binding sites and target gene networks in human B cells. *Proc Natl Acad Sci U S A* 2006;**103**:17 834–9.
103. Hummel M, Bentink S, Berger H, *et al.* A biologic definition of Burkitt's lymphoma from transcriptional and genomic profiling. *N Engl J Med* 2006;**354**:2419–30.
104. Dave SS, Fu K, Wright GW, *et al.* Molecular diagnosis of Burkitt's lymphoma. *N Engl J Med* 2006;**354**:2431–42.
105. Murphy SB, Bowman WP, Abromowitch M, *et al.* Results of treatment of advanced-stage Burkitt's lymphoma and B cell (SIg+) acute lymphoblastic leukemia with high-dose fractionated cyclophosphamide and coordinated high-dose methotrexate and cytarabine. *J Clin Oncol* 1986;**4**:1732–9.
106. Soussain C, Patte C, Ostronoff M, *et al.* Small noncleaved cell lymphoma and leukemia in adults. A retrospective study of 65 adults treated with the LMB pediatric protocols. *Blood* 1995;**85**: 664–74.
107. Thomas DA, Faderl S, O'Brien S, *et al.* Chemoimmunotherapy with HyperCVAD plus rituximab for the treatment of adult Burkitt and Burkitt-type lymphoma or acute lymphoblastic leukemia. *Cancer* 2006;**106**:1569–80.
108. Mead GM, Sydes MR, Walewski J, *et al.* An international evaluation of CODOX-M and CODOX-M alternating with IVAC in adult Burkitt's lymphoma: results of United Kingdom Lymphoma Group LY06 study. *Ann Oncol* 2002;**13**:1264–74.
109. Rizzieri DA, Johnson JL, Niedzwiecki D, *et al.* Intensive chemotherapy with and without cranial radiation for Burkitt leukemia and lymphoma: final results of Cancer and Leukemia Group B Study 9251. *Cancer* 2004;**100**: 1438–48.
110. Divine M, Casassus P, Koscielny S, *et al.* Burkitt lymphoma in adults: a prospective study of 72 patients treated with an adapted pediatric LMB protocol. *Ann Oncol* 2005;**16**:1928–35.
111. Hoelzer D, Hiddemann W, Baumann A, *et al.* High survival rate in adult Burkitt's lymphoma/leukemia and diffuse large B-cell lymphoma with mediastinal involvement. *ASH Annual Meeting Abstracts* 2007;**110**:518.
112. Gleissner B, Gokbuget N, Bartram CR, *et al.* Leading prognostic relevance of the BCR-ABL translocation in adult acute B-lineage lymphoblastic leukemia: a prospective study of the German Multicenter Trial Group and confirmed polymerase chain reaction analysis. *Blood* 2002;**99**:1536–43.
113. Moorman AV, Harrison CJ, Buck GA, *et al.* Karyotype is an independent prognostic factor in adult acute lymphoblastic leukemia (ALL): analysis of cytogenetic data from patients treated on the Medical Research Council (MRC) UKALLXII/Eastern Cooperative Oncology Group (ECOG) 2993 trial. *Blood* 2007;**109**:3189–97.
114. Dombret H, Gabert J, Boiron JM, *et al.* Outcome of treatment in adults with Philadelphia chromosome-positive acute lymphoblastic leukemia–results of the prospective multicenter LALA-94 trial. *Blood* 2002;**100**:2357–66.
115. Thomas DA, Faderl S, Cortes J, *et al.* Treatment of Philadelphia chromosome-positive acute

lymphocytic leukemia with HyperCVAD and imatinib mesylate. *Blood* 2004;**103**:4396–407.

116. Yanada M, Takeuchi J, Sugiura I, *et al.* High complete remission rate and promising outcome by combination of imatinib and chemotherapy for newly diagnosed BCR-ABL-positive acute lymphoblastic leukemia: a phase II study by the Japan Adult Leukemia Study Group. *J Clin Oncol* 2006;**24**:460–6.

117. de Labarthe A, Rousselot P, Huguet-Rigal F, *et al.* Imatinib combined with induction or consolidation chemotherapy in patients with de novo Philadelphia chromosome-positive acute lymphoblastic leukemia: results of the GRAAPH-2003 study. *Blood* 2007;**109**:1408–13.

118. Ottmann OG, Wassmann B, Pfeifer H, *et al.* Imatinib compared with chemotherapy as frontline treatment of elderly patients with Philadelphia chromosome-positive acute lymphoblastic leukemia (Ph+ALL). *Cancer* 2007;**109**:2068–76.

119. Vignetti M, Fazi P, Cimino G, *et al.* Imatinib plus steroids induces complete remissions and prolonged survival in elderly Philadelphia chromosome-positive patients with acute lymphoblastic leukemia without additional chemotherapy: results of the Gruppo Italiano Malattie Ematologiche dell'Adulto (GIMEMA) LAL0201-B protocol. *Blood* 2007;**109**:3676–8.

120. Lee S, Kim YJ, Min CK, *et al.* The effect of first-line imatinib interim therapy on the outcome of allogeneic stem cell transplantation in adults with newly diagnosed Philadelphia chromosome-positive acute lymphoblastic leukemia. *Blood* 2005;**105**:3449–57.

121. Schultz KR, Bowman WP, Slayton W, *et al.* Improved early event free survival (EFS) in children with Philadelphia chromosome-positive (Ph+) acute lymphoblastic leukemia (ALL) with intensive imatinib in combination with high dose chemotherapy: Children's Oncology Group (COG) Study AALL0031. *ASH Annual Meeting Abstracts* 2007;**110**:4.

122. Wassmann B, Pfeifer H, Goekbuget N, *et al.* Alternating versus concurrent schedules of imatinib and chemotherapy as frontline therapy for Philadelphia-positive acute lymphoblastic leukemia (Ph+ ALL). *Blood* 2006;**108**:1469–77.

123. Delannoy A, Ferrant A, Bosly A, *et al.* Acute lymphoblastic leukemia in the elderly. *Eur J Haematol* 1990;**45**:90–3.

124. Taylor PR, Reid MM, Bown N, *et al.* Acute lymphoblastic leukemia in patients aged 60 years and over: a population-based study of incidence and outcome. *Blood* 1992;**80**:1813–7.

125. Ferrari A, Annino L, Crescenzi S, *et al.* Acute lymphoblastic leukemia in the elderly: results of two different treatment approaches in 49 patients during a 25-year period. *Leukemia* 1995;**9**:1643–7.

126. Pagano L, Mele L, Casorelli I, *et al.* Acute lymphoblastic leukemia in the elderly. A twelve-year retrospective, single center study. *Haematologica* 2000;**85**:1327–9.

127. Delannoy A, Delabesse E, Lheritier V, *et al.* Imatinib and methylprednisolone alternated with chemotherapy improve the outcome of elderly patients with Philadelphia-positive acute lymphoblastic leukemia: results of the GRAALL AFR09 study. *Leukemia* 2006;**20**:1526–32.

128. Hofmann WK, Komor M, Hoelzer D, *et al.* Mechanisms of resistance to STI571 (Imatinib) in Philadelphia-chromosome positive acute lymphoblastic leukemia. *Leuk Lymphoma* 2004;**45**:655–60.

129. Deininger M, Buchdunger E, Druker BJ. The development of imatinib as a therapeutic agent for chronic myeloid leukemia. *Blood* 2005;**105**:2640–53.

130. Soverini S, Colarossi S, Gnani A, *et al.* Contribution of ABL kinase domain mutations to imatinib resistance in different subsets of Philadelphia-positive patients: by the GIMEMA Working Party on Chronic Myeloid Leukemia. *Clin Cancer Res* 2006;**12**:7374–9.

131. Branford S, Rudzki Z, Walsh S, *et al.* Detection of BCR-ABL mutations in patients with CML treated with imatinib is virtually always accompanied by clinical resistance, and mutations in the ATP phosphate-binding loop (P-loop) are associated with a poor prognosis. *Blood* 2003;**102**:276–83.

132. Soverini S, Martinelli G, Rosti G, *et al.* ABL mutations in late chronic phase chronic myeloid leukemia patients with up-front cytogenetic resistance to imatinib are associated with a greater likelihood of progression to blast crisis and shorter survival: a study by the GIMEMA Working Party on Chronic Myeloid Leukemia. *J Clin Oncol* 2005;**23**:4100–9.

133. Pfeifer H, Wassmann B, Pavlova A, *et al.* Kinase domain mutations of BCR-ABL frequently precede imatinib-based therapy and give rise to relapse in patients with de novo Philadelphia-positive acute lymphoblastic leukemia (Ph+ ALL). *Blood* 2007;**110**:727–34.

134. Talpaz M, Shah NP, Kantarjian H, *et al.* Dasatinib in imatinib-resistant Philadelphia chromosome-positive leukemias. *N Engl J Med* 2006;**354**:2531–41.

135. Foa R, Vignetti M, Vitale A, *et al.* Dasatinib as frontline monotherapy for the induction treatment of adult and elderly Ph+ acute lymphoblastic leukemia (ALL) patients: interim analysis of the GIMEMA Prospective Study LAL1205. *ASH Annual Meeting Abstracts* 2007;**110**:7.

136. Porkka K, Koskenvesa P, Lundan T, *et al.* Dasatinib crosses the blood-brain barrier and is an efficient therapy for central nervous system Philadelphia chromosome-positive leukemia. *Blood* 2008;**112**:1005–12.

137. Ravandi R, O'Brien S, Thomas DA, *et al.* First report of phase II study of dasatinib with hyperCVAD for the frontline treatment of patients with Philadelphia chromosome-positive (Ph+) acute lymphoblastic leukemia. *Blood* 2010; May 13 epub.

138. O'Hare T, Walters DK, Stoffregen EP, *et al.* In vitro activity of Bcr-Abl inhibitors AMN107 and BMS-354825 against clinically relevant imatinib-resistant Abl kinase domain mutants. *Cancer Res* 2005;**65**:4500–5.

139. Weisberg E, Manley PW, Breitenstein W, *et al.* Characterization of AMN107, a selective inhibitor of native and mutant Bcr-Abl. *Cancer Cell* 2005;**7**:129–41.

140. Larson R, Ottman O, Kantarjian H, *et al.* A phase II study of nilotinib administered to imatinib resistant or intolerant patients with chronic myelogenous leukemia (CML) in blast crisis (BC) or relapsed/refractory Ph+ acute lymphoblastic leukemia (ALL). *J Clin Oncol* (2007 ASCO Annual Meeting Proceedings Part I) 2007;**25** (18S):Abstract 7040.

141. Reiter A, Schrappe M, Ludwig WD, *et al.* Chemotherapy in 998 unselected

childhood acute lymphoblastic leukemia patients. Results and conclusions of the multicenter trial ALL-BFM 86. *Blood* 1994;**84**:3122–33.

142. Schrappe M, Reiter A, Zimmermann M, *et al.* Long-term results of four consecutive trials in childhood ALL performed by the ALL-BFM study group from 1981 to 1995. Berlin-Frankfurt-Munster. *Leukemia* 2000;**14**:2205–22.

143. Stock W, La M, Sanford B, *et al.* What determines the outcomes for adolescents and young adults with acute lymphoblastic leukemia treated on cooperative group protocols? A comparison of Children's Cancer Group and Cancer and Leukemia Group B studies. *Blood* 2008;**112**: 1646–54.

144. Boissel N, Auclerc MF, Lheritier V, *et al.* Should adolescents with acute lymphoblastic leukemia be treated as old children or young adults? Comparison of the French FRALLE-93 and LALA-94 trials. *J Clin Oncol* 2003;**21**:774–80.

145. de Bont JM, Holt B, Dekker AW, *et al.* Significant difference in outcome for adolescents with acute lymphoblastic leukemia treated on pediatric vs adult protocols in the Netherlands. *Leukemia* 2004;**18**:2032–5.

146. Testi AM, Valsecchi MG, Conter V, *et al.* Difference in outcome of adolescents with acute lymphoblastic leukemia (ALL) enrolled in pediatric (AIEOP) and adult (GIMEMA) protocols. *ASH Annual Meeting Abstracts* 2004;**104**:1954.

147. Ramanujachar R, Richards S, Hann I, *et al.* Adolescents with acute lymphoblastic leukaemia: outcome on UK national paediatric (ALL97) and adult (UKALLXII/E2993) trials. *Pediatr Blood Cancer* 2007;**48**:254–61.

148. Ribera JM, Oriol A, Sanz MA, *et al.* Comparison of the results of the treatment of adolescents and young adults with standard-risk acute lymphoblastic leukemia with the Programa Espanol de Tratamiento en Hematologia pediatric-based protocol ALL-96. *J Clin Oncol* 2008;**26**:1843–9.

149. DeAngelo DJ. The treatment of adolescents and young adults with acute lymphoblastic leukemia. *Am Soc Hematol Educ Prog* 2005:123–30.

150. Jeha S. Who should be treating adolescents and young adults with acute lymphoblastic leukaemia? *Eur J Cancer* 2003;**39**:2579–83.

151. Schiffer CA. Differences in outcome in adolescents with acute lymphoblastic leukemia: a consequence of better regimens? Better doctors? Both? *J Clin Oncol* 2003;**21**:760–1.

152. Barry E, DeAngelo DJ, Neuberg D, *et al.* Favorable outcome for adolescents with acute lymphoblastic leukemia treated on Dana-Farber Cancer Institute Acute Lymphoblastic Leukemia Consortium Protocols. *J Clin Oncol* 2007;**25**:813–19.

153. DeAngelo DJ, Dahlberg S, Silverman LB, *et al.* A multicenter phase II study using a dose intensified pediatric regimen in adults with untreated acute lymphoblastic leukemia. *ASH Annual Meeting Abstracts* 2007;**110**:587.

154. Kantarjian HM, O'Brien S, Smith T, *et al.* Acute lymphocytic leukaemia in the elderly: characteristics and outcome with the vincristine-adriamycin-dexamethasone (VAD) regimen. *Br J Haematol* 1994;**88**:94–100.

155. Bassan R, Di Bona E, Lerede T, *et al.* Age-adapted moderate-dose induction and flexible outpatient postremission therapy for elderly patients with acute lymphoblastic leukemia. *Leuk Lymphoma* 1996;**22**:295–301.

156. Thomas X, Olteanu N, Charrin C, *et al.* Acute lymphoblastic leukemia in the elderly: The Edouard Herriot Hospital experience. *Am J Hematol* 2001; **67**:73–83.

157. Robak T, Szmigielska-Kaplon A, Wrzesien-Kus A, *et al.* Acute lymphoblastic leukemia in elderly: the Polish Adult Leukemia Group (PALG) experience. *Ann Hematol* 2004; **83**:225–31.

158. Sancho JM, Ribera JM, Xicoy B, *et al.* Results of the PETHEMA ALL-96 trial in elderly patients with Philadelphia chromosome-negative acute lymphoblastic leukemia. *Eur J Haematol* 2007;**78**:102–10.

159. Spath-Schwalbe E, Heil G, Heimpel H. Acute lymphoblastic leukemia in patients over 59 years of age. Experience in a single center over a 10-year period. *Ann Hematol* 1994; **69**:291–6.

160. Pullarkat V, Slovak ML, Kopecky KJ, *et al.* Impact of cytogenetics on the outcome of adult acute lymphoblastic leukemia: results of Southwest Oncology Group 9400 study. *Blood* 2008;**111**:2563–72.

161. Hughes WT, Armstrong D, Bodey GP, *et al.* 2002 guidelines for the use of antimicrobial agents in neutropenic patients with cancer. *Clin Infect Dis* 2002;**34**:730–51.

162. Gafter-Gvili A, Fraser A, Paul M, *et al.* Antibiotic prophylaxis for bacterial infections in afebrile neutropenic patients following chemotherapy. *Cochrane Database Syst Rev* 2005;(4): CD004386.

163. Bow EJ, Laverdiere M, Lussier N, *et al.* Antifungal prophylaxis for severely neutropenic chemotherapy recipients: a meta analysis of randomized-controlled clinical trials. *Cancer* 2002;**94**:3230–46.

164. Sandherr M, Einsele H, Hebart H, *et al.* Antiviral prophylaxis in patients with haematological malignancies and solid tumours: Guidelines of the Infectious Diseases Working Party (AGIHO) of the German Society for Hematology and Oncology (DGHO). *Ann Oncol* 2006;**17**:1051–9.

165. Ottmann OG, Hoelzer D, Gracien E, *et al.* Concomitant granulocyte colony-stimulating factor and induction chemoradiotherapy in adult acute lymphoblastic leukemia: a randomized phase III trial. *Blood* 1995;**86**:444–50.

166. Geissler K, Koller E, Hubmann E, *et al.* Granulocyte colony-stimulating factor as an adjunct to induction chemotherapy for adult acute lymphoblastic leukemia–a randomized phase-III study. *Blood* 1997;**90**:590–6.

167. Thomas DA, O'Brien S, Cortes J, *et al.* Outcome with the HyperCVAD regimens in lymphoblastic lymphoma. *Blood* 2004;**104**:1624–30.

168. Coiffier B, Altman A, Pui CH, *et al.* Guidelines for the management of pediatric and adult tumor lysis syndrome: an evidence-based review. *J Clin Oncol* 2008;**26**:2767–78.

169. Bassan R, Lerede T, Barbui T. Strategies for the treatment of recurrent acute lymphoblastic leukemia in adults. *Haematologica* 1996;**81**:20–36.

170. Thomas DA, Kantarjian H, Smith TL, *et al.* Primary refractory and relapsed adult acute lymphoblastic leukemia: characteristics, treatment results, and prognosis with salvage therapy. *Cancer* 1999;**86**:1216–30.

171. Fielding AK, Richards SM, Chopra R, *et al.* Outcome of 609 adults after

relapse of acute lymphoblastic leukemia (ALL); an MRC UKALL12/ECOG 2993 study. *Blood* 2007;**109**:944–50.

172. Giona F, Annino L, Rondelli R, *et al.* Treatment of adults with acute lymphoblastic leukaemia in first bone marrow relapse: results of the ALL R-87 protocol. *Br J Haematol* 1997;**97**: 896–903.

173. Martino R, Brunet S, Sureda A, *et al.* Treatment of refractory and relapsed adult acute leukemia using a uniform chemotherapy protocol. *Leuk Lymphoma* 1993;**11**:393–8.

174. Weiss MA, Aliff TB, Tallman MS, *et al.* A single, high dose of idarubicin combined with cytarabine as induction therapy for adult patients with recurrent or refractory acute lymphoblastic leukemia. *Cancer* 2002;**95**:581–7.

175. Tavernier E, Boiron JM, Huguet F, *et al.* Outcome of treatment after first relapse in adults with acute lymphoblastic leukemia initially treated by the LALA-94 trial. *Leukemia* 2007;**21**:1907–14.

176. DeAngelo DJ, Yu D, Johnson JL, *et al.* Nelarabine induces complete remissions in adults with relapsed or refractory T-lineage acute lymphoblastic leukemia or lymphoblastic lymphoma: Cancer and Leukemia Group B study 19801. *Blood* 2007;**109**:5136–42.

177. Weiss MA. Treatment of adult patients with relapsed or refractory acute lymphoblastic leukemia (ALL). *Leukemia* 1997;**11** Suppl 4:S28–30.

178. Dunsmore K, Devidas M, Borowitz MJ, *et al.* Nelarabine in combination with intensive modified BFM AALL00P2: a pilot study for the treatment of high risk T-ALL, a report from the Children's Oncology Group. *J Clin Oncol* 2008 ASCO Annual Meeting Proceedings Part I 2008;**26** Abstract 10002.

179. Jeha S, Gaynon PS, Razzouk BI, *et al.* Phase II study of clofarabine in pediatric patients with refractory or relapsed acute lymphoblastic leukemia. *J Clin Oncol* 2006;**24**:1917–23.

180. Karp JE, Ricklis RM, Balakrishnan K, *et al.* A phase 1 clinical-laboratory study of clofarabine followed by cyclophosphamide for adults with refractory acute leukemias. *Blood* 2007;**110**:1762–9.

181. Leonetti C, Scarsella M, Semple SC, *et al.* In vivo administration of liposomal vincristine sensitizes drug-resistant human solid tumors. *Int J Cancer* 2004;**110**:767–74.

182. Thomas DA, Sarris AH, Cortes J, *et al.* Phase II study of sphingosomal vincristine in patients with recurrent or refractory adult acute lymphocytic leukemia. *Cancer* 2006;**106**:120–7.

183. Wetzler M, Sanford BL, Kurtzberg J, *et al.* Effective asparagine depletion with pegylated asparaginase results in improved outcomes in adult acute lymphoblastic leukemia: Cancer and Leukemia Group B Study 9511. *Blood* 2007;**109**:4164–7.

184. Avramis VI, Sencer S, Periclou AP, *et al.* A randomized comparison of native *Escherichia coli* asparaginase and polyethylene glycol conjugated asparaginase for treatment of children with newly diagnosed standard-risk acute lymphoblastic leukemia: a Children's Cancer Group study. *Blood* 2002;**99**:1986–94.

185. Golas JM, Arndt K, Etienne C, *et al.* SKI-606, a 4-anilino-3-quinolinecarbonitrile dual inhibitor of Src and Abl kinases, is a potent antiproliferative agent against chronic myelogenous leukemia cells in culture and causes regression of K562 xenografts in nude mice. *Cancer Res* 2003;**63**:375–81.

186. Kimura S, Naito H, Segawa H, *et al.* NS-187, a potent and selective dual Bcr-Abl/Lyn tyrosine kinase inhibitor, is a novel agent for imatinib-resistant leukemia. *Blood* 2005;**106**:3948–54.

187. Naito H, Kimura S, Nakaya Y, *et al.* In vivo antiproliferative effect of NS-187, a dual Bcr-Abl/Lyn tyrosine kinase inhibitor, on leukemic cells harbouring Abl kinase domain mutations. *Leuk Res* 2006;**30**:1443–6.

188. Giles FJ, Cortes J, Jones D, *et al.* MK-0457, a novel kinase inhibitor, is active in patients with chronic myeloid leukemia or acute lymphocytic leukemia with the T315I BCR-ABL mutation. *Blood* 2007;**109**:500–2.

189. Thomas DA, Kantarjian H, Cortes J, *et al.* Long-term outcome after HyperCVAD and rituximab chemoimmunotherapy for Burkitt (BL) or Burkitt-like (BLL) leukemia/lymphoma and mature B-cell acute lymphocytic leukemia (B-ALL). *ASH Annual Meeting Abstracts* 2007;**110**:2825.

190. Raetz EA, Cairo MS, Borowitz MJ, *et al.* Chemoimmunotherapy reinduction with epratuzumab in children with acute lymphoblastic leukemia in marrow relapse: a Children's Oncology Group Pilot Study. *J Clin Oncol* 2008;**26**:3756–62.

191. Stock W, Yu D, Sanford B, *et al.* Incorporation of alemtuzumab into frontline therapy of adult acute lymphoblastic leukemia (ALL) is feasible: a phase I/II study from the Cancer and Leukemia Group B (CALGB 10102). *ASH Annual Meeting Abstracts* 2005;**106**:145.

192. Staal FJ, Langerak AW. Signaling pathways involved in the development of T-cell acute lymphoblastic leukemia. *Haematologica* 2008;**93**:493–7.

193. DeAngelo DJ, Stone RM, Silverman LB, *et al.* A phase I clinical trial of the notch inhibitor MK-0752 in patients with T-cell acute lymphoblastic leukemia/lymphoma (T-ALL) and other leukemias. *J Clin Oncol* (*2006 ASCO Annual Meeting Proceedings Part I*) 2006;**24**(18S) Abstract 6585.

194. Wei G, Twomey D, Lamb J, *et al.* Gene expression-based chemical genomics identifies rapamycin as a modulator of MCL1 and glucocorticoid resistance. *Cancer Cell* 2006;**10**:331–42.

195. Teachey DT, Obzut DA, Cooperman J, *et al.* The mTOR inhibitor CCI-779 induces apoptosis and inhibits growth in preclinical models of primary adult human ALL. *Blood* 2006;**107**:1149–55.

196. Avellino R, Romano S, Parasole R, *et al.* Rapamycin stimulates apoptosis of childhood acute lymphoblastic leukemia cells. *Blood* 2005;**106**:1400–6.

197. Kharas MG, Janes MR, Scarfone VM, *et al.* Ablation of PI3K blocks BCR-ABL leukemogenesis in mice, and a dual PI3K/mTOR inhibitor prevents expansion of human BCR-ABL leukemia cells. *J Clin Invest* 2008;**118**:3038–50.

198. Jackman KM, Frye CB, Hunger SP. Flavopiridol displays preclinical activity in acute lymphoblastic leukemia. *Pediatr Blood Cancer* 2008;**50**:772–8.

199. Karp JE, Passaniti A, Gojo I, *et al.* Phase I and pharmacokinetic study of flavopiridol followed by 1-beta-D-arabinofuranosylcytosine and mitoxantrone in relapsed and refractory adult acute leukemias. *Clin Cancer Res* 2005;**11**:8403–12.

Chapter 4

Chronic myeloid leukemia

Elias Jabbour, Hagop M. Kantarjian, and Jorge E. Cortés

Introduction

Chronic myeloid leukemia (CML) is a relatively rare disease but is one of the most extensively studied and best understood neoplasms, and one for which a direct gene link has been found.[1–3] CML is characterized by a balanced genetic translocation, t(9;22)(q34;q11.2), involving a fusion of the Abelson oncogene (*ABL*) from chromosome 9q34 with the breakpoint cluster region (*BCR*) gene on chromosome 22q11.2. This rearrangement is known as the Philadelphia chromosome (Ph). The molecular consequence of this translocation is the generation of a *BCR-ABL* fusion oncogene, which in turn translates into a Bcr-Abl oncoprotein.[4,5] Bcr-Abl displays transforming activity owing to its constitutive kinase activity, which results in multiple signal transduction pathways leading to uncontrolled cell proliferation and reduced apoptosis and resulting in the malignant expansion of pluripotent stem cells in bone marrow.[6,7] CML is usually diagnosed in the chronic phase (CP) and, if not treated, progresses through an accelerated phase (AP) to a terminal blastic phase (BP).

Incidence, epidemiology, and etiology

CML accounts for 15% to 20% of cases of leukemia in the United States. There is a slight male preponderance. Its annual incidence is about 1 to 2 cases per 100 000 individuals. About 5000 to 6000 cases of CML are diagnosed annually. This incidence has not changed over the past few decades, and increases with age. The median age at CML diagnosis is 55 to 60 years; it is uncommon in children and adolescents. Before imatinib therapy, the prevalence of CML was about 25 000 cases in the United States. Now that the annual mortality following imatinib therapy has been reduced to 2%, the prevalence of CML will continue to rise, reaching a plateau (in the next 20 years) at about 250 000 cases (when the annual incidence will equal the annual mortality). This will change CML from an uncommon disorder to a prevalent one.

There are no known familial associations in CML. Its risk is not increased in monozygotic twins or in relatives of patients with CML. There are no known common etiologic agents incriminated in CML. Ionizing radiation (exposure to nuclear bombs or accidents; radiation treatment of ankylosing spondylitis and cervical cancer) has increased the risk of CML. Its peak incidence is 5 to 10 years after exposure and is dose related. The risk of CML is not increased in individuals working in the nuclear industry. Radiologists working without adequate protection (before 1940) had an increased risk of developing myeloid leukemia, but no such risk has been found in recent studies. Benzene exposure increases the risk of acute myeloid leukemia but not of CML. CML is not a frequent secondary leukemia following treatment of other cancers with radiation and/or alkylating agents.[8–11]

Pathogenesis

The hallmark of CML, and a subpopulation of patients with Philadelphia-positive acute lymphocytic leukemia (Ph+ ALL), is a genetic marker called the Philadelphia chromosome. This abnormality arises as a result of a rearrangement between genetic sequences from chromosomes 9 and 22 t(9;22)(q34; q11.2). This transposition juxtaposes the *BCR* adjacent to the *ABL* gene and codes for the Bcr-Abl fusion protein. Bcr-Abl is a tyrosine kinase that continuously functions and results in constitutive signaling in a variety of intracellular circuits.[12–14] Bcr-Abl expression has been shown to deregulate the cell growth, motility, angiogenic, and apoptotic mechanisms necessary for cellular transformation into a cancerous lesion. Some of the downstream signaling molecules activated by Bcr-Abl include Ras/Raf/mitogen-activated protein kinase (MAPK),[15–17] phosphatidylinositol 3 kinase (PI3K),[18–20] the STAT5/Janus kinase,[21–23] and c-Myc.[24–26] In addition to Bcr-Abl, these molecules also could serve as important targets for inhibition for drug development.

The transition from CP to advanced stages of CML is a poorly understood phenomenon. The pathogenesis of the disease may rely on the ability of Bcr-Abl to deregulate genomic replication, resulting in the acquisition of additional genetic changes. These mutations also may arise in the *BCR-ABL*

Management of Hematologic Malignancies, ed. Susan M. O'Brien, Julie M. Vose, and Hagop M. Kantarjian. Published by Cambridge University Press.

coding sequence itself, increasing mutagenic potential in a cell with an already unstable phenotype. The most common genetic mutations in patients in BP CML lie in p53, Rb, and INK41/arf genes.[27–29] These genes code for proteins critical in the maintenance of cellular homeostasis, and their modification has been repeatedly observed in a wide array of human cancers.[30] Therefore, directing inhibition of particular kinases and other signaling molecules in a specific and targeted manner has long been thought to represent an effective treatment strategy for CML.

Manifestations and staging

About 30–50% of patients with CML diagnosed in the United States are asymptomatic. The disease is found on routine physical examination or blood tests. CML can be classified into three disease phases: CP, AP, and BP. Diagnosis is most commonly made during the CP. Common signs and symptoms of CML in CP, when present, result from anemia and splenomegaly. These include fatigue, weight loss, malaise, easy satiety, and left upper quadrant fullness or pain. Rare manifestations include bleeding (associated with a low platelet count and/or platelet dysfunction), thrombosis (associated with thrombocytosis and/or marked leukocytosis), gouty arthritis (from elevated uric acid levels), priapism (usually with marked leukocytosis or thrombocytosis), retinal hemorrhages, and upper gastrointestinal ulceration and bleeding (from elevated histamine levels due to basophilia). Leukostatic symptoms (dyspnea, drowsiness, loss of coordination, confusion) due to sludging in the pulmonary or cerebral vessels are uncommon in the CP despite white blood cell (WBC) counts exceeding 100×10^9/L. Splenomegaly is the most consistent physical sign in CML, and is detected in 50% to 60% of cases. Hepatomegaly is less common (10–20%). Lymphadenopathy, and infiltration of skin or other tissues, is uncommon. When present, they favor Ph-negative CML or accelerated or blastic phases of CML. Headaches, bone pain, arthralgias, pain from splenic infarction, and fever are more frequent with CML transformation. Most patients evolve into AP prior to BP, but 20% transit into BP without warning. AP might be insidious or present with worsening anemia, splenomegaly, and organ infiltration. BP presents as an acute leukemia with worsening constitutional symptoms, bleeding, fever, and infections.

Diagnosis

The diagnosis of typical CML is simple and consists of documenting, in the setting of persistent unexplained leukocytosis (or occasionally thrombocytosis), the presence of the Ph chromosome abnormality, the t(9;22)(q34;q11), by routine cytogenetics, or the Ph-related molecular *BCR-ABL* abnormalities by fluorescent *in situ* hybridization (FISH) or by molecular studies.

A FISH analysis relies on the colocalization of large genomic probes specific to the *BCR* and *ABL* genes. Comparison of simultaneous marrow and blood samples by FISH analysis shows high concordance. FISH studies may have a false-positive range of 1% to 10% depending on the probes used.

Reverse transcriptase-polymerase chain reaction (RT-PCR) amplifies the region around the splice junction between *BCR* and *ABL*. It is highly sensitive for the detection of minimal residual disease. PCR testing can either be qualitative (QPCR), providing information about the presence of the *BCR-ABL* transcript, or quantitative, assessing the amount of *BCR-ABL* message. Qualitative PCR is useful for diagnosis of CML; quantitative PCR is ideal for monitoring residual disease. Simultaneous peripheral blood and marrow QPCR studies show a high level of concordance. False-positive and false-negative results can happen with PCR. False-negative results may be from poor-quality RNA or failure of the reaction; false-positive results can be due to contamination. A 0.5–1 log difference in some samples can occur depending on testing procedures, sample handling, and laboratory experience.[31,32]

The Ph chromosome is usually present in 100% of metaphases, often as the sole abnormality. Ten percent to 15% of patients have additional chromosomal changes (clonal evolution) involving trisomy 8, isochromosome 17, additional loss of material from 22q or double Ph, or others.

Eighty-five percent of patients have a typical t(9;22); 5% have variant translocations which can be simple (involving chromosome 22 and a chromosome other than chromosome 9), or complex (involving one or more chromosomes in addition to chromosomes 9 and 22). Patients with Ph variants have response to therapy and prognosis similar to Ph-positive CML.

Differential diagnosis

CML can be confused with leukemoid reactions. These are usually transient, have a temporal cause (severe infection, steroids, stress), show modest rises of WBC counts up to 50×10^9/L with toxic granulocytic vacuolation and Döhle bodies in the granulocytes, and a normal or increased leukocyte alkaline phosphatase (LAP) level. Corticosteroids can rarely cause self-limiting extreme neutrophilia with a left shift.

CML should be differentiated from other myelodysplastic or myeloproliferative syndromes like chronic myelomonocytic leukemia, proliferative myelodysplastic syndrome, agnogenic myeloid metaplasia, polycythemia rubra vera, and essential thrombocytosis. While the clinical syndromes may overlap, cytogenetic-molecular studies demonstrating the presence of the Ph chromosome or *BCR-ABL*-related abnormalities clarify the diagnosis.

A difficult diagnostic situation may arise in patients with a typical morphologic picture of CML (splenomegaly, leukocytosis) but who do not have the Ph chromosome. In some, the *BCR-ABL* hybrid gene can be demonstrated by molecular studies. Patients who are Ph negative and *BCR-ABL* negative often have chronic myelomonocytic leukemia. Patients may rarely have myeloid hyperplasia, with selective involvement of the neutrophil, eosinophil, or basophilic cell lineages. These are described as having chronic neutrophilic, eosinophilic, or basophilic leukemia and do not have evidence of the Ph chromosome or *BCR-ABL* gene. Occasionally, patients with Ph-positive CML may present like essential thrombocytosis (marked thrombocytosis without leukocytosis). Cytogenetic studies are required in all patients with essential thrombocytosis to identify the occasional patient with Ph-positive CML and essential thrombocytosis-like presentation.

Therapy

Treatment with imatinib

Historically, CML was treated with busulfan or hydroxyurea, and was associated with a poor prognosis.[33] These agents controlled the hematologic manifestations of the disease, but did not delay disease progression. Treatment with interferon alpha (IFN-α) induced complete cytogenetic responses in 5–25% of patients with CML in CP, and improved survival compared with previous treatments.[34] Combining IFN-α with cytarabine produced additional benefits.[35] Allogeneic stem cell transplantation (SCT) may be curative in CML, but it is applicable to only a fraction of CML patients and carries a significant risk of morbidity and mortality.

Imatinib (previously STI571), a small molecule tyrosine kinase inhibitor (TKI), was the first drug that targets Bcr-Abl to be developed[36] and it has become the standard frontline therapy for CML in early CP on the basis of the excellent response rates and favorable toxicity profile shown in numerous clinical trials. The International Randomized Study of Interferon and STI571 (IRIS) trial first demonstrated the benefits achieved with imatinib in this setting.[37] Recent 7-year update of the phase III IRIS trial confirmed the long-term efficacy and safety of imatinib.[38] After 7 years, the cumulative complete cytogenetic response rate for first-line imatinib-treated patients was 82%. The event-free survival (EFS) was 81%, and the estimated rate of freedom from progression to AP or BP was 93%, with a low annual rate of loss of response and transformation. The projected overall survival (OS) rate for patients treated with imatinib was 86%. At 7 years, 332 patients (60%) randomized to imatinib remained on treatment and on study.[37,38] Imatinib also was found to be well tolerated in the study, with the highest-grade adverse events (AEs) reported as cytopenias, elevated serum alanine or aspartate aminotransferase levels, pain, and nausea. Importantly, no new adverse events have occurred with long-term therapy.

The standard imatinib dose for patients treated in CP is 400 mg/day. However, the initial phase I, dose-finding trial in patients who had previously received IFN-α demonstrated no dose-limiting toxicities at imatinib doses up to 1000 mg/day,[39] and a dose–response relationship was observed. Based on these data, recent studies have assessed the efficacy of first-line therapy with high-dose imatinib, up to 800 mg/day. A single-arm study involving 114 patients with newly diagnosed CP-CML showed a complete hematologic response rate of 98% and a complete cytogenetic response rate of 90% in patients who received an imatinib dose of 800 mg/day.[39] These data compared favorably with historical controls from the same institution treated with the standard dose, with significantly higher complete cytogenetic response rates observed in patients who received 800 mg/day compared with those who received 400 mg/day (90% versus 74%, respectively; $p = 0.01$).

Randomized trials are now ongoing to assess whether high-dose imatinib may indeed improve the long-term outcome of patients with CML in CP. The Tyrosine kinase inhibitor *OP*timization and *S*electivity trial (TOPS) is a phase III study involving 476 patients with newly diagnosed CML in CP randomized in a 2:1 ratio to receive 800 or 400 mg/day imatinib.[40] Recent reports from this trial indicate that imatinib 800 mg/day showed a rapid response and trend of improved major molecular response rates at 3, 6, and 9 months compared with standard-dose imatinib therapy, although by 12 months the response rates were more similar. The European Leukemia Net study[41] compared 400 versus 800 mg/day imatinib in 215 high Sokal-risk patients, with a primary end point of complete cytogenetic response at 12 months. Results were similar to those in the TOPS trial. A trend toward higher rates of MMR with 800 mg/day compared with 400 mg/day was observed; however, the differences were not statistically significant.

Optimizing responses through careful monitoring

Throughout the course of therapy with imatinib, patients should be routinely assessed for their response to therapy, and the treatment should be optimized to maximize the response and ultimately the long-term outcome. In order to proactively identify patients with suboptimal responses or resistance to imatinib, adequate monitoring is recommended (Table 4.1).[42–45] Cytogenetic response is still the gold standard for adequate response to imatinib. Thus, monitoring of the bone marrow for cytogenetic response is recommended every 3–6 months until a complete cytogenetic response is achieved, and every 1 to 2 years thereafter. The *BCR-ABL* transcript levels should be monitored, preferably in peripheral blood, every 3 to 6 months until achievement of major molecular response. Patients with a stable major or complete molecular response can be monitored every 6 months. Although achieving the lowest possible levels of transcripts, and probably ideally undetectable, is desirable, persistence of detectable transcript levels in the context of a complete cytogenetic response is not an indication of failure of therapy. In some patients, transcript levels may increase. Some studies have suggested that an increase in transcript levels may increase the risk of developing mutations or failure of therapy. The magnitude of the increase that may predict for such events is variable, in part due to the variability of the testing in different laboratories. Most important is that a single elevation in transcript levels should first be confirmed in a subsequent determination and the magnitude of the increment should be determined to be greater than the variability of the test in the laboratory where it

Table 4.1. Recommended frequencies of response assessment in patients with chronic myeloid leukemia

Assessment method	Recommended frequencies of assessment	
	Initial monitoring (until at least CCyR achieved)	Subsequent monitoring (for patients with stable CCyR)
Hematologic	Every 2 weeks	Every 3 months once CHR is achieved
Cytogenetic	Every 3–6 months	Every 12–24 months once CCyR achieved
Molecular	Every 3 months	Every 3–6 months, increasing to monthly if a rising *BCR-ABL1* transcript level is detected[a]
Mutational assessment	Upon detection of failure, and possibly suboptimal response[b]	Upon detection of imatinib failure or rising *BCR-ABL1* transcript level[a]

Notes: [a] 5- to 10-fold increase of the *BCR-ABL1* transcript level.
[b] There is no use of measuring mutations before the start of therapy in newly diagnosed patients.
CCyR: complete cytogenetic response; CHR: complete hematologic response.

is being tested. The National Comprehensive Cancer Network (NCCN) recommends the following monitoring schedule: any 1-log increase in *BCR-ABL* transcripts should be repeated in 1 month; if the increase is confirmed on subsequent sampling, the frequency of monitoring should be increased from every 3 months to every month; and mutation assays can be considered in case of elevations in *BCR-ABL* transcripts. Still, most studies have demonstrated that the risk of relapse (or association with mutations) is mostly present when a sizeable increase (two- to five-fold) is associated with a loss of major molecular response (or occurs in a patient who had not achieved a major molecular response).

The early evaluation of response during the course of therapy is important to determine that response to therapy is progressing according to expectations that correlate with optimal outcome. It has been established that patients who do not achieve early responses have an increasing risk of eventual transformation and a decreasing probability of eventually achieving at least a complete cytogenetic response.[46] This is reflected in the current recommendations for the definition of failure and suboptimal response to imatinib therapy.[43]

Resistance to imatinib

The molecular mechanisms responsible for resistance are only partially understood. The most frequently identified mechanism of resistance is the development of Bcr-Abl kinase domain mutations. A mutation is identified in approximately 50% of patients with resistance to imatinib, and they are more common among patients with secondary resistance to imatinib than those with primary resistance. Up to now, more than 100 different mutants of Bcr-Abl have been described.[47–49] However, most of the clinically relevant mutations develop in a few residues in the P-loop (G250E, Y253F/H, and E255K/V), the contact site (T315I), and the catalytic domain (M351T and F359V).[48] In some patients, more than one mutation may be present at the same time. This phenomenon appears to increase in frequency after treatment with more than one tyrosine kinase inhibitor.

Another possible cause of resistance to imatinib is overexpression of Bcr-Abl. Although this was the most frequent cause of resistance identified in cell lines, and case reports have described clinical resistance to imatinib in association with Bcr-Abl amplification or multiple copies of the Ph chromosome, the frequency with which this mechanism is identified is not known, but is probably low.

The acquisition of additional chromosomal abnormalities in the Ph-positive cell population, generally referred to as clonal evolution, appears to be one of the main mechanisms associated with both disease progression and imatinib resistance. Multiple different chromosomes are involved in different patients. This has made identification of the molecular mechanisms behind these events complicated. Activation of members of the Src-kinase family or of other pathways downstream of Bcr-Abl (like the PI3K/AKT pathway) has been reported although the frequency of occurrence of these mechanisms is not known. It is increasingly becoming evident that multiple mechanisms and events can be involved in the development of imatinib-resistant subclones and most of these mechanisms are unknown.[47–50] Many of the mechanisms of resistance can be ascribed to the high degree of genomic instability characterizing the Ph-positive clone.[50] So far the molecular mechanisms leading to this instability are only in part understood and, although it has been suggested that Bcr-Abl activation is able to induce some degree of genomic instability, a preexisting genomic instability, probably at the level of the stem cell, cannot be excluded.

Imatinib dose escalation

Dose escalation can improve the response in some of the patients with resistance to standard dose imatinib and was the main option for managing suboptimal responses and treatment failures before the introduction of second-generation TKIs. In an analysis of patients enrolled in the IRIS trial, in whom imatinib dose was escalated due to resistance to standard-dose therapy, freedom-from-progression and OS rates were 89% and 84%, respectively, at 3 years from dose escalation.[51] In another study, 84 CP-CML patients were dose escalated to imatinib 600–800 mg/day after developing hematologic failure (n = 21), or cytogenetic failure (resistance: n = 30; relapse: n = 33) to imatinib 400 mg/day. Among patients that met the criteria for cytogenetic failure, 75%

(47/63) responded to imatinib dose escalation. Patients achieving major cytogenetic response after imatinib dose escalation had durable responses, with a sustained major cytogenetic response in 88% and 74% of patients at 2 and 3 years, respectively. In contrast, in patients where imatinib was dose escalated because of hematologic failure, 48% achieved a complete hematologic response and 14% (3/21) only attained a cytogenetic response.[52] Although dose escalation after failure with standard-dose imatinib is an important option for patients with imatinib resistance, it is likely to be useful only in a subset of patients with previous cytogenetic response to standard imatinib therapy. Even in this setting, second-generation TKIs have shown to be superior to dose escalation. Currently dose escalation is mainly used for instances of suboptimal response to imatinib, although there are limited data showing the value of this approach (or any other) in this setting.

Second-generation TKIs

Strategies to overcome imatinib resistance are a logical progression for improving the prognosis of patients with CML. These include novel and more potent multi-TKIs such as dasatinib (BMS-354825, Bristol-Myers Squibb), an orally bioavailable dual Bcr-Abl and Src inhibitor, and potent selective Bcr-Abl inhibitors such as nilotinib (Tasigna; AMN-107). Both nilotinib and dasatinib induced significant clinical responses and have been approved by the Food and Drug Administration (FDA) and European Medicines Agency (EMEA).

Dasatinib

Dasatinib is an orally available Abl kinase inhibitor with 325-fold greater in vitro selectivity for unmutated Bcr-Abl compared with imatinib.[53] It differs from imatinib in that it can bind to both the active and inactive conformations of the Abl kinase domain and also inhibits a distinct spectrum of kinases that overlaps with the array of kinases that imatinib inhibits. Targets of dasatinib include Src family kinases (SFKs), c-Kit, platelet-derived growth factor receptor, beta polypeptide (PDGFR-β), and ephrin A. Dasatinib has activity against many imatinib-resistant kinase domain mutations of Bcr-Abl. Bcr-Abl mutations associated with resistance to dasatinib have been characterized. In an in vitro mutagenesis study, mutations at six residues were found to form nine dasatinib-resistant Bcr-Abl mutants. However, only two (F317V and T315I) were isolated at intermediate drug concentrations, and T315I was the only mutant to be isolated at maximal achievable plasma concentrations.[54] Dasatinib was approved by the FDA on the basis of its efficacy and safety profiles shown in a series of phase II trials in patients who failed or were intolerant to first-line imatinib therapy (Table 4.2).[55–57] Dasatinib was initially approved at a dosage of 70 mg twice daily for all indications. The label has recently been changed such that 100 mg once daily is now the recommended starting dose for patients with CP-CML on the basis of a phase III dose-optimization study designed to evaluate the efficacy and safety of four different dasatinib doses in patients who had previously experienced imatinib failure. This study showed that the 100-mg once-daily dosage was efficaciously equivalent to 70 mg twice daily, with decreased rates of thrombocytopenia and pleural effusion.[58,59] Dasatinib was registered for the treatment of CP-CML based on results from the SRC/ABL Tyrosine kinase inhibition Activity Research Trials of dasatinib (START)-C trial, a phase II international study of dasatinib 70 mg twice daily which included 387 CP-CML patients with resistance or intolerance to imatinib.[56] Recent 24-month follow-up data demonstrated a 2-year major cytogenetic response rate of 62% and a complete cytogenetic response rate of 53%.[60] The progression-free survival (PFS) at 2 years was 80% and the OS rate was 94%. Responses to dasatinib in patients with imatinib-resistant CP-CML enrolled in phase II studies of dasatinib have been assessed by baseline mutational status.[61] Complete cytogenetic response rates were similar among patients with unmutated Bcr-Abl and those harboring mutations. Importantly, responses to dasatinib did not appear to be diminished among patients harboring the P-loop mutations. However, the activity was somewhat reduced in patients with the F317L mutation, a mutant that has required in vitro high concentrations of dasatinib to achieve some inhibition. As expected, no complete cytogenetic responses were achieved in patients harboring the T315I mutation. The most frequently detected mutations in patients exhibiting resistance to dasatinib are T315A/I, F317I/L, and V299L.[54,61–65] A randomized trial of dasatinib or dose increase of imatinib (to 800 mg daily) among patients who had failed prior therapy with imatinib (400–600 mg) demonstrated a significantly higher rate of response and PFS for patients receiving dasatinib, particularly among those who were already receiving imatinib 600 mg, those with Bcr-Abl mutations, and those who had never achieved a cytogenetic response with imatinib.[66,67]

Table 4.2. Phase II data for dasatinib second-line to imatinib failure

Disease	n	% Response			
		CHR	Cytogenetic response		Overall survival
			Major	Complete	
CML chronic	387	91	59	49	96% at 15 months
CML accelerated	174	50	43	31	76% at 10 months
CML myelo-blastic	109	26	34	27	11.8 months
CML lympho-blastic	48	29	52	46	5.3 months

Note: CHR: complete hematologic response.

Grade 3–4 toxicities included thrombocytopenia (49%) and neutropenia (50%), pleural effusion (9%), dyspnea (6%), bleeding (4%), diarrhea (3%), and fatigue (3%). Three percent of imatinib-intolerant patients developed similar grade 3–4 toxicities. The appearance of new higher-grade toxicity between 12 and 24 months was uncommon.[60]

Dasatinib has also demonstrated clinical efficacy and is approved for patients with AP- and BP-CML after failure with other therapies (Table 4.2). Dasatinib treatment for patients with AP-CML (n = 174) was examined in the START-A study.[57,68] After a median follow-up period of 14.1 months, 45% of patients had a complete hematologic response, 39% had a major cytogenetic response, and 32% had a complete cytogenetic response. The estimated 12-month PFS and OS were 66% and 82%, respectively. Treatment of patients with myeloid BP-CML (n = 109) and lymphoid BP-CML (n = 48) with dasatinib 70 mg twice daily was evaluated in the START-B and START-L trials, respectively.[69] After a follow-up period of up to 21 months, 27% of patients with myeloid BP-CML and 29% of patients with lymphoid BP-CML had a complete hematologic response. Major cytogenetic responses were achieved in 33% of patients with myeloid BP-CML and in 52% of patients with lymphoid BP-CML. The START-L study also included 48 patients with Ph+ ALL who had failed or were intolerant to imatinib.[70] With follow-up extending to 18.5 months, the complete hematologic response rate was 33%. Major cytogenetic response was achieved for 57% of patients; this was complete in all but one of these patients (54%).

Nilotinib

Nilotinib is an analog of imatinib with 10- to 50-fold greater potency against un-mutated Bcr-Abl than its parent compound, and has activity against all tested imatinib-resistant Bcr-Abl mutants except T315I.[71] It is approved at a schedule of 400 mg twice daily, and it should be administered on an empty stomach (without food for 2 hours prior to and 1 hour after administration) as food may significantly increase absorption increasing the plasma concentrations in unpredictable fashion. Nilotinib was approved following an open-label phase II study in patients with CML who failed or who were intolerant to imatinib therapy.[72,73] Follow-up data confirmed the effectiveness of this compound in CP-, AP-, and BP-CML (Table 4.3), although it is currently approved only for CP and AP after imatinib failure.[74–76] At least ten nilotinib-insensitive Bcr-Abl mutations have been identified. In a mutagenesis study, the P-loop mutations Y253H and E255V persisted at intermediate drug concentrations, and T315I was isolated at maximum achievable plasma concentrations.[54] In the key phase II study, a total of 321 CP-CML patients (71% imatinib-resistant; 29% imatinib-intolerant) were evaluated. Imatinib-intolerant patients could not have achieved prior major cytogenetic response on imatinib therapy. Complete hematologic response was overall reported in 94% of patients and in 76% among those with active disease at the beginning. Of all imatinib-resistant and -intolerant patients, 58% achieved major cytogenetic response, with 72% of patients having a baseline complete hematologic response achieving major cytogenetic response. The major cytogenetic response rate was 63% in imatinib-intolerant and 56% in imatinib-resistant patients, respectively. Overall, 42% of patients achieved a complete cytogenetic response (50% in imatinib-intolerant and 39% in imatinib-resistant patients, respectively). The median time to complete hematologic response and major cytogenetic response was 1.0 and 2.8 months, respectively. Responses were durable, with 84% of patients maintaining their major cytogenetic response at 18 months. Estimated OS rates at 12 and 18 months were 95% and 91%, respectively. Median duration of exposure was 465 days (15.5 months).[73]

Table 4.3. Phase II data for nilotinib second-line to imatinib failure

Disease	n	% Response			
		CHR	Cytogenetic response		Overall survival
			Major	Complete	
CML chronic	321	76[a]	58	42	91% (18 months)
CML accelerated	129	29	38	29	82% (12 months)
CML blastic	136	11	40	29	42% (12 months)

Note: [a] 76% of patients achieved a CHR among those with active disease. Overall 94% of patients achieved a CHR.
CHR: complete hematologic response.

Of 321 CP-CML patients, 281 (88%) had baseline mutation data available, and 41% had detectable Bcr-Abl mutations prior to nilotinib therapy. Fourteen percent of imatinib-resistant patients had three mutations that were less sensitive to nilotinib in vitro ($IC_{50} > 150$ nM; Y253H, E255K/V, and F359C/V) and another 15% had a total of 16 mutations with unknown sensitivity to nilotinib. Cytogenetic response rates in patients harboring mutations sensitive to nilotinib (major cytogenetic response 59%; complete cytogenetic response 41%) or mutations with unknown sensitivity to nilotinib (major cytogenetic response 63%; complete cytogenetic response 50%) were comparable to those for patients without baseline mutations (major cytogenetic response 60%; complete cytogenetic response 40%). Patients with mutations less sensitive to nilotinib in vitro had less favorable response after 12 months of therapy (23% major cytogenetic response). No complete cytogenetic responses were observed in patients harboring L248V, Y253H, or E255K/V mutations.[77] Mutations most frequently associated with progression were E255K/V (6/7) and F359C/V (9/11).

Investigational second-generation TKIs (Bosutinib [SKI-606])

Bosutinib (SKI-606), an orally available dual Src/Abl inhibitor, is 30 to 50 times more potent than imatinib against unmutated Bcr-Abl, with minimal inhibitory activity against c-Kit and

PDGFR. It has been suggested that the decreased off-target effects may lead to decreased toxicity, particularly myelosuppression and fluid retention. It has significant activity against most Bcr-Abl mutants tested, with the main exception being T315I.[78] The phase I study identified a recommended dose of 500 mg daily and showed evidence of clinical efficacy. The phase II study in patients with CP Ph+ CML who have failed imatinib and second-generation TKIs therapy is ongoing. Preliminary data for 302 treated patients have been reported. Among 69 patients who were resistant to imatinib and had received no other TKI, 45% achieved a major cytogenetic response, including 32% who had a complete cytogenetic response. Treatment was generally well tolerated with no pleural effusions and modest myelosuppression.[79] The most common adverse events were gastrointestinal (nausea, vomiting, diarrhea) that were usually grade 1–2, manageable and transient, diminishing in frequency and severity after the first 3–4 weeks of treatment.[79]

Multikinase inhibitors

Imatinib, dasatinib, nilotinib, and bosutinib are ATP-competitive inhibitors and not active against the T315I mutant. Compounds that target binding sites unrelated to the ATP kinase domain may overcome this problem.

XL228 (Exelixis Inc, San Francisco, USA) is a potent, multi-targeted kinase inhibitor with potent activity against wild-type and T315I isoforms of Bcr-Abl (wild-type Abl kinase, $IC_{50} = 5$ nM; Abl T315I, 1.4 nM), aurora A (3.1 nM), IGF-1R (1.6 nM), SRC (6.1 nM), and LYN (2 nM) kinases. A phase I dose escalation clinical trial in patients with CML or Ph+ ALL who are resistant or intolerant to at least two prior standard TKIs (including imatinib, dasatinib, and nilotinib) or have a known Bcr-Abl T315I mutation is ongoing. XL228 was administered as a 1-hour IV infusion either once weekly or twice weekly. XL228 has been generally well tolerated. Dose-limiting toxicities observed with once-weekly dosing included grade 3 syncope and hyperglycemia in two patients. Preliminary evidence of clinical activity has been observed in patients treated at doses of 3.6 mg/kg and higher, including stable or decreasing WBC count and/or platelet count within 2 months (14 patients, 5 with T315I), and/or >1 log reduction in Bcr-Abl levels by QPCR within 3 months (3 patients, 2 with T315I).[80]

PHA-739538 (Nerviano Medical Sciences, Nerviano, Italy) is an aurora kinase inhibitor with potent activity against native and mutated Bcr-Abl, including T315I.[81] Strong antiproliferative effects of PHA-739358 have been observed in CD34+ cells harvested from untreated CML patients and from imatinib-resistant individuals, including those with the T315I mutation.[81,82] Simultaneous short-term treatment with PHA-739358 in association with imatinib resulted in pronounced apoptosis of wild-type or low-grade imatinib-resistant Bcr-Abl expressing cells while no such effects were observed in Bcr-Abl negative or highly imatinib-resistant T315I mutants. In primary CD34+ cells of CML patients including non-dividing quiescent leukemic stem cells, combination therapy with imatinib and PHA-739358 revealed a synergistic antiproliferative activity which also affected immature CD34+38− cells. However, neither mono- nor combination therapy led to a significant induction of apoptosis in this population of cells. PHA-739358 did not affect quiescent stem cells, but resistance emerged less frequently after incubation with PHA-739358 than with imatinib.[82] Preliminary results of a multicenter phase II study have been reported. Among seven patients treated (one CP, one AP, five BP; six with T315I mutations), one patient with a T315I mutation achieved a complete cytogenetic response and a second patient achieved a minor cytogenetic response.[83]

Several other multikinase inhibitors have been progressed into clinical trials. MK-0457, a potent aurora kinase inhibitor, was the first agent to demonstrate clinical activity against the T315I phenotype and in a study of 14 evaluable patients with CML, 11 had an objective (hematologic, cytogenetic, and/or molecular) response, including 9 patients with T315I.[84] However, clinical development of MK-0457 was recently halted over toxicity concerns.

AP24534 is an oral, multitargeted kinase inhibitor with activity against native and kinase domain-mutant Bcr-Abl, including T315I. Mutagenesis screening revealed that single-agent AP24534 (40 nM) completely suppressed outgrowth of most Bcr-Abl mutants. This agent is being explored in patients with TKI failure.[85] Among the patients treated in the phase I trial, overall complete hematologic response was observed in 88% of patients in CP and major hematologic response in 2 of 4 AP patients. Cytogenetic responses were 4 complete and 2 partial. Of the 12 patients with T315I mutations, complete hematologic response was reported in 5 of 6 CP patients and major hematologic response in 2 of 2 AP patients. Cytogenetic responses were 2 complete and 1 partial. The treatment was overall well tolerated.

DCC-2036 is highly selective for ABL, FLT3, TIE2, and Src family kinases, and when dosed at 100 mg/kg per day by oral gavage, significantly prolonged the survival of mice with CML-like myeloproliferative disease induced by retroviral expression of *BCR-ABL* wild type and T315I in bone marrow.[86] This agent is being explored in phase I clinical trials.

Non-tyrosine kinase inhibitors

Omacetaxine mepesuccinate (Omacetaxine; homoharringtonine; HHT; ChemGenex Pharmaceuticals, Victoria, Australia), a cephalotaxine ester, is a multitargeted protein synthase inhibitor that has been in clinical development for several years. Omacetaxine shows clinical activity against Ph+ CML[87,88] with a mechanism of action independent of tyrosine kinase inhibition. Omacetaxine is currently in phase II/III development in patients with CML (all phases) who are resistant or intolerant to at least two prior TKIs (including imatinib, dasatinib, and nilotinib) or who carry T315I-mutated Bcr-Abl. Sixty-six patients with T315I have been treated, including 40 in

CP, 16 in AP, and 10 in BP. A complete hematologic response has been reported in 85%, 31%, and 20% of patients in CP, AP, and BP, respectively. Major cytogenetic response has been reported in 15% of patients in CP, and 6% in AP. In addition, the T315I-mutated clone became undetectable in 39% of all patients treated. The most frequently occurring grade 3–4 toxicities associated with Omacetaxine therapy were thrombocytopenia 58%, neutropenia 41%, and anemia 36%.[89] Recent reports suggest that Omacetaxine is able to affect the leukemic stem cell compartment, which would make it attractive for the potential of total elimination of the leukemic cells and potential cure.

Novel approaches to prevent resistance

Combination therapy

Rarely are human cancers cured by single-agent therapy. The availability of several agents with demonstrated clinical activity against CML has triggered interest in the use of combination therapy with the aim to reduce the development of resistance, improving the long-term outcome, and offering the perspective of cure for most patients. The current strategy in CML is sequential treatment. Molecularly targeted kinase inhibitor therapies are currently administered sequentially rather than simultaneously. Newly diagnosed patients receive imatinib, followed by Abl-second-generation inhibitors at time of resistance or intolerance. The rationale for this approach is partly historical, since imatinib was approved for CML therapy prior to others on the basis of a very high single-agent response rate, and partly based on a molecular understanding of resistance mechanisms that led to the evaluation of other TKIs in imatinib-resistant CML.

There is growing interest in testing the hypothesis that administration of multiple Abl kinase inhibitors, such as nilotinib, dasatinib, and imatinib, in early-phase patients could be used to delay or prevent the emergence of drug-resistant clones.[90,91] Both nilotinib and dasatinib hold promise for treating patients with imatinib-resistant CML. Cross-resistance between nilotinib and dasatinib is limited to T315I, which is also the only mutant isolated at drug concentrations equivalent to maximal achievable plasma trough levels.[91–94] Since the T315I mutation of Bcr-Abl is highly resistant to imatinib, nilotinib, and dasatinib, this approach needs to be extended to include inhibitors of T315I Bcr-Abl to prevent this mutation from becoming more prevalent. Alternatively, it is also important to explore the potential for synergy between TKI and other classes of inhibitors that work through mechanisms not involving inhibition of Abl tyrosine kinase activity.[92,93] The use of interferon in combination with TKI is attractive since interferon induced durable responses, and even some cures, in a small subset of patients. Early efforts at combining interferon with imatinib suggested the combination to be manageable in most patients although results, in single-arm trials, did not appear better than what had been reported with single-agent imatinib.[94] Recently randomized trials have been reported comparing imatinib alone or in combination with interferon. One report suggested a higher rate of molecular responses with the combination of pegylated interferon (PEG-IFN-α-2a) and standard-dose imatinib.[95] The long-term results have not been reported. In another study, the combination of pegylated interferon (PEG-IFN-α-2b) with high-dose imatinib did not result in any difference in response rate or long-term EFS or OS.[96] Despite these negative results, there is still considerable interest in the potential advantages of combining interferon with imatinib. This is because there is the suggestion that patients who have had exposure to interferon may have a decreased probability of recurrence after interruption of imatinib therapy,[97] and it has been suggested that interferon may act at the level of the leukemic stem cell, something that currently available TKIs are unable to do.

Second-generation TKIs as first-line therapy

Another important approach to optimizing therapy in patients with early CP-CML may be the use of second-generation TKIs as frontline therapy. Several phase II trials are underway studying nilotinib and dasatinib in this setting. The Italian GIMEMA CML Working Party enrolled 73 patients in a phase II study, having the achievement of complete cytogenetic response rate at 1 year as the primary end point.[98] All patients and 48/73 (66%) completed 3 and 6 months of treatment, respectively. The complete hematologic response rates were 100% and 98%, respectively; the complete cytogenetic response rates were 78% and 96%, respectively. A major molecular response was achieved by 59% after 3 months and 74% after 6 months. One patient progressed at 6 months to accelerated-blastic phase with the T315I mutation. A phase II study in patients with newly diagnosed CP-CML at the MD Anderson Cancer Center showed that nilotinib 400 mg twice daily induces a complete cytogenetic response in nearly all patients as early as 3 months after the start of therapy with a favorable toxicity profile.[99] Forty-nine patients have been treated for a median of 13 months. Complete cytogenetic responses were achieved, respectively, by 93% and by 100% of patients at 3- and 6-month evaluations. The rate of complete cytogenetic response at 3, 6, 12, 18, and 24 months compares favorably to those observed in historical controls treated with imatinib 400 mg or 800 mg daily. Major molecular response was observed in 45% at 6 months and 52% at 12 months. The estimated 24-month EFS is 95%. Preliminary data demonstrate that nilotinib was well tolerated with infrequent reports of grade 3 or 4 hematologic laboratory abnormalities and non-hematologic AEs. Dasatinib has also been evaluated as frontline therapy in a phase II study.[100] Patients with previously untreated CP-CML received dasatinib 50 mg twice daily (53%) or 100 mg once daily (47%). Complete cytogenetic response rates at 3 and 6 months were 78% and 94%, respectively. Major molecular response rates of 23% and 36% were observed at 3 and 6 months, respectively. Grade 3–4 hematologic toxicity included neutropenia (23%), thrombocytopenia

(11%), and anemia (7%) and pleural effusions occurred in 13% (grade 2) and 2% (grade 3) of patients.

Decision making

The primary goal of therapy for patients with CML is still achievement of complete cytogenetic response. Those who achieve this goal have a low probability of eventually progressing. Achieving a major molecular response is desirable as it further improves the long-term outcome, but patients who have a complete cytogenetic response are not considered to have failure to imatinib if they do not have a major molecular response. This is because the difference in EFS probability is small, although significant. The timing of this response is also important. Despite initial suggestions from the IRIS trial that a major molecular response at 12 months improved long-term outcome, compared to complete cytogenetic response but no major molecular response, the 7-year follow-up data have shown no difference in outcome using this hallmark. By 18 months, patients who have a complete cytogenetic response and major molecular response have a better probability of EFS than those with complete cytogenetic response but no major molecular response, but the difference is small (95% vs. 86%), and even smaller if considering only transformation to AP or BP or death as an event (99% vs. 96%).

The recommendations by the European Leukemia Net (ELN) have provided a clear framework for decision making and the significance of the definitions of failure and suboptimal response have been demonstrated in two independent series.[101,102] Patients with suboptimal response to therapy have an inferior outcome, although the significance appears to be heterogeneous, with a more profound adverse prognostic effect for patients with suboptimal response to therapy at earlier time points (6 months) than at later time points (18 months). It is however reasonable to consider treatment modifications for patients who have a suboptimal response to therapy. Treatment guidelines recommend dose escalation of imatinib to 600 or 800 mg/day in cases of suboptimal response.[42,43] However, it should be acknowledged that there are minimal data available regarding the effectiveness of this approach.[52,53] For patients with clear failure to imatinib therapy, the current approach is to change therapy to a second-generation TKI, although allogeneic SCT is also an option following treatment failure.[42,43] Clinical trial data have confirmed the efficacy of dasatinib and nilotinib in patients with imatinib resistance or intolerance and the superiority of dasatinib versus imatinib dose escalation following imatinib resistance.[66,67] It is possible that earlier treatment switch to second-line agents, that is after suboptimal response, could result in more favorable long-term outcomes than with dose-escalated imatinib, but there are currently no clinical data to support this hypothesis.

An important question now is what the response hallmarks are for patients receiving second-generation TKIs. A recent study has hinted at possible treatment goals for second-line treatment. Among patients with CP-CML receiving dasatinib ($n = 70$) or nilotinib ($n = 43$) after imatinib failure, those who achieved a major cytogenetic response within 12 months post-imatinib treatment had a significantly higher survival rate than patients with a minor cytogenetic response or complete hematologic response (1-year survival: 97% vs. 84%, respectively; $p = 0.02$).[103] Moreover, fewer than 10% of patients with no cytogenetic response of any level within 3–6 months went on to achieve a major cytogenetic response at 12 months, suggesting these patients might require switch to third-line treatment or to allogeneic SCT. However, additional studies are required to confirm these findings.

The selection of second-line TKI therapy should be individualized to each patient, carefully considering drug efficacy and toxicity, as well as patient mutation data. In many cases, a patient's Bcr-Abl genotype can serve as a prognostic factor to disease progression. Preliminary analysis from phase II studies suggested that levels of response to new TKIs depend on the type of Bcr-Abl kinase domain mutation. The outcome of patients receiving second-generation TKIs depends on the type of mutation, with mutations with predicted intermediate levels of sensitivity (i.e., higher IC_{50} in vitro) having decreased probability of response and EFS, particularly in CP.[104]

Therapy decision should also take into consideration the potential side effects, in relation to each patient characteristic. Patient compliance is another point to be considered. Finally, allogeneic SCT remains a potential therapeutic modality provided the patient is young, fit, has not achieved a major cytogenetic response with second-generation TKI therapy, and a donor match can be quickly identified.

Conclusions

For patients with CML, imatinib represented a significant breakthrough in first-line treatment. Resistance to imatinib monotherapy has emerged as an important clinical challenge. The recent availability of highly potent TKIs, dasatinib and nilotinib, has further broadened the treatment armamentarium against CML. With the advent of novel agents, the combination approaches, and possibly compounds with other mechanisms of action, both conventional and targeted, the treatment prospects of patients with CML are very hopeful.

References

1. Barnes DJ, Melo JV. Cytogenetic and molecular genetic aspects of chronic myeloid leukaemia. *Acta Haematol* 2002;**108**:180–202.
2. Faderl S, Talpaz M, Estrov Z, *et al.* Chronic myelogenous leukemia: biology and therapy. *Ann Intern Med* 1999;**131**:207–19.
3. Litzow MR. Imatinib resistance: obstacles and opportunities. *Arch Pathol Lab Med* 2006;**130**:669–79.
4. Rowley JD. Letter: A new consistent chromosomal abnormality in chronic myelogenous leukaemia identified by quinacrine fluorescence and Giemsa staining. *Nature* 1973;**243**:290–3.

5. Koptyra M, Falinski R, Nowicki MO, *et al.* BCR/ABL kinase induces self-mutagenesis via reactive oxygen species to encode imatinib resistance. *Blood* 2006;**108**:319–27.
6. Hu Y, Liu Y, Pelletier S, *et al.* Requirement of Src kinases Lyn, Hck and Fgr for BCR-ABL1-induced B-lymphoblastic leukemia but not chronic myeloid leukemia. *Nat Genet* 2004;**36**:453–61.
7. Bhatia R, Holtz M, Niu N, *et al.* Persistence of malignant hematopoietic progenitors in chronic myelogenous leukemia patients in complete cytogenetic remission following imatinib mesylate treatment. *Blood* 2003;**101**:4701–7.
8. Ries LAG, Eisner MP, Kosary CL, *et al.* *SEER Cancer Statistics Review, 1975–2000*. Bethesda, MD, National Cancer Institute, 2003.
9. Brown WM, Doll R. Mortality from cancer and other causes after radiotherapy for ankylosing spondylitis. *BMJ* 1965;**5474**:1327–32.
10. Boice JD Jr, Day NE, Andersen A, *et al.* Second cancers following radiation treatment for cervical cancer: an international collaboration among cancer registries. *J Natl Cancer Inst* 1985;**74**:955–75.
11. Kato H, Schull WJ. Studies of the mortality of A-bomb survivors: 7. Mortality, 1950–1978: Part I. Cancer mortality. *Radiat Res* 1982;**90**:395–432.
12. Nowell PC, Hungerford DA. A minute chromosome in human chronic granulocytic leukemia. *Science* 1960;**132**:1497.
13. Rowley JD. A new consistent abnormality in chronic myelogenous leukaemia identified by quinacrine fluorescence and Giemsa staining. *Nature* 1973;**243**:290–3.
14. Lugo TG, Pendergast AM, Muller AJ, *et al.* Tyrosine kinase activity and transformation potency of bcr-abl oncogene products. *Science* 1990;**247**:1079–82.
15. Pendergast AM, Quilliam LA, Cripe LD, *et al.* BCRABL-induced oncogenesis is mediated by direct interaction with the SH2 domain of the GRB-2 adaptor protein. *Cell* 1993;**75**:175–85.
16. Puil L, Liu J, Gish G, *et al.* Bcr-Abl oncoproteins bind directly to activators of the Ras signalling pathway. *EMBO J* 1994;**13**:764–73.
17. Marais R, Light Y, Paterson HF, *et al.* Ras remits Raf-I to the plasma membrane for activation by tyrosine phosphorylation. *EMBO J* 1995;**14**:3136–45.
18. Skorski T, Kanakaraj P, Nieborowska-Skorska M, *et al.* Phosphatidylinositol-3 kinase activity is regulated by BCR/ABL and is required for the growth of Philadelphia chromosome-positive cells. *Blood* 1995;**86**:726–36.
19. Skorski T, Bellacosa A, Nieborowska-Skorska M, *et al.* Transformation of hematopoietic cells by BCR/ABL requires activation of a PI-3k/Akt-dependent pathway. *EMBO J* 1997;**16**:6151–61.
20. Franke TF, Kaplan DR, Cantley LC. PI3K: downstream AKTion blocks apoptosis. *Cell* 1997;**88**:435–7.
21. Shuai K, Halpern J, ten Hoeve J, *et al.* Constitutive activation of STAT5 by the Bcr-Abl oncogene in chronic myelogenous leukemia. *Oncogene* 1996;**13**:247–54.
22. Haria RL Jr, Van Etten RA. P2IO and PI90(BCR/ABL) induce the tyrosine phosphorylation and DNA binding activity of multiple specific STAT family members. *J Biol Chem* 1996;**271**:31 704–10.
23. Klejman A, Schreiner SJ, Nieborowska-Skorska M, *et al.* The Src family kinase Hck couples BCR/ABL to STAT5 activation in myeloid leukemia cells. *EMBO J* 2002;**21**:5766–74.
24. Menssen A, Hermeking H. Characterization of the c-MYC-regulated transcriptome by SAGE: identification and analysis of c-MYC target genes. *Proc Natl Acad Sci U S A* 2002;**99**:6274–9.
25. Sawyers CL, Callahan W, Witte ON. Dominant negative MYC blocks transformation by ABL oncogenes. *Cell* 1992;**70**:901–10.
26. Alar DE, Goga A, McLaughlin J, *et al.* Differential complementation of Bcr-Abl point mutants with c-Myc. *Science* 1994;**264**:424–6.
27. Skorski T, Nieborowska-Skorska M, Wlodarski P, *et al.* Blastic transformation of p53-deficient bone marrow cells by p2lObcr/abl tyrosine kinase. *Proc Natl Acad Sci U S A* 1996;**93**:13 137–42.
28. Serrano M, Lee H, Chin L, *et al.* Role of the INK4a locus in tumor suppression and cell mortality. *Cell* 1996;**85**:27–37.
29. Beck Z, Kiss A, Tóth FD, *et al.* Alterations of P53 and RB genes and the evolution of the accelerated phase of chronic myeloid leukemia. *Leuk Lymphoma* 2000;**38**:587–97.
30. Sherr C, McCormick F. The RB and p53 pathways in cancer. *Cancer Cell* 2002;**2**:103–12.
31. Schoch C, Schnittger S, Bursch S, *et al.* Comparison of chromosome banding analysis, interphase- and hypermetaphase-FISH, qualitative and quantitative PCR for diagnosis and for follow-up in chronic myeloid leukemia: a study on 350 cases. *Leukemia* 2002;**16**:53–9.
32. Wang YL, Bagg A, Pear W, *et al.* Chronic myelogenous leukemia: laboratory diagnosis and monitoring. *Genes Chromosomes Cancer* 2001;**32**:97–111.
33. Faderl S, Talpaz M, Estrov Z, *et al.* The biology of chronic myeloid leukemia. *N Engl J Med* 1999;**341**:164–72.
34. Guilhot F, Chastang C, Michallet M, *et al.* Interferon Alfa-2b combined with cytarabine versus interferon alone in chronic myelogenous leukemia. *N Engl J Med* 1997;**337**:223–9.
35. Kantarjian HM, O'Brien S, Smith TL, *et al.* Treatment of Philadelphia chromosome-positive early chronic phase chronic myelogenous leukemia with daily doses of interferon alpha and low-dose cytarabine. *J Clin Oncol* 1999;**17**:284–92.
36. Deininger M, Buchdunger E, Druker BJ. The development of imatinib as a therapeutic agent for chronic myeloid leukemia. *Blood* 2005;**105**:2640–53.
37. Druker BJ, Guilhot F, O'Brien SG, *et al.* Five-year follow-up of patients receiving imatinib for chronic myeloid leukemia. *N Engl J Med* 2006;**355**:2408–17.
38. O'Brien SG, Guilhot F, Goldman JM, *et al.* International Randomized Study of Interferon Versus STI571 (IRIS) 7-year follow-up: sustained survival, low rate of transformation and increased rate of major molecular response (MMR) in patients (pts) with newly diagnosed chronic myeloid leukemia in chronic phase (CMLCP) treated with imatinib (IM). *ASH Annual Meeting Abstracts* 2008;**112**:186.
39. Kantarjian H, Talpaz M, O'Brien S, *et al.* High-dose imatinib mesylate therapy in newly diagnosed

Philadelphia chromosome-positive chronic phase chronic myeloid leukemia. *Blood* 2004;**103**:2873–8.

40. Cortes J, Baccarani M, Guilhot F, *et al.* A phase III, randomized, open-label study of 400 mg versus 800 mg of imatinib mesylate (IM) in patients (pts) with newly diagnosed, previously untreated chronic myeloid leukemia in chronic phase (CML-CP) using molecular endpoints: 1-year results of TOPS (Tyrosine Kinase Inhibitor Optimization and Selectivity) Study. *ASH Annual Meeting Abstracts* 2008;**112**:335.

41. Baccarani M, Rosti G, Castagnetti F, *et al.* Comparison of imatinib 400 mg and 800 mg daily in the front-line treatment of high-risk, Philadelphia-positive chronic myeloid leukemia: a European LeukemiaNet Study. *Blood* 2009;**113**:4497–504.

42. 2009. NccnNCpgioCMLV.

43. Baccarani M, Saglio G, Goldman J, *et al.* Evolving concepts in the management of chronic myeloid leukemia: recommendations from an expert panel on behalf of the European LeukemiaNet. *Blood* 2006;**108**:1809–20.

44. Hughes T, Branford S. Molecular monitoring of BCR-ABL as a guide to clinical management in chronic myeloid leukaemia. *Blood Rev* 2006;**20**:29–41.

45. Kantarjian H, O'Brien S, Shan J, *et al.* Cytogenetic and molecular responses and outcome in chronic myelogenous leukemia: need for new response definitions? *Cancer* 2008;**112**:837–45.

46. Quintas-Cardama A, Kantarjian H, Jones D, *et al.* Delayed achievement of cytogenetic and molecular response is associated with increased risk of progression among patients with chronic myeloid leukemia in early chronic phase receiving high-dose or standard-dose imatinib therapy. *Blood* 2009;**113**:6315–21.

47. Apperley JF. Part I: mechanisms of resistance to imatinib in chronic myeloid leukaemia. *Lancet Oncol* 2007;**8**:1018–29.

48. Soverini S, Colarossi S, Gnani A, *et al.* Contribution of ABL kinase domain mutations to imatinib resistance in different subsets of Philadelphia-positive patients: by the GIMEMA Working Party on Chronic Myeloid Leukemia. *Clin Cancer Res* 2006;**12**:7374–9.

49. Donato NJ, Wu JY, Stapley J, *et al.* Imatinib mesylate resistance through BCR-ABL independence in chronic myelogenous leukemia. *Cancer Res* 2004;**64**:672–7.

50. Penserga ET, Skorski T. Fusion tyrosine kinases: a result and cause of genomic instability. *Oncogene* 2007;**26**:11–20.

51. Kantarjian HM, Larson RA, Guilhot F, *et al.* Efficacy of imatinib dose escalation in patients with chronic myeloid leukemia in chronic phase. *Cancer* 2009;**115**:551–60.

52. Jabbour E, Kantarjian HM, Jones D, *et al.* Imatinib mesylate dose escalation is associated with durable responses in patients with chronic myeloid leukemia after cytogenetic failure on standard-dose imatinib therapy. *Blood* 2009;**113**:2154–60.

53. Lombardo LJ, Lee FY, Chen P, *et al.* Discovery of N-(2-chloro-6-methyl-phenyl)-2-(6-(4-(2-hydroxyethyl)-piperazin-1-yl)-2-methylpyrimidin-4-ylamino)thiazole-5-carboxamide (BMS-354825), a dual Src/Abl kinase inhibitor with potent antitumor activity in preclinical assays. *J Med Chem* 2004;**47**:6658–61.

54. Bradeen HA, Eide CA, O'Hare T, *et al.* Comparison of imatinib mesylate, dasatinib (BMS-354825), and nilotinib (AMN107) in an N-ethyl-N-nitrosourea (ENU)-based mutagenesis screen: high efficacy of drug combinations. *Blood* 2006;**108**:2332–8.

55. Guilhot F, Apperley J, Kim DW, *et al.* Dasatinib induces significant hematologic and cytogenetic responses in patients with imatinib-resistant or -intolerant chronic myeloid leukemia in accelerated phase. *Blood* 2007; **109**:4143–50.

56. Hochhaus A, Baccarani M, Deininger M, *et al.* Dasatinib induces durable cytogenetic responses in patients with chronic myelogenous leukemia in chronic phase with resistance or intolerance to imatinib. *Leukemia* 2008;**22**:1200–6.

57. Cortes J, Rousselot P, Kim DW, *et al.* Dasatinib induces complete hematologic and cytogenetic responses in patients with imatinib-resistant or -intolerant chronic myeloid leukemia in blast crisis. *Blood* 2007;**109**:3207–13.

58. Shah NP, Kim D-W, Kantarjian HM, *et al.* Dasatinib dose-optimization in chronic phase chronic myeloid leukemia (CML-CP): two-year data from CA180–034 show equivalent long-term efficacy and improved safety with 100 mg once daily dose. *ASH Annual Meeting Abstracts* 2008;**112**:3225.

59. Porkka K, Khoury HJ, Paquette R, *et al.* Dasatinib 100 mg once daily (QD) maintains long-term efficacy and minimizes the occurrence of pleural effusion: an analysis of 24-month data in patients with resistance, suboptimal response, or intolerance to imatinib (CA180–034). *ASH Annual Meeting Abstracts* 2008;**112**:3242.

60. Mauro MJ, Baccarani M, Cervantes F, *et al.* Dasatinib 2-year efficacy in patients with chronic-phase chronic myelogenous leukemia (CP-CML) with resistance or intolerance to imatinib (START-C). *J Clin Oncol (2008 ASCO Annual Meeting Proceedings)* 2008;**26**: Abstract 7009.

61. Hochhaus A, Mueller M, Cortes JE, *et al.* Dasatinib efficacy by dosing schedule across individual baseline BCR-ABL mutations in chronic phase chronic myelogenous leukemia (CP-CML) after imatinib failure. *J Clin Oncol* (*2008 ASCO Annual Meeting Proceedings*) 2008;**26**: Abstract 7014.

62. Soverini S, Colarossi S, Gnani A, *et al.* Resistance to dasatinib in Philadelphia-positive leukemia patients and the presence or the selection of mutations at residues 315 and 317 in the BCR-ABL kinase domain. *Haematologica* 2007;**92**:401–4.

63. Shah NP, Skaggs BJ, Branford S, *et al.* Sequential ABL kinase inhibitor therapy selects for compound drug-resistant BCR-ABL mutations with altered oncogenic potency. *J Clin Invest* 2007;**117**:2562–9.

64. Khorashad JS, Milojkovic D, Mehta P, *et al.* In vivo kinetics of kinase domain mutations in CML patients treated with dasatinib after failing imatinib. *Blood* 2008;**111**:2378–81.

65. Jabbour E, Kantarjian HM, Jones D, *et al.* Characteristics and outcome of chronic myeloid leukemia patients with F317L BCR-ABL kinase domain mutation after therapy with tyrosine kinase inhibitors. *Blood* 2008;**112**: 4839–42.

66. Kantarjian H, Pasquini R, Hamerschlak N, *et al.* Dasatinib or high-dose imatinib for chronic-phase chronic myeloid leukemia after failure of first-

line imatinib: a randomized phase 2 trial. *Blood* 2007;**109**:5143–50.

67. Kantarjian H, Pasquinin R, Levy V, *et al.* Dasatinib or high-dose imatinib for chronic-phase chronic myeloid leukemia resistant to imatinib at a dose of 400 to 600 milligrams daily: two-year follow-up of a randomized phase 2 study (START-R). *Cancer* 2009;**115**:4136–47.

68. Apperley JF, Cortes JE, Kim DW, *et al.* Dasatinib in the treatment of chronic myeloid leukemia in accelerated phase after imatinib failure: the START a trial. *J Clin Oncol* 2009;**27**(21):3472–9.

69. Martinelli G, Hochhaus A, Coutre S, *et al.* Dasatinib (SPRYCEL) efficacy and safety in patients (pts) with chronic myelogenous leukemia in lymphoid (CML-LB) or myeloid blast (CML-MB) phase who are imatinib-resistant (im-r) or -intolerant (im-i). *Blood* 2006;**108**: Abstract 745.

70. Ottmann O, Dombret H, Baccarani M, *et al.* Dasatinib induces rapid hematologic and cytogenetic responses in patients with Philadelphia chromosome-positive acute lymphoblastic leukemia with resistance or intolerance to imatinib: interim results of a phase II study. *Blood* 2007;**110**:2309–15.

71. Weisberg E, Manley PW, Breitenstein W, *et al.* Characterization of AMN107, a selective inhibitor of native and mutant Bcr-Abl. *Cancer Cell* 2005;**7**:129–41.

72. Kantarjian HM, Giles F, Gattermann N, *et al.* Nilotinib (formerly AMN107), a highly selective BCR-ABL tyrosine kinase inhibitor, is effective in patients with Philadelphia chromosome-positive chronic myelogenous leukemia in chronic phase following imatinib resistance and intolerance. *Blood* 2007;**110**:3540–6.

73. le Coutre P, Ottmann OG, Giles F, *et al.* Nilotinib (formerly AMN107), a highly selective BCR-ABL tyrosine kinase inhibitor, is active in patients with imatinib-resistant or -intolerant accelerated-phase chronic myelogenous leukemia. *Blood* 2008;**111**:1834–9.

74. Kantarjian HM, Giles F, Bhalla KN, *et al.* Nilotinib in chronic myeloid leukemia patients in chronic phase (CMLCP) with imatinib resistance or intolerance: 2-year follow-up results of a phase 2 study. *ASH Annual Meeting Abstracts* 2008;**112**:3238.

75. le Coutre PD, Giles F, Hochhaus A, *et al.* Nilotinib in chronic myeloid leukemia patients in accelerated phase (CML-AP) with imatinib resistance or intolerance: 2-year follow-up results of a phase 2 study. *ASH Annual Meeting Abstracts* 2008;**112**:3229.

76. Giles FJ, Larson RA, Kantarjian HM, *et al.* Nilotinib in patients with Philadelphia chromosome-positive chronic myelogenous leukemia in blast crisis (CML-BC) who are resistant or intolerant to imatinib. *J Clin Oncol (2008 ASCO Annual Meeting Proceedings)* 2008;**26**: Abstract 7017.

77. Hochhaus A, Kim D-W, Martinelli G, *et al.* Nilotinib efficacy according to baseline BCR-ABL mutations in patients with imatinib-resistant chronic myeloid leukemia in chronic phase (CP-CML). *ASH Annual Meeting Abstracts* 2008;**112**:3216.

78. Redaelli S, Piazza R, Rostagno R, *et al.* Activity of bosutinib, dasatinib, and nilotinib against 18 imatinib-resistant BCR/ABL mutants. *J Clin Oncol* 2009;**27**:469–71.

79. Cortes J, Kantarjian HM, Kim D-W, *et al.* Efficacy and safety of bosutinib (SKI-606) in patients with chronic phase (CP) Ph+ chronic myelogenous leukemia (CML) with resistance or intolerance to imatinib. *ASH Annual Meeting Abstracts* 2008;**112**:1098.

80. Cortes J, Paquette R, Talpaz M, *et al.* Preliminary clinical activity in a phase I trial of the BCR-ABL/IGF-1R/aurora kinase inhibitor XL228 in patients with Ph+ leukemias with either failure to multiple TKI therapies or with T315I mutation. *ASH Annual Meeting Abstracts* 2008;**112**:3232.

81. Gontarewicz A, Balabanov S, Keller G, *et al.* Simultaneous targeting of aurora kinases and Bcr-Abl by the small molecule inhibitor PHA-739358 is effective in imatinib-resistant mutations including T315I. *ASH Annual Meeting Abstracts* 2007;**110**:1042.

82. Gontarewicz A, Balabanov S, Keller G, *et al.* PHA-680626 exhibits anti-proliferative and pro-apoptotic activity on imatinib-resistant chronic myeloid leukemia cell lines and primary CD34+ cells by inhibition of both Bcr-Abl tyrosine kinase and aurora kinases. *ASH Annual Meeting Abstracts* 2007;**110**:4568.

83. Paquette RL, Shah NP, Sawyers CL, *et al.* PHA-739358, an aurora kinase inhibitor, induces clinical responses in chronic myeloid leukemia harboring T315I mutations of BCR-ABL. *ASH Annual Meeting Abstracts* **2007**;110:1030.

84. Giles FJ, Cortes J, Jones D, *et al.* MK-0457, a novel kinase inhibitor, is active in patients with chronic myeloid leukemia or acute lymphocytic leukemia with the T315I BCR-ABL mutation. *Blood* 2007;**109**:500–2.

85. Cortes J, Talpaz T, Deininger M, *et al.* A phase 1 trial of oral AP24534 in patients with refractory chronic myeloid leukemia and other hematologic malignancies: first results of safety and clinical activity against T315I and resistant mutations. *Blood* 2009;**114**:643.

86. Van Etten RA, Chan WW, Zaleskas VM, *et al.* Switch pocket inhibitors of the ABL tyrosine kinase: distinct kinome inhibition profiles and in vivo efficacy in mouse models of CML and B-lymphoblastic leukemia induced by BCR-ABL T315I. *Blood* 2008;**112**:576.

87. Kantarjian HM, Talpaz M, Santini V, *et al.* Homoharringtonine: history, current research, and future direction. *Cancer* 2001;**92**:1591–605.

88. O'Brien S, Kantarjian H, Keating M, *et al.* Homoharringtonine therapy induces responses in patients with chronic myelogenous leukemia in late chronic phase. *Blood* 1995;**86**:3322–6.

89. Cortes J, Khoury HJ, Corm S, *et al.* Safety and efficacy of subcutaneous (SC) omacetaxine mepesuccinate in imatinib (IM)-resistant chronic myeloid leukemia (CML) patients (pts) with the T315I mutation – results of an ongoing multicenter phase II study. *ASH Annual Meeting Abstracts* 2008;**112**:3239.

90. Shah NP, Nicoll JM, Branford S, *et al.* Molecular analysis of dasatinib resistance mechanisms in CML patients identifies novel BCR-ABL mutations predicted to retain sensitivity to imatinib: rationale for combination tyrosine kinase inhibitor therapy. *Blood* **2005**;106:1093.

91. Weisberg E, Catley L, Wright RD, *et al.* Beneficial effects of combining nilotinib and imatinib in preclinical models of BCR-ABL+ leukemias. *Blood* 2007;**109**:2112–20.

92. Fiskus W, Pranpat M, Bali P, *et al.* Combined effects of novel tyrosine kinase inhibitor AMN107 and histone

deacetylase inhibitor LBH589 against Bcr-Abl-expressing human leukemia cells. *Blood* 2006;**108**:645–52.

93. O'Hare T, Eide CA, Tyner JW, *et al.* SGX393 inhibits the CML mutant Bcr-AblT315I and preempts in vitro resistance when combined with nilotinib or dasatinib. *Proc Natl Acad Sci U S A* 2008;**105**:5507–12.

94. Baccarani M, Martinelli G, Rosti G, *et al.* Imatinib and pegylated human recombinant interferon alpha2b in early chronic-phase chronic myeloid leukemia. *Blood* 2004;**104**:4245–51.

95. Guilhot F, Mahon F, Guilhot J, *et al.* Randomized comparison of imatinib versus imatinib combination therapies in newly diagnosed chronic myeloid leukaemia (CML) patients in chronic phase (CP): first results of the phase III (SPIRIT) trial from the French CML Group (FI LMC) *Blood* 2008;**112**:183.

96. Quintas-Cardama A, Kantarjian HM, Ravandi F, *et al.* Immune modulation of minimal residual disease (MRD) in patients (pts) with chronic myelogenous leukemia (CML) in early chronic phase (CP): a randomized trial of frontline high-dose (HD) imatinib mesylate (IM) with or without pegylated-interferon (PEG-IFN) and GM-CSF. *Blood* 2006;**108**:2207.

97. Mahon F, Huguet F, Guilhot F, *et al.* Is it possible to stop imatinib in patients with chronic myeloid leukemia? An update from a French pilot study and first results from the multicentre "Stop Imatinib" (STIM) study. *Blood* 2008;**112**:187.

98. Rosti G, Castagnetti F, Poerio A, *et al.* High and early rates of cytogenetic and molecular response with nilotinib 800 mg daily as first line treatment of Ph-positive chronic myeloid leukemia in chronic phase: results of a phase 2 trial of the GIMEMA CML Working Party. *ASH Annual Meeting Abstracts* 2008;**112**:181.

99. Cortes J, O'Brien S, Jones D, *et al.* Efficacy of nilotinib (formerly AMN107) in patients (pts) with newly diagnosed, previously untreated Philadelphia chromosome (Ph)-positive chronic myelogenous leukemia in early chronic phase (CP-CML). *ASH Annual Meeting Abstracts* 2008;**112**:446.

100. Cortes J, O'Brien S, Borthakur G, *et al.* Efficacy of dasatinib in patients (pts) with previously untreated chronic myelogenous leukemia (CML) in early chronic phase (CML-CP). *ASH Annual Meeting Abstracts* 2008;**112**:182.

101. Marin D, Milojkovic D, Olavarria E, *et al.* European LeukemiaNet criteria for failure or suboptimal response reliably identify patients with CML in early chronic phase treated with imatinib whose eventual outcome is poor. *Blood* 2008;**112**:4437–44.

102. Alvarado Y, Kantarjian H, O'Brien S, *et al.* Significance of suboptimal response to imatinib, as defined by the European LeukemiaNet, in the long-term outcome of patients with early chronic myeloid leukemia in chronic phase. *Cancer* 2009;**115**: 3709–18.

103. Tam CS, Kantarjian H, Garcia-Manero G, *et al.* Failure to achieve a major cytogenetic response by 12 months defines inadequate response in patients receiving nilotinib or dasatinib as second or subsequent line therapy for chronic myeloid leukemia. *Blood* 2008;**112**:516–18.

104. Jabbour E, Kantarjian H, Jones D, *et al.* Long-term outcome of patients with chronic myeloid leukemia treated with second-generation tyrosine kinase inhibitors after imatinib failure is predicted by the in vitro sensitivity of BCR-ABL kinase domain mutations. *Blood* 2009;**114**:2037–43.

Chapter 5

Chronic lymphocytic leukemia/small lymphocytic lymphoma

Karen W. L. Yee and Susan M. O'Brien

Introduction

Chronic lymphocytic leukemia (CLL) is the most common form of leukemia in adults in the Western world, accounting for nearly 25% of all leukemias with an estimated annual age-adjusted incidence of 3 per 100 000 persons in the United States.[1,2] The median age at diagnosis is approximately 70 years, with 81% of the patients diagnosed when aged ≥ 60 years.[1] Under the World Health Organization (WHO) classification, CLL is a B-cell neoplasm and the entity T-cell CLL has been reclassified as T-cell prolymphocytic leukemia (PLL).[3] Recent data from the Surveillance, Epidemiology, and End Results (SEER) cancer statistics indicate that 5-year survival of patients with CLL is 73%.[4]

Significant changes in the understanding and management of CLL have occurred in the last two decades. With the advent of newer treatment modalities, such as purine analogs and monoclonal antibodies, substantial improvements have been made in achieving complete responses (CR), with a proportion achieving molecular remissions and durable responses. Despite the advances in the treatment of patients with CLL, the majority of patients will relapse after primary therapy.

Diagnosis

The current diagnosis of CLL is based on minor modifications of the criteria originally proposed by the National Cancer Institute (NCI) (Table 5.1).[5,6] A bone marrow evaluation is no longer required for diagnosis but is useful to determine the extent and pattern of involvement and to clarify the etiology of cytopenias.[6]

The morphology and immunophenotype are adequate for diagnosis and to distinguish CLL from other disorders (Table 5.2).[7] Although the typical B-cell CLL immunophenotype is CD5+, CD19+, CD23+, FMC7-, with weak or negative expression of CD22, CD79b, and surface membrane immunoglobulin, there can be some variability in the expression of these surface markers.[8–11] Therefore, an immunophenotypic scoring system is often used to aid in the diagnosis and differentiation from other B-cell malignancies (Table 5.3).[12–18]

Using a highly sensitive flow cytometric technique, a monoclonal B-cell lymphocytosis (MBL) can be detected in individuals with no other features of a B-cell lymphoproliferative disorder.[19,20] The B-cell clones may have a CLL-like immunophenotype or that of other B-cell lymphoproliferative disorders (Table 5.4). It is unclear whether the CLL-phenotype MBL is biologically indistinguishable from CLL B cells.[21,22] Monoclonal CLL-phenotype B cells can be detected in 2–5.5% of the general population with normal blood counts,[19,21,23,24] and in 13.9% of those with lymphocytosis.[24] A higher incidence of MBL (15–57.5%) has been observed in healthy first-degree relatives of individuals affected with CLL; of whom 13.5–18% have CLL-like immunophenotype.[25,26] Individuals with CLL-phenotype MBL and lymphocytosis may progress to frank CLL requiring treatment at a rate of 1–2% per year.[24]

The diagnosis of small lymphocytic lymphoma (SLL) requires the presence of adenopathy and/or splenomegaly. The number of B lymphocytes in the peripheral blood should not exceed 5×10^9/L. The diagnosis should be confirmed by histologic evaluation of a lymph node.

Prognosis

The natural history of CLL is highly variable. Survival has been shown to correlate with clinical staging. Patients can be classified into low-, intermediate-, and high-risk groups (i.e., Rai or Binet classifications) on the basis of presenting features (i.e., lymphadenopathy, hepatosplenomegaly, anemia, and thrombocytopenia) with median survivals of > 10, 7–9, and 2 years, respectively (Tables 5.5 and 5.6).[5,27,28] Both staging systems rely only on physical examination and laboratory tests and do not require imaging. However, there is still marked heterogeneity in outcome between different individuals within the same stage.[29]

Risk may be further refined by the presence of other adverse biologic prognostic factors, including a lymphocyte doubling time of < 12 months, atypical morphology, elevated serum β_2-microglobulin levels, high levels of soluble CD23, elevated serum thymidine kinase levels, and deletions or

Management of Hematologic Malignancies, ed. Susan M. O'Brien, Julie M. Vose, and Hagop M. Kantarjian. Published by Cambridge University Press.

Table 5.1. Diagnosis for chronic lymphocytic leukemia

Criteria	NCI-WG 1996[5]	IWCLL 2005[6,80]
Peripheral blood lymphocytes ($\times 10^9$/L)	>5	Not specified[a] (≥ 5)
Morphology	Not specified	Small mature lymphocytes without visible nucleoli; smudge cells are characteristic
Immunophenotype of lymphocytes	≥ 1 B-cell marker (CD19, CD20, or CD23) and CD5 positivity in the absence of other pan-T-cell marker. Monoclonal expression of either κ or κ chain low-density surface Ig (sIg)	≥ 1 B-cell marker (CD19, CD20, or CD23) and CD5 positivity in the absence of other pan-T-cell marker. Monoclonal expression of either γ or γ chain low-density surface Ig (sIg)
Atypical cells (e.g., prolymphocytes)	$<55\%$ and/or $<15 \times 10^9$/L	$<55\%$ and/or $<15 \times 10^9$/L
Duration of lymphocytosis	None required	Not specified but needs to be chronic
Bone marrow lymphocytes (%)	≥ 30	Bone marrow evaluation not required[b]

Notes: [a]Not specified initially in IWCLL, but mandated only that a chronic, absolute increase in blood lymphocytes with the characteristic morphology and immunophenotype be present; subsequently defined as $\geq 5 \times 10^9$/L.
[b]Bone marrow evaluation is no longer required for diagnosis but useful to determine extent and pattern of involvement and clarification of etiology of cytopenias.
Source: NCI-WG: National Cancer Institute-sponsored Working Group; IWCLL: International Workshop on Chronic Lymphocytic Leukemia.

mutations of the *p53* gene (Table 5.7).[13,30–46] Chromosomal abnormalities are detected in 30–50% and in over 80% of patients using cytogenetic or fluorescence *in situ* hybridization (FISH) analyses, respectively.[47,48] Median survivals for patients with 17p-, 11q-, trisomy 12q, normal karyotype, and 13q- as the sole abnormality were 32, 79, 114, 111, and 133 months, respectively.[48] On multivariate analysis, 17p- and 11q- were associated with shorter overall survival (OS).[48] However, recent data suggest that 17p- CLL is a clinically heterogeneous disease, with some patients experiencing an indolent course with prolonged survival.[49] Furthermore, complex chromosomal abnormalities and translocations may also be associated with advanced stage and inferior overall survival.[50,51] As cytogenetic abnormalities have prognostic significance and may influence treatment decisions, cytogenetics and/or FISH analyses should be performed prior to treating a patient. Moreover, as clonal evolution may occur during the course of the disease,[52,53] it would be prudent to repeat cytogenetic and/or FISH analyses prior to administering salvage therapy.

Table 5.2. Differential diagnosis

Benign causes
- B cell
  - Post-splenectomy
  - Hyper-reactive malarial splenomegaly
  - Persistent polyclonal B-cell lymphocytosis (e.g., smokers)
- T cell
  - Bacterial (e.g., tuberculosis, syphilis)
  - Viral (e.g., infectious mononucleosis, cytomegalovirus [CMV])
  - Serum sickness
  - Thyrotoxicosis
  - Addison's disease
  - Post-splenectomy

Malignant causes
- B cell
- Chronic lymphocytic leukemia
- Prolymphocytic leukemia
- Leukemic phase of non-Hodgkin lymphoma
  - Mantle cell lymphoma
  - Follicular small cleaved cell lymphoma
  - Splenic lymphoma with villous lymphocytes
  - Marginal zone lymphomas
  - Large cell lymphoma
  - Hairy cell leukemia
  - Waldenstrom's macroglobulinemia
- T cell
  - T-cell prolymphocytic leukemia
  - Adult T-cell leukemia/lymphoma
  - Sézary syndrome
  - Large granular lymphocytic leukemia
  - Peripheral T-cell lymphoma

Table 5.3. Scoring system for diagnosis of chronic lymphocytic leukemia[12–14]

Marker	Score for marker intensity	
	1	0
sIg	Weak	Strong
CD5	Positive	Negative
CD23	Positive	Negative
CD22 or CD79b	Weak	Strong
FMC7	Negative	Positive

Note: Diagnosis of CLL requires a score of >3 (with most cases of CLL having scores of 4 or 5), whereas in other B-cell malignancies, the scores are usually <3.
sIg: surface immunoglobulin.
Source: Reproduced from Oscier *et al.* 2004.[14]

Table 5.4. Diagnosis for monoclonal B-cell lymphocytosis (MBL)[19,20]

Criteria	
Immunophenotype of lymphocytes	Disease-specific immunophenotype; Monoclonal expression of either κ or γ chain; Absent or low-density surface Ig in > 25% B cells
Supplementary	Abnormal CD20/CD5 pattern; Heavy chain monoclonal *IGHV* rearrangements
Exclusion criteria	Lymphadenopathy and organomegaly, or Associated autoimmune/infectious disease, or B-lymphocyte count > 5 × 10^9/L, or any other feature diagnostic of a B-lymphoproliferative disorder (except possibly for a paraprotein which may be present or associated with MBL)
Duration of monoclonal B-cell population	3 months
Subclassification	CD5+ CD20Dim – corresponds to CLL phenotype CD5+ CD20Bright – corresponds with atypical CLL [exclude t(11;14)] CD5 – corresponds to non-CLL lymphoproliferative disease IgD-only

Table 5.5. Modified Rai clinical staging system[5,27]

Risk level	Stage	Clinical features	Median survival (yr)
Low	0	Lymphocytosis only (in blood and bone marrow)[a]	10
Intermediate	I	Lymphocytosis[a] with lymphadenopathy	7
	II	Lymphocytosis[a] with splenomegaly and/or hepatomegaly with or without lymphadenopathy	7
High	III	Lymphocytosis[a] with anemia[b] (hemoglobin < 110 g/L) with or without lymphadenopathy, splenomegaly, or hepatomegaly	1.5 to 4
	IV	Lymphocytosis[a] with thrombocytopenia[a] (platelets < 100 × 10^9/L) with or without anemia and/or lymphadenopathy, splenomegaly, or hepatomegaly	1.5 to 4

Notes: [a]Lymphocytes > 5 × 10^9/L in the peripheral blood and comprising > 30% of nucleated cells in the bone marrow.
[b]Excluding immune-mediated anemia or thrombocytopenia.

The presence of unmutated *IGHV* genes has been associated with high-risk cytogenetics,[54,55] a need for chemotherapy,[56] and shortened survival.[55–57] *IGHV* mutational status can also segregate the different stages of Binet's classification into distinct groups with different survival patterns.[55,57] However, it is unclear what degree of homology of *IGHV* genes to germline sequences (i.e., ≥ 95% or ≥ 98%) should be used to define an unmutated phenotype.[58] Recent data suggest that the use of specific *IGHV* gene segments, such as the V_H 3–21 gene, may be associated with an inferior outcome regardless of mutational status.[59,60]

In multivariate analysis, unmutated *IGHV* status, 17p deletion, 11q deletion, age, white blood cell (WBC) count, and lactate dehydrogenase (LDH) levels were independent prognostic factors for survival.[54] Two other series have indicated that unmutated *IGHV* status and mutation, loss, or dysfunction of p53 were independent adverse prognostic factors.[58,61] Patients with an unmutated *IGHV* status and/or high-risk interphase cytogenetics may have a shorter progression-free survival (PFS) and OS following therapy with a fludarabine-based regimen.[62–64]

Because of the difficulty sequencing *IGHV* genes in a clinical laboratory, surrogate markers for *IGHV* mutational status have been evaluated. CD38 expression correlates with unmutated *IGHV* gene, but is not a surrogate marker for *IGHV* mutational status; however, it may serve as an independent prognostic variable in patients with CLL.[56,58,61,65,66] The optimum cutoff level defining CD38-positivity remains unclear.[56,58,65,67] Furthermore, CD38 expression may vary during the course of the disease.[65]

Gene expression profiles of CLL cells with unmutated *IGHV* genes are similar to those with mutated *IGHV* genes, with a limited number of genes being differentially expressed.[68,69] One such gene is the intracellular protein tyrosine kinase ZAP-70, which plays a critical role in T-cell receptor signaling. The function of ZAP-70 in CLL is unclear, but postulated to enhance IgM signaling and thereby contribute to the aggressive clinical course of patients with CLL and unmutated *IGHV* genes.[70] ZAP-70 expression appears to correlate with an unmutated *IGHV* gene status and inferior outcome.[71–74] However, its validity as a surrogate marker for *IGHV* mutational status is unclear as (1) approximately 6–29% of cases show discordant status for ZAP-70 expression and *IGHV* mutational phenotype, (2) the optimum cutoff level defining ZAP-70-positivity remains to be defined, and (3) careful separation of T cells is required.[71–75] Furthermore, reproducible results between labs have been marred by technical difficulties with the standardization of flow cytometric methods for assessing ZAP-70 expression.[76]

Table 5.6. Binet classification[5,28]

Stage	Clinical features	Equivalent Rai staging	Median survival (yr)
A	Lymphocytosis (in blood and bone marrow)[a] with < 3 areas of nodal involvement.[b] No anemia or thrombocytopenia	0–II	12
B	Lymphocytosis[a] with ≥ 3 areas of nodal involvement[b], with or without splenomegaly and/or hepatomegaly. No anemia or thrombocytopenia	I–II	7
C	Lymphocytosis[a] with anemia[c] (hemoglobin < 110 g/L in men and < 100 g/L in women) or thrombocytopenia[c] (platelets < 100 × 10^9/L) regardless of the number of areas of nodal involvement, splenomegaly, or hepatomegaly	III–IV	2 to 4

Notes: [a]Lymphocytes > 5 × 10^9/L in the peripheral blood and comprising > 30% of total nucleated cells in the bone marrow.

[b]Each cervical, axillary, and inguinal area (whether unilateral or bilateral); spleen, and liver count as one area. Therefore, the number of areas of nodal involvement ranges from 1 to 5.

[c]Excluding immune-mediated anemia or thrombocytopenia.

A comprehensive review of other prognostic markers is beyond the scope of this chapter (reviewed in van Bockstaele *et al.* and Kay *et al.*).[77,78] A prognostic nomogram has been generated to predict survival.[36,37,46] However, with the exception of cytogenetics and FISH analyses, these prognostic markers and/or indices should not be used to influence therapeutic decisions. Prospective trials (such as the German CLL Study Group [GCLLSG] trial comparing fludarabine, cyclophosphamide, and rituximab with observation in untreated, Binet stage A, CLL patients at high risk of disease progression and the Cancer and Leukemia Group B [CALGB] study comparing early versus delayed fludarabine and rituximab therapy in asymptomatic, untreated, high-risk CLL patients) are required to verify and establish the role of these prognostic markers in determining the need for therapy, selecting the type of therapy,[79] and determining and/or predicting the response to therapy.

Indications for treatment

The indications for initiation of therapy in CLL remain those recommended by the NCI-sponsored Working Group (NCI-WG) (Table 5.8).[5,80] Criteria for therapy include B symptoms

Table 5.7. Prognostic factors[14,30]

Prognostic factor	Clinical risk	
	Low	High
Clinical features		
Gender	Female	Male
Clinical stage	Binet A/Rai 0	Binet C/Rai III–IV
Morphology		
Lymphocyte morphology	Typical	Atypical
Pattern of marrow trephine infiltration	Nodular or interstitial	Diffuse
Chromosomal abnormalities	Normal Trisomy 12 13q- (sole)	17p- 11q-
CD38 expression	< 20–30%	> 20–30%
ZAP-70 expression	< 20–30%	> 20–30%
IgV_H gene status	Mutated	Unmutated
Markers of tumor burden or proliferation		
Lymphocyte doubling time	> 12 months	≤ 12 months
β_2-microglobulin levels	Low or normal	High
Thymidine kinase (TK)	Low or normal	High
Lactate dehydrogenase (LDH)	Low or normal	High
Soluble CD23 levels	Low or normal	High
Markers of angiogenesis		
Microvessel density	Low or normal	High
Serum VEGF levels	Low or normal	High
Tumor suppressors or oncogenes p53	Normal	Loss or mutation/ dysfunction

Note: VEGF: vascular endothelial growth factor.
Source: Adapted from Oscier *et al.* 2004.[14]

(i.e., fevers, sweats, or weight loss), progressive enlargement of lymph nodes or hepatosplenomegaly, obstructive adenopathy, development of or worsening thrombocytopenia and anemia, immune hemolysis or thrombocytopenia not responsive to corticosteroids, and rapid lymphocyte doubling time. Hyperviscosity due to a high lymphocyte count is uncommon; therefore, a high lymphocyte count in the absence of a rapid doubling time is not an indication for therapy.

Assessment of response

The International Workshop on CLL (IWCLL)–NCI-WG[80,81] has refined the evaluation of response to therapy previously established by the NCI-WG,[5] with more precision of lymph node diameters (Table 5.9). Assessment of minimal residual disease (MRD), by either multiparametric flow cytometry based on the immunophenotype of the CLL cell or polymerase chain reaction (PCR)-based strategies using either the qualitative consensus IgH PCR or quantitative allele-specific oligonucleotide (to the complementarity determining region 3 [CDR3]) PCR,[82–84] should only be performed in a research setting. Techniques for assessing MRD have become standardized;[84] however, prospective clinical studies are required to validate the role of MRD-negativity as a surrogate marker for disease eradication and/or improved survival prior to its incorporation into routine clinical practice.

Table 5.8. Indications for treatment[5]

Disease-related systemic symptoms[a]
Weight loss ≥ 10% within the previous 6 months
Extreme fatigue
Fevers > 38 °C for ≥ 2 weeks
Night sweats
Progressive marrow failure with development or worsening of anemia and/or thrombocytopenia
Autoimmune cytopenias
Massive (> 6 cm below the costal margin) or progressive splenomegaly
Massive (> 10 cm) or progressive lymphadenopathy
Progressive lymphocytosis
> 50% increase over 2 months
Lymphocyte doubling time < 6 months

Note: [a]Exclude other causes, e.g., infection.

Therapeutic options for first-line therapy

Despite the failure of randomized trials to demonstrate an improvement in OS between the different treatment regimens and the paucity of data evaluating different therapeutic strategies and achievement of CR on patient quality of life (QoL), treatment rationales have been based on observations that patients achieving a CR are more likely to have a prolonged PFS and OS[85] and the assumption that prolonged time to treatment failure is associated with improved QoL. Therefore, frontline treatment decisions are usually geared to achieving a CR without increased toxicity.

Alkylating agents

An individual patient data meta-analysis indicated that immediate treatment with chlorambucil with or without corticosteroids did not have a survival advantage over deferred chemotherapy (10-year survival 44% vs. 47%, respectively, $p > 0.1$) in patients with early-stage disease (Rai stages I or II; Binet stage A).[86] Therefore, treatment of asymptomatic early-stage disease with alkylating agents is not warranted. At this time, it is unclear whether (1) early therapy with nucleoside analog combinations will be superior to observation in this

Table 5.9. Response criteria[80]

Criteria	Complete response (CR)	Partial response (PR)	Stable disease (SD)	Progressive disease (PD)
Symptoms	Absent	Absent or present	Absent or present	Absent or present
Lymphadenopathy[a]	None > 1 cm	≥ 50% reduction	Change of –49% to +49%	≥ 50% increase
Hepato- and/or splenomegaly	Absent	≥ 50% reduction	Change of –49% to +49%	≥ 50% increase
Neutrophils (× 10^9/L)	≥ 1.5	≥ 1.5 or ≥ 50% improvement from baseline	Any	Any
Lymphocytes (× 10^9/L)	Normal	≥ 50% reduction from baseline	Change of –49% to +49%	≥ 50% increase
Platelets (× 10^9/L)	> 100	> 100 or ≥ 50% improvement from baseline	Change of –49% to +49%	≥ 50% reduction from baseline
Hemoglobin (g/dL) (untransfused)	> 11	> 11 or ≥ 50% improvement from baseline	Increase < 11 or < 50% improvement from baseline, or decrease < 2	Decrease > 2 from baseline
Bone marrow aspirate and biopsy	Normocellular; < 30% lymphocytes; no B-lymphoid nodules	Hypocellular, or ≥ 30% lymphocytes, or B-lymphoid nodules, or not done	No change of marrow infiltrate	Increase of lymphocytes to > 30% from normal

Note: [a]Sum of the products of multiple lymph nodes (as evaluated by CT scans, ultrasound, or by physical exam).

group of patients or (2) asymptomatic patients with early-stage disease and leukemic cells expressing CD38, unmutated IGHV genes, ZAP-70, etc. should be treated.

This same meta-analysis also demonstrated that there was no difference in 5-year OS for previously untreated CLL patients (mostly Binet stages B or C disease) who received combination therapy (i.e., COP (cyclophosphamide, vincristine, and prednisone), CHOP (cyclophosphamide, doxorubicin, vincristine, and prednisone), or chlorambucil and epirubcin) compared with those who received chlorambucil with or without corticosteroids (48% vs. 48%, respectively, $p > 0.1$).[86] Early inclusion of an anthracycline did not improve 5-year survival.

Bendamustine

A phase III trial compared bendamustine, a potent alkylating agent, with chlorambucil in 319 untreated patients with advanced CLL.[87,88] The overall response (OR) rate was superior with bendamustine compared to chlorambucil (67% vs. 30%, respectively, $p < 0.0001$). After a median follow-up of 29.2 months, median PFS was 21.5 months with bendamustine and 8.3 months with chlorambucil ($p < 0.0001$). These results with bendamustine appear similar to those obtained with single-agent fludarabine.[89–96]

Purine analogs

Fludarabine

Four randomized trials comparing fludarabine monotherapy to alkylator-based chemotherapy (i.e., chlorambucil, mini-CHOP, and CAP) in previously untreated patients with active CLL consistently demonstrated higher OR and CR rates with fludarabine compared with alkylator-based chemotherapy regimens.[89–92] Therapy with fludarabine was associated with an improved PFS[90,91] but no differences in OS have been detected. The lack of survival difference may partly be due to (1) the permittance of crossover to the other arm if there was no response or disease progression,[89,91] (2) lack of significant high-quality responses achieved,[89–92] and (3) heterogeneity in other unmeasured prognostic variables (e.g., proportion of patients with CD38-positive leukemic cells and unmutated *IGHV* genes).

In an attempt to improve upon these response rates fludarabine has been combined with chemotherapeutic agents and/or monoclonal antibodies. Phase II studies evaluating fludarabine plus cyclophosphamide (FC), administered in a variety of different schedules and doses, in untreated patients with CLL demonstrated OR rates of 76–100% and CR rates of 21–60%,[94,97,98] with a higher proportion of complete responders lacking detectable disease by flow cytometry (i.e., < 1% CD5+/CD19+ cells).[98–100]

Five randomized trials comparing fludarabine alone to FC, fludarabine and epirubicin (FE), or fludarabine administered in conjunction with chlorambucil (F/CB) in untreated patients with active CLL have been reported.[91,93–96,101] FE and FC demonstrated superior response rates and PFS compared to single-agent fludarabine and/or single-agent chlorambucil.[93,95,96,101] In the United Kingdom (UK) CLL4 trial comparing single-agent chlorambucil, single-agent fludarabine, and FC, more hemolytic anemias were observed with chlorambucil therapy.[93] In the CALGB trial comparing single-agent fludarabine, single-agent chlorambucil, and F/CB, the F/CB arm was prematurely closed due to excessive rates of life-threatening toxicities, including major infections.[91,101] More recently, an increased frequency of therapy-related myelodysplasia (MDS) and/or acute myeloid leukemia (AML) has been observed in the patients treated with F/CB (0.5% vs. 0% vs. 3.5%, respectively) after a median follow-up of 4.2 years.[102] Similar findings have not been reported in trials employing combination fludarabine (or cladribine) and cyclophosphamide or cladribine and chlorambucil therapy;[93,94,98,99,103,104] but have been observed in patients treated with fludarabine, cyclophosphamide, and rituximab, with a 2.8% risk of developing MDS at 6 years.[100,105]

Treatment with fludarabine and mitoxantrone (FM) does not appear to yield higher response rates (OR = 83%; CR = 20%)[106] compared to historical results achievable with single-agent fludarabine, FC, or FE. In contrast, treatment of 69 untreated patients with CLL with combination fludarabine, cyclophosphamide, and mitoxantrone (FCM) yielded an OR rate of 90% (MRD-negative CR = 26%; MRD-positive CR = 38%; nodular partial remission [NPR] = 14%; PR = 12%).[107] Median response duration was 37 months. It remains to be determined whether FCM is truly superior to therapy with FC.

Cladribine (2-chlorodeoxyadenosine, 2-CdA)

Cladribine with or without corticosteroids has been evaluated in previously untreated CLL patients with OR rates of 49–86% (CR = 10–47%).[108–111] These results are comparable to those obtained with single-agent fludarabine.

A randomized phase III trial compared single-agent cladribine with chlorambucil monotherapy and fludarabine monotherapy in 221 previously untreated CLL patients.[112] OR rates were similar in all three arms. CR rates were not reported. Median time-to-progression (TTP) was significantly prolonged in patients receiving cladribine compared with fludarabine or chlorambucil (25 months vs. 10 months vs. 9 months, respectively, $p = 0.0003$).

A phase III trial compared single-agent cladribine with cladribine plus cyclophosphamide (2-CdA/C) and cladribine plus cyclophosphamide and mitoxantrone (2-CdA/CM).[110] Significantly higher CR rates were obtained in the 2-CdA/CM arm compared with cladribine alone (36% vs. 21%, respectively, $p = 0.004$), whereas only a trend for higher CR was observed with 2-CdA/C compared with cladribine (29% vs. 21%, respectively, $p = 0.08$). Eradication of MRD, as evaluated by immunophenotyping, was higher in the 2-CdA/CM arm compared with cladribine alone (23% vs. 14%, respectively, $p = 0.042$). There were no detectable differences in OR, PFS, and OS between the three groups.

Pentostatin (deoxycoformycin)

Limited data are available on the usage of single-agent pentostatin in untreated patients with CLL (OR = 46%; CR = 0%).[113] Use of pentostatin in combination with cyclophosphamide and rituximab is more efficacious than single-agent therapy (vida infra).

Rituximab (Rituxan)

Rituximab induction therapy

Previously untreated CLL/SLL patients who received single-agent rituximab, a chimeric human–murine anti-CD20 monoclonal antibody, as first-line and maintenance therapy achieved OR rates of 57% (CR = 9%).[114,115] Higher response rates (OR = 90%; CR = 19%) were obtained when standard-dose rituximab was administered for 8 weeks, instead of 4 weeks, in untreated patients with low tumor burden (Rai stage 0 to II).[116]

Although CRs are rarely observed in CLL patients treated with either single-agent rituximab or high-dose methylprednisolone (HDMP),[117–119] the combination of rituximab and HDMP (R-HDMP) has shown activity in relapsed or refractory CLL, with tolerable side effects.[120–122]

The combination of fludarabine, cyclophosphamide, and rituximab (FCR) has been assessed in 300 previously untreated patients with CLL.[100,105] OR was 95% (CR = 70%; NPR = 10%; PR = 13%) with 82% and 42% of complete responders having no MRD (i.e., < 1% CD5+/CD19+ cells in the marrow) by immunophenotyping and PCR analysis, respectively. After a median follow-up of 72 months, the actuarial 6-year OS and failure-free survival (FFS) were 71% and 51%, respectively. Median TTP was 80 months with a projected 6-year PFS of 60%. Pretreatment characteristics independently associated with inferior response were age ≥ 70 years, β_2-microglobulin levels ≥ twice the upper limit of normal, WBC $\geq 150 \times 10^9$/L, abnormal chromosome 17, and LDH ≥ twice the upper limit of normal. The risk of serious or opportunistic infection was 10% and 4% for the first and second years of remission, respectively, and < 1.5% per year for the third year onwards. The 6-year risks of transformation to Richter's syndrome and development of MDS were 2.5% and 2.8%, respectively. The proportion of patients achieving a CR and < 1% CD5+/CD19+ cells was significantly higher than that historically achieved with FC therapy alone.[99] The addition of three doses of rituximab to FC (FCR-3), in lieu of the single dose administered in the FCR regimen, did not appear to improve responses.[123]

A phase III GCLLSG trial compared therapy with FC and FCR as frontline therapy in 817 previously untreated patients with advanced CLL.[124] OR and CR rates were superior in the FCR arm compared to the FC arm (95% and 52% vs. 88% and 27%, respectively, $p \leq 0.001$). PFS at 2 years was significantly improved in the FCR arm (76.6% vs. 62.3%, $p < 0.0001$). There was a trend to an increased 2-year OS rate in the FCR arm (91% vs. 88%, $p = 0.18$). However, FCR treatment does not appear to overcome the poor prognosis associated with 17p– genomic aberrations.[125] Treatment with FCR was associated with more grade 3 and 4 adverse events (62% vs. 47%). Although FCR therapy caused more neutropenia (33.6% vs. 20.9%, respectively, $p = 0.001$), the incidence of severe infections was not increased. A recent update shows that FCR therapy was associated with improved OS. The OS rate at 38 months was 84.1% in the FCR arm versus 79% in the FC arm ($p = 0.01$).[126] A formal comparison of FCR with FR therapy[127,128] is still needed to determine which regimen is more efficacious without increased toxicity. Furthermore, because of encouraging results obtained with bendamustine and rituximab (BR) in patients with relapsed or refractory CLL,[129] the GCLLSG conducted a phase II trial evaluating BR in patients with untreated CLL.[130] The OR rate was 91% with 33% clinical CR. After 18 months 76% of patients were still in remission; median PFS had not been reached. Based on this data the GCLLSG is conducting a phase III trial of BR versus FCR as frontline therapy for CLL.

The combination of pentostatin, cyclophosphamide, and rituximab (PCR) appears to yield comparable OR rates (91%), but lower CR rates (41%) compared with FCR, with eradication of MRD in some patients.[131]

Rituximab induction and consolidation therapy

The CALGB conducted a randomized phase II trial of fludarabine with concurrent versus sequential treatment with rituximab in 104 symptomatic, previously untreated CLL patients.[127] Patients were randomized to either six cycles of fludarabine alone or six cycles of FR. After a 2-month observation period, patients with ≥ stable disease (SD) were treated with rituximab for 4 weeks. The OR and CR rates after induction therapy were 90% and 33% vs. 77% and 15%, respectively. These responses increased to 90% and 47% vs. 77% and 28%, respectively, after consolidation with rituximab. Median follow-up was 43 months. The estimated 2-year PFS was 70% for each arm. OS was similar in both arms.

Using data generated from the above study[127] and a prior randomized trial,[91] a retrospective comparison of fludarabine monotherapy to FR (sequential and concurrent) in previously untreated CLL patients was performed by CALGB.[132] Baseline features of the patients were similar. Therapy with FR was associated with significantly more ORs (84% vs. 63%, respectively, $p = 0.0003$) and CRs (38% vs. 20%, respectively, $p = 0.002$). There was a significant difference in PFS (67% vs. 45%, respectively, $p < 0.0001$) and OS (93% vs. 81%, respectively, $p = 0.0006$) at 2 years in favor of FR.

Alemtuzumab (Campath)

Alemtuzumab induction therapy

Subcutaneous alemtuzumab, a humanized anti-CD52 monoclonal antibody, produces OR rates of 87% (CR 19%) as frontline therapy in patients with CLL.[133] The majority of patients (95%) cleared CLL cells from the blood. Although 86% of patients with adenopathy had a response, only 29% achieved a CR (all of whom had lymph nodes of < 2 cm in diameter). Most responses occurred after 18 weeks of therapy. First-dose reactions typically associated with intravenous administration (i.e., rash, nausea, dyspnea, and hypotension) were absent.

A phase III trial indicated that superior responses were obtained with single-agent intravenous alemtuzumab compared with chlorambucil as first-line therapy for patients with CLL and active disease (OR 83% vs. 55%, respectively, $p < 0.001$; CR 24% vs. 2%, respectively, $p < 0.0001$).[134] Elimination of MRD occurred in 11 of 36 complete responders to alemtuzumab versus none to chlorambucil. Median PFS was significantly prolonged for patients receiving alemtuzumab (14.6 months vs. 11.7 months, respectively, $p = 0.001$). Higher incidences of grade 3 or 4 neutropenia were observed in the alemtuzumab arm, but did not translate to increased incidence of neutropenic fever or sepsis. More infusion-related events and CMV infections were noted in patients receiving alemtuzumab.

The CFAR regimen, where alemtuzumab is combined with the FCR regimen,[135] was evaluated as frontline therapy in 60 patients with high-risk CLL, including those with deletion 17p abnormalities.[136] Twenty-eight percent of patients had the deletion 17p abnormality. The OR and CR rates were 94% and 69%, respectively. For the 13 patients with deletion 17p, OR and CR rates were 77% and 54%, respectively. CFAR was associated with more myelosuppression and fewer patients completing all six intended cycles of therapy compared to a historical high-risk group treated with FCR. With a median follow-up of only 16 months, there was no difference in OS, TTP, or infectious complications between the two groups.

Alemtuzumab consolidation therapy

Consolidation with single-agent alemtuzumab appears to improve responses (i.e., PR or better) obtained with fludarabine in patients with CLL.[137] Alemtuzumab was administered a median of 4 months after fludarabine therapy. Six of seven patients were converted from NPR to CR, and 12 of 15 patients in PR to either a NPR ($n = 3$) or CR ($n = 9$). Nineteen of the 27 (56%) patients in CR after alemtuzumab therapy achieved a molecular CR.

The efficacy of alemtuzumab for the treatment of MRD following single-agent fludarabine therapy has been evaluated further in two phase II trials; alemtuzumab was administered (intravenously or subcutaneously) for 6 weeks following 4 months of standard dose and schedule fludarabine.[138,139] Retrospective analyses indicated an increased frequency of infections requiring hospitalization and/or parenteral antibiotics in patients receiving fludarabine followed by alemtuzumab compared with single-agent fludarabine or FR therapy (38% vs. 23% vs. 20%, respectively, $p \leq 0.01$).[140] CMV reactivation occurred in 20% of patients receiving intravenous or subcutaneous alemtuzumab.[138–140] Alemtuzumab was able to convert a proportion of patients with SD or PR after fludarabine to PRs and/or CRs.

The GCLLSG assessed the safety and efficacy of alemtuzumab consolidation in patients with CLL in first remission.[141,142] Twenty-three patients responding to first-line therapy with fludarabine or FC were randomized to either standard-dose alemtuzumab for 12 weeks or observation. Of the 21 evaluable patients, 11 were randomized to the alemtuzumab arm before the study was prematurely stopped due to grade 3 to 4 infections (64%) and grade 4 hematologic toxicities in the alemtuzumab arm (36%). All infections were successfully treated. Five of six patients in the alemtuzumab arm achieved a molecular remission in the peripheral blood compared to none of three patients in the observation arm ($p = 0.048$). After a median follow-up of 48 months, PFS was superior in the alemtuzumab arm compared to the observation arm (i.e., not reached vs. 20.6 months, respectively, $p = 0.004$).

The increased incidence of non-CMV infections observed in the GCLLSG[141,142,] and the CALGB[138,139] studies compared to the Italian[137] and MD Anderson[143,144] studies (27% and 33% vs. < 10%, respectively) may be due to the shorter interval between chemotherapy and alemtuzumab administration, 2 months vs. 5–6 months, respectively. In an attempt to decrease the risk of infections associated with alemtuzumab consolidation therapy, the French Cooperative Group on Chronic Lymphocytic Leukemia and Waldenstrom Macroglobulinemia (FCGCLL/WM) limited the number of cycles of FC induction chemotherapy to three and the duration of alemtuzumab therapy to 8 weeks,[145] whereas the CALGB increased the interval between completion of FR induction therapy (up to six cycles) and alemtuzumab consolidation therapy to 3 months, with alemtuzumab being administered for a total of 6 weeks.[146] In the FCGCLL/WM trial, only 16 of 42 patients completed alemtuzumab therapy, with 5 patients discontinuing therapy due to CMV reactivation.[145] In the CALGB study, 17 of 51 patients (33%) developed unacceptable toxicity attributable to alemtuzumab, including 5 deaths due to infectious complications. Therefore, although all studies have shown improvement in response rates with alemtuzumab consolidation, the optimal regimen remains to be determined and its safety and efficacy need to be verified in a randomized trial.

Therapeutic options for salvage therapy

Choice of salvage therapy is guided by factors such as age, performance status, prior therapy, response and duration of response to such therapy, and the goal of salvage therapy. Based on retrospective data indicating that response to salvage therapy appears to be strongly associated with response to prior therapies and most patients have been or will be treated with fludarabine or fludarabine-based regimens, relapsed patients have generally been classified into two groups based on prior response or exposure to fludarabine: fludarabine-naïve or -sensitive and fludarabine-refractory. However, the choice of appropriate salvage therapy in relapsed patients is hampered by (1) the lack of randomized trials, including those involving stem cell transplantation (SCT), in patients who will have been previously exposed to purine analog-based regimens and monoclonal antibodies, (2) incomplete data in the currently reported phase II studies with respect to prior sensitivity or resistance to purine analog- and/or monoclonal antibody-based treatment regimens, and (3) usually inclusion of both purine analog-sensitive and -resistant patients and/or alkylator-sensitive and -resistant patients in the same clinical trial.

Fludarabine (purine analog)-naïve or fludarabine (purine analog)-sensitive patients

Alkylating agents

Although retreatment of patients who have received prior therapy with an alkylating agent with an alkylator-based regimen may induce responses in 21–62% of patients, the quality of responses is poor (CR = 0–31%) and the duration of responses usually short (2–18 months).[90,147–150]

Purine analogs

Fludarabine

In the majority of patients who have failed therapy with an alkylator-based regimen, OR rates of 12–58% with CR rates of 0–26% can be obtained with single agent fludarabine.[151–156] OS strongly correlated with quality of response achieved (i.e., CR vs. PR vs. no response [NR]).[153,154] Long-term follow-up of 174 patients who received first-line therapy with single agent fludarabine indicated that 67% of patients who relapse will respond to salvage therapy with a fludarabine-based regimen, with 74% of patients responding to rechallenge with single-agent fludarabine.[85]

Several phase II studies have evaluated the efficacy of fludarabine in combination with alkylators (e.g., fludarabine and cyclophosphamide [FC]),[99,157–160] anthracyclines/anthraquinones (e.g., fludarabine and doxorubicin [FDox] or fludarabine and mitoxantrone [FM]),[106,161,162] both alkylators and anthracyclines/anthraquinones (e.g., fludarabine, cyclophosphamide, and mitoxantrone [FCM]),[163,164] or other nucleoside analogs. Therapy with FC yielded OR rates of 60–94% (CR = 10–29%) in previously treated patients, a proportion of whom had received prior fludarabine (14–79%).[99,157,158] Treatment with FDox[161] or FM[106] appears to yield inferior results compared to those obtained with FC. However, the majority (72–83%) of these patients had received prior fludarabine in contrast to patients treated with FC. Treatment with FCM appears to yield similar response rates in patients who have not received prior fludarabine, but may be associated with more myelosuppression.[163] While fludarabine, cytarabine (cytosine arabinoside; Ara-C), mitoxantrone, and dexamethasone (FAND) chemotherapy can induce CRs of 60% in previously treated patients (87% of whom had received prior fludarabine, with at least 19% being fludarabine-refractory), granulocyte colony-stimulating factor (G-CSF) was required to treat severe myelosuppression.[165]

Cladribine

Cladribine with or without corticosteroids can induce OR rates of 31–68% with CRs of 0–31% in previously treated patients with CLL.[111,166–169] These results appear to be comparable to single-agent fludarabine.

A small number of patients with CLL received therapy with cladribine and cyclophosphamide (2-CdA/C) or cladribine, cyclophosphamide, and mitoxantrone (2-CdA/CM).[170–172] Treatment with 2-CdA/C yielded OR rates of 45–62% (CR 8–15%),[170,172] which are similar to those obtained with FC therapy. Therapy with 2-CdA/CM appears to be inferior to both 2-CdA/C and FCM with an OR of only 37% (CR 5%) and median response duration of 5 months.[171]

Pentostatin

Minimal efficacy was seen when pentostatin monotherapy was used in previously treated patients with CLL (OR = 15–29%; CR = 0–8%).[113,173,174] However, 59% of the patients in at least one study had been exposed to prior fludarabine.[174] Twenty-one patients with CLL were treated with pentostatin plus cyclophosphamide (PC).[175] OR was 81% (CR 19%) with median response duration of only 7 months. Similar to what has been observed with fludarabine-based regimens, response to salvage therapy with cladribine- or pentostatin-based regimens appears to be affected by prior fludarabine exposure.

Rituximab

Rituximab induction therapy

Single-agent rituximab administered at the standard dose and schedule yielded unimpressive responses in previously treated CLL/SLL patients (OR = 0–35%; CR = 0%).[176–179] Alternative doses (up to 2250 mg/m^2 per week) and schedules of administration (thrice weekly) have improved response rates of single-agent rituximab therapy (OR 36% and 52% and CR 0% and 4%, respectively) with median TTP of 8–11 months.[180,181]

The combination of rituximab and HDMP or high-dose dexamethasone (HDD) can yield responses (OR = 75–93%; CR = 8–36%) in patients with relapsed or refractory CLL with tolerable side effects.[120–122,182] Rituximab was administered in combination with bendamustine (BR) to 81 patients with relapsed or refractory CLL.[129] Major toxicities included myelosuppression and infections. In the 62 evaluable patients, the OR rate was 77% (CR = 14%; PR = 63%). Inferior results were obtained when rituximab was combined with either pentostatin or cladribine.[183]

Fludarabine, cyclophosphamide, and rituximab (FCR) therapy has been evaluated in 143 previously treated patients with CLL.[184] An OR of 73% (CR = 25%; NPR = 16%; PR = 32%) was obtained. Twenty-five of 35 (71%) patients in CR had < 1% CD5+/CD19+ cells in the marrow by flow cytometry and 12 of 37 (32%) patients in CR achieved a molecular remission. With a follow-up of 28 months, the estimated median survival was 42 months. These results were compared to those seen in historical controls treated with FC and fludarabine with or without prednisone (F+/–P).[185] ORs and CRs for FC and F+/–P were 67% and 12% and 59% and 13%, respectively. Estimated median survival was 31 months and 19 months, respectively. Multivariate analysis showed that the FCR group had a significantly higher CR rate and longer survival compared to FC and F+/−P ($p = 0.0001$ and $p < 0.0001$, respectively). Median survival for the non-responders was similar for all three groups suggesting that improved supportive care over time did not have a major impact on survival.

A multicenter, phase III trial compared FCR with FC in 552 previously treated patients with CLL.[186] A median of one prior therapy had been administered, consisting of single-agent alkylator therapy (66%), single-agent purine analog (16%), or combination therapy (CHOP, COP, or fludarabine-containing; 18%). Patients with prior FC combination treatment or prior rituximab were not eligible. OR and CR rates were superior in the FCR arm compared to the FC arm (70% and 24% vs. 58% and 13%, respectively, $p \leq 0.0034$). PFS was significantly improved in the FCR arm (30.6 months vs. 20.6 months, $p = 0.0002$).

Therapy with pentostatin, cyclophosphamide, and rituximab (PCR) yielded OR rates of 75% (CR = 25%).[187] Median response duration and TTF were 25 months and 40 months, respectively. Median survival was 44 months. Although response frequencies were similar between patients treated with the PCR regimen and the PC regimen, response duration and OS with PCR appeared superior to results historically obtained with PC.[175,183] Results with PCR appear to be comparable to those obtained with FCR therapy, although a relatively small number of patients were treated with PCR compared to those treated with FCR.[184] Comparable OR rates (78%) were obtained with cladribine, cyclophosphamide, and rituximab (2-CdA/CR).[188]

Alemtuzumab

Alemtuzumab induction therapy

Alemtuzumab was initially approved by the US Food and Drug Administration (FDA) for the treatment of patients with refractory CLL.[191] The majority of these patients had advanced-stage disease, had received prior fludarabine (55–100%), and ≤3 prior therapies. Standard-dose alemtuzumab was administered intravenously in all except one study[189] until a maximum response was achieved or for a maximum of 12 weeks.[190–197] The OR rates were 31–70% with CRs of 0–30%. Patients were less likely to respond if they had high-risk disease, enlarged lymph nodes, especially > 5 cm in diameter, WHO performance status of 2, and > 5 prior therapeutic regimens. The higher quality of the responses (CR 30% and 36%, with no detectable bone marrow disease by immunophenotyping in 20% of patients) achieved in two trials may be due to differences in patient characteristics and the duration of therapy with alemtuzumab. Median OS was reported only in three studies and ranged from 16 months to 27.5 months. Median OS and treatment-free survival may be significantly longer for patients with MRD-negative CR compared to those achieving a MRD-positive CR, PR, or non-responders. Major toxicities were infusion-related, infections (including CMV reactivation), neutropenia, and thrombocytopenia.

Based on promising preliminary results with fludarabine and alemtuzumab in patients with fludarabine-refractory CLL,[197] the efficacy and safety of this combination was further evaluated in 36 patients with relapsed or refractory CLL.[198] Twenty-five percent were fludarabine-refractory. Most toxicities were infusion-related (predominantly with initial alemtuzumab doses); myelosuppression was also seen. The OR rate was 83% (CR = 30%; PR = 53%). With a median follow-up time of 15 months, the median OS for all patients was 35.6 months with a median TTP of 12.97 months.

In an attempt to improve upon results obtained with FCR in previously treated patients, alemtuzumab was added to the FCR regimen (CFAR).[135] Of 74 evaluable patients, the OR rate was 65% (CR = 24%; NPR = 3%; PR = 38%). Among the fludarabine-refractory patients, the OR rate was 51% (CR = 13%; PR = 38%). Responses were also observed in patients with unfavorable cytogenetics; 44% of patients with del(17p) responded. Estimated median TTP for all responders and OS for all patients were 26 months and 19 months, respectively. Toxicities included grade 3 or 4 neutropenia and thrombocytopenia. CMV reactivation occurred in 12 patients.

Three studies have evaluated the efficacy and safety of alemtuzumab combined with rituximab in patients with relapsed or refractory CLL (OR = 0–67%; CR = 0–44%).[199–202] Responses may be higher in patients who are not fludarabine/purine analog-refractory and have less advanced disease. CMV reactivation occurred in up to 27% of patients.

Fludarabine-refractory patients

Treatment of fludarabine-refractory patients has met with limited success. Furthermore, a significant proportion (40–89%) of these patients will develop serious infections.[203–205] Historically, OR rates of 22% (CR 1%) with a median survival of 10–13 months have been obtained after first salvage therapy with a variety of agents.[203–205]

The mechanisms implicated in resistance to purine analogs include (1) a low intracellular deoxycytidine kinase (dCK) to 5'-nucleotidase (5'NT) ratio leading to decreased phosphorylation of the purine analogs, (2) mutations, deletions, and/or epigenetic silencing via promoter methylation of the tumor suppressor protein p53 which is required for apoptosis, and (3) overexpression of the antiapoptotic *BCL2* family members which can impair p53 activity.[206]

Purine analogs

Cladribine

Although structurally similar, cladribine and fludarabine differ in their mechanism of inducing apoptosis. Unfortunately, this has not translated into clinical benefit for fludarabine-refractory patients.[207] In a very select group of fludarabine-refractory patients (i.e. intermediate stage, good baseline hematologic parameters, ≤3 prior types of therapy, ≤6 cycles of fludarabine), a modest response was seen (OR = 32%; CR = 0%) with an OS of 26 months with single-agent cladribine.[208] However, few patients will fulfill these characteristics, as demonstrated by an accrual time of 4 years for 28 patients.

Rituximab

The OFAR regimen, consisting of oxaliplatin, fludarabine, Ara-C, and rituximab, can induce responses in 33% of fludarabine-refractory patients (CR = 7%; PR = 27%), including those patients with 17p abnormalities.[209] The 6-month OS was 89%.

Alemtuzumab

Single-agent alemtuzumab given either intravenously or subcutaneously can induce OR rates of 31–46% (CR = 0–29%) in this group of patients.[189–194,210,211] Response duration ranged from 8.7 to 15.4 months[188] with reported median OS for all patients being 16–27.5 months.

In a small pilot trial of only six patients the combination of alemtuzumab and fludarabine (FCam) yielded responses even in patients refractory to single-agent alemtuzumab and single-agent fludarabine.[197] A phase II study conducted by the United Kingdom National Cancer Research Institute (NCRI) involving 50 patients with fludarabine-refractory CLL confirmed that OR rates of 45% (CR = 16%; PR = 29%) can be achieved with single-agent alemtuzumab; however, only 2 of 11 (18%) patients who were refractory to both fludarabine and single-agent alemtuzumab achieved a PR with oral fludarabine and subcutaneous alemtuzumab combination therapy.[212]

The combination of fludarabine, cyclophosphamide, alemtuzumab, and rituximab (CFAR) had activity in patients with fludarabine-refractory CLL (OR = 51%; CR = 13%; PR = 38%).[135] Responses were observed in patients who had previously been treated with FCR and FC combination chemotherapy.

Patients who are both fludarabine- and alemtuzumab-refractory (defined as failure to achieve a response following at least 8 weeks of single-agent alemtuzumab or an alemtuzumab-based regimen or disease progression within 3 months of completing therapy) have a poor outcome. Salvage therapy with a variety of agents induced OR rates of only 20% (CR 0%) with a median survival of 8 months.[213] Major infections occurred in 60% of patients during first salvage therapy.

Recently ofatumumab, a humanized antibody targeting CD20 at a different epitope from rituximab, produced a response rate of 58% in patients with CLL refractory to both fludarabine and alemtuzumab. Side effects were predominantly infusion-related and mild. The significant activity of this agent in a high-risk population led to FDA approval of ofatumumab in 2009.[214]

BCL2 family-targeted therapies

Oblimersen sodium

One of the mechanisms implicated in resistance to purine analogs is overexpression of the anti-apoptotic *BCL2* family members.[206] Therefore, in an attempt to reduce *BCL2* levels and render cells more susceptible to apoptosis-inducing agents, a randomized phase III trial evaluating FC with or without oblimersen sodium in 241 patients with relapsed or refractory CLL was conducted.[215] Oblimersen sodium (OBL) is a first-generation phosphorothioate antisense oligodeoxynucleotide of 18 nucleotides in length that is directed against the first six codons of the open reading frame of the *BCL2* mRNA.

The OR rate was similar for both groups. However, a higher proportion of patients who were treated with OBL-FC achieved a major response (i.e., CR or NPR [17% vs. 7%, respectively; $p = 0.025$]). For responders (i.e., CR or NPR), the median response duration was significantly shorter in the FC-only arm compared to the OBL-FC arm (20 months vs. not reached, respectively; $p = 0.002$). As observed for TTP, in patients achieving a response, the 5-year survival rates were 47% in the OBL-FC arm compared with 24% in the FC-only arm ($p = 0.038$).[216] Furthermore, among fludarabine-sensitive patients, the addition of OBL to FC chemotherapy resulted in a significant survival benefit ($p = 0.004$).

Hematopoietic stem cell transplantation

Autologous stem cell transplantation

The rationale behind autologous SCT (ASCT) is the linear dose efficacy observed with some chemotherapeutic agents, with higher doses resulting in higher tumor kill. However, limitations include potential for re-infusion of the tumor cells, development of secondary MDS, lack of graft-versus-leukemia (GVL) effect, and recent improvements in response rates and remission durations with chemoimmunotherapy alone.

Several randomized trials are underway comparing autotransplant to chemotherapy in previously untreated patients with advanced CLL (http://www.ebmt.org/5workingparties/clwp/clwp6.html).[217,218] Preliminary results from two of these trials in younger (i.e., < 60–66 years of age) patients with advanced CLL have been reported.[217,218] Only one reported event-free survival (EFS) outcomes in favor of autotransplant (median of 63.1 months vs. 23.6 months, respectively; $p < 0.001$) and none reported OS. Furthermore, up to 30% of patients did not receive the intended autotransplant.[218] Analysis of mutational *IGHV* status is ongoing for both trials, as it is unclear whether autologous SCT is superior to standard treatment, especially in patients at high risk, for example unmutated *IGHV* gene status.[219] Longer-term follow-up is required to determine impact of autotransplant in patients with advanced-stage and/or high-risk disease. Currently, the use of autotransplant is not recommended outside of a clinical trial.

Allogeneic stem cell transplantation

The underlying principles behind the application of allogeneic SCT are the higher antitumor activity with increased

Table 5.10. Selected non-myeloablative stem cell transplantation trials

Investigator, y (references)	Patient characteristics					Median F/U	Response and toxicity		
	Median age (y)	n	Time from diagnosis to SCT (range, mo)	Status prior to SCT (%)	MUD (%)		TRM (%)	Disease control	Overall survival
Dreger 2003 [237] (EBMTR)	54	77	49 (8–146)	CR (10); PR (55)	18	1.5 yr	TRM_{1yr} 18%	CR 69% PR 22% EFS_{2yr} 56%	OS_{2yr} 73%
Schetelig 2003 [241]	50	30[a]	48 (12–204)	Refractory (46)	50	2 yr	NRM_{2yr} 15%	CR 40% PR 53% PFS_{2yr} 67%	OS_{2yr} 72%
Khouri 2004 [229]	54	17	67 (22–168)	Refractory (53)	0	1.8 yr	0% at 100-day; TRM_{2yr} 22%	CR 71% PR 24% PFS_{2yr} 60%	OS_{2yr} 80%
Sorror 2005 [239]	56	64[b]	52.8 (7.2–300)	Refractory (53)	31	2 yr	NRM_{2y} 22%	CR 50% DFS_{2yr} 52%	OS_{2yr} 60%
Caballero 2005 [240]	53	30[c]	44 (6–201)	Refractory (20); CR (17); PR (63)	0	3.9 yr	$NRM_{5.7yr}$ 22%	DFS_{5yr} 93%	OS_{5yr} 72%
Schetelig 2004 [238]	54	20	NR	NR	80	1.1 yr	NR	PFS_{1yr} 50%	OS_{1yr} 75%
Brown 2005 [233]	53	50	76.8 (2.4–176.4)	Refractory (6); CR (16); PR (26)	62	1 yr[d]	NR	PFS_{2yr} 28%[d]	OS_{2yr} 48%[d]
Delgado 2006 [230]	54	41	54 (10–164)	Refractory (17); CR (12); PR (70)	42	1.2 yr	5% at 100-day; TRM_{2yr} 26%	PFS_{2yr} 45%	OS_{2y} 51%
Michallet 2006 [225] (SFGM-TC)	49[e]	158[e]	51[e]	CR + PR (51)[e]	89[e]	40 mo[e]	NRM_{1yr} 29% [e]	NR[e]	OS_{8yr} 35%[e]
Brown 2008 [232]	55	62	NR	CR + PR (56)	66	3.3 yr	TRM_{3yr} 15%	PFS_{3yr} 54%	OS_{3yr} 65%

Notes: [a]Includes 1 patient with PLL.
[b]Includes patients with CLL/SLL (n = 5) and CLL/PLL (n = 3)
[c]Includes 2 patients with Richter's syndrome.
[d]Surviving patients only (n = 31).
[e]Includes 73 patients who received NMA SCT.
EBMTR: European Bone Marrow Transplant Registry; MUD: matched unrelated donor; F/U: follow-up; TRM: treatment-related mortality; NRM: non-relapse mortality; NR: not reported.

doses of chemotherapy, the GVL effect, and the lack of stem cell contamination. However, allogeneic SCT is associated with morbidity and mortality due to toxicities from the conditioning regimen, the presence of graft-versus-host disease (GVHD), and infectious complications. Furthermore, feasibility is limited by age restrictions and donor availability. As first-degree relatives of patients with CLL may harbor a monoclonal population of B cells with a CLL-like immunophenotype,[25,26] all potential HLA-identical related donors should have peripheral blood evaluated by flow cytometry.

In contrast to ASCT, allotransplant is associated with a plateau in disease-free survival (DFS) and OS,[220–225] suggesting that allotransplantation may be curative for some patients. Allogeneic SCT may also be superior to standard treatment and/or autotransplant in patients with CLL and an unmutated *IGHV* gene status or 17p deletion.[226,227] Recent data suggest that patients with negative MRD status have an improved survival compared to those with MRD-positivity.[195] However, it is unclear whether allergenic SCT offers any additional benefit to patients who have already achieved MRD-negativity after chemoimmunotherapy.[226] There are no published randomized trials comparing allogeneic SCT to standard chemotherapy and/or ASCT in patients with CLL. The optimal source of stem cells (i.e., bone marrow versus peripheral blood), the best conditioning regimen, the timing of the transplant, and patient selection remain to be defined.

Non-myeloablative stem cell transplantation

Non-myeloablative (NMA) allogeneic SCT was developed in order to minimize the toxicity of the preparative regimen and to exploit the potential for immune-mediated GVL effect. The low-dose NMA preparative regimen (often fludarabine-based) is designed not to eradicate the leukemia but to provide sufficient immunosuppression to allow engraftment of donor stem cells and development of a GVL effect. This strategy allows for treatment of patients who are older and/or have comorbidities that prevent use of standard, ablative conditioning regimens.

Although follow-up is relatively short, NMA SCT is associated with a much lower cumulative and 100-day transplant-related mortality (TRM) compared with myeloablative SCTs (16–26% and 0–5%, respectively, vs. 38–50%, and 11–29%, respectively), but potentially higher relapse rates (Table 5.10).[220–222,224,225,228–232] However, the incidences of grade 2 to 4 acute GVHD and chronic GVHD appear to be comparable in patients receiving either NMA or myeloablative SCTs (9–63% and 33–75%, respectively, vs. 37–56% and 40–85%, respectively).[220,224,228–230,233–238] Data suggest NMA SCT may overcome the negative prognostic impact of ZAP-70-positivity, unmutated *IGHV* gene status, and/or chromosomal abnormalities.[240–242] The optimal conditioning regimen and strategy for prophylaxis of GVHD are unknown. Longer follow-up is required to determine if remissions are durable, whether rates of relapse or disease progression are comparable to those achieved with myeloablative SCT, and whether the use of donor leukocyte infusions (DLIs) to either achieve full donor chimerism or control disease post-transplant is effective. In view of these uncertainties, NMA SCTs should be performed in the context of a clinical trial.

Conclusions

Significant changes in the understanding and management of CLL have occurred in the last two decades. With the advent of newer treatment modalities, such as purine chemoimmunotherapy, substantial improvements have been made in achieving CRs, with a proportion of patients achieving molecular remissions and durable responses, which may translate into prolonged survival for these patients. Several questions remain unanswered in patients with symptomatic previously untreated CLL, including (1) the value of new prognostic testing in guiding initial therapy, (2) the optimal first-line therapy, (3) the role of maintenance therapy, and (4) the role of allogeneic SCT. Furthermore, despite the advances made in the understanding and treatment of CLL, the majority of patients will relapse after initial therapy. There is a paucity of data to guide choice of appropriate salvage therapy in patients with relapsed or refractory CLL.

Also, prior to the development of the revised IWCLL-NCI-WG guidelines, there was no widely accepted definition for relapsed and refractory CLL. This lack of a standardized definition for relapse or refractory disease has impeded comparability between studies and the evaluation of the clinical significance of new therapeutic agents.

Allogeneic myeloablative and NMA SCT may be reasonable and feasible options in the setting of patients with relapsed and/or refractory CLL. However, responses and remission durations are not satisfactory with the currently available salvage therapies. Novel agents need to be evaluated and newer treatment strategies need to be developed in order to circumvent or overcome resistance, optimize responses, and potentially cure CLL. In the absence of data to guide salvage therapy in these patients, enrollment onto a clinical trial should be considered.

References

1. Diehl LF, Karnell LH, Menck HR. The American College of Surgeons Commission on Cancer and the American Cancer Society. The National Cancer Data Base report on age, gender, treatment, and outcomes of patients with chronic lymphocytic leukemia. *Cancer* 1999;**86**:2684–92.
2. Group USCSW. *United States Cancer Statistics: 2000 Incidence*. Atlanta, GA, Department of Health and Human Services, Centers for Disease Control and Prevention and National Cancer Institute, 2003.
3. Jaffe ES, Harris N, Stein H, *et al.* (eds.) *World Health Organization Classification of Tumours: Pathology and Genetics of Tumours of Haematopoietic and Lymphoid Tissues*. Lyon, France, IARC Press, 2001.
4. Jemal A, Clegg LX, Ward E, *et al.* Annual report to the nation on the status of cancer, 1975–2001, with a special feature regarding survival. *Cancer* 2004;**101**:3–27.
5. Cheson BD, Bennett JM, Grever M, *et al.* National Cancer Institute-sponsored Working Group guidelines for chronic lymphocytic leukemia: revised guidelines for diagnosis and treatment. *Blood* 1996;**87**:4990–7.
6. Binet JL, Caligaris-Cappio F, Catovsky D, *et al.* Perspectives on the use of new diagnostic tools in the treatment of chronic lymphocytic leukemia. *Blood* 2006;**107**:859–61.
7. Harris NL, Jaffe ES, Stein H, *et al.* A revised European-American

classification of lymphoid neoplasms: a proposal from the International Lymphoma Study Group. *Blood* 1994;**84**:1361–92.

8. Geisler CH, Larsen JK, Hansen NE, *et al.* Prognostic importance of flow cytometric immunophenotyping of 540 consecutive patients with B-cell chronic lymphocytic leukemia. *Blood* 1991;**78**:1795–802.
9. Monaghan SA, Peterson LC, James C, *et al.* Pan B-cell markers are not redundant in analysis of chronic lymphocytic leukemia (CLL). *Cytometry B Clin Cytom* 2003;**56**:30–42.
10. Criel A, Michaux L, De Wolf-Peeters C. The concept of typical and atypical chronic lymphocytic leukemia. *Leuk Lymphoma* 1999;**33**:33–45.
11. Kurec AS, Threatte GA, Gottlieb AJ, *et al.* Immunophenotypic subclassification of chronic lymphocytic leukemia (CLL). *Br J Haematol* 1992;**81**:45–51.
12. Moreau EJ, Matutes E, A'Hern RP, *et al.* Improvement of the chronic lymphocytic leukemia scoring system with the monoclonal antibody SN8 (CD79b). *Am J Clin Pathol* 1997;**108**:378–82.
13. Matutes E, Polliack A. Morphological and immunophenotypic features of chronic lymphocytic leukemia. *Rev Clin Exp Hematol* 2000;**4**:22–47.
14. Oscier D, Fegan C, Hillmen P, *et al.* Guidelines on the diagnosis and management of chronic lymphocytic leukemia. *Br J Haematol* 2004; **125**:294–317.
15. Gascoyne RD. Differential diagnosis of the chronic B-cell lymphoid leukemias. In: Cheson BD, ed. *Chronic Lymphoid Leukemias*, 2nd edn. New York, Marcel Dekker Inc. 2001; 209–30.
16. Rozman C, Montserrat E, Vinolas N. Serum immunoglobulins in B-chronic lymphocytic leukemia. Natural history and prognostic significance. *Cancer* 1988;**61**:279–83.
17. DiGiuseppe JA, Borowitz MJ. Clinical utility of flow cytometry in the chronic lymphoid leukemias. *Semin Oncol* 1998;**25**:6–10.
18. Johnston JB. Chronic lymphocytic leukemia. In: Greer JP, Foerster JF, Lukens JN, *et al.*, eds. *Wintrobe's Clinical Hematology* Vol. 2, 11th edn. Philadelphia, PA, Lippincott Williams & Wilkins. 2004; 2429–63.
19. Marti GE, Rawstron AC, Ghia P, *et al.* Diagnostic criteria for monoclonal B-cell lymphocytosis. *Br J Haematol* 2005;**130**:325–32.
20. Marti G, Abbasi F, Raveche E, *et al.* Overview of monoclonal B-cell lymphocytosis. *Br J Haematol* 2007;**139**:701–8.
21. Rawstron AC, Green MJ, Kuzmicki A, *et al.* Monoclonal B lymphocytes with the characteristics of "indolent" chronic lymphocytic leukemia are present in 3.5% of adults with normal blood counts. *Blood* 2002;**100**:635–9.
22. Rossi D, Sozzi E, Puma A, *et al.* The prognosis of clinical monoclonal B cell lymphocytosis differs from prognosis of Rai 0 chronic lymphocytic leukemia and is recapitulated by biological risk factors. *Br J Haematol* 2009;**146**:64–75.
23. Ghia P, Prato G, Scielzo C, *et al.* Monoclonal CD5+ and CD5- B-lymphocyte expansions are frequent in the peripheral blood of the elderly. *Blood* 2004;**103**:2337–42.
24. Rawstron AC, Bennett FL, O'Connor SJ, *et al.* Monoclonal B-cell lymphocytosis and chronic lymphocytic leukemia. *N Engl J Med* 2008;**359**: 575–83.
25. Rawstron AC, Yuille MR, Fuller J, *et al.* Inherited predisposition to CLL is detectable as subclinical monoclonal B-lymphocyte expansion. *Blood* 2002;**100**:2289–90.
26. Marti GE, Carter P, Abbasi F, *et al.* B-cell monoclonal lymphocytosis and B-cell abnormalities in the setting of familial B-cell chronic lymphocytic leukemia. *Cytometry B Clin Cytom* 2003;**52**:1–12.
27. Rai KR, Sawitsky A, Cronkite EP, *et al.* Clinical staging of chronic lymphocytic leukemia. *Blood* 1975;**46**:219–34.
28. Binet JL, Auquier A, Dighiero G, *et al.* A new prognostic classification of chronic lymphocytic leukemia derived from a multivariate survival analysis. *Cancer* 1981;**48**:198–206.
29. Dighiero G, Maloum K, Desablens B, *et al.* Chlorambucil in indolent chronic lymphocytic leukemia. French Cooperative Group on Chronic Lymphocytic Leukemia. *N Engl J Med* 1998;**338**:1506–14.
30. Shanafelt TD, Geyer SM, Kay NE. Prognosis at diagnosis: integrating molecular biologic insights into clinical practice for patients with CLL. *Blood* 2004;**103**:1202–10.
31. Melo JV, Catovsky D, Gregory WM, *et al.* The relationship between chronic lymphocytic leukaemia and prolymphocytic leukaemia. IV. Analysis of survival and prognostic features. *Br J Haematol* 1987;**65**:23–9.
32. Zenz T, Krober A, Scherer K, *et al.* Monoallelic TP53 inactivation is associated with poor prognosis in chronic lymphocytic leukemia: results from a detailed genetic characterization with long-term follow-up. *Blood* 2008;**112**:3322–9.
33. Hallek M, Langenmayer I, Nerl C, *et al.* Elevated serum thymidine kinase levels identify a subgroup at high risk of disease progression in early, nonsmoldering chronic lymphocytic leukemia. *Blood* 1999;**93**:1732–7.
34. Reinisch W, Willheim M, Hilgarth M, *et al.* Soluble CD23 reliably reflects disease activity in B-cell chronic lymphocytic leukemia. *J Clin Oncol* 1994;**12**:2146–52.
35. Sarfati M, Chevret S, Chastang C, *et al.* Prognostic importance of serum soluble CD23 level in chronic lymphocytic leukemia. *Blood* 1996;**88**:4259–64.
36. Wierda WG, O'Brien S, Wang X, *et al.* Prognostic nomogram and index for overall survival in previously untreated patients with chronic lymphocytic leukemia. *Blood* 2007;**109**:4679–85.
37. Wierda WG, O'Brien S, Wang X, *et al.* Characteristics associated with important clinical end points in patients with chronic lymphocytic leukemia at initial treatment. *J Clin Oncol* 2009;**27**:1637–43.
38. Magnac C, Porcher R, Davi F, *et al.* Predictive value of serum thymidine kinase level for Ig-V mutational status in B-CLL. *Leukemia* 2003;**17**:133–7.
39. Matthews C, Catherwood MA, Morris TC, *et al.* Serum TK levels in CLL identify Binet stage A patients within biologically defined prognostic subgroups most likely to undergo disease progression. *Eur J Haematol* 2006;**77**:309–17.
40. Montserrat E, Sanchez-Bisono J, Vinolas N, *et al.* Lymphocyte doubling time in chronic lymphocytic leukaemia: analysis of its prognostic significance. *Br J Haematol* 1986;**62**:567–75.
41. Molica S, Alberti A. Prognostic value of the lymphocyte doubling time in

chronic lymphocytic leukemia. *Cancer* 1987;**60**:2712–6.

42. Vallespi T, Montserrat E, Sanz MA. Chronic lymphocytic leukaemia: prognostic value of lymphocyte morphological subtypes. A multivariate survival analysis in 146 patients. *Br J Haematol* 1991;**77**:478–85.
43. Dhodapkar M, Tefferi A, Su J, *et al.* Prognostic features and survival in young adults with early/intermediate chronic lymphocytic leukemia (B-CLL): a single institution study. *Leukemia* 1993;**7**:1232–5.
44. Molica S, Reverter JC, Alberti A, *et al.* Timing of diagnosis and lymphocyte accumulation patterns in chronic lymphocytic leukemia: analysis of their clinical significance. *Eur J Haematol* 1990;**44**:277–81.
45. Bergmann MA, Eichhorst BF, Busch R, *et al.* Prospective evaluation of prognostic parameters in early stage chronic lymphocytic leukemia (CLL): results of the CLL1-protocol of the German CLL Study Group (GCLLSG). *Blood* 2007;**110**:193a.
46. Shanafelt TD, Jenkins G, Call TG, *et al.* Validation of a new prognostic index for patients with chronic lymphocytic leukemia. *Cancer* 2009;**115**:363–72.
47. Juliusson G, Merup M. Cytogenetics in chronic lymphocytic leukemia. *Semin Oncol* 1998;**25**:19–26.
48. Dohner H, Stilgenbauer S, Benner A, *et al.* Genomic aberrations and survival in chronic lymphocytic leukemia. *N Engl J Med* 2000;**343**:1910–16.
49. Tam CS, Shanafelt TD, Wierda WG, *et al.* De novo deletion 17p13.1 chronic lymphocytic leukemia shows significant clinical heterogeneity: the MD Anderson and Mayo Clinic experience. *Blood* 2009;**114**:957–64.
50. Mayr C, Speicher MR, Kofler DM, *et al.* Chromosomal translocations are associated with poor prognosis in chronic lymphocytic leukemia. *Blood* 2006;**107**:742–51.
51. Haferlach C, Dicker F, Schnittger S, *et al.* Comprehensive genetic characterization of CLL: a study on 506 cases analysed with chromosome banding analysis, interphase FISH, IgV (H) status and immunophenotyping. *Leukemia* 2007;**21**:2442–51.
52. Stilgenbauer S, Sander S, Bullinger L, *et al.* Clonal evolution in chronic lymphocytic leukemia: acquisition of high-risk genomic aberrations associated with unmutated VH, resistance to therapy, and short survival. *Haematologica* 2007;**92**:1242–5.
53. Shanafelt TD, Witzig TE, Fink SR, *et al.* Prospective evaluation of clonal evolution during long-term follow-up of patients with untreated early-stage chronic lymphocytic leukemia. *J Clin Oncol* 2006;**24**:4634–41.
54. Krober A, Seiler T, Benner A, *et al.* V (H) mutation status, CD38 expression level, genomic aberrations, and survival in chronic lymphocytic leukemia. *Blood* 2002;**100**:1410–16.
55. Hamblin TJ, Davis Z, Gardiner A, *et al.* Unmutated Ig V(H) genes are associated with a more aggressive form of chronic lymphocytic leukemia. *Blood* 1999;**94**:1848–54.
56. Damle RN, Wasil T, Fais F, *et al.* Ig V gene mutation status and CD38 expression as novel prognostic indicators in chronic lymphocytic leukemia. *Blood* 1999;**94**:1840–7.
57. Vasconcelos Y, Davi F, Levy V, *et al.* Binet's staging system and VH genes are independent but complementary prognostic indicators in chronic lymphocytic leukemia. *J Clin Oncol* 2003;**21**:3928–32.
58. Lin K, Sherrington PD, Dennis M, *et al.* Relationship between p53 dysfunction, CD38 expression, and IgV(H) mutation in chronic lymphocytic leukemia. *Blood* 2002;**100**:1404–9.
59. Tobin G, Thunberg U, Johnson A, *et al.* Somatically mutated Ig V(H)3–21 genes characterize a new subset of chronic lymphocytic leukemia. *Blood* 2002;**99**:2262–4.
60. Thorselius M, Krober A, Murray F, *et al.* Strikingly homologous immunoglobulin gene rearrangements and poor outcome in VH3–21-using chronic lymphocytic leukemia patients independent of geographic origin and mutational status. *Blood* 2006;**107**:2889–94.
61. Oscier DG, Gardiner AC, Mould SJ, *et al.* Multivariate analysis of prognostic factors in CLL: clinical stage, IGVH gene mutational status, and loss or mutation of the p53 gene are independent prognostic factors. *Blood* 2002;**100**:1177–84.
62. Byrd JC, Gribben JG, Peterson BL, *et al.* Select high-risk genetic features predict earlier progression following chemoimmunotherapy with fludarabine and rituximab in chronic lymphocytic leukemia: justification for risk-adapted therapy. *J Clin Oncol* 2006;**24**:437–43.
63. Grever MR, Lucas DM, Dewald GW, *et al.* Comprehensive assessment of genetic and molecular features predicting outcome in patients with chronic lymphocytic leukemia: results from the US Intergroup Phase III Trial E2997. *J Clin Oncol* 2007;**25**:799–804.
64. Lin KI, Tam CS, Keating MJ, *et al.* Relevance of the immunoglobulin VH somatic mutation status in patients with chronic lymphocytic leukemia treated with fludarabine, cyclophosphamide, and rituximab (FCR) or related chemoimmunotherapy regimens. *Blood* 2009;**113**:3168–71.
65. Hamblin TJ, Orchard JA, Ibbotson RE, *et al.* CD38 expression and immunoglobulin variable region mutations are independent prognostic variables in chronic lymphocytic leukemia, but CD38 expression may vary during the course of the disease. *Blood* 2002;**99**:1023–9.
66. Thunberg U, Johnson A, Roos G, *et al.* CD38 expression is a poor predictor for VH gene mutational status and prognosis in chronic lymphocytic leukemia. *Blood* 2001;**97**:1892–4.
67. Gentile M, Mauro FR, Calabrese E, *et al.* The prognostic value of CD38 expression in chronic lymphocytic leukaemia patients studied prospectively at diagnosis: a single institute experience. *Br J Haematol* 2005;**130**:549–57.
68. Rosenwald A, Alizadeh AA, Widhopf G, *et al.* Relation of gene expression phenotype to immunoglobulin mutation genotype in B cell chronic lymphocytic leukemia. *J Exp Med* 2001;**194**:1639–47.
69. Klein U, Tu Y, Stolovitzky GA, *et al.* Gene expression profiling of B cell chronic lymphocytic leukemia reveals a homogeneous phenotype related to memory B cells. *J Exp Med* 2001;**194**:1625–38.
70. Chen L, Apgar J, Huynh L, *et al.* ZAP-70 directly enhances IgM signaling in chronic lymphocytic leukemia. *Blood* 2005;**105**:2036–41.
71. Orchard JA, Ibbotson RE, Davis Z, *et al.* ZAP-70 expression and prognosis in

chronic lymphocytic leukaemia. *Lancet* 2004;**363**:105–11.

72. Rassenti LZ, Huynh L, Toy TL, *et al.* ZAP-70 compared with immunoglobulin heavy-chain gene mutation status as a predictor of disease progression in chronic lymphocytic leukemia. *N Engl J Med* 2004;**351**: 893–901.

73. Crespo M, Bosch F, Villamor N, *et al.* ZAP-70 expression as a surrogate for immunoglobulin-variable-region mutations in chronic lymphocytic leukemia. *N Engl J Med* 2003;**348**: 1764–75.

74. Wiestner A, Rosenwald A, Barry TS, *et al.* ZAP-70 expression identifies a chronic lymphocytic leukemia subtype with unmutated immunoglobulin genes, inferior clinical outcome, and distinct gene expression profile. *Blood* 2003;**101**:4944–51.

75. Orchard J, Ibbotson R, Best G, *et al.* ZAP-70 in B cell malignancies. *Leuk Lymphoma* 2005;**46**:1689–98.

76. Kay S, Herishanu Y, Pick M, *et al.* Quantitative flow cytometry of ZAP-70 levels in chronic lymphocytic leukemia using molecules of equivalent soluble fluorochrome. *Cytometry B Clin Cytom* 2006;**70**:218–26.

77. Van Bockstaele F, Verhasselt B, Philippe J. Prognostic markers in chronic lymphocytic leukemia: a comprehensive review. *Blood Rev* 2009;**23**:25–47.

78. Kay NE, O'Brien SM, Pettitt AR, *et al.* The role of prognostic factors in assessing 'high-risk' subgroups of patients with chronic lymphocytic leukemia. *Leukemia* 2007;**21**:1885–91.

79. Stilgenbauer S, Kröber A, Busch R, *et al.* 17p deletion predicts for inferior overall survival after fludarabine-based first line therapy in chronic lymphocytic leukemia: first analysis of genetics in the CLL4 trial of the GCLLSG. *Blood* 2005;**106**:212a.

80. Eichhorst B, Hallek M. Revision of the guidelines for diagnosis and therapy of chronic lymphocytic leukemia (CLL). *Best Pract Res Clin Haematol* 2007;**20**:469–77.

81. Hallek M, Cheson BD, Catovsky D, *et al.* Guidelines for the diagnosis and treatment of chronic lymphocytic leukemia: a report from the International Workshop on Chronic Lymphocytic Leukemia updating the National Cancer Institute-Working Group 1996 guidelines. *Blood* 2008;**111**:5446–56.

82. Bottcher S, Ritgen M, Pott C, *et al.* Comparative analysis of minimal residual disease detection using four-color flow cytometry, consensus IgH-PCR, and quantitative IgH PCR in CLL after allogeneic and autologous stem cell transplantation. *Leukemia* 2004;**18**:1637–45.

83. Moreno C, Villamor N, Colomer D, *et al.* Clinical significance of minimal residual disease, as assessed by different techniques, after stem cell transplantation for chronic lymphocytic leukemia. *Blood* 2006;**107**:4563–9.

84. Rawstron AC, Villamor N, Ritgen M, *et al.* International standardized approach for flow cytometric residual disease monitoring in chronic lymphocytic leukaemia. *Leukemia* 2007;**21**:956–64.

85. Keating MJ, O'Brien S, Lerner S, *et al.* Long-term follow-up of patients with chronic lymphocytic leukemia (CLL) receiving fludarabine regimens as initial therapy. *Blood* 1998;**92**:1165–71.

86. Chemotherapeutic options in chronic lymphocytic leukemia: a meta-analysis of the randomized trials. CLL Trialists' Collaborative Group. *J Natl Cancer Inst* 1999;**91**:861–8.

87. Knauf WU, Lissichkov T, Aldaoud A, *et al.* Bendamustine versus chlorambucil in treatment-naive patients with B-cell chronic lymphocytic leukemia (B-CLL): results of an international phase III study. *Blood* 2007;**110**:609a.

88. Knauf WU, Lissichkov T, Aldaoud A, *et al.* Bendamustine versus chlorambucil as first-line treatment in B cell chronic lymphocytic leukemia: an updated analysis from an international phase III study. *J Clin Oncol* 2009;**27**:4378–84.

89. Leporrier M, Chevret S, Cazin B, *et al.* Randomized comparison of fludarabine, CAP, and CHOP in 938 previously untreated stage B and C chronic lymphocytic leukemia patients. *Blood* 2001;**98**:2319–25.

90. Johnson S, Smith AG, Loffler H, *et al.* Multicentre prospective randomised trial of fludarabine versus cyclophosphamide, doxorubicin, and prednisone (CAP) for treatment of advanced-stage chronic lymphocytic leukaemia. The French Cooperative Group on CLL. *Lancet* 1996;**347**: 1432–8.

91. Rai KR, Peterson BL, Appelbaum FR, *et al.* Fludarabine compared with chlorambucil as primary therapy for chronic lymphocytic leukemia. *N Engl J Med* 2000;**343**:1750–7.

92. Eichhorst BF, Busch R, Stauch M, *et al.* No significant clinical benefit of first line therapy with fludarabine (F) in comparison to chlorambucil (Clb) in elderly patients (pts) with advanced chronic lymphocytic leukemia (CLL): results of a phase III study of the German CLL Study Group (GCLLSG). *Blood* 2007;**110**:194–2.

93. Catovsky D, Richards S, Matutes E, *et al.* Assessment of fludarabine plus cyclophosphamide for patients with chronic lymphocytic leukaemia (the LRF CLL4 Trial): a randomised controlled trial. *Lancet* 2007;**370**:230–9.

94. Eichhorst BF, Busch R, Hopfinger G, *et al.* Fludarabine plus cyclophosphamide versus fludarabine alone in first-line therapy of younger patients with chronic lymphocytic leukemia. *Blood* 2006;**107**:885–91.

95. Flinn IW, Neuberg DS, Grever MR, *et al.* Phase III trial of fludarabine plus cyclophosphamide compared with fludarabine for patients with previously untreated chronic lymphocytic leukemia: US Intergroup Trial E2997. *J Clin Oncol* 2007;**25**:793–8.

96. Rummel MJ, Stilgenbauer S, Gamm H, *et al.* Fludarabine versus fludarabine plus epirubicin in the treatment of chronic lymphocytic leukemia – final results of a German randomized phase-III study. *Blood* 2005;**106**:600a.

97. Weiss MA, Glenn M, Maslak P, *et al.* Consolidation therapy with high-dose cyclophosphamide improves the quality of response in patients with chronic lymphocytic leukemia treated with fludarabine as induction therapy. *Leukemia* 2000;**14**:1577–82.

98. Cazin B, Divine M, Lepretre S, *et al.* High efficacy with five days schedule of oral fludarabine phosphate and cyclophosphamide in patients with previously untreated chronic lymphocytic leukaemia. *Br J Haematol* 2008;**143**:54–9.

99. O'Brien SM, Kantarjian HM, Cortes J, *et al.* Results of the fludarabine and cyclophosphamide combination

regimen in chronic lymphocytic leukemia. *J Clin Oncol* 2001; **19**:1414–20.

100. Keating MJ, O'Brien S, Albitar M, *et al.* Early results of a chemoimmunotherapy regimen of fludarabine, cyclophosphamide, and rituximab as initial therapy for chronic lymphocytic leukemia. *J Clin Oncol* 2005;**23**:4079–88.
101. Morrison VA, Rai KR, Peterson BL, *et al.* Impact of therapy with chlorambucil, fludarabine, or fludarabine plus chlorambucil on infections in patients with chronic lymphocytic leukemia: Intergroup Study Cancer and Leukemia Group B 9011. *J Clin Oncol* 2001; **19**:3611–21.
102. Morrison VA, Rai KR, Peterson BL, *et al.* Therapy-related myeloid leukemias are observed in patients with chronic lymphocytic leukemia after treatment with fludarabine and chlorambucil: results of an intergroup study, cancer and leukemia group B 9011. *J Clin Oncol* 2002;**20**:3878–84.
103. Tefferi A, Levitt R, Li CY, *et al.* Phase II study of 2-chlorodeoxyadenosine in combination with chlorambucil in previously untreated B-cell chronic lymphocytic leukemia. *Am J Clin Oncol* 1999;**22**:509–16.
104. Tefferi A, Li CY, Reeder CB, *et al.* A phase II study of sequential combination chemotherapy with cyclophosphamide, prednisone, and 2-chlorodeoxyadenosine in previously untreated patients with chronic lymphocytic leukemia. *Leukemia* 2001;**15**:1171–5.
105. Tam CS, O'Brien S, Wierda W, *et al.* Long-term results of the fludarabine, cyclophosphamide, and rituximab regimen as initial therapy of chronic lymphocytic leukemia. *Blood* 2008;**112**:975–80.
106. Tsimberidou AM, Keating MJ, Giles FJ, *et al.* Fludarabine and mitoxantrone for patients with chronic lymphocytic leukemia. *Cancer* 2004;**100**:2583–91.
107. Bosch F, Ferrer A, Villamor N, *et al.* Fludarabine, cyclophosphamide, and mitoxantrone as initial therapy of chronic lymphocytic leukemia: high response rate and disease eradication. *Clin Cancer Res* 2008;**14**:155–61.
108. Saven A, Lemon RH, Kosty M, *et al.* 2-Chlorodeoxyadenosine activity in patients with untreated chronic lymphocytic leukemia. *J Clin Oncol* 1995;**13**:570–4.
109. Robak T, Blonski JZ, Kasznicki M, *et al.* Cladribine with prednisone versus chlorambucil with prednisone as first-line therapy in chronic lymphocytic leukemia: report of a prospective, randomized, multicenter trial. *Blood* 2000;**96**:2723–9.
110. Robak T, Blonski JZ, Gora-Tybor J, *et al.* Cladribine alone and in combination with cyclophosphamide or cyclophosphamide plus mitoxantrone in the treatment of progressive chronic lymphocytic leukemia: report of a prospective, multicenter, randomized trial of the Polish Adult Leukemia Group (PALG CLL2). *Blood* 2006;**108**:473–9.
111. Robak T, Blonski JZ, Kasznicki M, *et al.* Cladribine with or without prednisone in the treatment of previously treated and untreated B-cell chronic lymphocytic leukaemia – updated results of the multicentre study of 378 patients. *Br J Haematol* 2000;**108**:357–68.
112. Karlsson KA, Strömberg M, Jönsson V, *et al.* Cladribine (CdA) gives longer response duration than fludarabine (F) and high-dose intermittent chlorambucil (Chl) as first-line treatment of symptomatic chronic lymphocytic leukemia (CLL). First results from the international randomized phase III trial. *Blood* 2007;**110**:194a.
113. Dillman RO, Mick R, McIntyre OR. Pentostatin in chronic lymphocytic leukemia: a phase II trial of Cancer and Leukemia group B. *J Clin Oncol* 1989;**7**:433–8.
114. Hainsworth JD, Burris HA 3rd, Morrissey LH, *et al.* Rituximab monoclonal antibody as initial systemic therapy for patients with low-grade non-Hodgkin lymphoma. *Blood* 2000;**95**:3052–6.
115. Hainsworth JD, Litchy S, Barton JH, *et al.* Single-agent rituximab as first-line and maintenance treatment for patients with chronic lymphocytic leukemia or small lymphocytic lymphoma: a phase II trial of the Minnie Pearl Cancer Research Network. *J Clin Oncol* 2003;**21**:1746–51.
116. Thomas DA, O'Brien S, Giles FJ, *et al.* Single agent rituxan in early stage chronic lymphocytic leukemia (CLL). *Blood* 2001;**98**:364a.
117. Bosanquet AG, McCann SR, Crotty GM, *et al.* Methylprednisolone in advanced chronic lymphocytic leukaemia: rationale for, and effectiveness of treatment suggested by DiSC assay. *Acta Haematol* 1995;**93**:73–9.
118. Thornton PD, Hamblin M, Treleaven JG, *et al.* High dose methyl prednisolone in refractory chronic lymphocytic leukaemia. *Leuk Lymphoma* 1999;**34**:167–70.
119. Thornton PD, Matutes E, Bosanquet AG, *et al.* High dose methylprednisolone can induce remissions in CLL patients with p53 abnormalities. *Ann Hematol* 2003;**82**:759–65.
120. Castro JE, Sandoval-Sus JD, Bole J, *et al.* Rituximab in combination with high-dose methylprednisolone for the treatment of fludarabine refractory high-risk chronic lymphocytic leukemia. *Leukemia* 2008;**22**:2048–53.
121. Bowen DA, Call TG, Jenkins GD, *et al.* Methylprednisolone-rituximab is an effective salvage therapy for patients with relapsed chronic lymphocytic leukemia including those with unfavorable cytogenetic features. *Leuk Lymphoma* 2007;**48**:2412–17.
122. Dungarwalla M, Evans SO, Riley U, *et al.* High dose methylprednisolone and rituximab is an effective therapy in advanced refractory chronic lymphocytic leukemia resistant to fludarabine therapy. *Haematologica* 2008;**93**:475–6.
123. O'Brien S, Wierda WG, Faderl S, *et al.* FCR-3 as frontline therapy for patients with chronic lymphocytic leukemia (CLL). *Blood* 2005;**106**:599a.
124. Hallek M, Fingerle-Rowson G, Fink A-M, *et al.* Immunochemotherapy with fludarabine (F), cyclophosphamide (C), and rituximab (R) (FCR) versus fludarabine and cyclophosphamide (FC) improves response rates and progression-free survival (PFS) of previously untreated patients (pts) with advanced chronic lymphocytic leukemia (CLL). *Blood* 2008;**112**:
125. Stilgenbauer S, Zenz T, Winkler D, *et al.* Genomic aberrations, VH mutation status and outcome after fludarabine and cyclophosphamide (FC) or FC plus rituximab (FCR) in the CLL8 trial. *Blood* 2008;**112**:
126. Hallek M, Fingerle-Rowson G, Fink A-M, *et al.* First-line treatment with

fludarabine (F), cyclophosphamide (C), and rituximab (R) (FCR) improves overall survival (OS) in previously untreated patients (pts) with advanced chronic lymphocytic leukemia (CLL): results of a randomized phase III trial on behalf of an international group of investigators and the German CLL Study Group. *Blood* 2009;**144**: 223–4.

127. Byrd JC, Peterson BL, Morrison VA, *et al.* Randomized phase 2 study of fludarabine with concurrent versus sequential treatment with rituximab in symptomatic, untreated patients with B-cell chronic lymphocytic leukemia: results from Cancer and Leukemia Group B 9712 (CALGB 9712). *Blood* 2003;**101**:6–14.

128. Schulz H, Klein SK, Rehwald U, *et al.* Phase 2 study of a combined immunochemotherapy using rituximab and fludarabine in patients with chronic lymphocytic leukemia. *Blood* 2002;**100**:3115–20.

129. Fischer K, Stilgenbauer S, Schweighofer CD, *et al.* Bendamustine in combination with rituximab (BR) for patients with relapsed chronic lymphocytic leukemia (CLL): a multicentre phase II trial of the German CLL Study Group (GCLLSG). *Blood* 2008;**112**:128.

130. Fischer K, Cramer P, Stilgenbauer S, *et al.* Bendamustine combined with rituximab (BR) in first-line therapy of advanced CLL: a multicenter phase II trial of the German CLL Study Group (GCLLSG). *ASH Annual Meeting Abstracts* 2009;**114**:89.

131. Kay NE, Geyer SM, Call TG, *et al.* Combination chemoimmunotherapy with pentostatin, cyclophosphamide, and rituximab shows significant clinical activity with low accompanying toxicity in previously untreated B chronic lymphocytic leukemia. *Blood* 2007;**109**:405–11.

132. Byrd JC, Rai K, Peterson BL, *et al.* Addition of rituximab to fludarabine may prolong progression-free survival and overall survival in patients with previously untreated chronic lymphocytic leukemia: an updated retrospective comparative analysis of CALGB 9712 and CALGB 9011. *Blood* 2005;**105**:49–53.

133. Lundin J, Kimby E, Bjorkholm M, *et al.* Phase II trial of subcutaneous anti-CD52 monoclonal antibody alemtuzumab (Campath-1H) as first-line treatment for patients with B-cell chronic lymphocytic leukemia (B-CLL). *Blood* 2002;**100**:768–73.

134. Hillmen P, Skotnicki AB, Robak T, *et al.* Alemtuzumab compared with chlorambucil as first-line therapy for chronic lymphocytic leukemia. *J Clin Oncol* 2007;**25**:5616–23.

135. Wierda WG, O'Brien S, Faderl S, *et al.* Combined cyclophosphamide, fludarabine, alemtuzumab, and rituximab (CFAR), an active regimen for heavily treated patients with CLL. *Blood* 2006;**108**:14a.

136. Wierda WG, O'Brien SM, Faderl SH, *et al.* CFAR, an active frontline regimen for high-risk patients with CLL, including those with del 17p. *Blood* 2008;**112**:729.

137. Montillo M, Tedeschi A, Miqueleiz S, *et al.* Alemtuzumab as consolidation after a response to fludarabine is effective in purging residual disease in patients with chronic lymphocytic leukemia. *J Clin Oncol* 2006;**24**: 2337–42.

138. Rai KR, Byrd JC, Peterson BL, *et al.* A phase II trial of fludarabine followed by alemtuzumab (Campath-1H) in previously untreated chronic lymphocytic leukemia (CLL) patients with active disease: Cancer and Leukemia Group B (CALGB) study 19901. *Blood* 2002;**100**:205a.

139. Rai KR, Byrd JC, Peterson BL, *et al.* Subcutaneous alemtuzumab following fludarabine for previously untreated patients with chronic lymphocytic leukemia (CLL): Cancer and Leukemia Group B (CALGB) study 19901. *Blood* 2003;**102**:676a.

140. Morrison VA, Peterson BL, Rai KR, *et al.* Alemtuzumab increases serious infections in patients with previously untreated chronic lymphocytic leukemia (CLL) receiving fludarabine-based therapy: a comparative analysis of 3 Cancer and Leukemia Group B studies (CALGB 9011, 9712, 19901). *Blood* 2007;**110**:233a.

141. Wendtner CM, Ritgen M, Schweighofer CD, *et al.* Consolidation with alemtuzumab in patients with chronic lymphocytic leukemia (CLL) in first remission–experience on safety and efficacy within a randomized multicenter phase III trial of the German CLL Study Group (GCLLSG). *Leukemia* 2004;**18**:1093–101.

142. Schweighofer CD, Ritgen M, Eichhorst BF, *et al.* Consolidation with alemtuzumab improves progression-free survival in patients with chronic lymphocytic leukaemia (CLL) in first remission: long-term follow-up of a randomized phase III trial of the German CLL Study Group (GCLLSG). *Br J Haematol* 2009;**144**:95–8.

143. O'Brien SM, Kantarjian HM, Thomas DA, *et al.* Alemtuzumab as treatment for residual disease after chemotherapy in patients with chronic lymphocytic leukemia. *Cancer* 2003;**98**:2657–63.

144. O'Brien SM, Gribben JG, Thomas DA, *et al.* Alemtuzumab for minimal residual disease in CLL. *Blood* 2003;**102**:109a.

145. Delmer A, Leprêtre S, Cazin B, *et al.* Consolidation therapy with subcutaneous alemtuzumab following induction treatment with oral FC (fludarabine and cyclophosphamide) in previously untreated patients aged 65–70 years with advanced stage chronic lymphocytic leukemia (CLL): a phase II trial of the FCGCLL/MW. *Blood* 2006;**108**:801a.

146. Lin TS, Donohue KA, Lucas MS, *et al.* Consolidation therapy with subcutaneous (sc) alemtuzumab results in severe infectious toxicity in previously untreated CLL patients who achieve a complete response (CR) after fludarabine and rituximab (FR) induction therapy: interim safety analysis of the CALGB study 10101. *Blood* 2007;**110**:232a–3a.

147. Sawitsky A, Rai KR, Glidewell O, *et al.* Comparison of daily versus intermittent chlorambucil and prednisone therapy in the treatment of patients with chronic lymphocytic leukemia. *Blood* 1977;**50**:1049–59.

148. Montserrat E, Alcala A, Alonso C, *et al.* A randomized trial comparing chlorambucil plus prednisone vs cyclophosphamide, melphalan, and prednisone in the treatment of chronic lymphocytic leukemia stages B and C. *Nouv Rev Fr Hematol* 1988;**30**:429–32.

149. Itala M, Remes K. The COP regimen is not a feasible treatment for advanced, refractory chronic lymphocytic leukemia. *Leuk Lymphoma* 1996;**23**:137–41.

150. Liepman M, Votaw ML. The treatment of chronic lymphocytic leukemia with COP chemotherapy. *Cancer* 1978;**41**:1664–9.

151. Grever MR, Kopecky KJ, Coltman CA, *et al.* Fludarabine monophosphate: a potentially useful agent in chronic lymphocytic leukemia. *Nouv Rev Fr Hematol* 1988;**30**:457–9.

152. Puccio CA, Mittelman A, Lichtman SM, *et al.* A loading dose/continuous infusion schedule of fludarabine phosphate in chronic lymphocytic leukemia. *J Clin Oncol* 1991;**9**:1562–9.

153. Keating MJ, O'Brien S, Kantarjian H, *et al.* Long-term follow-up of patients with chronic lymphocytic leukemia treated with fludarabine as a single agent. *Blood* 1993;**81**:2878–84.

154. Kemena A, O'Brien S, Kantarjian H, *et al.* Phase II clinical trial of fludarabine in chronic lymphocytic leukemia on a weekly low-dose schedule. *Leuk Lymphoma* 1993;**10**:187–93.

155. Sorensen JM, Vena DA, Fallavollita A, *et al.* Treatment of refractory chronic lymphocytic leukemia with fludarabine phosphate via the group C protocol mechanism of the National Cancer Institute: five-year follow-up report. *J Clin Oncol* 1997;**15**:458–65.

156. Zinzani PL, Bendandi M, Magagnoli M, *et al.* Long-term follow-up after fludarabine treatment in pretreated patients with chronic lymphocytic leukemia. *Haematologica* 2000;**85**:1135–9.

157. Hallek M, Schmitt B, Wilhelm M, *et al.* Fludarabine plus cyclophosphamide is an efficient treatment for advanced chronic lymphocytic leukaemia (CLL): results of a phase II study of the German CLL Study Group. *Br J Haematol* 2001;**114**:342–8.

158. Gonzalez H, Maloum K, Tezenas du Montcel S, *et al.* Fludarabine + cyclophosphamide in chronic lymphoproliferative disorders. *Blood* 2003;**102**:357b.

159. Marotta G, Bigazzi C, Lenoci M, *et al.* Low-dose fludarabine and cyclophosphamide in elderly patients with B-cell chronic lymphocytic leukemia refractory to conventional therapy. *Haematologica* 2000;**85**:1268–70.

160. Schiavone EM, De Simone M, Palmieri S, *et al.* Fludarabine plus cyclophosphamide for the treatment of advanced chronic lymphocytic leukemia. *Eur J Haematol* 2003;**71**:23–8.

161. Robertson LE, O'Brien S, Kantarjian H, *et al.* Fludarabine plus doxorubicin in previously treated chronic lymphocytic leukemia. *Leukemia* 1995;**9**:943–5.

162. Rummel MJ, Kafer G, Pfreundschuh M, *et al.* Fludarabine and epirubicin in the treatment of chronic lymphocytic leukaemia: a German multicenter phase II study. *Ann Oncol* 1999;**10**:183–8.

163. Bosch F, Ferrer A, Lopez-Guillermo A, *et al.* Fludarabine, cyclophosphamide and mitoxantrone in the treatment of resistant or relapsed chronic lymphocytic leukaemia. *Br J Haematol* 2002;**119**:976–84.

164. Schmitt B, Franke A, Burkhard O, *et al.* Fludarabine, mitoxantrone and cyclophosphamide combination therapy in relapsed chronic lymphocytic leukemia (CLL) with or without G-CSF: results of the first interim analysis of a phase III study of the German CLL Study Group (GCLLSG). *Blood* 2002;**100**:364b.

165. Mauro FR, Foa R, Meloni G, *et al.* Fludarabine, ara-C, novantrone and dexamethasone (FAND) in previously treated chronic lymphocytic leukemia patients. *Haematologica* 2002;**87**:926–33.

166. Tallman MS, Hakimian D, Zanzig C, *et al.* Cladribine in the treatment of relapsed or refractory chronic lymphocytic leukemia. *J Clin Oncol* 1995;**13**:983–8.

167. Juliusson G, Liliemark J. Long-term survival following cladribine (2-chlorodeoxyadenosine) therapy in previously treated patients with chronic lymphocytic leukemia. *Ann Oncol* 1996;**7**:373–9.

168. Rondelli D, Lauria F, Zinzani PL, *et al.* 2-Chlorodeoxyadenosine in the treatment of relapsed/refractory chronic lymphoproliferative disorders. *Eur J Haematol* 1997;**58**:46–50.

169. Betticher DC, Ratschiller D, Hsu Schmitz SF, *et al.* Reduced dose of subcutaneous cladribine induces identical response rates but decreased toxicity in pretreated chronic lymphocytic leukaemia. Swiss Group for Clinical Cancer Research (SAKK). *Ann Oncol* 1998;**9**:721–6.

170. Van Den Neste E, Louviaux I, Michaux JL, *et al.* Phase I/II study of 2-chloro-2'-deoxyadenosine with cyclophosphamide in patients with pretreated B cell chronic lymphocytic leukemia and indolent non-Hodgkin's lymphoma. *Leukemia* 2000;**14**:1136–42.

171. Robak T, Gora-Tybor J, Lech-Maranda E, *et al.* Cladribine in combination with mitoxantrone and cyclophosphamide (CMC) in the treatment of heavily pre-treated patients with advanced indolent lymphoid malignancies. *Eur J Haematol* 2001;**66**:188–94.

172. Montillo M, Tedeschi A, O'Brien S, *et al.* Phase II study of cladribine and cyclophosphamide in patients with chronic lymphocytic leukemia and prolymphocytic leukemia. *Cancer* 2003;**97**:114–20.

173. Ho AD, Thaler J, Stryckmans P, *et al.* Pentostatin in refractory chronic lymphocytic leukemia: a phase II trial of the European Organization for Research and Treatment of Cancer. *J Natl Cancer Inst* 1990;**82**:1416–20.

174. Johnson SA, Catovsky D, Child JA, *et al.* Phase I/II evaluation of pentostatin (2'-deoxycoformycin) in a five day schedule for the treatment of relapsed/refractory B-cell chronic lymphocytic leukaemia. *Invest New Drugs* 1998;**16**:155–60.

175. Weiss MA, Maslak PG, Jurcic JG, *et al.* Pentostatin and cyclophosphamide: an effective new regimen in previously treated patients with chronic lymphocytic leukemia. *J Clin Oncol* 2003;**21**:1278–84.

176. McLaughlin P, Grillo-Lopez AJ, Link BK, *et al.* Rituximab chimeric anti-CD20 monoclonal antibody therapy for relapsed indolent lymphoma: half of patients respond to a four-dose treatment program. *J Clin Oncol* 1998;**16**:2825–33.

177. Foran JM, Rohatiner AZ, Cunningham D, *et al.* European phase II study of rituximab (chimeric anti-CD20 monoclonal antibody) for patients with newly diagnosed mantle-cell lymphoma and previously treated mantle-cell lymphoma, immunocytoma, and small B-cell lymphocytic lymphoma. *J Clin Oncol* 2000;**18**:317–24.

178. Huhn D, von Schilling C, Wilhelm M, *et al.* Rituximab therapy of patients with B-cell chronic lymphocytic leukemia. *Blood* 2001;**98**:1326–31.

179. Itala M, Geisler CH, Kimby E, *et al.* Standard-dose anti-CD20 antibody rituximab has efficacy in chronic lymphocytic leukaemia: results from a Nordic multicentre study. *Eur J Haematol* 2002;**69**:129–34.

180. Byrd JC, Murphy T, Howard RS, *et al.* Rituximab using a thrice weekly dosing schedule in B-cell chronic lymphocytic leukemia and small lymphocytic lymphoma demonstrates clinical activity and acceptable toxicity. *J Clin Oncol* 2001;**19**:2153–64.

181. O'Brien SM, Kantarjian H, Thomas DA, *et al.* Rituximab dose-escalation trial in chronic lymphocytic leukemia. *J Clin Oncol* 2001;**19**:2165–70.

182. Quinn JP, Mohamedbhai S, Chipperfield K, *et al.* Efficacy of rituximab in combination with steroids in refractory chronic lymphocytic leukemia. *Leuk Lymphoma* 2008;**49**:1995–8.

183. Drapkin R, Di Bella NJ, Cuasay LC, *et al.* Phase II multicenter trial of pentostatin and rituximab in patients with previously treated or untreated chronic lymphocytic leukemia. *Blood* 2002;**100**:803a.

184. Wierda W, O'Brien S, Wen S, *et al.* Chemoimmunotherapy with fludarabine, cyclophosphamide, and rituximab for relapsed and refractory chronic lymphocytic leukemia. *J Clin Oncol* 2005;**23**:4070–8.

185. Wierda W, O'Brien S, Faderl S, *et al.* A retrospective comparison of three sequential groups of patients with Recurrent/Refractory chronic lymphocytic leukemia treated with fludarabine-based regimens. *Cancer* 2006;**106**:337–45.

186. Robak T, Moiseev SI, Dmoszynska A, *et al.* Rituximab, fludarabine, and cyclophosphamide (R-FC) prolongs progression free survival in relapsed or refractory chronic lymphocytic leukemia (CLL) compared with FC alone: final results from the international randomized phase III REACH trial. Blood 2008, 112.

187. Lamanna N, Kalaycio M, Maslak P, *et al.* Pentostatin, cyclophosphamide, and rituximab is an active, well-tolerated regimen for patients with previously treated chronic lymphocytic leukemia. *J Clin Oncol* 2006;**24**:1575–81.

188. Robak T, Smolewski P, Cebula B, *et al.* Rituximab plus cladribine with or without cyclophosphamide in patients with relapsed or refractory chronic lymphocytic leukemia. *Eur J Haematol* 2007;**79**:107–13.

189. Ciolli S, Gigli F, Mannelli F, *et al.* High response rates and reduced first-dose reactions with subcutaneous alemtuzumab in patients with relapsed and refractory CLL. *Blood* 2003;**102**:357b.

190. Ferrajoli A, O'Brien SM, Cortes JE, *et al.* Phase II study of alemtuzumab in chronic lymphoproliferative disorders. *Cancer* 2003;**98**:773–8.

191. Keating MJ, Flinn I, Jain V, *et al.* Therapeutic role of alemtuzumab (Campath-1H) in patients who have failed fludarabine: results of a large international study. *Blood* 2002;**99**:3554–61.

192. Rai KR, Coutre S, Rizzieri D, *et al.* Efficacy and safety of alemtuzumab (Campath-1H) in refractory B-CLL patients treated on a compassionate basis. *Blood* 2001;**98**:365a.

193. Rai KR, Freter CE, Mercier RJ, *et al.* Alemtuzumab in previously treated chronic lymphocytic leukemia patients who also had received fludarabine. *J Clin Oncol* 2002;**20**:3891–7.

194. Rai KR, Keating MJ, Coutre S, *et al.* Patients with refractory B-CLL and T-PLL treated with alemtuzumab (Campath®) on a compassionate basis. A report on efficacy and safety of CAM 511 trial. *Blood* 2002;**100**:802a.

195. Moreton P, Kennedy B, Lucas G, *et al.* Eradication of minimal residual disease in B-cell chronic lymphocytic leukemia after alemtuzumab therapy is associated with prolonged survival. *J Clin Oncol* 2005;**23**:2971–9.

196. Anderson JR, Neuberg DS. Analysis of outcome by response flawed. *J Clin Oncol* 2005;**23**:8122–3; author reply 8123–4.

197. Kennedy B, Rawstron A, Carter C, *et al.* Campath-1H and fludarabine in combination are highly active in refractory chronic lymphocytic leukemia. *Blood* 2002;**99**:2245–7.

198. Elter T, Borchmann P, Schulz H, *et al.* Fludarabine in combination with alemtuzumab is effective and feasible in patients with relapsed or refractory B-cell chronic lymphocytic leukemia: results of a phase II trial. *J Clin Oncol* 2005;**23**:7024–31.

199. Faderl S, Ferrajoli A, Wierda WG, *et al.* The combination of alemtuzumab [continuous intravenous infusion (civ) followed by subcutaneous injection (sc)] plus rituximab has activity in patients (pts) with relapsed chronic lymphocytic leukemia (CLL) *Blood* 2006;**108**:800a.

200. Faderl S, Thomas DA, O'Brien S, *et al.* Experience with alemtuzumab plus rituximab in patients with relapsed and refractory lymphoid malignancies. *Blood* 2003;**101**:3413–15.

201. Nabhan C, Patton D, Gordon LI, *et al.* A pilot trial of rituximab and alemtuzumab combination therapy in patients with relapsed and/or refractory chronic lymphocytic leukemia (CLL). *Leuk Lymphoma* 2004;**45**:2269–73.

202. Faderl S, Ferrajoli A, Wierda W, *et al.* Continuous infusion/subcutaneous alemtuzumab (Campath-1H) plus rituximab is active for patients with relapsed/refractory chronic lymphocytic leukemia (CLL). *Blood* 2005;**106**:831a.

203. Eichhorst BF, Busch R, Stauch M, *et al.* Fludarabine (F) induces higher response rates in first line therapy of older patients (pts) with advanced chronic lymphocytic leukemia (CLL) than chlormabucil: interim analysis of a phase III study of the German CLL Study Group (GCLLSG). *Blood* 2003;**102**:109a.

204. Keating MJ, O'Brien S, Kontoyiannis D, *et al.* Results of first salvage therapy for patients refractory to a fludarabine regimen in chronic lymphocytic leukemia. *Leuk Lymphoma* 2002;**43**:1755–62.

205. Perkins JG, Flynn JM, Howard RS, *et al.* Frequency and type of serious infections in fludarabine-refractory B-cell chronic lymphocytic leukemia and small lymphocytic lymphoma: implications for clinical trials in this patient population. *Cancer* 2002;**94**:2033–9.

206. Pettitt AR. Mechanism of action of purine analogues in chronic lymphocytic leukaemia. *Br J Haematol* 2003;**121**:692–702.

207. O'Brien S, Kantarjian H, Estey E, *et al.* Lack of effect of 2-chlorodeoxyadenosine therapy in patients with chronic lymphocytic leukemia refractory to fludarabine therapy. *N Engl J Med* 1994;**330**:319–22.

208. Byrd JC, Peterson B, Piro L, *et al.* A phase II study of cladribine treatment for fludarabine refractory B cell chronic lymphocytic leukemia: results from CALGB Study 9211. *Leukemia* 2003;**17**:323–7.

209. Tsimberidou AM, Wierda WG, Plunkett W, *et al.* Phase I-II study of

oxaliplatin, fludarabine, cytarabine, and rituximab combination therapy in patients with Richter's syndrome or fludarabine-refractory chronic lymphocytic leukemia. *J Clin Oncol* 2008;**26**:196–203.

210. Stilgenbauer S, Zenz T, Winkler D, *et al.* Subcutaneous alemtuzumab (Campath) in fludarabine-refractory CLL: final results of the CLL2H trial of the GCLLSG and comprehensive analysis of prognostic markers. *J Clin Oncol* 2009;**27**:3994–4001.

211. Lozanski G, Heerema NA, Flinn IW, *et al.* Alemtuzumab is an effective therapy for chronic lymphocytic leukemia with p53 mutations and deletions. *Blood* 2004;**103**:3278–81.

212. Sayala HA, Moreton P, Jones RA, *et al.* Final report of the UKCLL02 trial: a phase II study of subcutaneous alemtuzumab plus fludarabine in patients with fludarabine refractory CLL (on behalf of the NCRI CLL Trials Sub-Group) *Blood* 2006;**108**:14a–15a.

213. Tam CS, O'Brien S, Lerner S, *et al.* The natural history of fludarabine-refractory chronic lymphocytic leukemia patients who fail alemtuzumab or have bulky lymphadenopathy. *Leuk Lymphoma* 2007;**48**:1931–9.

214. Osterborg A, Kipps T, Mayer J, *et al.* Ofatumumab (HuMax-CD20), a novel CD20 monoclonal antibody, is an active treatment for patients with CLL refractory to both fludarabine and alembuzumab or bulky fludarabine-refractory disease: results from the planned interim analysis of an international pivotal trial. *Blood* 2008;**111**:126.

215. O'Brien S, Moore JO, Boyd TE, *et al.* Randomized phase III trial of fludarabine plus cyclophosphamide with or without oblimersen sodium (Bcl-2 antisense) in patients with relapsed or refractory chronic lymphocytic leukemia. *J Clin Oncol* 2007;**25**:1114–20.

216. O'Brien S, Moore JO, Boyd TE, *et al.* 5-year survival in patients with relapsed or refractory chronic lymphocytic leukemia in a randomized, phase III trial of fludarabine plus cyclophosphamide with or without oblimersen. *J Clin Oncol* 2009;**27**:5208–12.

217. Brion A, Mahe B, Kolb B, *et al.* Preliminary results of a prospective randomized study comparing first line conventional therapy versus high dose therapy with autologous CD34+ purified progenitor cell support in B CLL patients with B and C Binet stages: the GOELAMS LLC98 study. *Blood* 2005;**106**:48a.

218. Sutton L, Diviné M, Travade P, *et al.* Autologous stem cell transplantation (ASCT) versus standard treatments for CLL patients: first interim analysis of a prospective randomized study from the French Cooperative Study Group on CLL. *Blood* 2005;**106**:455b.

219. Moreno C, Villamor N, Colomer D, *et al.* Allogeneic stem-cell transplantation may overcome the adverse prognosis of unmutated VH gene in patients with chronic lymphocytic leukemia. *J Clin Oncol* 2005;**23**:3433–8.

220. Michallet M, Van Biezen A, Bandini G, *et al.* Allotransplants and autotransplants in chronic lymphocytic leukemia (CLL). *Bone Marrow Transplant* 1999;**23**:S53.

221. Pavletic ZS, Arrowsmith ER, Bierman PJ, *et al.* Outcome of allogeneic stem cell transplantation for B cell chronic lymphocytic leukemia. *Bone Marrow Transplant* 2000;**25**:717–22.

222. Doney KC, Chauncey T, Appelbaum FR. Allogeneic related donor hematopoietic stem cell transplantation for treatment of chronic lymphocytic leukemia. *Bone Marrow Transplant* 2002;**29**:817–23.

223. Toze CL, Galal A, Barnett MJ, *et al.* Myeloablative allografting for chronic lymphocytic leukemia: evidence for a potent graft-versus-leukemia effect associated with graft-versus-host disease. *Bone Marrow Transplant* 2005;**36**:825–30.

224. Pavletic SZ, Khouri IF, Haagenson M, *et al.* Unrelated donor marrow transplantation for B-cell chronic lymphocytic leukemia after using myeloablative conditioning: results from the Center for International Blood and Marrow Transplant research. *J Clin Oncol* 2005;**23**:5788–94.

225. Michallet M, Lê Q-H, Vernant JP, *et al.* Allogeneic hematopoietic stem cell transplantation cures CLL: a retrospective analysis from the SFGM-TC registry. *Blood* 2006;**108**:848a.

226. Ritgen M, Stilgenbauer S, von Neuhoff N, *et al.* Graft-versus-leukemia activity may overcome therapeutic resistance of chronic lymphocytic leukemia with unmutated immunoglobulin variable heavy-chain gene status: implications of minimal residual disease measurement with quantitative PCR. *Blood* 2004;**104**:2600–2.

227. Schetelig J, van Biezen A, Brand R, *et al.* Allogeneic hematopoietic stem-cell transplantation for chronic lymphocytic leukemia with 17p deletion: a retrospective European Group for Blood and Marrow Transplantation analysis. *J Clin Oncol* 2008;**26**:5094–100.

228. Khouri IF, Keating MJ, Saliba RM, *et al.* Long-term follow-up of patients with CLL treated with allogeneic hematopoietic transplantation. *Cytotherapy* 2002;**4**:217–21.

229. Khouri IF, Lee MS, Saliba RM, *et al.* Nonablative allogeneic stem cell transplantation for chronic lymphocytic leukemia: impact of rituximab on immunomodulation and survival. *Exp Hematol* 2004;**32**:28–35.

230. Delgado J, Thomson K, Russell N, *et al.* Results of alemtuzumab-based reduced-intensity allogeneic transplantation for chronic lymphocytic leukemia: a British Society of Blood and Marrow Transplantation Study. *Blood* 2006;**107**:1724–30.

231. Dreger P, Brand R, Milligan D, *et al.* Reduced-intensity conditioning lowers treatment-related mortality of allogeneic stem cell transplantation for chronic lymphocytic leukemia: a population-matched analysis. *Leukemia* 2005;**19**:1029–33.

232. Brown JR, Stevenson K, Kim HT, *et al.* Comparative outcome of myeloablative and reduced intensity allogeneic stem cell transplantation for chronic lymphocytic leukemia. *Blood* 2008;**112**:257–8.

233. Brown JR, Li S, Kim H, *et al.* High levels of early donor chimerism and treatment-responsive disease predict improved progression-free survival following non-myeloablative transplantation for advanced CLL. *Blood* 2005;**106**:166a–7a.

234. Brown JR, Kim HT, Li S, *et al.* Predictors of improved progression-free survival after nonmyeloablative allogeneic stem cell transplantation for advanced chronic lymphocytic leukemia. *Biol Blood Marrow Transplant* 2006;**12**:1056–64.

235. Horowitz MM, Montserrat E, Sobocinski K, *et al.* Haematopoietic

stem cell transplantation for chronic lymphocytic leukemia. *Blood* 2000;**96**:522a.

236. Michallet M, Archimbaud E, Bandini G, *et al.* HLA-identical sibling bone marrow transplantation in younger patients with chronic lymphocytic leukemia. European Group for Blood and Marrow Transplantation and the International Bone Marrow Transplant Registry. *Ann Intern Med* 1996;**124**:311–15.

237. Dreger P, Brand R, Hansz J, *et al.* Treatment-related mortality and graft-versus-leukemia activity after allogeneic stem cell transplantation for chronic lymphocytic leukemia using intensity-reduced conditioning. *Leukemia* 2003;**17**:841–8.

238. Schetelig J, Bornhaeuser M, Thiede C, *et al.* Reduced-intensity conditioning (RIC) with busulfan, fludarabine and Campath-1H is complicated by a high rate of graft failure and severe viral complications in patients with CLL. *Blood* 2004;**104**:353b.

239. Sorror ML, Maris MB, Sandmaier BM, *et al.* Hematopoietic cell transplantation after nonmyeloablative conditioning for advanced chronic lymphocytic leukemia. *J Clin Oncol* 2005;**23**:3819–29.

240. Caballero D, Garcia-Marco JA, Martino R, *et al.* Allogeneic transplant with reduced intensity conditioning regimens may overcome the poor prognosis of B-cell chronic lymphocytic leukemia with unmutated immunoglobulin variable heavy-chain gene and chromosomal abnormalities (11q- and 17p-). *Clin Cancer Res* 2005;**11**:7757–63.

241. Schetelig J, Thiede C, Bornhauser M, *et al.* Evidence of a graft-versus-leukemia effect in chronic lymphocytic leukemia after reduced-intensity conditioning and allogeneic stem-cell transplantation: the Cooperative German Transplant Study Group. *J Clin Oncol* 2003;**21**:2747–53.

242. Khouri IF, Saliba RM, Admirand J, *et al.* Graft-versus-leukaemia effect after non-myeloablative haematopoietic transplantation can overcome the unfavourable expression of ZAP-70 in refractory chronic lymphocytic leukaemia. *Br J Haematol* 2007;**137**:355–63.

Chapter 6

Myelodysplastic syndromes (MDS)

Stefan H. Faderl, Guillermo Garcia-Manero, and Hagop M. Kantarjian

Introduction

Myelodysplastic syndromes (MDS) are a heterogeneous group of hematopoietic stem cell disorders which are distinguished by cytopenias in the face of hypercellular marrows and dysplastic hematopoietic cell lines.[1] Up into the 1970s MDS have been called "preleukemia" expressing the proximity of MDS to acute myeloid leukemia (AML), and their capacity to evolve into AML over time. Although MDS is the currently accepted term, the pathophysiology of MDS varies widely extending from abnormalities of apoptosis and differentiation to proliferation and maturation arrest. It is nowadays also better understood that there are notable differences between MDS and AML, a separation which is also underlined by the clinical manifestations and prognosis of MDS, which are primarily determined by cytopenias and not leukemic transformation.[2] The complexity of pathophysiology and resultant heterogeneity of prognosis have led to several recent attempts to fine tune criteria for diagnosis and classification. In addition, recent years have also seen important advances of treatment with respect to hematopoietic growth factors, iron chelation, and particularly epigenetic therapy and immunomodulatory inhibitory derivatives (e.g., lenalidomide). These developments have made the care of patients with MDS more demanding but at the same time more satisfying as the possibilities for patients with MDS are now larger than before.

Epidemiology and etiology

MDS occurs with an incidence of 3.5–12.6 per 100 000 per year in the United States and is more frequent in men than women. The incidence increases with age however, and can amount to as high as 20–50 per 100 000 in individuals over 60 years, but may yet remain under diagnosed in a substantial number of patients.[3,4] A recent analysis of a Medicare claims database puts the incidence of MDS as high as 41 per 100 000 population emphasizing the significant economic implications of MDS based on the high incidence of cardiac, pulmonary, and endocrine (diabetes) complications for transfusion-dependent patients.[5] Reasons for underdiagnosing MDS in the past may have included a lack of reporting, overlap with other disorders (e.g., aplastic anemia, myeloproliferative diseases, or AML), or simply a perceived lack of effective therapeutic intervention (e.g., in older patients with comorbidities).

The etiology of MDS remains unknown in most patients. A relationship to predisposing factors is found in only 20–30%.[6,7] In addition to factors such as smoking, use of hair dyes, exposure to agricultural and industrial toxins, occupational exposures to stone and cereal dusts, or exposure to ionizing radiation (atomic bomb survivors in Japan, decontamination workers following the Chernobyl nuclear plant accident, chronic exposure to low-dose radiation such as with radiopharmaceuticals), one of the most striking forms of secondary MDS is treatment-related MDS (t-MDS).[8] The incidence of t-MDS is increasing because of better outcome for tumors that formerly lacked effective therapy and can nowadays be as high as 10–15% at 10 years following the primary malignancy (e.g., in Hodgkin lymphoma, non-Hodgkin lymphoma, or breast cancer).[9] Risk factors associated with t-MDS include the cumulative dose of alkylating agents (e.g., cyclophosphamide, melphalan) or topoisomerase II inhibitors (e.g., etoposide), previous radiation exposure, older age, and use of radiotherapy prior to transplantation. t-MDS following alkylator therapy has a latency period of 3–8 years and is often associated with abnormalities of chromosomes 5 and 7, whereas the latency period following topoisomerase II inhibitors is shorter (e.g., 2–3 years), and cytogenetic-molecular abnormalities more frequently involve rearrangements of the *MLL* gene on chromosome 11q23.

Secondary and t-MDS are distinguishable from primary MDS by an earlier age of onset, more prominent dysplasia, more severe cytopenias, more rapid progression to AML, and worse outcome.

Clinical and laboratory features

Most frequently, patients present with fatigue, pallor, exertional dyspnea, infections, and easy bruising and bleeding.

Management of Hematologic Malignancies, ed. Susan M. O'Brien, Julie M. Vose, and Hagop M. Kantarjian. Published by Cambridge University Press.

Table 6.1. Morphologic criteria of dysplasia

Dyserythropoiesis	Dysmyelopoiesis	Dysmegakaryopoiesis
– Anisocytosis	– Hypogranulation	– Large abnormally granular platelets or hypogranular platelets
– Poikilocytosis	– Hyposegmentation (Pelger-Huët-like)	
– Macrocytosis		
– Marrow dyserythropoiesis including ringed sideroblasts, asynchronous maturation, abnormal nuclear shapes, and chromatin clumping		– Marrow micromegakaryocytes

Lymphadenopathy and hepatosplenomegaly (10–20%) and central nervous system involvement are rare.

Among laboratory abnormalities, anemia is most common followed by neutropenia and thrombocytopenia. Monocytosis exceeding 1×10^9/L in the blood favors a diagnosis of chronic myelomonocytic leukemia, CMML). Marrow and blood smears demonstrate dysplasia of varying severity in one or more cell lines (Table 6.1). It should be noted that dysplastic changes are not pathognomonic for MDS and can be seen in many other conditions. Dyserythropoiesis in particular is a common manifestation of secondary dysplasia and other conditions associated with dysplasias and cytopenias need to be excluded: B12 or folic acid deficiencies; nutritional deficiencies in general (anorexia nervosa); exposure to antibiotics, chemotherapy, ethanol, benzene, or lead; regenerating bone marrow following a hypoplastic phase induced by drugs or infections; HIV-positive disease; chronic inflammation and tuberculosis; liver disorders; hypersplenism; Hodgkin disease, lymphomas, and metastatic disease to the marrow.[10] In some situations, follow-up testing and an observation period will help to clarify the diagnosis.

The marrow in MDS is typically hypercellular, although hypocellular variants may occur occasionally. In the latter case, a significant overlap with aplastic anemia or other disorders based on autoimmune-mediated mechanisms may exist and these patients may benefit from immunomodulatory therapies.

The role of cytochemical stains is more limited in MDS than AML, but they may play a role in some situations such as (1) iron to assess iron content and to identify ringed sideroblasts; (2) reticulin to define the degree of fibrosis; and (3) platelet antibodies to highlight micromegakaryocytes.

Additional abnormalities observed in MDS include polyclonal gammopathies in up to one-third of patients, monoclonal gammopathies or hypogammaglobulinemia, the presence of autoimmune antibodies, and B- or T-cell abnormalities.

Pathogenesis

Models of MDS pathogenesis assume a multistep process manifested as ineffective hematopoiesis from increased apoptosis and impaired differentiation and additional molecular hits leading to genomic instability, karyotypic evolution, proliferation, and maturation arrest. Identification of specific, identifiable molecular abnormalities of the hematopoietic cells in MDS remains limited and therefore the impact of the microenvironment and other components of the non-hematopoietic cell milieu have been emphasized more recently. Some aspects of the process have been elucidated, opening the way to therapeutic interventions.

The hallmark of MDS is ineffective hematopoiesis associated with dysplasia.[11] Dysplasia is considered to reflect apoptosis of hematopoietic progenitors. According to one hypothesis, the early stages of MDS are characterized by excessive proapoptotic signals, which are counterbalanced by a compensatory phase of excessive hematopoiesis, hence the apparent paradox of peripheral cytopenias in the presence of hypercellular marrows.[12] Increased apoptosis has also been demonstrated in cells of the microenvironment, suggesting that the primitive stem cell involved may be a progenitor to both hematopoietic and stromal cells. Several cytokines and intracellular proteins have been implicated: (1) overexpression of the proapoptotic BCL2 family members in early stages of MDS and the reverse observation in later stage MDS and secondary AML;[13] and (2) high levels of tumor necrosis factor alpha (TNF-α) with induction of Fas expression. TNF-α mRNA is overexpressed in marrows from MDS, but not in normal marrows or marrows from AML. Similar to the activity of BCL2 family proteins, TNF-α overproduction seems to be restricted to earlier MDS phases.[14] Heterogeneity of the behavior of MDS is furthermore promoted by the contribution of additional processes such as abnormal marrow environment, immune dysregulation, increased function of macrophages, and changes in microvessel density and expression of angiogenic factors and their receptors, respectively.

Of particular interest are recurrent cytogenetic abnormalities, some of which have been associated with specific clinical syndromes.[15] To underline biologic differences with AML, deletions, numerical abnormalities, and unbalanced translocations are more commonly observed in MDS, whereas translocations specifically associated with MDS are rare. Chromosomes frequently involved are 3 (*MDS1-EVI-1*), 5 (e.g., 5q-), 7 (e.g., monosomy 7 and 7q-), 8 (e.g., trisomy 8), 20 (e.g., monosomy 20, 20q-), and complex abnormalities (Figure 6.1).[16] The prognostic significance of cytogenetic abnormalities in MDS is substantial, not inferior in its significance to a high blast percentage, and therefore underestimated in the currently used clinical prognostication tables (see IPSS below) (Table 6.2).[17] Of interest are abnormalities of chromosome 5, as several genes involved in hematopoiesis have been mapped to this region (e.g., macrophage colony-stimulating factor [M-CSF], granulocyte-monocyte colony-stimulating factor [GM-CSF], interleukin

Table 6.2. Karyotype and survival in MDS

Karyotype	Median survival (months)
9q-, 15q-, t(15q), 12p-, +21, 5q-	≥77
-X, diploid, -Y, t(1q), t(7q), t(11q), -21	32–56
11q-, +8, +19, 7q-/-7, complex[a]	14–26
Complex,[a] t(5q)	4.4–8.7

Note: [a] ≥3 abnormalities.
Source: Modified from Haase *et al.*[17]

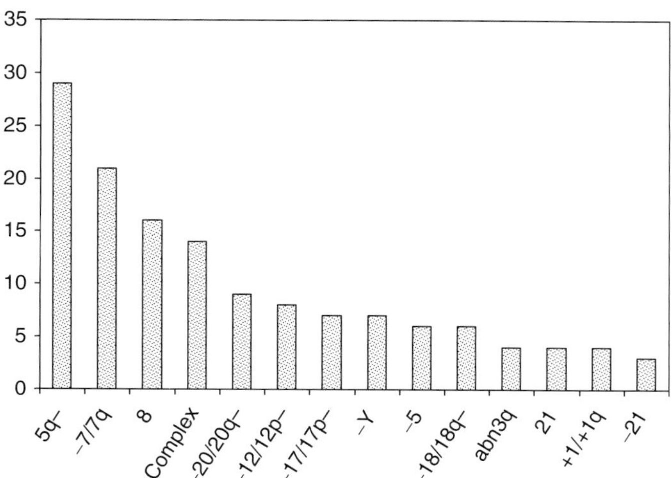

Figure 6.1 Karyotype and survival in MDS.

Table 6.3. Clinical and pathologic characteristics of the 5q- syndrome

Demographics
• Younger age
• Female gender
Clinicopathologic features
• Isolated del(5)(q31-q33)
• Macrocytosis, erythroid hypoplasia, mono- or hypolobated megakaryocytes
• Normal or elevated platelet count
Disease course
• Low rate of AML transformation (5–10%)
• Long median survival (> 5 yrs)
• Prolonged packed red blood cell (PRBC) transfusion needs (risk of iron overload)
Therapy
• Lenalidomide ± hematopoietic growth factors
• High rate of transfusion independence (> 60%)
• Durable response duration (median ~2 yrs)

[IL]-4 and IL-5, CD14, interferon regulatory factor [IRF]-1, the receptors for platelet-derived growth factor [PDGF], and others). Some MDS patients with an interstitial deletion of chromosome 5 meet the definition of the 5q- syndrome (Table 6.3).[18] The most commonly involved deleted region affects segment 5q13-q31. Although identification of a critical gene has long evaded scientific enquiry, more recently decreased expression (haploinsufficiency) of a ribosomal protein, RPS 14, was found to inhibit erythroid growth, and promote megakaryocytic colony growth and erythroid apoptosis.[19]

Genomic instability and numerous additional molecular hits (*RAS, FLT3, KIT, PDGFRβ, FMS, JAK2, CTNN1*, and others) have been observed in MDS and characterize the transition from excess apoptosis to increased proliferation and maturation arrest.[20,21] Implication of *CTNN1*, located on 5q31 and part of the heme biosynthesis pathway, is interesting as it links abnormal mitochondrial iron regulation to some forms of MDS (such as RARS, see below). Abnormal methylation of DNA promoter areas and deacetylation of histones (protein complexes that form part of the chromatin structure of genes) have been linked to silencing of genomic regions including tumor suppressor genes. Hypermethylation of *SOCS1* (suppressor of cytokine signaling) has been observed in almost half of the patients with high-risk MDS, but only in 20% of patients with early-stage disease.[22] *SOCS1* methylation was associated with *RAS* gene mutations, with adverse karyotype, and with a higher risk of leukemic transformation.

A hypothetical model of the pathobiology of MDS starts with suppression of normal hematopoiesis by polyclonal, unaffected CD8-positive T cells and other cytotoxic suppressor cells through production of proapoptotic cytokines (e.g., TNF-α, the Fas/Fas ligand system, transforming growth factor beta [TGF-β]). An exaggerated immune response following injury to hematopoietic progenitors thus provides the rationale for the use of immunomodulatory therapy in MDS (e.g., antithymocyte globulins [ATG], ciclosporin, corticosteroids) or antiapoptotic mediators. As proliferation continues, genomic instability and additional molecular hits may shift the balance from excessive apoptosis towards maturation arrest and unchecked proliferation as can be seen more commonly in advanced stages of MDS.

The role of the marrow microenvironment and non-hematopoietic cellular components has long been underestimated, but has recently received renewed support by the success of immunomodulatory, antiangiogenic, and microenvironment-oriented therapies such as lenalidomide in at least some subtypes of MDS.

The classification of MDS

Historically, the classification of MDS has been heavily focused on morphologic criteria and in that sense, the classification by the French–American–British (FAB) group provides the basis for all subsequent classifications.[23] It categorizes patients based on percentage of blood and marrow blasts, the presence of

Table 6.4. The International Prognostic Scoring System (IPSS) for MDS

Prognostic variable	Score value				
	0	0.5	1	1.5	2.0
Marrow blasts (%)	<5	5–10	–	11–20	21–30
Karyotype[a]	Good	Intermediate	Poor		
Cytopenias[b]	0/1	2/3			
Combined score	**IPSS risk group**	**Survival (%)[c]**	**Progression to AML (%)[c]**		
0	Low	55	15		
0.5–1	Int-1	35	30		
1.5–2	Int-2	7	65		
>2	High	0	100		

Notes: Int, intermediate.
[a]Good: diploid, -Y, del(5q), del(20q); Poor: complex, chromosome 7 abnormalities; Intermediate: others.
[b]Hemoglobin < 10 g/dL, neutrophils < 1.5×10^9/L, platelets < 100×10^9/L.
[c]At 5 years.
Source: Modified from Greenberg *et al.*[26]

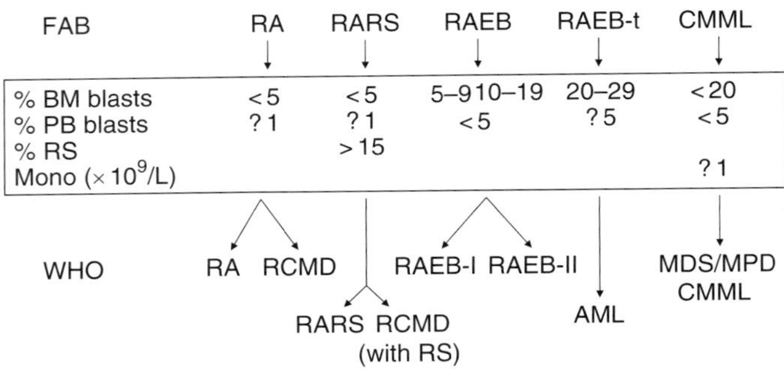

Figure 6.2 FAB and World Health Organization (WHO) classification: diagnostic criteria. BM: bone marrow; PB: peripheral blood; RS: ringed sideroblasts; Mono: monocytes; RCMD: refractory cytopenia with multilineage dysplasia; MPD: myeloproliferative disease.

marrow ringed sideroblasts, the number of peripheral monocytes, and the presence of Auer rods. Five subtypes are defined (Figure 6.2): refractory anemia (RA), refractory anemia with ringed sideroblasts (RARS), refractory anemia with excess of blasts (RAEB), refractory anemia with excess of blasts in transformation (RAEB-t), and CMML.

Although time-tested and valuable, a number of limitations of the FAB classification led to a new proposal by the World Health Organization (WHO), which tried to integrate biologic, immunophenotypic, and genetic information in addition to morphologic criteria.[18,24] Although morphologic criteria remain a cornerstone of the WHO system, important differences compared to FAB exist (Figure 6.2): (1) RA and RARS are divided by unilineage and multilineage dysplasia; (2) RAEB is separated into RAEB-I (5–10% blasts) and RAEB-II (11–19% blasts); (3) RAEB-t has been eliminated and patients with ≥ 20% blasts are now diagnosed to have AML; (4) CMML is not part of MDS any longer, but a separate entity characterized by either myelodysplastic or myeloproliferative features; and (5) there is now a group of unclassifiable MDS. The WHO categories have correlated better with prognosis and response to therapy than the FAB system.[25] Attempts at a molecular classification of MDS and identification of genetic abnormalities in morphologic subgroups (e.g., *JAK2* mutations in refractory anemia with ringed sideroblasts and thrombocytosis [RARS-T]) are in early stages, but will undoubtedly expand rapidly in the years to come leading to revisions of the WHO as it is known today.

The International Prognostic Scoring System (IPSS) was developed in 1996 based on a multivariate analysis of 816 patients with de novo, untreated (except for supportive care) MDS.[26] Calculating from the time of diagnosis, three variables were significant for survival and AML transformation: percent of marrow blasts, cytogenetic abnormalities, and severity of blood cytopenias. It assigns points to each of the factors and divides patients into low-, intermediate-1-, intermediate-2-, and high-risk groups with a corresponding decline of median survival times and increase of the risk of AML transformation, respectively (Table 6.4). Given the characteristics of the patients based on whom the IPSS was developed it should be kept in mind that expectations for survival and AML transformation may not apply to other patients, such as previously treated patients or those referred to tertiary care centers. For example, the median survival of patients with IPSS low and intermediate-1 groups referred to MD Anderson Cancer Center was only 2.1 and 1.2 years, respectively.[27] Furthermore, the IPSS undervalues poor prognostic cytogenetic abnormalities and does not take into account the significance of bad neutropenia and/or thrombocytopenia. Refinements of the IPSS therefore continue to be proposed. The WPSS (WHO-based prognostic scoring system) includes transfusion dependency, which has been associated with poorer prognosis in MDS, cytogenetic risk group, and criteria of the WHO classification.[28]

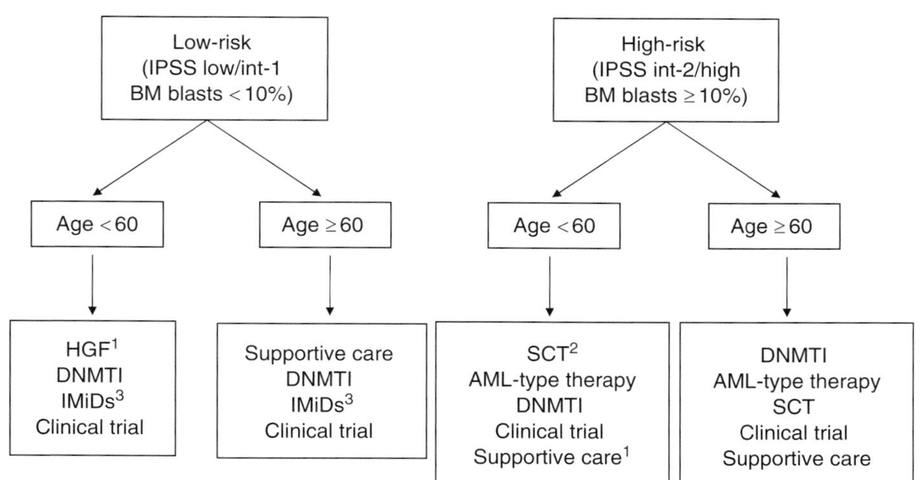

Figure 6.3 Possible treatment algorithm for MDS. Decision of low- versus high-intensity treatment based on IPSS score, age, and performance status. [1]Growth factors/supportive care in patients with poor performance status; [2]SCT especially for younger patients with matched-related sibling donor; [3]5q- MDS. HGF: hematopoietic growth factors; BM: bone marrow; DNMTI: DNA methyltransferase inhibitor (azacitidine, decitabine); IMiD: immunomodulatory inhibitory drug (lenalidomide); SCT: stem cell transplantation.

The MD Anderson group published a new prognostic model accounting for duration of MDS and prior therapy.[29] It was based on almost 2000 patients with MDS of whom only about one-quarter had primary MDS without any prior therapy and to whom the original IPSS would have been applicable. Based on a multivariate analysis, four prognostic groups of patients could be identified with significantly different outcomes.

Other groups of MDS

Hypocellular MDS

Rather than hypercellular, a few patients with MDS present with hypocellular marrows, a situation which is not always easy to distinguish from aplastic anemia.[30] Both conditions share common features such as T-cell-mediated myelosuppression, presence of parokysmal nocturnal hemoglobinuria (PNH)-type clones, and responsiveness to immunomodulation. Distinctive features based on antigen expression patterns of CD34-positive cells by flow cytometry or immunohistochemistry have been suggested.[31] In practice, however, therapy may often be similar.

MDS with myelofibrosis

About 15% of patients with MDS have sufficient reticulin fibrosis to warrant the diagnosis. Minimal diagnostic criteria include diffuse, coarse reticulin fibrosis and dysplasia in at least two cell lineages. Depending on blast percentage and other clinical features, the differential diagnostic considerations include acute panmyelosis with fibrosis (APMF), acute megakaryocytic leukemia (FAB M7), malignant lymphomas, or hairy cell leukemia. Marrow fibrosis identifies a distinct subgroup of MDS associated with high transfusion requirements and poor prognosis.[32]

Myelodysplastic syndromes/myeloproliferative neoplasms (MDS/MPN)

This category includes myeloid disorders, which are difficult to unambiguously assign to a purely dysplastic or proliferative entity as they share characteristics of each. CMML serves as a good example to highlight some of the controversies.[33] Formerly part of the FAB classification and counted among MDS, it has since become a separate disease entity with some distinct features. Cytogenetic abnormalities are less frequent than in MDS and, when present, involve monosomy 7, trisomy 8, or other structural changes including 12p. Among molecular abnormalities disruptions of the *PDGFRβ* gene located on chromosome 5q33 were first described as the result of the reciprocal translocation t(5;12). The resulting TEL-PDGFRβ fusion tyrosine kinase leads to constitutive and ligand-independent stimulation of the tyrosine kinase activity of PDGFRβ and to a phenotype more consistent with a MPD than MDS. Several translocations lead to fusions of *PDGFRβ* with other genes, and ultimately result in the same consequences.[34,35]

RARS-T (Refractory anemia with ringed sideroblasts and thrombocytosis)

RARS-T is a fairly recently defined subgroup of MDS. On a molecular level, it is characterized by a mutation of *JAK2*, which is typically found in patients with MPD (mostly polycythemia vera). The *JAK2* mutation is thought to drive the thrombocytosis.

Therapy

For many years supportive care was the only available therapy for MDS except for "active therapy" in the form of AML-type chemotherapy or stem cell transplant (SCT) in the case of advanced stages or progression to AML. This situation has changed radically as new drugs became available in recent years, which combine activity with acceptable toxicity and tolerability. Treatment decisions in MDS have hence become even more challenging as therapeutic decisions are also determined by other factors such as age and performance status, the IPSS score, and disease-specific characteristics (e.g., abnormalities of 5q-). Specific criteria and guidelines which help in the decision-making process have been established and are constantly revised (Figure 6.3). It is important to be clear about the goals of therapy in MDS, which differ from those in other hematologic malignancies. MDS is often a chronic ailment that creates morbidity

Table 6.5. Therapy in MDS

Low-risk	High-risk
• Hematopoietic growth factors	• DNMT inhibitors
– Erythropoietin ± filgrastim/ pegfilgrastim	– azacitidine
	–decitabine
• Immunomodulation	• Intensive chemotherapy (younger patients, diploid cytogenetics)
– Antithymocyte globulins ± ciclosporin, ± steroids	
• Lenalidomide for 5q-	• Allogeneic stem cell transplantation
• Imatinib mesylate for translocations involving 5q33, e.g., t(5;12)	• Investigational
• DMNT inhibitors	
– azacitidine	
– decitabine	
• Investigational (histone deacetylase inhibitors)	

and mortality because of refractory cytopenias and not, for most patients, from progression to AML. For practical purposes, patients are therefore usually divided into those with lower- versus those with higher-risk disease (based on IPSS alone or in some cases based on $< 10\%$ versus $\geq 10\%$ marrow blasts). Patients with low-risk MDS can sometimes be observed as long as they are asymptomatic, have few marrow blasts, and are not transfusion-dependent. At any sign of progression they can then be assessed for therapeutic intervention as outlined in Table 6.5. Because of the more rapid pace of disease and poorer prognosis with high-risk MDS, prompt therapy is usually recommended. In either case, efforts should be made to enroll patients in clinical trials. The goal of low-intensity programs is to produce improvement of hematologic indices and quality of life, whereas high-intensity programs are aimed at achieving remissions and therefore changing the natural history of the MDS.

As there has been considerable heterogeneity among interpretation of clinical trials in the past, adherence to a proposed set of standardized response criteria for clinical trials in MDS has largely facilitated reporting of responses and continues to be crucial in the evaluation of patients with MDS on therapy (Table 6.6).[36,37]

Supportive and low-intensity therapy

If the goal is hematologic improvement while at least maintaining an acceptable quality of life the possibilities include transfusions of blood products, administration of hematopoietic growth factors, and use of antibiotics. For some patients, immune suppression (ATG, cyclosporine), immunomodulatory inhibitory derivatives (lenalidomide), or hypomethylating agents (azacitidine or decitabine) may be appropriate. Supportive care and other forms of MDS-specific therapy are therefore not mutually exclusive, and used in combination may be synergistic.

Iron chelation therapy

Clinically significant iron accumulation may be expected in patients who have received 5 g of iron or the equivalent of 25 units of packed red blood cells. Iron accumulation is of concern in patients with more indolent forms of MDS who are likely to require transfusion support over several years (e.g., in 5q- syndrome). Iron overload can be effectively managed with iron chelation therapy. Desferioxamine (Desferal) has been in use for many years and is administered either subcutaneously or intravenously on up to 5-7 days/week. Deferasirox (Exjade) is a once-daily oral iron chelator, which has recently been approved in the United States for treatment of transfusional iron overload in adult and pediatric patients. Use of iron chelation in patients with MDS has shown to result in improvement of survival in lower-risk MDS with low transfusion needs (less than 2 units per month).[38,39]

Hematopoietic growth factors

Erythropoietin or darbepoietin (a modified form of erythropoietin with prolonged serum half-life and increased in vivo biologic activity requiring less frequent dosing) alone or with granulocyte colony-stimulating factor (G-CSF; filgrastim) can result in erythroid responses in 40–50% of patients, particularly those with low endogenous erythropoietin levels, which are durable for a median of 2 to 2.5 years. Low pretreatment serum erythropoietin levels ($<$ 200–500 mU/mL), infrequent transfusion requirements ($<$ 2 units packed red blood cells per month), and favorable IPSS group have been predictive for response.[40,41] The combination of erythropoietin plus filgrastim achieves durable responses (median duration of up to 29 months in responding patients) and not only improves anemia, but also survival for patients with above defined characteristics.[42] Higher doses of erythropoietins may improve response rates.

Patients with severe neutropenia present a bigger challenge and/or thrombocytopenia as response rates under those circumstances are lower than in patients with predominantly anemia. Patients with neutropenia should be counseled about the risk of infections and be aware of the telltale signs and symptoms in order to seek prompt medical attention when necessary. Filgrastim (or its pegylated variant pegfilgrastim) or GM-CSF (sargramostim) should be used in patients with neutropenic fever or to boost response rates in combination with erythropoietins as outlined above. Either agent may improve neutropenia in up to 70% of patients, but no data exist to prove that they would reduce the number of infectious episodes,

Table 6.6. Modified International Working Group response criteria in MDS

Criteria for altering the natural history of MDS	
Category	**Response criteria (responses must last at least 4 weeks)**
Complete remission (CR)	• Marrow:
	$\leq$ 5% blasts with normal maturation of all cell lines
	• Blood:
	Hemoglobin $\geq$ 11 g/dL, platelets $\geq 100 \times 10^9$/L, neutrophils $\geq 1 \times 10^9$/L, blasts 0%
Partial remission	All CR criteria if abnormal before treatment except:
	• Marrow:
	Blasts decreased by $\geq$ 50% over pretreatment but still > 5% (cellularity and morphology not relevant)
Cytogenetic response	• Complete:
	Disappearance of the chromosomal abnormality without appearance of new ones
	• Partial:
	At least 50% reduction of the chromosomal abnormality
Criteria for hematologic improvement	
Category	**Response criteria (responses must last at least 8 weeks)**
Erythroid response[a]	• Hemoglobin increase by $\geq$ 1.5 g/dL
	• Relevant reduction of units of red blood cell (RBC) transfusions by an absolute number of at least 4 RBC transfusions/8 wk compared with the pretreatment transfusion number in the previous 8 wk[b]
Platelet response[a]	• Absolute increase of $\geq 30 \times 10^9$/L for patients starting with $> 20 \times 10^9$/L platelets
	• Increase from $< 20 \times 10^9$/L to $> 20 \times 10^9$/L and by at least 100%
Neutrophil response[a]	• At least 100% increase and an absolute increase $> 0.5 \times 10^9$/L

Notes: [a]Hematologic improvement is measured in patients with the following pretreatment abnormal values: hemoglobin < 11g/dL or RBC-transfusion dependence, platelet count $< 100 \times 10^9$/L or platelet-transfusion dependence, absolute neutrophil count $< 1 \times 10^9$/L. Pretreatment counts are averages of at least 2 measurements (not influenced by transfusions) $\geq$ 1 week apart.
[b]Only RBC transfusions given for a hemoglobin of $\leq$ 9 g/dL pretreatment will count in the RBC transfusion response evaluation.
Source: Modified from Cheson *et al.*[37]

prolong survival, or influence the rate of transformation to AML.

Severe thrombocytopenia (platelet count $< 20 \times 10^9$/L) can be expected to occur in almost a fifth of MDS patients, with hemorrhagic complications ranging from 3% to 53% (depending on therapy administered), and the frequency of hemorrhagic deaths ranging from 14% to 24%.[43] Recombinant human IL-11 (oprelvekin) is a megakaryocytic growth factor that stimulates proliferation and maturation of megakaryocytic progenitor cells and has been approved by the US Food and Drug Administration (FDA) for prevention of severe thrombocytopenia following myelosuppressive chemotherapy. However, adverse events (arrhythmias, fluid retention) may be severe, especially in elderly patients, and response rates in up to a third of patients (mainly with platelet counts $< 20 \times 10^9$/L) are rather low.[44] Recently, two new drugs have emerged on the market which both work via the thrombopoietin (TPO) receptor site, thus stimulating proliferation and differentiation of marrow megakaryocytes. Eltrombopag is an orally available small molecule binding to the TPO (c-mpl) receptor thereby activating Jak-Stat signaling pathways.[45] Romiplostim is a fusion protein analog (peptibody) which shares two peptide residues with four TPO receptor binding sites.[46] Both drugs received FDA approval in idiopathic thrombocytopenic purpura (ITP). Although they have both raised interest in MDS therapy, their role in MDS remains undefined at this point.[47]

Immune modulation therapy

Immunosuppression

Some patients with MDS may benefit from immunosuppressive therapy with antithymocyte (ATG) or antilymphocyte (ALG) globulins and ciclosporin with or without corticosteroids. Responses of immunosuppressive therapy vary widely and have been reported to be between 16% and 50%.[48,49] Expression of D-related human leukemic antigen 15 (HLA-DR15), a CD59-deficient phenotype, marrow hypocellularity, low-risk MDS in the absence of cytogenetic abnormalities, and a short history of transfusion dependence have been correlated with a higher likelihood of response to immunosuppression. Recent larger studies, however, have challenged the predictive value of these factors.[50,51] Among 68 patients with MDS treated with ATG, the only independent variable for response and survival was a more favorable IPSS score.[50] Combining ATG with ciclosporin leads to higher responses than ATG alone.[51] Response durations are in the range of up to 1 year and in general shorter than can be achieved in aplastic anemia.[52] ATG are derived from horses, goats, and other animals, so that problems with serum sickness and other toxicities are frequent, especially in older patients. Selection of appropriate patients is therefore essential. The current consensus seems to favor younger patients with low-risk MDS and possibly with shorter MDS duration.

Immunomodulatory inhibitory drugs (IMiDs)

Lenalidomide (a 4-amino-glutarimide analog of thalidomide) stimulates T lymphocytes to shift from Th-1 to Th-2 responses and enhances cell-mediated immunity. In addition, it has an anticytokine effect and inhibits basic fibroblast growth factor (bFGF) and vascular endothelial growth factor (VEGF)-induced angiogenesis. Its precise mechanism of action is unclear and may be a combination of any of the ones described. In a combined phase I/II trial of 43 patients with transfusion-dependent or symptomatic anemia, lenalidomide (25 mg or 10 mg daily or 10 mg daily for 21 days with a one-week rest) produced response rates of 56% including 47% of patients with sustained independence from transfusions.[53] Of particular interest was the observation that among those patients with 5q- syndrome, the response rate was as high as 83%. These results were confirmed in an expanded phase II trial of patients with lower-risk MDS, transfusion dependence, and chromosome 5q deletion where the rate of transfusion independence was 67% accompanied by a median rise of hemoglobin by 5.3 g/dL.[54] The median time to response was 4.6 weeks and the median duration of transfusion independence 2.2 years. Moreover, 45% of evaluable patients achieved a complete cytogenetic remission. Severe neutropenia and thrombocytopenia occurred in 50% to 60% of the patients requiring frequent treatment interruptions or dose adjustments. Response rates (transfusion independence) in patients with similar clinical characteristics but without del(5q) were 26%.[55] Furthermore the median increase of hemoglobin levels was lower, and response durations shorter (median of 41 weeks).

Lenalidomide is FDA approved for patients with low-risk MDS who are transfusion-dependent and have a detectable del (5q) and should be considered standard therapy for this group. Its role in other settings of MDS remains investigational.

Epigenetic therapy

Global and gene-specific hypermethylation of promoter-associated CpG islands in combination with deacetylation and methylation of nucleosome-associated histone tails leads to silencing of gene expression critical for cell growth and differentiation.[56] On the other hand, reversal of abnormal methylation patterns or inhibition of deacetylase activity of histone proteins can trigger a permissive gene expression state and reactivate aberrantly silenced genes leading to leukemic suppression of the MDS clone. Hypomethylating agents covalently bind to DNA methyltransferase (DNMT) inhibitors after phosphorylation and incorporation into DNA where they inhibit their function leading to progressive hypomethylation. This association has led to great interest in hypomethylating agents as well as histone deacetylase (HDAC) inhibitors, which have become a mainstay of MDS treatment. The two most important drugs to date are azacitidine and 5-aza-2'-deoxycytidine (decitabine).

The clinical development of azacitidine, a pyrimidine nucleoside analog, in MDS dates back to the early 1980s. Following encouraging results in initial studies of patients with MDS the Cancer and Leukemia Group B (CALGB) conducted a randomized study of observation ($n = 92$) versus subcutaneous azacitidine (75 mg/m^2 subcutaneously daily $\times$ 7 days every 4 weeks) ($n = 99$) in patients with high-risk MDS.[57] The results significantly favored azacitidine. Sixty-three percent (6% complete response [CR], 10% partial response [PR], 47% hematologic improvement) of patients responded to azacitidine versus 7% in the observation arm. Median time to leukemia transformation (21 months versus 13 months, $p < 0.01$) and median survival (20 months versus 14 months, $p = 0.01$) were also more favorable for azacitidine-treated patients. Furthermore, quality-of-life parameters such as fatigue, dyspnea, physical functioning, positive affect, and psychological distress improved significantly on the treatment arm. A larger phase III follow-up study randomly assigned 358 patients to receive azacitidine or conventional care regimens (best supportive care, low-dose cytarabine, or intensive chemotherapy).[58] After a median follow-up of 21.1 months, median overall survival was 24.5 months in the azacitidine group compared to 15 months for the conventional care group. This non-crossover study is thus the first to demonstrate a survival advantage of a therapeutic intervention in MDS.

Decitabine, a deoxycytidine analog with close relationship to azacitidine, has been tested in similar types of patients. When used at higher doses of 1500–2250 mg/m^2 per course it was associated with severe and prolonged myelosuppression. More recent in vitro data, however, demonstrated that at lower doses, the cytotoxic effect of decitabine was minimal while still markedly inhibiting DNMT activity.

At the lower dose schedule of 15 mg/m^2 three times daily for 3 days every 6 weeks (145 mg/m^2 per course), 49% of 177 patients with MDS and a median age of 70 years responded.[59] The median response duration was 36 weeks and median survival 15 months. Using the same dose and schedule, in a randomized study of decitabine versus best supportive care, decitabine-treated patients had higher response rates (17% overall including 9% complete responders compared to 0%, $p < 0.001$) and a trend toward a longer median time to AML progression or death (12.1 months versus 7.8 months, p

= 0.16).[60] Responses were durable and associated with transfusion independence. The favorable results with lower-dose schedules led to further trials to optimize the decitabine dose schedule. In one study 95 patients with advanced MDS (including CMML) were randomized to receive decitabine 20 mg/m^2 intravenously daily for 5 days, 20 mg/m^2 subcutaneously daily for 5 days, and 10 mg/m^2 intravenously daily for 10 days every 4 weeks (rather than 6 weeks as in previous studies).[61] Sixty-nine patients (73%) had an objective response (including 34% complete responders). The 5-day intravenous schedule had the highest CR rate (39%). These single-center results have recently been confirmed in a multicenter study.[62] A low-dose but dose-intense schedule of decitabine may thus be able to optimize clinical responses in MDS. In an international phase III study, 233 patients over 60 years with primary or secondary MDS or CMML were randomized to decitabine or supportive care.[63] Up to eight cycles of decitabine were permitted with overall survival as the primary end point. Both the response rate (34%) and progression-free survival (0.55 versus 0.25 years, p = 0.004) were significantly better with decitabine. However, overall survival was not significantly different.

Both azacitidine and decitabine are now approved for use in patients with MDS and CMML. Both drugs may alter the natural history of MDS, but need to be administered for a minimum of three to six cycles to ensure adequate exposure for patients to demonstrate a clinical response.[64] Many questions remain: (1) optimal dose and schedule: there is a trend to use lower doses to emphasize biologic activity at the cost of untoward toxicity; (2) combination partners: current clinical trials are evaluating whether the combination of a DNMT inhibitor with a HDAC inhibitor enhances gene reactivation and clinical responses. Numerous HDAC inhibitors are available in clinical trials with no clear picture yet as of a preferred agent and the advantage of the combinations over single-agent DNMT inhibitor therapy; and (3) how to approach patients who fail DNMT inhibitors. A small study suggested response rates of 30–40% for patients treated with decitabine after failing azacitidine.[65] However, most patients are not likely to benefit from this strategy and it hence raises the specter of intensive therapy (including SCT) and other investigational drugs.

Investigational therapies

Arsenic trioxide has multiple mechanisms of action including apoptosis, tumor cell differentiation, and inhibition of proliferation of leukemic cells. There are two large multicenter phase II trials of arsenic trioxide in MDS. In the European study, 115 patients with a median age of 68 years received arsenic trioxide 0.3 mg/kg per day for 5 days followed by a maintenance dose of 0.25 mg/kg twice weekly for 15 weeks.[66] The overall rate of hematologic improvement was 19% with higher response rates in lower-risk patients (26% versus 17%). Median response duration was only 3.4 months. In the US trial, 76 patients received arsenic trioxide 0.25 mg/kg per day on 5 consecutive days per week for 2 weeks, followed by 2 weeks' rest.[67] The overall rate of hematologic improvement was in the range of 20% with a median duration of hematologic improvement of 6.8 months. Only one patient with higher-risk MDS achieved CR. The activity of arsenic trioxide has therefore been modest and could not establish itself in MDS treatment algorithms.

The activity of tyrosine kinase inhibitors has been restricted to MDS cases with specific molecular abnormalities (e.g., fusion of the *PDGFRβ* gene on chromosome 5q33 to the *ETV6* gene in translocation t(5;12)).[68] As these are rare in MDS and more frequent in patients with a proliferative variant such as in CMML, only a few MDS patients will be eligible.

Ezatiostat is a small molecule glutathione analog, which stimulates blood stem cell colony formation in vitro. In a phase I/II study of ezatiostat in MDS (74% low and intermediate-1), several dose schedules were explored, whereby 600 mg/m^2 intravenously daily for 3 days in cycles of 21 days was well tolerated.[69] Of 43 evaluable patients, 27 (63%) achieved hematologic improvement in one or more cell lineages. Other schedules are since being explored and an oral compound of ezatiostat is in development.

Obatoclax is a small molecule antagonist of the BH3-binding groove of the BCL2 family of antiapoptotic proteins. In an exploratory study, patients with a variety of hematologic malignancies were treated at doses of 7–40 mg/m^2 intravenously over 24 hours every 2 weeks.[70] Three of eight patients with MDS achieved hematologic improvement characterized by red blood cell or platelet transfusion independence.

Clofarabine is a new deoxyadenosine nucleoside analog with activity in AML and MDS. Results from currently ongoing phase II studies of intravenous and oral clofarabine at different dose levels in patients with higher-risk MDS have recently been reported.[71] The overall response was 47% including 30% of patients achieving CR. Responses were lower in patients who had failed prior hypomethylating agents. Myelosuppression and hospitalizations for neutropenic fever together with nausea, vomiting, skin rashes, hyperbilirubinemia, and transaminase elevations were frequent. Although clofarabine has shown activity in patients with higher-risk MDS, the optimal dose and schedule, especially for the oral formulation, remain to be defined.

High-intensity therapy

Either AML-type regimens or SCT can change the natural course of MDS leading to long-term benefit for some patients. Given the demographics of MDS, however, either approach will only be relevant for a few patients. The availability of lenalidomide and epigenetic therapy makes judicious selection of patients for high-intensity approaches even more crucial and challenging. When comparing the outcome of patients with high-risk MDS treated with decitabine versus cytarabine-based chemotherapy, complete responses were comparable (43%

versus 46%), whereas mortality at 6 weeks (3% versus 12%, $p = 0.002$) and 3 months (7% versus 22%) and estimated 2-year survival (47% versus 25%, $p < 0.001$) were significantly in favor of decitabine.[72]

A multivariate analysis based on 394 newly diagnosed patients with high-risk MDS addressed the outcome and relative merits of the following chemotherapy combinations: (1) idarubicin plus cytarabine; (2) fludarabine plus cytarabine; (3) fludarabine, cytarabine, plus idarubicin; (4) topotecan plus cytarabine; and (5) cyclophosphamide, cytarabine, plus topotecan).[73] The CR rate was 58% and was significantly associated with karyotype, performance status, age, duration of antecedent hematologic disorder, and treatment in laminar air flow rooms. There was no difference in CR rate based on the regimen used. Topotecan-based regimens had the lowest induction mortality, especially in patients > 65 years. Overall survival was similar to that of patients treated with idarubicin and cytarabine.

Improvement in outcome is therefore unlikely to come from further intensification of therapy. Innovative post-remission strategies (availability of "targeted" therapies, immunomodulation, epigenetic therapy) and exploration of new drugs (e.g., novel nucleoside analogs such as clofarabine, or new topoisomerase I inhibitors) are more likely to be promising.

Although potentially curative with long-term disease-free survival rates of 30-70%, allogeneic SCT is applicable to only a small fraction of patients because of age, concomitant medical conditions, and donor availability. Treatment-related morbidity and mortality remain substantial impediments to SCT. Outcome is most favorable in patients who may need transplant the least, for example younger patients with low-risk MDS.[74] In an update of the International Bone Marrow Transplant Registry (IBMTR), 452 recipients of HLA-identical sibling transplants with a median age of 34 years and high-risk MDS in almost two-thirds were reviewed.[75] Overall survival at 3 years was 42%. Survival was more favorable in younger patients and those with platelet counts $> 100 \times 10^9$/L. Relapse risk was higher in patients with high percentages of marrow blasts at transplantation, with high IPSS scores, and with T-cell depleted transplants. When patients were evaluated by the IPSS, the disease-free survival was 60% in the low-risk, 36% in the intermediate-1-risk, and 28% in the intermediate-2-risk groups. This compared to 5-year survival rates of 55%, 35%, and 7%, respectively for unselected patients not receiving SCT suggesting a benefit of SCT mostly for high-risk MDS patients.

A key question is therefore the optimal timing of SCT. Many patients may enjoy relatively long periods of stable disease following diagnosis, so that the risks of transplant-related complications outweigh any possible benefit. Using a Markov decision model, three transplant strategies were compared with each other: (1) SCT at diagnosis; (2) SCT at the time of progression to leukemia; and (3) SCT some time after diagnosis but prior to progression.[76] In both the low and intermediate-1 IPSS groups, delayed transplantation maximized overall survival, whereas earlier transplantation improved survival in intermediate-2 and high IPSS groups. Reduced intensity conditioning (RIC) SCT is one way to get around excessive toxicity in older and pretreated patients. The European Blood and Marrow Transplantation Group has reported a retrospective comparison of 836 patients with MDS who received RIC (215 patients) or a standard conditioning regimen (621 patients).[77] The RIC group showed a significantly higher 3-year relapse rate and lower 3-year non-relapse mortality rate, which translated into a similar progression-free (33% in RIC versus 39% with standard conditioning, $p = 0.9$) and overall survival (41% versus 45%, $p = 0.8$).

Results from matched unrelated donor programs lag behind those of matched related sibling transplants, although better results (3-year relapse-free survival rate of 59%) have been reported by the Seattle group using conditioning regimens with targeted busulfan and cyclophosphamide.[78] Autologous SCT has a limited role in MDS and is restricted to patients in CR, who could be harvested, and were candidates for the procedure. Few data exist to evaluate the impact of other investigational transplant approaches such as umbilical cord blood transplants in MDS.

Conclusion

There is no doubt that progress has been made over the last few years in the management of patients with MDS. Most notably, the high activity of lenalidomide in 5q-syndrome and the encouraging outcome of epigenetic therapy in most other MDS scenarios have significantly altered the therapeutic field where supportive therapy was once the preferred approach. Therapeutic nihilism is therefore not justified any longer. Undoubtedly, many more drugs will appear in the years to come. As the biology of MDS becomes better understood, classification and prognostic schemes will become more sophisticated, new drugs will come to the market, and further progress can be expected.

References

1. Heaney M, Golde D. Myelodysplasia. *New Engl J Med* 1999;**340**:1649–60.
2. Albitar M, Manshouri T, Shen Y, *et al.* Myelodysplastic syndrome is not merely "preleukemia." *Blood* 2002;**100**:791–8.
3. Kuendgen A, Strupp C, Avivado M, *et al.* Myelodysplastic syndromes in patients younger than age 50. *J Clin Oncol* 2006;**24**:5358–65.
4. Rollison DE, Hayat M, Smith M, *et al.* First report of national estimates of the incidence of myelodysplastic syndromes and chronic myeloproliferative disorders from the U.S. SEER Program. *Blood* 2006;**108**:77a.
5. Goldberg SL, Mody-Patel N, Chen ER. Clinical and economic consequences of myelodysplastic syndromes in the United States: an analysis of the Medicare database. *Blood* 2008;**112**:237.

6. Nagata C, Shimizu H, Hirashima K, *et al.* Hair dye use and occupational exposure to organic solvents as risk factors for myelodysplastic syndrome. *Leuk Res* 1999;**23**:57–62.

7. Kimura A, Takeuchi Y, Tanaka H, *et al.* Atomic bomb radiation increases the risk of MDS. *Leuk Res* 2001;**25**:S13.

8. Park DJ, Koeffler HP. Therapy-related myelodysplastic syndromes. *Semin Hematol* 1996;**33**:256–73.

9. Armitage JO, Carbone PP, Connors JM, *et al.* Treatment-related myelodysplasia and acute leukemia in non-Hodgkin's lymphoma patients. *J Clin Oncol* 2003;**21**:897–906.

10. Bowen D, Culligan D, Jowitt S, *et al.* of the UK MDS Guidelines Group. Guidelines for the diagnosis and therapy of adult myelodysplastic syndromes. *Br J Haematol* 2003; **120**:187–200.

11. Rosenfeld C, List A. A hypothesis for the pathogenesis of myelodysplastic syndromes: implications for new therapies. *Leukemia* 2000;**14**:2–8.

12. Testa LJ. Apoptotic mechanisms in the control of erythropoiesis. *Leukemia* 2004;**18**:1176–99.

13. Parker JE, Mufti GJ, Rasool F, *et al.* The role of apoptosis, proliferation, and the BCL2-related proteins in the myelodysplastic syndromes and acute myeloid leukemia secondary to MDS. *Blood* 2000;**96**:3932–8.

14. Campioni D, Secchiero P, Corallini F, *et al.* Evidence for a role of TNF-related apoptosis-inducing ligand (TRAIL) in the anemia of myelodysplastic syndromes. *Am J Pathol* 2005; **166**:557–63.

15. Bruce Galili N, Mehdi M, Mumtaz J, *et al.* Can molecular profiling of cytogenetic subgroups draw a roadmap for individualizing therapy in myelodysplastic syndromes? *Future Oncol* 2006;**2**:407–15.

16. Haase D, Steidl D, Schanz J, *et al.* Correlation of cytogenetic findings with morphology, clinical course, and prognosis in 2124 patients with MDS. *Blood* 2005;**106**:232a.

17. Haase D, Germing U, Schanz J, *et al.* New insights into the prognostic impact of the karyotype in MDS and correlation with subtypes: evidence from a core dataset of 2124 patients. *Blood* 2007;**110**:4385–95.

18. Vardiman JW, Harris NL, Brunning RD. The World Health Organization (WHO) classification of the myeloid neoplasms. *Blood* 2002;**100**: 2292–302.

19. Ebert B, Pretz J, Bosco J, *et al.* Identification of RPS14 as a 5q- syndrome gene by RNA interference screen. *Nature* 2008;**451**:335–9.

20. Hirai H, Kobayashi Y, Mano H, *et al.* A point mutation at codon 13 of the N-ras oncogene in myelodysplastic syndrome. *Nature* 1987;**327**:430–32.

21. Liu E, Hjelle B, Morgan R, *et al.* Mutations of the Kirsten-ras proto-oncogene in human preleukaemia. *Nature* 1987;**330**:186–8.

22. Wu S-J, Chou W-C, Yao M, *et al.* *SOCS1* methylation predicts a high risk of acute leukemic transformation in primary myelodysplastic syndrome. *Blood* 2006;**108**:742a.

23. Bennett JM, Catovsky D, Daniel MT, *et al.* Proposals for the classification of the myelodysplastic syndromes. *Br J Haematol* 1982;**51**:189–99.

24. Verhoef GEG, Pittaluga S, Wolfe-Peters CDE, *et al.* FAB classification of myelodysplastic syndromes: merits and controversies. *Ann Hematol* 1995;**71**:3–11.

25. Germing U, Strupp C, Kuendgen A, *et al.* Prospective validation of the WHO proposals for the classification of myelodysplastic syndromes. *Haematologica* 2006;**91**:1596–604.

26. Greenberg P, Cox C, LeBeau MM, *et al.* International scoring system for evaluating prognosis in myelodysplastic syndromes. *Blood* 1997;**89**:2079–88.

27. Estey E, Keating M, Pierce S, *et al.* Application of the international scoring system for myelodysplasia to MD Anderson patients. *Blood* 1997;**90**:2843–4.

28. Cazzola M, Malcovati L. Myelodysplastic syndromes: coping with ineffective hematopoiesis. *N Engl J Med* 2005;**352**:536–8.

29. Kantarjian H, O'Brien S, Ravandi F, *et al.* Proposal for a new risk model in myelodysplastic syndrome that accounts for events not considered in the original International Prognostic Scoring System. *Cancer* 2008;**113**:1351–61.

30. Wong KF, So CC. Hyoplastic myelodysplastic syndrome – a clinical, morphologic, or genetic diagnosis? *Cancer Genet Cytogenet* 2002; **138**:85–8.

31. Matsui WH, Brodksy RA, Smith BD, *et al.* Quantitative analysis of bone marrow CD34 cells in aplastic anemia and hypoplastic myelodysplastic syndromes. *Leukemia* 2006; **20**:458–62.

32. Della Porta MG, Malcovati L, Boveri E, *et al.* Clinical clusters of bone marrow fibrosis and CD34-positive cell clusters in primary myelodysplastic syndromes. *J Clin Oncol* 2009;**27**:754–62.

33. Bowen DT. Chronic myelomonocytic leukemia: lost in classification? *Hematol Oncol* 2005;**23**:26–33.

34. Remacha AF, Nomdedéu JF, Puget G, *et al.* Occurrence of the *JAK2* V617F mutation in the WHO provisional entity: myelodysplastic/ myeloproliferative disease, unclassifiable-refractory anemia with ringed sideroblasts associated with marked thrombocytosis. *Haematologica* 2006;**91**:719–20.

35. David M, Cross NCP, Burgstaller S, *et al.* Durable responses to imatinib in patients with *PDGFRB* fusion gene-positive and *BCR-ABL*-negative chronic myeloproliferative disorders. *Blood* 2007;**109**:61–4.

36. Cheson BD, Bennett JM, Kantarjian HM, *et al.* Report of an international working group to standardize response criteria for myelodysplastic syndromes. *Blood* 2000;**96**:3671–4.

37. Cheson BD, Greenberg PL, Bennett JM, *et al.* Clinical application and proposal for modification of the International Working Group (IWG) response criteria in myelodysplasia. *Blood* 2006;**108**:419–25.

38. Gattermann N, Schmid M, Della Porta M, *et al.* Efficacy and safety of Deferasirox (Exjade®) during 1 year of treatment in transfusion-dependent patients with myelodysplastic syndromes: results from EPIC trial. *Blood* 2008;**112**:235.

39. List AF, Baer MR, Steensma D, *et al.* Iron chelation with Deferasirox (Exjade®) improves iron burden in patients with myelodysplastic syndromes (MDS). *Blood* 2008; **112**:236.

40. Hellström-Lindberg E, Gulbrandsen N, Lindberg G, *et al.* A validated decision model for treating the anaemia of myelodysplastic syndromes with

erythropoietin + granulocyte colony-stimulating factor: significant effects on quality of life. *Br J Haematol* 2003;**120**:1037–46.

41. Park S, Kelaidi C, Grabar S, *et al.* Prognostic factors and response duration in 419 MDS treated with erythropoietin ± G-CSF: The GFM experience. *Blood* 2006;**108**:158a.
42. Jädersten M, Montgomery SM, Dybedal I, *et al.* Long-term outcome of treatment of anemia in MDS with erythropoietin and G-CSF. *Blood* 2005;**106**:803–11.
43. Kantarjian HM, Giles F, List AF, *et al.* The incidence and impact of thrombocytopenia in myelodysplastic syndrome (MDS). *Blood* 2006; **108**:739a.
44. Montero AJ, Estrov Z, Freireich EJ, *et al.* Phase II study of low-dose interleukin-11 in patients with myelodysplastic syndrome. *Leuk Lymphoma* 2006;**47**:2049–54.
45. Bussel JB, Cheng G, Saleh MN, *et al.* Eltrombopag for the treatment of chronic idiopathic thrombocytopenic purpura. *N Engl J Med* 2007;**357**:2237–47.
46. Bussel JB, Kuter DJ, George JN, *et al.* AMG 531, a thrombopoiesis-stimulating protein, for chronic ITP. *N Engl J Med* 2006;**355**:2054.
47. Kantarjian H, Fenaux P, Sekeres MA, *et al.* Phase 1/2 study of AMG 531 in thrombocytopenic patients (Pts) with low-risk myelodysplastic syndrome (MDS): update including extended treatment. *Blood* 2007;**110**:81a.
48. Molldrem JJ, Leifer E, Bahceci E, *et al.* Antithymocyte globulin for treatment of the bone marrow failure associated with myelodysplastic syndromes. *Ann Intern Med* 2002;**137**:156–63.
49. Stadler M, Germing U, Kliche K-O, *et al.* A prospective, randomized, phase II study of horse antithymocyte globulin *vs* rabbit antithymoycte globulin as immune-modulating therapy in patients with low-risk myelodysplastic syndrome. *Leukemia* 2004;**18**:460–5.
50. Lim Z, Killick S, Cavenagh J, *et al.* European multi-centre study on the use of anti-thymocyte globulin in the treatment of myelodysplastic syndromes. *Blood* 2005;**106**:707a.
51. Sloand EM, Wu C, Greenberg P, *et al.* Factors affecting response and survival in patients with myelodysplasia treated with immunosuppressive therapy. *J Clin Oncol* 2008;**26**:2505–11.
52. Paquette RL, Tebyani N, Frane M, *et al.* Long-term outcome of aplastic anemia in adults treated with antithymocyte globulin: comparison with bone marrow transplantation. *Blood* 1995;**85**:283–90.
53. List A, Kurtin S, Roe DJ, *et al.* Efficacy of lenalidomide in myelodysplastic syndromes. *N Engl J Med* 2005;**352**:549–57.
54. List A, Dewald G, Bennett J, *et al.* Lenalidomide in the myelodysplastic syndrome with chromosome 5q deletion. *N Engl J Med* 2006;**355**:1456–65.
55. Raza A, Reeves JA, Feldman EJ, *et al.* Phase 2 study of lenalidomide in transfusion-dependent, low-risk, and intermediate-1 risk myelodysplastic syndromes with karyotypes other than deletion 5q. *Blood* 2008;**111**:86–93.
56. Issa J-P. Optimizing therapy with methylation inhibitors in myelodysplastic syndromes: dose, duration, and patient selection. *Nat Clin Pract Oncol* 2005;**2** Suppl 1:S24–9.
57. Silverman LR, Demakos EP, Peterson BL, *et al.* Randomized controlled trial of azacitidine in patients with the myelodysplastic syndrome: a study of the cancer and leukemia group B. *J Clin Oncol* 2002;**20**:2429–40.
58. Fenaux P, Mufti GJ, Hellstrom-Lindberg E, *et al.* Efficacy of azacitidine compared with that of conventional care regimens in the treatment of higher-risk myelodysplastic syndromes: a randomized, open-label, phase III study. *Lancet Oncol* 2009;**10**:223–32.
59. Wijermans P, Lübbert M, Verhoef G, *et al.* An epigenetic approach to the treatment of advanced MDS; the experience with the DNA demethylating agent 5-aza-2'-deoxycytidine (decitabine) in 177 patients. *Ann Hematol* 2005;**84**:9–17.
60. Kantarjian H, Issa J-P, Rosenfeld CS, *et al.* Decitabine improves patient outcome in myelodysplastic syndrome. *Cancer* 2006;**106**:1794–803.
61. Kantarjian H, Oki Y, Garcia-Manero G, *et al.* Results of a randomized study of 3 schedules of low-dose decitabine in higher-risk myelodysplastic syndrome and chronic myelomonocytic leukemia. *Blood* 2007;**109**:52–7.
62. Steensma DP, Baer MR, Slack JL, *et al.* Preliminary results of a phase II study of decitabine administered daily for 5 days every 4 weeks to adults with myelodysplastic syndrome (MDS). *Blood* 2007;**110**:434a.
63. Wijermans P, Suciu S, Baila L, *et al.* Low dose decitabine versus best supportive care in elderly patients with intermediate or high risk MDS not eligible for intensive chemotherapy: final results of the randomized phase III study (06011) of the EORTC leukemia and German MDS Study Groups. *Blood* 2008;**112**:90.
64. Silverman LR, McKenzie DR, Peterson BL, *et al.* Further analysis of trials with azacitidine in patients with myelodysplastic syndrome: studies 8421, 8921, and 9221 by the Cancer and Leukemia Group B. *J Clin Oncol* 2006;**24**:3895–902.
65. Borthakur G, Ahdab SE, Ravandi F, *et al.* Activity of decitabine in patients with myelodysplastic syndrome previously treated with azacitdine. *Leuk Lymphoma* 2008;**49**:650–1.
66. Vey N, Bosly A, Guerci A, *et al.* Arsenic trioxide in patients with myelodysplastic syndromes: a phase II multicenter study. *J Clin Oncol* 2006;**24**:2465–72.
67. Schiller GJ, Slack J, Hainsworth JD, *et al.* Phase II multicenter study of arsenic trioxide in patients with myelodysplastic syndromes. *J Clin Oncol* 2006;**24**:2456–64.
68. Cain JA, Grisolano JL, Laird AD, *et al.* Complete remission of TEL-PDGFRB-induced myeloproliferative disease in mice by receptor tyrosine kinase inhibitor SU11657. *Blood* 2004; **104**:561–4.
69. Raza A, Callander N, Ochoa L, *et al.* Hematologic improvement (HI) by TLK199 (Telintra™), a novel glutathione analog, in myelodysplastic syndrome: phase 2 study results. *Blood* 2005;**106**:708a.
70. Borthakur G, O'Brien S, Ravandi-Kashani F, *et al.* A phase I trial of the small molecule pan-BCL2 family inhibitor Obatoclax (GX15-070) administered by 24 hour infusion every 2 weeks to patients with myeloid malignancies and chronic lymphocytic leukemia (CLL). *Blood* 2006;**108**:750a.
71. Faderl S, Garcia-Manero G, Ravandi F, *et al.* Oral (po) and intravenous (iv) clofarabine for patients (pts) with myelodysplastic syndrome (MDS). *Blood* 2008;**112**:89.

72. Jabbour E, Kantarjian HM, Cortes J, *et al.* Survival benefit with decitabine compared to historical experience with intensive chemotherapy in patients with high risk myelodysplastic syndrome (MDS). *Blood* 2006;**108**:749a.

73. Beran M, Shen Y, Kantarjian H, *et al.* High-dose chemotherapy in high-risk myelodysplastic syndrome – covariate-adjusted comparison of five regimens. *Cancer* 2001;**92**:1999–2015.

74. Deeg HJ, Appelbaum FR. Hematopoietic stem cell transplantation in patients with myelodysplastic syndrome. *Leuk Res* 2000;**24**:653–63.

75. Sierra J, Perez WS, Rozman C, *et al.* Bone marrow transplantation from HLA-identical siblings as treatment for myelodsyplasia. *Blood* 2002; **200**:1997–2004.

76. Cutler CS, Lee SJ, Greenberg P, *et al.* A decision analysis of allogeneic bone marrow transplantation for the myelodysplastic syndromes: delayed transplantation for low-risk myelodysplasia is associated with improved outcome. *Blood* 2004;**104**:579–85.

77. Martino R, Iacobelli S, Brand R, *et al.* Retrospective comparison of reduced-intensity conditioning and conventional high-dose conditioning for allogeneic hematopoietic stem cell transplantation using HLA-identical sibling donors in myelodysplastic syndromes. *Blood* 2006;**108**:836–46.

78. Deeg HJ, Storer B, Slattery JT, *et al.* Conditioning with targeted busulfan and cyclophosphamide for hemopoietic stem cell transplantation from related and unrelated donors in patients with myelodysplastic syndrome. *Blood* 2002;**100**:1201–7.

Chapter 7

Hairy cell leukemia

Darren S. Sigal and Alan Saven

Introduction

Hairy cell leukemia (HCL) is a rare, chronic lymphoproliferative disorder characterized by splenomegaly, pancytopenia, bone marrow fibrosis, and frequent infectious complications. Its hallmark is the hairy cell, a small- to medium-sized mononuclear cell with a typical serrated border and cytoplasmic projections.[1] Although the World Health Organization (WHO) has codified the appellation "hairy cell leukemia," "leukemic reticuloendotheliosis" was its historical reference in the literature.[2] Ewald first used this term for a disease more consistent with acute monocytic leukemia.[3] In 1958, Bouroncle *et al.* used "leukemic reticuloendotheliosis" to describe the clinical entity now recognizable as HCL.[4] Eight years later, Schrek and Donnelly also reported on the same disease and commented on "peculiar cells" that had numerous short villi and were arbitrarily called "hairy cells" on phase contrast microscopy.[5] "Hairy cell leukemia" gained popular and official recognition.

Epidemiology

HCL constitutes approximately 2% of all lymphoid leukemias.[4] It is predominantly a male disease, with the male:female ratio ranging from 4:1 to 7:1.[4,6] The vast majority of affected people are white, with Ashkenazi Jews being an overrepresented group.[7] The median age of onset is in the early fifth decade.

Etiology

HCL has no known cause and risk factors are poorly characterized. Farming or woodworking, or occupational exposure to organic solvents, resulted in a higher relative risk for developing HCL.[7] Infectious mononucleosis has been associated with HCL, but a pathogenic role for Epstein–Barr virus has been disputed.[7–9] Studies evaluating radiation exposure as a HCL risk factor have also produced conflicting results.[7,10]

Multiple case reports have documented the existence of a rare familial HCL. Specific HLA haplotypes have been associated with some cases of familial HCL, but each family's HLA haplotype was unique.[11,12] There has been no identification of a common HLA haplotype among cases of unrelated HCL.[11] Fluorescence *in situ* hybridization techniques have detected clonal chromosomal abnormalities in up to 67% of HCL patients.[13] Gain or loss of alleles on chromosomes 5 and 14 were common findings. Mutations of specific bands on chromosomes 1, 2, and 5 were unique to hairy cells from other lymphoid neoplasms. However, it is not clear how or if these changes culminate in HCL.[13,14]

Biology

A central tenet in the study of malignant hematology posits that neoplastic cells are derived from normal cell counterparts. Identification of these normal cells can elucidate the biology and ontogeny of the neoplasm. A persistent search for the normal counterpart of the hairy cell has not yielded definitive answers. Bouroncle's description of hairy cells possessing pseudopods first suggested a common lineage with monocytes.[4] Hairy cells behave like monocytes, performing phagocytosis, producing a fibronectin matrix, and stimulating T-lymphocyte colonies in semi-solid agar cultures.[15–17] They also resemble monocytes, displaying cell surface Fc receptors and sharing overlapping electrophoretic mobility distributions.[18,19] Implicit in the association of monocytopenia with HCL is the erroneous notion that the hairy cell is an abnormal monocyte. A proliferation of clonal monocytes could suppress normal monocyte development and manifest as monocytopenia.[20] Other papers have demonstrated hairy cells to have morphology, functionality, and cell surface markers consistent with T lymphocytes.[21–23]

Korsmeyer *et al.* resolved some of the controversy surrounding hairy cell ontogeny when they demonstrated that they possess immunoglobulin heavy and light chain gene rearrangements. Hairy cells were clearly placed in the B-lymphocyte lineage since T lymphocytes do not exhibit immunoglobulin light chain gene rearrangement and monocytes have neither heavy nor light chain rearrangement.[24] Light chain-restricted surface immunoglobulin was displayed

Management of Hematologic Malignancies, ed. Susan M. O'Brien, Julie M. Vose, and Hagop M. Kantarjian. Published by Cambridge University Press.

on 90–100% of hairy cells, reinforcing a B-lymphocyte ancestry.[25,26] Hairy cells also displayed the pan-B-cell markers CD19, CD20, and CD22.[27]

In the schema of B-cell ontogeny, the hairy cell can be considered an activated, late-stage, pre-plasma cell B lymphocyte. Activation refers to cellular changes that occur in the germinal center following antigen exposure and demonstrates late B-cell maturation. Hairy cell transit through the germinal center is supported by the presence of BCL6 mutations.[28] Further evidence for hairy cell activation is the "hairy" border itself. The cytoskeletal arrangement of actin and spectrin necessary to scaffold the "hairy" border resembles that of an activated B cell.[29,30] Hairy cell overexpression of the *src* proto-oncogene is also found in hematologic malignancies of later stages of B-cell development.[31] Early B-cell markers, such as CD21 and CD24, not present on activated B lymphocytes are also absent from hairy cells.[32] Hairy cells display the activation antigens CD11c, CD22, CD25, HC2, and PCA-1.[24,27,33,34] B lymphocytes transiently exhibit HC2, before developing into plasma cells; PCA-1 is only found on plasma cells. Coexpression of HC2 and PCA-1 places the hairy cell in a transitional developmental location between an activated B lymphocyte and a plasma cell. Lack of affinity maturation markers excludes the possibility that the hairy cell arises from a plasma cell.[35]

Despite having a B-cell ancestry, the hairy cell has several key features that distinguish it from any other B-cell lymphoproliferative disorder. Hairy cell shape and antigen expression, as discussed above, are unique. Hairy cells display immunoglobulins that are light-chain restricted, but have multiple heavy-chain isotypes. One paper reported a cell with IgM, IgD, IgA, and IgG on its surface, despite no evidence of deletional recombination beyond the IgM isotype.[26,36] This can occur because of post-transcriptional mRNA splicing of a common V_HDJ_H transcript.[36] Chronic lymphocytic leukemia (CLL) and poorly differentiated lymphocytic lymphoma have a very different isotype profile and do not display more than two isotypes on any cell.[25] Hairy cells preferentially express the IgG3 subclass that was not found on any IgG-positive non-Hodgkin lymphoma cells.[37] Up to 75% of hairy cells have p53 mutations, a marker traditionally associated with poor prognosis in lymphoid hematologic disorders.[38] Such a high rate of p53 mutations in an indolent disease is surprising.[39] The 7% of CLL cases with p53 mutations or deletions have a significantly worse prognosis, and do not benefit from chemoimmunotherapy.[40–42]

The monocytoid B lymphocyte (MBL) emerged as a tempting candidate for the normal hairy cell counterpart. The term monocytoid is a misnomer describing a polyclonal proliferation of B lymphocytes in reactive lymph nodes that morphologically resemble monocytes. MBLs have a striking morphologic resemblance to hairy cells.[43] Immunohistochemistry and flow cytometry reveal shared antigenic expression, including CD11c and CD20, between hairy cells and MBLs.[43–45] Surface immunoglobulin is displayed on both cells. Like hairy cells, MBLs may also represent a pre-plasma cell.[43,44] However, it has become clear that MBLs are much more tightly bound to a different lymphoproliferative neoplasia: monocytoid B-cell lymphoma (MBCL, known as splenic marginal zone lymphoma by current WHO criteria).[2] The immunophenotype of MBL and MBCL are identical.[43] Large cells found among MBLs in reactive lymph nodes are indistinguishable from MBCL and serve as the bridge linking the benign and malignant conditions.[46] Key differences between MBCL and HCL further refute any direct relationship between MBLs and hairy cells. MBCL stains actin and epithelial membrane antigen (EMA), HCL does not; HCL expresses tartrate-resistant acid phosphatase (TRAP), CD25, and PCA-1, while MBCL does not.[44,45]

Hairy B-cell lymphoproliferative disorder has been proposed as the benign counterpart to a rare HCL variant. However, a clear, direct HCL precursor cell analogous to the relationship of MBL with MBCL remains elusive.[47] An interesting consideration was Burthem's hypothesis that the hairy cell derives from a B cell activated by T-cell-independent mechanisms, or resembles such a cell after an unknown oncogenic event.[48] B cells activated by T-cell-independent pathways produce antigen-specific antibodies of all isotypes except IgE, preferentially produce the IgG3 subclass, and colocalize with macrophages in the splenic red pulp.[49,50] All three observations have been made in HCL.[26,37,51]

Pathology

Clinical features (see Table 7.1)

HCL usually has an insidious onset.[1,4,6,16,52] The most common symptoms leading to diagnosis were infectious episodes (29%), weakness and fatigue (27%), bleeding complications (16%), and abdominal pain or fullness (15%).[6,52] Twenty-six percent of patients were asymptomatic and discovered to have HCL on routine hemograms or as an incidental finding on physical exam.[52] Most of the bleeding complications were from petechiae or echymoses.[6] Severe hemorrhage was rare and was usually associated with a poor overall condition. About 70% of patients with severe hemorrhage had platelet counts greater than 50 000/mm^3 suggesting that a qualitative platelet defect, not absolute platelet numbers, was the culprit.[52]

Well over 90% of patients have splenomegaly at presentation, with the vast majority described as moderate or massive. In fact, the diagnosis of HCL should be questioned in patients without splenomegaly.[1,53] Hepatomegaly affected up to 50% of patients and was often associated with splenomegaly.[4,6,52] Palpable lymphadenopathy has been reported to occur in 0–35% of patients, but was rarely considered clinically significant.[1,4,6] Autopsy series reported discordance between palpable peripheral lymphadenopathy and internal lymphadenopathy.[54] Bulky or massive abdominal lymphadenopathy occurred in patients with longer disease duration and in patients with a splenectomy.[55,56]

Infections frequently led to the diagnosis of HCL or accompanied its diagnosis.[52] Some form of serious infection eventually developed in over 50% of patients and was the most common cause of death in patients with HCL.[6] Unusual infections have been chronicled in HCL patients, including

Table 7.1. HCL presenting features

Symptoms	Laboratory
Infections (29%)	Pancytopenia (79%)
Constitutional (27%)	Monocytopenia (always)
Asymptomatic (26%)	Neutropenia (75%)
Bleeding (16%)	Polyclonal hypergammaglobulinemia (22%)
Abdominal pain/fullness (15%)	Monoclonal proteins (rare)
Signs	Platelet function abnormalities
Splenomegaly (> 90%)	High LAP score
Hepatomegaly (50%)	Accelerated ESR
Palpable lymphadenopathy (rare)	Hypocholesterolemia
	Chemistry panel and liver function usually normal

Notes: ESR: erythrocyte sedimentation rate; LAP: leukocyte alkaline phosphatase.

Mycobacterium kansasii, *Mycobacterium tuberculosis*, *Cryptococcus neoformans*, *Aspergillus* species, *Legionella pneumophila*, and superficial and necrotizing herpes simplex virus. *Pseudomonas*, *Escherichia coli*, and *Enterococcus* have also been cultured from patients.[1,6,16,53,54] Aside from neutropenia and monocytopenia, several other factors may explain the immunodeficiency of HCL.[20,52] HCL patients have deficient granulocyte reserve and leukocyte mobilization;[57] impaired microbicidal functioning;[58] deficiencies in natural killer cell activity;[59] and poor interferon alpha production.[60] Hairy cells have also been found to secrete soluble interleukin-2 (IL-2) receptor that may absorb IL-2 released from T cells, blunting an adaptive immune response.[61]

In comparison to the National Cancer Institute's Surveillance, Epidemiology, and End Results Program, HCL patients have 4.33 relative risk increase for either hematologic or solid tumor secondary neoplasms. In one report, the relative risk was 40 for hematologic malignancies alone. The secondary cancers were aggressive with a median survival of only 8.8 months after diagnosis.[62] HCL has also been rarely associated with vasculitic syndromes and hairy cell infiltration of cortical bone.[63–65]

Laboratory features (see Table 7.1)

General

Routine chemistry and liver function panels do not demonstrate any striking abnormalities.[16,66] Markedly increased leukocyte alkaline phosphatase and accelerated erythrocyte sedimentation rates have been reported.[67] Serum protein electrophoresis detected polyclonal hypergammaglobulinemia in 22% of patients. Rare monoclonal spikes were also found.[16,52] Hypocholesterolemia was a manifestation of HCL.[68]

Blood

Pancytopenia was reported in up to 79% of patients with one-quarter of these cases having severe pancytopenia (hemoglobin [Hb] < 8.5 g/dL, platelet count [Plt] $< 100 \times 10^9$/L, and absolute neutrophil count [ANC] $< 0.5 \times 10^9$/L).[52] Neutropenia was present in over 75% of patients, frequently with an absolute neutrophil count of $< 0.5 \times 10^9$/L. Monocytopenia was a consistent finding.[6,20] Anemia was usually normochromic and normocytic without evidence of a myelophthisic process.[6] One report documented abnormal platelet function in eight out of ten patients.[69] Leukopenia was the most common white blood cell finding, but leukocytosis did infrequently occur. The percentage of circulating hairy cells was highly variable, ranging from 0% to 99%.[6] In Romanovsky-stained preparations, hairy cells are medium sized (10–20 μm) with a characteristically serrated border and cytoplasmic projections occasionally visualized. The nucleus is eccentric and round or bilobed with a spongy appearance; nucleoli may be present (Figure 7.1).[1,6]

Splenic size on exam and at splenectomy correlated poorly with the cytopenias.[52,70] However, it is clear that blood counts improved after splenectomy, indicating that hypersplenism is one explanation for peripheral blood cytopenias.[53] Hairy cell infiltration of the marrow causing marrow failure also occurs.[71] Sometimes marked pancytopenia can occur with only minimal hairy cell infiltration of the marrow. Increased secretion of tumor necrosis factor alpha, an inhibitor of hematopoiesis, from hairy cells can account for this finding.[70]

Bone marrow

HCL invariably involves the bone marrow; however, attempts at aspiration were only successful in 20–50% of patients.[1,6,72] In contrast, bone marrow core biopsies were almost always diagnostic.[16] Hairy cells synthesize and assemble an insoluble fibronectin matrix that was always present, making marrow aspiration difficult.[16,17] Hairy cell infiltration of the marrow can be either patchy, focal, or diffuse with complete marrow replacement.[73] It may be that earlier disease is associated with the former.[1] Even with heavy infiltration, hairy cells do not appear packed due to a finely reticulated zone of abundant cytoplasm separating the nuclei (Figure 7.2).[72] Hairy cell nuclei could be round to ovoid, convoluted, or indented.[73] Mitosis is rare.[72]

Spleen, liver, and lymph nodes

Splenomegaly is one of the hallmark clinical findings in HCL. The weight of splenectomy specimens ranged from 335 to 4000 g with nearly half of the spleens weighing more than 2000 g.[1] Cut sections demonstrated the parenchyma to be fleshy and congested. Microscopic examination revealed replacement of the splenic architecture by hairy cells filling the red pulp cords and sinuses, displacing the white pulp. Nuclear indentation was more obvious than in the bone marrow.[6] On gross section, distended blood-filled spaces occurred in the red pulp forming "blood lakes" or

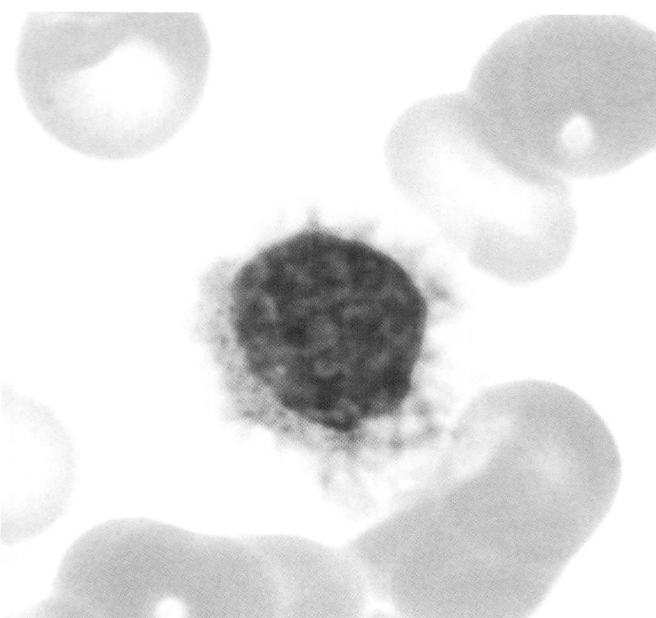

Figure 7.1 Classic hairy cell with a round nucleus, partially condensed chromatin, small nucleolus, and ample rim of blue, agranular cytoplasm with frayed margins. (Wright–Giemsa, × 1000.)

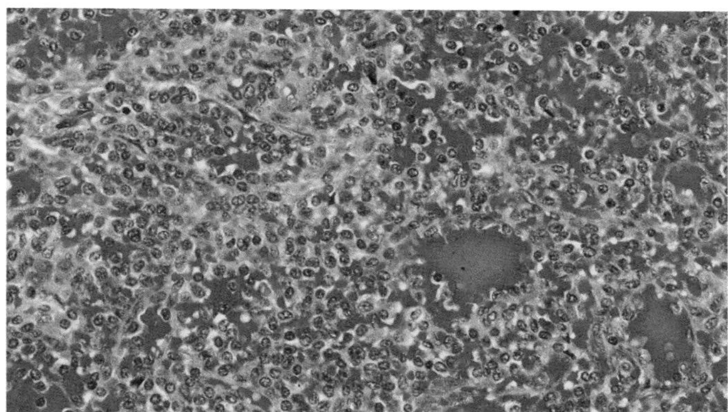

Figure 7.3 Hairy cell leukemic involvement of the splenic red pulp. Note the presence of several blood-filled spaces lined by leukemic cells known as "blood lakes," a distinctive feature of splenic hairy cell leukemia. (H&E, × 200.)

hemangiomas (Figure 7.3). These were presumably collections of pseudosinuses, luminal structures lined by hairy cells and filled with erythrocytes and leukocytes.[6,51] Pseudosinuses, as opposed to normal sinuses, were devoid of ringed fibers and had an increased reticulin network.[51]

Liver specimens usually had mild to moderate enlargement. Hairy cells were diffusely present in the sinusoids and portal tracts, only occasionally involving the liver parenchyma.[1] Hepatic architecture was generally preserved, but hairy cell-lined angiomatous lesions, resembling splenic pseudosinuses, can be found in the sinusoids and portal tracts.[6,51]

Despite negligible palpable peripheral lymph node involvement, an autopsy series noted lymph node involvement in

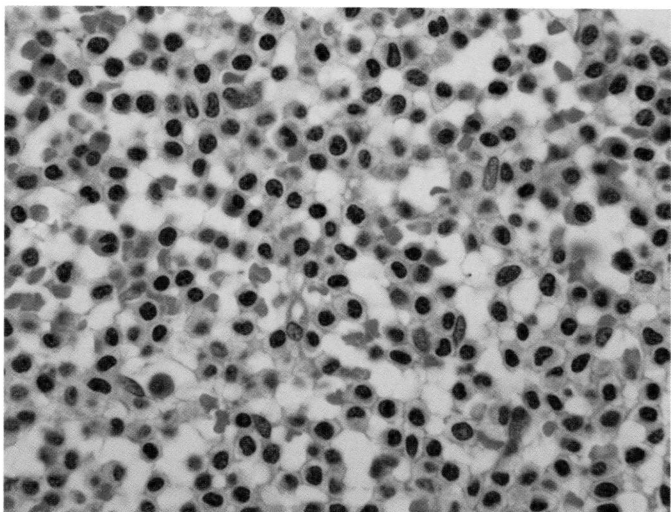

Figure 7.2 Typical histologic appearance of hairy cell leukemia characterized by a monotonous population of lymphoid cells with abundant cytoplasm imparting a well-spaced appearance to the centrally placed nuclei. (Hematoxylin and eosin [H&E], × 400.)

20 of 20 patients.[54] Microscopy documented focal aggregation to complete replacement of lymph node architecture by hairy cells.[1]

Hairy cells have a predilection for the bone marrow, spleen, liver, and lymph nodes. They only rarely involve other organ systems.[54] As the main motility-inducing integrin on hairy cells, $\alpha_V\beta_3$ facilitates hairy cell infiltration of the spleen via vitronectin and of the lymph nodes and liver via laminin and collagen.[74,75] CD44 homes hairy cells to the bone marrow by binding to hyaluronan, triggering fibronectin generation.[76]

Cytochemistry

Li *et al.* first demonstrated that acid phosphatase isoenzyme 5 was highly specific for HCL and was tartaric acid resistant (Figure 7.4).[77] It was proposed that TRAP activity could distinguish hairy cells and be used as a marker for diagnosis.[78] However, the percentage of TRAP-positive cells varied considerably and occasionally HCL patients were TRAP negative.[53] It has subsequently become evident that TRAP activity is also present in CLL, Hodgkin lymphoma, normal B lymphocytes, and even in myeloid cells.[79]

Electron microscopy

Electron microscopy defined the ultrastructural features of hairy cells. Cytoplasmic projections ranged from 0.5 to 4 μm and were diffusely present on the cell. In contrast, splenic marginal zone lymphoma cells have polarized cytoplasmic projections.[6,80] The nucleus measured 8–12 μm in diameter, was oval, and frequently indented. Nucleoli were present in about 50% of cells. The rough endoplasmic reticulum was limited to several short strands.[6] Ribosome-lamella complexes have been found in 50% of patients with HCL.[67] They are cylindrical cytoplasmic inclusion bodies, although their exact

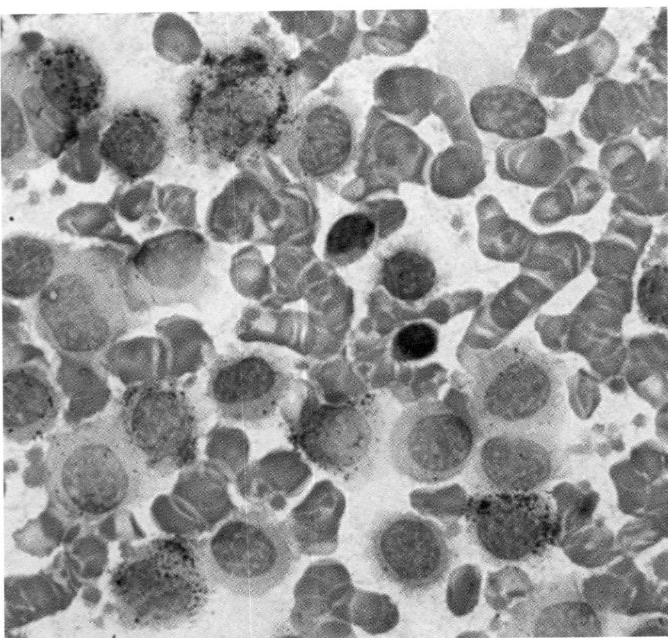

Figure 7.4 Tartrate-resistant acid phosphatase staining in hairy cell leukemia. Note the presence of cells with intense cytoplasmic positivity (red granules). (Acid phosphatase with tartrate, × 1000.)

Table 7.2. HCL immunophenotype

Fluorescence activated cell sorting
(FACS) antigens
CD11c, CD25, CD103, CD5 (4%), CD10 (26%), HLA-DR, CD19, CD20, CD22
Fixative-resistant monoclonal antibodies
DBA.44, L26 (anti-CD20 antibody), anti-T-bet antibody

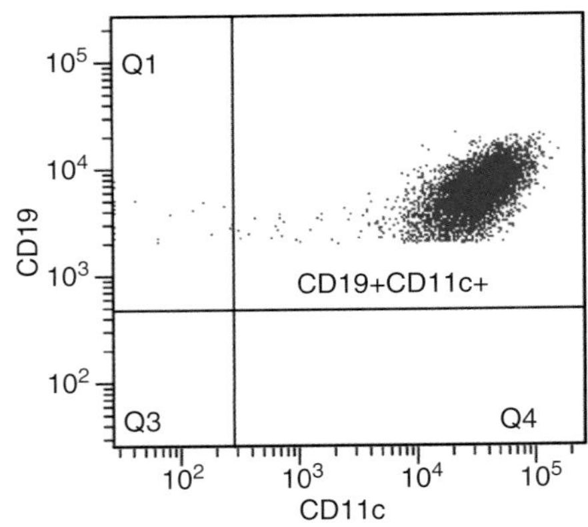

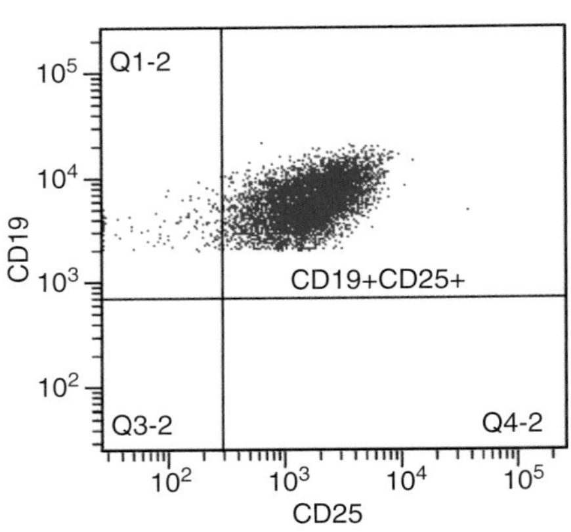

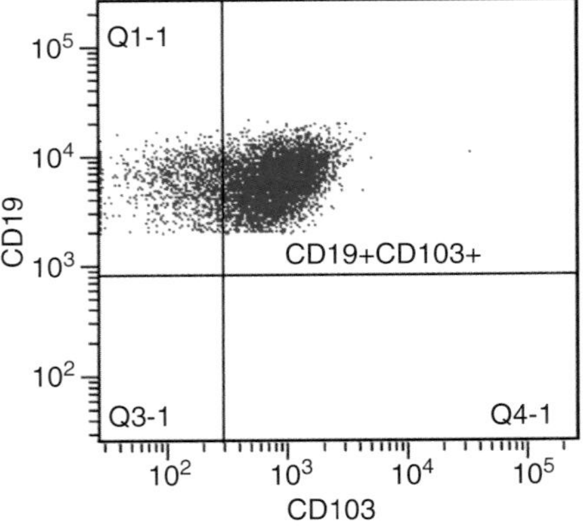

Figure 7.5 The characteristic immunophenotypic profile of hairy cell leukemia with expression of CD11c (bright), CD25, and CD103.

cellular role remains to be defined.[81] Ribosome-lamella complexes have also been rarely identified in other hematologic malignancies, including myeloid leukemia, Waldenstrom's macroglobulinemia, and CLL.[82]

Immunophenotype (see Table 7.2)

Snap-frozen bone marrow or soft-tissue specimens were used to discern the immunophenotype of hairy cells. HLA-DR, CD19, CD20, and CD22 were pan-B-cell antigens expressed on hairy cells.[34,83,84] An antigenic profile of CD11c, CD25, and CD103 served to distinguish hairy cells from other lymphoproliferative disorders. CD103 was the most specific marker.[85] Routine preparation of bone marrow specimens does not include snap-freezing. Instead, samples are formalin-fixed, decalcified, and paraffin-embedded. This process damages the cluster of differentiation antigens diminishing the utility of these monoclonal antibodies in clinical practice.[86] DBA.44 and L26 (an anti-CD20 antibody) are fixative-resistant monoclonal antibodies that were sensitive for hairy cells, although not specific.[45,87] Formalin-resistant antibodies have been raised against T-bet, a T-cell-associated transcription factor. Antibodies against T-bet strongly and uniformly stained hairy cells, exposing even minimal residual disease in bone marrow specimens. Weak non-specific staining to other B-cell lymphomas was easily distinguished.[88]

Two-color flow cytometry was able to detect hairy cells constituting $< 1\%$ of peripheral blood lymphocytes. Coexpression of CD11c, CD25, and CD103 reliably separated HCL from CLL (Figure 7.5). CD11c and CD25 binding was relatively non-specific. However, their expression intensities on flow cytometry conferred very specific characteristics: CD11c and CD25 had 30-fold and 6-fold higher intensities in HCL than in CLL, respectively. CD103 was the most specific marker, without any expression on CLL cells.[27]

However, CD103 is now known to occur on intraepithelial T lymphocytes as the α^E subunit of the $\alpha^E\beta7$ integrin.[89] CD5 and CD10, antigens used to exclude HCL as a diagnostic possibility, were actually expressed on 4% and 26% of hairy cells, respectively.[27]

Differential diagnosis

The differential diagnosis of lymphoproliferative disorders with splenomegaly and no peripheral lymphadenopathy includes splenic lymphoma with villous lymphocytes, HCL-variant, and prolymphocytic leukemia.

HCL-variant is a very rare B-cell lymphoproliferative disorder with features distinct from typical HCL. Patients present with vague symptoms, massive splenomegaly, and a markedly elevated white blood cell count. Mild cytopenias occur, but monocytopenia and neutropenia are absent.[90,91] HCL-variant is probably a hybrid disease between typical HCL and B-cell prolymphocytic leukemia (B-PLL). The cells have a round, centrally located nucleus, a nucleolus, and peripheral condensation of the chromatin, as in B-PLL. Their evenly distributed numerous broad-based cytoplasmic projections resemble typical HCL. The nuclear:cytoplasmic ratio is intermediate between typical HCL and B-PLL.[92] HCL-variant cells have variable TRAP staining and are CD11c positive and CD25 negative.[91,92] Bone marrow aspiration is easily obtained and reticulin is not increased on core biopsy.[90,91] Splenectomy specimens reveal red pulp infiltration, but "blood lakes" are not observed. Patients usually follow a chronic course, but have poor responses to standard HCL therapies.[91,93] An aggressive blastic variant form has been described.[94]

Splenic lymphoma with villous lymphocytes (SLVL) is a marginal zone lymphoma that also has an insidious onset, often massive splenomegaly, and cytopenias. SLVL patients have an absolute lymphocytosis and a frequent monoclonal protein spike.[80,95] SLVL cells resemble those of HCL except for a more condensed chromatin and a moderate degree of cytoplasmic basophilia without ribosome-lamella complexes (Figure 7.6). Their thin cytoplasmic projections have a unique polar distribution. SLVL cells commonly express CD11c and CD25, but only rarely display CD103. They are TRAP negative.[80,96] Bone marrow aspiration is easily obtained. Splenic infiltration is mainly in the white pulp.[80]

B-cell prolymphocytic leukemia (B-PLL) is mainly a disease of elderly men presenting with vague symptoms. Exam reveals massive splenomegaly without peripheral lymphadenopathy. Median absolute lymphocyte counts are greater than 350×10^9/L with anemia and thrombocytopenia.[97] B-PLL cells have scant cytoplasm, a centrally placed nucleus with a large nucleolus, and peripheral chromatin condensation.[53]

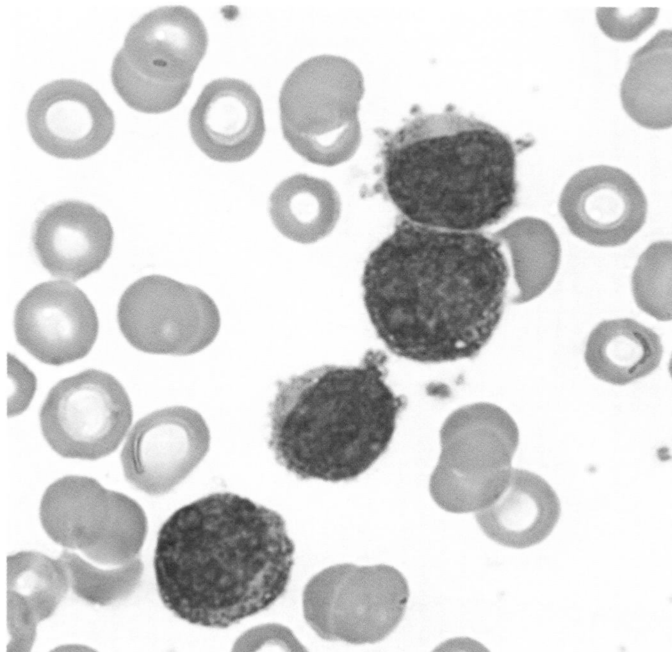

Figure 7.6 The neoplastic cells of splenic marginal zone lymphoma (also known as splenic lymphoma with villous lymphocytes) bear a superficial resemblance to hairy cells but have more cytoplasmic basophilia without the characteristic textured appearance of hairy cell cytoplasm. While the cytoplasm may display coarse villous projections it lacks the frayed margins typical of hairy cells. (Wright–Giemsa, × 1000.)

Therapy

Before the introduction of active therapies, most HCL patients had a chronic disorder with survival extending over several years. A small group of patients with neutropenia, thrombocytopenia, and a rapid deterioration of general health experience an aggressive course.[52] Splenectomy was utilized early on to palliate symptoms, but also potentially altered the natural history of disease. Interferon alpha was the first systemic therapy to demonstrate significant activity. Pentostatin and cladribine were progressive improvements in therapy, extending survival by inducing very protracted remissions. Treatment is reserved for patients with symptoms or cytopenias. These include an ANC $\leq 1.5 \times 10^9$/L, Hb ≤ 10 g/dL, Plt $\leq 100 \times 10^9$/L, symptomatic splenomegaly, recurrent infections, or bone lesions. About 80% of patients at diagnosis will require therapy.

Splenectomy

Bouroncle's initial description of HCL included a patient with pancytopenia who had a rapid normalization of his peripheral blood counts after splenectomy.[4] Many other case series have since confirmed the beneficial effects of splenectomy in HCL.[6,52,53,66,71,98] Patients who had a splenectomy were cytopenic, in their fifth decade, and were recently diagnosed with HCL.[52,53,98,99] Complete response (CR) rates after splenectomy, as defined by Catovsky's criteria (Hb > 11 g/dL, ANC $> 1.0 \times 10^9$/L, and Plt $> 100 \times 10^9$/L), were 40–60%, with overall responses (OR) approaching 100%.[6,52,53,98] Responses were brisk, occurring within one to two weeks post-splenectomy; platelets were the most common cell line to normalize.[53,99] Interestingly, spleen size at splenectomy did not correlate with blood count responses.[52,71,98] Splenectomy was associated with a decreased risk for infection in HCL patients.[98] Partial responses (PRs) relapsed more quickly and had a shortened survival when compared to CRs.[53,98] In a large retrospective multicenter analysis with matched controls, splenectomy conferred a statistically significant survival benefit. Median survival for splenectomized patients had not been reached at 96 months, while non-splenectomized patients had a median survival less than 24 months.[99] However, whether splenectomy actually improves survival in HCL is moot.[6,66] Splenectomy was only found to affect survival in patients with cytopenias (Hb < 12 g/dL, ANC $< 0.5 \times 10^9$/L, or Plt $< 100 \times 10^9$/L) or spleens more than 4 cm below the costal margin.[52,99]

Interferon

Quesada *et al.* first reported on the activity of interferon alpha in HCL. Of seven patients (five with a prior splenectomy), there were three CRs, four PRs, and an OR rate of 100%.[100] Six other studies included heavily pre-treated patients (over three-quarters with prior splenectomy or chemotherapy) with a median age in the early fifth decade. They reported a CR range of 0–30%, a PR range of 24–92%, and an OR range of 52–93% (see Tables 7.3 and 7.4).[101–107] Surprisingly, in a large intergroup study randomizing untreated patients to either interferon alpha or pentostatin, the interferon alpha group only had 11% CRs, 27% PRs, and an OR rate of 38%.[103] Variability in response criteria may help explain this discrepancy, as some studies documented CRs even with detectable bone marrow hairy cells.[105,108] Also, the intergroup study had the lowest median baseline platelet count suggesting a worse prognosis for these patients.[52,99,103] Finally, the intergroup study included actively infected patients who did not respond as well to therapy.

Time to blood count normalization after therapy for platelets, hemoglobin, and neutrophils were 4–8 weeks, 4 months, and 5 months, respectively. Monocytopenia continued to improve over one year. Hairy cells were rapidly cleared from the peripheral blood, but persisted in the bone marrow for months.[100,108] Disease-free survival (DFS) ranged from 6 months to 2 years, but long-term DFS was observed in a small group of interferon alpha-treated patients.[101,103–105] One study that randomized patients treated with one year of interferon alpha to another 6 months of treatment or observation noted that the additional therapy only delayed relapses, but did not reduce them.[109] CRs and PRs appeared to relapse at the same rate.[104,105] With over 7 years of follow-up, overall survival was about 90%.[101,104,105] The intergroup study noted equivalent survival between interferon alpha and pentostatin, but the study had a crossover design.[103] Fatigue, malaise, myalgias, and mild bone marrow suppression were the main toxicities. Infections did not occur beyond 8 weeks of interferon alpha therapy, and patients suffered from fewer infections after therapy started.[100,104,108]

Table 7.3. HCL therapies

Cladribine: 0.1 mg/kg per day by continuous intravenous infusion for seven consecutive days
Pentostatin: 4 mg/m^2 intravenously every other week for two cycles beyond maximum response for 6 to 12 months
Interferon alpha-2a: 3 million IU subcutaneously daily for 16 to 24 weeks, then maintenance at 3 million IU three times per week
Interferon alpha-2b: 2 million IU/m^2 subcutaneously three times per week for 6 months

Purine nucleoside analogs

In 1972, Giblett *et al.* described a pediatric condition with clinical immunodeficiency, lymphopenia, and adenosine deaminase (ADA) deficiency.[110] ADA-deficient immunodeficiency produces dramatic elevations of deoxyadenosine 5′-triphosphate (dATP).[111,112] All tissues lack ADA, but only lymphocytes are susceptible to the toxic effects of dATP.[113,114] Carson *et al.* reasoned that ADA-resistant deoxyadenosine

Table 7.4. Interferon studies

Study	Patients (n)		Untreated patients (n)	Median age (years)	Responses (%)		Median DFS (months)
	Overall	Evaluable			OR	CR	
Berman *et al.*[101]	35	23	10	54	69	0	24
Foon *et al.*[102]	15	14	5	52	93	1	NR
Grever *et al.*[103]	159	159	159	53	38	11	20
Quesada *et al.*[104]	30	30	7	48	87	30	> 10
Ratain *et al.*[105]	69	68	8	53	75	13	25
Rai *et al.*[106]	42	25	42	NR	52	28	NR
Golomb *et al.*[107]	195	195	NR	NR	82	4	NR
Median values	42	30	9	53	75	11	> 22

Notes: DFS: disease-free survival; NR: not reported.

Table 7.5. Pentostatin studies

Study	Patients (n)		Untreated patients (n)	Median age (years)	Responses (%)		Median DFS (months)
	Overall	Evaluable			OR	CR	
Cassileth *et al.*[122]	62	50	19	NR	84	64	> 39
Else *et al.*[123]	185	185	76	52	96	81	180
Flinn *et al.*[124]	154	154	154	57	79[a]	76[a]	> 120
Grem *et al.*[125]	66	66	NR	57	91	65	>6
Kraut *et al.*[126]	23	23	10	54	91	87	13.5
Median values	66	66	47.5	55.5	91	73	> 39

Note: [a]Data from Grever *et al.*[103]
NR: not reported.

analogs would be specifically lymphotoxic. With a chlorine substitution at position 2 of the purine ring of 2′-deoxyadenosine, cladribine (2-chlorodeoxyadenosine) is resistant to ADA deamination.[115] Therefore, the relative activities of deoxcytidine kinase and 5′-nucleotidase regulate the intracellular concentrations of phosphorylated cladribine.[116,117] Lymphocytes are unique for constitutively expressing deoxycytidine kinase, rendering them specifically susceptible to cladribine.[118] Pentostatin (2-deoxycoformycin), another purine nucleoside analog, directly inhibits ADA producing a lymphotoxic build-up of dATP.[119]

Pentostatin

Spiers *et al.* first reported on the dramatic activity of pentostatin in two HCL patients with pancytopenia, splenomegaly, and bone marrows that could not be aspirated. Within 4 weeks, peripheral blood counts normalized, spleen size corrected, and the marrow was aspirable.[120,121] Several much larger series included heavily pre-treated patients (over half with splenectomy and/or interferon alpha) with a median age in the mid-fifth decade. CRs ranged from 64% to 87%, PRs ranged from 3% to 26%, and ORs ranged from 79% to 96% (see Tables 7.3 and 7.5).[122–126] A large cohort of previously untreated patients had 76% CRs, 3% PRs, and 79% OR.[103] Hematologic values corrected over a matter of weeks.[121,127,128] ORs to pentostatin were equivalent among patients who had received prior therapy and those who had not.[122,125] CRs were achieved after six to ten cycles (each cycle was 2 weeks).[122,125,126] Relapse-free survival extended beyond 10 years, but a plateau had not been reached for late relapses.[122,124–126,129] Most relapses occurred within 2 years of therapy and did not require retreatment at the time of relapse.[122,126] With nearly 10 years median follow-up the overall survival was 80%.[124] Patients who achieved CR had statistically improved overall survival compared to patients whose best response was a PR.[129]

Pentostatin-treated patients developed bacterial and opportunistic infections.[122,124,125] Infection-related deaths occurred in several studies, usually within the first two cycles of therapy.[103,122,125] Delayed infections were also reported, mainly localized herpes zoster. Pentostatin has divergent effects on the immune system. Prolonged suppression of T-cell subsets contributes to delayed toxicities. However, pentostatin also normalizes the total white blood cell count, monocyte count, and natural killer (NK)-cell activity. [130,131] Other drug toxicities were usually mild, including nausea and vomiting, skin rash, and keratoconjunctivitis. Neutropenic fever was common, but resolved rapidly together with other cytopenias. Severe liver and neurotoxicity was rarely reported at treatment doses, with one death attributed to neurologic toxicity.[122,125,126]

Cladribine

Cladribine has been generally accepted as the first-line treatment of HCL for several reasons: brief treatment regimen, high response rates that are durable, and a favorable toxicity profile. Scripps Clinic initiated the first phase I clinical study of cladribine in February of 1981, establishing the standard dose at 0.1 mg/kg per day by continuous infusion for seven consecutive days.[132] Investigators there later reported on the first use of cladribine for HCL in 12 patients; 11 patients achieved a CR and 1 patient a PR.[133] Additional series included heavily pre-treated patients (at least half with prior splenectomy, interferon, or pentostatin) with a median age in the early- to mid-fifth decade, and administered the standard 0.1 mg/kg per day by continuous infusion for seven consecutive days. CRs ranged from 75% to 91%, PRs ranged from 0% to 24%, and ORs ranged from 75% to 100% (see Tables 7.3 and 7.6).[123,134–140] Four of the six studies had OR rates of 98% to 100%.[123,134,137,139] The largest series of cladribine in HCL, reported by Saven *et al.*, included 358 patients, more than all other cladribine studies combined, and reported 91% CRs and 7% PRs for an OR rate of 98%.[139] Alternative regimens using oral, subcutaneous, or weekly bolus schedules have achieved results similar to standard infusional cladribine, but these studies are small and with limited follow-up.[141–144] Response rates to cladribine were independent of prior therapies.[139,140]

Most patients had normalization of their peripheral blood counts within 7 weeks, heralded by resolution of thrombocytopenia.[135,137–139] Hairy cells began clearing from

Table 7.6. Cladribine studies

Study	Patients (n)		Untreated patients (n)	Median age (years)	Responses (%)		Median DFS (months)
	Overall	Evaluable			OR	CR	
Else *et al.*[123]	34	34	18	52	100	82	> 132
Chadha *et al.*[134]	86	85	60	49	100	79	> 115
Estey *et al.*[135]	46	46	27	51	89	78	> 30[a]
Hoffman *et al.*[137]	49	49	21	51	100	76	> 55
Juliusson *et al.*[138]	16	16	3	48	75	75	12
Saven *et al.*[139]	358	349	179	53	98	91	98[b]
Median values	47.5	47.5	24	51	99	78.5	> 76.5

Note: [a]Data from Seymour *et al.*[140]
[b]Data from Goodman *et al.*[136]

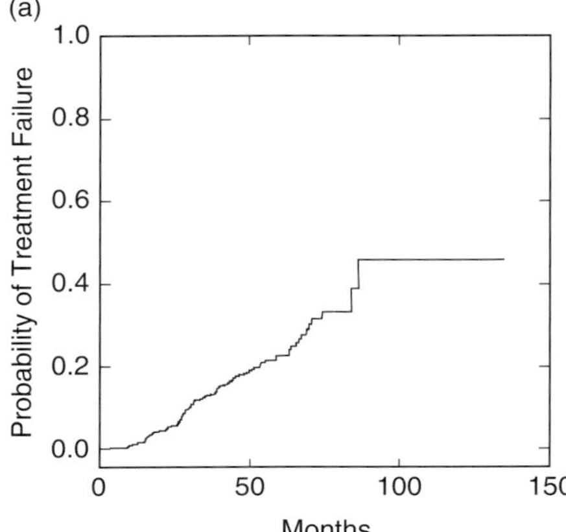

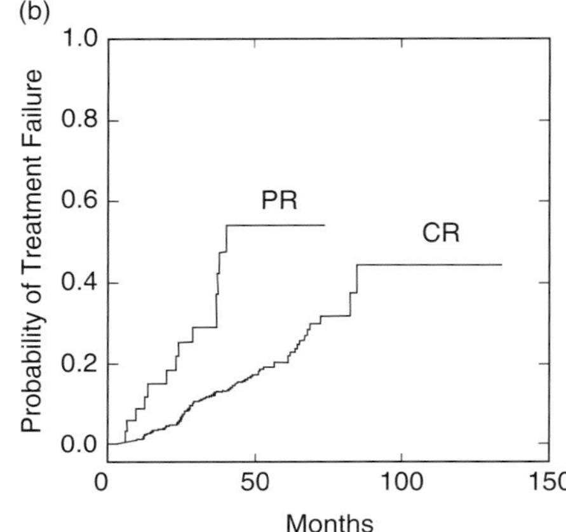

Figure 7.7 (a) Time-to-treatment failure for all 341 patients who achieved a response. (b) Time-to-treatment failure for patients achieving a complete response or partial response. This research was originally published in *Blood*. Saven A, Burian C, Koziol JA, Piro L. Long-term follow-up of patients with hairy cell leukemia after cladribine treatment. 1998;**92**:1918–26.[139] © the American Society of Hematology. Reproduced with kind permission from *Blood*.

the peripheral blood within days, splenomegaly corrected within 3 months, and the bone marrow cleared over 6 months.[138] Median time to first relapse for CRs ranged from 30 to 35 months and for PRs ranged from 10.5 to 24 months.[134,139] Relapse-free survival at 10 years was 64%, with CRs having longer relapse-free survival than PRs. There was no plateau in the curve, questioning the potential curability of HCL with cladribine (Figure 7.7).[134,136] Recent follow-up of the Scripps' patients found no evidence of bone marrow hairy cells even 18 years after treatment, indicating that some patients may perhaps be cured.[145] Overall survival with follow-up of 9 and 12 years was 97% and 87%, respectively.[134,136]

Patients developed bacterial and opportunistic infections, including oral herpes simplex virus, dermatomal and disseminated herpes zoster, and cytomegalovirus.[139] Infectious deaths to *Candida* (two patients) and aspergillosis (one patient) were reported within 4 weeks of cladribine.[135,138] In comparison to pentostatin, cladribine had many fewer early infection-related deaths despite more patients being enrolled on cladribine studies. This is probably related to active infection being an exclusion criterion in the cladribine studies. Delayed infections occurred, but were very uncommon.[139] Cladribine causes suppression of CD4+ lymphocytes for extended periods of time.[141] This is balanced against a restoration of mononuclear cell interferon alpha production and a rapid regeneration of certain lymphocyte subsets, possibly contributing to the rarity of delayed infections.[60,146]

Myelosuppression and culture-negative fevers were the most common acute toxicities. Culture-negative fevers were frequent, occurring in 42% of patients. Due to this, patients with neutropenic fever were not routinely given antibiotics unless associated with fever > 38.5°C, shaking chills or rigors, or an inability to maintain oral hydration despite acetominophen.[129,139,147] Filgrastim did not alter the rate of culture-negative fevers and is not recommended for routine use in this setting.[148] Four patients developed peripheral neuropathies of which two were reversible.[139,147]

Salvage therapies

An approach to salvage therapy after the first cycle of cladribine will be presented. Indications for salvage therapy are the same as the indications for initial therapy (see above).

Most patients who relapse do not require salvage therapy at the time of relapse.

Retreatment with a purine analog or interferon

After first relapse, 60 patients were treated with a second course of cladribine producing a CR and PR in 73% (44 patients) and 17% (10) of patients, respectively, with a median response duration of 35 months. After a second relapse, ten patients received a third course of cladribine producing a CR and PR in 60% (6) and 20%[131] of patients, respectively, with a median response duration of 20 months. Finally, two patients received a fourth course of cladribine resulting in one durable CR of 42 months.[136] Although response rates appear similar, subsequent lines of therapy are of diminishing duration.[123] Pentostatin and interferon alpha have been used as salvage therapy in small numbers of patients and each have elicited responses, including complete and partial remissions.[139,140]

Rituximab

Rituximab has been an effective salvage therapy for relapsed and/or refractory HCL. One study treated 24 HCL-relapsed patients with rituximab 375 mg/m^2 weekly for four consecutive weeks, producing an OR rate of 26% that was evenly split between CRs and PRs. Two of six patients relapsed at 14 and 16 months, including one CR and one PR.[149] Another study treated 15 relapsed and/or refractory patients with the same dose of rituximab for eight consecutive weeks. OR rate was 80%, including eight CRs, two CRs with minimal residual disease, and two PRs. Five patients relapsed between 8 and 39 months from starting therapy. Of eight CRs, only one relapsed at 18 months.[150]

A retrospective study evaluated eight patients who had relapsed HCL to prior purine analog therapy. All eight patients received salvage therapy with rituximab in combination (either sequential or concomitant) with a purine analog. The OR rate was 100%, including 87.5% CRs. Median progression-free survival has not been reached with 29-month median follow-up. The recurrence rate at 2 years was 20%.[151]

BL-22 recombinant immunotoxin

BL-22 is a recombinant immunotoxin composed of an anti-CD22 variable domain fused to a fragment of pseudomonas exotoxin. Sixteen heavily pretreated HCL patients received BL-22 as salvage therapy. All patients had received multiple prior regimens and had relapsed and/or progressive disease after cladribine. Eleven patients had a CR and two patients experienced a PR. Six patients had a CR after one cycle, while five patients required two to nine cycles. Three patients relapsed (two with HCL-variant) within 12 months, but achieved another CR after retreatment. Patients received concomitant rofecoxib and infliximab to prevent a cytokine-release syndrome. Reversible hemolytic-uremic syndrome occurred in two patients requiring plasmapheresis.[152] Fatal hemolytic-uremic syndrome was reported with a different construct of the anti-CD22 immunotoxin.[153] BL-22 is currently available for research patients at the National Cancer Institute.

Minimal residual disease

CR requires the absence of bone marrow hairy cells, which has historically been determined by histology and TRAP staining. These techniques are not reliable for identifying minimal residual disease (MRD), the very small numbers of cells that can persist after definitive therapy. More sensitive methods using DBA.44 and L26 (anti-CD20 antibody) immunohistochemical stains have detected residual hairy cells in half the bone marrow samples from patients considered in CR by standard morphologic techniques.[154] Another study has suggested that the presence of MRD predicts for relapse, which would hold therapeutic and surveillance implications.[155] MRD can also remain stable for extended periods of time and even fluctuate.[154,155] Much longer follow-up is necessary to better define the importance of MRD in HCL. Scripps Clinic recently reviewed the bone marrows of patients who were in a continuous hematologic complete remission, up to 18 years after a single course of cladribine, for evidence of MRD. Using highly sensitive multi-color flow cytometry for CD11c, CD25, CD103, and a pan-B-cell marker, the immunohistochemical stains DBA.44 and L26, and standard histology, half of the patients had no evidence of residual bone marrow hairy cells and may be potentially cured. The other half of patients had MRD without ever experiencing a clinical relapse.[145] This suggests that MRD may not be a major end point in HCL and undermines the rationale for eliminating MRD or performing surveillance bone marrow biopsies.

Diagnosis and treatment strategy

Patients presenting with cytopenias, including monocytopenia, splenomegaly, and minimal lymphadenopathy should be evaluated for HCL. B lymphocytes coexpressing CD11c, CD25, and CD103, with a pan-B-cell marker, on two-color flow cytometry of peripheral blood is diagnostic of HCL. Confirmatory bone marrow biopsies should also be performed.

Treatment is limited to patients with symptoms or cytopenias, including an ANC $\leq 1.0 \times 10^9$/L, Hb ≤ 10 g/dL, Plt $\leq 100 \times 10^9$/L, symptomatic splenomegaly, recurrent infections, or bone lesions. Most patients will require therapy at presentation. However, at first relapse, most patients will not require treatment and can be observed. Cladribine delivered at a dose of 0.1 mg/kg per day by continuous infusion for seven consecutive days is generally considered standard frontline therapy.

Special circumstances

- Actively infected or severely thrombocytopenic patients: Splenectomy may be the most appropriate therapy for this group of patients because of the infectious and cytopenic risks with systemic therapy.

- Patients ≤ 50 years old: Younger patients will enjoy longer life expectancy exposing them to a greater potential for delayed adverse effects from any frontline therapy. They are also more likely to require second- and third-line therapies. For these reasons, consideration should be given to starting therapy with single-agent rituximab. Rituximab is a relatively innocuous therapy with proven activity as a second-line agent, even if perhaps less active than the purine analogs.
- Relapse ≥ 18 months after first-line cladribine: In this situation, cladribine will likely produce a second remission that is again relatively durable.
- Relapse < 18 months after first-line cladribine: A variety of reasonable approaches are possible, including single-agent rituximab given weekly for eight consecutive weeks; use of a pentostatin; use of interferon; or splenectomy.
- Second relapse and beyond: Depending on the duration of the first two remissions, the status of hematopoiesis, and a patient's performance status, therapeutic options include pentostatin, rituximab (depending on prior therapy), splenectomy, interferon, or BL-22 (on study). Case reports have also documented the roles of alemtuzumab and bone marrow transplantation.[156,157]

Acknowledgements

The authors would like to thank and acknowledge the gracious help offered by Dr. Robert Sharpe in compiling and interpreting the hematopathology sections and flow cytometry plots.

References

1. Katayama I, Finkel HE. Leukemic reticuloendotheliosis. A clinicopathologic study with review of the literature. *Am J Med* 1974;**57**:115–26.
2. Farcet JP, Dehoulle C. Hairy cell leukemia. In: Jaffe EJ, Harris NL, Stein H, *et al.*, eds. *World Health Organization Classification of Tumours: Pathology and Genetics of Haematopoietic and Lymphoid Tissues*. Lyon, France, IARC Press. 2001; 188–90.
3. Ewald O. Die leukamische reticuloendotheliose. *Deutsch Arch Klin Med* 1923;**142**:222–8.
4. Bouroncle BA, Wiseman BK, Doan CA. Leukemic reticuloendotheliosis. *Blood* 1958;**13**:609–30.
5. Schrek R, Donnelly WJ. "Hairy" cells in blood in lymphoreticular neoplastic disease and " flagellated" cells of normal lymph nodes. *Blood* 1966;**27**:199–211.
6. Turner A, Kjeldsberg CR. Hairy cell leukemia: a review. *Medicine (Baltimore)* 1978;**57**:477–99.
7. Oleske D, Golomb HM, Farber MD, *et al.* A case-control inquiry into the etiology of hairy cell leukemia. *Am J Epidemiol* 1985;**121**:675–83.
8. Wolf BC, Martin AW, Neiman RS, *et al.* The detection of Epstein-Barr virus in hairy cell leukemia cells by in situ hybridization. *Am J Pathol* 1990;**136**:717–23.
9. Chang KL, Chen YY, Weiss LM. Lack of evidence of Epstein-Barr virus in hairy cell leukemia and monocytoid B-cell lymphoma. *Hum Pathol* 1993;**24**:58–61.
10. Stewart DJ, Keating MJ. Radiation exposure as a possible etiologic factor in hairy cell leukemia (leukemic reticuloendotheliosis). *Cancer* 1980;**46**:1577–80.
11. Colovic MD, Jankovic GM, Wiernik PH. Hairy cell leukemia in first cousins and review of the literature. *Eur J Haematol* 2001;**67**:185–8.
12. Wylin RF, Greene MH, Palutke M, *et al.* Hairy cell leukemia in three siblings: an apparent HLA-linked disease. *Cancer* 1982;**49**:538–42.
13. Haglund U, Juliusson G, Stellan B, *et al.* Hairy cell leukemia is characterized by clonal chromosome abnormalities clustered to specific regions. *Blood* 1994;**83**:2637–45.
14. Sambani C, Trafalis DT, Mitsoulis-Mentzikoff C, *et al.* Clonal chromosome rearrangements in hairy cell leukemia: personal experience and review of literature. *Cancer Genet Cytogenet* 2001;**129**:138–44.
15. Farcet JP, Gourdin MF, Testa U, *et al.* Expression of an accessory cell phenotype by hairy cells during lymphocyte colony formation in agar culture. *Leuk Res* 1983;**7**:87–95.
16. Golomb HM. Hairy cell leukemia: an unusual lymphoproliferative disease: a study of 24 patients. *Cancer* 1978;**42**:946–56.
17. Burthem J, Cawley JC. The bone marrow fibrosis of hairy-cell leukemia is caused by the synthesis and assembly of a fibronectin matrix by the hairy cells. *Blood* 1994;**83**:497–504.
18. Jaffe ES, Shevach EM, Frank MM, *et al.* Leukemic reticuloendotheliosis: presence of a receptor for cytophilic antibody. *Am J Med* 1974;**57**:108–14.
19. Petty HR, Ware BR, Liebes LF, *et al.* Electrophoretic mobility distributions distinguish hairy cells from other mononuclear blood cells and provide evidence for the heterogeneity of normal monocytes. *Blood* 1981;**57**:250–5.
20. Seshadri RS, Brown EJ, Zipursky A. Leukemic reticuloendotheliosis. A failure of monocyte production. *N Engl J Med* 1976;**295**:181–4.
21. Cawley JC, Burns GF, Nash TA, *et al.* Hairy-cell leukemia with T-cell features. *Blood* 1978;**51**:61–9.
22. Guglielmi P, Preud'homme JL, Flandrin G. Phenotypic changes of phytohaemagglutinin-stimulated hairy cells. *Nature* 1980;**286**:166–8.
23. Hanson CA, Ward PC, Schnitzer B. A multilobular variant of hairy cell leukemia with morphologic similarities to T-cell lymphoma. *Am J Surg Pathol* 1989;**13**:671–9.
24. Korsmeyer SJ, Greene WC, Cossman J, *et al.* Rearrangement and expression of immunoglobulin genes and expression of Tac antigen in hairy cell leukemia. *Proc Natl Acad Sci U S A* 1983;**80**:4522–6.
25. Golomb HM, Davis S, Wilson C, *et al.* Surface immunoglobulins on hairy cells of 55 patients with hairy cell leukemia. *Am J Hematol* 1982;**12**:397–401.
26. Burns GF, Cawley JC, Worman CP, *et al.* Multiple heavy chain isotypes on the surface of the cells of hairy cell leukemia. *Blood* 1978;**52**:1132–47.
27. Robbins BA, Ellison DJ, Spinosa JC, *et al.* Diagnostic application of

two-color flow cytometry in 161 cases of hairy cell leukemia. *Blood* 1993;**82**:1277–87.

28. Capello D, Vitolo U, Pasqualucci L, *et al.* Distribution and pattern of BCL-6 mutations throughout the spectrum of B-cell neoplasia. *Blood* 2000;**95**:651–9.
29. Caligaris-Cappio F, Bergui L, Tesio L, *et al.* Cytoskeleton organization is aberrantly rearranged in the cells of B chronic lymphocytic leukemia and hairy cell leukemia. *Blood* 1986;**67**:233–9.
30. Evans SS, Wang WC, Gregorio CC, *et al.* Interferon-alpha alters spectrin organization in normal and leukemic human B lymphocytes. *Blood* 1993;**81**:759–66.
31. Lynch SA, Brugge JS, Fromowitz F, *et al.* Increased expression of the src proto-oncogene in hairy cell leukemia and a subgroup of B-cell lymphomas. *Leukemia* 1993;**7**:1416–22.
32. Knapp W, Dörken B, Gilks WR, *et al.* *White Cell Differentiation Antigens*. Oxford, Oxford University Press, 1989.
33. Posnett DN, Wang CY, Chiorazzi N, *et al.* An antigen characteristic of hairy cell leukemia cells is expressed on certain activated B cells. *J Immunol* 1984;**133**:1635–40.
34. Anderson KC, Boyd AW, Fisher DC, *et al.* Hairy cell leukemia: a tumor of pre-plasma cells. *Blood* 1985;**65**:620–9.
35. Wagner SD, Martinelli V, Luzzatto L. Similar patterns of V kappa gene usage but different degrees of somatic mutation in hairy cell leukemia, prolymphocytic leukemia, Waldenstrom's macroglobulinemia, and myeloma. *Blood* 1994;**83**:3647–53.
36. Forconi F, Sahota SS, Raspadori D, *et al.* Tumor cells of hairy cell leukemia express multiple clonally related immunoglobulin isotypes via RNA splicing. *Blood* 2001;**98**:1174–81.
37. Kluin-Nelemans HC, Krouwels MM, Jansen JH, *et al.* Hairy cell leukemia preferentially expresses the IgG3-subclass. *Blood* 1990;**75**:972–5.
38. Vallianatou K, Brito-Babapulle V, Matutes E, *et al.* p53 gene deletion and trisomy 12 in hairy cell leukemia and its variant. *Leuk Res* 1999;**23**:1041–5.
39. Konig EA, Kusser WC, Day C, *et al.* p53 mutations in hairy cell leukemia. *Leukemia* 2000;**14**:706–11.
40. Byrd JC, Gribben JG, Peterson BL, *et al.* Select high-risk genetic features predict earlier progression following chemoimmunotherapy with fludarabine and rituximab in chronic lymphocytic leukemia: justification for risk-adapted therapy. *J Clin Oncol* 2006;**24**:437–43.
41. Dohner H, Stilgenbauer S, Benner A, *et al.* Genomic aberrations and survival in chronic lymphocytic leukemia. *N Engl J Med* 2000;**343**:1910–16.
42. Stilgenbauer S, Alexander K, Busch R, *et al.* 17p deletion predicts for inferior overall survival after fludarabine-based first line therapy in chronic lymphocytic leukemia: first analysis of genetics in the CLL4 trial of the GCLLSG. *Blood* 2005;**106** Suppl: Abstract 715.
43. Burke JS, Sheibani K. Hairy cells and monocytoid B lymphocytes: are they related? *Leukemia* 1987;**1**:298–300.
44. Traweek ST, Sheibani K, Winberg CD, *et al.* Monocytoid B-cell lymphoma: its evolution and relationship to other low-grade B-cell neoplasms. *Blood* 1989;**73**:573–8.
45. Stroup R, Sheibani K. Antigenic phenotypes of hairy cell leukemia and monocytoid B-cell lymphoma: an immunohistochemical evaluation of 66 cases. *Hum Pathol* 1992;**23**:172–7.
46. Plank L, Hansmann ML, Fischer R. The cytological spectrum of the monocytoid B-cell reaction: recognition of its large cell type. *Histopathology* 1993;**23**:425–31.
47. Machii T, Yamaguchi M, Inoue R, *et al.* Polyclonal B-cell lymphocytosis with features resembling hairy cell leukemia-Japanese variant. *Blood* 1997;**89**:2008–14.
48. Burthem J, Zuzel M, Cawley JC. What is the nature of the hairy cell and why should we be interested? *Br J Haematol* 1997;**97**:511–14.
49. Renshaw BR, Fanslow WC 3rd, Armitage RJ, *et al.* Humoral immune responses in CD40 ligand-deficient mice. *J Exp Med* 1994;**180**:1889–900.
50. Liu YJ, Zhang J, Lane PJ, *et al.* Sites of specific B cell activation in primary and secondary responses to T cell-dependent and T cell-independent antigens. *Eur J Immunol* 1991;**21**:2951–62.
51. Nanba K, Soban EJ, Bowling MC, *et al.* Splenic pseudosinuses and hepatic angiomatous lesions. Distinctive features of hairy cell leukemia. *Am J Clin Pathol* 1977;**67**:415–26.
52. Flandrin G, Sigaux F, Sebahoun G, *et al.* Hairy cell leukemia: clinical presentation and follow-up of 211 patients. *Semin Oncol* 1984;**11**:458–71.
53. Catovsky D. Hairy-cell leukaemia and prolymphocytic leukaemia. *Clin Haematol* 1977;**6**:245–68.
54. Vardiman JW, Golomb HM. Autopsy findings in hairy cell leukemia. *Semin Oncol* 1984;**11**:370–80.
55. Hakimian D, Tallman MS, Hogan DK, *et al.* Prospective evaluation of internal adenopathy in a cohort of 43 patients with hairy cell leukemia. *J Clin Oncol* 1994;**12**:268–72.
56. Mercieca J, Matutes E, Moskovic E, *et al.* Massive abdominal lymphadenopathy in hairy cell leukaemia: a report of 12 cases. *Br J Haematol* 1992;**82**:547–54.
57. Yam LT, Chaudhry AA, Janckila AJ. Impaired marrow granulocyte reserve and leukocyte mobilization in leukemic reticuloendotheliosis. *Ann Intern Med* 1977;**87**:444–6.
58. Child JA, Cawley JC, Martin S, *et al.* Microbicidal function of the neutrophils in hairy-cell leukaemia. *Acta Haematol* 1979;**62**:191–8.
59. Ruco LP, Procopio A, Maccallini V, *et al.* Severe deficiency of natural killer activity in the peripheral blood of patients with hairy cell leukemia. *Blood* 1983;**61**:1132–7.
60. Siegal FP, Shodell M, Shah K, *et al.* Impaired interferon alpha response in hairy cell leukemia is corrected by therapy with 2-chloro-2′-deoxyadenosine: implications for susceptibility to opportunistic infections. *Leukemia* 1994;**8**:1474–9.
61. Steis RG, Marcon L, Clark J, *et al.* Serum soluble IL-2 receptor as a tumor marker in patients with hairy cell leukemia. *Blood* 1988;**71**:1304–9.
62. Kampmeier P, Spielberger R, Dickstein J, *et al.* Increased incidence of second neoplasms in patients treated with interferon alpha 2b for hairy cell leukemia: a clinicopathologic assessment. *Blood* 1994;**83**:2931–8.
63. Arkel YS, Lake-Lewin D, Savopoulos AA, *et al.* Bone lesions in hairy cell leukemia. A case report and response of bone pains to steroids. *Cancer* 1984;**53**:2401–3.
64. Dorsey JK, Penick GD. The association of hairy cell leukemia with unusual immunologic disorders. *Arch Intern Med* 1982;**142**:902–3.

65. Lembersky BC, Ratain MJ, Golomb HM. Skeletal complications in hairy cell leukemia: diagnosis and therapy. *J Clin Oncol* 1988;**6**:1280–4.

66. Golomb HM, Catovsky D, Golde DW. Hairy cell leukemia: a clinical review based on 71 cases. *Ann Intern Med* 1978;**89**:677–83.

67. Katayama I, Li CY, Yam LT. Ultrastructural characteristics of the "hairy cells" of leukemic reticuloendotheliosis. *Am J Pathol* 1972;**67**:361–70.

68. Juliusson G, Vitols S, Liliemark J. Disease-related hypocholesterolemia in patients with hairy cell leukemia. Positive correlation with spleen size but not with tumor cell burden or low density lipoprotein receptor activity. *Cancer* 1995;**76**:423–8.

69. Levine PH, Katayama I. The platelet in leukemic reticuloendotheliosis. Functional and morphological evidence of a qualitative disorder. *Cancer* 1975;**36**:1353–8.

70. Lindemann A, Ludwig WD, Oster W, *et al.* High-level secretion of tumor necrosis factor-alpha contributes to hematopoietic failure in hairy cell leukemia. *Blood* 1989; **73**:880–4.

71. Golomb HM, Vardiman JW. Response to splenectomy in 65 patients with hairy cell leukemia: an evaluation of spleen weight and bone marrow involvement. *Blood* 1983;**61**:349–52.

72. Burke JS. The value of the bone-marrow biopsy in the diagnosis of hairy cell leukemia. *Am J Clin Pathol* 1978;**70**:876–84.

73. Bartl R, Frisch B, Hill W, *et al.* Bone marrow histology in hairy cell leukemia. Identification of subtypes and their prognostic significance. *Am J Clin Pathol* 1983;**79**:531–45.

74. Burthem J, Baker PK, Hunt JA, *et al.* Hairy cell interactions with extracellular matrix: expression of specific integrin receptors and their role in the cell's response to specific adhesive proteins. *Blood* 1994;**84**:873–82.

75. Burthem J, Baker PK, Hunt JA, *et al.* The function of c-fms in hairy-cell leukemia: macrophage colony-stimulating factor stimulates hairy-cell movement. *Blood* 1994;**83**:1381–9.

76. Aziz KA, Till KJ, Zuzel M, *et al.* Involvement of CD44-hyaluronan interaction in malignant cell homing and fibronectin synthesis in hairy cell leukemia. *Blood* 2000;**96**:3161–7.

77. Li CY, Yam LT, Lam KW. Studies of acid phosphatase isoenzymes in human leukocytes: demonstration of isoenzyme cell specificity. *J Histochem Cytochem* 1970;**18**:901–10.

78. Yam LT, Li CY, Lam KW. Tartrate-resistant acid phosphatase isoenzyme in the reticulum cells of leukemic reticuloendotheliosis. *N Engl J Med* 1971;**284**:357–60.

79. Drexler HG, Gaedicke G, Minowada J. Isoenzyme studies in human leukemia-lymphoma cells lines–II. Acid phosphatase. *Leuk Res* 1985;**9**:537–48.

80. Melo JV, Robinson DS, Gregory C, *et al.* Splenic B cell lymphoma with "villous" lymphocytes in the peripheral blood: a disorder distinct from hairy cell leukemia. *Leukemia* 1987;**1**:294–8.

81. Rosner MC, Golomb HM. Ribosome-lamella complex in hairy cell leukemia. Ultrastructure and distribution. *Lab Invest* 1980;**42**:236–47.

82. Brunning RD, Parkin J. Ribosome-lamella complexes in neoplastic hematopoietic cells. *Am J Pathol* 1975;**79**:565–78.

83. Falini B, Schwarting R, Erber W, *et al.* The differential diagnosis of hairy cell leukemia with a panel of monoclonal antibodies. *Am J Clin Pathol* 1985;**83**:289–300.

84. Hsu SM, Yang K, Jaffe ES. Hairy cell leukemia: a B cell neoplasm with a unique antigenic phenotype. *Am J Clin Pathol* 1983;**80**:421–8.

85. Visser L, Shaw A, Slupsky J, *et al.* Monoclonal antibodies reactive with hairy cell leukemia. *Blood* 1989;**74**:320–5.

86. al Saati T, Caspar S, Brousset P, *et al.* Production of anti-B monoclonal antibodies (DBB.42, DBA.44, DNA.7, and DND.53) reactive on paraffin-embedded tissues with a new B-lymphoma cell line grafted into athymic nude mice. *Blood* 1989;**74**:2476–85.

87. Hounieu H, Chittal SM, al Saati T, *et al.* Hairy cell leukemia. Diagnosis of bone marrow involvement in paraffin-embedded sections with monoclonal antibody DBA.44. *Am J Clin Pathol* 1992;**98**:26–33.

88. Johrens K, Stein H, Anagnostopoulos I. T-bet transcription factor detection facilitates the diagnosis of minimal hairy cell leukemia infiltrates in bone marrow trephines. *Am J Surg Pathol* 2007;**31**:1181–5.

89. Cepek KL, Parker CM, Madara JL, *et al.* Integrin alpha E beta 7 mediates adhesion of T lymphocytes to epithelial cells. *J Immunol* 1993;**150**:3459–70.

90. Cawley JC, Burns GF, Hayhoe FG. A chronic lymphoproliferative disorder with distinctive features: a distinct variant of hairy-cell leukaemia. *Leuk Res* 1980;**4**:547–59.

91. Sainati L, Matutes E, Mulligan S, *et al.* A variant form of hairy cell leukemia resistant to alpha-interferon: clinical and phenotypic characteristics of 17 patients. *Blood* 1990;**76**:157–62.

92. Catovsky D, O'Brien M, Melo JV, *et al.* Hairy cell leukemia (HCL) variant: an intermediate disease between HCL and B prolymphocytic leukemia. *Semin Oncol* 1984;**11**:362–9.

93. Tetreault SA, Robbins BA, Saven A. Treatment of hairy cell leukemia-variant with cladribine. *Leuk Lymphoma* 1999;**35**:347–54.

94. Diez Martin JL, Li CY, Banks PM. Blastic variant of hairy-cell leukemia. *Am J Clin Pathol* 1987;**87**:576–83.

95. Troussard X, Valensi F, Duchayne E, *et al.* Splenic lymphoma with villous lymphocytes: clinical presentation, biology and prognostic factors in a series of 100 patients. Groupe Francais d'Hematologie Cellulaire (GFHC). *Br J Haematol* 1996;**93**:731–6.

96. Matutes E, Morilla R, Owusu-Ankomah K, *et al.* The immunophenotype of splenic lymphoma with villous lymphocytes and its relevance to the differential diagnosis with other B-cell disorders. *Blood* 1994;**83**:1558–62.

97. Galton DA, Goldman JM, Wiltshaw E, *et al.* Prolymphocytic leukaemia. *Br J Haematol* 1974;**27**:7–23.

98. Mintz U, Golomb HM. Splenectomy as initial therapy in twenty-six patients with leukemic reticuloendotheliosis (hairy cell leukemia). *Cancer Res* 1979;**39**:2366–70.

99. Jansen J, Hermans J. Splenectomy in hairy cell leukemia: a retrospective multicenter analysis. *Cancer* 1981;**47**:2066–76.

100. Quesada JR, Reuben J, Manning JT, *et al.* Alpha interferon for induction of remission in hairy-cell leukemia. *N Engl J Med* 1984;**310**:15–18.

101. Berman E, Heller G, Kempin S, *et al.* Incidence of response and long-term

follow-up in patients with hairy cell leukemia treated with recombinant interferon alfa-2a. *Blood* 1990;**75**:839–45.

102. Foon KA, Maluish AE, Abrams PG, *et al.* Recombinant leukocyte A interferon therapy for advanced hairy cell leukemia. Therapeutic and immunologic results. *Am J Med* 1986;**80**:351–6.

103. Grever M, Kopecky K, Foucar MK, *et al.* Randomized comparison of pentostatin versus interferon alfa-2a in previously untreated patients with hairy cell leukemia: an intergroup study. *J Clin Oncol* 1995;**13**:974–82.

104. Quesada JR, Hersh EM, Manning J, *et al.* Treatment of hairy cell leukemia with recombinant alpha-interferon. *Blood* 1986;**68**:493–7.

105. Ratain MJ, Golomb HM, Vardiman JW, *et al.* Relapse after interferon alfa-2b therapy for hairy-cell leukemia: analysis of prognostic variables. *J Clin Oncol* 1988;**6**:1714–21.

106. Rai K, Mick R, Ozer H, *et al.* Alpha-interferon therapy in untreated active hairy cell leukemia: a Cancer and Leukemia Group B (CALGB) study. *J Clin Oncol* 1987;**6** Suppl: Abstract 159.

107. Golomb HM, Fefer A, Golde D, *et al.* Survival experience of 195 patients with hairy cell leukemia treated in a multi-institutional study with interferon-alpha 2b. *Leuk Lymphoma* 1991;**4**:9–102.

108. Golomb HM, Jacobs A, Fefer A, *et al.* Alpha-2 interferon therapy of hairy-cell leukemia: a multicenter study of 64 patients. *J Clin Oncol* 1986;**4**:900–5.

109. Golomb HM, Ratain MJ, Fefer A, *et al.* Randomized study of the duration of treatment with interferon alfa-2B in patients with hairy cell leukemia. *J Natl Cancer Inst* 1988;**80**:369–73.

110. Giblett ER, Anderson JE, Cohen F, *et al.* Adenosine-deaminase deficiency in two patients with severely impaired cellular immunity. *Lancet* 1972;**2**:1067–9.

111. Cohen A, Hirschhorn R, Horowitz SD, *et al.* Deoxyadenosine triphosphate as a potentially toxic metabolite in adenosine deaminase deficiency. *Proc Natl Acad Sci U S A* 1978;**75**:472–6.

112. Polmar SH, Wetzler EM, Stern RC, *et al.* Restoration of in-vitro lymphocyte responses with exogenous adenosine deaminase in a patient with severe combined immunodeficiency. *Lancet* 1975;**2**:743–6.

113. Carson DA, Kaye J, Seegmiller JE. Lymphospecific toxicity in adenosine deaminase deficiency and purine nucleoside phosphorylase deficiency: possible role of nucleoside kinase(s). *Proc Natl Acad Sci U S A* 1977;**74**: 5677–81.

114. Hirschhorn R, Levytaka V, Pollara B, *et al.* Evidence for control of several different tissue-specific isozymes of adenosine deaminase by a single genetic locus. *Nat New Biol* 1973;**246**:200–2.

115. Carson DA, Wasson DB, Kaye J, *et al.* Deoxycytidine kinase-mediated toxicity of deoxyadenosine analogs toward malignant human lymphoblasts in vitro and toward murine L1210 leukemia in vivo. *Proc Natl Acad Sci U S A* 1980;**77**:6865–9.

116. Carson DA, Wasson DB, Taetle R, *et al.* Specific toxicity of 2-chlorodeoxyadenosine toward resting and proliferating human lymphocytes. *Blood* 1983;**62**:737–43.

117. Kawasaki H, Carrera CJ, Piro LD, *et al.* Relationship of deoxycytidine kinase and cytoplasmic 5'-nucleotidase to the chemotherapeutic efficacy of 2-chlorodeoxyadenosine. *Blood* 1993;**81**:597–601.

118. Arner ES, Flygar M, Bohman C, *et al.* Deoxycytidine kinase is constitutively expressed in human lymphocytes: consequences for compartmentation effects, unscheduled DNA synthesis, and viral replication in resting cells. *Exp Cell Res* 1988;**178**:335–42.

119. Saven A, Piro L. Newer purine analogues for the treatment of hairy-cell leukemia. *N Engl J Med* 1994; **330**:691–7.

120. Spiers AS, Parekh SJ. Complete remission in hairy cell leukaemia achieved with pentostatin. *Lancet* 1984;**1**:1080–1.

121. Spiers AS, Parekh SJ, Bishop MB. Hairy-cell leukemia: induction of complete remission with pentostatin (2'-deoxycoformycin). *J Clin Oncol* 1984;**2**:1336–42.

122. Cassileth PA, Cheuvart B, Spiers AS, *et al.* Pentostatin induces durable remissions in hairy cell leukemia. *J Clin Oncol* 1991;**9**:243–6.

123. Else M, Ruchlemer R, Osuji N, *et al.* Long remissions in hairy cell leukemia with purine analogs: a report of 219 patients with a median follow-up of 12.5 years. *Cancer* 2005;**104**:2442–8.

124. Flinn IW, Kopecky KJ, Foucar MK, *et al.* Long-term follow-up of remission duration, mortality, and second malignancies in hairy cell leukemia patients treated with pentostatin. *Blood* 2000;**96**:2981–6.

125. Grem JL, King SA, Cheson BD, *et al.* Pentostatin in hairy cell leukemia: treatment by the special exception mechanism. *J Natl Cancer Inst* 1989;**81**:448–53.

126. Kraut EH, Bouroncle BA, Grever MR. Pentostatin in the treatment of advanced hairy cell leukemia. *J Clin Oncol* 1989;**7**:168–72.

127. Johnston JB, Glazer RI, Pugh L, *et al.* The treatment of hairy-cell leukaemia with 2'-deoxycoformycin. *Br J Haematol* 1986;**63**:525–34.

128. Spiers AS, Moore D, Cassileth PA, *et al.* Remissions in hairy-cell leukemia with pentostatin (2'-deoxycoformycin). *N Engl J Med* 1987;**316**:825–30.

129. Dearden CE, Matutes E, Hilditch BL, *et al.* Long-term follow-up of patients with hairy cell leukaemia after treatment with pentostatin or cladribine. *Br J Haematol* 1999;**106**:515–19.

130. Kraut EH, Neff JC, Bouroncle BA, *et al.* Immunosuppressive effects of pentostatin. *J Clin Oncol* 1990;**8**:848–55.

131. Urba WJ, Baseler MW, Kopp WC, *et al.* Deoxycoformycin-induced immunosuppression in patients with hairy cell leukemia. *Blood* 1989;**73**:38–46.

132. Carson DA, Wasson DB, Beutler E. Antileukemic and immunosuppressive activity of 2-chloro-2'-deoxyadenosine. *Proc Natl Acad Sci U S A* 1984;**81**:2232–6.

133. Piro LD, Carrera CJ, Carson DA, *et al.* Lasting remissions in hairy-cell leukemia induced by a single infusion of 2-chlorodeoxyadenosine. *N Engl J Med* 1990;**322**:1117–21.

134. Chadha P, Rademaker AW, Mendiratta P, *et al.* Treatment of hairy cell leukemia with 2-chlorodeoxyadenosine (2-CdA): long-term follow-up of the Northwestern University experience. *Blood* 2005;**106**:241–6.

135. Estey EH, Kurzrock R, Kantarjian HM, *et al.* Treatment of hairy cell leukemia with 2-chlorodeoxyadenosine (2-CdA). *Blood* 1992;**79**:882–7.

136. Goodman GR, Burian C, Koziol JA, *et al.* Extended follow-up of patients with hairy cell leukemia after treatment

with cladribine. *J Clin Oncol* 2003;**21**:891–6.

137. Hoffman MA, Janson D, Rose E, *et al.* Treatment of hairy-cell leukemia with cladribine: response, toxicity, and long-term follow-up. *J Clin Oncol* 1997;**15**:1138–42.
138. Juliusson G, Liliemark J. Rapid recovery from cytopenia in hairy cell leukemia after treatment with 2-chloro-2'-deoxyadenosine (CdA): relation to opportunistic infections. *Blood* 1992;**79**:888–94.
139. Saven A, Burian C, Koziol JA, *et al.* Long-term follow-up of patients with hairy cell leukemia after cladribine treatment. *Blood* 1998;**92**:1918–26.
140. Seymour JF, Kurzrock R, Freireich EJ, *et al.* 2-chlorodeoxyadenosine induces durable remissions and prolonged suppression of CD4+ lymphocyte counts in patients with hairy cell leukemia. *Blood* 1994;**83**:2906–11.
141. Juliusson G, Christiansen I, Hansen MM, *et al.* Oral cladribine as primary therapy for patients with B-cell chronic lymphocytic leukemia. *J Clin Oncol* 1996;**14**:2160–6.
142. Juliusson G, Heldal D, Hippe E, *et al.* Subcutaneous injections of 2-chlorodeoxyadenosine for symptomatic hairy cell leukemia. *J Clin Oncol* 1995;**13**:989–95.
143. Lauria F, Bocchia M, Marotta G, *et al.* Weekly administration of 2-chlorodeoxyadenosine in patients with hairy-cell leukemia: a new treatment schedule effective and safer in preventing infectious complications. *Blood* 1997;**89**:1838–9.
144. Zinzani PL, Tani M, Marchi E, *et al.* Long-term follow-up of front-line treatment of hairy cell leukemia with 2-chlorodeoxyadenosine. *Haematologica* 2004;**89**:309–13.
145. Sigal D, Sharpe R, Burian C, *et al.* Very long-term eradication of minimal residual disease in patients with hairy cell leukemia after a single course of cladribine. *Blood* 2010;**115**:1893–6.
146. Juliusson G, Lenkei R, Liliemark J. Flow cytometry of blood and bone marrow cells from patients with hairy cell leukemia: phenotype of hairy cells and lymphocyte subsets after treatment with 2-chlorodeoxyadenosine. *Blood* 1994;**83**:3672–81.
147. Tallman MS, Hakimian D, Rademaker AW, *et al.* Relapse of hairy cell leukemia after 2-chlorodeoxyadenosine: long-term follow-up of the Northwestern University experience. *Blood* 1996;**88**:1954–9.
148. Saven A, Burian C, Adusumalli J, *et al.* Filgrastim for cladribine-induced neutropenic fever in patients with hairy cell leukemia. *Blood* 1999;**93**:2471–7.
149. Nieva J, Bethel K, Saven A. Phase 2 study of rituximab in the treatment of cladribine-failed patients with hairy cell leukemia. *Blood* 2003;**102**:810–13.
150. Thomas DA, O'Brien S, Bueso-Ramos C, *et al.* Rituximab in relapsed or refractory hairy cell leukemia. *Blood* 2003;**102**:3906–11.
151. Else M, Osuji N, Forconi F, *et al.* The role of rituximab in combination with pentostatin or cladribine for the treatment of recurrent/refractory hairy cell leukemia. *Cancer* 2007;**110**:2240–7.
152. Kreitman RJ, Wilson WH, Robbins D, *et al.* Responses in refractory hairy cell leukemia to a recombinant immunotoxin. *Blood* 1999;**94**:3340–8.
153. Messmann RA, Vitetta ES, Headlee D, *et al.* A phase I study of combination therapy with immunotoxins IgG-HD37-deglycosylated ricin A chain (dgA) and IgG-RFB4-dgA (Combotox) in patients with refractory CD19(+), CD22(+) B cell lymphoma. *Clin Cancer Res* 2000;**6**:1302–13.
154. Ellison DJ, Sharpe RW, Robbins BA, *et al.* Immunomorphologic analysis of bone marrow biopsies after treatment with 2-chlorodeoxyadenosine for hairy cell leukemia. *Blood* 1994;**84**:4310–15.
155. Wheaton S, Tallman MS, Hakimian D, *et al.* Minimal residual disease may predict bone marrow relapse in patients with hairy cell leukemia treated with 2-chlorodeoxyadenosine. *Blood* 1996;**87**:1556–60.
156. Fietz T, Rieger K, Schmittel A, *et al.* Alemtuzumab (Campath 1H) in hairy cell leukaemia relapsing after rituximab treatment. *Hematol J* 2004;**5**:451–2.
157. Cheever MA, Fefer A, Greenberg PD, *et al.* Identical twin bone marrow transplantation for hairy cell leukemia. *Semin Oncol* 1984;**11**:511–13.

Acute promyelocytic leukemia: pathophysiology and clinical results update

Francesco Lo-Coco, Massimo Breccia, and Syed Khizer Hasan

Introduction

Acute promyelocytic leukemia (APL) is a distinct subset of acute myeloid leukemia (AML) associated with unique features and requiring specific management. The disease was initially recognized in 1957 by Hillestad,[1] who described three patients with a rapidly fatal acute leukemia characterized by an abundant number of abnormal promyelocytes infiltrating the marrow and a severe hemorrhagic syndrome. In the following decades, APL has become a well-recognized entity, characterized as the M3 subtype of AML within the French–American–British (FAB) morphologic classification accounting for approximately 10% of cases of AML.[2]

Clinically, APL is associated with a bleeding diathesis due to excessive fibrinolysis, which worsens during initial administration of chemotherapy. Most patients present with a low white blood cell (WBC) count, but 10% to 30% have a WBC count greater than 10 000/μL, with increased risk of serious and potentially fatal hemorrhages into the central nervous system and lungs. The disease is initiated by a malignant transformation of an immature myeloid cell followed by block in differentiation at the promyelocyte stage. The promyelocytes and blasts in > 95% of APL cases harbor a balanced, reciprocal translocation involving the long arms of chromosomes 15 and 17 that is often the only cytogenetic abnormality present.[3,4]

In spite of being an infrequent disease, APL represents one of the most successful examples of translational research in medicine. Over the past two decades, considerable progress has been made in the treatment of this leukemia, such that it has been converted nowadays into the most frequently curable adult leukemia.[5,6] Moreover, the APL model provides an extraordinary opportunity to investigate key mechanisms of leukemogenesis and a paradigm for innovative treatments including differentiation therapy and the use of chromatin remodeling agents and antibody-directed therapy.

Molecular architecture of the t(15;17)

In 1977, Rowley *et al.*[7] from the University of Chicago reported on the consistent occurrence of a chromosomal translocation t(15;17)(q22;q21) in APL. This aberration was subsequently found to be uniquely associated to and therefore pathognomonic of the disease. Upon cloning of the translocation in the late 1980s, it was shown that chromosome breakpoints lie within the *RARα* locus on chromosome 17 and the *PML* locus on chromosome 15, resulting in the fusion of the two genes.[8,9] Based on the location of breakpoints within the *PML* locus, the *PML-RARα* transcript isoforms Bcr1, Bcr2, and Bcr3 may be formed. The Bcr1, Bcr2, and Bcr3 transcripts derive from *PML* breakpoints in intron 6, exon 6, and intron 3 and are referred to as long (L) isoform, variable (V) isoform, and short (S) isoform, respectively.[4] Breakpoints in *RARα* invariably occur in all patients in intron 2. *PML-RARα* L isoform accounts for approximately 55% of APL cases, while the S and V isoforms are detected in approximately 35% and 8% of patients, respectively. The *PML-RARα* fusion is detectable by fluorescence *in situ* hybridization (FISH) or reverse transcriptase-polymerase chain reaction (RT-PCR) in > 95% of APLs morphologically defined by FAB criteria, while in the remaining cases several variant rearrangements have been described that constantly involve *RARα* and partner genes other than *PML*[4] (described in more detail below).

Structure and function of PML and RARα

The human *PML* gene is comprised of nine exons with exons 7 to 9 having potential to generate by alternative splicing a number of C-terminally divergent PML isoforms.[10] The exact functions of these isoforms are not clear at present. PML belongs to a family of proteins containing a distinctive C_3HC_4 zinc-binding domain referred to as RING (really interesting new gene) finger. Similarly to other members of this family, such as BRCA1, PML acts as a tumor suppressor and has been implicated in the control of genomic stability.[11] PML controls p53-dependent apoptosis, growth suppression, and cellular senescence in response to ionizing radiation and oncogenic transformation.[12] In the nucleus PML co-localizes with other proteins such as p53, pRb, Daxx, and CBP[12,13] and organizes into a multiprotein complex termed "PML nuclear bodies" through its ability to form homomultimers. The PML

Management of Hematologic Malignancies, ed. Susan M. O'Brien, Julie M. Vose, and Hagop M. Kantarjian. Published by Cambridge University Press.

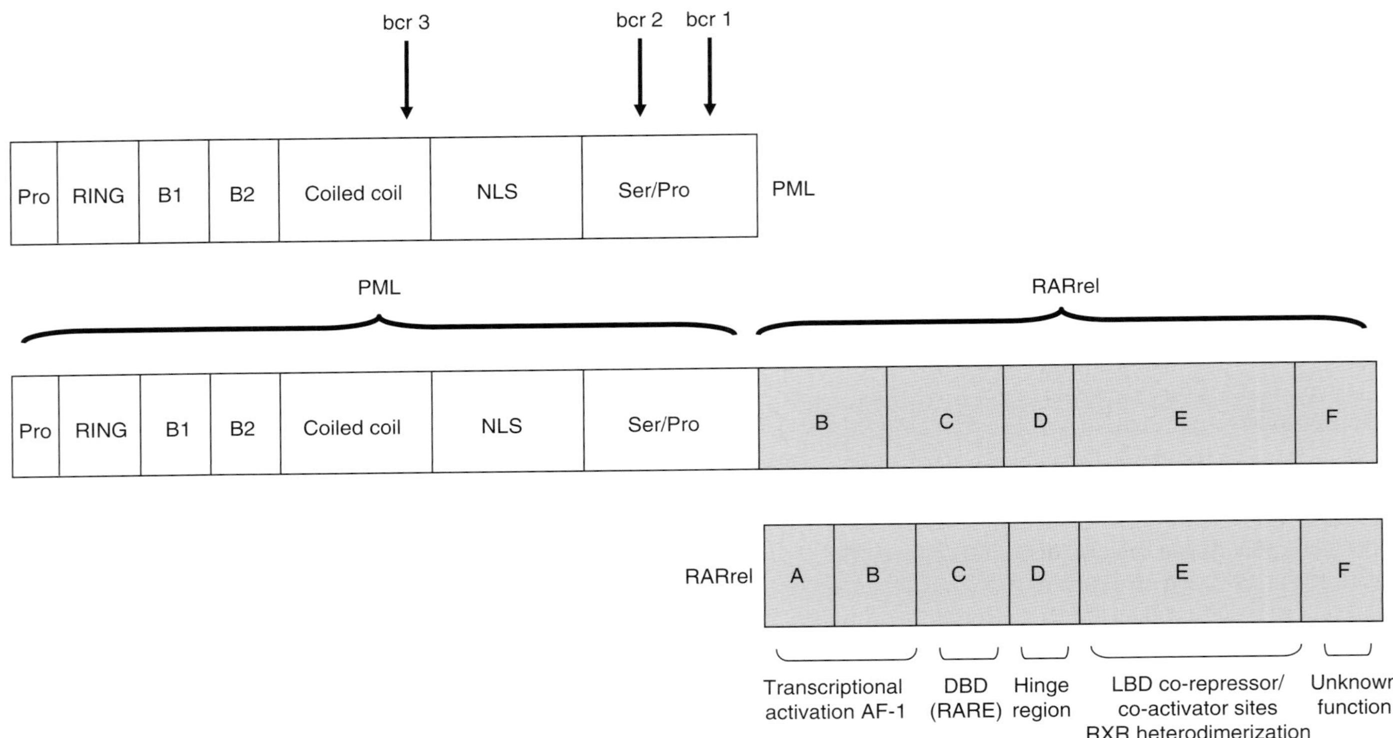

Figure 8.1 Schematic representation of PML-RARα fusion protein. PML regions labeled as RING, B1, and B2 represent cysteine–histidine-rich domains; coiled-coil region, nuclear localization signal (NLS), and an acidic C-terminal Ser/Pro-rich domain, positions of three breakpoint cluster regions indicated by arrows (upper panel); A–F: RARα functional domains; DBD: DNA binding domain; RARE: retinoic acid response element; LBD: ligand binding domain; RXR: retinoid X receptor (lower panel). In the fusion protein (middle panel), RING finger, the B boxes, and the coiled-coil regions are consistently retained, whereas the C-terminal portion of PML varies depending on alternative splicing of the *PML* exons. RARα is fused through B to F domain.

protein has a modular structure with several domains (Figure 8.1). These include the following: a cysteine-rich region (aa 57–222) composed of three zinc finger-like structures. The first is a Zn^{2+} binding motif, RING finger. The following two are called B-box zinc fingers (aa 140–161 and aa 189–222). RING finger/B-box proteins often are linked to a coiled-coil (CC) domain and comprise a subfamily of RING proteins (RBCC for **R**ING-**B** Box-**C**oiled-**C**oil). In addition to the RBCC motif, a nuclear localization signal (NLS) which is required for biologic activity of protein and an acidic Ser/Pro-rich region of unknown function is present within the C-terminal portion of PML. The RING finger/B-box region is involved in localization of PML into nuclear bodies (NB). The CC motif mediates oligomerization of PML-RARα and its interaction with wild type PML.[8,9,10,14,15]

RARα is a member of the retinoic acid (RA) nuclear receptor family serving as a ligand-inducible transcription factor by binding through its DNA binding domain "C" to specific retinoic acid response elements (RARE) which are located in the promoters of many genes, including those of RARα, RARβ, and RARγ. The RARE are composed of hexanucleotide direct repeats with a variable number of spacer nucleotides between the repeated motifs. As shown in Figure 8.1, RARα contains two domains, AF-1 (A/B domain) and AF-2 (E domain), which can cooperate to activate transcription. RA-RARα pathway indeed plays an important role in the control of the myeloid cell differentiation. In the absence of ligand, RARα forms heterodimers with the retinoid X receptor (RXR) through its ligand binding domain "E" and recruits a corepressor complex containing histone deacetylase (HDAC) activities that induces chromatin condensation and transcriptional repression.[16]

Retinoids, natural or synthetic derivatives of vitamin A, are necessary dietary constituents that exert profound effects on development, cell proliferation and differentiation in normal cells and various cancer cells by regulating the expression of specific genes. RARs (α, β, γ,) are activated by both all-*trans* retinoic acid (ATRA, also called tretinoin, which is an acid form of vitamin A) and 9-cis-RA, whereas RXRs (α, β, γ,) are activated by 9-cis-RA only. Physiologic concentrations of RA (1×10^{-9} M) are able to release the nuclear corepressors complex from the RAR-RXR and recruit coactivators with histone acetyltransferase activities (HAT). This results in hyperacetylation of histones at RARE sites, chromatin remodeling, and transcriptional activation of RARα-target genes.[17–19]

Both the PML and RARα moiety of the PML-RARα fusion protein have functional domains from each of the two native proteins. The N-terminal proline-rich domain together with the RING finger, the B boxes, and the coiled-coil (RBCC) motifs of PML are fused to domains B through to F of RARα.[16]

Biologic effects of PML-RARα

The t(15;17) translocation results in two fusion gene products, *PML-RARα* and *RARα-PML* on the 15q+ and 17q- derivatives, respectively. Whereas *PML-RARα* is invariably expressed in all patients, the reciprocal *RARα-PML* fusion is detectable only in ~70% of cases[4,20,21] suggesting that the former hybrid is the one contributing a major role in disease pathogenesis.

Both in vivo studies in transgenic animals and in vitro analysis in hematopoietic cells have demonstrated that the PML-RARα fusion protein contributes to the leukemic phenotype by inhibiting differentiation and promoting survival of hematopoietic precursors. In the PML-RARα fusion protein, oligomerization of RARα through the coiled-coil domain of PML is responsible for the oncogenic activity.[22] As a consequence of heterodimerization through the RING finger domain of wild-type PML with PML-RARα, wild-type PML becomes delocalized into micro-speckled nuclear particles. This variation in subcellular distribution of PML in APLs bearing the PML-RARα rearrangement is clinically relevant as it allows rapid diagnosis through immunostaining techniques.[21,23] PML-RARα protein alters the intranuclear distribution of PML and other nuclear-body-associated proteins and is a stronger transcriptional repressor than RARα. This results from its increased affinity for the SMRT (silencing mediator for retinoid and thyroid hormone receptors) corepressor and nuclear receptor corepressor (N-CoR).[24,25]

The corepressors N-CoR and SMRT are part of a multiprotein complex that includes HDACs. In the absence of ligand, both wild-type RARα and PML-RARα repress transcription by increasing recruitment of corepressors and HDAC complex to the promoter region of RA target genes resulting in deacetylation of histones. Deacetylated histones alter the conformation of chromatin and its accessibility to the transcriptional machinery, resulting in transcriptional silencing.[19,26] Pharmacologic doses of RA are able to release the interaction between HDACs and corepressors, favoring recruitment of coactivators leading to active transcription on the DNA of target genes. In turn, these molecular events overcome the maturation arrest of leukemic promyelocytes resulting in in vivo differentiation of blasts and clinical remission.

Variant *RARα* translocations

In the vast majority of FAB-defined M3 cases, the classical t(15;17) is detected;[27] however, a series of variant chromosomal aberrations have been reported, including t(11;17)(q23;q21), t(5;17)(q35;q12-q21), t(11;17)(q13;q21), and der(17), whereby *RARα* is fused to the *PLZF*, *NPM*, *NuMA*, and *STAT5b* genes, respectively.[28–31] In common with *PML-RARα*-associated APL, patients with fusion genes involving *NPM* and *NuMA* appear to be sensitive to ATRA. In contrast, APL associated with a *PLZF-RARα* rearrangement is characterized by lack of a differentiation response to retinoids, and patients harboring this variant translocation treated with ATRA alone have a poor prognosis.[32] At pharmacologic levels of ATRA, the corepressor complex is released from the retinoid receptor moiety of PML-RARα, NPM-RARα, PLZF-RARα, and presumably NuMA-RARα fusion proteins; however, the PLZF moiety of the PLZF-RARα fusion protein contains a BTB/POZ repression domain that binds the N-CoR and SMRT corepressors in a retinoid-independent manner so that transcriptional repression is not relieved by ATRA. This latter phenomenon has been proposed to account for the lack of response to ATRA that characterizes cases of APL with the t(11;17)(q23;q21).

Molecular basis for response to all-*trans* retinoic acid (ATRA) and arsenic trioxide (ATO)

PML-RARα in its basal state interacts with N-CoR and SMRT corepressors that mediate transcriptional silencing. Transcriptional activation by PML-RARα in response to pharmacologic doses of ATRA (10^{-6}–10^{-7} M) occurs via a conformational shift that releases these corepressors and instead recruits coactivator proteins. This coregulator exchange model (replacement of corepressors by coactivators) is supported by recent transcriptome and proteome analyses[33] with modulation of a large number of genes involved in the initiation/promotion of granulocytic differentiation, such as the upregulation of granulopoiesis-associated transcription factors *C/EBPs* and cytokines/cytokine receptors, as well as their corresponding post-receptor signal transduction molecules. Furthermore ATRA induces the degradation of the PML-RARα chimeric protein by triggering caspase-mediated cleavage.[34] Further studies on the pathways involved in PML-RARα catabolism led to the discovery of a ubiquitin/proteasome-mediated degradation of PML-RARα and RARα, which was dependent on the binding of 26S proteasome regulatory subunit 1 (SUG-1) in the AF-2 transactivation domain of RARα.[35,36] Indeed, a number of components of the proteasome pathway that appear to be necessary for the degradation of PML-RARα can be significantly enhanced upon ATRA.[37]

Arsenic trioxide (ATO) exerts dose-dependent effects on APL cells.[38] At high concentration ($1–2 \times 10^{-6}$ M), ATO induces apoptosis, mainly through activating the mitochondria-mediated intrinsic apoptotic pathway. At low concentrations ($0.25–0.5 \times 10^{-6}$ M) and with a longer treatment course, ATO tends to promote differentiation of APL cells. Several mechanisms have been implicated in the action of arsenic in APL. One of the most intensively studied mechanisms is the induction of reactive oxygen species (ROS) in cells treated with arsenic.[39,40] ROS species include hydrogen peroxide and superoxide, which could be scavenged by systems that include glutathione, glutathione-S-transferase, catalase, and *N*-acetylcysteine (NAC). These systems can decrease arsenic-induced cell death.[41,42] ROS production can induce phosphorylation and activate Jun N-terminal kinase (JNK), which in turn triggers apoptosis.[43,44]

Other biologic features of APL and their impact on therapy

In addition to PML-RARα, other biologic features of APL account for its unique phenotype and provide potential targets for tailored treatment. As concerning their surface markers, APL cells are characterized by a virtually absent or minimally expressed gp-170, i.e., the main effector of the multidrug resistance phenotype that is found in a high proportion of AML. Immunophenotypic studies have also shown that APL is featured by a distinctive antigen profile that includes strong positivity for CD33; expression of CD13 and CD117; infrequent expression of HLA-DR and CD34; and lack of CD7, CD11a, CD11b, CD14, and CD18.[45,46] In addition, leukemic promyelocytes frequently show aberrant expression of the T-cell-associated antigen CD2 and low or negative CD34 expression.[46,47] A negative impact on outcome has been suggested for CD2 and CD56 expression although studies in large series of patients receiving modern ATRA plus chemotherapy regimens have not confirmed these associations.[6,47] CD33 is detected in virtually 100% of APL cases at high density and homogeneously. This may account, together with lack of gp-170 expression, for the optimal therapeutic response observed with the anti-CD33 monoclonal antibody (mAb) gemtuzumab ozogamicin (GO), a compound which may induce molecular remission even if used as single agent and/or in advanced disease.[48,49] The cytotoxic agent of GO is N-acetyl gamma calicheamicin dimethyl hydrazide, a derivative of gamma calicheamicin.[50] Binding of GO to the CD33 antigen is followed by endocytosis, cleavage of the covalent link between the mAb and calicheamicin in lysosomes by acid hydrolysis, and release of calicheamicin. Glutathione reduction produces a reactive intermediate of calicheamicin which in turn causes DNA double-strand breaks.[51–56] GO allows delivery of an anthracycline-like compound (calicheamicin) directly to leukemia blasts. Although at present only a few reports have been published on GO treatment for APL, it is presumable that its use in this leukemic subset will be expanded in the near future and most investigators believe that APL represents an ideal target disease for GO.

The FLT3 receptor is involved in the proliferation and differentiation of hemopoietic stem cells. Following binding to its ligand, the FLT3 receptor activates several intracellular signaling pathways which ultimately lead to cell proliferation. FLT3 receptor internal tandem duplications (ITD) in the juxtamembrane domain and point mutations in the tyrosine kinase II domain have been reported to occur in up to 45% of APL cases. This suggests that targeted therapies using FLT3 inhibitors may prove effective in APL. Both ITD and mutations in the tyrosine kinase II domain have been correlated with higher WBC count at presentation, and ITD mutations have been more frequently detected in cases harboring the S-type *PML-RARα*.[57,58] Expression profile studies in patients with mutated FLT3 have shown increased expression of genes involved in cell growth, cell cycle control, cell adhesion and migration, suggesting a role of these alterations in the pathogenesis of the disease and its clinical manifestations.[57,59] As concerning their prognostic significance, a presumed negative impact of FLT3 mutations on treatment outcome has not been confirmed in the large clinical studies with modern ATRA and chemotherapy reported by the GIMEMA and Medical Research Council (MRC) groups.[57,58] Although FLT3 inhibitors have been successfully used in APL mouse models,[59] due to the availability of several other effective agents no clinical trials have been conducted so far in patients.

Treatment of newly diagnosed APL

Standard induction therapy and supportive measures

The current standard approach for induction in newly diagnosed patients includes the simultaneous administration of ATRA and anthracycline-based chemotherapy, which leads to complete remission (CR) in 90% to 95% of patients.[60] Initial studies on ATRA monotherapy highlighted the need for consolidation therapy to avoid clinical relapse:[61] two subsequent randomized studies (European APL group and North American Intergroup)[62,63] demonstrated the significantly better outcomes of patients who received ATRA and chemotherapy compared to patients treated with chemotherapy alone, in terms of relapse rate. A subsequent randomized European APL group study[64] clearly showed that simultaneous administration of ATRA and chemotherapy improved the outcome of APL patients. Based on these studies, a consensus has been reached to establish the concomitant combination of ATRA plus chemotherapy as the standard approach for frontline induction[65–70] (Table 8.1). As to the type of anthracyclines, comparable CR rates have been reported using ATRA plus daunorubicin and cytarabine[64] and ATRA plus idarubicin alone,[67,69] while no apparent advantage was observed by using other cytotoxic agents in addition to anthracyclines (e.g., cytarabine). A recent randomized study of the European APL group[71] showed an increased risk of relapse when cytarabine was omitted from a schedule using daunorubicin both in induction and consolidation therapy; however, this study was unable to demonstrate differences in terms of CR or induction failure rates.

Possible modifications of the standard approach, based on poor recognized prognostic factors, such as CD56 expression, short *PML-RARα* isoform, or FLT3 mutations, are not supported by data on large cohorts of patients treated with ATRA and idarubicin schedule.

In addition to the specific antileukemic treatment, supportive care is critical for the successful outcome of therapy. Once a suspicion of APL is established on the basis of morphologic criteria, the disease should be treated as a medical emergency, even before a genetic diagnosis is made, in order to reduce the risk of fatal hemorrhages due to coagulopathy.[6,72] Treatment of the hemorrhagic diathesis should be based on transfusion of

Table 8.1. Outcomes of newly diagnosed APL patients treated with simultaneous ATRA and chemotherapy

Reference/ Cooperative group	Induction regimen	No. treated patients	CR (%)	DFS (%)	CIR (%)	OS (%)
Mandelli *et al.*, 1997[67] GIMEMA	ATRA + idarubicin	253	95	79	NA	87 (2 yrs)
Sanz *et al.*, 1999[69] PETHEMA	ATRA + idarubicin	123	89	92	NA	82 (2 yrs)
Burnett *et al.*, 1999[65] MRC	ATRA + anthracycline + cytarabine ± etoposide	120	87	72	20	71 (4 yrs)
Sanz *et al.*, 2004[66] PETHEMA	ATRA + idarubicin (risk-adapted)	251	90	90	7.5	85 (3 yrs)
Lengfelder *et al.*, 2009[70] AMLCG	ATRA + daunorubicin + cytarabine + thioguanine	142	92	81.8	8.1	82 (6 yrs)
Kelaidi *et al.*, 2009[64]	ATRA + daunorubicin + cytarabine					
European APL 93[a]		571	81.8–94	NA	18.4–59.2	36.4–77.3
European APL 2000[a]		331	91.4–93.9	NA	24.1–18.9	88.6–95.6

Note: DFS: disease-free survival; CIR: cumulative incidence of relapse; OS: overall survival; NA: not applicable.
[a]results are expressed only for patients with WBC counts ranging from > 50 000/μl to 10 000/μl

frozen plasma and platelet support to maintain the fibrinogen level above 150 mg/dL and platelet counts above 30–50 × 10^9/L. These supportive measures should be more intensive in patients considered at higher risk of lethal hemorrhages due to the presence at diagnosis of adverse prognostic features, such as older age, hyperleukocytosis, or increased levels of creatinine.[72] On the other hand, use of heparin or other anticoagulants to attenuate the risk of bleeding remains questionable.[72] Particular attention must be paid to early symptoms or signs suggestive of the APL differentiation syndrome (DS) in patients treated with either ATRA or ATO. The diagnosis of DS should be suspected in the presence of one of the following symptoms/signs: dyspnea, fever, weight gain, peripheral edema, hypotension, acute renal failure, and pulmonary infiltrates at chest X-rays. Treatment with dexamethasone at a dose of 10 mg twice daily should be promptly started in suspected DS. Differentiating agents could be maintained unless progression to overt syndrome or lack of response to dexamethasone is observed. At the present time, no evidence of morbidity and mortality rates reduction with use of prophylactic corticosteroids has been reported.[73]

ATO in newly diagnosed patients

Several studies conducted in China, India, and the USA have explored the role of ATO as frontline therapy. The results of these trials reported clinical remission rates of more than 80% and a high incidence of molecular remission using ATO alone or in combination with ATRA[73–78] (Table 8.2). Based on these encouraging findings, the ongoing trial of the Italian cooperative group GIMEMA compares the standard AIDA (all-*trans* retinoic acid and IDArubicin) versus an ATO plus ATRA-based regimen first developed at the MD Anderson Cancer Center in Houston.[78]

As to its toxicity profile, ATO therapy may result in development of DS in up to 25% of cases. Moreover, treatment with ATO is frequently associated with QT prolongation that may in turn lead to fatal torsade de pointes. Physicians caring for APL patients treated with ATO should therefore maintain serum potassium above 4.0 mEq/L and serum magnesium above 1.8 mEq/L and withhold the drug in case of significant QTc interval prolongation.[73]

Consolidation therapy

Current consensus on consolidation exists on the need of using at least two cycles of intensive anthracycline-containing therapy and on the adoption of a risk-adapted strategy whereby treatment intensity is modulated according to the predefined risk of relapse.[66,73] Although no randomized studies proved in the long term the benefit of adding ATRA to chemotherapy during consolidation therapy, two independent trials (GIMEMA and PETHEMA) showed a statistically significant improvement in outcomes when ATRA was added in the first 15 days of each consolidation course.[66,79]

As to the role of cytarabine, a recent randomized study of the European APL group demonstrated an increased risk of relapse when this agent was omitted from the consolidation schedule.[71] A recent joint analysis of the PETHEMA and European APL groups showed a significantly lower cumulative incidence of relapse in younger patients with low WBC count (< 10 × 10^9/L) treated with anthracycline as a single agent in the Spanish LAP99 trial as compared to patients treated in the European APL2000 trial, which included cytarabine.

Table 8.2. Outcomes of APL patients treated with arsenic trioxide as frontline therapy

Reference	No. APL patients	Induction therapy	CR (%)	Molecular remission (%)	OS (%)	DFS (%)
Lazo *et al.*, 2003[74]	12	ATO 0.15 mg/kg	100	90	80 (2 yrs)	80 (2 yrs)
Shen *et al.*, 2004[75]	61	ATRA vs. ATO vs. ATRA + ATO	95 vs. 90 vs. 95	NA	NA	68 vs. 85 vs. 100 (2 yrs)
Mathews *et al.*, 2006[76]	72	ATO 10 mg	86	76	81 (2.5 yrs)	86 (2.5 yrs)
Ghavamzadeh *et al.*, 2006[77]	111	ATO 0.16 mg/kg	86	92	88 (3 yrs)	64 (2 yrs)
Ravandi *et al.*, 2009[78]	82	ATRA + ATO 0.15 mg/kg (+GO 19 patients)	92	100	85 (3 yrs)	78 (3 yrs)

The possible reasons underlying these discrepancies could be due to the different type and/or dosing schedule of the anthracyclines used.[80] Both the PETHEMA and GIMEMA groups suggested a potential benefit in using cytarabine in consolidation therapy in the high-risk relapse group.

The role of ATO therapy in consolidation is currently being explored not only in patients treated with ATO in induction but also in patients treated with standard approaches. The above-mentioned studies that used ATO as induction and post-remission therapy demonstrated a high efficacy of this agent.[75–79] In a recent large trial of the US Intergroup, patients who entered CR after standard ATRA plus chemotherapy were randomized to receive or not two courses of ATO before classic post-remission therapy with daunorubicin and ATRA.[81] Patients in the ATO arm had better overall survival and event-free survival compared to patients treated with the standard approach; however, while this study clearly shows a benefit in adding ATO as post-remission therapy, it has to be emphasized that the standard arm resulted in inferior survival rates as compared to those reported from other studies using conventional ATRA plus chemotherapy schedule.

The achievement of molecular remission after post-remission therapy represents a major treatment objective according to International Working Group criteria response in AML.[82] Patients persistently PCR positive at the end of consolidation confirmed in two consecutive low-sensitivity assays will invariably relapse and should be considered, according to recent European LeukemiaNet (ELN) guidelines[73] for allogeneic stem cell transplantation (SCT). Patients with molecular persistence, who are not candidates for SCT, should be considered for rescue therapy with ATO or GO.

Stem cell transplantation

In light of the high cure rates that are obtained with upfront ATRA and chemotherapy, there is no role for SCT in patients who are in first remission at the end of consolidation. SCT is instead recommended for the small fraction of APL patients with molecular persistence of residual disease at this time point, as well as for patients in second CR with unavailable HLA-identical donor remaining PCR positive after salvage therapy with ATO. Recent ELN guidelines indicate autologous SCT as a valid alternative for patients ineligible for allogeneic transplant, provided that molecular remission is achieved after salvage therapy. All published studies regarding allogeneic SCT were based on the use of ablative conditioning regimens and data following reduced intensity conditioning are currently lacking.[73]

Maintenance therapy

The role of maintenance in APL patients is still a matter of debate: two randomized trials have proved the benefit of ATRA-based regimens as post-consolidation therapy,[63,64] whereas two additional and more recent randomized trials did not report substantial benefit from two different maintenance regimens.[83,84] The GIMEMA group[83] and the Japanese group[84] failed to demonstrate an improvement in terms of relapse rate and survival. These apparently contradictory findings suggest that the effectiveness of maintenance would be inversely related to the intensity of prior induction and consolidation therapy. Although the role and type of maintenance therapy is still being investigated at present, particularly with respect to its optimal schedule and target patient population, the majority of groups have incorporated maintenance into their APL therapeutic programs.

Treatment of relapsed APL

The benefit of early intervention at the time of molecular relapse as compared to treatment started at the time of frank hematologic relapse has been demonstrated by two studies carried out in the pre-ATO era.[85,86] These investigations provided the rationale for sequential molecular monitoring after consolidation therapy for a minimum period of three years in APL patients. The improvement of survival and hematologic relapse risk remains to be proven with ATO-based relapse therapy. The recommendations for management of documented molecular relapse, in the absence of specific data, are identical to those for patients with hematologic relapse. In the pre-ATO era, salvage therapy in this latter subset consisted of the re-administration of ATRA and chemotherapy followed by

SCT. Preliminary studies with ATO as salvage therapy conducted by the Shangai and by the Western group[75] and confirmed by recent studies[75,87] showed a CR rate of 80–90% with 50–70% of patients alive at 3 years. As suggested by recent ELN guidelines, the use of at least two cycles of ATO results in the achievement of a second molecular remission in nearly 80% of cases.[73] In addition, GO appears to induce a high rate of molecular responses as a single agent in advanced disease,[48] even when used at low doses.[88] After ATO rescue to obtain second CR, there are no current guidelines as regards the choice of autologous or allogeneic SCT in second CR. As previously detailed in the section on SCT role in APL, allogeneic SCT is highly recommended at the present time only for patients failing to achieve a second molecular remission whereas for patients unfit for SCT, the available options include repeated cycles of ATO with or without ATRA and GO.[73]

Conclusions and future perspectives

Elucidation of the pathophysiology of APL by identification of the specific PML-RARα oncoprotein and of its biochemical functions has provided relevant information to unravel key mechanisms of leukemogenesis in this disease. In particular, recruitment of the corepressor complex by a fusion protein leading to transcription inhibition and maturation arrest represents a frequent finding in AML pathogenesis and provides a rationale for transcription therapeutic targeting. Moreover, molecular insights into APL have proved extremely useful to improve rapid and specific diagnosis of this leukemia and to sensitively monitor minimal residual disease. Tailored treatment with ATRA and chemotherapy results in cure of nearly 80% of APL patients and attempts to substitute cytotoxic therapy with combinatorial ATRA plus ATO are currently underway. In spite of this progress, the therapeutic benefit achieved in APL through targeted therapy has not yet been translated into other leukemic subsets which remain essentially unresponsive to differentiating agents. Further studies on the mechanisms underlying the maturation block of AML and to unravel relevant pathways for therapeutic targeting are warranted to improve treatment results in the other AML subsets.

References

1. Hillestad LK. Acute promyelocytic leukemia. *Acta Med Scand* 1957; **159**:189–94.
2. Bennett JM, Catovsky D, Daniel MT, *et al.* Proposed revised criteria for the classification of acute myeloid leukemia. A report of the French-American-British Cooperative Group. *Ann Intern Med* 1985;**103**:620–5.
3. Melnick A, Licht JD. Deconstructing a disease: RARalpha, its fusion partners, and their roles in the pathogenesis of acute promyelocytic leukemia. *Blood* 1999;**93**:3167–215.
4. Grimwade D. The pathogenesis of acute promyelocytic leukaemia: evaluation of the role of molecular diagnosis and monitoring in the management of the disease. *Br J Haematol* 1999;**106**:591–613.
5. Tallman MS, Nabhan C, Feusner JH, *et al.* Acute promyelocytic leukemia: evolving therapeutic strategies. *Blood* 2002;**99**:759–67.
6. Sanz MA, Tallman MS, Lo-Coco F. Tricks of the trade for the appropriate management of newly diagnosed acute promyelocytic leukemia. *Blood* 2005;**105**:3019–25.
7. Rowley JD, Golomb HM, Dougherty C. 15/17 translocation, a consistent chromosomal change in acute promyelocytic leukaemia. *Lancet* 1977;**1**:549–50.
8. de The H, Chomienne C, Lanotte M, *et al.* The t(15;17) translocation of acute promyelocytic leukaemia fuses the retinoic acid receptor alpha gene to a novel transcribed locus. *Nature* 1990;**347**:558–61.
9. Kakizuka A, Miller WH Jr, Umesono K, *et al.* Chromosomal translocation t (15;17) in human acute promyelocytic leukemia fuses RAR alpha with a novel putative transcription factor, PML. *Cell* 1991;**66**:663–74.
10. Fagioli M, Alcalay M, Pandolfi PP, *et al.* Alternative splicing of PML transcripts predicts coexpression of several carboxy-terminally different protein isoforms. *Oncogene* 1992;**7**:1083–91.
11. Salomoni P, Pandolfi PP. p53 de-ubiquitination: at the edge between life and death. *Nat Cell Biol* 2002;**4**: E152–3.
12. Gurrieri C, Capodieci P, Bernardi R, *et al.* Loss of the tumor suppressor PML in human cancers of multiple histologic origins. *J Natl Cancer Inst* 2004; **96**:269–79.
13. Jensen K, Shiels C, Freemont PS. PML protein isoforms and the RBCC/TRIM motif. *Oncogene* 2001;**20**:7223–33.
14. Goddard AD, Borrow J, Freemont PS, *et al.* Characterization of a zinc finger gene disrupted by the t(15;17) in acute promyelocytic leukemia. *Science* 1991;**254**:1371–4.
15. de The H, Lavau C, Marchio A, *et al.* The PML-RAR alpha fusion mRNA generated by the t(15;17) translocation in acute promyelocytic leukemia encodes a functionally altered RAR. *Cell* 1991;**66**:675–84.
16. Mistry AR, Pedersen EW, Solomon E, *et al.* The molecular pathogenesis of acute promyelocytic leukaemia: implications for the clinical management of the disease. *Blood Rev* 2003;**17**:71–97.
17. Chambon P. A decade of molecular biology of retinoic acid receptors. *FASEB J* 1996;**10**:940–54.
18. Mangelsdorf DJ, Evans RM. The RXR heterodimers and orphan receptors. *Cell* 1995;**83**:841–50.
19. Minucci S, Ozato K. Retinoid receptors in transcriptional regulation. *Curr Opin Genet Dev* 1996;**6**:567–74.
20. Alcalay M, Zangrilli D, Fagioli M, *et al.* Expression pattern of the RAR alpha-PML fusion gene in acute promyelocytic leukemia. *Proc Natl Acad Sci USA* 1992;**89**:4840–4.
21. Grimwade D, Howe K, Langabeer S, *et al.* Establishing the presence of the t (15;17) in suspected acute promyelocytic leukaemia: cytogenetic, molecular and PML immunofluorescence assessment of patients entered into the M.R.C. ATRA trial. M.R.C. Adult Leukaemia Working Party. *Br J Haematol* 1996;**94**:557–73.

22. Wang ZY, Chen Z. Acute promyelocytic leukemia: from highly fatal to highly curable. *Blood* 2008;**111**:2505–15.

23. Falini B, Flenghi L, Fagioli M, *et al.* Immunocytochemical diagnosis of acute promyelocytic leukemia (M3) with the monoclonal antibody PG-M3 (anti-PML). *Blood* 1997;**90**:4046–53.

24. Lin RJ, Evans RM. Acquisition of oncogenic potential by RAR chimeras in acute promyelocytic leukemia through formation of homodimers. *Mol Cell* 2000;**5**:821–30.

25. Minucci S, Maccarana M, Cioce M, *et al.* Oligomerization of RAR and AML1 transcription factors as a novel mechanism of oncogenic activation. *Mol Cell* 2000;**5**:811–20.

26. Grignani F, De Matteis S, Nervi C, *et al.* Fusion proteins of the retinoic acid receptor-α recruit histone deacetylase in promyelocytic leukaemia. *Nature* 1998;**391**:815–18.

27. Larson RA, Kondo K, Vardiman JW, *et al.* Evidence for a 15;17 translocation in every patient with acute promyelocytic leukemia. *Am J Med* 1984;**76**:827–41.

28. Arnould C, Philippe C, Bourdon V, *et al.* The signal transducer and activator of transcription STAT5b gene is a new partner of retinoic acid receptor alpha in acute promyelocytic-like leukaemia. *Hum Mol Genet* 1999;**8**:1741–9.

29. Chen Z, Brand NJ, Chen A, *et al.* Fusion between a novel Kruppel-like zinc finger gene and the retinoic acid receptor-alpha locus due to a variant t (11;17) translocation associated with acute promyelocytic leukaemia. *EMBO J* 1993;**12**:1161–7.

30. Redner RL, Rush EA, Faas S, *et al.* The t (5;17) variant of acute promyelocytic leukemia expresses a nucleophosmin-retinoic acid receptor fusion. *Blood* 1996;**87**:882–6.

31. Wells RA, Catzavelos C, Kamel-Reid S. Fusion of retinoic acid receptor alpha to NuMA, the nuclear mitotic apparatus protein, by a variant translocation in acute promyelocytic leukaemia. *Nat Genet* 1997;**17**:109–13.

32. Licht JD, Chomienne C, Goy A, *et al.* Clinical and molecular characterization of a rare syndrome of acute promyelocytic leukemia associated with translocation (11;17). *Blood* 1995;**85**:1083–94.

33. Zheng PZ, Wang KK, Zhang QY, *et al.* Systems analysis of transcriptome and proteome in retinoic acid/arsenic trioxide-induced cell differentiation/apoptosis of promyelocytic leukemia. *Proc Natl Acad Sci USA* 2005;**102**:7653–8.

34. Nervi C, Ferrara FF, Fanelli M, *et al.* Caspases mediate retinoic acid-induced degradation of the acute promyelocytic leukemia PML/RARalpha fusion protein. *Blood* 1998;**92**:2244–51.

35. Brown D, Kogan S, Lagasse E, *et al.* A PMLRARalpha transgene initiates murine acute promyelocytic leukemia. *Proc Natl Acad Sci USA* 1997; **94**:2551–6.

36. vom Baur E, Zechel C, Heery D, *et al.* Differential ligand-dependent interactions between the AF-2 activating domain of nuclear receptors and the putative transcriptional intermediary factors mSUG1 and TIF1. *EMBO J* 1996;**15**:110–24.

37. Zhu J, Gianni M, Kopf E, *et al.* Retinoic acid induces proteosome-dependent degradation of retinoic acid receptor α (RARα) and oncogenic RARα fusion proteins. *Proc Natl Acad Sci USA* 1999;**96**:14 807–12.

38. Chen GQ, Shi XG, Tang W, *et al.* Use of arsenic trioxide (As_2O_3) in the treatment of acute promyelocytic leukemia (APL): I. As_2O_3 exerts dose-dependent dual effects on APL cells. *Blood* 1997;**89**:3345–53.

39. Hei TK, Filipic M. Role of oxidative damage in the genotoxicity of arsenic. *Free Radic Biol Med* 2004;**37**:574–81.

40. Hei TK, Liu SX, Waldren C. Mutagenicity of arsenic in mammalian cells: role of reactive oxygen species. *Proc Natl Acad Sci USA* 1998; **95**:8103–7.

41. Chou WC, Jie C, Kenedy AA, *et al.* Role of NADPH oxidase in arsenic-induced reactive oxygen species formation and cytotoxicity in myeloid leukemia cells. *Proc Natl Acad Sci USA* 2004;**101**:4578–83.

42. Zhou L, Jing Y, Styblo M, *et al.* Glutathione-S-transferase pi inhibits As_2O_3-induced apoptosis in lymphoma cells: involvement of hydrogen peroxide catabolism. *Blood* 2005;**105**:1198–203.

43. Davison K, Mann KK, Waxman S, *et al.* JNK activation is a mediator of arsenic trioxide-induced apoptosis in acute promyelocytic leukemia cells. *Blood* 2004;**103**:3496–502.

44. Huang C, Ma WY, Li J, *et al.* Arsenic induces apoptosis through a c-Jun NH2-terminal kinase-dependent, p53-independent pathway. *Cancer Res* 1999;**59**:3053–8.

45. Paietta E. Expression of cell-surface antigens in acute promyelocytic leukaemia. *Best Pract Res Clin Haematol* 2003;**16**:369–85.

46. Paietta E, Goloubeva O, Neuberg D, *et al.* A surrogate marker profile for PML/RAR alpha expressing acute promyelocytic leukemia and the association of immunophenotypic markers with morphologic and molecular subtypes. *Cytometry B Clin Cytom* 2004;**59**:1–9.

47. Albano F, Mestice A, Pannunzio A, *et al.* The biological characteristics of CD34+ CD2+ adult acute promyelocytic leukemia and the CD34 CD2 hypergranular (M3) and microgranular (M3v) phenotypes. *Haematologica* 2006;**91**:311–16.

48. Lo-Coco F, Cimino G, Breccia M, *et al.* Gemtuzumab ozogamicin (Mylotarg) as a single agent for molecularly relapsed acute promyelocytic leukemia. *Blood* 2004;**104**:1995–9.

49. Gale RE, Hills R, Pizzey AR, *et al.* Relationship between FLT3 mutation status, biologic characteristics, and response to targeted therapy in acute promyelocytic leukemia. *Blood* 2005;**106**:3768–76.

50. Sievers E, Larson R, Stadmauer E, *et al.* Efficacy and safety of gemtuzumab ozogamicin in patients with CD33-positive acute myeloid leukemia in first relapse. *J Clin Oncol* 2001;**19**:3244–54.

51. Wellhausen SR, Peiper SC. CD33: biochemical and biological characterization and evaluation of clinical relevance. *J Biol Regul Homeost Agents* 2002;**16**:139–43.

52. Dedon PC, Salzberg AA, Xu J. Exclusive production of bistranded DNA damage by calicheamicin. *Biochemistry* 1993;**32**:3617–22.

53. LaMarr WA, Yu L, Nicolaou KC, *et al.* Supercoiling affects the accessibility of glutathione to DNA-bound molecules: positive supercoiling inhibits calicheamicin-induced DNA damage. *Proc Natl Acad Sci USA* 1998;**95**:102–7.

54. Yu L, Goldberg IH, Dedon PC. Enediyne-mediated DNA damage in

nuclei is modulated at the level of the nucleosome. *J Biol Chem* 1994;**269**:4144–51.

55. Kumar RA, Ikemoto N, Patel DJ. Solution structure of the calicheamicin gamma 1I-DNA complex. *J Mol Biol* 1997;**265**:187–201.

56. Zein N, Sinha AM, McGahren WJ, *et al.* Calicheamicin gamma 1I: an antitumor antibiotic that cleaves double-stranded DNA site specifically. *Science* 1988;**240**:1198–201.

57. Noguera NI, Breccia M, Divona M, *et al.* Alterations of the FLT3 gene in acute promyelocytic leukemia: association with diagnostic characteristics and analysis of clinical outcome in patients treated with the Italian AIDA protocol. *Leukemia* 2002;**16**:2185–9.

58. Marasca R, Maffei R, Zucchini P, *et al.* Gene expression profiling of acute promyelocytic leukaemia identifies two subtypes mainly associated with flt3 mutational status. *Leukemia* 2006;**20**:103–14.

59. Kelly LM, Kutok JL, Williams IR, *et al.* PML/RARalpha and FLT3-ITD induce an APL-like disease in a mouse model. *Proc Natl Acad Sci USA* 2002;**99**:8283–8.

60. Sanz MA. Treatment of acute promyelocytic leukemia. *Hematology Am Soc Hematol Educ Program* 2006; 147–55.

61. Tallmann MS, Nabhan CH, Feusner JH, *et al.* Acute promyelocytic leukemia: evolving therapeutic strategies. *Blood* 2002;**99**:759–67.

62. Fenaux P, Le Deley MC, Castaigne S, *et al.* Effect of all transretinoic acid in newly diagnosed acute promyelocytic leukemia. Results of a multicenter randomized trial. European APL 91 Group. *Blood* 1993;**82**:3241–9.

63. Tallman MS, Andersen JW, Schiffer CA, *et al.* All-trans-retinoic acid in acute promyelocytic leukemia. *N Engl J Med* 1997;**337**:1201–8.

64. Kelaidi C, Chevret S, De Botton S, *et al.* Improved outcome of acute promyelocytic leukemia with high WBC counts over the last 15 years: the European APL Group experience. *J Clin Oncol* 2009;**27**:2668–76.

65. Burnett AK, Grimwade D, Solomon E, *et al.* Presenting white blood cell count and kinetics of molecular remission predict prognosis in acute promyelocytic leukemia treated with all-trans retinoic acid: result of the Randomized MRC Trial. *Blood* 1999;**93**:4131–43.

66. Sanz MA, Martín G, González M, *et al.* Risk-adapted treatment of acute promyelocytic leukemia with all-trans-retinoic acid and anthracycline monochemotherapy: a multicenter study by the PETHEMA group. *Blood* 2004;**103**:1237–43.

67. Mandelli F, Diverio D, Avvisati G, *et al.* Molecular remission in PML/RAR alpha-positive acute promyelocytic leukemia by combined all-trans retinoic acid and idarubicin (AIDA) therapy. Gruppo Italiano-Malattie Ematologiche Maligne dell'Adulto and Associazione Italiana di Ematologia ed Oncologia Pediatrica Cooperative Groups. *Blood* 1997;**90**:1014–21.

68. Asou N, Adachi K, Tamura J, *et al.* Analysis of prognostic factors in newly diagnosed acute promyelocytic leukemia treated with all-trans retinoic acid and chemotherapy. Japan Adult Leukemia Study Group. *J Clin Oncol* 1998;**16**:76–85.

69. Sanz MA, Martín G, Rayón C, *et al.* A modified AIDA protocol with anthracycline-based consolidation results in high antileukemic efficacy and reduced toxicity in newly diagnosed PML/RARalpha-positive acute promyelocytic leukemia. PETHEMA group. *Blood* 1999; **94**:3015–21.

70. Lengfelder E, Haferlach C, Saussele S, *et al.* High dose ara-C in the treatment of newly diagnosed acute promyelocytic leukemia: long-term results of the German AMLCG. *Leukemia* 2009;**23**:2248–58.

71. Adès L, Chevret S, Raffoux E, *et al.* Is cytarabine useful in the treatment of acute promyelocytic leukemia? Results of a randomized trial from the European Acute Promyelocytic Leukemia Group. *J Clin Oncol* 2006;**24**:5703–10.

72. Sanz MA, Grimwade D, Tallman MS, *et al.* Management of acute promyelocytic leukemia: recommendations from an expert panel on behalf of the European LeukemiaNet. *Blood* 2009;**113**:1875–91.

73. Sanz MA, Lo Coco F. Arsenic trioxide. Its use in the treatment of acute promyelocytic leukemia. *Am J Cancer* 2006;**5**:183–91.

74. Lazo G, Kantarjian H, Estey E, *et al.* Use of arsenic trioxide (As_2O_3) in the treatment of patients with acute promyelocytic leukemia: the M. D. Anderson experience. *Cancer* 2003;**97**:2218–24.

75. Shen ZX, Shi ZZ, Fang J, *et al.* All-trans retinoic acid/As_2O_3 combination yields a high quality remission and survival in newly diagnosed acute promyelocytic leukemia. *Proc Natl Acad Sci USA* 2004;**101**:5328–35.

76. Mathews V, George B, Lakshmi KM, *et al.* Single-agent arsenic trioxide in the treatment of newly diagnosed acute promyelocytic leukemia: durable remissions with minimal toxicity. *Blood* 2006;**107**:2627–32.

77. Ghavamzadeh A, Alimoghaddam K, Ghaffari SH, *et al.* Treatment of acute promyelocytic leukemia with arsenic trioxide without ATRA and/or chemotherapy. *Ann Oncol* 2006;**17**:131–4.

78. Ravandi F, Estey E, Jones D, *et al.* Effective treatment of acute promyelocytic leukemia with all-trans-retinoic acid, arsenic trioxide, and gemtuzumab ozogamicin. *J Clin Oncol* 2009;**27**:504–10.

79. Lo Coco F, Avvisati G, Vignetti M, *et al.* Front-line treatment of acute promyelocytic leukaemia with AIDA induction followed by risk-adapted consolidation: results of the AIDA2000 trial of the Italian GIMEMA group. *Blood* 2004;**104**:392a.

80. Adès L, Sanz MA, Chevret S, *et al.* Treatment of newly diagnosed acute promyelocytic leukemia (APL): a comparison of French-Belgian-Swiss and PETHEMA results. *Blood* 2008;**111**:1078–84.

81. Powell BL. Effect of consolidation with arsenic trioxide (As_2O_3) on event free survival (EFS) and overall survival (OS) among patients with newly diagnosed acute promyelocytic leukemia (APL): North Intergroup Protocol C9710. *J Clin Oncol (2007 ASCO Annual Meeting Proceedings Part 1)* 2007;**25**(185): Abstract 2.

82. Cheson BD, Bennett JM, Kopecky KJ, *et al.* Revised recommendations of the International Working Group for Diagnosis, Standardization of Response Criteria, Treatment Outcomes, and Reporting Standards for Therapeutic

Trials in Acute Myeloid Leukemia. *J Clin Oncol* 2003;**21**:4642–9.

83. Avvisati G, Petti MC, Lo Coco F, *et al.* AIDA: the Italian way of treating acute promyelocytic leukemia, final act. *Blood* 2003;**102**:142a.

84. Asou N, Kishimoto Y, Kiyoi H, *et al.* A randomized study with or without intensified maintenance chemotherapy in patients with acute promyelocytic leukemia who have become negative for PML-RARalpha transcript after consolidation therapy: the Japan Adult Leukemia Study Group (JALSG) APL97 study. *Blood* 2007;**110**:59–66.

85. Lo Coco F, Diverio D, Avvisati G, *et al.* Therapy of molecular relapse in acute promyelocytic leukemia. *Blood* 1999;**94**:2225–9.

86. Esteve J, Escoda L, Martín G, *et al.* Outcome of patients with acute promyelocytic leukemia failing to front-line treatment with all-trans retinoic acid and anthracycline-based chemotherapy (PETHEMA protocols LPA96 and LPA99): benefit of an early intervention. *Leukemia* 2007;**21**:446–52.

87. Tallman MS. Treatment of relapsed or refractory acute promyelocytic leukemia. *Best Pract Res Clin Haematol* 2007;**20**:57–65.

88. Breccia M, Cimino G, Diverio D, *et al.* Sustained molecular remission after low dose gemtuzumab-ozogamicin in elderly patients with advanced acute promyelocytic leukemia. *Haematologica* 2007;**92**:1273–4.

Chapter 9

Myeloproliferative neoplasms

Ayalew Tefferi

Introduction

The 2008 World Health Organization (WHO) classification system for hematologic malignancies uses histology and genetic information to organize myeloid neoplasms into five operational categories: acute myeloid leukemia (AML), myelodysplastic syndromes (MDS), myeloproliferative neoplasms (MPN), "MDS/MPN," and "myeloid/lymphoid neoplasms associated with eosinophilia and rearrangements of platelet-derived growth factor receptor α/β or fibroblast growth factor receptor 1" (Table 9.1).[1] The MPN category is in turn subclassified into eight separate entities: chronic myelogenous leukemia (CML), polycythemia vera (PV), essential thrombocythemia (ET), primary myelofibrosis (PMF), systemic mastocytosis (SM), chronic eosinophilic leukemia, not otherwise specified (CEL-NOS), chronic neutrophilic leukemia, and "MPN, unclassifiable." The first four are referred to as "classic" MPN and further subclassified into *BCR-ABL*-positive (CML) and *BCR-ABL*-negative classic MPN. This chapter will focus on the latter.

Historical perspective

In 1951, William Dameshek (1900–69) grouped the four classic MPN (CML, PV, ET, and PMF), along with DiGuglielmo's syndrome (erythroleukemia), under the rubric of "myeloproliferative disorders (MPD)."[2] However, the history of MPD antedates Dameshek by more than a century. In 1879, Gustav Heuck (1854–1940) described PMF under the title of "Two cases of leukemia with peculiar blood and bone marrow findings."[3] In 1904, Max Askanazy (1865–1940) reported another PMF case with substantial EMH of the liver and diffuse bone marrow fibrosis.[4] In 1907, Herbert Assmann (1882–1950) described a similar case ("Heuck–Assmann syndrome"), which he called "osteosclerotic anemia."[5] PMF is also known as agnogenic myeloid metaplasia (a term first used in 1940),[6] chronic idiopathic myelofibrosis (a term used in the 2001 WHO document on the classification of hematologic malignancies),[7] and myelofibrosis with myeloid metaplasia. In 2006, the International Working Group for Myelofibrosis Research and Treatment (IWG-MRT) reached a consensus to exclusively use the term PMF.[8]

Louis Henri Vaquez (1860–1936) was the first to describe PV in 1892 in a 40-year-old man with chronic "cyanosis", distended veins, vertigo, dyspnea, palpitations, hepatosplenomegaly, and marked erythrocytosis.[9] In 1903, William Osler (1849–1919) published a landmark, descriptive case series consisting of four patients with "Chronic cyanosis, with polycythemia and enlarged spleen: a new clinical entity."[10] Osler distinguished PV from both relative polycythemia and secondary polycythemia associated with heart and lung diseases. By 1908, Osler had reviewed 18 cases of what he referred to as "Vaquez's disease" or "polycythemia with cyanosis."[11]

ET is the last of the classic MPN to be formally described (as "hemorrhagic thrombocythemia") in 1934 by Emil Epstein (1875–1951) and Alfred Goedel.[12] Their patient presented with extreme thrombocytosis, slight erythrocytosis, and recurrent mucocutaneous bleeding. Similar cases of thrombocythemia associated with bone marrow megakaryocytic hyperplasia, splenomegaly, thrombosis, or hemorrhage had subsequently appeared in the literature under different names: hemorrhagic thrombocythemia, idiopathic thrombocythemia, thrombocythemia, essential thrombocythemia, megakaryocytic leukemia, thromboblasthemia, and piastrinemia. In a 1954 review of these cases,[13] the authors made note of the distinction between idiopathic and secondary thrombocythemia and suggested the former to be a manifestation of a primary bone marrow proliferative disorder that is distinct from both PV and "megakaryocytic leukemia."

Classification and morphology

The 2008 WHO classification system for hematologic malignancies includes five categories of myeloid neoplasms (Table 9.1): AML, MDS, "MDS/MPN", MPN, and "*PDGFR*- or *FGFR1*-rearranged myeloid/lymphoid neoplasms associated with eosinophilia."[14]

Management of Hematologic Malignancies, ed. Susan M. O'Brien, Julie M. Vose, and Hagop M. Kantarjian. Published by Cambridge University Press.

Table 9.1. The World Health Organization classification of myeloid neoplasms

1. **Acute myeloid leukemia and related neoplasms**
   a. Acute myeloid leukemia with recurrent genetic abnormalities[a]
   b. Acute myeloid leukemia with myelodysplasia-related changes (includes therapy-related myeloid neoplasms)
   c. Acute myeloid leukemia, not otherwise specified[b]
   d. Myeloid sarcoma
   e. Myeloid proliferations related to Down syndrome[c]
   f. Blastic plasmacytoid dendritic cell neoplasms
   g. Acute leukemias of ambiguous lineage[d]
2. **Myeloproliferative neoplasms**
   a. Chronic myelogenous leukemia, *BCR-ABL1*+
   b. Neutrophilic leukemia
   c. Polycythemia vera
   d. Primary myelofibrosis
   e. Essential thrombocythemia
   f. Chronic eosinophilic leukemia, not otherwise specified
   g. Mastocytosis
   h. Myeloproliferative neoplasms, unclassifiable
3. **Myeloid/lymphoid neoplasms associated with eosinophilia and abnormalities of *PDGFRA, PDGFRB*, or *FGFR1***
4. **Myelodysplastic/Myeloproliferative neoplasms**
   a. Chronic myelomonocytic leukemia
   b. Atypical chronic myeloid leukemia, *BCR-ABL1* negative
   c. Juvenile myelomonocytic leukemia
   d. Myelodysplastic/Myeloproliferative neoplasm, unclassifiable (includes the provisional entity of refractory anemia with ring sideroblast and thrombocytosis)
5. **Myelodysplastic syndrome**
   a. Refractory cytopenia with uni-lineage dysplasia (could be mono- or bi-cytopenia)
      i. Refractory anemia (ring sideroblasts < 15% of erythroid precursors)
      ii. Refractory neutropenia
      iii. Refractory thrombocytopenia
   b. Refractory anemia with ring sideroblasts (dysplasia limited to erythroid lineage)
   c. Refractory cytopenia with multi-lineage dysplasia (regardless of ring sideroblast %)
   d. Refractory anemia with excess blasts
   e. Myelodysplastic syndrome with isolated del(5q) (requires < 5% marrow blast count)
   f. Myelodysplastic syndrome, unclassifiable
   g. Childhood myelodysplastic syndrome (includes the provisional entity of refractory cytopenia of childhood)

Notes: [a]The recurrent genetic abnormalities include t(8;21)(q22;q22), inv(16)(p13.1q22) or t(16;16)(p13.1;q22), t(15;17)(q22;q12), t(9;11)(p22;q23), t(6;9)(p23;q34), inv(3)(q21q26.2) or t(3;3)(q21;q26.2), t(1;22)(p13;q13), and the provisional entity of AML with mutated *NPM1* or *CEBPA*.
[b]Subclassified into AML with minimal differentiation, without or with maturation and acute myelomonocytic, monoblastic/monocytic, erythroid, megakaryoblastic, or basophilic leukemia; also includes acute panmyelosis with myelofibrosis.
[c]Includes transient abnormal myelopoiesis and acute myeloid leukemia associated with Down syndrome.
[d]Includes acute undifferentiated leukemia, mixed phenotype acute leukemia with t(9;22)(q34;q11.2), mixed phenotype acute leukemia with t(v;11q23), mixed B/myeloid phenotype acute leukemia-NOS, mixed T/myeloid phenotype acute leukemia-NOS, and the provisional entity of natural killer cell lymphoblastic leukemia/lymphoma.

Table 9.2. The 2008 World Health Organization diagnostic criteria for polycythemia vera (PV), essential thrombocythemia (ET), and primary myelofibrosis (PMF)

2008 WHO diagnostic criteria			
	PV[a]	ET[a]	PMF[a]
Major criteria	1 Hb > 18.5 g/dL (men) > 16.5 g/dL (women) *or* Hb > 17 g/dL (men), or > 15 g/dL (women) if associated with a sustained increase of ≥ 2 g/dL from baseline that cannot be attributed to correction of iron deficiency *or*[b]	1 Platelet count ≥ 450 × 10^9/L	1 Megakaryocyte proliferation and atypia[c] accompanied by either reticulin and/or collagen fibrosis *or* in the absence of reticulin fibrosis, the megakaryocyte changes must be accompanied by increased marrow cellularity, granulocytic proliferation, and often decreased erythropoiesis (i.e., pre-fibrotic PMF)
	2 Presence of *JAK2*V617F or similar mutation	2 Megakaryocyte proliferation with large and mature morphology No or little granulocyte or erythroid proliferation	2 Not meeting WHO criteria for CML, PV, MDS, or other myeloid neoplasm
		3 Not meeting WHO criteria for CML, PV, PMF, MDS, or other myeloid neoplasm	3 Demonstration of *JAK2*V617F or other clonal marker *or* no evidence of reactive marrow fibrosis
		4 Demonstration of *JAK2*V617F or other clonal marker *or* no evidence of reactive thrombocytosis	
Minor criteria	1 BM trilineage myeloproliferation		1 Leukoerythroblastosis
	2 Subnormal serum Epo level		2 Increased serum LDH
	3 EEC growth		3 Anemia
			4 Palpable splenomegaly

Notes: [a]Diagnosis of PV requires meeting either both major criteria and one minor criterion ***or*** the first major criterion and two minor criteria.
[a]Diagnosis of ET requires meeting all four major criteria.
[a]Diagnosis of PMF requires meeting all three major criteria and two minor criteria.
[b]***or*** Hb or Hct > 99th percentile of reference range for age, sex, or altitude of residence *or* red cell mass > 25% above mean normal predicted.
[c]Small to large megakaryocytes with aberrant nuclear/cytoplasmic ratio and hyperchromatic and irregularly folded nuclei and dense clustering.
Hb: hemoglobin; Hct: hematocrit; BM: bone marrow; Epo: erythropoietin; EEC: endogenous erythroid colony; WHO: World Health Organization; CML: chronic myelogenous leukemia; MDS: myelodysplastic syndrome; LDH: lactate dehydrogenase.
Source: Jaffe *et al.*[7]

AML is defined by the presence of ≥ 20% peripheral blood or bone marrow blasts *or* t(8;21)(q22;q22), inv(16)(p13.1q22)/t(16;16)(p13.1;q22), t(15;17)(q22;q12), *or* extramedullary myeloid sarcoma. MDS is typically characterized by cytopenia(s) and trilineage myeloid dysplasia. The MDS/MPN category includes chronic myeloid neoplasms that display laboratory features of both MDS and MPN (Table 9.1).[15]

MPN is distinguished from MDS and MDS/MPN by the absence of dyserythropoiesis, dysgranulopoiesis, and monocytosis (≥ 1 × 10^9/L). Within the MPN category, specific diagnosis is not based on isolated histologic findings but on comprehensive assessment of multiple clinical and laboratory features (Table 9.2). Bone marrow megakaryocyte cluster formation is a characteristic feature of ET, PV, and PMF. Megakaryocytes in ET and PV are large and mature-appearing (Figure 9.1a). Megakaryocytes in PMF have hyperchromatic and irregularly folded bulky nuclei (Figure 9.1b). In PV and PMF, there is histologic evidence of trilineage proliferation. CML is characterized by small and hypolobulated megakaryocytes.

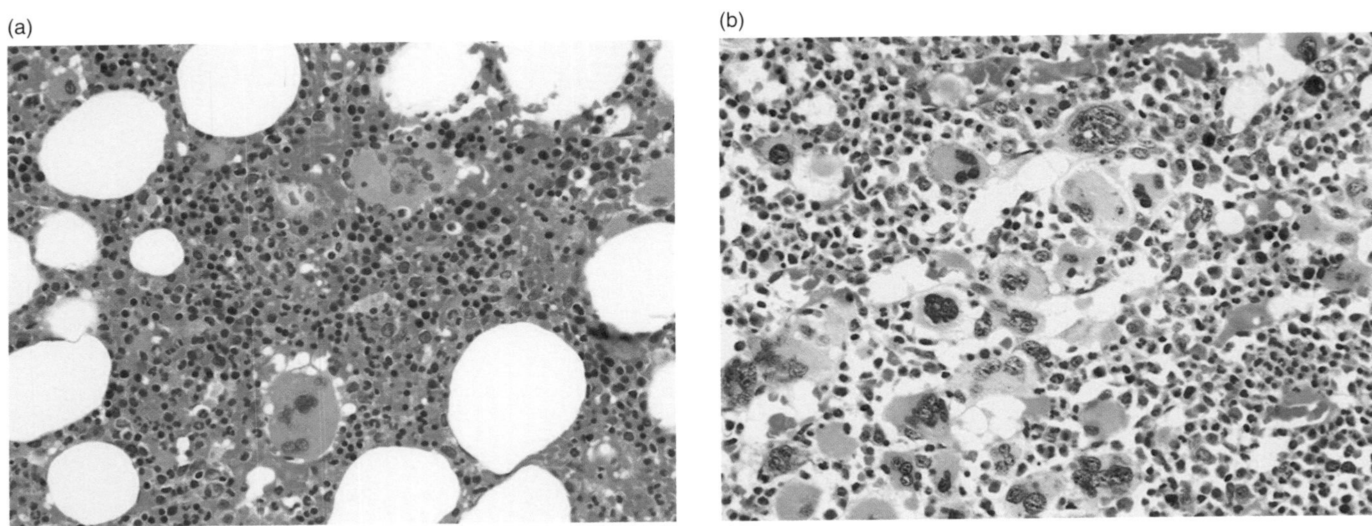

Figure 9.1 Megakaryocyte morphology in essential thrombocythemia (a) as opposed to primary myelofibrosis (b). From Tefferi *et al.*[16]

Cytogenetic findings

Cytogenetic abnormalities are seen in approximately 33% of patients with PMF,[17] 11% of patients with PV,[18] and 7% of those with ET.[19] The type of cytogenetic abnormalities seen in PMF, PV, and ET are similar and the most frequent are del(20q), del(13q), +8, +9, and chromosome 1 abnormalities.[17–20] Of note, abnormalities of chromosomes 5 and 7, which are prevalent in MDS, also occur in MPN.[21] On the other hand, +9 and del(13q), which are frequently seen in MPN, are rarely seen in MDS whereas del(20q) is seen in both MPN and MDS.[22,23] Chromosomal breakpoint regions seen with del(20q) include q11.2-q13·1, with del(13q) q12-q22 and with chromosome 1 anomalies q10-q25/p10-q31.

Molecular pathogenesis

JAK2, *MPL*, and *TET2* mutations are recurrent in PV, ET, and PMF but their precise pathogenetic contribution has not been fully elucidated. *JAK2*V617F is most prevalent in PV, ET, and PMF but also occurs in other myeloid neoplasms;[23,24] mutational frequency is estimated at ~95% in PV, ~60% in ET or PMF, and less than 20% in other myeloid neoplasms.[25,26] *JAK2*V617F allele burden in patients with ET is significantly lower than that seen in patients with either PV or PMF in whom mutant allele homozygosity has been ascribed to mitotic recombination leading to uniparental disomy.[27] Most of the approximately 5% of patients with *JAK2*V617F-negative PV carry *JAK2* exon 12 mutations.[28] Among the latter, N542-E543del is the most frequent.[29] PV patients with *JAK2* exon 12 mutation are younger and might present with apparently "isolated" erythrocytosis.

MPN-associated *MPL* mutations are much less frequent than *JAK2* mutations and have been described in *JAK2*V617F-negative patients with ET or PMF. Specific *MPL* mutations include *MPL*W515L, *MPL*W515K, *MPL*W515S, and *MPL*S505N.) *MPL*515 mutational frequency is estimated at 4% for ET and 11% for PMF.[30–34] *TET2* mutations occur in ~14% of patients with *JAK2*V617F-positive PV, ET, or PMF.[35] Additional studies have demonstrated *TET2* mutations also in *JAK2*V617F-negative MPN as well as in SM, MPN-U, chronic myelomonocytic leukemia (CMML), MDS, MDS/MPN, and AML.[36–38] Furthermore, *TET2* mutations have been shown to coexist with other pathogenetically relevant mutations including *PML-RARA*, *MPL*W515L, *JAK2*V617F, or *KIT*D816V.[36–38]

JAK2, *MPL*, and *TET2* mutations all originate from a primitive hematopoietic stem cell but do not necessarily represent the primary oncogenic event. Expression of *JAK2*V617F, *JAK2* exon 12 mutant, or *MPL*W515L in mice has been shown to induce a PV-like or PMF-like phenotype.[39] Recent studies suggest genetic susceptibility for the acquisition of *JAK2*V617F.[40–43]

Diagnosis

In suspected PV, diagnostic evaluation begins with peripheral blood *JAK2*V617F mutation screen and measurement of serum erythropoietin (Epo) level (Figure 9.2). The presence of *JAK2*V617F is expected in > 95% of patients with PV and excludes the possibility of secondary polycythemia. The presence of subnormal serum Epo level, which is expected in > 90% of patients with PV, further confirms the diagnosis.[44,45] In the absence of *JAK2*V617F, a normal or elevated serum Epo level makes the diagnosis of PV highly unlikely and evaluation for secondary polycythemia should be considered (Figure 9.3). If serum Epo level is subnormal, however, the possibility of PV associated with a *JAK2* exon 12 mutation should be entertained (Figure 9.2). The 2008 WHO diagnostic criteria for PV are outlined in Table 9.2.

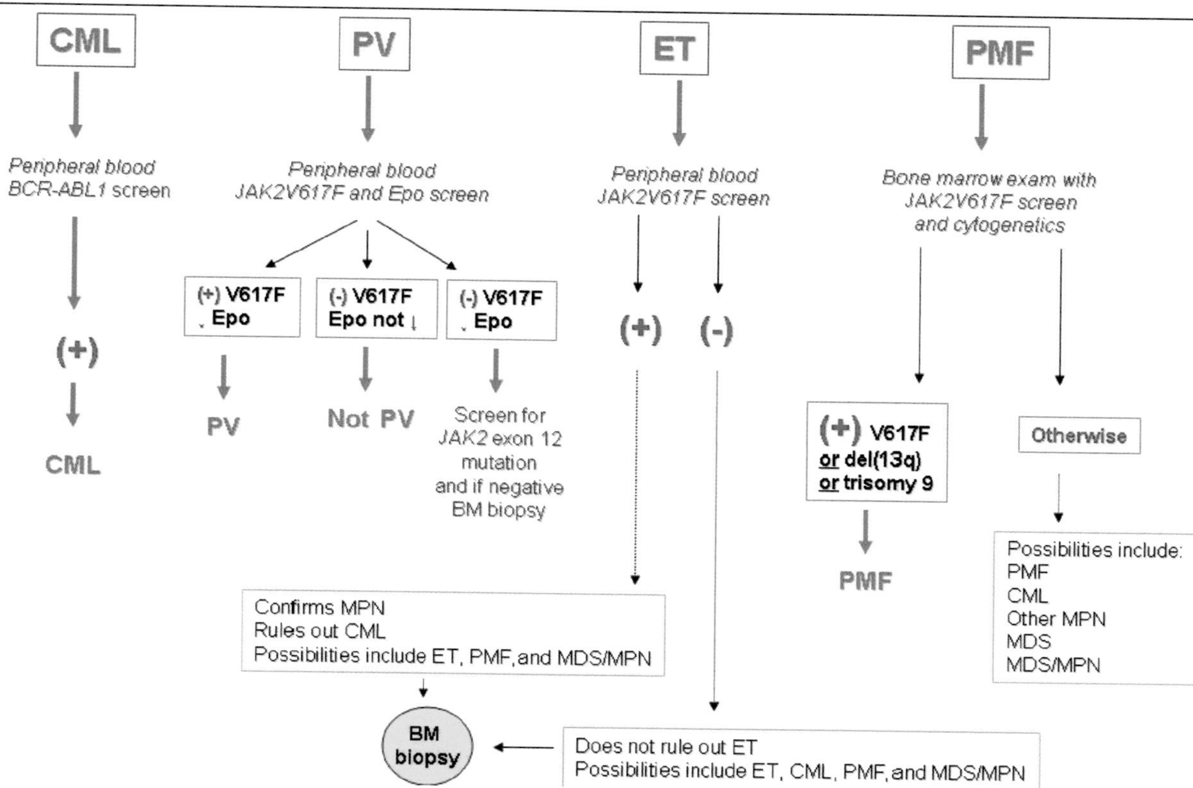

Figure 9.2 Diagnostic algorithm in chronic myelogenous leukemia (CML), polycythemia vera (PV), essential thrombocythemia (ET), and primary myelofibrosis (PMF). MDS: myelodysplastic syndrome; MPN: myeloproliferative neoplasm; Epo: serum erythropoietin; BM: bone marrow. From Tefferi *et al.*[16]

According to the 2008 WHO criteria, the platelet threshold for the diagnosis of ET has been lowered from 600×10^9/L to 450×10^9/L (Table 9.2).[46] After excluding obvious cases of reactive thrombocytosis, it is reasonable to screen peripheral blood for *JAK2*V617F since the mutation is detected in the majority of patients with ET (Figure 9.2).[47] The presence of *JAK2*V617F confirms clonal thrombocytosis but specific diagnosis is made after careful review of bone marrow histology. It is important to always consider the possibility of CML or prefibrotic PMF in patients presenting with "isolated" thrombocythemia; the presence of *BCR-ABL1* or dwarf megakaryocytes supports a diagnosis of CML whereas the presence of leukoerythroblastosis or increased lactate dehydrogenase (LDH) suggests PMF.[48]

Epidemiology

There appears to be a higher incidence of PV, ET, and PMF in persons of Jewish ancestry.[49] Reported incidence figures in PV range from 0.5–2.6/100 000.[50,51] ET is the most frequent among the classic *BCR-ABL*-negative MPN with an annual incidence of between 0.2 and 2.5/100 000.[49,52–57] Incidence figures in PMF range from 0.4 to 1.5/100 000.[53–56,58] Median age at diagnosis of PV is approximately 60 years with a slight (1.2:1) male preponderance.[59] Approximately 7% of patients are diagnosed before age 40.[59] In ET, median age at presentation is approximately 55 years and the disease is more prevalent in women by a factor of approximately 2. Based on a large Mayo Clinic database of well-documented cases, median age at diagnosis in PMF was approximately 57 years with a male to female ratio of 1.6. The same database revealed approximately 2%, 9%, and 29% prevalence rates of patients diagnosed before age 30, 40, and 50 years, respectively (unpublished).

Clinical manifestations

Clinical features in PV and ET include microvascular disturbances (headaches, lightheadedness, atypical chest discomfort, paresthesias, and erythromelalgia), aquagenic pruritus, constitutional symptoms (fatigue, night sweats, low-grade fever), and thrombohemorrhagic complications. Erythromelalgia represents painful and burning sensation of the feet or hands associated with erythema and warmth. Aquagenic pruritus occurs in 48% of patients with PV but is infrequent in ET.[60]

Incidences of major thrombosis at diagnosis range from 9.7% to 29.4% for ET and 34% to 38.6% for PV; the corresponding figures for major thrombosis during follow-up are 8%

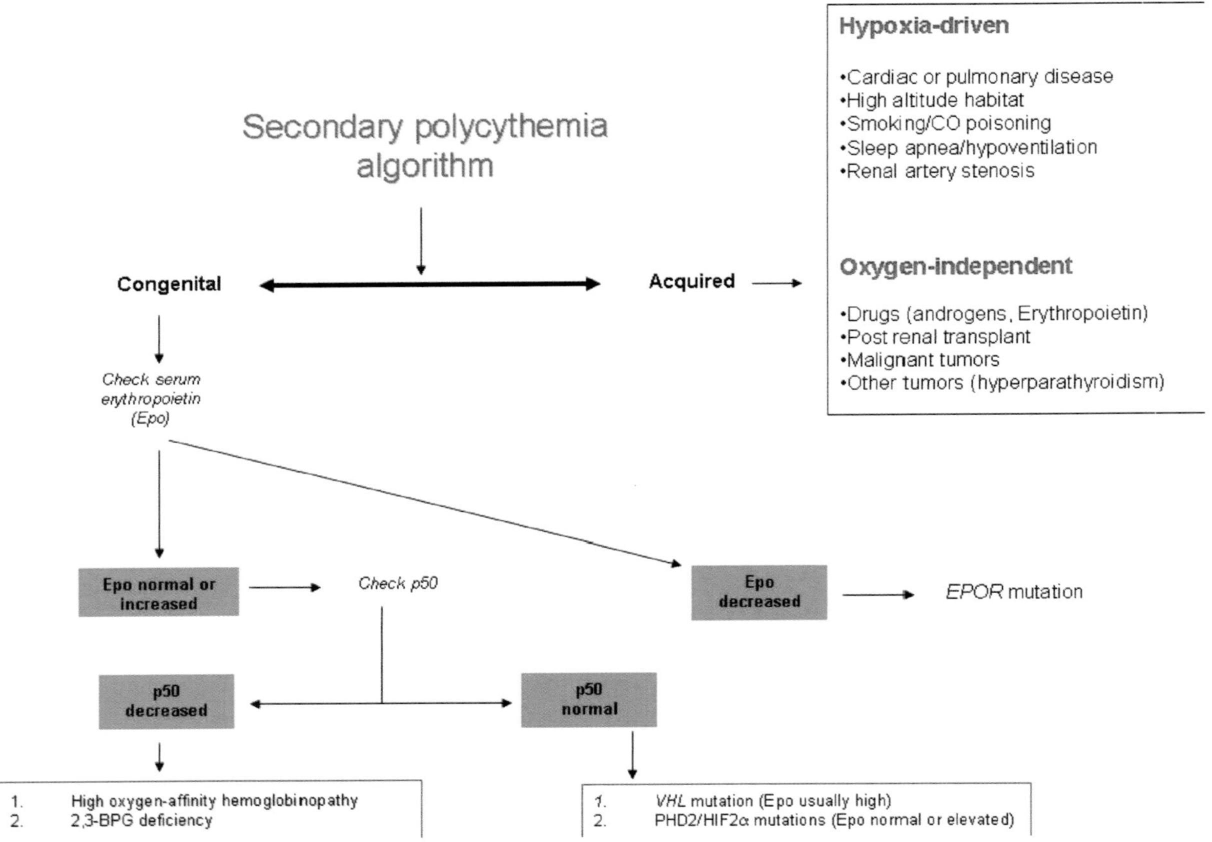

Figure 9.3 A contemporary approach to the diagnosis of secondary polycythemia. CO: carbon monoxide; p50: the partial pressure of oxygen in blood at which 50% of the hemoglobin is saturated with oxygen; EPOR: erythropoietin receptor; BPG: biphosphoglycerate; PHD: prolyl hydroxylase domain-containing enzyme; VHL: the von Hippel-Lindau tumor suppressor protein; HIF: hypoxia-inducible factor. From Tefferi *et al.*[16]

to 30.7% for ET and 8.1% to 19% for PV.[61] In almost all instances, arterial events are more prevalent than venous events and thrombosis in general is more frequent than major bleeding. Venous thrombosis in PV and ET includes sometimes catastrophic abdominal vein thrombosis (AVT). The prevalence of MPN-associated AVT might be higher than the reported ~5% figure since a substantial proportion of "idiopathic" AVT might represent latent MPN, as has been recently indicated by *JAK2*V617F mutational analysis of such cases.[62–64] Other disease manifestations in PV and ET include splenomegaly, ill-defined constitutional symptoms, and first-trimester miscarriages.[65]

Bleeding diathesis in PV and ET is currently believed to involve an acquired von Willebrand syndrome (AvWS) that becomes apparent in the presence of extreme thrombocytosis. The mechanism of AvWS in MPN is currently believed to involve a platelet count-dependent increased proteolysis of high molecular weight von Willebrand protein.[66] Other qualitative platelet defects in PV and ET are believed to play a minor role in disease-associated hemorrhage and include defects in epinephrine-, collagen-, and ADP-induced platelet aggregation, decreased ATP secretion, and acquired storage pool deficiency that results from abnormal in-vivo platelet activation.

The typical features of PMF are anemia, marked hepatosplenomegaly, and constitutional symptoms. Cachexia develops over the disease course with profound weight loss primarily affecting muscle mass. Other symptoms include left upper quadrant discomfort, early satiety, pruritus, easy bruising, peripheral edema, lymphadenopathy, and ascites. Some patients may experience splenic infarcts with severe pain that may be referred to the left shoulder. Hepatosplenomegaly in PMF is secondary to extramedullary hematopoiesis (EMH) that might also involve other organs: lymph nodes (lymphadenopathy), pleura (effusion), peritoneum (ascites), lung (interstitial process), and the paraspinal and epidural spaces (spinal cord and nerve root compression).

Laboratory features

Erythrocytosis in PV and thrombocytosis in ET are essential components of the two diseases. Approximately a third of the patients in addition display mature (i.e., not left-shifted) leukocytosis. The peripheral blood smear in PV and ET does not show substantial qualitative changes. Bone marrow examination in ET is equally unremarkable with the exception of the presence of megakaryocyte clusters. In contrast, the bone marrow is hypercellular in PV and shows trilineage proliferation, in addition to megakaryocyte clusters.

The most characteristic peripheral blood finding in PMF is leukoerythroblastosis (presence of nucleated red blood cells, metamyelocytes, myelocytes, myeloblasts, or megakaryocytes) and dacryocytosis. Anemia is present at diagnosis in the majority of the patients. Other peripheral blood findings include leukocytosis or leukopenia, thrombocytosis or thrombocytopenia, presence of circulating blasts, and increased serum levels of LDH. Bone marrow biopsy often yields a "dry tap." Both "cellular phase" and "overtly fibrotic" stages of the disease are recognized. In general, increased proliferation of granulocytic and megakaryocytic lineage cells is accompanied by reduced erythropoietic elements. Reticulin fibrosis in PMF is sometimes accompanied by dilated sinuses, intra-sinusoidal hematopoiesis, and/or osteosclerosis.

Prognosis

Patients with ET and PV display a shortened life expectancy, which becomes apparent after the first decade of the disease.[67,68] In both instances, shortened survival has been ascribed to delayed disease transformation into AML or MF but deaths from thrombohemorrhagic complications can also occur. In addition, over the course of the disease, there is an increased risk of both thrombosis and bleeding.

Two recent Mayo Clinic studies have described prognostic factors in ET and PV.[69,70] Median survival in ET was 23.2 years in the absence of advanced age, anemia, and leukocytosis and 9 years in the presence of two of these three factors. Also, anemia and extreme thrombocytosis predicted a significantly higher risk of leukemic transformation, which was 0.4% in the absence of these risk factors and 6.5% in the presence of both risk factors. In PV, advanced age, leukocytosis, and arterial thrombosis at diagnosis predicted of inferior survival. In the absence of the first two risk factors, median survival was projected at 23 years as opposed to 9 years in the presence of both risk factors. Leukocytosis in PV was also identified as an independent predictor of leukemic transformation.

Risk factors for thrombosis in ET and PV are well-defined and most investigators agree on what constitutes "high-risk" and "low-risk" in this instance.[61] Several studies have consistently identified advanced age (>60 years) and thrombosis history as risk factors for thrombosis in both PV[70–72] and ET.[67,73,74] Whether or not the presence of cardiovascular risk factors confers additional risk is uncertain.[61,75,76] What is no longer controversial is the lack of prognostic relevance attached to platelet count.[70,77] Instead, recent studies have suggested that leukocytosis predicts a higher risk of thrombosis in both ET and PV but an even more recent study in low-risk disease could not confirm these observations.[78] The frequently cited association of extreme thrombocytosis with gastrointestinal bleeding is based on anecdotal observation and may, in some instances, be attributed to occult acquired von Willebrand syndrome.[79]

PMF is associated with shortened survival (median ~69 months)[80] and causes of death include progression into blast phase disease. A subset of patients with either PV or ET progress into a clinical phenotype that is similar to PMF and such post-PV or post-ET MF is managed like PMF. The International Prognostic Scoring System (IPSS) for PMF utilizes five independent predictors of inferior survival (age >65 years, hemoglobin <10 g/dL, leukocyte count $>25\times10^9$/L, circulating blasts $\geq1\%$, and presence of constitutional symptoms) to stratify patients into low- (no risk factors), intermediate-1- (one risk factor), intermediate-2- (two risk factors), and high- (≥3 risk factors) risk categories; the respective median survivals are estimated at 135, 95, 48, and 27 months.[80] More recently, red blood cell transfusion requirement at diagnosis (median survival ~20 months)[81] and the presence of "unfavorable" cytogenetic abnormalities (median survival ~50 months)[17] were reported to carry an IPSS-independent adverse prognostic effect.

*JAK2*V617F and prognosis in myeloproliferative neoplasms

In ET, the presence of *JAK2*V617F has been associated with advanced age, higher hemoglobin level, increased leukocyte count, decreased platelet count, and venous thrombosis.[82] Furthermore, in mutation-positive patients with ET, a Mayo Clinic study has demonstrated a direct correlation between bone marrow mutant allele burden and both leukocyte and platelet count.[47] The aforementioned study from the Mayo Clinic also showed a higher prevalence of palpable splenomegaly and venous thrombosis in patients with a higher mutant allele burden. More importantly, however, overall survival or transformation rates to MF or AML were not affected by either the presence of the mutation or its allele burden.[47] In another Italian ET study, *JAK2*V617F "homozygous" patients, compared to those with a wild-type or "heterozygous" mutational status, displayed older age, higher leukocyte count, higher hemoglobin level, larger spleen size, and higher incidences of thrombosis and fibrotic transformation.[83]

In PV, the first study that compared *JAK2*V617F "homozygous" and "heterozygous" patients associated the former with higher hemoglobin level, presence of pruritus, and higher rate of fibrotic transformation.[84] A subsequent study confirmed these findings and also demonstrated a higher leukocyte count and lower platelet count in homozygous patients.[83] The later group of investigators also showed that a high mutant allele burden correlated with higher hemoglobin level and leukocyte count, larger spleen size, presence of pruritus, and an increased propensity to require chemotherapy or experience cardiovascular events.[85] A Mayo Clinic PV study using bone marrow-derived DNA for allele burden measurement also found a correlation with leukocyte count and pruritus, but not with hemoglobin level, spleen size, thrombotic complications, or need for cytoreductive therapy.[86]

Table 9.3. Current management and risk stratification in essential thrombocythemia (ET) and polycythemia vera (PV)

Risk categories		
	ET	PV
Low	Low-dose aspirin	Low-dose aspirin + phlebotomy
Low but with extreme thrombocytosis[a]	Low-dose aspirin[b]	Low-dose aspirin[c] + phlebotomy
High	Low-dose aspirin + hydroxyurea	Low-dose aspirin + phlebotomy + hydroxyurea

Notes: [a]Extreme thrombocytosis is defined as a platelet count of 1000 × 10^9/L or more.
[b]Clinically significant acquired von Willebrand syndrome (ristocetin cofactor activity < 30%) should be excluded before the use of aspirin in patients with a platelet count of over 1000 × 10^9/L.
[c]RIC, reduced intensity conditioning.
Risk stratification for ET and PV:
High risk: age ≥ 60 years *or* previous thrombosis.
Low risk: neither of the above.

In PMF, the first Mayo Clinic study showed an association between *JAK2*V617F and older age, history of thrombosis, and pruritus.[87] The particular study did not identify *JAK2*V617F mutational status as an independent prognostic factor for survival. Subsequently, an Italian study found that *JAK2*V617F "homozygous" patients with PMF displayed a higher leukocyte count; larger spleen size; and were more likely to experience pruritus, leukemic transformation, and require chemotherapy or splenectomy.[88] In a most recent Mayo Clinic study, significantly shortened overall and leukemia-free survivals were associated with a low *JAK2*V617F allele burden.[89] In contrast, the outcome of patients with higher mutant allele burden was not significantly different than that of *JAK2*V617F-negative cases.

Treatment

ET and PV

There are a limited number of controlled studies that guide treatment decisions in PV and ET. Controlled studies have demonstrated the value of low-dose aspirin in all patients with PV and hydroxyurea in high-risk patients with ET for preventing thrombotic complications.[90,91] Other randomized studies in PV include (1) hydroxyurea vs. pipobroman (similar survival, thrombosis risk, and leukemic transformation rate),[92] (2) phlebotomy alone vs. phlebotomy plus oral chlorambucil or radiophosphorus (results favored treatment with phlebotomy alone in terms of survival),[71] (3) radiophosphorus vs. oral busulfan (results favored busulfan in terms of survival),[93] and (4) radiophosphorus alone vs. radiophosphorus plus hydroxyurea (no difference in survival).[92] In ET, another randomized study showed hydroxyurea (plus aspirin) to be superior to anagrelide (plus aspirin) in terms of preventing arterial thrombosis and severe bleeding complications.[94] In the same study, although anagrelide performed better in terms of venous thrombosis, it was generally less tolerated and was associated with a higher incidence of fibrotic transformation.

In addition to the above-listed randomized studies, there is general agreement, although not evaluated in a controlled setting, to employ phlebotomy in all patients with PV.[95] In this regard, I recommended a hematocrit target of below 45% in men and 42% in women although I do not object to higher hematocrit targets of up to 50%, if necessary for one reason or another.[77] Also in PV, uncontrolled studies have provided convincing evidence that hydroxyurea benefits high-risk patients with PV, as is the case with high-risk ET.[96] Uncontrolled studies have also shown the value of pipobroman and interferon alpha (IFN-α) for both PV and ET, sometimes associated with modest reductions in *JAK2*V617F allele burden in the case of IFN-α.[97–105] The latter drug can also be useful in patients with PV-associated pruritus; other treatment approaches for pruritus include serotonin reuptake inhibitors[106] and phototherapy.[72]

Considering the above, I recommend phlebotomy and low-dose aspirin in all patients with PV. In addition, I recommend instituting hydroxyurea therapy in high-risk disease.[107] This treatment strategy, with the exception of phlebotomy, also applies to ET – low-dose aspirin in all patients[75,108,109] and the addition of hydroxyurea for high-risk disease.[110,111] However, the use of aspirin in both PV and ET requires the absence of clinically relevant acquired von Willebrand syndrome, which might occur in patients with extreme thrombocytosis;[66] I recommend screening for ristocetin cofactor activity in patients with platelet counts that exceed one million per microliter and holding aspirin if the results are below 30%. It is reasonable to consider IFN-α, pipobroman, or busulfan as second-line therapy in hydroxyurea-intolerant or -refractory cases but randomized studies are needed to establish their role as first-line therapy. Of note, there is no hard evidence to implicate hydroxyurea as being leukemogenic in the treatment of PV or ET.[69,70,112]

Myelofibrosis

At present, allogeneic hematopoietic stem cell transplantation (allo-SCT) is the only treatment approach in MF that is potentially curative.[113] However, such therapy is marred by high treatment-related mortality (TRM) and morbidity. In a recent review of the literature,[114] the estimated 1-year TRM associated with conventional intensity conditioning (CIC) allo-SCT was ~30% and overall survival ~50%. Overall outcome is similar for reduced intensity conditioning (RIC) allo-SCT (5-year median survival of 45%).[115] In the latter study of RIC allo-SCT in MF, treatment-related and relapse-related death rates were each ~41%. By comparison, in a recent study of transplant-eligible patients with PMF who were not transplanted, the 1- and 3-year survival rates ranged from 71% to

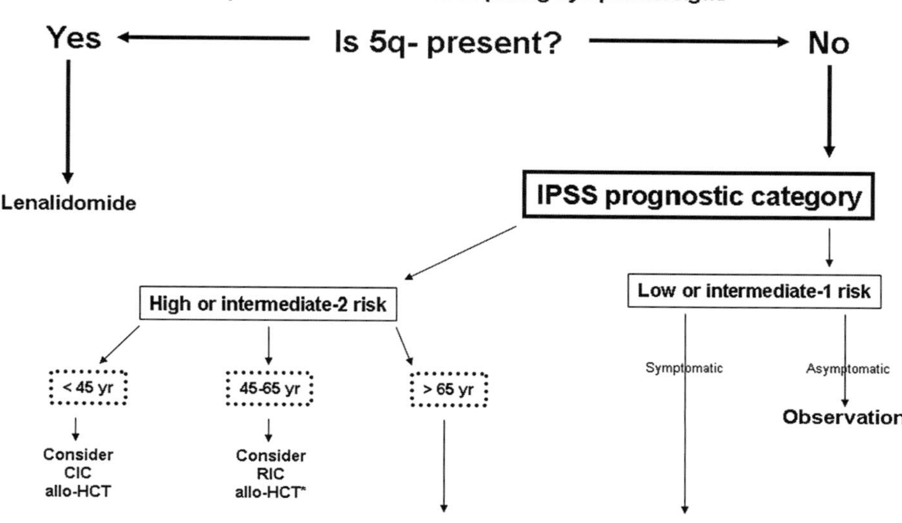

Figure 9.4 A treatment approach for the symptomatic patient with myelofibrosis. IPSS: International Prognostic Scoring System for primary myelofibrosis; CIC: conventional intensity conditioning; RIC: reduced intensity conditioning; allo-SCT: allogeneic hematopoietic cell transplantation. *Alternatively, one could consider investigational drug therapy in the presence of risk factors for poor transplant outcome (e.g., presence of marked splenomegaly or absence of an HLA-identical sibling donor). From Tefferi. *Bone Marrow Transplant*, in press.

95% and 55% to 77%, respectively.[114] Furthermore, although a substantial number of patients who survive allo-SCT achieve complete hematologic, histologic, and molecular remissions,[116] approximately 60% experience extensive, treatment-requiring chronic graft-versus-host disease.[113]

Considering the above, I am currently recommending allo-SCT in transplant-eligible patients with PMF whose median survival is estimated at less than 5 years: (1) IPSS[80] high- (median survival ~27 months) or intermediate-2-risk patients (median survival ~48 months), (2) red blood cell transfusion-dependent patients (median survival ~20 months),[81] and (3) patients with unfavorable cytogenetic abnormalities (median survival ~40 months).[117] I also prefer pre-transplant splenectomy for patients with marked splenomegaly, in the setting of RIC allo-SCT.

Drug therapy in PMF has not been shown to improve survival and is usually considered in the presence of either symptomatic anemia or splenomegaly. Conventional therapy for the former include androgen preparations,[118] prednisone,[118] erythropoiesis stimulating agents,[119–121] and danazol.[122,123] Each one of these options results in response rates of 10% to 20% and response durations of 6 to 18 months. Low-dose thalidomide in combination with prednisone has recently been identified as an effective drug for MF-associated anemia, thrombocytopenia, and splenomegaly with an approximately 50% overall response rate.[124–128] Lenalidomide, a thalidomide analog, has also been evaluated in MF where 20% to 30% response rates in both anemia and splenomegaly were documented.[129] Lenalidomide response rates were higher and quality of responses most impressive in MF patients with the del(5q) abnormality.[130] The therapeutic value of thalidomide is undermined by its neurotoxicity and that of lenalidomide by its myelotoxicity.

Pomalidomide (not US Food and Drug Administration [FDA] approved at this time) is another second-generation immunomodulatory agent (IMiD) created by chemical modification of thalidomide with the intent to reduce toxicity and enhance therapeutic activity. Pomalidomide and lenalidomide are more potent than thalidomide in their antiangiogenic, antitumor necrosis factor alpha (TNF-α), and T-cell costimulatory activity. In an international phase II randomized study, 84 patients were randomized to one of four treatment arms: pomalidomide (2 mg/day) + placebo (n = 22), pomalidomide (2 mg/day) + prednisone (n = 19), pomalidomide (0.5 mg/day) + prednisone (n = 22), and prednisone + placebo (n = 21).[131] Response rates among the four treatment arms were 23% (pomalidomide 2 mg/day + placebo), 16% (pomalidomide 2 mg/day + prednisone), 36% (pomalidomide 0.5 mg/day + prednisone), and 19% (prednisone + placebo). The drug was well tolerated and neuropathy and severe myelosuppression did not appear to be an issue. Longer follow-up and additional studies are required to define the role of pomalidomide in the treatment of MF.

Hydroxyurea is the current drug of choice for controlling splenomegaly, leukocytosis, or thrombocytosis in PMF.[132] Other drugs that have been used in a similar setting include busulfan,[133] melphalan,[134] and 2-chlorodeoxyadenosine.[135] In contrast, IFN-α has limited therapeutic value in MF.[136] Splenectomy is a viable treatment option for drug-refractory symptomatic splenomegaly and may also result in red blood cell transfusion-independence in approximately 25% of patients.[137] Radiation therapy is most useful in the treatment of non-hepatosplenic EMH whereas splenic irradiation offers only transient benefit and might be associated with severe myelosuppression.[138,139]

Management during pregnancy

There is an increased rate of first-trimester miscarriages (approximately 30%) in both ET and PV.[65,140,141] There is no controlled evidence to suggest that specific treatment influences outcome.[65,142] Therefore, at present, I recommend that low-risk pregnant patients with ET or PV be managed the same way as their non-pregnant counterparts. A most recent study suggested the value of aspirin therapy in reducing first trimester miscarriage risk in low-risk ET.[143] In high-risk disease, IFN-α is the drug of choice in women of childbearing age wishing to be pregnant, because of the theoretical risk of teratogenicity associated with the use of other cytoreductive agents.[98]

Conclusions

Recent descriptions of *JAK2*, *MPL*, and *TET2* mutations in PMF and related MPN have raised the prospect of molecularly targeted therapy.[36,144,145] Several anti-JAK2 drugs are currently in active clinical trials. TG101348 is a potent and selective orally bioavailable JAK2 inhibitor with excellent in vitro[146] and in vivo[147] activity against *JAK2*V617F-driven neoplasia. Preliminary results in humans suggest favorable effects in splenomegaly, leukocytosis, and constitutional symptoms.[148] Similar treatment effects have also been shown with another JAK2/JAK1 inhibitor, INCB018424.[149] Other drugs that are currently in clinical trials or soon will be include both ATP mimetics (XL019, CYT387,[150] AZD1480, SB1518) and histone deacetylase (HDAC) inhibitors (ITF2357, MK0683, LBH589). Only time will tell how much an anti-JAK2 therapeutic approach will affect survival and quality of life in MPN.

References

1. Tefferi A, Thiele J, Orazi A, *et al.* Proposals and rationale for revision of the World Health Organization diagnostic criteria for polycythemia vera, essential thrombocythemia, and primary myelofibrosis: recommendations from an ad hoc international expert panel. *Blood* 2007;**110**:1092–7.
2. Dameshek W. Some speculations on the myeloproliferative syndromes. *Blood* 1951;**6**:372–5.
3. Heuck G. Zwei Falle von Leukamie mit eigenthumlichem Blut-resp. Knochenmarksbefund (Two cases of leukemia with peculiar blood and bone marrow findings, respectively). *Arch Pathol Anat Physiol Virchows* 1879;**78**:475–96.
4. Askanazy M. Ueber extrauterine Bildung von Blutzellen in der Leber. *Verh Dtsch Pathol Ges* 1904;**7**:58–65.
5. Assmann H. Beitrage zur osteosklerotischen anamie. *Beitr Pathol Anat Allgemeinen Pathologie (Jena)* 1907;**41**:565–95.
6. Jackson H Jr, Parker FJ, Lemon HM. Agnogenic myeloid metaplasia of the spleen: a syndrome simulating other more definite hematological disorders. *N Engl J Med* 1940;**222**:985–94.
7. Jaffe ES, Harris NL, Stein H, *et al.* (eds.) *World Health Organization Classification of Tumours: Pathology and Genetics of Haematopoietic and Lymphoid Tissues.* Lyon, France, IARC Press. 2001; 1–351.
8. Mesa RA, Verstovsek S, Cervantes F, *et al.* Primary myelofibrosis (PMF), post polycythemia vera myelofibrosis (post-PV MF), post essential thrombocythemia myelofibrosis (post-ET MF), blast phase PMF (PMF-BP): consensus on terminology by the international working group for myelofibrosis research and treatment (IWG-MRT). *Leuk Res* 2007;**31**:737–40.
9. Vaquez H. Sur une forme speciale de cyanose s'accompanant d'hyperglobulie excessive et peristente (On a special form of cyanosis accompanied by excessive and persistent erythrocytosis). *Compt rend Soc de biol* and suppl note, *Bull et mem Soc med d'hop de Paris, 3 ser* 1895;**12**:60. 1892;**4**:384–8.
10. Osler W. Chronic cyanosis, with polycythemia and enlarged spleen: a new clinical entity. *Am J Med Sci* 1903;**126**:187–201.
11. Osler W. A clinical lecture on erythraemia (polycythaemia with cyanosis, maladie de Vaquez). *Lancet* 1908;**1**:143–6.
12. Epstein E, Goedel A. Hamorrhagische thrombozythamie bei vasculärer schrumpfmilz (Hemorrhagic thrombocythemia with a vascular, sclerotic spleen). *Virchows Arch A Pathol Anat Histopathol* 1934;**293**:233–48.
13. Fanger H, Cella LJ Jr, Litchman H. Thrombocythemia; report of three cases and review of literature. *N Engl J Med* 1954;**250**:456–61.
14. Vardiman JW, Brunning RD, Arber DA, *et al.* Introduction and overview of the classification of the myeloid neoplasms. In: Swerdlow SH, Campo E, Harris NL, *et al.*, eds. *WHO Classification of Tumours of Haematopoietic and Lymphoid Tissues*, Vol. 2, 4th edn. Lyon, France, IARC Press. 2008:18–30.
15. Vardiman JW, Brunning RD, Harris NL. WHO histological classification of chronic myeloproliferative diseases. In: Jaffe ES, Harris NL, Stein H, *et al.*, eds. *World Health Organization Classification of Tumours: Pathology and Genetics of Tumours of the Haematopoietic and Lymphoid tissues.* Lyon, France, IARC Press. 2001; 17–44.
16. Tefferi A, Skoda R, Vardiman JW. Myeloproliferative neoplasms: contemporary diagnosis using histology and genetics. *Nat Rev Clin Oncol* 2009;**6**:627–37.
17. Hussein K, Huang J, Lasho T, *et al.* Karyotype complements the International Prognostic Scoring System for primary myelofibrosis. *Eur J Haematol* 2009;**82**:255–9.
18. Gangat N, Strand J, Lasho TL, *et al.* Cytogenetic studies at diagnosis in polycythemia vera: clinical and JAK2V617F allele burden correlates. *Eur J Haematol* 2008;**80**:197–200.
19. Gangat N, Tefferi A, Thanarajasingam G, *et al.* Cytogenetic abnormalities in essential thrombocythemia: prevalence and prognostic significance. *Eur J Haematol* 2009;**83**:17–21.
20. Hussein K, Van Dyke DL, Tefferi A. Conventional cytogenetics in myelofibrosis: literature review and discussion. *Eur J Haematol* 2009;**82**:329–38.
21. Santana-Davila R, Holtan SG, Dewald GW, *et al.* Chromosome 5q deletion: specific diagnoses and cytogenetic details among 358 consecutive cases from a single institution. *Leuk Res* 2008;**32**:407–11.
22. Bacher U, Schnittger S, Kern W, *et al.* Distribution of cytogenetic abnormalities in myelodysplastic syndromes, Philadelphia negative myeloproliferative neoplasms, and the overlap MDS/MPN category. *Ann Hematol* 2009;**88**:1207–13.

23. Steensma DP, Dewald GW, Lasho TL, *et al.* The JAK2 V617F activating tyrosine kinase mutation is an infrequent event in both "atypical" myeloproliferative disorders and myelodysplastic syndromes. *Blood* 2005;**106**:1207–9.

24. Jones AV, Kreil S, Zoi K, *et al.* Widespread occurrence of the JAK2 V617F mutation in chronic myeloproliferative disorders. *Blood* 2005;**106**:2162–8.

25. Renneville A, Quesnel B, Charpentier A, *et al.* High occurrence of JAK2 V617 mutation in refractory anemia with ringed sideroblasts associated with marked thrombocytosis. *Leukemia* 2006;**20**:2067–70.

26. Schmitt-Graeff AH, Teo SS, Olschewski M, *et al.* JAK2V617F mutation status identifies subtypes of refractory anemia with ringed sideroblasts associated with marked thrombocytosis. *Haematologica* 2008;**93**:34–40.

27. Kralovics R, Passamonti F, Buser AS, *et al.* A gain-of-function mutation of JAK2 in myeloproliferative disorders. *N Engl J Med* 2005;**352**:1779–90.

28. Scott LM, Tong W, Levine RL, *et al.* JAK2 exon 12 mutations in polycythemia vera and idiopathic erythrocytosis. *N Engl J Med* 2007;**356**:459–68.

29. Pietra D, Li S, Brisci A, *et al.* Somatic mutations of JAK2 exon 12 in patients with JAK2 (V617F)-negative myeloproliferative disorders. *Blood* 2008;**111**:1686–9.

30. Pardanani AD, Levine RL, Lasho T, *et al.* MPL515 mutations in myeloproliferative and other myeloid disorders: a study of 1182 patients. *Blood* 2006;**108**:3472–6.

31. Schnittger S, Haferlach C, Beelen DW, *et al.* Detection of three different MPLW515 mutations in 10.1% of all JAK2 V617 unmutated ET and 9.3% of all JAK2 V617F unmutated OMF: a study of 387 patients. *ASH Annual Meeting Abstracts* 2007;**110**:2546.

32. Vannucchi AM, Antonioli E, Pancrazzi A, *et al.* The clinical phenotype of patients with essential thrombocythemia harboring MPL 515W>L/K mutation. *ASH Annual Meeting Abstracts* 2007;**110**:678.

33. Guglielmelli P, Pancrazzi A, Bergamaschi G, *et al.* Anaemia characterises patients with myelofibrosis harbouring Mpl mutation. *Br J Haematol* 2007;**137**:244–7.

34. Beer PA, Campbell PJ, Scott LM, *et al.* MPL mutations in myeloproliferative disorders: analysis of the PT-1 cohort. *Blood* 2008;**112**:141–9.

35. Delhommeau F, Dupont S, James C, *et al.* TET2 is a novel tumor suppressor gene inactivated in myeloproliferative neoplasms: identification of a pre-JAK2 V617F event. *ASH Annual Meeting Abstracts* 2008;**112**:lba-3. Late-Breaking Abstract.

36. Tefferi A, Pardanani A, Lim KH, *et al.* TET2 mutations and their clinical correlates in polycythemia vera, essential thrombocythemia and myelofibrosis. *Leukemia* 2009;**23**:905–11.

37. Tefferi A, Levine RL, Lim KH, *et al.* Frequent TET2 mutations in systemic mastocytosis: clinical, KITD816V and FIP1L1-PDGFRA correlates. *Leukemia* 2009;**23**:900–4.

38. Tefferi A, Lim KH, Abdel-Wahab O, *et al.* Detection of mutant TET2 in myeloid malignancies other than myeloproliferative neoplasms: CMML, MDS, MDS/MPN and AML. *Leukemia* 2009;**23**:1343–5. doi:101038/leu200959. 2009.

39. Wernig G, Mercher T, Okabe R, *et al.* Expression of Jak2V617F causes a polycythemia vera-like disease with associated myelofibrosis in a murine bone marrow transplant model. *Blood* 2006;**107**:4274–81.

40. Pardanani A, Fridley BL, Lasho TL, *et al.* Host genetic variation contributes to phenotypic diversity in myeloproliferative disorders. *Blood* 2008;**111**:2785–9.

41. Jones AV, Chase A, Silver RT, *et al.* JAK2 haplotype is a major risk factor for the development of myeloproliferative neoplasms. *Nat Genet* 2009;**41**:446–9.

42. Kilpivaara O, Mukherjee S, Schram AM, *et al.* A germline JAK2 SNP is associated with predisposition to the development of JAK2(V617F)-positive myeloproliferative neoplasms. *Nat Genet* 2009;**41**: 455–9.

43. Olcaydu D, Harutyunyan A, Jager R, *et al.* A common JAK2 haplotype confers susceptibility to myeloproliferative neoplasms. *Nat Genet* 2009;**41**:450–4.

44. Messinezy M, Westwood NB, El-Hemaidi I, *et al.* Serum erythropoietin values in erythrocytoses and in primary thrombocythaemia. *Br J Haematol* 2002;**117**:47–53.

45. Mossuz P, Girodon F, Donnard M, *et al.* Diagnostic value of serum erythropoietin level in patients with absolute erythrocytosis. *Haematologica* 2004;**89**:1194–8.

46. Tefferi A, Vardiman JW. Classification and diagnosis of myeloproliferative neoplasms: the 2008 World Health Organization criteria and point-of-care diagnostic algorithms. *Leukemia* 2008;**22**:14–22.

47. Kittur J, Knudson RA, Lasho TL, *et al.* Clinical correlates of JAK2V617F allele burden in essential thrombocythemia. *Cancer* 2007;**109**:2279–84.

48. Vardiman JW, Thiele J, Arber DA, *et al.* The 2008 revision of the WHO classification of myeloid neoplasms and acute leukemia: rationale and important changes. *Blood* 2009;**114**:937–51.

49. Chaiter Y, Brenner B, Aghai E, *et al.* High incidence of myeloproliferative disorders in Ashkenazi Jews in northern Israel. *Leuk Lymphoma* 1992;**7**:251–5.

50. Ania BJ, Suman VJ, Sobell JL, *et al.* Trends in the incidence of polycythemia vera among Olmsted County, Minnesota residents, 1935–1989. *Am J Hematol* 1994;**47**:89–93.

51. Berglund S, Zettervall O. Incidence of polycythemia vera in a defined population. *Eur J Haematol* 1992;**48**:20–6.

52. Jensen MK, de Nully Brown P, Nielsen OJ, *et al.* Incidence, clinical features and outcome of essential thrombocythaemia in a well defined geographical area. *Eur J Haematol* 2000;**65**:132–9.

53. Ridell B, Carneskog J, Wedel H, *et al.* Incidence of chronic myeloproliferative disorders in the city of Goteborg, Sweden 1983–1992. *Eur J Haematol* 2000;**65**:267–71.

54. McNally RJ, Rowland D, Roman E, *et al.* Age and sex distributions of hematological malignancies in the U.K. *Hematol Oncol* 1997;**15**:173–89.

55. Heudes D, Carli PM, Bailly F, *et al.* Myeloproliferative disorders in the department of Cote d'Or between 1980 and 1986. *Nouv Rev Fr Hematol* 1989;**31**:375–8.

56. Mesa RA, Silverstein MN, Jacobsen SJ, *et al.* Population-based incidence and

survival figures in essential thrombocythemia and agnogenic myeloid metaplasia: an Olmsted County study, 1976–1995. *Am J Hematol* 1999;**61**:10–15.

57. Johansson P, Kutti J, Andreasson B, *et al.* Trends in the incidence of chronic Philadelphia chromosome negative (Ph-) myeloproliferative disorders in the city of Goteborg, Sweden, during 1983–99. *J Intern Med* 2004;**256**:161–5.

58. Woodliff HJ, Dougan L. Myelofibrosis in Western Australia: an epidemiological study of 29 cases. *Med J Aust* 1976;**1**:523–5.

59. Anonymous. Polycythemia vera: the natural history of 1213 patients followed for 20 years. Gruppo Italiano Studio Policitemia. *Ann Intern Med* 1995;**123**:656–64.

60. Diehn F, Tefferi A. Pruritus in polycythaemia vera: prevalence, laboratory correlates and management. *Br J Haematol* 2001;**115**:619–21.

61. Tefferi A, Elliott M. Thrombosis in myeloproliferative disorders: prevalence, prognostic factors, and the role of leukocytes and JAK2V617F. *Semin Thromb Hemost* 2007;**33**:313–20.

62. Patel RK, Lea NC, Heneghan MA, *et al.* Prevalence of the activating JAK2 tyrosine kinase mutation V617F in the Budd-Chiari syndrome. *Gastroenterology* 2006;**130**:2031–8.

63. Colaizzo D, Amitrano L, Tiscia GL, *et al.* The JAK2 V617F mutation frequently occurs in patients with portal and mesenteric venous thrombosis. *J Thromb Haemost* 2007;**5**:55–61.

64. Boissinot M, Lippert E, Girodon F, *et al.* Latent myeloproliferative disorder revealed by the JAK2-V617F mutation and endogenous megakaryocytic colonies in patients with splanchnic vein thrombosis. *Blood* 2006;**108**:3223–4.

65. Wright CA, Tefferi A. A single institutional experience with 43 pregnancies in essential thrombocythemia. *Eur J Haematol* 2001;**66**:152–9.

66. Budde U, Schaefer G, Mueller N, *et al.* Acquired von Willebrand's disease in the myeloproliferative syndrome. *Blood* 1984;**64**:981–5.

67. Wolanskyj AP, Schwager SM, McClure RF, *et al.* Essential thrombocythemia beyond the first decade: life expectancy, long-term complication rates, and prognostic factors. *Mayo Clin Proc* 2006;**81**:159–66.

68. Passamonti F, Rumi E, Pungolino E, *et al.* Life expectancy and prognostic factors for survival in patients with polycythemia vera and essential thrombocythemia. *Am J Med* 2004;**117**:755–61.

69. Gangat N, Wolanskyj AP, McClure RF, *et al.* Risk stratification for survival and leukemic transformation in essential thrombocythemia: a single institutional study of 605 patients. *Leukemia* 2007;**21**:270–6.

70. Gangat N, Strand J, Li CY, *et al.* Leucocytosis in polycythaemia vera predicts both inferior survival and leukaemic transformation. *Br J Haematol* 2007;**138**:354–8.

71. Berk PD, Wasserman LR, Fruchtman SM, *et al.* Treatment of polycythemia vera: a summary of clinical trials conducted by the polycythemia vera study group. In: Wasserman LR, Berk PD, Berlin NI, eds. *Polycythemia Vera and the Myeloproliferative Disorders.* Philadelphia, W.B. Saunders. 1995; 166–94.

72. Tefferi A. Polycythemia vera: a comprehensive review and clinical recommendations. *Mayo Clin Proc* 2003;**78**:174–94.

73. Cortelazzo S, Viero P, Finazzi G, *et al.* Incidence and risk factors for thrombotic complications in a historical cohort of 100 patients with essential thrombocythemia. *J Clin Oncol* 1990;**8**:556–62.

74. Carobbio A, Finazzi G, Guerini V, *et al.* Leukocytosis is a risk factor for thrombosis in essential thrombocythemia: interaction with treatment, standard risk factors, and Jak2 mutation status. *Blood* 2007;**109**:2310–13.

75. Barbui T, Barosi G, Grossi A, *et al.* Practice guidelines for the therapy of essential thrombocythemia. A statement from the Italian Society of Hematology, the Italian Society of Experimental Hematology and the Italian Group for Bone Marrow Transplantation. *Haematologica* 2004;**89**:215–32.

76. Elliott MA, Tefferi A. Thrombosis and haemorrhage in polycythaemia vera and essential thrombocythaemia. *Br J Haematol* 2005;**128**:275–90.

77. Di Nisio M, Barbui T, Di Gennaro L, *et al.* The haematocrit and platelet target in polycythemia vera. *Br J Haematol* 2007;**136**:249–59.

78. Gangat N, Wolanskyj A, Schwager S, *et al.* Leukocytosis at diagnosis and the risk of subsequent thrombosis in low-risk essential thrombocythemia and polycythemia vera. *ASH Annual Meeting Abstracts* 2008;**112**:1751.

79. Fabris F, Casonato A, Grazia del Ben M, *et al.* Abnormalities of von Willebrand factor in myeloproliferative disease: a relationship with bleeding diathesis. *Br J Haematol* 1986;**63**:75–83.

80. Cervantes F, Dupriez B, Pereira A, *et al.* New prognostic scoring system for primary myelofibrosis based on a study of the International Working Group for Myelofibrosis Research and Treatment. *Blood* 2009;**113**:2895–901.

81. Tefferi A, Mesa RA, Pardanani A, *et al.* Red blood cell transfusion need at diagnosis adversely affects survival in primary myelofibrosis-increased serum ferritin or transfusion load does not. *Am J Hematol* 2009;**84**:265–7.

82. Campbell PJ, Scott LM, Buck G, *et al.* Definition of subtypes of essential thrombocythaemia and relation to polycythaemia vera based on JAK2 V617F mutation status: a prospective study. *Lancet* 2005;**366**:1945–53.

83. Vannucchi AM, Antonioli E, Guglielmelli P, *et al.* Clinical profile of homozygous JAK2 617V>F mutation in patients with polycythemia vera or essential thrombocythemia. *Blood* 2007;**110**:840–6.

84. Tefferi A, Lasho TL, Schwager SM, *et al.* The clinical phenotype of wild-type, heterozygous, and homozygous JAK2V617F in polycythemia vera. *Cancer* 2006;**106**:631–5.

85. Vannucchi AM, Antonioli E, Guglielmelli P, *et al.* Prospective identification of high-risk polycythemia vera patients based on JAK2(V617F) allele burden. *Leukemia* 2007;**21**: 1952–9.

86. Tefferi A, Strand JJ, Lasho TL, *et al.* Bone marrow JAK2V617F allele burden and clinical correlates in polycythemia vera. *Leukemia* 2007;**21**:2074–5.

87. Tefferi A, Lasho TL, Schwager SM, *et al.* The JAK2 tyrosine kinase mutation in myelofibrosis with myeloid metaplasia: lineage specificity and clinical correlates. *Br J Haematol* 2005;**131**:320–8.

88. Barosi G, Bergamaschi G, Marchetti M, *et al.* JAK2 V617F mutational status predicts progression to large splenomegaly and leukemic transformation in primary myelofibrosis. *Blood* 2007;**110**:4030–6.

89. Tefferi A, Lasho TL, Huang J, *et al.* Low JAK2V617F allele burden in primary myelofibrosis, compared to either a higher allele burden or unmutated status, is associated with inferior overall and leukemia-free survival. *Leukemia* 2008;**22**:756–61.

90. Landolfi R, Marchioli R, Kutti J, *et al.* Efficacy and safety of low-dose aspirin in polycythemia vera. *N Engl J Med* 2004;**350**:114–24.

91. Cortelazzo S, Finazzi G, Ruggeri M, *et al.* Hydroxyurea for patients with essential thrombocythemia and a high risk of thrombosis. *N Engl J Med* 1995;**332**:1132–6.

92. Najean Y, Rain JD. Treatment of polycythemia vera – the use of hydroxyurea and pipobroman in 292 patients under the age of 65 years. *Blood* 1997;**90**:3370–7.

93. Anonymous. Treatment of polycythaemia vera by radiophosphorus or busulphan: a randomized trial. "Leukemia and Hematosarcoma" Cooperative Group, European Organization for Research on Treatment of Cancer (E.O.R.T.C.). *Br J Cancer* 1981;**44**:75–80.

94. Harrison CN, Campbell PJ, Buck G, *et al.* Hydroxyurea compared with anagrelide in high-risk essential thrombocythemia. *N Engl J Med* 2005;**353**:33–45.

95. Chievitz E, Thiede T. Complications and causes of death in polycythemia vera. *Acta Med Scand* 1962;**172**:513–23.

96. Berk PD, Goldberg JD, Donovan PB, *et al.* Therapeutic recommendations in polycythemia vera based on Polycythemia Vera Study Group protocols. *Semin Hematol* 1986;**23**:132–43.

97. Silver RT. Interferon alfa: effects of long-term treatment for polycythemia vera. *Semin Hematol* 1997;**34**:40–50.

98. Elliott MA, Tefferi A. Interferon-alpha therapy in polycythemia vera and essential thrombocythemia. *Semin Thromb Hemost* 1997;**23**:463–72.

99. Silver RT. Long-term effects of the treatment of polycythemia vera with recombinant interferon-alpha. *Cancer* 2006;**107**:451–8.

100. Samuelsson J, Hasselbalch H, Bruserud O, *et al.* A phase II trial of pegylated interferon alpha-2b therapy for polycythemia vera and essential thrombocythemia: feasibility, clinical and biologic effects, and impact on quality of life. *Cancer* 2006;**106**:2397–405.

101. Kiladjian JJ, Cassinat B, Turlure P, *et al.* High molecular response rate of polycythemia vera patients treated with pegylated interferon alpha-2a. *Blood* 2006;**108**:2037–40.

102. Jones AV, Silver RT, Waghorn K, *et al.* Minimal molecular response in polycythemia vera patients treated with imatinib or interferon alpha. *Blood* 2006;**107**:3339–41.

103. Passamonti F, Malabarba L, Orlandi E, *et al.* Pipobroman is safe and effective treatment for patients with essential thrombocythaemia at high risk of thrombosis. *Br J Haematol* 2002;**116**:855–61.

104. De Sanctis V, Mazzucconi MG, Spadea A, *et al.* Long-term evaluation of 164 patients with essential thrombocythaemia treated with pipobroman: occurrence of leukaemic evolution. *Br J Haematol* 2003;**123**:517–21.

105. Passamonti F, Brusamolino E, Lazzarino M, *et al.* Efficacy of pipobroman in the treatment of polycythemia vera: long-term results in 163 patients. *Haematologica* 2000;**85**:1011–18.

106. Tefferi A, Fonseca R. Selective serotonin reuptake inhibitors are effective in the treatment of polycythemia vera-associated pruritus. *Blood* 2002;**99**:2627.

107. Finazzi G, Barbui T. How I treat patients with polycythemia vera. *Blood* 2007;**109**:5104–111.

108. Barbui T, Finazzi G. When and how to treat essential thrombocythemia. *N Engl J Med* 2005;**353**:85–6.

109. van Genderen PJ, Mulder PG, Waleboer M, *et al.* Prevention and treatment of thrombotic complications in essential thrombocythaemia: efficacy and safety of aspirin. *Br J Haematol* 1997;**97**:179–84.

110. Finazzi G, Ruggeri M, Rodeghiero F, *et al.* Second malignancies in patients with essential thrombocythaemia treated with busulphan and hydroxyurea: long-term follow-up of a randomized clinical trial. *Br J Haematol* 2000;**110**:577–83.

111. Finazzi G, Ruggeri M, Rodeghiero F, *et al.* Efficacy and safety of long-term use of hydroxyurea in young patients with essential thrombocythemia and a high risk of thrombosis. *Blood* 2003;**101**:3749.

112. Finazzi G, Caruso V, Marchioli R, *et al.* Acute leukemia in polycythemia vera. An analysis of 1,638 patients enrolled in a prospective observational study. *Blood* 2005;**105**:2664–70.

113. Kerbauy DM, Gooley TA, Sale GE, *et al.* Hematopoietic cell transplantation as curative therapy for idiopathic myelofibrosis, advanced polycythemia vera, and essential thrombocythemia. *Biol Blood Marrow Transplant* 2007;**13**:355–65.

114. Siragusa S, Passamonti F, Cervantes F, *et al.* Survival in young patients with intermediate-/high-risk myelofibrosis: estimates derived from databases for non transplant patients. *Am J Hematol* 2009;**84**:140–3.

115. Bacigalupo A, Soraru M, Dominietto A, *et al.* Allogenic hematopoietic stem-cell transplant for patients with primary myelofibrosis: a predictive transplant score based on transfusion requirement, spleen size and donor type. *Bone Marrow Transplant* 2010;**45**:419–21.

116. Kroger N, Badbaran A, Holler E, *et al.* Monitoring of the JAK2-V617F mutation by highly sensitive quantitative real-time PCR after allogeneic stem cell transplantation in patients with myelofibrosis. *Blood* 2007;**109**:1316–21.

117. Hussein K, Van Dyke DL, Tefferi A. Conventional cytogenetics in myelofibrosis: literature review and discussion. *Eur J Haematol* 2009;**82**:329–38.

118. Silverstein MN. *Agnogenic Myeloid Metaplasia.* Acton Mass, Publishing Science Group. 1975; 126.

119. Rodriguez JN, Martino ML, Dieguez JC, *et al.* rHuEpo for the treatment of anemia in myelofibrosis with myeloid metaplasia. Experience in 6 patients and meta-analytical approach. *Haematologica* 1998;**83**:616–21.

120. Cervantes F, Alvarez-Larran A, Hernandez-Boluda JC, *et al.* Darbepoetin-alpha for the anaemia of myelofibrosis with myeloid metaplasia. *Br J Haematol* 2006;**134**:184–6.

121. Cervantes F, Alvarez-Larran A, Hernandez-Boluda JC, *et al.*

Erythropoietin treatment of the anaemia of myelofibrosis with myeloid metaplasia: results in 20 patients and review of the literature. *Br J Haematol* 2004;**127**:399–403.

122. Cervantes F, Hernandez-Boluda JC, Alvarez A, *et al.* Danazol treatment of idiopathic myelofibrosis with severe anemia. *Haematologica* 2000;**85**:595–9.

123. Cervantes F, Alvarez-Larran A, Domingo A, *et al.* Efficacy and tolerability of danazol as a treatment for the anaemia of myelofibrosis with myeloid metaplasia: long-term results in 30 patients. *Br J Haematol* 2005;**129**:771–5.

124. Tefferi A, Elliot MA. Serious myeloproliferative reactions associated with the use of thalidomide in myelofibrosis with myeloid metaplasia. *Blood* 2000;**96**:4007.

125. Elliott MA, Mesa RA, Li CY, *et al.* Thalidomide treatment in myelofibrosis with myeloid metaplasia. *Br J Haematol* 2002;**117**:288–96.

126. Marchetti M, Barosi G, Balestri F, *et al.* Low-dose thalidomide ameliorates cytopenias and splenomegaly in myelofibrosis with myeloid metaplasia: a phase II trial. *J Clin Oncol* 2004;**22**:424–31.

127. Mesa RA, Elliott MA, Schroeder G, *et al.* Durable responses to thalidomide-based drug therapy for myelofibrosis with myeloid metaplasia. *Mayo Clin Proc* 2004;**79**:883–9.

128. Mesa RA, Steensma DP, Pardanani A, *et al.* A phase 2 trial of combination low-dose thalidomide and prednisone for the treatment of myelofibrosis with myeloid metaplasia. *Blood* 2003;**101**:2534–41.

129. Tefferi A, Cortes J, Verstovsek S, *et al.* Lenalidomide therapy in myelofibrosis with myeloid metaplasia. *Blood* 2006;**108**:1158–64.

130. Tefferi A, Lasho TL, Mesa RA, *et al.* Lenalidomide therapy in del(5)(q31)-associated myelofibrosis: cytogenetic and JAK2V617F molecular remissions. *Leukemia* 2007;**21**:1827–8.

131. Tefferi A, Verstovsek S, Barosi G, *et al.* Pomalidomide therapy in anemic patients with myelofibrosis: results from a phase-2 randomized multicenter study. *ASH Annual Meeting Abstracts* 2008;**112**:663.

132. Lofvenberg E, Wahlin A. Management of polycythaemia vera, essential thrombocythaemia and myelofibrosis with hydroxyurea. *Eur J Haematol* 1988;**41**:375–81.

133. Naqvi T, Baumann MA. Myelofibrosis: response to busulfan after hydroxyurea failure. *Int J Clin Pract* 2002;**56**:312–13.

134. Petti MC, Latagliata R, Spadea T, *et al.* Melphalan treatment in patients with myelofibrosis with myeloid metaplasia. *Br J Haematol* 2002;**116**:576–81.

135. Tefferi A, Silverstein MN, Li CY. 2-Chlorodeoxyadenosine treatment after splenectomy in patients who have myelofibrosis with myeloid metaplasia. *Br J Haematol* 1997;**99**:352–7.

136. Tefferi A, Elliot MA, Yoon SY, *et al.* Clinical and bone marrow effects of interferon alfa therapy in myelofibrosis with myeloid metaplasia. *Blood* 2001;**97**:1896.

137. Tefferi A, Mesa RA, Nagorney DM, *et al.* Splenectomy in myelofibrosis with myeloid metaplasia: a single-institution experience with 223 patients. *Blood* 2000;**95**:2226–33.

138. Koch CA, Li CY, Mesa RA, *et al.* Nonhepatosplenic extramedullary hematopoiesis: associated diseases, pathology, clinical course, and treatment. *Mayo Clin Proc* 2003;**78**:1223–33.

139. Elliott MA, Chen MG, Silverstein MN, *et al.* Splenic irradiation for symptomatic splenomegaly associated with myelofibrosis with myeloid metaplasia. *Br J Haematol* 1998;**103**:505–11.

140. Passamonti F, Randi ML, Rumi E, *et al.* Increased risk of pregnancy complications in patients with essential thrombocythemia carrying the JAK2 (617V>F) mutation. *Blood* 2007;**110**:485–9.

141. Griesshammer M, Struve S, Harrison CM. Essential thrombocythemia/polycythemia vera and pregnancy: the need for an observational study in Europe. *Semin Thromb Hemost* 2006;**32**:422–9.

142. Elliott MA, Tefferi A. Thrombocythaemia and pregnancy. *Best Pract Res Clin Haematol* 2003;**16**:227–42.

143. Gangat N, Wolanskyj AP, Schwager S, *et al.* Predictors of pregnancy outcome in essential thrombocythemia: a single institution study of 63 pregnancies. *Eur J Haematol* 2009;**82**:350–3.

144. James C, Ugo V, Le Couedic JP, *et al.* A unique clonal JAK2 mutation leading to constitutive signalling causes polycythaemia vera. *Nature* 2005;**434**:1144–8.

145. Pikman Y, Lee BH, Mercher T, *et al.* MPLW515L is a novel somatic activating mutation in myelofibrosis with myeloid metaplasia. *PLoS Med* 2006;**3**:e270.

146. Lasho TL, Tefferi A, Hood JD, *et al.* TG101348, a JAK2-selective antagonist, inhibits primary hematopoietic cells derived from myeloproliferative disorder patients with JAK2V617F, MPLW515K or JAK2 exon 12 mutations as well as mutation negative patients. *Leukemia* 2008;**22**:1790–2.

147. Wernig G, Kharas MG, Okabe R, *et al.* Efficacy of TG101348, a selective JAK2 inhibitor, in treatment of a murine model of JAK2V617F-induced polycythemia vera. *Cancer Cell* 2008;**13**:311–20.

148. Pardanani AD, Gotlib J, Jamieson C, *et al.* A phase I study of TG101348, an orally bioavailable JAK2-selective inhibitor, in patients with myelofibrosis. *ASH Annual Meeting Abstracts* 2008;**112**:97.

149. Verstovsek S, Kantarjian HM, Pardanani AD, *et al.* The JAK inhibitor, INCB018424, demonstrates durable and marked clinical responses in primary myelofibrosis (PMF) and post-polycythemia/essential thrombocythemia myelofibrosis (post PV/ETMF). *ASH Annual Meeting Abstracts* 2008;**112**:1762.

150. Pardanani A, Lasho T, Smith G, *et al.* CYT387, a selective JAK1/JAK2 inhibitor: in vitro assessment of kinase selectivity and preclinical studies using cell lines and primary cells from polycythemia vera patients. *Leukemia* 2009;**23**:1441–5.

151. Tefferi A, Huang J, Schwager S, *et al.* Validation and comparison of contemporary prognostic models in primary myelofibrosis: analysis based on 334 patients from a single institution. *Cancer* 2007;**109**:2083–8.

Chapter

10 Monoclonal gammopathy of undetermined significance, smoldering multiple myeloma, and multiple myeloma

S. Vincent Rajkumar and Suzanne R. Hayman

Introduction

The plasma cell dyscrasias are a diverse group of disorders characterized by the presence of a monoclonal plasma cell population in the bone marrow. The most common plasma cell disorders include monoclonal gammopathy of undetermined significance (MGUS), solitary plasmacytoma, smoldering myeloma (SMM), multiple myeloma (MM), primary (AL or immunoglobulin light chain) amyloidosis, and Waldenström's macroglobulinemia (WM) (Table 10.1). This chapter is focused on the pathogenesis, clinical features, diagnosis, and management of MGUS, SMM, and MM.

Laboratory testing for monoclonal proteins

Monoclonal immunoglobulins are commonly referred to as monoclonal proteins, M proteins, or paraproteins. The presence of an M protein is indicative of an underlying clonal plasma cell proliferative disorder, although further testing is required to distinguish among the various plasma cell disorders.

Serum protein electrophoresis and immunofixation

Agarose gel serum protein electrophoresis (SPEP) and serum immunofixation (IF) are the main methods of detection of serum M proteins (Figure 10.1a and b). M proteins appear as localized bands on SPEP.[1] Although presence of a localized band on SPEP is suggestive of M protein, IF is necessary for confirmation as well as to determine the heavy- and light-chain classes of the M protein. In addition, serum IF is more sensitive than SPEP and can detect smaller amounts of M protein, and should therefore be performed whenever MM or a related disorder is suspected. The size of the M protein is measured using the SPEP; small M proteins < 1 g/dL on SPEP and M proteins that are apparent only on serum IF are considered "unmeasurable."

Quantitative immunoglobulin studies

Quantitation of serum immunoglobulins is performed with a rate nephelometer in patients in whom M proteins are detected. It is an added parameter that can be followed, particularly in patients with MM and WM where, at times, the M protein size estimated on SPEP may be unreliable (e.g., small beta migrating proteins, and IgA/IgM proteins that tend to polymerize).

Urine protein electrophoresis and immunofixation

Typically, screening for suspected monoclonal gammopathies should include urine protein electrophoresis (UPEP) and urine IF in addition to the serum studies discussed earlier. Urine studies are important because approximately 15–20% of patients with plasma cell disorders secrete free monoclonal light chain M protein (Bence-Jones protein) that is excreted freely by the kidney. These proteins are usually not present in sufficient quantities in the serum to be detected by either SPEP or serum IF. In such patients, the diagnosis of a plasma cell dyscrasia would be missed if urine studies were not performed. A 24-hour urine specimen is therefore required for UPEP and urine IF. Urine M protein levels measured on UPEP are used in monitoring disease progression and response to therapy in the same manner as serum M protein levels. Urine M protein levels > 200 mg/day are considered measurable. If patients have measurable disease in the serum and urine, it is important to follow both the serum and urine M protein levels to monitor disease status.

Serum free light chain assay

Measurement of serum free light chains by the free light chain (FLC) assay (Freelite™, The Binding Site Limited, Birmingham, UK) may obviate the need for UPEP and urine IF in some circumstances. It provides a more convenient method of measuring serum light chains.[2] The FLC test is an automated nephelometric assay that quantitates free kappa (κ) and

Management of Hematologic Malignancies, ed. Susan M. O'Brien, Julie M. Vose, and Hagop M. Kantarjian. Published by Cambridge University Press.

Table 10.1. Diagnostic criteria for plasma cell disorders

Disorder	Disease definition	References
Monoclonal gammopathy of undetermined significance (MGUS)	All 3 criteria must be met: 1. Serum monoclonal protein < 3 g/dL 2. Clonal bone marrow plasma cells < 10%, and 3. Absence of end-organ damage such as hypercalcemia, *r*enal insufficiency, *a*nemia, and *b*one lesions (CRAB) that can be attributed to the plasma cell proliferative disorder	47
Smoldering multiple myeloma (also referred to as asymptomatic multiple myeloma)	Both criteria must be met: 1. Serum monoclonal protein (IgG or IgA) ≥ 3 g/dL and/or clonal bone marrow plasma cells ≥ 10%, and 2. Absence of end-organ damage such as lytic bone lesions, anemia, hypercalcemia, or renal failure that can be attributed to a plasma cell proliferative disorder	47
Multiple myeloma	All 3 criteria must be met except as noted: 1. Clonal bone marrow plasma cells ≥ 10% 2. Presence of serum and/or urinary monoclonal protein (except in patients with true non-secretory multiple myeloma), and 3. Evidence of end-organ damage that can be attributed to the underlying plasma cell proliferative disorder, specifically o Hypercalcemia: serum calcium ≥ 11.5 mg/dL o Renal insufficiency: serum creatinine > 1.73 mmol/L o Anemia: normochromic, normocytic with a hemoglobin value of > 2 g/dL below the lower limit of normal, or a hemoglobin value < 10 g/dL o Bone lesions: lytic lesions, severe osteopenia or pathologic fractures	47,228
Waldenstrom's macroglobulinemia	Both criteria must be met: 1. IgM monoclonal gammopathy (regardless of the size of the M protein), and 2. > 10% bone marrow lymphoplasmacytic infiltration (usually intertrabecular) by small lymphocytes that exhibit plasmacytoid or plasma cell differentiation and a typical immunophenotype (e.g., surface IgM+, CD5+/−, CD10−, CD19+, CD20+, CD23−) that satisfactorily excludes other lymphoproliferative disorders including chronic lymphocytic leukemia and mantle cell lymphoma **Note:** IgM MGUS is defined as • Serum IgM monoclonal protein < 3 g/dL, and bone marrow lymphoplasmacytic infiltration < 10%, and • No evidence of anemia, constitutional symptoms, hyperviscosity, lymphadenopathy, or hepatosplenomegaly Smoldering Waldenstrom's macroglobulinemia (also referred to as indolent or asymptomatic Waldenstrom's macroglobulinemia) is defined as	229–233

Table 10.1. *(cont.)*

Disorder	Disease definition	References
	• Serum IgM monoclonal protein ≥ 3 g/dL and/or bone marrow lymphoplasmacytic infiltration ≥ 10%, and • No evidence of end-organ damage such as anemia, constitutional symptoms, hyperviscosity, lymphadenopathy, or hepatosplenomegaly that can be attributed to a lympho-plasma cell proliferative disorder	
Solitary plasmacytoma	All 4 criteria must be met: 1. Biopsy proven solitary lesion of bone or soft tissue with evidence of clonal plasma cells 2. Normal bone marrow with no evidence of clonal plasma cells 3. Normal skeletal survey and MRI of spine and pelvis (except for the primary solitary lesion) 4. Absence of end-organ damage such as hyper*c*alcemia, *r*enal insufficiency, *a*nemia, or *b*one lesions (CRAB) that can be attributed to a lympho-plasma cell proliferative disorder	49,234
Systemic AL amyloidosis	All 4 criteria must be met: 1. Presence of an amyloid-related systemic syndrome (such as renal, liver, heart, gastrointestinal tract, or peripheral nerve involvement) 2. Positive amyloid staining by Congo red in any tissue (e.g., fat aspirate, bone marrow, or organ biopsy) 3. Evidence that amyloid is light-chain related established by direct examination of the amyloid (immunohistochemical staining, direct sequencing, etc.), and 4. Evidence of a monoclonal plasma cell proliferative disorder (serum or urine M protein, abnormal free light chain ratio, or clonal plasma cells in the bone marrow) **Note:** Approximately 2–3 percent of patients with AL amyloidosis will not meet the requirement for evidence of a monoclonal plasma cell disorder listed above; the diagnosis of AL amyloidosis must be made with caution in these patients	235
POEMS syndrome	All 3 criteria must be met: 1. Presence of a monoclonal plasma cell disorder 2. Peripheral neuropathy, and 3. At least one of the following seven features: osteosclerotic bone lesions, Castleman's disease, organomegaly, endocrinopathy (excluding diabetes mellitus or hypothyroidism), edema, typical skin changes, and papilledema **Note:** Not every patient meeting the above criteria will have POEMS syndrome; the features should have a temporal relationship to each other and no other attributable cause. The absence of osteosclerotic lesions should make the diagnosis suspect. Elevations in plasma or serum levels of vascular endothelial growth factor and thrombocytosis are common features of the syndrome and are helpful when the diagnosis is difficult	236

Source: Modified, reproduced with permission from Rajkumar SV, Dispenzieri A, Kyle RA. *Mayo Clinic Proc* 2006;**81**:693–703. © Mayo Clinic Proceedings.[235]

lambda (λ) chains (i.e., light chains that are not bound to intact immunoglobulin) secreted by plasma cells. An abnormal κ:λ FLC ratio is indicative of an excess of one light chain type versus the other, and is interpreted as a surrogate for clonal expansion. The assay is performed on automated chemistry analyzers, is widely available, and is commonly used to monitor patients with oligo-secretory MM and AL, as well as patients with the light chain-only form of MM.[3–5]

The normal serum free κ level is 3.3–19.4 mg/L and the normal free λ level is 5.7–26.3 mg/L.[6] The normal ratio for FLC κ:λ is 0.26–1.65. The normal reference range in the FLC assay reflects a higher serum level of free λ light chains than would be expected given the usual κ:λ ratio of 2 for intact immunoglobulins. This occurs because the renal excretion of free κ (usually existing in a monomeric state) is much faster than for free λ (which is usually in a dimeric state).[2,3] Patients with a κ:λ FLC ratio < 0.26 are typically defined as having monoclonal λ FLC and those with ratios > 1.65 are defined as having a monoclonal κ FLC.

Monoclonal gammopathy of undetermined significance (MGUS)

MGUS is a premalignant clonal plasma cell proliferative disorder defined as the presence of a serum M protein < 3 g/dL, bone marrow monoclonal plasma cells $< 10\%$, plus absence of anemia, hypercalcemia, lytic bone lesions, or renal failure that can be attributed to the plasma cell proliferative disorder.[7,8] It is the most common plasma cell dyscrasia, prevalent in approximately 3% of the general population ≥ 50 years of age.[9] The prevalence increases with age; 1.7% in those 50–59 years of age, and over 5% in those $>$ age 70. The age-specific incidence is higher in males than in females. MGUS is also twice as common in African-Americans compared to whites.[10]

MGUS is associated with a life-long risk of progression to MM or a related disorder. The overall rate of progression of MGUS is 1% per year[11,12] and the risk of progression does not diminish over time.[11,13] However, the true lifetime probability of progression is significantly lower when competing causes of death are taken into account, approximately 11% at 25 years.[14]

Pathogenesis

Pathogenesis of MGUS

Antigenic stimulation and immunosuppression

MGUS is the precursor lesion from which almost all cases of MM and related disorders are felt to evolve. It is characterized by evidence for genomic instability on molecular genetic testing. What initiates this instability is not well understood, but antigenic stimulation may be a key factor (Figure 10.2). Aberrant response to antigenic stimulation may be mediated by Toll-like receptors (TLRs) which normally aid in recognition of infectious agents and pathogen-associated molecular patterns (PAMP) and initiate the host-defense response.[15–17] Human MM cell lines and primary MM cells express a broad range of TLRs, unlike normal plasma cells. Another possible factor is enhanced activation of the interleukin (IL)-6 pathway in plasma cells. IL-6 is a major plasma cell growth factor[18] and there is overexpression of CD126 (IL-6 receptor alpha-chain) in MGUS compared to normal plasma cells.[19,20] During aberrant response to antigenic stimulation, plasma cells may acquire one of the various cytogenetic alterations that result in the limited clonal plasma cell proliferative process of MGUS (Figure 10.2).

Another factor that may increase the risk of MGUS is immunosuppression. Monoclonal proteins have been reported in the context of immunosuppressive states such as human immunodeficiency virus (HIV) and bone marrow/stem cell and organ transplantation.[21–24] Patients undergoing renal transplantation can develop monoclonal proteins dependent on their levels of immunosuppression.[24]

Cytogenetic changes

Over 90% of MGUS is associated with cytogenetic changes, likely during IGH switch recombination or somatic hypermutation.[25] We classify MGUS into two types: IGH translocated and IGH non-translocated. Approximately 50% of all patients with MGUS have IGH translocated MGUS with primary translocations in the clonal plasma cells involving the immunoglobulin heavy chain (IGH) locus on the long arm of chromosome 14 (q32) (Figure 10.2).[25,26] The most common partner chromosome loci and the genes dysregulated in these translocations are: 11q13 (*CCND1* [cyclin D1 gene]), 4p16.3 (*FGFR-3* and *MMSET*), 6p21 (*CCND3* [cyclin D3 gene]), 16q23 (c-*maf*), and 20q11 (*maf*-B).[27–29] It is likely that these translocations play an important pathogenetic role in the resulting limited clonal proliferation that manifests as MGUS.

Categories of MGUS which lack evidence of IGH translocations are referred to as IGH non-translocated MGUS. Most of these exhibit hyperdiploidy, usually of the odd-numbered chromosomes, with the exception of chromosome 13. A small proportion of MGUS does not have evidence of either IGH translocations or hyperdiploidy.[8,25,30–34] Deletion of chromosome 13, a major prognostic factor in MM, is seen in up to 50% of patients with MGUS by interphase fluorescent *in situ* hybridization (FISH); thus the presence of this abnormality cannot be used to differentiate MGUS from MM.[29]

Pathogenesis of myeloma

The progression of MGUS to MM or a related disease occurs at a rate of approximately 1% per year, and the fixed rate of progression is strongly suggestive of a simple, random, two-hit genetic model of malignancy.[11] In other words, the risk of progression is similar, regardless of the known duration of antecedent MGUS,

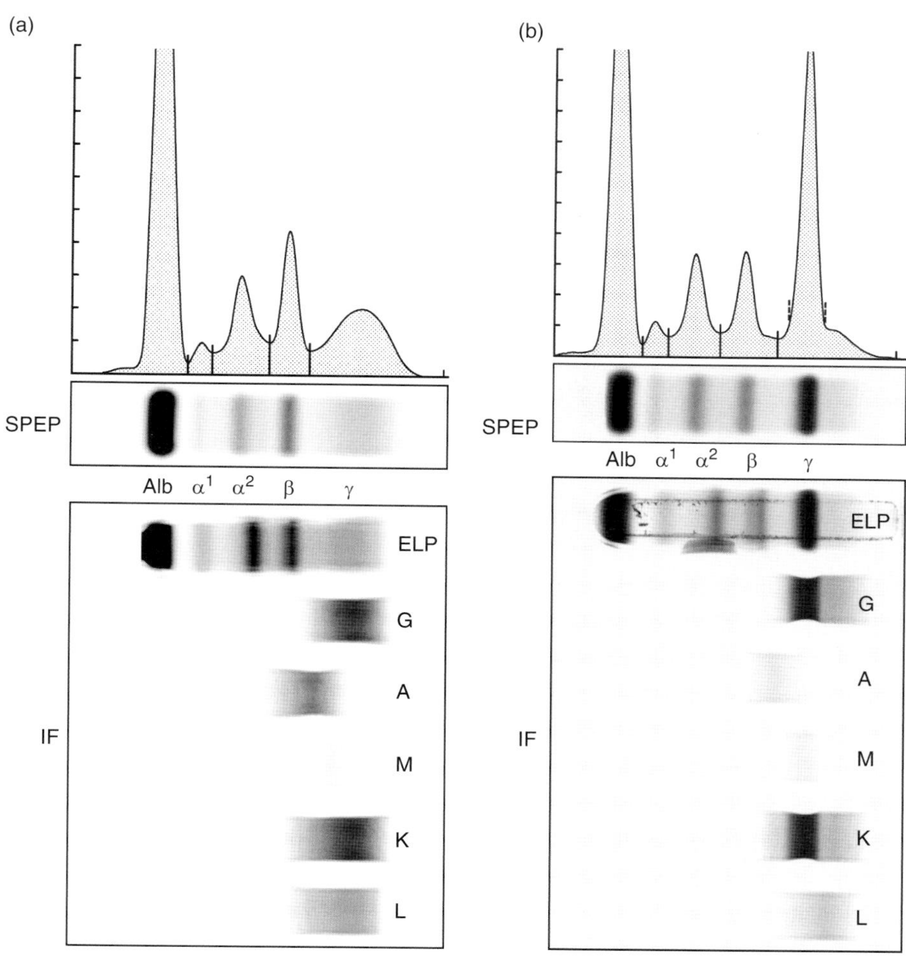

Figure 10.1 (a) Serum protein electrophoresis (SPEP) and immunofixation (IF) showing a normal pattern with no evidence of monoclonal protein. (b) Serum protein electrophoresis (SPEP) showing a monoclonal (M) protein in the gamma region, which is IgG lambda on immunofixation (IF).

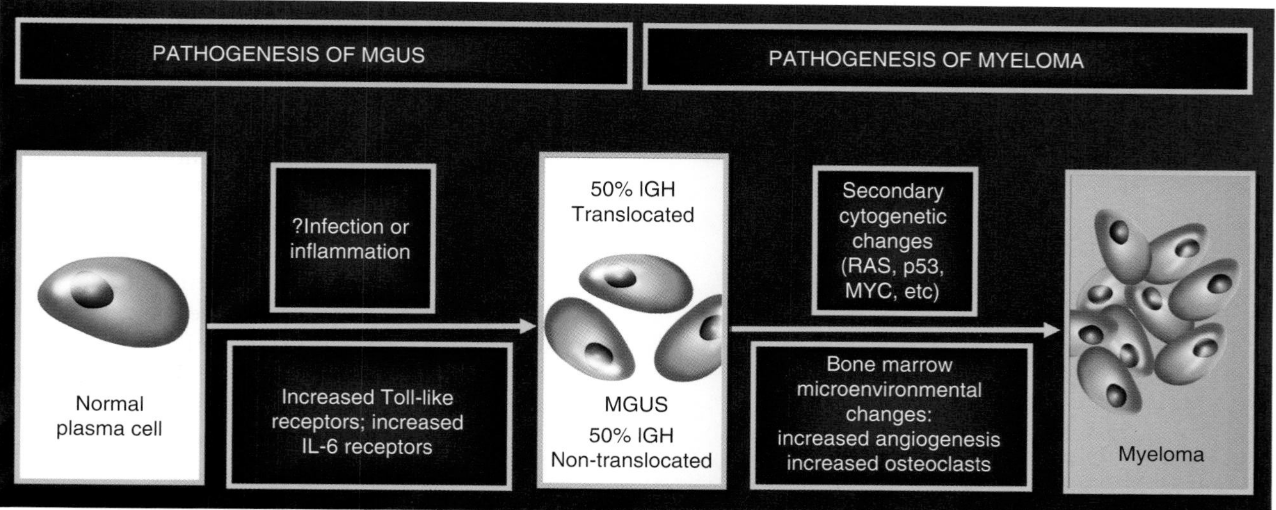

Figure 10.2 Pathogenesis of myeloma. MGUS: monoclonal gammopathy of undetermined significance; IL-6: interleukin 6.

suggesting that the second-hit responsible for progression is a random event, and not a consequence of cumulative damage.

The exact pathogenesis is unknown. Abnormalities in plasma cells and the microenvironment have been detected with progression, but little is known about the precise sequence of events (Figure 10.2). *RAS* mutations, p16 methylation, abnormalities involving the *c-MYC* family of oncogenes, secondary translocations, and p53 mutations have all been identified in clonal plasma cells in association with progression to a symptomatic stage.[27] It is possible that the second-hit responsible for disease progression may be different in IGH translocated versus non-translocated MGUS, and even within the various subtypes of IGH translocated MGUS, depending on the partner chromosome involved. For example, amplification of chromosome 1q21 has been found in $>40\%$ of patients with SMM and MM compared to 0% in MGUS,[35] suggesting that such amplification (e.g., by trisomy 1) may play a role in progression, perhaps in non-IGH translocated MGUS.

The bone marrow microenvironment undergoes marked changes with progression, including induction of angiogenesis,[36] suppression of cell-mediated immunity,[37] and paracrine loops involving cytokines such as IL-6 and vascular endothelial growth factor (VEGF).[38] As in solid tumors, the transition from MGUS to MM may involve an angiogenic switch. In a solitary plasmacytoma, which can be considered analogous to a localized stage I solid tumor, induction of angiogenesis at the time of diagnosis has been shown to be a predictor of progression to MM, suggesting a pathogenetic role.[39] There is also a gradual increase in degree of bone marrow angiogenesis along the disease spectrum of MGUS to SMM to symptomatic MM.[36] In one study, approximately 60% of MM bone marrow plasma samples stimulated angiogenesis in an in vitro angiogenesis assay, compared to 0% of SMM and 7% of MGUS, $P < 0.001$.[40]

The increased angiogenesis seen in MM may be related to the expressions of pro-angiogenic cytokines.[41] However, no significant differences are seen in the expressions of VEGF, basic fibroblast growth factor (b-FGF), or their receptors among MGUS, SMM, and MM. Loss of angiogenesis inhibitory activity has been noted with disease progression from MGUS to MM, which may, in part, account for the increase in angiogenesis that occurs in MM.[40,42]

New blood vessel formation may contribute to disease progression by ensuring an adequate tumor nutrient supply, as well as by paracrine stimulation of tumor growth. The role of angiogenesis in MM has triggered an interest in antiangiogenic therapy. Studies show that while increased microvessel density (MVD) in MM may not regress following conventional-dose or high-dose chemotherapy, regression has been noted in responders with thalidomide, a therapeutic agent with known antiangiogenic properties.[43] Clinical trials are ongoing to test the hypothesis that therapy with antiangiogenic agents may inhibit angiogenesis and delay progression in SMM.

Clinical features and differential diagnosis

MGUS usually is asymptomatic, although there is a group of MGUS-associated disorders (non-malignant and malignant) that can be symptomatic (see Chapter 11 on amyloidosis and other rare plasma cell dyscrasias). MGUS is differentiated from MM and related disorders based on the presence or absence of end-organ damage that can be attributed to the plasma cell disorder. The differentiation of MGUS from MM or the other plasma cell disorders can be difficult at the time of initial presentation because MGUS is relatively common in the general population in those over the age of 50 years, and some clinical and laboratory abnormalities may be coincidental. The typical laboratory studies necessary to differentiate MGUS from other plasma cell disorders are a complete blood count (CBC); serum electrolytes, including calcium, albumin, and creatinine; liver function tests; and a complete roentgenographic bone survey. If abnormalities are detected on the above tests, additional studies to determine the causes of these abnormalities are required; only patients in whom the abnormalities are felt to be related to the plasma cell proliferative disorder can be considered to have myeloma or a related process. A bone marrow aspirate and biopsy is indicated when the M protein is ≥ 1.5 g/dL, in a non-IgG MGUS, when the serum FLC ratio is abnormal (see below), and when abnormalities are noted on the CBC, serum creatinine, serum calcium, or radiographic bone survey. A bone marrow should also be considered in any patient with presumed MGUS in whom there is doubt about the diagnosis.

Prognosis

In a large population-based study of MGUS involving 1384 patients, only the size and type of M protein (IgM and IgA subtypes) were predictive of progression to MM or a related malignancy.[11] In another study, a bone marrow plasma cell percentage of 6–9% carried twice the risk of progression compared to having $\leq 5\%$ marrow involvement.[44] The presence of circulating peripheral blood plasma cells detected using a sensitive slide-based immunofluorescent assay is also a risk factor for progression.[45] This suggests that alterations in the expressions of adhesion molecules may be involved in the progression of MGUS to MM; alternatively, the presence of circulating plasma cells may be a marker of plasma cell proliferative rate. However, the clinical application of this test is limited by its lack of widespread availability in clinical practice.

An abnormal serum FLC ratio as determined by the serum FLC assay is an important risk factor for progression of MGUS. In a study of 1148 patients, the risk of progression with an abnormal FLC ratio at the time of diagnosis of MGUS was over three times higher compared to a normal ratio, and was independent of the size and type of the serum M protein.[14] The risk of progression to MM or related malignancy at 10 years was 17% with an abnormal ratio compared to 5% with a normal ratio. Based on three known risk factors (size of the serum M protein, the type of immunoglobulin, and the serum FLC ratio), a simple risk stratification system can be used to predict the risk of progression of MGUS (Table 10.2).[14] Patients with three adverse risk factors, namely an abnormal serum FLC ratio, non-IgG MGUS, and a high serum M protein level (≥ 15 g/L), have a 58% risk of progression at 20 years (high-risk MGUS), compared to 37% with any two risk factors present (high-intermediate-risk MGUS), 21% with one risk factor present (low-intermediate risk MGUS), and 5% when none of the risk factors are present (low-risk MGUS). The low-risk MGUS subset (constituting almost 40% of the cohort) has a life time risk of only 2% when competing causes of death are taken into account.

Management

The current standard of care for MGUS without an associated disorder is observation alone, without therapy.[26,46] Patients with MGUS may benefit from risk stratification as discussed above to guide follow-up. Patients with low-risk MGUS can be rechecked in 6 months, and then once every 2 years, or only at the time of symptoms for evidence of progression.[14] All other subsets of patients need to be rechecked in 6 months, and then yearly thereafter.

Smoldering multiple myeloma (SMM)

Introduction

SMM is defined by the presence of a serum IgG or IgA M protein ≥ 3 g/dL and/or bone marrow plasma cells $\geq 10\%$, plus absence of anemia, hypercalcemia, lytic bone lesions, or renal failure that can be attributed to the plasma cell proliferative disorder.[47,48] SMM accounts for approximately 15% of all cases of newly diagnosed MM.[7,49] SMM is a clinical entity separated from MGUS mainly to aid clinical management. There are no good data to suggest that SMM is a true, discrete, pathogenetic stage. The SMM phenotype likely comprises of patients with MGUS (i.e., no biologic malignant transformation has occurred) and early-stage MM (malignant transformation has occurred). As a result, the risk of progression of SMM is highest in the first 5 years when the subset of patients with preclinical early-stage myeloma develop overt disease, and decreases with time as the cohort becomes enriched with patients who have biologic MGUS. The risk of progression to MM or related malignancy is much higher in SMM compared to MGUS, 10–20% per year versus 1% per year, respectively. Therefore, patients with SMM and MGUS should be managed differently in terms of frequency of follow-up, development of chemopreventive strategies, and enrollment into clinical trials. Similar to MGUS and active MM, almost all patients with SMM appear to have evidence of genomic instability manifested as IGH translocations or aneuploidy on molecular genetic testing.[50]

Clinical features and differential diagnosis

By definition, SMM is asymptomatic. Testing to differentiate SMM from active MM is the same as described for MGUS. Most patients with SMM eventually develop symptomatic disease.[49] The time to progression (TTP) to symptomatic disease is approximately 3–4 years, but differs greatly depending on the definition used for SMM.[51] In the subset of SMM patients having bone marrow plasma cells $\geq 10\%$, the median TTP is approximately 2–3 years.[52]

The natural history of SMM was recently characterized by a large study from the Mayo Clinic.[53] During 2204 cumulative years of follow-up, the overall rate of progression at 10 years was 62%; median TTP was 5.5 years. Patients were categorized into three groups: Group 1, serum M protein ≥ 3 g/dL and bone marrow containing $\geq 10\%$ plasma cells ($n = 113$, 38%); Group 2, bone marrow plasma cells $\geq 10\%$, but serum M protein < 3 g/dL ($n = 158$, 52%); Group 3, serum M protein ≥ 3 g/dL, but bone marrow plasma cells $< 10\%$ ($n = 30$, 10%). The median TTP was 2.4, 9.2, and 19 years in groups 1, 2, and 3 respectively; correspondingly at 10 years, progression occurred in 76%, 59%, and 32%, respectively.

Prognosis

Similar to the results in MGUS, abnormal peripheral blood monoclonal plasma cell studies, defined as an increase in the number or proliferative rate of circulating plasma cells by slide-based immunofluorescent assays, have been shown to indicate a higher risk of progression in SMM.[52] However, this test is not widely available in clinical practice.

The presence of occult bone lesions on magnetic resonance imaging (MRI) increases the risk of progression in patients otherwise defined as having SMM.[49] In a recent study, Wang and colleagues estimated risk of progression in 72 patients with SMM in whom an MRI of the spine was also performed.[51] The median TTP was significantly shorter with an abnormal MRI compared to normal MRI, 1.5 years versus 5 years, respectively.

Risk stratification of SMM

Weber and colleagues have shown that similar to MGUS, the size and type of the involved immunoglobulin are important predictors of progression in SMM.[54] Patients with a serum M protein ≤ 3 g/dL and IgG type (comprising about 45% of patients with SMM) had a median TTP > 4 years. In contrast, patients with a serum M protein > 3 g/dL or of the IgA type (about 45% of patients) had a median TTP of approximately 2 years, while a small subset of patients with > 3 g/dL IgA SMM had a median TTP of 9 months.

Management

The standard of care is observation alone until evidence of progression to active MM.[26] Patients with SMM need more frequent follow-up than those with MGUS; at least every

Table 10.2. Risk-stratification models to predict progression of monoclonal gammopathy of undetermined significance to myeloma or related disorders

Risk group	No. of patients	Relative risk	Absolute risk of progression at 20 years	Absolute risk of progression at 20 years accounting for death as a competing risk
Risk stratification model incorporating all 3 predictive factors				
Low-risk (Serum M protein < 1.5 g/dL, IgG subtype, normal FLC ratio (0.26–1.65))	449	1	5%	2%
Low-intermediate-risk (Any 1 factor abnormal)	420	5.4	21%	10%
High-intermediate-risk (Any 2 factors abnormal)	226	10.1	37%	18%
High-risk (All 3 factors abnormal)	53	20.8	58%	27%

Source: This table was originally published in *Blood*. Rajkumar SV *et al.* Serum free light chain ratio is an independent risk factor for progression in monoclonal gammopathy of undetermined significance (MGUS). *Blood* 2005;**106**;812–17.[14] © The American Society of Hematology.

3–4 months.[8] Two small randomized trials have shown no benefit of early therapy compared to therapy at the time of symptomatic progression.[55,56]

There are preliminary data that thalidomide may delay TTP,[57,58] but data are needed from randomized trials before such therapy can be recommended, particularly given the adverse effects associated with the drug. A randomized phase III trial at Mayo Clinic is currently testing thalidomide plus zoledronic acid versus zoledronic acid alone in patients with SMM. The results of this study will help determine the utility of thalidomide in this setting. Outside of a clinical trial, routine therapy with bisphosphonates is not recommended.

With the increasing availability of novel targeted therapies for MM,[59–61] clinical trials are ongoing to determine if the early use of these newer agents or bisphosphonates can delay progression of SMM.

Multiple myeloma

Introduction

The diagnosis of active MM requires ≥ 10% monoclonal plasma cells on bone marrow examination (or a biopsy proven plasmacytoma), M protein in the serum and/or urine (except in patients with true non-secretory myeloma), and evidence of end-organ damage (hypercalcemia, renal insufficiency, anemia, or bone lesions) attributable to the underlying plasma cell disorder. Almost all MM is felt to evolve from an antecedent MGUS.

MM accounts for approximately 10% of hematologic malignancies.[26,62] The annual incidence, age-adjusted to the 2000 United States population, is 4.3 per 100 000.[63] Almost 20 000 new cases and 11 000 new deaths were estimated to occur in the United States in 2007.[64] MM is twice as common in African–Americans compared to whites, and slightly more common in males than females. The median age at diagnosis is 66 years,[65] and only 2% of patients are < 40 years of age.

Clinical features

The most common presenting symptoms of MM are fatigue and bone pain.[65] Osteolytic bone lesions and/or compression fractures are hallmarks of the disease, which can be detected on routine radiographs, MRI, or computed tomographic (CT) scans, and may cause significant morbidity. Bone pain may present as an area of persistent pain or migratory bone pain, often in the lower back and pelvis. Pain may be sudden in onset when associated with a pathological fracture, and is often precipitated by movement. Extramedullary expansion of bone lesions may cause nerve root or spinal cord compression. Anemia occurs in 70% of patients at diagnosis and is the primary cause of fatigue. Hypercalcemia is found in one-fourth of patients, while the serum creatinine is elevated in almost one-half.

Diagnosis

Laboratory studies

A CBC with differential, liver function tests, urinalysis, serum electrolytes, including serum creatinine and calcium, β2-microglobulin, albumin, C-reactive protein, and lactate dehydrogenase (LDH) are needed for diagnosis, prognosis, and staging. In addition, patients require SPEP/IF, UPEP/IF, and serum FLC to quantify and identify the involved monoclonal protein. An M protein can be detected by SPEP in 82% of patients with MM, and by serum IF in 93%.[65] Up to 20% of patients with MM lack heavy-chain expression in the M protein, and are considered to have light-chain MM. The M protein in these patients is always detected in the urine, but can be absent in the serum, even by IF, making it necessary that serum and urine protein electrophoreses and IF are always done in all patients in whom MM is suspected. The addition of a UPEP/IF will increase the sensitivity of detecting monoclonal proteins in patients with MM to 97%. A 24-hour urine for UPEP/IF that quantifies the amount of monoclonal protein, as well as the total protein, is frequently beneficial for diagnosis.

If the proteinuria determined on a 24-hour collection is not predominantly monoclonal, it is not consistent with MM, and other proteinuric diseases should be considered, including AL, hypertension, diabetes mellitus, membranoproliferative glomerulonephritis, or other renal parenchymal disease. The presence of a MGUS in this case may or may not be related to the pathologic renal process. Most (60%) of the remaining patients who are negative for monoclonal protein on serum and urine electrophoreses and IF studies will have evidence of a paraprotein by the serum FLC assay. Only 1–2% of patients with MM will have no detectable M on any of these tests, and these patients have true non-secretory MM.

Bone marrow studies

A unilateral bone marrow aspiration and biopsy is indicated in all patients with MM. By definition, all patients should have bone marrow involvement with $\geq$ 10% clonal plasma cells. If a lesser extent of involvement is detected, one is either dealing with an erroneous diagnosis or there is a sampling error due to patchy marrow involvement, in which case, a repeat bone marrow biopsy is indicated. Occasionally, an entity called "multiple" solitary plasmacytomas may be present in which there are clearly multiple plasmacytomas on clinical and radiographic examination, but marrow involvement is either minimal or absent. The monotypic nature of the bone marrow plasma cells then is established by the demonstration of an abnormal κ:λ ratio by immunohistochemistry or flow cytometry. Myeloma cells typically stain positive for CD38, CD56, and CD138, and are usually negative for surface immunoglobulin and CD19 on flow cytometry. Up to 20% stain positively for CD20.

Given the impact of MM cell cytogenetic abnormalities on prognosis (see Prognosis below), bone marrow plasma cells should be studied using conventional karyotyping and FISH studies to detect specific chromosome abnormalities, such as t (11;14), t(4;14), t(14;16), monosomy 13, interstitial deletion of 14q32, and 17p-. A bone marrow plasma cell DNA labeling index, another prognostic indicator, also should be performed, if available. The test must be performed on fresh marrow and is a double immunofluorescence technique in which the sample is incubated in vitro with 5-bromo-2-deoxyuridine. BU-1, a fluorescent monoclonal antibody, identifies cells synthesizing DNA, and by using fluorescein-conjugated immunoglobulin antisera (κ or λ), the plasma cell population is then identified.

Identification of bone disease

Plain radiographic examination of all bones, including long bones (skeletal survey), is the usual method for detecting lytic bone lesions in MM. Conventional roentgenograms show skeletal abnormalities in almost 80% of patients with MM; often these lesions have a characteristic punched-out appearance (Figure 10.3). Osteoporosis and/or fractures may also be detected by conventional radiography. Occasionally, osteosclerotic lesions can occur. CT and MRI scans are more sensitive than conventional radiography in detecting bone disease. In asymptomatic MM patients with normal roentgenograms, up to 50% have tumor-related abnormalities on MRI of the lower spine. CT and/or MRI studies are indicated when symptomatic areas show no abnormality on routine radiographs. Their routine use in assessing extent of bone disease in addition to skeletal radiographs is unclear.[18] F-fluoro deoxyglucose positron emission tomography (FDG-PET) has shown promise in the evaluation of bone disease and in the staging of MM (Figure 10.4). However, the routine use of this method and its specific role in disease management requires further investigation.

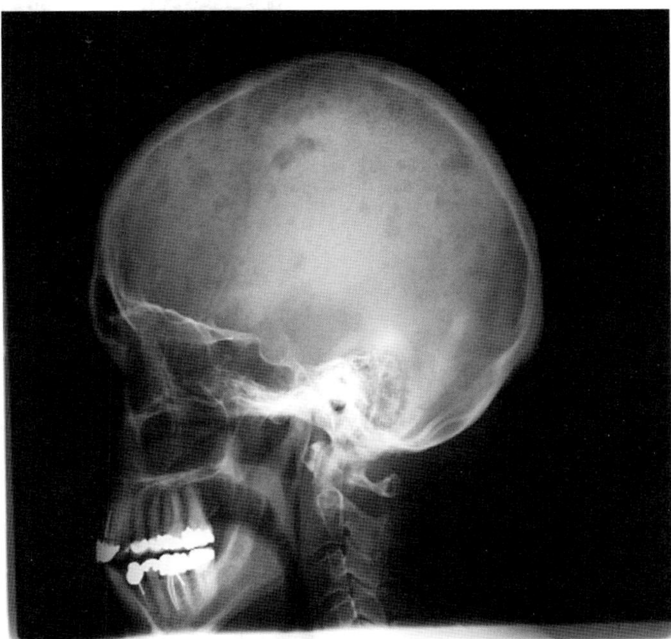

Figure 10.3 Osteolytic lesions in the skull on plain radiographs in a patient with myeloma.

The use of nuclear bone scans is not indicated, as this imaging modality is more sensitive for the detection of osteoblastic rather than osteolytic lesions. The role of bone mineral density studies in MM and their use in identifying patients at risk for pathologic fractures and those for whom prophylactic bisphosphonate therapy might be considered also remains unresolved.

Pathogenesis of bone lesions

The lytic bone lesions in MM are caused by an imbalance between the activities of osteoclasts and osteoblasts. There is an increase in RANKL (receptor activator of nuclear factor-kappa B ligand) expression by osteoblasts (and possibly plasma cells) accompanied by a reduction in the level of its decoy receptor, osteoprotegerin (OPG).[66,67] This leads to an increase in the RANKL/OPG ratio, which causes osteoclast activation and bone resorption. In addition, increased levels of macrophage inflammatory protein-1α (MIP-1α), IL-3, and IL-6 produced by marrow stromal cells contribute to osteoclast over activity.

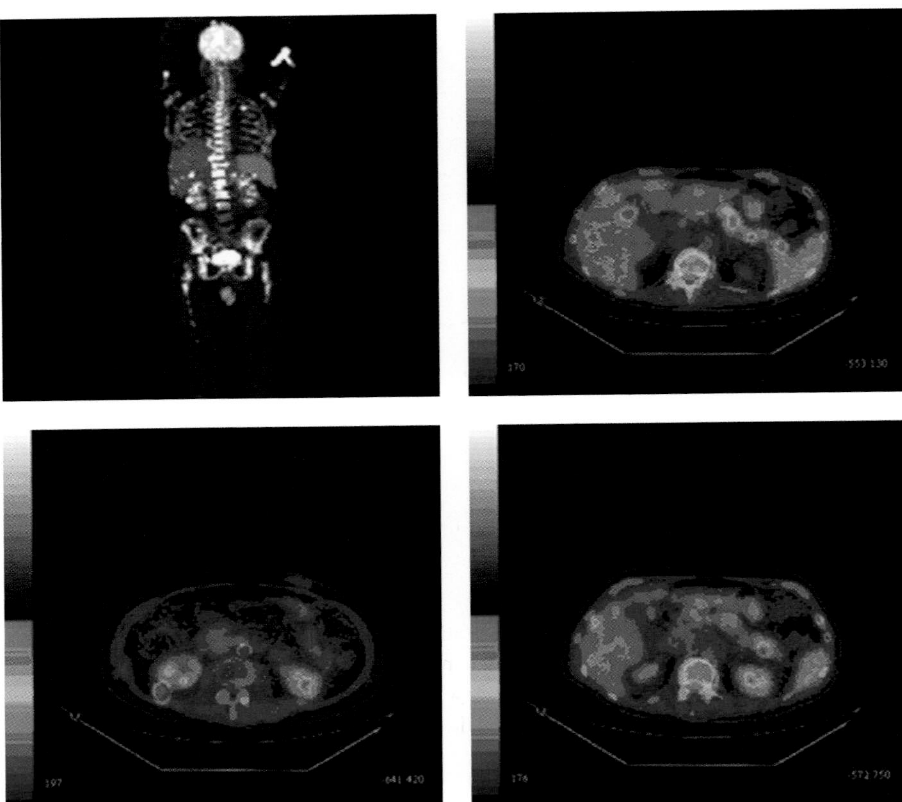

Figure 10.4 FDG-PET/CT imaging of a myeloma patient with disease involvement of the spine, extremities, ribs, pelvis, liver, gallbladder, pancreas, and right kidney.

Concurrently, increased levels of IL-3, IL-7, and dickkopf 1 (DKK1) inhibit osteoblast differentiation in MM. Myeloma cells express DKK1 and increased expression of DKK1 by these cells has been associated with the presence of focal bone lesions in MM.[68] The combination of osteoclast activation and inhibition of osteoblast differentiation is believed to be the mechanism behind the development of osteolytic lesions in MM.

Differential diagnosis

In patients with evidence of monoclonal proteins, the main differential diagnoses are among MM, MGUS, SMM, WM, and primary (AL) amyloidosis. In patients with a marrow plasmacytosis, monoclonal plasma cell disorders can be differentiated from a polyclonal reactive plasmacytosis based on κ/λ staining. A reactive plasmacytosis can be seen in autoimmune diseases, metastatic carcinoma, chronic liver disease, acquired immunodeficiency syndrome (AIDS), or chronic infection. In monoclonal plasma cell disorders, the monoclonal cells express either κ or λ, resulting in a markedly abnormal $\kappa:\lambda$ ratio. In contrast, both κ and λ staining plasma cells (usually in a $\kappa:\lambda$ ratio of approximately 2:1) are seen in disorders in which there is a reactive plasmacytosis.

Bone lesions in a patient with MGUS due to an unrelated metastatic carcinoma may be mistaken for MM. The presence of a small M protein and $< 10\%$ plasma cells in the bone marrow makes metastatic carcinoma with an unrelated MGUS more likely. If there is any doubt, a biopsy of one of the lytic lesions is needed.

Prognosis

Stage

Historically, although median overall survival (OS) has been approximately 3–4 years,[65] some patients may live longer than 10 years.[69–72] Survival partially depends on disease stage, and since 1975, the Durie–Salmon staging system has been used to stratify patients with MM.[73] However, this staging system has limitations, especially in the categorization of bone lesions.[74,75] The International Staging System (ISS) has subsequently been developed, a collaborative effort by investigators from 17 institutions worldwide and based on data from 11 171 patients.[76] The ISS overcomes the limitations of the Durie–Salmon staging, and has prognostic relevance. It divides patients into three distinct stages and prognostic groups, based solely on the $\beta 2$-microglobulin and serum albumin levels (Table 10.3).

Prognostic factors

Several independent prognostic factors are used in addition to disease stage to help predict outcome in MM (Table 10.3).[25,74,77–79] Facon *et al.* have shown that patients undergoing stem cell transplantation can be grouped into three clear prognostic categories using two prognostic factors; median OS was 25 months if patients had a high $\beta 2$-microglobulin and deletion

Table 10.3. Major prognostic factors in myeloma

• Advanced age
• Poor performance status
• International Staging System Stage
o Stage I (serum β_2 microglobulin < 3.5 mg/L and albumin ≥ 3.5 g/dL)
o Stage II (not fitting stage I or II)
o Stage III (serum β_2 microglobulin ≥ 5.5 mg/L)
• Durie–Salmon Stage
• Risk-stratification factors
o Deletion 13 or hypodiploidy by karyotyping
o Translocations t(4;14) or t(14;16) on fluorescent *in situ* hybridization (FISH)
o Deletion 17p on FISH
o Bone marrow plasma cell labeling index (PCLI) 3% or greater
• Elevated serum lactate dehydrogenase (LDH)
• Plasmablastic morphology

of chromosome 13 by FISH.[80] Patients with only one abnormal factor had a median OS of 47 months, while OS was > 111 months in patients in whom both factors were normal.

Age, hemoglobin, creatinine, calcium, albumin, immunoglobulin isotype, plasmablastic morphology, and extent of bone marrow involvement have also demonstrated prognostic value.[74,77,79] However, they possess limited predictive value, once the ISS and the independent prognostic factors discussed earlier are known.[81,82]

Risk stratification

The most compelling and powerful prognostic factors for survival in MM, whether alone or in combination with other factors, remain particular MM plasma cell cytogenetic abnormalities that form the basis for disease risk stratification. At the Mayo Clinic, newly diagnosed MM is stratified as either standard-risk (75% of patients) or high-risk disease (25%). This stratification often guides treatment and refines the estimates for survival, with patients with standard risk having a median OS of 6–7 years, and those with high-risk disease having a median OS of < 2–3 years, even in patients having undergone previous tandem autologous stem cell transplantation (ASCT).[62] Having one or more of the following places the disease in the high-risk category: PCLI $\geq 3\%$; by FISH: t(14;16), and/or deletion 17p, and/or t(4;14); by conventional cytogenetics (karyotype): monosomy 13, or hypodiploidy.

Management

Since the 1960s, the mainstay of therapy for myeloma had been conventional chemotherapy, particularly with oral melphalan and prednisone (MP). High-dose therapy with ASCT was then found to prolong survival compared to conventional chemotherapy. ASCT is now routinely incorporated into the treatment strategy either early in the disease course or at the time of relapse in eligible patients. In the last decade the treatment of myeloma has undergone remarkable advances with the emergence of thalidomide,[83] bortezomib,[84,85] and lenalidomide[86,87] as effective agents.

Initial therapy depends on eligibility for SCT and risk-stratification. Eligibility for SCT is determined by age, performance status, and coexisting comorbidities. Risk stratification is based on the presence or absence of high-risk factors.[88] The approach to treatment of symptomatic newly diagnosed MM at Mayo Clinic is outlined in Figure 10.5. Table 10.4 lists the most common regimens used in the treatment of newly diagnosed myeloma. Response to therapy is assessed using the International Myeloma Working Group Uniform Response Criteria (Table 10.5).[89]

Initial therapy in patients eligible for ASCT

It is important to avoid prolonged melphalan-based therapy in patients with newly diagnosed MM who are considered eligible for ASCT, as it can interfere with adequate stem cell mobilization, regardless of whether an early or delayed transplant is contemplated. Typically, patients are treated with approximately 2–4 cycles of induction therapy prior to stem cell harvest. This includes patients who are transplant candidates, but who wish to reserve ASCT as a delayed option for relapsed refractory disease. Such patients can resume induction therapy following stem cell collection until a plateau phase is reached, reserving ASCT for relapse.

Vincristine, doxorubicin, dexamethasone (VAD), used for many years as pre-transplant induction therapy, is no longer recommended. Cavo and colleagues, in a matched case–control study of 200 patients, demonstrated that response rates with VAD were significantly lower compared to thalidomide plus dexamethasone (Thal/Dex); 76% versus 52%, respectively.[90] Preliminary results from a randomized trial from France confirmed these findings.[91] Similarly, high-dose pulsed dexamethasone alone dosed at 40 mg orally on days 1–4, 9–12, and 17–20 every 4–5 weeks is also no longer recommended. Objective response rates with high-dose dexamethasone are low, approximately 45%.[92] More importantly, in randomized trials, the early mortality rate associated with dexamethasone is over 10% within the first 4 months of therapy, reflecting the high toxicity of this regimen.[93,94]

The main choices for initial therapy currently are either immunomodulatory agents (IMiDs) plus dexamethasone, i.e., Thal/Dex or lenalidomide-dexamethasone (Rev/Dex), or bortezomib-containing regimens. The role of other pre-transplant induction regimens besides the ones discussed below, such as those containing doxorubicin or liposomal doxorubicin, need to be weighed in terms of the added side effects that can affect quality of life, and should be considered investigational until future studies show that the addition of these agents improves long-term outcome.

Table 10.4. Selected regimens for the treatment of newly diagnosed multiple myeloma

Regimen	Usual dosing schedule*
Melphalan-Prednisone (MP)(7-day schedule)[26]	Melphalan 8–10 mg oral days 1–7
	Prednisone 60 mg/day oral days 1–7
	Repeated every 6 weeks until plateau
Melphalan-Prednisone (MP)(4-day schedule)[111]	Melphalan 0.25 mg/kg (9 mg/m^2) oral days 1–4
	Prednisone 2 mg/kg oral days 1–4
	Repeated every 4–6 weeks until plateau
Thalidomide-Dexamethasone (Thal/Dex)[92]	Thalidomide 200 mg oral days 1–28
	Dexamethasone 40 mg oral days 1–4, 9–12, 17–20
	Reduce dexamethasone to days 1–4 after first 4 cycles
	Repeated every 4 weeks × 4 cycles as pre-transplant induction therapy; or continued till plateau or progression if used as primary therapy
Lenalidomide-Dexamethasone (Rev/Dex)[86,98]	Lenalidomide 25 mg oral days 1–21 every 28 days
	Dexamethasone 40 mg oral days 1–4, 9–12, 17–20 every 28 days
	Reduce dexamethasone to days 1–4 after first 4 cycles
	Repeated every 4 weeks × 4 cycles as pre-transplant induction therapy; or continued till plateau or progression if used as primary therapy
Lenalidomide-Dexamethasone (Rev/low-dose Dex)[98]	Lenalidomide 25 mg oral days 1–21 every 28 days
	Dexamethasone 40 mg oral days 1, 8, 15, 22 every 28 days
	Repeated every 4 weeks × 4 cycles as pre-transplant induction therapy; or continued till plateau or progression if used as primary therapy
Bortezomib-Dex (Vel/Dex)[103]	Bortezomib 1.3 mg/m^2 intravenous days 1, 4, 8, 11
	Dexamethasone 40 mg oral days 1–4, 9–12
	Reduce dexamethasone to days 1–4 after first 2 cycles
	Repeated every 3 weeks × 4 cycles as pre-transplant induction therapy
Melphalan-Prednisone-Thalidomide (MPT)[111]	Melphalan 0.25 mg/kg oral days 1–4
	Prednisone 2 mg/kg oral days 1–4
	Thalidomide 100–200 mg oral days 1–28
	Repeated every 6 weeks × 12 cycles
Melphalan-Prednisone-Bortezomib (MPV)[113]	Melphalan 9 mg/m^2 oral days 1–4
	Prednisone 60 mg/m^2 oral days 1 to 4
	Bortezomib 1.3 mg/m^2 intravenous days 1, 4, 8, 11, 22, 25, 29, 32
	Repeated every 42 days × 4 cycles followed by maintenance therapy as given below:
	Melphalan 9 mg/m^2 oral days 1–4
	Prednisone 60 mg/m^2 oral days 1 to 4
	Bortezomib 1.3 mg/m^2 intravenous days 1, 8, 15, 22
	Repeated every 35 days × 5 cycles
Melphalan-Prednisone-Lenalidomide (MPR)	Melphalan 0.18 mg/kg oral days 1–4
	Prednisone 2 mg/kg oral days 1–4
	Lenalidomide 10 mg oral days 1–28
	Repeated every 4–6 weeks × 9 cycles
Bortezomib-Thalidomide-Dexamethasone (VTD)[237]	Bortezomib 1.3 mg/m^2 intravenous days 1, 4, 8, 11
	Thalidomide 100–200 mg oral days 1–21
	Dexamethasone 20 mg/m^2 oral days 1–4, 9–12, 17–20
	Reduce dexamethasone to days 1–4 after first 2 cycles
	Repeated every 4 weeks × 4 cycles as pre-transplant induction therapy

Note: *Starting and subsequent doses need to be adjusted for performance status, renal function, blood counts, and other toxicities.
Source: Reproduced with permission from Rajkumar SV, Lacy MQ. *ASCO Education Book* 2006 © ASCO.

Table 10.5. Response criteria for multiple myeloma

Response subcategory	Response criteria
Complete response (CR)	• Negative immunofixation of serum and urine, and
	• Disappearance of any soft tissue plasmacytomas, and
	• < 5% plasma cells in bone marrow
Stringent complete response (sCR)	CR as defined above plus
	• Normal FLC ratio, and
	• Absence of clonal cells in bone marrow by immunohistochemistry or immunofluorescence
Very good partial response (VGPR)	• Serum and urine M-component detectable by immunofixation but not on electrophoresis, or
	• ≥ 90% reduction in serum M-component plus urine M-component < 100 mg per 24 h
Partial response (PR)	• ≥ 50% reduction of serum M-protein and reduction in 24-h urinary M-protein by ≥ 90% or to < 200 mg per 24 h
	• If the serum and urine M-protein are unmeasurable a ≥ 50% decrease in the difference between involved and uninvolved FLC levels is required in place of the M-protein criteria
	• If serum and urine M-protein are unmeasurable, and serum free light chain assay is also unmeasurable, ≥ 50% reduction in bone marrow plasma cells is required in place of M-protein, provided baseline percentage was ≥ 30%
	• In addition to the above criteria, if present at baseline, ≥ 50% reduction in the size of soft tissue plasmacytomas is also required
Stable disease (SD)	• Not meeting criteria for CR, VGPR, PR, or progressive disease
Progressive disease (PD)	Increase of 25% from lowest response value in any one or more of the following:
	• Serum M-component (absolute increase must be ≥ 0.5 g/dL)[c] and/or
	• Urine M-component (absolute increase must be ≥ 200 mg per 24 h) and/or
	• Only in patients without measurable serum and urine M-protein levels: the difference between involved and uninvolved FLC levels (absolute increase must be > 10 mg/L)
	• Bone marrow plasma cell percentage (absolute % must be ≥ 10%)
	• Definite development of new bone lesions or soft tissue plasmacytomas or definite increase in the size of existing bone lesions or soft tissue plasmacytomas
	• Development of hypercalcemia (corrected serum calcium > 11.5 mg/dL) that can be attributed solely to the plasma cell proliferative disorder

Note: All response categories (CR, sCR, VGPR, PR) require two consecutive assessments made at any time before the institution of any new therapy; CR and PR and SD categories also require no known evidence of progressive or new bone lesions if radiographic studies were performed. Radiographic studies are not required to satisfy these response requirements. Bone marrow assessments need not be confirmed.

Source: Adapted with permission from Durie *et al.* International uniform response criteria for multiple myeloma. *Leukemia* 2006;**20**:1467–73.[89]

Thalidomide, dexamethasone (Thal/Dex)

The finding of increased angiogenesis in MM and the recognition of the antiangiogenic properties of thalidomide led to its evaluation in MM. In the last few years, Thal/Dex has emerged as the most commonly used induction regimen for the treatment of newly diagnosed MM in the United States. The upfront use of Thal/Dex was initially based on three phase II clinical trials.[58,95,96] Response rates with Thal/Dex range from 64–76% in these studies.

The Eastern Cooperative Oncology Group (ECOG) reported the results of a randomized trial comparing Thal/Dex to dexamethasone in 202 patients.[92] The best response within four cycles of therapy was significantly higher with Thal/Dex compared to dexamethasone alone; 63% versus 41%, respectively, $p = 0.0017$. Stem cell harvest was successful in 90% of patients in each arm. Deep vein thrombosis (DVT) was more frequent with Thal/Dex (17% vs. 3%). Overall, grade 3 or higher non-hematologic toxicities were seen in 67% of patients within four cycles with Thal/Dex, and 43% with dexamethasone alone ($p < 0.001$). Early mortality (first 4 months) was 7% with Thal/Dex and 11% with dexamethasone alone. Based on this trial, the United States Food and Drug Administration (FDA) granted accelerated approval for Thal/Dex for the treatment of newly diagnosed myeloma.

Another randomized, double-blind, placebo-controlled study compared Thal/Dex versus dexamethasone alone as primary therapy in 470 patients with newly diagnosed myeloma.[94] As in the ECOG trial, response rates were

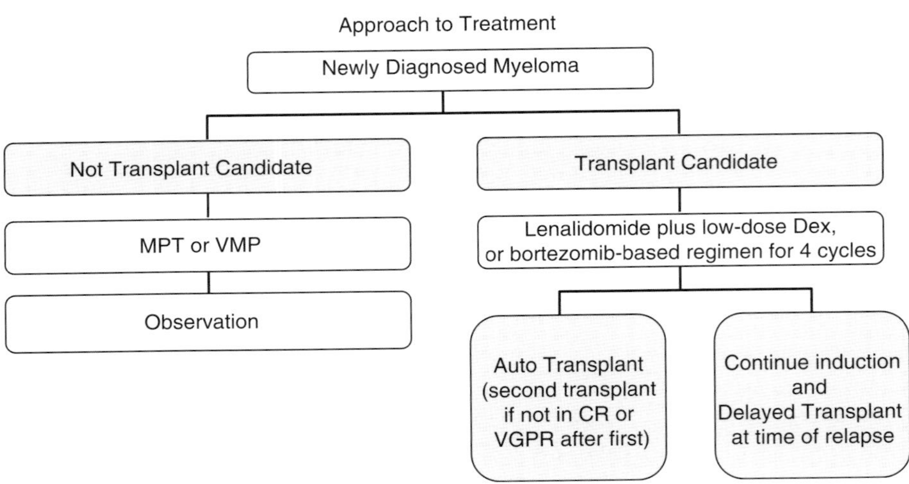

Figure 10.5 Approach to the treatment of newly diagnosed myeloma. MPT: melphalan, prednisone, thalidomide; VMP, bortezomib, melphalan, prednisone; Dex: dexamethasone; CR: complete response; VGPR: very good partial response.

significantly higher with Thal/Dex compared to placebo/dex, 63% versus 46%, respectively, $p < 0.001$. The TTP also was superior with Thal/Dex versus placebo/dex 22.6 versus 6.5 months, $p < 0.001$. DVT and other grade 3–4 events were more frequent with Thal/Dex (30.3% vs. 22.8%).

Lenalidomide, dexamethasone (Rev/Dex)

Lenalidomide, a thalidomide analog, is a second-generation IMiD. It appears safer and more effective than thalidomide in preclinical and clinical studies. Rev/Dex is currently approved by the FDA for the treatment of MM in patients who have failed one prior therapy. In newly diagnosed MM, a phase II trial conducted at the Mayo Clinic demonstrated remarkably high activity with the Rev/Dex regimen. Thirty-one of 34 patients (91%) achieved an objective response.[86] With longer follow-up, 56% of patients achieved VGPR or better.[97] The rate of grade 3 or higher non-hematologic toxicity (50%) was lower than Thal/Dex. The OS rate at 3 years was remarkably high at 88%.[97]

A recent randomized trial (E4A03) compared Rev/standard-dose Dex (dexamethasone dosed at 40 mg days 1–4, 9–12, 17–20) versus Rev/low-dose Dex (40 mg dexamethasone once weekly).[98] Preliminary results showed lower toxicity, lower early mortality, and superior OS at 1 and 2 years with Rev/low-dose Dex. DVT rates were also low with Rev/low-dose Dex making this one of the safest pre-transplant induction regimens for MM. Based on these data, Rev/low-dose Dex is currently the regimen of choice in the Mayo Stratification for Myeloma and Risk-adapted Therapy (mSMART) protocol for the treatment of standard-risk MM in patients who are candidates for ASCT outside the setting of a clinical trial (Figure 10.5).[88]

Although Rev/low-dose Dex appears to be an excellent pre-transplant induction regimen, there is evidence to suggest that it may impact negatively on the collection of peripheral blood stem cells for transplant.[99,100] A total of 376 patients over a 5-year period were evaluated at the Mayo Clinic, Rochester. In those patients mobilized with granulocyte colony-stimulating factor (G-CSF) alone, there were fewer total CD34+ stem cells collected ($p < 0.001$), a decrease in the average daily and day 1 collections (both $p < 0.001$), and an increase in the number of aphereses ($p = 0.004$), compared to those who previously had been induced with dexamethasone alone, Thal/Dex, or VAD.[99] These findings largely were reproduced by Mazumder *et al.*[100] It remains unclear whether longer duration of therapy or interval from the last dose of lenalidomide ultimately impacts collection. Stem cell mobilization may still be successful with chemotherapy-containing mobilization regimens, such as cyclophosphamide and G-CSF. Once AMD-3100, the CXCR4 inhibitor mobilizing agent, becomes available, its utility in this setting will also be evaluated.

Bortezomib-based regimens

Bortezomib is a proteasome inhibitor FDA approved for the treatment of patients with relapsed and refractory MM. In newly diagnosed MM, bortezomib has shown response rates of approximately 40% as a single agent.[101] Significantly higher response rates (approximately 70–90%) have been observed with bortezomib plus dexamethasone (Vel/Dex),[102,103] bortezomib, thalidomide, dexamethasone (VTD), and other bortezomib-based combinations. The CR plus VGPR rate was approximately 25–30% with Vel/Dex in one study. No adverse effect on stem cell mobilization was noted. The most common grade 2 or higher adverse events in one study were sensory neuropathy (31%), constipation (28%), myalgias (28%), and fatigue (25%).[102]

Harousseau and colleagues reported preliminary results of a randomized trial comparing VAD versus Vel/Dex as pre-transplant induction therapy.[104] With over 400 patients enrolled, the preliminary results show superior response rates and long-term outcome with Vel/Dex compared to VAD. DVT risk was low with bortezomib (< 5%).

The major drawback of bortezomib-based regimens is the need for intravenous therapy and the risk of neurotoxicity early in the disease course. However, bortezomib-based regimens e.g., VTD are of particular value in patients with renal failure, in whom it has been found to be safe and effective,[105] and in patients with high-risk MM (see below).

Initial therapy in patients ineligible for ASCT

Melphalan, prednisone (MP)

MP has been used in the treatment of MM for over 40 years.[106,107] The response rate with MP is approximately 50%. The median survival is approximately 3–4 years. A meta-analysis of 26 randomized trials found superior response rates but no survival benefit with combination chemotherapy regimens compared with MP prior to the arrival of thalidomide and bortezomib.[107] MP is well tolerated, but responses can sometimes take 6 months to occur. The substitution of dexamethasone in place of prednisone improves response rate and the speed of response, but does not improve OS.

Melphalan, prednisone, thalidomide (MPT)

Four randomized studies have shown that MPT (melphalan, prednisone, thalidomide) improves response and event-free survival (EFS) compared to MP;[108–110] an OS advantage has been observed in the two Intergroupe Francophone Myelome (IFM) trials.[109,111]

Palumbo *et al.* randomized compared MP for 6 months versus MPT for 6 months followed by maintenance thalidomide.[112] Overall response rates were significantly higher with the MPT compared to MP (76% versus 48%) as was the CR plus near CR rate (28% versus 7%). MPT resulted in superior 2-year progression-free survival (PFS) rates (54% versus 27%, $p < 0.001$), and a trend toward an improved 3-year OS. Facon *et al.* randomized 447 patients (ages 65–75) to MP versus MPT versus tandem ASCT with reduced-dose melphalan (100 mg/m^2; MEL100).[108] PFS was superior with MPT compared to either MP or tandem MEL100 groups, median PFS 28 months, 18 months, and 19 months, respectively, $p < 0.001$. There was also a significant survival advantage with MPT; median OS 52 months, 33 months, and 38 months, respectively. Early (first 3 months) mortality rate was 8% with MP compared to 3% with MPT.

Hulin *et al.* confirmed a survival advantage with MPT compared to MP in a randomized trial in 232 patients over the age of 75, median survival 45 versus 28 months respectively, $p = 0.03$.[109] This trial showed that the benefit of MPT over MP persists in patients up to at least age 85, but it is important to note that patients received a lower dose of thalidomide of 100 mg/day. In contrast to the three MPT randomized trials discussed so far, Waage and colleagues found no benefit with MPT compared with MP in a randomized placebo-controlled trial.[110] The reasons for this discrepancy are not clear, but may be related to the use of high doses of thalidomide (400 mg) in an elderly patient population resulting in increased early mortality particularly among those over the age of 75.

As a result of the above studies, MPT has emerged as the current standard of care for patients not eligible for ASCT (Figure 10.5). MPT therapy is associated with greater toxicity than MP. Therefore, not all elderly patients may be able to tolerate the regimen. Grade 3–4 adverse events occur in approximately 55% of patients treated with MPT, compared to 22% with MP.[112] As with Thal/Dex, there is a significant (20%) risk of DVT with MPT in the absence of thromboprophylaxis. However, this rate drops to approximately 3% with the use of thromboprophylaxis (e.g., enoxaparin).[112]

Melphalan, prednisone, bortezomib (VMP)

Mateos *et al.* found a response rate of 89%, with a remarkably high CR rate of 32% with the VMP regimen in a phase II study.[113] A recent randomized trial compared VMP to MP in 682 patients, median age 71 years.[114] In this trial, VMP had a significantly superior response rate compared to MP (71% versus 35%, $p < 0.001$), as well as a superior CR rate (30% versus 4%). TTP was significantly superior with VMP compared to MP, 24 versus 17 months respectively, $p < 0.001$. The 2-year OS rate was 83% with VMP versus 70% with MP respectively, $p < 0.001$. Importantly, VMP appeared to overcome adverse cytogenetic features; there was no significant difference in TTP or OS with VMP in patients with and without high-risk myeloma. Neuropathy is a significant risk with VMP therapy; grade 3 neuropathy occurred in 13% of patients versus 0% with MP. Neuropathy of any grade with VMP occurred in 44% of patients; grade 2 or higher in 30%. Based on this trial, VMP is an alternative to MPT for the treatment of patients with newly diagnosed myeloma not eligible for ASCT, especially those with high-risk features (Figure 10.5).

Melphalan, prednisone, lenalidomide (MPR)

Palumbo and colleagues studied the addition of lenalidomide to MP in newly diagnosed patients > 65 years of age.[115] Fifty-four patients were studied. The overall response rate was 85%, with 42% of patients achieving at least VGPR or better, and 17% of patients achieving a CR. PFS was 87% at 16 months; and similar to VMP, therapy with MPR appeared to overcome the adverse effect of deletion 13.[115] Major grade 3–4 adverse events were neutropenia (66%), thrombocytopenia (34%), anemia (17%), rash (10%), and febrile neutropenia (8%). All patients received prophylactic aspirin; DVT was uncommon, occurring in three patients (6%), including two after aspirin discontinuation. Based on this trial, MPR appears to be a very effective oral regimen for the treatment of elderly patients with MM who are not candidates for ASCT. An ECOG randomized trial (E1A06) is comparing MPR to MPT.

Hematopoietic stem cell transplantation

Autologous stem cell transplantation (ASCT)

Although not curative, ASCT improves CR rates and prolongs median OS in MM by approximately 12 months).[116–119] The mortality rate is 1–2%. Melphalan 200 mg/m^2 is the most widely used preparative (conditioning) regimen for ASCT. Melphalan 140 mg/m^2 and 8 Gy total body irradiation (TBI) is inferior and is not recommended.[120] Studies are ongoing to determine if the conditioning regimen can be improved with the addition of radioactive compounds (holmium [^{166}Ho-DOTMP] or samarium [^{153}Sm-EDTMP])[121, 122] or bortezomib.

Three randomized trials show that survival is similar whether ASCT is done early (immediately following four cycles of induction therapy) or delayed (at the time of relapse as salvage therapy).[123–125] In a Spanish randomized trial, patients responding to induction therapy had similar OS and PFS when ASCT was compared with eight cycles of chemotherapy.[126] The results of this trial suggest that the greatest benefit from ASCT may be in those with disease refractory to induction therapy.[127,128]

There is little doubt that ASCT prolongs survival in MM, but its timing (early versus delayed) is controversial.[118] Given the new, effective, and well-tolerated agents to treat MM, some patients and physicians may choose to delay the procedure.

Tandem autologous transplantation

With tandem (double) ASCT, patients receive a second planned ASCT after recovery from the first procedure.[71,129] The IFM 94 randomized trial found significantly better EFS and OS in recipients of double versus single ASCT.[130] A similar benefit was also demonstrated in a randomized trial conducted in Italy;[131] two other randomized trials have yet to show significant improvement in OS with tandem ASCT, but they have shorter follow-up.[132,133] In both the French and Italian trials, the benefit of a second ASCT was restricted to patients failing to achieve a CR or VGPR with the first procedure. Based on these results, we now routinely collect enough stem cells for two transplants in all eligible patients, but we do not routinely offer tandem ASCT. Patients achieving a CR or VGPR with the first transplant are just observed or offered clinical trials investigating maintenance therapy, reserving the second ASCT for relapse.[134] Patients not achieving such a response are offered a second ASCT.

Allogeneic transplantation

Allogeneic transplantation is supported in myeloma by the presence of a graft-versus-myeloma effect.[135,136] However, only 5–10% of patients are candidates because of age, availability of a HLA-matched sibling donor, and adequate organ function. Further, the high treatment-related mortality (TRM), mainly related to graft-versus-host disease (GVHD) has made conventional allogeneic transplants unacceptable for most patients with MM.

Several recent trials have been conducted using non-myeloablative conditioning regimens (mini-allogeneic transplantation).[137] Initial trials evaluating this approach included relapsed or refractory patients, which were thought to account at least in part for the poor outcomes. It also became apparent that this approach was less useful in patients who had significant residual tumor burden at the time of the non-myeloablative transplant, which led to the concept of a planned ASCT followed by a planned reduced intensity conditioning allogeneic stem cell transplant (RIC SCT) a couple of months later.[138] The initial studies had treatment-related mortalities approaching 25%; 3-year OS and PFS rates were 41% and 21%, respectively.[138] Adverse OS was associated with chemoresistant disease, more than one prior transplantation, and absence of chronic GVHD. Using the planned tandem autologous/non-myeloablative allogeneic SCT approach, outcomes have been better with TRM of 15%, and 2-year OS approaching 75%.[139] However, there is also a high risk of acute and chronic GVHD, and the occurrence of GVHD appears necessary for disease control.

There are published data from only one randomized trial that addresses allogeneic SCT in high-risk patients, as defined by the presence of deletion 13 by FISH and of a β2 microglobulin > 3 mg/L.[140] Based on biologic randomization, patients were allocated to either double ASCT or to a single ASCT followed by a RIC allogeneic SCT. Although patients did better than expected in both arms, with median OS of 41 and 35 months, respectively, there was no significant difference between the two arms with a median follow-up of 24 months. The major criticisms of this study have been that the criteria used to select 'high-risk' disease did not select for the highest-risk patients, and that the reduced intensity conditioning used may have been too immunosuppressive, thereby abrogating the graft-versus-myeloma effect.

At this time, mini-allogeneic transplantation remains investigational. It should only be considered in the context of clinical trials in standard-risk MM because current results with the tandem ASCT strategy described earlier yield 7-year survival rates in excess of 40%. In these patients, the TRM and GVHD rates with non-myeloablative allogeneic transplantation are unacceptably high.

Treatment of high-risk myeloma

Patients with high-risk MM tend to do poorly with a median OS of approximately 2 years, even with tandem ASCT. Options for these patients should include novel therapeutic strategies.[62,88] For example, bortezomib-containing regimens can be considered early in the disease course as primary therapy, with ASCT reserved for relapse. In at least three separate studies, bortezomib appears to overcome the adverse effect of deletion 13.[113,141,142] Thus for initial therapy in transplant candidates, a bortezomib-containing regimen should be considered; similarly for non-transplant candidates, VMP should be preferred over MPT.

Allogeneic approaches may be an option in selected patients; for example, ASCT followed by non-myeloablative allogeneic transplantation. However, as mentioned above, the IFM 99 trial in patients with deletion 13 and high β2-microglobulin levels did not show significant benefit with this strategy compared to tandem ASCT.[140] We generally do not advocate early ASCT in high-risk myeloma. If ASCT is done (early or delayed), routine maintenance therapy could be considered given the high risk for early relapse. Clearly, clinical trials and new agents specifically designed for high-risk MM are needed.

Maintenance therapy

Maintenance therapy with interferon alpha is of limited value and is seldom used.[143] Results from the phase III US Intergroup Trial S9321 showed no benefit with interferon as maintenance therapy after ASCT.[144] A study by Berenson and colleagues suggests that prednisone may be useful for maintenance therapy.[145] PFS (14 vs. 5 months) and OS (37 vs. 26 months) were significantly longer with 50 mg versus 10 mg of prednisone orally every other day. As this comparison included only those who responded initially to steroid-based therapy, and patients did not receive ASCT, it is difficult to generalize these results to current practice.

A French trial (IFM 99–02) randomized 597 patients (age < 65) following tandem ASCT to no maintenance (arm A), pamidronate (arm B), or pamidronate plus thalidomide (arm C).[146] There was a significant improvement in EFS with maintenance thalidomide plus pamidronate; the 3-year EFS rate from the time of randomization was 36% in arm A, 37% in arm B, and 52% in arm C ($p < 0.009$). The corresponding 4-year OS rates were 77%, 74%, and 87%, respectively ($p < 0.04$). Results of a few other studies are also showing benefit with maintenance thalidomide, but questions still remain if all patients in the control arm had timely access to thalidomide off-study.[147] Studies addressing the use of lenalidomide and other agents post-ASCT are ongoing. At present, we do not recommend routine maintenance therapy in myeloma except for high-risk patients.

Treatment of relapsed multiple myeloma

Almost all patients with MM eventually relapse. If relapse occurs more than 6 months after stopping therapy, the initial treatment regimen should be re-instituted. Patients who have cryopreserved stem cells early in the disease course can derive significant benefit from ASCT as salvage therapy.[148] In general, patients who have an indolent relapse can often be treated with single agents with or without low-dose corticosteroids. These patients present with asymptomatic increases in serum and urine monoclonal protein levels, progressive anemia, or a few small lytic bone lesions. In contrast, patients with more aggressive relapse often require therapy with a combination of active agents. Given the non-curative nature of myeloma, patients with relapsed disease typically continue on one drug/regimen until relapse or toxicity and then try the next option.

Corticosteroids and conventional chemotherapeutic agents

High-dose pulsed dexamethasone or intravenous methylprednisolone are reasonable options, particularly if the patient has had an initial response to corticosteroids and was off high-dose corticosteroids when the relapse occurred.[149,150] Patients relapsing more than 6–12 months following an ASCT can respond to MP or MPT, since most would not have been exposed to this regimen as induction therapy. Conventional combination chemotherapy regimens such as VBMCP (vincistine, carmustine [BCN4], melphalan, cyclophosphamide, and prednisone), VAD, or other alkylator-based regimens can be effective in relapsed and refractory disease. Intravenous melphalan at a dose of 25 mg/m^2 is another active regimen, but usually requires transfusion and growth factor support.

Thalidomide and thalidomide-based regimens

Thalidomide has a response rate of 25% in heavily pre-treated patients with relapsed and refractory disease.[83,151] Several studies have confirmed the activity of thalidomide in relapsed, refractory MM.[152–156] The median duration of response is approximately one year. Thalidomide is usually given in a dosage of 100–200 mg daily. After a response is achieved, the dose should be adjusted to the lowest dose that can achieve and maintain a response in order to minimize long-term toxicity.

Thal/Dex with or without cyclophosphamide has significant activity in the treatment of relapsed MM. Studies show that response rates in relapsed disease are about 50% with the combination of thalidomide and corticosteroids,[157] and increase to over 65% with an oral three-drug combination of thalidomide, corticosteroids, steroids, and cyclophosphamide (CTD).[158–160] Several other combination chemotherapy regimens containing thalidomide are being studied, including VDT-PACE (bortezomib, dexamethasone, thalidomide, cisplatin, doxorubicin [Adriamycin], cyclophosphamide, and etoposide), BLT-D (clarithromycin, low-dose thalidomide, and dexamethasone), and MTD (melphalan, thalidomide, and dexamethasone).[161]

Bortezomib and bortezomib-based regimens

Bortezomib is approved for the treatment of patients with relapsed and refractory MM.[162,163] Approximately one-third of patients with relapsed refractory myeloma respond to bortezomib therapy, with an average response duration of one year.[84,164] In a phase III trial, PFS was superior with bortezomib compared to dexamethasone alone in patients with relapsed, refractory MM.[85] With extended follow-up the median OS with bortezomib was 29.8 months versus 23.7 months for dexamethasone, despite significant crossover from the dexamethasone to bortezomib arm.[165]

Bortezomib with or without dexamethasone is an active regimen for the treatment of aggressive relapse; bortezomib has also been combined with intravenous liposomal doxorubicin with a high response rate.[166] In a randomized trial, this combination yielded a superior TTP (9.3 versus 6.5 months) as compared to single-agent bortezomib; this promising result, however, has not yet translated into a better OS.[167]

Zangari *et al.* reported their experience with bortezomib, thalidomide, and dexamethasone (VTD) in a phase I trial.[168] The overall response rate was 55%; EFS and OS were 9 and 22 months, respectively. Myelosuppression was the most common grade 3–4 toxicity. Peripheral neuropathy worsened above baseline in 5–9% of these heavily pre-treated patients.

Lenalidomide

Lenalidomide first showed promising activity in MM in two phase I trials.[169,170] Richardson *et al.* reported activity in a multicenter randomized phase II trial that enrolled 102 patients with relapsed/refractory MM.[87] The overall response rate with single-agent lenalidomide was 17%.

Two large phase III trials have since shown significantly superior TTP with Rev/Dex compared to placebo plus dexamethasone in relapsed MM.[171,172] In these trials, grade 3–4 neutropenia was more frequently seen with the combination of Rev/Dex; the frequency of grade 3–4 infections was similar in both arms.

Other drugs

There is a continued search for other active agents based on advances in myeloma biology.[173] There are preliminary data suggesting modest efficacy with arsenic trioxide,[174] but further confirmation is needed. CC-4047 (pomalidomide, another thalidomide analog) has also shown promising activity.[175]

Disease complications

Hypercalcemia

Aggressive hydration with isotonic saline and corticosteroids are effective in most cases. A single dose of pamidronate, 60–90 mg intravenously over 2–4 hours,[176] or zoledronic acid, 4 mg intravenously over 15 minutes,[177] will normalize the calcium levels within 24–72 hours in most patients.

Skeletal lesions

Surgical fixation of fractures or impending fractures of long bones may be needed. Local radiation should be limited to patients with disabling pain who have a well-defined focal process that has not responded to analgesics and/or chemotherapy. The administration of bisphosphonates significantly reduces the number of skeletal events (pathologic fracture, need for irradiation or surgery on bone, and spinal cord compression).[178] In a randomized trial of 392 patients with at least one lytic lesion, skeletal events (pathologic fracture, radiation or surgery to bone, and spinal cord compression) after 9 months of therapy were significantly fewer with pamidronate compared to placebo, 24% versus 41%, respectively, $p < 0.001$.[178] More recently, zoledronic acid has been shown to have comparable efficacy to pamidronate.[179,180] Either pamidronate (90 mg intravenously over at least 2 hours every 4 weeks) or zoledronic acid (4 mg intravenously over 15–30 minutes every 4 weeks) is recommended in patients with MM who have one or more lytic lesions on skeletal roentgenograms.[179,181]

The typical recommendation initially was to continue bisphosphonates indefinitely at monthly intervals.[181] However, by 2003, avascular osteonecrosis of jaw (ONJ) was described as a new complication associated with their use.[182–186] The etiology of ONJ is unclear, but is likely multifactorial in origin. Although most patients who develop ONJ have had recent dental or oral surgical procedures (70%), the remainder develop spontaneous ONJ.[186] Proposed mechanisms include that inhibition of osteoclast activity reduces bone turnover and remodeling and that bisphosphonates prevent release of bone-specific factors that promote bone formation.[187]

The incidence of ONJ ranges from 4.4% to 21%, depending on the type and duration of bisphosphonate use.[187,188] The risk increases with duration of therapy, and likely with the use of zoledronic acid compared to pamidronate or other lower intensity bisphosphonates. A Mayo Clinic consensus statement recommends pamidronate instead of zoledronic acid as the bisphosphonate of choice for long-term therapy.[187] It also recommends 2 years of monthly bisphosphonate therapy for patients with MM bone disease, followed by either cessation of therapy in patients who are off active treatment for their myeloma or continuation of therapy every 3 months for those who are receiving MM therapy. These recommendations are bolstered by two recent observations. The first is that the rates of MM bone disease in the pre-bisphosphonate era were highest during the first 2 years after diagnosis.[189] The second supporting observation is the recent finding that pamidronate use after tandem transplant did not provide any significant reduction in skeletal events.[146]

Calcium supplementation should be given in those with MM, without hypercalcemia, at 500–600 mg twice daily. Vitamin D deficiency is very common in MM patients and levels should be drawn upon diagnosis and repletion instituted accordingly. Daily vitamin D supplementation in the absence of frank deficiency should be approximately 800–1000 IU in addition to calcium to optimize bone health. Myeloma patients with severe renal impairment or end-stage renal disease on dialysis benefit from a formal endocrinology evaluation in a bone clinic, given the prevalence of other metabolic bone diseases in this group. The use of intravenous and oral bisphosphonates in the dialysis population remains controversial.[190] The recommendations for calcium and vitamin D supplementation listed above also do not apply to this population.

Vertebroplasty (injection of methylmethacrylate into a collapsed vertebral body) and kyphoplasty (introduction of an inflatable bone tamp into the vertebral body and after inflation the injection of methylmethacrylate into the cavity) have been successfully used to decrease pain and help restore height.[191] Pain relief is generally rapid, and can be long-lasting in eligible patients.

Spinal cord compression from an extramedullary plasmacytoma should be suspected in patients with severe back pain, weakness or paresthesias of the extremities, bladder or bowel dysfunction, or incontinence. The standard treatment for cord or cauda equina compression are corticosteroids (dexamethasone 10 mg to 40 mg intravenously, followed by 4 mg orally/intravenously four times daily) and radiation therapy. On rare occasions, surgical decompression may be necessary if the spine is deemed unstable.

Renal insufficiency

Non-steroidal anti-inflammatory agents can precipitate renal failure and should generally be avoided.[192,193] Volume depletion, infection, and radiographic contrast media may also contribute to acute renal failure. Maintenance of a high urinary output (3 L/day) is important in preventing renal failure in those with high levels of monoclonal light chains in the urine. A trial of plasmapheresis should be considered in patients with acute or subacute renal failure due to light-chain cast nephropathy in an attempt to prevent irreversible renal damage.[194] This should be followed by a rapid-acting bortezomib-containing combination therapy, such as bortezomib, dexamethasone, and thalidomide (VDT), bortezomib, doxorubicin, and dexamethasone (VDD), cyclophosphamide, bortezomib, and dexamethasone (CyBor-D), or bortezomib, doxorubicin, and dexamethasone (PAD).

Anemia

Iron, folate, or B12 deficiencies may contribute to the anemia seen with MM as well and must be recognized and treated. Treatment of the underlying disease and renal failure often leads to improvement in the hemoglobin level. Erythropoietin (40 000 units subcutaneously weekly) or darbepoietin (200 mcg subcutaneously every 2 weeks) are useful in patients with persistent symptomatic anemia,[195,196] but should be used cautiously because of a higher risk of DVT when used in combination with thalidomide or lenalidomide. In addition, the recent data concerning erythropoiesis-stimulating agents and their possible roles in tumor progression, including in the hematologic malignancies, need to be taken into consideration as well. Blood transfusions are indicated for patients with symptomatic anemia who do not obtain benefit from other therapies.

Infections

Patients should receive pneumococcal and influenza vaccinations. Intravenous gamma globulin every 3–4 weeks is only indicated if patients have recurrent serious infections associated with severe hypogammaglobulinemia. The use of prophylactic antibiotics in patients receiving chemotherapy for myeloma has not been settled. Prophylaxis against *Pneumocystis jiroveci* pneumonia (previously known as *Pneumocystis carinii* or PCP) should be considered in all patients receiving high-dose corticosteroid therapy. A small randomized placebo-controlled trial of trimethoprim and sulfamethoxazole in 57 patients with newly diagnosed MM demonstrated benefit with routine prophylaxis administered with the first two cycles of chemotherapy.[197] Trimethoprim-sulfamethoxazole should be avoided in patients receiving Thal/Dex therapy due to the risk of serious skin toxicity. Prophylaxis with other antibiotics (such as ciprofloxacin, levofloxacin, or cephalosporins), alternative agents for *Pneumocystis jiroveci* prophylaxis, should be considered. A US randomized trial, URCC 1099, comparing no prophylaxis, trimethoprim plus sulfamethoxazole, and ciprofloxacin in patients with newly diagnosed MM receiving chemotherapy recently completed accrual; however, its results are not yet available. It has been recognized that bortezomib increases the risk for activation of herpes zoster and antiviral prophylaxis is recommended.

Hyperviscosity syndrome

Infrequently, patients with MM with an IgA or IgG isotype develop hyperviscosity syndrome. Plasmapheresis is indicated and relieves the symptoms. Plasmapheresis should be performed regardless of the viscosity level if the patient has signs or symptoms of hyperviscosity.[198] It is a temporizing measure which should be followed by prompt systemic therapy.

Side effects associated with novel agents

IMiDs

Increased risk for venous thromboembolism (VTE)

As a single agent, neither thalidomide nor lenalidomide increases the incidence of VTE in patients with newly diagnosed or previously treated MM. The incidence of VTE with thalidomide alone is 3–4% in new MM[57,199] and 2–4% in refractory disease.[200] However, the addition of dexamethasone, especially at high dose, to either IMiD markedly increases the risk, particularly in those with new disease. In newly diagnosed MM, the incidence of VTE with Thal/Dex is 14–26%[92,95,96] and 2–8% in those with relapsed/refractory disease without thromboprophylaxis.[201] The risk increases to about 25% in patients receiving the Thal/Dex in combination with other cytotoxic chemotherapeutic agents, particularly doxorubicin.[152,200,202–204] Other risk factors associated with an increased VTE risk include concurrent erythropoietin administration and dose of dexamethasone. Data arising from the E4A03 ECOG protocol evaluating lenalidomide and either low-dose dexamethasone (160 mg/month) or high-dose dexamethasone (480 mg/month) showed VTE rates of 8% and 23%, respectively.[205] Prophylactic anticoagulation strategies have not been systematically evaluated in randomized trials, but include aspirin, low molecular weight heparin, and warfarin. Based on limited data, a recent consensus was published on behalf of the International Myeloma Working Group recommending varying strategies based on a risk assessment model.[201]

Teratogenicity

The use of thalidomide, lenalidomide, and other IMiDs in pregnancy is absolutely contraindicated and the System for Thalidomide Education and Prescribing Safety Program (STEPS) must be followed to prevent teratogenicity.[206]

Rash

The use of IMiDs can result in a rash, which can often be dose-related rather than due to a true drug allergy. The rash can be mild and fleeting or extensive and desquamating. No dosing changes are likely to be necessary with mild (grade 1) rashes, as often they resolve spontaneously despite continuation of treatment.

For those patients with grade 2–3 skin toxicity, it is advisable to hold the IMiD until the rash resolves and then restart the drug at a lower dose. Patients with grade 4 toxicity should not receive further drug, regardless of dose. Medications being administered concurrently with the IMiD, such as a sulfonamide or allopurinol, may increase the risk for and severity of the rash and should be avoided, if possible. Rarely, a life-threatening hypersensitivity reaction, toxic epidermal necrolysis, has been reported with the use of thalidomide.[207]

Hypothyroidism

Thyroid function tests should be performed prior to treatment with an IMiD, with periodic monitoring thereafter, every 3–4 months. Multiple reports of the development of hypothyroidism in patients on thalidomide have been published.[208,209] More recently, thyroid dysfunction with lenalidomide has also been reported.[210,211]

Peripheral neuropathy

An autonomic neuropathy (5%) may be seen with the use of thalidomide and may manifest as sinus bradycardia and/or hypotension, with occasional syncope. Modifications in dose may reduce the severity of the symptoms, although at times, the drug may need to be completely discontinued.

The development of a peripheral neuropathy while taking thalidomide is much more common than an autonomic neuropathy. It is the most common side effect for which thalidomide is either held or dose reduced, and occurs in $> 50\%$ of patients.[212] Initial symptoms typically are numbness and tingling in the hands and feet, but can progress to more severe manifestations such as ataxia and motor dysfunction.

Constipation

Constipation is the most common gastrointestinal side effect ($> 50\%$) seen with the use of thalidomide. It can be severe and is exacerbated by other medications such as narcotics. A bowel regimen should be initiated when treatment with thalidomide is started. If constipation is severe, a dose reduction in thalidomide should be considered as the constipation may be dose dependent. When constipation is seen with lenalidomide, it is usually mild and dose reductions are not usually necessary.

Myelosuppression

Thaldomide is not associated with significant myelosuppression. Mild leukopenia and neutropenia may be seen in a minority of patients and are usually not significant enough to warrant a change in dose. Lenalidomide, by comparison, is associated much more frequently with a reduction in blood counts, and myelosuppression is its most frequent side effect, with rates depending on whether or not a patient has been previously treated. Dose modifications are frequently necessary as a result.

Use of IMiDs in patients with renal dysfunction

The pharmacokinetics of thalidomide have been reported as similar in patients with normal renal function and in those with significant renal impairment, as has the frequency of drug side effects in these two groups of patients.[213] Dose reductions in thalidomide in the setting of renal insufficiency and dialysis are not necessary. This is in contradistinction to lenalidomide, which is renally excreted, where total and renal clearance significantly decrease with progressively worsening renal function.[214] Dose adjustments are recommended for patients with a creatinine clearance < 50 mL/min.[214] Lenalidomide should be administered after dialysis if used in that setting.

Bortezomib

Bortezomib is cleared by the liver and those with severe hepatic dysfunction should not be given the drug. Some of the most common side effects associated with bortezomib are gastrointestinal, such as nausea (64%), vomiting (36%), constipation (43%), and diarrhea (51%), which usually can be readily managed with supportive care measures. Cytopenias are also not unusual, particularly thrombocytopenia (43%), for which a dose reduction or holding a dose may be indicated. The development of a predominantly sensory, often painful peripheral neuropathy develops in approximately 40%. It most often begins in the feet and lower extremities, but can go on to affect the upper extremities. A dose reduction should be instituted promptly if symptoms develop. The neuropathy can improve with the discontinuation of the drug, but potentially can take months. Bortezomib is not associated with an increased risk for venous thromboembolism.

IgM myeloma

The majority of MM is associated with an IgA or IgG isotype. IgM myeloma represents a distinct entity, but comprises $< 0.5\%$ of all MM.[215] The differential diagnosis to be made is between IgM MM and WM, the distinction of which is important based on differing clinical courses, prognoses, and treatments. The distinction may be clinically straightforward, with IgM MM demonstrating $> 10\%$ marrow involvement with a clonal plasma cell population and one or more of the following: lytic bone lesions, hypercalcemia, and/or renal insufficiency. However, in more ambiguous cases where a diagnosis cannot be made on clinical grounds, immunophenotyping, chromosomal, and FISH analyses may be of particular value. Karyotyping is usually normal in both diseases; however, $\geq 50\%$ of WM cases by FISH show chromosome 6q-, not found in MM.[216–219] In addition, IGH translocations commonly seen in MM are rarely seen with WM.[216,219,220]

Plasma cell leukemia

Definition

Plasma cell leukemia (PCL) is a variant of MM characterized by a fulminant course and poor prognosis. It is the most aggressive of the plasma cell neoplasms. It may arise as a primary process, de novo (pPCL), or secondarily (sPCL) as a leukemic transformation from a previously diagnosed MM.

These two forms of PCL are different with respect to immunophenotypic and genetic features, history, and OS. The current, clinically derived definition of PCL is the presence of an absolute peripheral blood plasma cell count of $> 2 \times 10^9$/L or a differential with > 20% plasma cells.[221]

Epidemiology

Primary PCL represents approximately 2–4% of newly diagnosed MM[221,222] and sPCL has a similar incidence.[223] The median age at diagnosis of pPCL in a recent study was 54.5 years compared to 65.7 years for those with sPCL.[223] Secondary PCL often has been characterized as a late manifestation of MM; however, a recent study noted that the median time to leukemic transformation from an underlying MM was approximately 20.8 months from the time of the MM diagnosis.[223]

Cytogenetics

The genetic and molecular bases for both forms of PCL are not well understood.

Primary PCL tumors compared to sPCL or MM more often have hypodiploid or pseudodiploid karyotypes.[223,224,225] The prevalence of IGH translocations in both pPCL (87%) and sPCL (82%)[223] is higher than reported for MM (50%),[25,26] and is consistent with the positive correlation between these translocations and non-hyperdiploidy.[226,227] The prevalences of the common IGH translocations have been reported as significantly different between pPCL and sPCL. Tiedemann *et al.* noted that 71% of pPCL versus 23% of sPCL had t(11;14), p = 0.03.[223] The increased prevalence of t(11;14) in pPCL compared to MM has been previously noted (33% versus 13%), although its significance has not been delineated fully.[225] Deletion of 13q is believed to be a negative prognostic factor in MM, especially if detected by karyotyping. The prevalence of this deletion was found to be 42% in MM in one study,[225] 68–85% in pPCL,[223,225] and 67% in sPCL.[223] Loss or inactivation of 17p13.1 confers a poor prognosis in MM, although it is found in a minority of MM cases, approximately 10%. Allelic TP53 inactivation in pPCL and sPCL has been reported as 50% and 75%, respectively.[223] This same study, however, did not find that 17p and deletion 13 in PCL significantly affected OS.[223] Clearly, the relative importance and interrelationships among the cytogenetic abnormalities in both forms of PCL remain largely unknown.

Prognosis

The prognosis for PCL is poor, although significantly better for pPCL compared to sPCL, 7–11 months[222–225] versus 1.3 months, respectively, p = <0.001.[223]

Treatment

There is no one first-line therapy recommended for pPCL, as there are relatively few patients and there are no randomized trials. Therapy is extrapolated from the MM literature. Before the development of IMiDs and bortezomib, treatment with combination chemotherapy versus the use of melphalan and corticosteroids alone resulted in a significant OS benefit in PCL, unlike in MM. Whether OS will improve in both PCL categories with the use of the newer therapeutic agents, alone or in combination, remains to be seen. Although there are no data suggesting that allogeneic SCT is superior to ASCT in this group of patients, allogeneic transplant is often considered in younger, eligible patients given the otherwise poor prognosis.

References

1. Kyle RA, Rajkumar SV. Monoclonal gammopathy of undetermined significance. *Br J Haematol* 2006;**134**:573–89.
2. Katzmann JA, Clark RJ, Abraham RS, *et al.* Serum reference intervals and diagnostic ranges for free kappa and free lambda immunoglobulin light chains: relative sensitivity for detection of monoclonal light chains. *Clin Chem* 2002;**48**:1437–44.
3. Bradwell AR, Carr-Smith HD, Mead GP, *et al.* Serum test for assessment of patients with Bence Jones myeloma. *Lancet* 2003;**361**:489–91.
4. Drayson M, Tang LX, Drew R, *et al.* Serum free light-chain measurements for identifying and monitoring patients with nonsecretory multiple myeloma. *Blood* 2001;**97**:2900–2.
5. Lachmann HJ, Gallimore R, Gillmore JD, *et al.* Outcome in systemic AL amyloidosis in relation to changes in concentration of circulating free immunoglobulin light chains following chemotherapy. *Br J Haematol* 2003;**122**:78–84.
6. Abraham RS, Clark RJ, Bryant SC, *et al.* Correlation of serum immunoglobulin free light chain quantification with urinary Bence Jones protein in light chain myeloma. *Clin Chem* 2002;**48**:655–7.
7. Kyle RA, Rajkumar SV. Plasma cell disorders. In: Goldman L, Ausiello D, eds. *Cecil Textbook of Medicine*, 22nd edn. Philadelphia, W.B. Saunders. 2004; 1184–95.
8. Rajkumar SV. MGUS and smoldering multiple myeloma: update on pathogenesis, natural history, and management. *Hematology (Am Soc Hematol Educ Program)* 2005;340–5.
9. Kyle RA, Therneau TM, Rajkumar SV, *et al.* Prevalence of monoclonal gammopathy of undetermined significance (MGUS) among Olmsted County, MN residents 50 years of age. *Blood* 2003;**102**:934a (A3476).
10. Landgren O, Gridley G, Turesson I, *et al.* Risk of monoclonal gammopathy of undetermined significance (MGUS) and subsequent multiple myeloma among African American and white veterans in the United States. *Blood* 2006;**107**:904–6.
11. Kyle RA, Therneau TM, Rajkumar SV, *et al.* A long-term study of prognosis of monoclonal gammopathy of undetermined significance. *N Engl J Med* 2002;**346**:564–9.
12. Kyle RA, Therneau TM, Rajkumar SV, *et al.* Long-term follow-up of 241 patients with monoclonal gammopathy of undetermined significance: the original Mayo Clinic series 25 years later.[see comment]. *Mayo Clin Proc* 2004;**79**:859–66.

13. Kyle RA. "Benign" monoclonal gammopathy–after 20 to 35 years of follow-up. *Mayo Clin Proc* 1993; **68**:26–36.

14. Rajkumar SV, Kyle RA, Therneau TM, *et al.* Serum free light chain ratio is an independent risk factor for progression in monoclonal gammopathy of undetermined significance (MGUS). *Blood* 2005;**106**:812–17.

15. Jego G, Bataille R, Geffroy-Luseau A, *et al.* Pathogen-associated molecular patterns are growth and survival factors for human myeloma cells through Toll-like receptors. *Leukemia* 2006;**20**:1130–7.

16. Bohnhorst J, Rasmussen T, Moen SH, *et al.* Toll-like receptors mediate proliferation and survival of multiple myeloma cells. *Leukemia* 2006;**20**:1138–44.

17. Mantovani A, Garlanda C. Inflammation and multiple myeloma: the Toll connection. *Leukemia* 2006;**20**:937–8.

18. van de Donk NW, Lokhorst HM, Bloem AC. Growth factors and antiapoptotic signaling pathways in multiple myeloma. *Leukemia* 2005;**19**: 2177–85.

19. Perez-Andres M, Almeida J, Martin-Ayuso M, *et al.* Clonal plasma cells from monoclonal gammopathy of undetermined significance, multiple myeloma and plasma cell leukemia show different expression profiles of molecules involved in the interaction with the immunological bone marrow microenvironment. *Leukemia* 2005;**19**:449–55.

20. Rawstron AC, Fenton JA, Ashcroft J, *et al.* The interleukin-6 receptor alpha-chain (CD126) is expressed by neoplastic but not normal plasma cells. *Blood* 2000;**96**:3880–6.

21. Zent CS, Wilson CS, Tricot G, *et al.* Oligoclonal protein bands and Ig isotype switching in multiple myeloma treated with high-dose therapy and hematopoietic cell transplantation. *Blood* 1998;**91**:3518–23.

22. Amara S, Dezube BJ, Cooley TP, *et al.* HIV-associated monoclonal gammopathy: a retrospective analysis of 25 patients. *Clin Infect Dis* 2006;**43**:1198–205.

23. Dezube BJ, Aboulafia DM, Pantanowitz L. Plasma cell disorders in HIV-infected patients: from benign gammopathy to multiple myeloma. *AIDS Reader* 2004;**14**:372–4.

24. Passweg J, Thiel G, Bock HA. Monoclonal gammopathy after intense induction immunosuppression in renal transplant patients. *Nephrol Dial Transplant* 1996;**11**:2461–5.

25. Fonseca R, Barlogie B, Bataille R, *et al.* Genetics and cytogenetics of multiple myeloma: a workshop report. *Cancer Res* 2004;**64**:1546–58.

26. Kyle RA, Rajkumar SV. Multiple myeloma. *N Engl J Med* 2004; **351**:1860–73.

27. Kuehl WM, Bergsagel PL. Multiple myeloma: evolving genetic events and host interactions. *Nat Rev Cancer* 2002;**2**:175–87.

28. Bergsagel PL, Kuehl WM. Chromosome translocations in multiple myeloma. *Oncogene* 2001;**20**:5611–22.

29. Fonseca R, Bailey RJ, Ahmann GJ, *et al.* Genomic abnormalities in monoclonal gammopathy of undetermined significance. *Blood* 2002;**100**:1417–24.

30. Drach J, Angerler J, Schuster J, *et al.* Interphase fluorescence in situ hybridization identifies chromosomal abnormalities in plasma cells from patients with monoclonal gammopathy of undetermined significance. *Blood* 1995;**86**:3915–21.

31. Fonseca R, Aguayo P, Ahmann GJ, *et al.* Translocations at 14q32 are common in patients with the monoclonal gammopathy of undetermined significance (MGUS) and involve several partner chromosomes. *Blood* 1999;**94** Suppl 1:663a (A 2943).

32. Chng WJ, Van Wier SA, Ahmann GJ, *et al.* A validated FISH trisomy index demonstrates the hyperdiploid and nonhyperdiploid dichotomy in MGUS. *Blood* 2005;**106**:2156–61.

33. Magrangeas F, Lode L, Wuilleme S, *et al.* Genetic heterogeneity in multiple myeloma. *Leukemia* 2005;**19**:191–4.

34. Kaufmann H, Ackermann J, Baldia C, *et al.* Both IGH translocations and chromosome 13q deletions are early events in monoclonal gammopathy of undetermined significance and do not evolve during transition to multiple myeloma. *Leukemia* 2004;**18**:1879–82.

35. Hanamura I, Stewart JP, Huang Y, *et al.* Frequent gain of chromosome band 1q21 in plasma-cell dyscrasias detected by fluorescence in situ hybridization: incidence increases from MGUS to relapsed myeloma and is related to prognosis and disease progression following tandem stem-cell transplantation. *Blood* 2006;**108**: 1724–32.

36. Rajkumar SV, Mesa RA, Fonseca R, *et al.* Bone marrow angiogenesis in 400 patients with monoclonal gammopathy of undetermined significance, multiple myeloma, and primary amyloidosis. *Clin Cancer Res* 2002;**8**:2210–16.

37. Galea HR, Cogne M. GM-CSF and IL-12 production by malignant plasma cells promotes cell-mediated immune responses against monoclonal Ig determinants in a light chain myeloma model. *Clin Exp Immunol* 2002;**129**:247–53.

38. Vacca A, Ria R, Ribatti D, *et al.* A paracrine loop in the vascular endothelial growth factor pathway triggers tumor angiogenesis and growth in multiple myeloma. *Haematologica* 2003;**88**:176–85.

39. Kumar S, Fonseca R, Dispenzieri A, *et al.* Prognostic value of angiogenesis in solitary bone plasmacytoma. *Blood* 2003;**101**:1715–17.

40. Kumar S, Witzig TE, Timm M, *et al.* Bone marrow angiogenic ability and expression of angiogenic cytokines in myeloma: Evidence favoring loss of marrow angiogenesis inhibitory activity with disease progression. *Blood* 2004;**104**:1159–65.

41. Kumar S, Witzig TE, Timm M, *et al.* Expression of VEGF and its receptors by myeloma cells. *Leukemia* 2003;**17**:2025–31.

42. Vacca A, Scavelli C, Serini G, *et al.* Loss of inhibitory semaphorin 3A (SEMA3A) autocrine loops in bone marrow endothelial cells of patients with multiple myeloma. *Blood* 2006;**108**:1661–7.

43. Kumar S, Witzig TE, Wellik L, *et al.* Effect of thalidomide therapy on bone marrow angiogenesis in multiple myeloma. *Leukemia* 2004;**18**:624–7.

44. Cesana C, Klersy C, Barbarano L, *et al.* Prognostic factors for malignant transformation in monoclonal gammopathy of undetermined significance and smoldering multiple myeloma. *J Clin Oncol* 2002;**20**:1625–34.

45. Kumar S, Rajkumar SV, Kyle RA, *et al.* Prognostic value of circulating plasma

cells in monoclonal gammopathy of undetermined significance. *J Clin Oncol* 2005;**23**:5668–74.

46. Barosi G, Boccadoro M, Cavo M, *et al.* Management of multiple myeloma and related-disorders: guidelines from the Italian Society of Hematology (SIE), Italian Society of Experimental Hematology (SIES) and Italian Group for Bone Marrow Transplantation (GITMO). *Haematologica* 2004;**89**:717–41.
47. The International Myeloma Working Group. Criteria for the classification of monoclonal gammopathies, multiple myeloma and related disorders: a report of the International Myeloma Working Group. *Br J Haematol* 2003; **121**:749–57.
48. Rajkumar SV, Dispenzieri A, Fonseca R, *et al.* Thalidomide for previously untreated indolent or smoldering multiple myeloma. *Leukemia* 2001;**15**:1274–6.
49. Dimopoulos MA, Moulopoulos LA, Maniatis A, *et al.* Solitary plasmacytoma of bone and asymptomatic multiple myeloma. *Blood* 2000;**96**:2037–44.
50. Ross FM, Ibrahim AH, Vilain-Holmes A, *et al.* Age has a profound effect on the incidence and significance of chromosome abnormalities in myeloma. *Leukemia* 2005;**19**:1634–42.
51. Wang M, Alexanian R, Delasalle K, *et al.* Abnormal MRI of spine is the dominant risk factor for early progression of asymptomatic multiple myeloma. *Blood* 2003;**102**:687a.
52. Witzig TE, Kyle RA, O'Fallon WM, Greipp PR. Detection of peripheral blood plasma cells as a predictor of disease course in patients with smoldering multiple myeloma. *Br J Haematol* 1994;**87**:266–72.
53. Kyle R, Remstein E, Therneau T, *et al.* The natural history of smoldering (asymptomatic) multiple myeloma. *Blood* 2005;**106**:949a (A3396).
54. Weber D, Wang LM, Delasalle K, *et al.* Risk factors for early progression of asymptomatic multiple myeloma. *Hematol J* 2003;**4** Suppl 1:S31.
55. Hjorth M, Hellquist L, Holmberg E, *et al.* Initial versus deferred melphalan-prednisone therapy for asymptomatic multiple myeloma stage I–a randomized study. Myeloma Group of Western Sweden. *Eur J Haematol* 1993;**50**:95–102.
56. Riccardi A, Mora O, Tinelli C, *et al.* Long-term survival of stage I multiple myeloma given chemotherapy just after diagnosis or at progression of the disease: a multicentre randomized study. Cooperative Group of Study and Treatment of Multiple Myeloma. *Br J Cancer* 2000;**82**:1254–60.
57. Rajkumar SV, Gertz MA, Lacy MQ, *et al.* Thalidomide as initial therapy for early-stage myeloma. *Leukemia* 2003;**17**:775–9.
58. Weber DM, Gavino M, Delasalle K, *et al.* Thalidomide alone or with dexamethasone for multiple myeloma. *Blood* 1999;**94** Suppl 1:604a (A2686).
59. Bruno B, Giaccone L, Rotta M, *et al.* Novel targeted drugs for the treatment of multiple myeloma: from bench to bedside. *Leukemia* 2005;**19**: 1729–38.
60. Richardson PG, Mitsiades CS, Hideshima T, *et al.* Novel biological therapies for the treatment of multiple myeloma. *Best Pract Res Clin Hematol* 2005;**18**:619–34.
61. Kumar S, Raje N, Hideshima T, *et al.* Antimyeloma activity of two novel N-substituted and tetraflourinated thalidomide analogs. *Leukemia* 2005;**19**:1253–61.
62. Rajkumar SV, Kyle RA. Multiple myeloma: diagnosis and treatment. *Mayo Clin Proc* 2005;**80**:1371–82.
63. Kyle RA, Therneau TM, Rajkumar SV, *et al.* Incidence of multiple myeloma in Olmsted County, Minnesota: trend over 6 decades. *Cancer* 2004;**101**: 2667–74.
64. Jemal A, Siegel R, Ward E, *et al.* Cancer statistics, 2007. *CA Cancer J Clin* 2007;**57**:43–66.
65. Kyle RA, Gertz MA, Witzig TE, *et al.* Review of 1,027 patients with newly diagnosed multiple myeloma. *Mayo Clinic Proc* 2003;**78**:21–33.
66. Roodman GD. Role of the bone marrow microenvironment in multiple myeloma. *J Bone Miner Res* 2002;**17**:1921–5.
67. Roodman GD. Mechanisms of bone metastasis. *N Engl J Med* 2004;**350**:1655–64.
68. Tian E, Zhan F, Walker R, *et al.* The role of the Wnt-signaling antagonist DKK1 in the development of osteolytic lesions in multiple myeloma. *N Engl J Med* 2003;**349**:2483–94.
69. Kyle RA. Long-term survival in multiple myeloma. *N Engl J Med* 1983;**308**:314–16.
70. Attal M, Payen C, Facon T, *et al.* Single versus double transplant in myeloma: a randomized trial of the "Inter Groupe Francais du Myelome" (IFM). *Blood* 1997;**90** Suppl 1:418a.
71. Barlogie B, Jagannath S, Desikan KR, *et al.* Total therapy with tandem transplants for newly diagnosed multiple myeloma. *Blood* 1999; **93**:55–65.
72. Desikan R, Barlogie B, Sawyer J, *et al.* Results of high-dose therapy for 1000 patients with multiple myeloma: durable complete remissions and superior survival in the absence of chromosome 13 abnormalities. *Blood* 2000;**95**:4008–10.
73. Durie BG, Salmon SE. A clinical staging system for multiple myeloma. Correlation of measured myeloma cell mass with presenting clinical features, response to treatment, and survival. *Cancer* 1975;**36**:842–54.
74. Kyle RA. Prognostic factors in multiple myeloma. *Stem Cells* 1995;**2**:56–63.
75. Rapoport BL, Falkson HC, Falkson G. Prognostic factors affecting the survival of patients with multiple myeloma. A retrospective analysis of 86 patients. *S Afr Med J* 1990;**79**:65–7.
76. Greipp PR, San Miguel JF, Durie BG, *et al.* International staging system for multiple myeloma. *J Clin Oncol* 2005;**23**:3412–20.
77. Rajkumar SV, Greipp PR. Prognostic factors in multiple myeloma. *Hematol Oncol Clin North Am* 1999;**13**:1295–314.
78. Tricot G, Sawyer JR, Jagannath S, *et al.* Unique role of cytogenetics in the prognosis of patients with myeloma receiving high-dose therapy and autotransplants. *J Clin Oncol* 1997;**15**:2659–66.
79. Greipp PR. Prognosis in myeloma. [75 refs]. *Mayo Clin Proc* 1994;**69**: 895–902.
80. Facon T, Avet-Loiseau H, Guillerm G, *et al.* Chromosome 13 abnormalities identified by FISH analysis and serum beta2-microglobulin produce a powerful myeloma staging system for patients receiving high-dose therapy. *Blood* 2001;**97**:1566–71.
81. Greipp PR, Leong T, Bennett JM, *et al.* Plasmablastic morphology–an

independent prognostic factor with clinical and laboratory correlates: Eastern Cooperative Oncology Group (ECOG) myeloma trial E9486 report by the ECOG Myeloma Laboratory Group. *Blood* 1998;**91**:2501–7.

82. Greipp PR, Lust JA, O'Fallon WM, *et al.* Plasma cell labeling index and beta 2-microglobulin predict survival independent of thymidine kinase and C-reactive protein in multiple myeloma [see comments]. *Blood* 1993; **81**:3382–7.

83. Singhal S, Mehta J, Desikan R, *et al.* Antitumor activity of thalidomide in refractory multiple myeloma. *N Engl J Med* 1999;**341**:1565–71.

84. Richardson PG, Barlogie B, Berenson J, *et al.* A phase 2 study of bortezomib in relapsed, refractory myeloma. *N Engl J Med* 2003;**348**:2609–17.

85. Richardson PG, Sonneveld P, Schuster MW, *et al.* Bortezomib or high-dose dexamethasone for relapsed multiple myeloma. *N Engl J Med* 2005;**352**: 2487–98.

86. Rajkumar SV, Hayman SR, Lacy MQ, *et al.* Combination therapy with lenalidomide plus dexamethasone (Rev/Dex) for newly diagnosed myeloma. *Blood* 2005;**106**:4050–3.

87. Richardson PG, Blood E, Mitsiades CS, *et al.* A randomized phase 2 study of lenalidomide therapy for patients with relapsed or relapsed and refractory multiple myeloma. *Blood* 2006;**108**:3458–64.

88. Dispenzieri A, Rajkumar SV, Gertz MA, *et al.* Treatment of newly diagnosed multiple myeloma based on Mayo Stratification of Myeloma and Risk-adapted Therapy (mSMART): consensus statement. *Mayo Clin Proc* 2007;**82**:323–41.

89. Durie BGM, Harousseau J-L, Miguel JS, *et al.* International uniform response criteria for multiple myeloma. *Leukemia* 2006;**20**:1467–73.

90. Cavo M, Zamagni E, Tosi P, *et al.* Superiority of thalidomide and dexamethasone over vincristine-doxorubicindexamethasone (VAD) as primary therapy in preparation for autologous transplantation for multiple myeloma. *Blood* 2005; **106**:35–9.

91. Fermand J-P, Jaccard A, Macro M, *et al.* A randomized comparison of dexamethasone + thalidomide (Dex/Thal) vs dex + placebo (Dex/P) in patients (pts) with relapsing multiple myeloma (MM). *Blood* 2006;**108**:3563–.

92. Rajkumar SV, Blood E, Vesole DH, *et al.* Phase III clinical trial of thalidomide plus dexamethasone compared with dexamethasone alone in newly diagnosed multiple myeloma: a clinical trial coordinated by the Eastern Cooperative Oncology Group. *J Clin Oncol* 2006;**24**:431–6.

93. Rajkumar SV, Hussein M, Catalano J, *et al.* A randomized, double-blind, placebo-controlled trial of thalidomide plus dexamethasone versus dexamethasone alone as primary therapy for newly diagnosed multiple myeloma. *Blood* 2006;**108**:795.

94. Rajkumar SV, Rosiñol L, Hussein M, *et al.* A multicenter, randomized, double-blind, placebo-controlled study of thalidomide plus dexamethasone versus dexamethasone as initial therapy for newly diagnosed multiple myeloma. *J Clin Oncol* 2008;**26**:2171–7.

95. Rajkumar SV, Hayman S, Gertz MA, *et al.* Combination therapy with thalidomide plus dexamethasone for newly diagnosed myeloma. *J Clin Oncol* 2002;**20**:4319–23.

96. Cavo M, Zamagni E, Tosi P, *et al.* First-line therapy with thalidomide and dexamethasone in preparation for autologous stem cell transplantation for multiple myeloma. *Haematologica* 2004;**89**:826–31.

97. Lacy MQ, Gertz MA, Dispenzieri AA, *et al.* Long-term results of response to therapy, time to progression, and survival with lenalidomide plus dexamethasone in newly diagnosed myeloma. *Mayo Clin Proc* 2007;**82**:1179–84.

98. Rajkumar SV, Jacobus S, Callander N, *et al.* A randomized phase III trial of lenalidomide plus high-dose dexamethasone versus lenalidomide plus low-dose dexamethasone in newly diagnosed multiple myeloma (E4A03): a trial coordinated by the Eastern Cooperative Oncology Group. *Blood* 2006;**108**:799.

99. Kumar S, Dispenzieri A, Lacy MQ, *et al.* Impact of lenalidomide therapy on stem cell mobilization and engraftment post-peripheral blood stem cell transplantation in patients with newly diagnosed myeloma. *Leukemia* 2007;**21**:2035–42.

100. Mazumder A, Kaufman J, Niesvizky R, *et al.* Effect of lenalidomide therapy on mobilization of peripheral blood stem cells in previously untreated multiple myeloma patients. *Leukemia* 2008;**22**:1280–1; author reply 1281–2.

101. Richardson PG, Chanan-Khan A, Schlossman RL, *et al.* Phase II trial of single agent bortezomib (VELCADE®) in patients with previously untreated multiple myeloma (MM). *Blood* 2004;**104**:100a (A336).

102. Jagannath S, Durie BG, Wolf J, *et al.* Bortezomib therapy alone and in combination with dexamethasone for previously untreated symptomatic multiple myeloma. *Br J Haematol* 2005;**129**:776–83.

103. Harousseau J, Attal M, Leleu X, *et al.* Bortezomib plus dexamethasone as induction treatment prior to autologous stem cell transplantation in patients with newly diagnosed multiple myeloma: results of an IFM phase II study. *Haematologica* 2006;**91**:1498–505.

104. Harousseau J-L, Marit G, Caillot D, *et al.* VELCADE/dexamethasone (Vel/Dex) versus VAD as induction treatment prior to autologous stem cell transplantation (ASCT) in newly diagnosed multiple myeloma (MM): an interim analysis of the IFM 2005-01 randomized multicenter phase III trial. *Blood* 2006;**108**:56.

105. San-Miguel J, Harousseau JL, Joshua D, *et al.* Individualizing treatment of patients with myeloma in the era of novel agents. *J Clin Oncol* 2008;**26**:2761–6.

106. Kyle RA, Rajkumar SV. Multiple myeloma. *Blood* 2008;**111**:2962–72.

107. Myeloma Trialists' Collaborative Group. Combination chemotherapy versus melphalan plus prednisone as treatment for multiple myeloma: an overview of 6,633 patients from 27 randomized trials. *J Clin Oncol* 1998;**16**:3832–42.

108. Facon T, Mary JY, Hulin C, *et al.* Melphalan and prednisone plus thalidomide versus melphalan and prednisone alone or reduced-intensity autologous stem cell transplantation in elderly patients with multiple myeloma (IFM 99-06): a randomised trial. *Lancet* 2007;**370**:1209–18.

109. Hulin C, Facon T, Rodon P, *et al.* Melphalan-prednisone-thalidomide (MP-T) demonstrates a significant survival advantage in elderly patients $\geq$ 75 years with multiple myeloma compared with melphalan-prednisone (MP) in a randomized, double-blind, placebo-controlled trial, IFM 01/01. *ASH Annual Meeting Abstracts* 2007;**110**:75.

110. Waage A, Gimsing P, Juliusson G, *et al.* Melphalan-prednisone-thalidomide to newly diagnosed patients with multiple myeloma: a placebo controlled randomised phase 3 trial. *ASH Annual Meeting Abstracts* 2007; **110**:78.

111. Facon T, Mary JY, Hulin C, *et al.* Major superiority of melphalan–prednisone (MP) + thalidomide (THAL) over MP and autologous stem cell transplantation in the treatment of newly diagnosed elderly patients with multiple myeloma. *Blood* 2005;**106**:230a (A780).

112. Palumbo A, Bringhen S, Caravita T, *et al.* Oral melphalan and prednisone chemotherapy plus thalidomide compared with melphalan and prednisone alone in elderly patients with multiple myeloma: randomised controlled trial. *Lancet* 2006;**367**:825–31.

113. Mateos M-V, Hernandez J-M, Hernandez M-T, *et al.* Bortezomib plus melphalan and prednisone in elderly untreated patients with multiple myeloma: results of a multicenter phase 1/2 study. *Blood* 2006;**108**:2165–72.

114. San Miguel JF, Schlag R, Khuageva NK, *et al.* Bortezomib plus melphalan and prednisone for initial treatment of multiple myeloma. *N Engl J Med* 2008;**359**:906–17.

115. Palumbo A, Falco P, Corradini P, *et al.* Melphalan, prednisone, and lenalidomide treatment for newly diagnosed myeloma: a report from the GIMEMA Italian Multiple Myeloma Network. *J Clin Oncol* 2007;**25**:4459–65.

116. Attal M, Harousseau JL, Stoppa AM, *et al.* A prospective, randomized trial of autologous bone marrow transplantation and chemotherapy in multiple myeloma. Intergroupe Francais du Myelome. *N Engl J Med* 1996;**335**:91–7.

117. Child JA, Morgan GJ, Davies FE, *et al.* High-dose chemotherapy with hematopoietic stem-cell rescue for multiple myeloma. *N Engl J Med* 2003;**348**:1875–83.

118. Blade J, Vesole DH, Gertz M. Transplantation for multiple myeloma: who, when, how often? *Blood* 2003;**102**:3469–77.

119. Kumar A, Loughran T, Alsina M, *et al.* Management of multiple myeloma: a systematic review and critical appraisal of published studies. *Lancet Oncol* 2003;**4**:293–304.

120. Moreau P, Facon T, Attal M, *et al.* Comparison of 200 mg/m^2 melphalan and 8 Gy total body irradiation plus 140 mg/m^2 melphalan as conditioning regimens for peripheral blood stem cell transplantation in patients with newly diagnosed multiple myeloma: final analysis of the Intergroupe Francophone du Myélome 9502 randomized trial. *Blood* 2002;**99**:731–5.

121. Bensinger W, Giralt S, Holmberg L, *et al.* 166H0-DOTMP and high-dose melphalan before autologous peripheral blood stem cell transplantation in patients with multiple myeloma. *Hematol J* 2003;**4** Suppl 1:S215–16.

122. Dispenzieri A, Wiseman GA, Lacy MQ, *et al.* A phase II study of high dose 153-samarium EDMTP (153-Sm EDMTP) and melphalan for peripheral stem cell transplantation (PBSCT) in multiple myeloma (MM). *Blood* 2003;**102**:982a.

123. Fermand JP, Ravaud P, Chevret S, *et al.* High-dose therapy and autologous peripheral blood stem cell transplantation in multiple myeloma: up-front or rescue treatment? Results of a multicenter sequential randomized clinical trial. *Blood* 1998;**92**:3131–6.

124. Facon T, Mary JY, Harousseau JL, *et al.* Front-line or rescue autologous bone marrow transplantation (ABMT) following a first course of high dose melphalan (HDM) in multiple myeloma (MM). Preliminary results of a prospective randomized trial (CIAM) protocol. *Blood* 1996;**88** Suppl 1:685a.

125. Barlogie B, Kyle R, Anderson K, *et al.* Comparable survival in multiple myeloma (MM) with high dose therapy (HDT) employing MEL 140 mg/m^2 + TBI 12 Gy autotransplants versus standard dose therapy with VBMCP and no benefit from interferon (IFN) maintenance: results of Intergroup Trial S9321. *Blood* 2003;**102**:42a.

126. Blade J, Sureda A, Ribera JM, *et al.* High-dose therapy autotransplantation/intensification versus continued conventional chemotherapy in multiple myeloma patients responding to initial chemotherapy. Definitive results from PETHEMA after a median follow-up of 66 months. *Blood* 2003;**102**:42a.

127. Rajkumar SV, Fonseca R, Lacy MQ, *et al.* Autologous stem cell transplantation for relapsed and primary refractory myeloma. *Bone Marrow Transplant* 1999;**23**:1267–72.

128. Blade J, Esteve J. Treatment approaches for relapsing and refractory multiple myeloma. [44 refs]. *Acta Oncologica* 2000;**39**:843–7.

129. Barlogie B, Jagannath S, Vesole DH, *et al.* Superiority of tandem autologous transplantation over standard therapy for previously untreated multiple myeloma. *Blood* 1997;**89**:789–93.

130. Attal M, Harousseau JL, Facon T, *et al.* Double autologous transplantation improves survival of multiple myeloma patients: final analysis of a prospective randomized study of the "Intergroupe Francophone du Myelome" (IFM 94). *Blood* 2002;**100**:5a.

131. Cavo M, Cellini C, Zamagni E, *et al.* Superiority of double over single autologous stem cell transplantation as first-line therapy for multiple myeloma. *Blood* 2004;**104**:155a (A536).

132. Fermand JP, Alberti C, Marolleau JP. Single versus tandem high dose therapy (HDT) supported with autologous blood stem cell (ABSC) transplantation using unselected or CD34-enriched ABSC: results of a two by two designed randomized trial in 230 young patients with multiple myeloma (MM). *Hematol J* 2003;**4** Suppl 1:S59.

133. Goldschmidt H. Single vs. tandem autologous transplantation in multiple myeloma: the GMMG experience. *Hematol J* 2003;**4** Suppl 1:S61.

134. Sirohi B, Powles R, Singhal S, *et al.* High-dose melphalan and second autografts for myeloma relapsing after one autograft: results equivalent to tandem autotransplantation. *Blood* 2001;**98**:402a (A1690).

135. Mehta J, Singhal S. Graft-versus-myeloma. *Bone Marrow Transplant* 1998;**22**:835–43.

136. Gahrton G, Svensson H, Cavo M, *et al.* Progress in allogenic bone marrow and peripheral blood stem cell transplantation for multiple myeloma: a

comparison between transplants performed 1983–93 and 1994–8 at European Group for Blood and Marrow Transplantation centres. *Br J Haematol* 2001;**113**:209–16.

137. Einsele H, Schafer HJ, Hebart H, *et al.* Follow-up of patients with progressive multiple myeloma undergoing allografts after reduced-intensity conditioning. *Br J Haematol* 2003;**121**:411–18.

138. Crawley C, Lalancette M, Szydlo R, *et al.* Outcomes for reduced-intensity allogeneic transplantation for multiple myeloma: an analysis of prognostic factors from the Chronic Leukaemia Working Party of the EBMT. *Blood* 2005;**105**:4532–9.

139. Maloney DG, Molina AJ, Sahebi F, *et al.* Allografting with nonmyeloablative conditioning following cytoreductive autografts for the treatment of patients with multiple myeloma. *Blood* 2003;**102**:3447–54.

140. Garban F, Attal M, Michallet M, *et al.* Prospective comparison of autologous stem cell transplantation followed by dose-reduced allograft (IFM99-03 trial) with tandem autologous stem cell transplantation (IFM99-04 trial) in high-risk de novo multiple myeloma. *Blood* 2006;**107**:3474–80.

141. Jagannath S, Richardson PG, Sonneveld P, *et al.* Bortezomib appears to overcome the poor prognosis conferred by chromosome 13 deletion in phase 2 and 3 trials. *Leukemia* 2006;**21**:151–7.

142. Sagaster V, Ludwig H, Kaufmann H, *et al.* Bortezomib in relapsed multiple myeloma: response rates and duration of response are independent of a chromosome 13q-deletion. *Leukemia* 2006;**21**:164–8.

143. Myeloma Trialists' Collaborative Group. Interferon as therapy for multiple myeloma: an individual patient data overview of 24 randomized trials and 4012 patients. *Br J Haematol* 2001;**113**:1020–34.

144. Barlogie B, Kyle RA, Anderson KC, *et al.* Standard chemotherapy compared with high-dose chemoradiotherapy for multiple myeloma: final results of phase III US Intergroup Trial S9321. *J Clin Oncol* 2006;**24**:929–36.

145. Berenson JR, Crowley JJ, Grogan TM, *et al.* Maintenance therapy with alternate-day prednisone improves survival in multiple myeloma patients. *Blood* 2002;**99**:3163–8.

146. Attal M, Harousseau J-L, Leyvraz S, *et al.* Maintenance therapy with thalidomide improves survival in patients with multiple myeloma. *Blood* 2006;**108**:3289–94.

147. Abdelkefi A, Ladeb S, Torjman L, *et al.* Single autologous stem-cell transplantation followed by maintenance therapy with thalidomide is superior to double autologous transplantation in multiple myeloma: results of a multicenter randomized clinical trial. *Blood* 2008;**111**: 1805–10.

148. Gertz MA, Lacy MQ, Inwards DJ, *et al.* Early harvest and late transplantation as an effective therapeutic strategy in multiple myeloma. *Bone Marrow Transplant* 1999;**23**:221–6.

149. Alexanian R, Barlogie B, Dixon D. High-dose glucocorticoid treatment of resistant myeloma. *Ann Intern Med* 1986;**105**:8–11.

150. Gertz MA, Garton JP, Greipp PR, *et al.* A phase II study of high-dose methylprednisolone in refractory or relapsed multiple myeloma. *Leukemia* 1995;**9**:2115–18.

151. Barlogie B, Spencer T, Tricot G, *et al.* Long term follow up of 169 patients receiving a phase II trial of single agent thalidomide for advanced and refractory multiple myeloma (MM). *Blood* 2000;**96**:514a (A2213).

152. Dimopoulos MA, Anagnostopoulos A, Weber D. Treatment of plasma cell dyscrasias with thalidomide and its derivatives. *J Clin Oncol* 2003; **21**:4444–54.

153. Kumar S, Witzig TE, Rajkumar SV. Thalidomide – current role in the treatment of non-plasma cell malignancies. *J Clin Oncol* 2004;**22**:2477–88.

154. Richardson P, Schlossman R, Jagannath S, *et al.* Thalidomide for patients with relapsed multiple myeloma after high-dose chemotherapy and stem cell transplantation: results of an open-label multicenter phase 2 study of efficacy, toxicity, and biological activity. *Mayo Clin Proc* 2004;**79**:875–82.

155. Kumar S, Gertz MA, Dispenzieri A, *et al.* Response rate, durability of response, and survival after thalidomide therapy for relapsed multiple myeloma. [comment]. *Mayo Clin Proc* 2003;**78**:34–9.

156. Juliusson G, Celsing F, Turesson I, *et al.* Thalidomide frequently induces good partial remission and best response ever in patients with advanced multiple myeloma and prior high dose melphalan and autotransplant. *Blood* 1999;**94** Suppl 1:124a (A546).

157. Anagnostopoulos A, Weber D, Rankin K, *et al.* Thalidomide and dexamethasone for resistant multiple myeloma. *Br J Haematol* 2003; **121**:768–71.

158. Dimopoulos MA, Hamilos G, Zomas A, *et al.* Pulsed cyclophosphamide, thalidomide and dexamethasone: an oral regimen for previously treated patients with multiple myeloma. *Hematol J* 2004;**5**:112–17.

159. Garcia-Sanz R, Gonzalez-Fraile MI, Sierra M, *et al.* The combination of thalidomide, cyclophosphamide and dexamethasone (ThaCyDex) is feasible and can be an option for relapsed/ refractory multiple myeloma. *Hematol J* 2002;**3**:43–8.

160. Kropff MH, Lang N, Bisping G, *et al.* Hyperfractionated cyclophosphamide in combination with pulsed dexamethasone and thalidomide (HyperCDT) in primary refractory or relapsed multiple myeloma. *Br J Haematol* 2003;**122**:607–16.

161. Coleman M, Leonard J, Lyons L, *et al.* BLT-D (clarithromycin [Biaxin], low-dose thalidomide, and dexamethasone) for the treatment of myeloma and Waldenstrom's macroglobulinemia. *Leuk Lymphoma* 2002;**43**:1777–82.

162. Adams J. Proteasome inhibitors as new anticancer drugs. *Curr Opin Oncol* 2002;**14**:628–34.

163. Rajkumar SV, Richardson PG, Hideshima T, *et al.* Proteasome inhibition as a novel therapeutic target in human cancer. *J Clin Oncol* 2004;**23**:630–9.

164. Berenson JR, Jagannath S, Barlogie B, *et al.* Experience with long-term therapy using the proteasome inhibitor, bortezomib, in advanced multiple myeloma (MM). *Proc Am Soc Clin Oncol* 2003;**22**:581.

165. Richardson PG, Sonneveld P, Schuster M, *et al.* Extended follow-up of a phase 3 trial in relapsed multiple myeloma: final time-to-event results

of the APEX trial. *Blood* 2007;**110**: 3557–60.

166. Orlowski RZ, Voorhees PM, Garcia R, *et al.* Phase I study of the proteasome inhibitor bortezomib and pegylated liposomal doxorubicin in patients with refractory hematologic malignancies. *Proc Am Soc Clin Oncol* 2003;**22**:200.

167. Orlowski RZ, Zhuang SH, Parekh T, *et al.* The DOXIL-MMY-3001 Study Investigators. The combination of pegylated liposomal doxorubicin and bortezomib significantly improves time to progression of patients with relapsed/refractory multiple myeloma compared with bortezomib alone: results from a planned interim analysis of a randomized phase III study. *ASH Annual Meeting Abstracts* 2006; **108**:404.

168. Zangari M, Barlogie B, Burns MJ, *et al.* Velcade (V)-thalidomide (T)-dexamethasone (D) for advanced and refractory multiple myeloma (MM): long-term follow-up of phase I-II trial UARK 2001-37: superior outcome in patients with normal cytogenetics and no prior T. *ASH Annual Meeting Abstracts* 2005;**106**:2552.

169. Zangari M, Tricot G, Zeldis J, *et al.* Results of phase I study of CC-5013 for the treatment of multiple myeloma (MM) patients who relapse after high dose chemotherapy (HDCT). *Blood* 2001:775a (A3226).

170. Richardson PG, Schlossman RL, Weller E, *et al.* Immunomodulatory drug CC-5013 overcomes drug resistance and is well tolerated in patients with relapsed multiple myeloma. *Blood* 2002;**100**:3063–7.

171. Dimopoulos MA, Spencer A, Attal M, *et al.* Study of lenalidomide plus dexamethasone versus dexamethasone alone in relapsed or refractory multiple myeloma (MM): results of a phase 3 study (MM-010). *Blood* 2005;**106**:6.

172. Weber DM, Chen C, Niesvizky R, *et al.* Lenalidomide plus high-dose dexamethasone provides improved overall survival compared to high-dose dexamethasone alone for relapsed or refractory multiple myeloma (MM): results of a North American phase III study (MM-009). *Proc Am Soc Clin Oncol* 2006;**24**:A7521.

173. Hideshima T, Chauhan D, Podar K, *et al.* Novel therapies targeting the myeloma cell and its bone marrow microenvironment. *Semin Oncol* 2001;**28**:607–12.

174. Munshi NC. Arsenic trioxide: an emerging therapy for multiple myeloma. *Oncologist* 2001;**6** Suppl 2:17–21.

175. Streetly M, Jones RW, Knight R, *et al.* An update of the use and outcomes of the new immunomodulatory agent CC-4047 (actimid) in patients with relapsed/refractory myeloma. *Blood* 2003;**102**:236a.

176. Gucalp R, Theriault R, Gill I, *et al.* Treatment of cancer-associated hypercalcemia. Double-blind comparison of rapid and slow intravenous infusion regimens of pamidronate disodium and saline alone. *Arch Intern Med* 1994;**154**:1935–44.

177. Major P, Lortholary A, Hon J, *et al.* Zoledronic acid is superior to pamidronate in the treatment of hypercalcemia of malignancy: a pooled analysis of two randomized, controlled clinical trials. *J Clin Oncol* 2001; **19**:558–67.

178. Berenson JR, Lichtenstein A, Porter L, *et al.* Efficacy of pamidronate in reducing skeletal events in patients with advanced multiple myeloma. Myeloma Aredia Study Group. [see comments]. *N Engl J Med* 1996;**334**:488–93.

179. Berenson JR, Rosen LS, Howell A, *et al.* Zoledronic acid reduces skeletal-related events in patients with osteolytic metastases. [Erratum appears in *Cancer* 2001 May 15;**91**(10):1956.] *Cancer* 2001;**91**:1191–200.

180. Rosen LS, Gordon D, Kaminski M, *et al.* Zoledronic acid versus pamidronate in the treatment of skeletal metastases in patients with breast cancer or osteolytic lesions of multiple myeloma: a phase II, double blind, comparative trial. *Cancer J* 2001;**7**:377–87.

181. Berenson JR, Hillner BE, Kyle RA, *et al.* American Society of Clinical Oncology Clinical Practice Guidelines: The role of bisphosphonates in multiple myeloma. *J Clin Oncol* 2002;**20**:3719–36.

182. Marx RE. Pamidronate (Aredia) and zoledronate (Zometa) induced avascular necrosis of the jaws: a growing epidemic.[see comment]. *J Oral Maxillofac Surg* 2003;**61**: 1115–17.

183. Kademani D, Koka S, Lacy MQ, *et al.* Primary surgical therapy for osteonecrosis of the jaw secondary to bisphosphonate therapy. *Mayo Clin Proc* 2006;**81**:1100–3.

184. Badros A, Weikel D, Salama A, *et al.* Osteonecrosis of the jaw in multiple myeloma patients: clinical features and risk factors. *J Clin Oncol* 2006;**24**:945–52.

185. Durie BG, Katz M, Crowley J. Osteonecrosis of the jaw and bisphosphonates. *N Engl J Med* 2005;**353**:99–102; discussion 99–102.

186. Ruggiero SL, Mehrotra B, Rosenberg TJ, *et al.* Osteonecrosis of the jaws associated with the use of bisphosphonates: a review of 63 cases. *J Oral Maxillofac Surg* 2004;**62**:527–34.

187. Lacy MQ, Dispenzieri A, Gertz MA, *et al.* Mayo clinic consensus statement for the use of bisphosphonates in multiple myeloma. *Mayo Clin Proc* 2006;**81**:1047–53.

188. Dimopoulos MA, Kastritis E, Anagnostopoulos A, *et al.* Osteonecrosis of the jaw in patients with multiple myeloma treated with bisphosphonates: evidence of increased risk after treatment with zoledronic acid. *Haematologica* 2006;**91**:968–71.

189. Melton LJ, 3rd, Kyle RA, Achenbach SJ, *et al.* Fracture risk with multiple myeloma: a population-based study. *J Bone Miner Res* 2005;**20**:487–93.

190. Miller PD. Treatment of osteoporosis in chronic kidney disease and end-stage renal disease. *Curr Osteoporos Rep* 2005;**3**:5–12.

191. Fourney DR, Schomer DF, Nader R, *et al.* Percutaneous vertebroplasty and kyphoplasty for painful vertebral body fractures in cancer patients. *J Neurosurg* 2003;**98**:21–30.

192. Yussim E, Schwartz E, Sidi Y, *et al.* Acute renal failure precipitated by non-steroidal anti-inflammatory drugs (NSAIDs) in multiple myeloma. *Am J Hematol* 1998;**58**:142–4.

193. Wu MJ, Kumar KS, Kulkarni G, *et al.* Multiple myeloma in naproxen-induced acute renal failure. *N Engl J Med* 1987;**317**:170–1.

194. Johnson WJ, Kyle RA, Pineda AA, *et al.* Treatment of renal failure associated with multiple myeloma. Plasmapheresis, hemodialysis, and chemotherapy. *Arch Intern Med* 1990;**150**:863–9.

195. Garton JP, Gertz MA, Witzig TE, *et al.* Epoetin alfa for the treatment of the anemia of multiple myeloma.

A prospective, randomized, placebo-controlled, double-blind trial. *Arch Intern Med* 1995;**155**:2069–74.

196. Dammacco F, Castoldi G, Rodjer S. Efficacy of epoetin alfa in the treatment of anaemia of multiple myeloma. [Erratum appears in *Br J Haematol* 2001 Sep;**114**(3):738.] *Br J Haematol* 2001;**113**:172–9.

197. Oken MM, Pomeroy C, Weisdorf D, *et al.* Prophylactic antibiotics for the prevention of early infection in multiple myeloma. *Am J Med* 1996;**100**:624–8.

198. Gertz MA, Kyle RA. Hyperviscosity syndrome. *J Intensive Care Med* 1995;**10**:128–41.

199. Weber D, Rankin K, Gavino M, *et al.* Thalidomide alone or with dexamethasone for previously untreated multiple myeloma. *J Clin Oncol* 2003;**21**:16–19.

200. Barlogie B, Desikan R, Eddlemon P, *et al.* Extended survival in advanced and refractory multiple myeloma after single-agent thalidomide: identification of prognostic factors in a phase 2 study of 169 patients. *Blood* 2001;**98**:492–4.

201. Palumbo A, Rajkumar SV, Dimopoulos MA, *et al.* Prevention of thalidomide- and lenalidomide-associated thrombosis in myeloma. *Leukemia* 2008;**22**:414–23.

202. Osman K, Comenzo R, Rajkumar SV. Deep vein thrombosis and thalidomide therapy for multiple myeloma. *N Engl J Med* 2001;**344**:1951–2.

203. Zangari M, Anaissie E, Barlogie B, *et al.* Increased risk of deep-vein thrombosis in patients with multiple myeloma receiving thalidomide and chemotherapy. *Blood* 2001;**98**:1614–15.

204. Zangari M, Siegel E, Barlogie B, *et al.* Thrombogenic activity of doxorubicin in myeloma patients receiving thalidomide: implications for therapy. *Blood* 2002;**100**:1168–71.

205. Rajkumar SV, Blood E. Lenalidomide and venous thrombosis in multiple myeloma. *N Engl J Med* 2006;**354**: 2079–80.

206. Zeldis JB, Williams BA, Thomas SD, *et al.* S.T.E.P.S.: a comprehensive program for controlling and monitoring access to thalidomide. *Clin Ther* 1999;**21**:319–30.

207. Rajkumar SV, Gertz MA, Witzig TE. Life-threatening toxic epidermal necrolysis with thalidomide therapy for myeloma. *N Engl J Med* 2000; **343**:972–3.

208. Dimopoulos MA, Eleutherakis-Papaiakovou V. Adverse effects of thalidomide administration in patients with neoplastic diseases. *Am J Med* 2004;**117**:508–15.

209. Badros AZ, Siegel E, Bodenner D, *et al.* Hypothyroidism in patients with multiple myeloma following treatment with thalidomide. *Am J Med* 2002;**112**:412–13.

210. Menon S, Habermann T, Witzig T. Lenalidomide-associated hypothyroidism. *Leuk Lymphoma* 2007;**48**:2465–7.

211. Stein EM, Rivera C. Transient thyroiditis after treatment with lenalidomide in a patient with metastatic renal cell carcinoma. *Thyroid* 2007;**17**:681–3.

212. Kastritis E, Dimopoulos MA. Thalidomide in the treatment of multiple myeloma. *Best Pract Res Clin Haematol* 2007;**20**:681–99.

213. Eriksson T, Hoglund P, Turesson I, *et al.* Pharmacokinetics of thalidomide in patients with impaired renal function and while on and off dialysis. *J Pharm Pharmacol* 2003;**55**:1701–6.

214. Chen N, Lau H, Kong L, *et al.* Pharmacokinetics of lenalidomide in subjects with various degrees of renal impairment and in subjects on hemodialysis. *J Clin Pharmacol* 2007;**47**:1466–75.

215. De Gramont A, Grosbois B, Michaux JL, *et al.* Myelome a IgM: 6 observations et revue de la litterature. *Rev Med Interne* 1990;**11**:13–18.

216. Mansoor A, Medeiros LJ, Weber DM, *et al.* Cytogenetic findings in lymphoplasmacytic lymphoma/ Waldenstrom macroglobulinemia. Chromosomal abnormalities are associated with the polymorphous subtype and an aggressive clinical course. *Am J Clin Pathol* 2001; **116**:543–9.

217. Wong KF, So CC. Waldenstrom macroglobulinemia with karyotypic aberrations involving both homologous 6q. *Cancer Genet Cytogenet* 2001;**124**:137–9.

218. Jankovic GM, Colovic MD, Wiernik PH, *et al.* Multiple karyotypic aberrations in a polymorphous variant of Waldenstrom macroglobulinemia. *Cancer Genet Cytogenet* 1999; **111**:77–80.

219. Schop RF, Jalal SM, Van Wier SA, *et al.* Deletions of 17p13.1 and 13q14 are uncommon in Waldenstrom macroglobulinemia clonal cells and mostly seen at the time of disease progression. *Cancer Genet Cytogenet* 2002;**132**:55–60.

220. Avet-Loiseau H, Garand R, Lode L, *et al.* 14q32 translocations discriminate IgM multiple myeloma from Waldenstrom's macroglobulinemia. *Semin Oncol* 2003;**30**:153–5.

221. Blade J, Kyle RA. Nonsecretory myeloma, immunoglobulin D myeloma, and plasma cell leukemia. *Hematol Oncol Clin North Am* 1999;**13**:1259–72.

222. Dimopoulos MA, Palumbo A, Delasalle KB, *et al.* Primary plasma cell leukaemia. *Br J Haematol* 1994; **88**:754–9.

223. Tiedemann RE, Gonzalez-Paz N, Kyle RA, *et al.* Genetic aberrations and survival in plasma cell leukemia. *Leukemia* 2008;**22**:1044–52.

224. Garcia-Sanz R, Orfao A, Gonzalez M, *et al.* Primary plasma cell leukemia: clinical, immunophenotypic, DNA ploidy, and cytogenetic characteristics. *Blood* 1999;**93**:1032–7.

225. Avet-Loiseau H, Gerson F, Magrangeas F, *et al.* Rearrangements of the c-myc oncogene are present in 15% of primary human multiple myeloma tumors. *Blood* 2001;**98**:3082–6.

226. Saez B, Martin-Subero JI, Guillen-Grima F, *et al.* Chromosomal abnormalities clustering in multiple myeloma reveals cytogenetic subgroups with nonrandom acquisition of chromosomal changes. *Leukemia* 2004;**18**:654–7.

227. Smadja NV, Bastard C, Brigaudeau C, *et al.* Groupe Francais de Cytogenetique Hématologique. Hypodiploidy is a major prognostic factor in multiple myeloma. *Blood* 2001;**98**: 2229–38.

228. Rajkumar SV, Kyle RA. Multiple myeloma: diagnosis and treatment. *Mayo Clin Proc* 2005;**80**: 1371–82.

229. Kyle RA, Therneau TM, Rajkumar SV, *et al.* Long-term follow-up of IgM monoclonal gammopathy of

undetermined significance. *Blood* 2003;**102**:3759–64.

230. Gobbi PG, Baldini L, Broglia C, *et al.* Prognostic validation of the international classification of immunoglobulin M gammopathies: a survival advantage for patients with immunoglobulin M monoclonal gammopathy of undetermined significance? *Clin Cancer Res* 2005;**11**:1786–90.

231. Kyle RA, Therneau TM, Rajkumar SV, *et al.* Long-term follow-up of IgM monoclonal gammopathy of undetermined significance. *Semin Oncol* 2003;**30**:169–71.

232. Baldini L, Goldaniga M, Guffanti A, *et al.* Immunoglobulin M monoclonal gammopathies of undetermined significance and indolent Waldenstrom's macroglobulinemia recognize the same determinants of evolution into symptomatic lymphoid disorders: proposal for a common prognostic scoring system. *J Clin Oncol* 2005;**23**:4662–8.

233. Owen RG, Treon SP, Al-Katib A, *et al.* Clinicopathological definition of Waldenstrom's macroglobulinemia: consensus panel recommendations from the Second International Workshop on Waldenstrom's Macroglobulinemia. *Semin Oncol* 2003;**30**:110–15.

234. Dimopoulos MA, Kiamouris C, Moulopoulos LA. Solitary plasmacytoma of bone and extramedullary plasmacytoma. *Hematol Oncol Clin North Am* 1999;**13**:1249–57.

235. Rajkumar SV, Dispenzieri A, Kyle RA. Monoclonal gammopathy of undetermined significance, Waldenstrom macroglobulinemia, AL amyloidosis, and related plasma cell disorders: diagnosis and treatment. *Mayo Clin Proc* 2006;**81**:693–703.

236. Dispenzieri A, Kyle RA, Lacy MQ, *et al.* POEMS syndrome: definitions and long-term outcome. *Blood* 2003;**101**: 2496–506.

237. Wang M, Delasalle K, Giralt S, *et al.* Rapid control of previously untreated multiple myeloma with bortezomib-thalidomide-dexamethasone followed by early intensive therapy. *Blood* 2005;**106**:784.

Chapter 11

Amyloidosis and other rare plasma cell dyscrasias

Angela Dispenzieri and Suzanne R. Hayman

Introduction

The spectrum of plasma cell disorders is vast. From a proliferation standpoint, the spectrum extends from the premalignant monoclonal gammopathy of undetermined significance (MGUS) to multiple myeloma, to plasma cell leukemia. The picture, however, is much more complex because there are also low tumor burden and low proliferation plasma cell diseases responsible for a clinical phenotype ranging from troublesome to fatal. These conditions are rare, but must be recognized in order to reduce morbidity and mortality. For most of these diseases, the pathogenesis is not well understood.

The discussion will begin with the three more common and potentially life-threatening disorders, light chain amyloidosis (AL), POEMS syndrome (polyradiculoneuropathy, organomegaly, endocrinopathy, monoclonal protein, skin changes), and cryoglobulinemia. Subsequently, the monoclonal gammopathy-associated disease entities will be parsed according to their dominant clinical feature – neuropathy, dermopathy, and nephropathy – and will include: MGUS-associated peripheral neuropathy, scleromyxedema, xanthogranulosum necrobiotica, and Schnitzler's syndrome.

Immunoglobulin light chain amyloidosis

Immunoglobulin light chain amyloidosis (AL) is a low tumor burden plasma cell disorder characterized by deposition of insoluble fibrils composed of immunoglobulin light chains. Without treatment, it has an inexorable progressive course due to uncontrolled tissue damage. Not all amyloidosis is related to a plasma cell dyscrasia. Although AL is the most common form of systemic amyloidosis, with an incidence of approximately 1 case per 100 000 person-years in Western countries,[1] there are other forms of systemic amyloidosis as well (Table 11.1). It is imperative that the amyloid be typed to ascertain which type of amyloidosis is present in order to direct the treatment plan accordingly.

Diagnosis

There are four essential steps in diagnosing amyloidosis: (1) consider the diagnosis; (2) make the diagnosis by tissue biopsy; (3) determine the precursor protein; and (4) define the extent of involvement. Perhaps the biggest challenge for patients with AL is having the diagnosis considered in timely fashion. Often it is a physician other than a hematologist/oncologist who is charged with thinking about diagnosis. Although features like periorbital purpura and macroglossia are nearly pathognomonic, they are rare and cannot be relied upon to trigger consideration of a diagnosis of AL. The most commonly affected organs resulting in symptoms are the heart, kidneys, skin, peripheral nerves, autonomic nerves, and liver. Although the gastrointestinal tract is commonly biopsy positive, it is relatively uncommon for patients to have symptoms referable to it. As shown in Figure 11.1 the dominant symptomatic organ system involved varies among different practices.[3]

Once the diagnosis is suspected, a monoclonal protein in the serum and the urine should be sought and a tissue biopsy performed. Screening for a monoclonal protein is done by serum immunoglobulin free light chain measurement and immunofixation studies of the serum and urine, although an important part of the workup, serum and 24-hour urine protein electrophoresis, are insufficient as screening tools. The biopsy may be of the tissue causing symptoms or of a more accessible tissue, like fat or bone marrow. The sensitivity of a biopsy of a symptomatic organ is much higher than that of the more accessible tissues, i.e., more than 95% for symptomatic tissue, 75–80% for fat, and 50–65% for bone marrow. A diagnosis of amyloidosis is not made by hematoxylin and eosin staining alone; rather special stains like Congo red, thioflavin T, and sulfated Alcian blue are required. Congo red avidity is not sufficient; apple-green birefringence under polarized light is essential for a diagnosis. Electron microscopy is also helpful to identify the 8–11 nanometer non-branching fibrils. Once a diagnosis of amyloidosis is made, typing is required by subjecting the amyloid to direct sequencing,

Management of Hematologic Malignancies, ed. Susan M. O'Brien, Julie M. Vose, and Hagop M. Kantarjian. Published by Cambridge University Press.

Table 11.1. Classification of the most common amyloidoses

Type of amyloidosis	Precursor protein component	Clinical presentation
AL amyloidosis[a] (previously referred to as primary amyloidosis)	κ or λ immunoglobulin light chain	Primary or localized; see text for syndromes
AA amyloidosis (previously referred to as secondary amyloidosis)	Serum amyloid A protein	Renal presentation most common; associated with chronic inflammatory conditions; typically acquired, but hereditary in case of familial Mediterranean fever
ATTR amyloidosis		
[b]Mutated TTR (commonly referred to as familial amyloid polyneuropathy)	Mutant TTR	Hereditary; peripheral neuropathy and/or cardiomyopathy
Wild-type TTR[b] (senile amyloidosis)	Normal TTR	Restrictive cardiomyopathy; carpal tunnel syndrome
β_2-microglobulin amyloidosis (associated with long-term dialysis)	β_2-microglobulin	Carpal tunnel syndrome
Aβ amyloidosis	Aβ protein precursor	Alzheimer disease
Other hereditary amyloidosis		
A fibrinogen (also called familial renal amyloidosis)	Fibrinogen α-chain	Renal presentation
Lysozyme	Lysozyme	Renal presentation most common
Apolipoprotein A-I	A-I apolipoprotein	Renal presentation most common

Notes: [a]AL amyloidosis is the only form of amyloidosis that is secondary to a clonal plasma cell disorder. AL amyloidosis can be associated with multiple myeloma in approximately 10% of patients.
[b]TTR refers to transthyretin, which is commonly referred to as prealbumin.
Source: Printed from Rajkumar *et al.* with permission.[2]

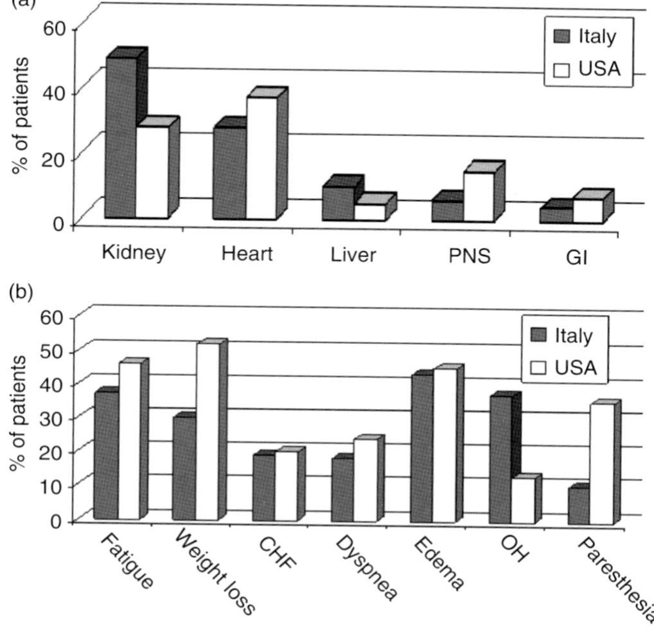

Figure 11.1 AL amyloidosis organ involvement and symptomatology. (a) Dominant organ involvement at presentation. (b) Symptoms at presentation. PNS: peripheral nervous system; GI: gastrointestinal; CHF: congestive heart failure; OH: orthostatic hypotension. Based on data from Palladini G, *et al.*[3]

immunogold, immunofluorescence, or immunohistochemistry because even the presence of serum or urine monoclonal protein does not assure a diagnosis of AL.[4,5]

Finally, a thorough assessment of extent of involvement is required in order to develop a treatment plan.[6] It is at this time that the distinction between localized and systemic AL is made. The designation "localized" applies to those cases of AL in which the precursor protein (the immunoglobulin light chain) is made at the site of amyloid deposition[7] and is typically not associated with a detectable circulating monoclonal protein in the serum or urine. The classic examples of localized AL are tracheobronchial, urinary tract, cutaneous, lymph node, and nodular cutaneous involvement. Establishing the extent of disease is achieved by a thorough review of systems and physical examination and by performing the tests shown in Table 11.2: these are required to assess prognosis and plan follow-up. The definitions of organ involvement are listed in Table 11.3.

Treatment

At present, all treatments are directed at destroying the underlying plasma cell clone, which in turn reduces or eliminates the amyloidogenic clonal immunoglobulin light chain. It had been assumed that the amyloid fibrils detected in tissue biopsies

Table 11.2. Tests required for diagnosis and staging of AL

All patients	
Tissue biopsy	Congo red stain with apple-green birefringence Type amyloid protein
Blood tests	Alkaline phosphatase
	Bilirubin
	Creatinine
	Albumin
	Troponin
	Brain natriuretic peptide or N-terminal brain natriuretic peptide
	Immunoglobulin free light chain
	Serum protein electrophoresis with immunofixation
	Factor X
24-hour urine	Protein electrophoresis with immunofixation
Echocardiogram	Assess for heart size and diastolic dysfunction
As clinically indicated	
Diagnostic imaging of liver and spleen	
Fecal fat measurements	
Serum carotene levels	
Nerve conduction studies	

were the source of tissue injury and dysfunction and that chemotherapy produced improvement in organ function by shifting the equilibrium from fibril formation and favored fibril dissolution. More recently, that hypothesis has been challenged with the hypothesis that the clonal amyloidogenic light chains form toxic intermediates responsible for the tissue damage.[9] In every day clinical practice, this debate is less important since currently there are no drugs that directly attack and/or dissolve the amyloid.

Nearly all cases of systemic AL will require therapy. Determining the extent of organ involvement helps estimate the risk associated with different treatment options. Which parameters will be followed to modulate ongoing treatment decisions should also be defined. This last recommendation cannot be overemphasized; patients with AL are complex, often very ill, and have multiple disease parameters to follow, making it difficult to track a patient's progress in a busy clinical practice. The goal in these patients is to achieve a reduction in the precursor protein (monoclonal protein), ideally complete disappearance of it; however, for some patients a mere 50% reduction of the monoclonal protein is sufficient to both halt the progression of organ damage and to allow for significant improvement of organ function (Table 11.3).[10] A priori, it is unclear which patients will require the complete hematologic response or the partial hematologic response. Therefore, the ultimate challenge in managing these patients is balancing treatment-related toxicity and efficacy.

Figure 11.2 illustrates the current treatment strategy employed for patients with systemic AL seen at the Mayo Clinic. The three most important questions relating to therapy of AL are: (1) the role of high-dose chemotherapy with peripheral blood stem cell transplantation (SCT); (2) the role of novel therapies; and (3) the relative importance of complete remission.

High-dose chemotherapy with stem cell transplant

In routine practice, the first question asked is whether a patient is a candidate for high-dose chemotherapy with SCT. Risk factors include physiologic age, performance status, cardiac function as determined by serum troponin T and functional class, and numbers of organs involved.[11–13] Capitalizing on the improved overall survival observed with patients with myeloma undergoing high-dose chemotherapy with peripheral blood SCT, SCT has been widely applied to patients with AL, and over 1000 patients have been reported in the literature. The most common conditioning regimen is melphalan 200 mg/m^2. Hematologic responses have been reported anywhere from 32% to 68% and complete hematologic responses from 16% to 50%.[13–18] Organ response is time dependent and a median time to response can take up to one year, but organ responses, the most important outcome, range anywhere from 31% to 64%. Patients with the deepest hematologic responses are more likely to have long-term overall survival.[10] The treatment-related mortality is quoted from 6% to 27% at day 100 with the majority of deaths due to cardiac causes, but patients also succumb to multiorgan failure, hepatic insufficiency, hemorrhage, and sepsis.[13–18] At Mayo Clinic, the day-100 mortality is 11%, and the median survival of patients with three-organ involvement is 30 months, with two-organ involvement 68 months, and 98 months for patients with one-organ involvement.[13] Overall survival of 337 patients is a projected median of 82 months.

A small, prospective randomized controlled trial comparing melphalan and dexamethasone to SCT did not demonstrate any improvement in overall survival for the SCT arm over the conventional chemotherapy arm (see below).[17] In contrast, a case–control study comparing overall survival of 63 AL patients undergoing SCT with 63 patients not undergoing transplantation was performed.[19] For SCT and control groups, respectively, the 1-, 2-, and 4-year overall survival rates were 89% and 71%; 81% and 55%; and 71% and 41%. Allogeneic SCT should be considered experimental in these patients. The European Group for Blood and Marrow Transplantation (EBMT) registry reported 19 patients with AL who underwent allogeneic (n = 15) or syngeneic (n = 4) SCT between 1991 and 2003.[20] With a median follow-up time of 19 months, overall and progression-free survival were 60% and 53% at 1 year, respectively. Overall, 40% of patients died of transplant-related mortality.

Table 11.3. Defining amyloid organ involvement and response to therapy

Organ system	Involvement[a]	Improvement	Worsening
Kidney	24-hour urine protein > 0.5 g/day, predominantly albumin	50% reduction in 24-hour urine protein excretion (at least 0.5 g/day) without worsening of creatinine or creatinine clearance by 25% over baseline	50% increase in urinary protein loss (at least 1 g/24 hours), or 25% worsening of creatinine or creatinine clearance
Heart	Echo: mean wall thickness > 12 mm, no other cardiac cause	≥ 2 mm reduction in the interventricular septal (IVS) thickness by echocardiogram, or	Increase in cardiac wall thickness by ≥ 2 mm (2-D ECHO), or
		Improvement of ejection fraction by ≥ 20%, or	Increase in New York Heart Association class by 1 grade with a decreasing ejection fraction of ≥ 10%
		Improvement by 2 New York Heart Association classes without an increase in diuretic use or in wall thickness	
Liver	Total liver span > 15 cm in the absence of heart failure or alkaline phosphatase > 1.5 times institutional upper limit of normal	≥ 50% decrease in an initially elevated alkaline phosphatase level, or Decrease in liver size by at least 2 cm (radiographic determination)	≥ 50% increase of alkaline phosphatase above lowest level
Nerve, peripheral	Clinical symmetric lower extremity sensorimotor peripheral neuropathy	Improvement in electromyogram nerve conduction velocity (rare)	Not defined
Nerve, autonomic	Gastric-emptying disorder, pseudo-obstruction, voiding dysfunction not related to direct organ infiltration	Not defined	Not defined
Gastrointestinal tract	Direct biopsy verification with symptoms	Not defined	Not defined
Lung	Direct biopsy verification with symptoms Interstitial radiographic pattern	Not defined	Not defined
Soft tissue	Tongue enlargement, clinical Arthropathy Claudication, presumed vascular amyloid Skin Myopathy by biopsy or pseudohypertrophy Lymph node (may be localized) Carpal tunnel	Not defined	Not defined
Hematologic		Complete response (CR): Serum and urine negative for monoclonal protein by immunofixation Free light chain ratio normal Marrow < 5% plasma cells Partial response (PR): If serum M component > 0.5 g/dL, a 50% reduction If urine light chain in urine with a visible peak and > 100 mg/day and 50% reduction If free light chain > 10 mg/dL and 50% reduction	Progression from CR: Any detectable monoclonal protein or abnormal free light chain ratio (light chain must double) Progression from PR or stable disease: 50% increase in serum M protein to > 0.5 g/dL or 50% increase in urine M protein to > 200 mg/day, or free light chain increase of 50% to > 10 mg/dL

Note: [a]Biopsy of affected organ or biopsy at an alternate site with clinical involvement.
Source: Reprinted from Gertz *et al.* with permission.[8]

Table 11.4. Standard chemotherapy for AL

	n	Hematologic response (%)	Organ response (%)	Median survival (mo)
MP[23–26]	~200	28	20–30	18–29
VBMCP[27]	49	29	31	29
Melphalan IV (25 mg/m^2 every 4–6 weeks)[28]		50	Not stated	~50
Melphalan-Dex[17,29]	96	52–67	39–48	57–60
Dex[30,31]	77	Not stated	15–35	12–21
Dex-IFN[32]	93	33	Not stated	29
VAD[28,33–37]	~100	42–50	Not stated	Not stated

Note: MP: melphalan and prednisone; VBMCP: vincinstine, carmustine (BCNU), melphalan, cyclophosphamide, and prednisone; Dex: dexamethasone; IFN: interferon; VAD: vincinstine, doxorubicin, and dexamethasone.

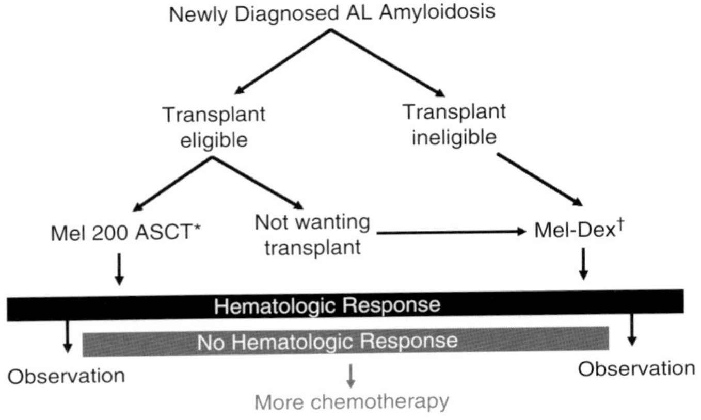

Figure 11.2 Mayo Clinic treatment algorithm.
*Consider second-line therapy if either hematologic partial response not achieved at day +100 or organ progression at 6 months.
†Treat to max response +2 (no more than ten cycles), and consider second-line therapy if hematologic minimal response not seen after four cycles or organ progression at 6 months.

Standard chemotherapy

The successful use of cytotoxic chemotherapy to produce regression of AL was reported over 30 years ago,[21–23] and its value was verified in a double-blinded prospective randomized study of melphalan and prednisone versus placebo in 1978.[24] Melphalan and prednisone doubled the overall survival as compared to colchicine in two subsequent randomized trials, making it the standard therapy for most patients with AL until the mid-2000s[25,26] (Table 11.4). The median time to response was 1 year. Although only 18% of patients responded to melphalan and prednisone, responders enjoyed a median survival of 89 months, whereas non-responders had a median survival of 15 months. Nephrotic-only patients with a normal serum creatinine enjoyed an organ response rate of 39%; whereas patients with cardiomyopathy had organ response rates of only 15%.[38] Other treatments like single-agent dexamethasone and VAD (vincristine, doxorubicin [Adriamycin], and dexamethasone) may produce responses in patients.[28,30–37]

Multiagent alkylator-based therapy did not improve overall survival,[27] but replacing the prednisone with dexamethasone is associated with higher response rates and better overall survival. In 2004, Palladini *et al.* reported their experience treating 41 patients who were not transplant candidates with melphalan and dexamethasone. Hematologic response rates of 67%, including 33% complete responses, and organ response rates of 48% were reported.[29] In a 3-year update, these patients had an overall median survival of 5.1 years and progression-free survival of 3.8 years.[39] A total of 21 patients – 13 non-responders and 8 responders – died after a median of 1.6 years (range, 0.1–5.7 years). Death was not amyloid-related in four patients who responded to melphalan and dexamethasone, whereas it was due to progressive cardiac amyloidosis in the remaining cases. The lower than expected rate of myelodysplasia (2.4%) seen in this study was attributed to the modest total dose of melphalan administered (median, 288 mg; range, 48–912 mg), even considering the additional cycles delivered in four relapsing patients. In a separate retrospective study of 153 amyloid patients receiving melphalan/prednisone regimens, bone marrow damage consistent with alkylator-induced myelodysplasia was seen in 7% of the total patient population, with a 42 month actuarial risk of myelodysplasia or acute leukemia of 21%.[40]

The value of melphalan and dexamethasone was further validated in a prospective randomized study of 100 patients randomized to autologous SCT (ASCT) with melphalan compared to oral melphalan and dexamethasone which showed no difference between the two arms for hematologic responses. The landmark analysis performed to correct for early mortality associated with transplant also showed no difference in overall survival.[17] On an intention-to-treat basis, the median survival for melphalan and dexamethasone was 57 months vs. 22 months for the SCT arm. This important study is limited by its very small size for a disease that is very heterogeneous in its extent. Among the 50 patients randomized to receive SCT, only 37 actually made it to transplant and then 9 of those died

Table 11.5. Immune modulatory derivatives and proteosome inhibitors in patients with AL

Regimen	n	No prior Rx (%)	≥2 organs (%)	Cardiac (%)	Heme response (%)	Organ response (%)	Median f/u (mo)	Grade 3–4 AE (%)
Thal 200–800 mg[41]	16	6	31	25	25	0	NR	50
Thal/Dex [42]	31	42	61	38	48	26	32	65
Thal 200–800 mg[43]	12	58	67	42	0	11	2.3[a]	58
Thal 50–200 mg[44]	18	28	50	67	0	11	5.6[a]	75
CTX/Thal/Dex[45]	75	59	33	16	48	26	18	NR
Len ± Dex[46]	22	43	57	65	43	26	17	83
Len ± Dex[47]	34	NR	NR	NR	47	21	NR	>35
Bortez ± Dex[48]	18	61	61	84	94 (44 CR)	28	9.5	NR
Bortez ± Dex[49]	20	NR	NR	60	80 (ISCR)	30	11	NR
Bortez[50]	31	0	55	19	50 (20 CR)	NR	NR	52

Note: [a]Median time on treatment.
Rx: treatment; AE: adverse events; Cardiac: cardiac involvement; Dex: dexamethasone; f/u: follow-up; mo: months; Thal: thalidomide; Len: lenalidomide; CTX: cyclophosphamide; Bortez: bortezomib; NR: not reported.

within 100 days, a 24% treatment-related mortality, leaving only 28 patients for their landmark analysis. In contrast, of the 50 patients randomized to melphalan and dexamethasone, 43 patients received three or more cycles of therapy.

Novel therapies for AL

New therapies for AL involving incorporation of novel agents have also been described. Thalidomide, as a single agent, has a heightened toxicity in patients with AL and in most studies no hematologic or organ responses have been reported (Table 11.5).[41,44,51] In contrast, in combination with dexamethasone, 48% of 31 patients achieved hematologic response, with 8 (26%) organ responses. Median time to response was 3.6 months (range, 2.5–8.0 months). Treatment-related toxicity was frequent (65%), and symptomatic bradycardia was a common (26%) adverse reaction.[42] Wechalekar *et al.* have treated 75 patients with a cyclophosphamide, thalidomide, dexamethasone combination.[45] A hematologic response occurred in 48 (74%) of 65 evaluable patients including complete hematologic responses in 14 (22%). With a median follow-up of 22 months, median estimated overall survival from commencement of treatment was 41 months.

Lenalidomide has been combined with dexamethasone for the treatment of AL. In a trial of 23 patients, one patient had a hematologic and organ response with lenalidomide alone.[46] Eleven patients also received dexamethasone after three cycles of lenalidomide, and overall response rates of 12 who completed more than three cycles of therapy were 10/12 with 9/12 hematologic and 5/12 organ responses. Of interest, ten patients did not complete three cycles of therapy, and analysis demonstrated that the cardiac troponin T level was highly predictive of patients being able to complete protocol therapy. In a similar study, with more restrictive eligibility entry criteria, of 24 evaluable patients, the overall hematologic response rate was 67%, including a 29% hematologic complete response.[47]

There have been three published manuscripts on the role of bortezomib, only one of which was a prospective clinical trial.[50] In the phase I study authored by Reece *et al.* two schedules were tested: bortezomib (0.7–1.6 mg/m^2) days 1, 8, 15, and 22 every five weeks and days 1, 4, 8, and 11 every three weeks (0.7–1.3 mg/m^2).[50] Of these 31 patients who had a relapsed AL, 50% had a hematologic response to therapy. Most commonly reported toxicities included gastrointestinal events, fatigue, and nervous system disorders. Maximum tolerated dose was not defined but grade 3 congestive heart failure was observed in two patients. The once weekly schedule was better tolerated. Of the two non-clinical trial reports, the first of these was that of Kastritis *et al.*[48] Patients received standard dose bortezomib plus dexamethasone 40 mg days 1–4 every 21 days. Grade 3 non-hematologic toxicities included neurotoxicity, fatigue, peripheral edema, constipation, and exacerbation of postural hypotension. Among 16 evaluable patients 94% had a hematologic response and 44% had a hematologic complete response. Five patients (28%) had a response in at least one affected organ. The median number of administered cycles was five. Among the 12 patients who received fewer than the proscribed six courses of therapy, the reasons were progression in 1 patient, death in 3 patients and toxicity in 8 patients. In the other retrospective study looking at 20 patients who were treated with bortezomib with or without dexamethasone, the median numbers of cycles administered was three with a range of 1–6. Among the 16 patients who had hematologic response, 25% of these patients had relapsed at 9 months. Treatment was discontinued early in 40% of the patients due to toxicity.[49]

Using prognostic factors to make treatment decisions

There have been many prognostic factors identified in these patients including β-2 microglobulin and level of circulating immunoglobulin free light chains.[52,53] One of the most commonly applied prognostic factors applied in the past decade has been the numbers of organs involved.[54] Although useful, more important than "number" of organs involved is the "extent" of organs involved. Because the most important determinant of survival is the extent of cardiac involvement,[55] echocardiogram has been an important test in characterizing cardiac involvement.[56] However, these measurements do not detect early involvement and there are issues with interobserver variability. More recently, cardiac biomarkers (troponin T, troponin I, N-terminal brain natriuretic factor [NT-BNP], and brain natriuretic factor [BNP]) that can be measured in the blood have been shown to be excellent predictors of prognosis (Figure 11.3).[12,57–59] These routine laboratory tests are reproducible and relatively inexpensive.

Troponin T is also a powerful predictor of treatment-related mortality for patients undergoing SCT. Among 271 patients, those with troponin levels of 0.06 mg/L or higher had a day-100 all-cause mortality rate of 28% as compared to patients with troponin levels less than 0.06 mg/L who had a day-100 all-cause mortality rate of 7% ($p < 0.001$) despite risk-adapted dose modification of melphalan.[60]

Because the immunoglobulin free light chain is an important prognostic factor in AL patients in terms of both baseline value and extent of reduction,[28,53,61] investigators at Memorial Sloan Kettering have looked at treating those patients who did not achieve a complete hematologic response at 3 months after their SCT with adjuvant thalidomide and dexamethasone. Thirty-one patients began adjuvant therapy, with 16 (52%) completing 9 months of treatment and 13 (42%) achieving an improvement in hematologic response. By intention-to-treat, overall hematologic response rate was 71% (36% complete response), with 44% having organ responses. With a median follow-up of 31 months, 2-year survival was 84% (95% confidence interval: 73%, 94%).[62]

Treating localized amyloidosis

The location of the amyloid is an important clue in recognizing the amyloid as being localized. The most frequent sites of localized amyloid are respiratory tract, genitourinary tract, and skin.[63] Pulmonary amyloid can be subdivided into nodular, laryngeal/tracheobronchial, or diffuse interstitial. Only the third represents a manifestation of systemic AL.[64,65] The nodular form of amyloid presents as solitary pulmonary nodules or multiple nodules. This does not represent the systemic form of AL.[66] These nodules are not calcified and often require resection to exclude a diagnosis of malignancy. The usual treatment for tracheobronchial AL is yttrium-aluminum-garnet (YAG) laser resection of the tissue and more recently electron beam radiation therapy (EBRT).[67] Obstructive ureterovesicular amyloidosis is always localized. Patients present with hematuria or obstruction.[68] Surgery[69] and dimethylsulfoxide instillation[70] are the standard approaches.

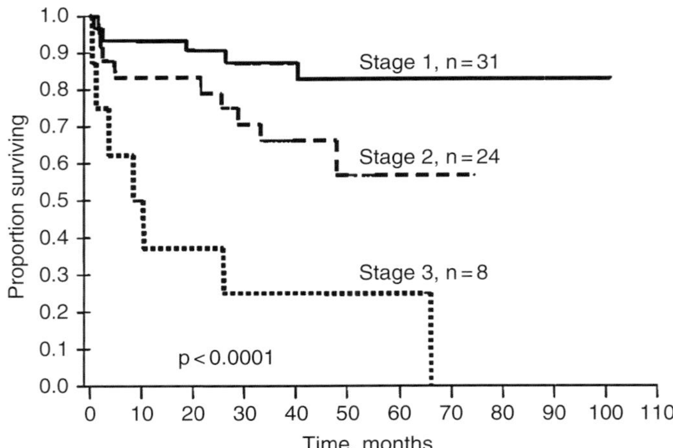

Figure 11.3 Predicting outcome post autologous peripheral blood stem cell transplant based on cardiac biomarker staging system. Stage 1, both biomarkers below cutoff; Stage 2, one of the two biomarkers below cutoff; and Stage 3, both biomarkers above cutoffs. Cutoffs troponin T < 0.035 μg/L and NT-proBNP < 332 ng/L (39 pmol/L). Results updated from original publication published in *Blood* 2004;**104**:1881–7.[12] Median follow-up of surviving patients is 35.5 months.

POEMS syndrome

POEMS syndrome is an acronym referable to 5 of the 12 important features of a fascinating paraneoplastic syndrome: *p*olyradiculoneuropathy; *o*rganomegaly; *e*ndocrinopathy; *m*onoclonal protein; *s*kin changes. The other six include: *p*apilledema; *e*xtravascular volume overload; *s*clerotic bone lesions; *t*hrombocytosis (PEST); high levels of *v*ascular *e*ndothelial *g*rowth *f*actor (VEGF); and abnormal pulmonary function tests (Table 11.6). The major clinical feature of the syndrome is a chronic progressive polyradiculoneuropathy with a predominant motor disability.[71–73] Other names for the syndrome include osteosclerotic myeloma, Crow–Fukase syndrome, and Takatsuki syndrome.[73,74] Although the majority of patients have osteosclerotic myeloma, these same patients usually have only 5% bone marrow plasma cells or less (almost always monoclonal lambda), and rarely have anemia, hypercalcemia, or renal insufficiency. Castleman's disease may also be a part of the disease. These characteristics and the superior median survival differentiate POEMS syndrome from multiple myeloma.

The pathogenesis of this multisystem disease is complex. Elevation of VEGF and proangiogenic and proinflammatory cytokines is a hallmark of the disorder.[75] Little is known about the plasma cells except that more than 95% of the time they are lambda light chain restricted. Plasma and serum levels of VEGF are markedly elevated in patients with POEMS[76–78] and correlate with the activity of the disease.[77,79,80] During the median follow-up period of 11 months, there was a total of four deaths and three progressions.

Table 11.6. Criteria for the diagnosis of POEMS syndrome[a]

Major criteria	1. Polyradiculoneuropathy
	2. Monoclonal plasma cell proliferative disorder (almost always λ)
	3. Sclerotic bone lesions
	4. Castleman's disease
	5. Vascular endothelial growth factor elevation
Minor criteria	6. Organomegaly (splenomegaly, hepatomegaly, or lymphadenopathy)
	7. Extravascular volume overload (edema, pleural effusion, or ascites)
	8. Endocrinopathy (adrenal, thyroid,[b] pituitary, gonadal, parathyroid, pancreatic[b])
	9. Skin changes (hyperpigmentation, hypertrichosis, glomeruloid hemangiomata, plethora, acrocyanosis, flushing, white nails)
	10. Papilledema
	11. Thrombocytosis/polycythemia[c]
Other symptoms and signs	Clubbing, weight loss, hyperhidrosis, pulmonary hypertension/restrictive lung disease, thrombotic diatheses, diarrhea, low vitamin B_{12} values
Possible associations	Arthralgias, cardiomyopathy (systolic dysfunction), and fever

Note: [a]Polyradiculoneuropathy and monoclonal plasma cell disorder present in all patients; to make diagnosis *at least* one other major criterion and one minor criterion is required after exclusion of other causes.
[b]Because of the high prevalence of diabetes mellitus and thyroid abnormalities, this diagnosis alone is not sufficient to meet this minor criterion.
[c]Anemia and/or thrombocytopenia are distinctively unusual in this syndrome unless Castleman's disease is present.
POEMS: polyradiculoneuropathy, organomegaly, endocrinopathy, M protein, skin changes.

The peak incidence of the POEMS syndrome is in the fifth and sixth decades of life, one to two decades earlier than patients with multiple myeloma. Symptoms of peripheral neuropathy (PN) usually dominate the clinical picture.[81] Patients will usually present with complaint of tingling, paresthesias, and coldness beginning in the feet. Motor involvement follows the sensory symptoms. Severe weakness occurs in more than one-half of patients and results in inability to climb stairs, arise from a chair, or grip objects firmly with their hands. The course is usually progressive and patients may be confined to a wheelchair. Impotence occurs but autonomic symptoms are not a feature. The cranial nerves are not involved except for papilledema. Hyperpigmentation is common. Coarse black hair may appear on the extremities. Other skin changes include skin thickening, rapid accumulation of glomeruloid angiomata, flushing, dependent rubor or acrocyanosis, white nails, and clubbing. Testicular atrophy and gynecomastia may be present. Pitting edema of the lower extremities is common. Ascites and pleural effusion occur in approximately one-third of patients. The liver is palpable in almost one-half of patients but splenomegaly and lymphadenopathy is found in fewer patients. Bone pain and fractures rarely occur. Weight loss and fatigue are common features as the disease progresses. Because patients become so restricted in their movement due to their neuropathy, it is rare for them to report dyspnea despite markedly abnormal pulmonary testing.

Thrombocytosis is common, and polycythemia may be seen.[72,81] Anemia and thrombocytopenia are not characteristic unless there is coexisting Castleman's disease. The size of the M protein on electrophoresis is small (median 1.1 g/dL) and is rarely more than 3.0 g/dL. The M protein is usually IgG or IgA and almost always of the lambda type.[72,73] Bone marrow usually contains $< 5\%$ plasma cells, and when clonal cells are found they are almost always monoclonal lambda. Protein levels in the cerebrospinal fluid are elevated in virtually all patients. Osteosclerotic lesions occur in approximately 95% of patients, and can be confused with benign bone islands, aneurysmal bone cysts, non-ossifying fibromas, and fibrous dysplasia. Lesions may be densely sclerotic, be lytic with a sclerotic rim, have a mixed soap-bubble appearance, or any such combination (Figure 11.4). Bone windows of CT body images are often very informative. 18-fluoro-deoxyglucose (FDG)-avidity is variable.

Endocrinopathy is a central but poorly understood feature of POEMS. In a recent large series from the Mayo Clinic,[82] approximately 84% of patients have a recognized endocrinopathy, with hypogonadism as the most common endocrine abnormality, followed by thyroid abnormalities, glucose metabolism abnormalities, and lastly by adrenal insufficiency. The majority of patients had evidence of multiple endocrinopathies in the four major endocrine axes (gonadal, thyroid, glucose, and adrenal).

Renal dysfunction is usually not a dominant feature of this syndrome, and it is more likely to occur in the context of coexisting Castleman's disease. In our experience approximately 9% of patients have proteinuria exceeding

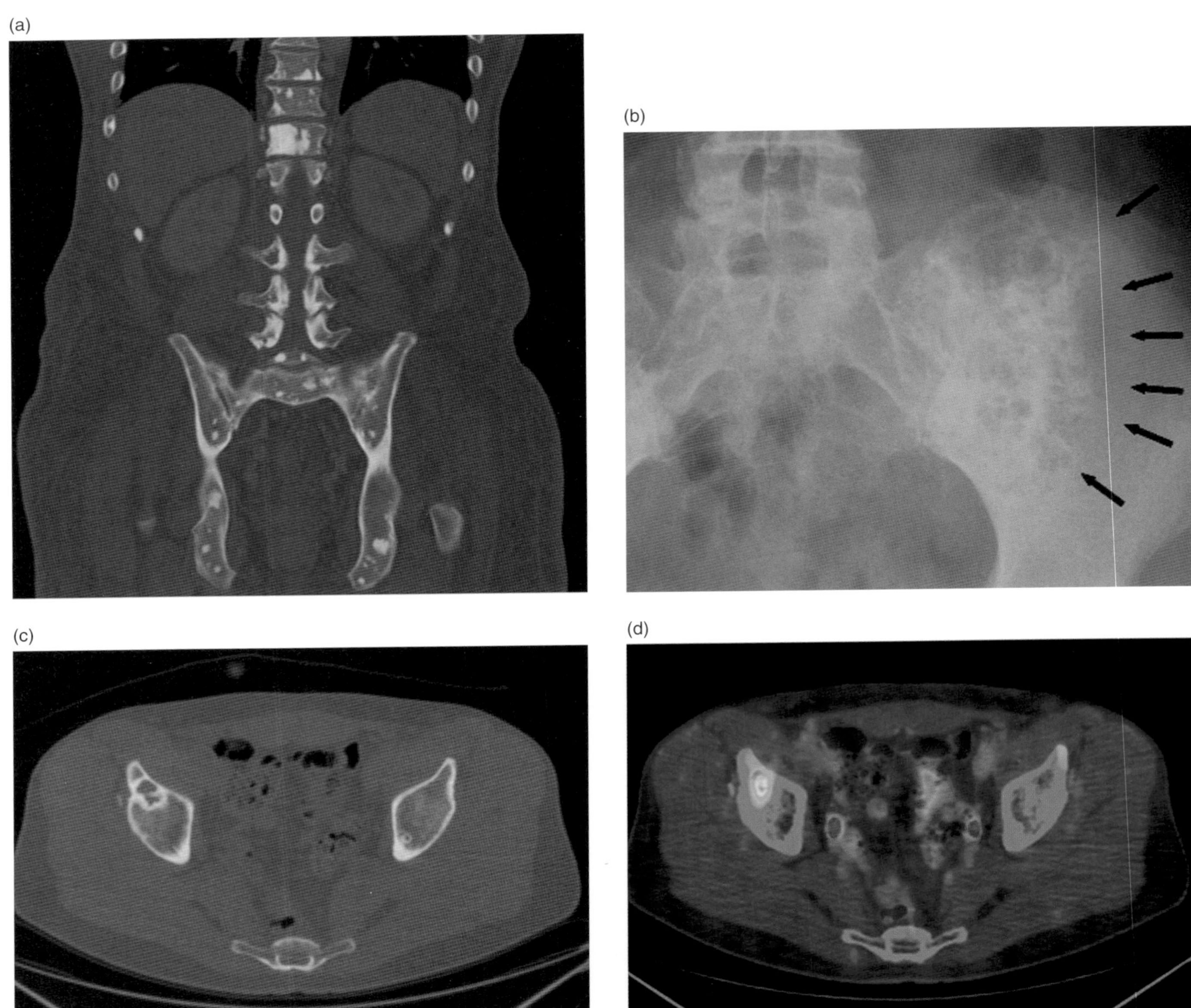

Figure 11.4 Bone lesions in POEMS syndrome. (a) Diffuse sclerotic lesions seen on bone windows of CT scan. (b) Mixed lytic and sclerotic lesion, "soap-bubble lesion." (c and d) Lytic lesion with sclerotic rim on right ischium on CT (c) and ^{18}F-fluorodeoxyglucose (FDG-PET) (d). With permission from *Blood Reviews*. Dispenzieri *Blood Reviews* 2007;**21**:285–99.[75]

0.5 g/24 hours and only 6% have a serum creatinine greater than or equal to 1.5 mg/dL.[72] The renal histology is diverse with membranoproliferative features and evidence of endothelial injury being most common.[83]

On lymph node biopsy, the histology is frequently angiofollicular lymph node hyperplasia (Castleman's disease) or Castleman's disease-like.[72,74] Between 11% and 30% of POEMS patients have documented Castleman's disease or Castleman's-like disease.[74,84] This estimate may be conservative since most patients do not undergo lymph node biopsies.

Nerve conduction studies and electromyelography demonstrate a polyradiculoneuropathy with prominent demyelination as well as features of axonal degeneration, which are similar to the findings of patients with chronic inflammatory demyelinating polyradiculoneuropathy (CIDP). The dominant feature of this syndrome is typically the PN, and not infrequently patients are initially diagnosed with CIDP or, less frequently, Guillain–Barre syndrome.

Patients may develop arterial and/or venous thromboses during their course. Lesprit *et al.* observed 4/20 patients to have arterial occlusion.[85] In the Mayo series, there were 18 patients suffering serious events such as stroke, myocardial infarction, and Budd–Chiari syndrome.[72] Affected vessels include carotid, iliac, celiac, subclavian, mesenteric, and femoral.[86–89] Gangrene of lower extremities can occur.[88]

The pulmonary manifestations are protean, including pulmonary hypertension, restrictive lung disease, impaired neuromuscular respiratory function, and impaired diffuse capacity of carbon monoxide, but improve with effective therapy.[90–94]

Treatment and prognosis

The course of POEMS syndrome is chronic and patients typically survive for more than a decade in contrast to multiple myeloma. In our experience, the median survival was 13.8 years.[72] In one French study, at least 7/15 patients were alive for more than 5 years.[84] In Nakanishi *et al.*'s series of 102 patients, the median survival was 33 months[74] though in Takatsuki *et al.*'s study of 109 patients, the authors stated that the "clinical course is very chronic ... some patients survived greater than 10 years."[73] In our experience, only fingernail clubbing and extravascular volume overload, i.e., effusions, edema, and ascites, were significantly associated with a shorter overall survival.[72] More recently, we have identified respiratory symptoms to be predictive of adverse outcome.[90] In the French series, patients without plasmocytoma or bone lesions had a worse prognosis than those with other types of plasma cell dyscrasia in the absence of bone lesions.[84]

Additional features typically arise over time if treatment is unsuccessful or if the diagnosis is delayed.[72] The most common causes of death are cardiorespiratory failure, progressive inanition, infection, capillary-leak-like syndrome, and renal failure. Even those patients with multiple bone lesions or more than 10% plasma cells do not progress to classic multiple myeloma.

There are no randomized controlled trials in patients with POEMS. Information about benefits of therapy is most typically derived retrospectively (Table 11.7). Given these limitations, however, there are therapies which benefit patients with POEMS syndrome, including radiation therapy, alkylator-based therapies, and corticosteroids.[75] Intensive supportive care measures must also be instituted. Single or multiple osteosclerotic lesions in a limited area should be treated with radiation. If a patient has widespread osteosclerotic lesions or diffuse bone marrow plasmacytosis, systemic therapy is warranted. In contrast to CIDP, plasmapheresis and intravenous immunoglobulin do not produce clinical benefit. High-dose chemotherapy with peripheral blood transplant is yielding very promising results.[107] When the selected therapy is effective, response of systemic symptoms and skin changes typically precede those of the neuropathy, with the former beginning to respond within a month, and the latter within 3–6 months with maximum benefit frequently not seen before 2–3 years. Clinical response to therapy correlates better with VEGF level than M-protein level,[108,109] and complete hematologic response is not required to derive substantial clinical benefit.

Melphalan is among the most effective agents against plasmaproliferative disorders. Based on retrospective data approximately 40% of patients with POEMS syndrome will response to melphalan and prednisone.[73] The optimal duration of therapy has not been established, but borrowing from the experience of multiple myeloma, 6–12 months of treatment is reasonable. Limiting the melphalan exposure is important because secondary myelodysplastic syndrome or acute leukemia can occur. Cyclophosphamide is another alkylator that can control the disease in a limited number of patients. If the patient is considered to be a candidate for peripheral blood SCT, melphalan-containing regimens should be avoided until after stem cell harvest.

High-dose chemotherapy with peripheral blood SCT is an emerging therapy for patients with POEMS.[107] All patients had improvement of their neuropathy over time; as in the case with radiation therapy and other chemotherapy, improvement of the PN takes months to years. Other clinical features improve after SCT, including levels of VEGF in several of the patients studied.[110,111] Patients with POEMS appear to be at higher risk for peri-engraftment syndrome, and intensive care unit stays can be avoided with prompt institution of corticosteroids in the context of high fever, rash, edema, and pulmonary infiltrates days 8–15 post-stem cell infusion.[107]

Other treatments which have been reported are shown in Table 11.7, and include plasmapheresis, intravenous immunoglobulin, interferon alpha (IFN-α), tamoxifen, all-*trans* retinoic acid, thalidomide, ticlopidine, argatroban, strontium-89, bevacizumab, and lenalidomide. Plasmapheresis is not an effective treatment in this disorder.[75] Those reports purporting efficacy of plasma exchange combine the treatment with corticosteroids and/or other therapies, confounding interpretation. Intravenous immunoglobulin also cannot be recommended based on our experience or on a review of the literature. Once again the few reports claiming effectiveness simultaneously use other immunosuppressants or treatments. Although there is a theoretical rationale (anti-VEGF and antitumor necrosis factor effects) for using thalidomide in POEMS patients, enthusiasm for its use should be tempered by the high rate of PN induced by the drug.[112] In contrast, the next-generation immune modulatory drug, lenalidomide, has a much lower risk of PN. We have observed dramatic improvements in one patient treated with this drug.[106] Bevacizumab has been tried with mixed results. Two patients who had also received alkylator during and/or predating the bevacizumab had benefit. One who received it after radiation died.[104,105]

The physical limitations of the patient should not be overlooked while evaluating and/or treating the underlying plasma cell disorder. As always a multidisciplinary, thoughtful treatment program will improve a complex patient's treatment outcome. A physical therapy and occupational therapy program is essential to maintain flexibility and assist in lifestyle management despite the neuropathy. In those patients with respiratory muscle weakness and/or pulmonary hypertension, overnight oxygen or continuous positive airway pressure (CPAP) may be useful.

Table 11.7. POEMS syndrome response to therapy

Response to standard therapies[75]

Treatment	Improvement rates
Radiation	≥ 50%
Standard-dose alkylator-based therapy	≥ 40%
Corticosteroids	≥ 15%
High-dose chemotherapy with PBSCT	≥ 90%

Response to experimental therapies

Ref	Treatment	n	Outcomes
95	Tamoxifen	1	Disappearance of edema, effusions, and regression of PN
96	Ticlopidine	1	Improved edema, ascites, effusions, and VEGF for "several months"; no improvement in PN, other labs, or thyroid function
97	Argatroban	2	1 improvement; 1 no response
98	Interferon + argatroban	2	Improvement in paraprotein, neuropathy, and coagulation parameters – doing well at 2 years
99	Interferon α	1	POEMS + CD: Begun after radiation. Remarkable improvement of PN and organomegaly and lymphadenopathy after 3 months
100	Trans-retinoic acid	1	Improved cytokines and platelet count, but worsening PN
101	Strontium-89	1	Improvement of LA, hepatomegaly, peripheral neuropathy, platelets
102	Thalidomide + dexamethasone	1	POEMS + CD: Improved PN, ascites, pleural effusion, dyspnea, creatinine, CBC, IL-6 w/in 2 months
103	Thalidomide	1[a]	Improved ascites, anemia, leukopenia, thrombocytopenia, ESR, and sense of well-being
104	Bevacizumab	1	Patient also receiving melphalan + dexamethasone; improved edema, pain, weakness, VEGF
105	Bevacizumab	1	Worsening PN, anasarca, MOF; died of pneumonia 5 weeks after treatment
105	Bevacizumab	1	Initial worsening; dose repeated with cyclophosphamide resulted in improvement of pulmonary HTN, anasarca, skin changes
106	Lenalidomide plus low-dose dexamethasone	1	Improvement in ascites, performance status, peripheral neuropathy, VEGF levels, testosterone levels, pulmonary function tests

Notes: [a]POEMS (normal IL-6 and no bone lesions), but CD-like since anemia, leukopenia, thrombocytopenia, incr. erythrocyte sedimentation rate (ESR).
CD: Castleman's disease; HTN: hypertension; IL-6: interleukin-6; LA: lymphadenopathy; PN: peripheral neuropathy; MOF: multiorgan failure; VEGF, vascular endothelial growth factor; PBSCT: peripheral blood stem cell transplant; CBC: complete blood count.

Cryoglobulinemia

The term "cryoglobulin" was coined by Lerner and Watson in 1947 referring to precipitation of immunoglobulins in the cold.[113] Meltzer and others delineated a distinct syndrome of purpura, arthralgias, asthenia, renal disease, and neuropathy – often occurring with immune complex deposition or vasculitis, or both.[114] Brouet *et al.* popularized a system of classifying cryoglobulinemia on the basis of the components of the cryoprecipitate: type I, isolated monoclonal immunoglobulins; type II, a monoclonal component, usually IgM, possessing activity toward polyclonal immunoglobulins, usually IgG; and type III, polyclonal immunoglobulins of more than one isotype.[115] This classification provided a framework by which clinical correlations could be made. Associated conditions, such as lymphoproliferative disorders, connective tissue disorders, infection, and liver disease were observed in some patients. In several large series, 34–71% of cryoglobulinemia cases were not associated with other specific disease states and were termed "essential" or primary cryoglobulinemia.[115–117] In 1990, hepatitis C virus (HCV) was recognized as an etiologic factor for the majority of these cases.[118,119]

Cryoglobulinemia is driven primarily by four classes of disease: liver disease (predominantly HCV), infection (again, predominantly HCV), connective tissue disease, and lymphoproliferative disease. These diseases induce a seemingly non-specific stimulation of B cells, frequently resulting in polyclonal hypergammaglobulinemia. Although only a minority of patients with serum cryoglobulins have symptoms referable to them, cryoglobulins may be found in patients with cirrhosis (up to 45%), alcoholic hepatitis (32%), autoimmune hepatitis (40%), subacute bacterial endocarditis (90%), rheumatoid arthritis (47%), IgG myeloma (10%), and Waldenstrom's macroglobulinemia (19%).[113]

The median age at diagnosis is the early to mid 50s. In some studies, the female predominance for cryoglobulinemia is greater than 2:1. No racial preference has been noted, but the incidence is higher in regions where HCV occurs at higher frequencies (e.g., southern Europe). Involvement of the skin, peripheral nerves, kidneys, and liver is common. Lymphadenopathy is present in approximately 17% of patients.[114,116] On autopsy, widespread vasculitis involving small and medium vessels in the heart, gastrointestinal tract, central nervous system, muscles, lungs, and adrenal glands may also be seen.[116,120] The interval between the onset of symptoms and the time of diagnosis varies considerably (range, 0–10 years).[116] Type I cryoglobulinemia is usually asymptomatic. When symptomatic, it most commonly causes occlusive symptoms rather than the vasculitis of types II and III.[114,116] Symptoms of hyperviscosity may occur. Type II cryoglobulinemia is more frequently symptomatic (61% of patients) than type III (21% of patients).[121]

Purpura is the most frequent symptom of mixed (type II and type III) cryoglobulinemia. The incidence varies from 15% to 33% in type I, from 60% to 93% in type II, and from 70% to 83% in type III.[122] Petechiae and palpable purpura are the most common lesions, although ecchymoses, erythematous spots, and dermal nodules occur in as many as 20% of patients. Bullous or vesicular lesions are distinctly uncommon.[115] Occasionally the arms are involved, but the face and trunk are generally spared.[115] Head and mucosal involvement, livedoid vasculitis, and cold-induced acrocyanosis of the helices of the ears are more frequently observed in type I; infarction, hemorrhagic crusts, or ulcers occur in 10–25% of all patients with mixed cryoglobulinemia.[123] Showers of purpura last for 1–2 weeks and occur once or twice a month. Cold precipitates these types of lesions in only 10–30% of the patients.[115,123] Skin necrosis, urticaria, and livedo, which are all rare, are more commonly associated with exposure to cold.

Approximately 21–39% of patients with mixed cryoglobulinemia have renal involvement.[115,124,125] The incidence of renal injury is highest in patients with type II cryoglobulins.[117,126] Although cryopathic membranoproliferative glomerulonephritis portends a poor prognosis[116,126–129] progression to end-stage renal failure due to sclerosing nephritis is uncommon.[1] Among patients with mixed cryoglobulinemia-associated membranoproliferative glomerulonephritis followed up for a median of 11 years, 15% had disease progression to end-stage renal failure, and 43% died of cardiovascular, hepatic, or infectious causes.[128]

PN is the more common presentation, although central nervous system involvement may occur. In the largest clinical series, peripheral nerve involvement is described in 12–56% of patients.[115–117,125,130] Signs and symptoms of sensory neuropathy usually precede those of motor neuropathy.[115,131] The presentation may be an acute or subacute distal symmetric polyneuropathy or a mononeuritis multiplex[131–133] with a chronic or chronic-relapsing evolution.[134] The neuropathy in essential mixed cryoglobulinemia is most often characterized by axonal degeneration. Even when other manifestations of mixed cryoglobulinemia are stable over time, there is typically worsening of the PN.[135]

The type or quantity of the cryoglobulin does not reliably predict the presence or nature of symptoms. On serum protein electrophoresis, polyclonal hypergammaglobulinemia is the most common finding, although normal patterns or hypogammaglobulinemia may also be seen.[114,116,136] Even among patients with type II cryoglobulinemia, only 15% have a visible monoclonal spike on serum protein electrophoresis. Hyperviscosity occurs only occasionally. Marked depression of complement CH50, C1q, and C4 in the presence of relatively normal C3 levels is usual.[116,125,137] Neither C4 concentrations nor cryoglobulin levels correlate with overall clinical severity, although for individual patients the cryoglobulin level can sometimes serve as a marker for disease activity.[116,137–139] Rheumatoid factor activity – that is, anti-Fc activity – is detectable in the sera in 87–100% of patients with mixed cryoglobulinemia,[114,115,140] and levels may decrease with response to therapy.[141] An elevated erythrocyte sedimentation rate and a mild normochromic, normocytic anemia are fairly common.[116,139]

Treatment and prognosis

It is well recognized that cryoglobulinemia has a fluctuating course with spontaneous exacerbation and remission. In a large series by Ferri *et al.* of 231 patients seen from 1972 to 2001, the mixed cryoglobulinemia syndrome followed a relatively benign clinical course in over 50% of cases, whereas a moderate-severe clinical course was observed in one-third of patients whose prognosis was severely affected by renal and/or liver failure. For 15% of individuals the disease was complicated by malignancy: B cell more common than hepatocellular and thyroid malignancies. Ten-year overall survival was 56%. Lower survival rates were seen in males and in individuals with renal involvement.[142] The most common causes of death include renal failure, infection, lymphoproliferative disorders, liver failure, cardiovascular complications, and hemorrhage.[115–117,130,143]

With the exception of the IFN-α trials of the 1990s[144–148] and the small low-antigen diet trial performed in the 1980s,[149] the remainder of the information about the treatment of symptomatic cryoglobulinemia is anecdotal. The standard treatment of mild symptomatic cryoglobulinemia (purpura, asthenia, arthralgia, and mild sensory neuropathy) has included bed rest, analgesics, low-dose corticosteroid therapy, low-antigen-content diet, and protective measures against cold; the treatment of severe disease (glomerulonephritis, motor neuropathy, and systemic vasculitis) has included plasmapheresis, high-dose corticosteroid therapy, and cytotoxic therapy.[150–152] Plasma exchange or plasmapheresis alone can reverse serious complications, but most authors have reported use of these procedures in combination with cytotoxic agents or corticosteroids for more durable responses.[138,153–155] According to case reports, responses may be seen in 60–100% of patients.[138,153–155]

Since the association was made between HCV and mixed cryoglobulinemia, immunosuppressive therapy has been viewed less favorably, and IFN is generally considered to be first-line therapy for HCV-positive patients who are in non-emergent situations.[144–148,156] There is mounting evidence that the ribavirin and IFN-α combination is effective in the setting of renal disease.[151,157] One should be cognisant of reports of peripheral neuropathy (personal observation and Casato *et al.*[158]), nephritis,[159] vasculitis,[160] and ischemic manifestations being exacerbated by IFN-α.[161]

For patients with symptomatic type I cryoglobulinemia, anti-CD20 therapy and/or cytotoxic therapy appropriate for the lymphoproliferative disorder remains the therapy of choice. Anti-CD20 therapy with rituximab has been shown to produce responses in patients with all types of cryoglobulinemia;[162–164] however, those patients with HCV are at risk for increased HCV replication.[162,163] Zaja *et al.* reported on 15 patients with type II mixed cryoglobulinemia (HCV-related in 12 of 15) who were treated with rituximab. Skin vasculitis manifestations (ulcers, purpura, or urticaria), subjective symptoms of PN, low-grade B-cell lymphoma, arthralgias, and fever improved and nephritis of recent onset went into remission in one case. Laboratory features, that is, significantly decreased serum rheumatoid factor and cryoglobulins and increased C4, were consistent with the clinical efficacy.[162] In another report, Sansonno *et al.* treated 20 patients with mixed cryoglobulinemia and HCV-positive chronic active liver disease, resistant to IFN-α therapy, with rituximab. Sixteen patients (80%) showed a complete response, characterized by rapid improvement of clinical signs (disappearance of purpura and weakness arthralgia and improvement of PN), and decline of cryocrit. Complete response was associated with a significant reduction of rheumatoid factor activity and anti-HCV antibody titers. However, HCV RNA increased to approximately twice the baseline levels in the responders, whereas it remained much the same in the non-responders.[163] Others have seen similar clinical results.[164,165] Basse *et al.* studied seven patients with type III cryoglobulin-related renal graft dysfunction, five of whom were HCV positive. Rituximab resulted in a dramatic improvement in all renal parameters, but two patients experienced serious infectious complications as well.[166] The initial increase in the cryoglobulin level after rituximab therapy for type II cryoglobulinemia secondary to Waldenstrom's macroglobulinemia does not indicate failure of response.[167]

Although not formally studied, high-dose therapy with ASCT may be considered for patients with symptomatic, refractory cryoglobulinemia that results from a plasmaproliferative disorder. There is an increased risk of lethal veno-occlusive disease in patients with chronic hepatitis C who are undergoing SCT;[168] for these patients, there are no data to support implementation of this therapy.

Dramatic reductions in the cryocrit and the cryoglobulinemic symptoms, including membranoproliferative glomerulonephritis, have been reported in several patients who underwent splenectomy for hypersplenism.[169,170] In contrast, in the series reported by Meltzer and Franklin the one patient who underwent splenectomy died of acute renal failure.[171] Because this intervention has not been studied thoroughly, and because of the high risk involved, it should not be considered as a standard therapy but rather as a potential option for patients without cirrhosis who have disease that is difficult to manage because of cytopenias resulting from hypersplenism.

MGUS-associated peripheral neuropathy

MGUS is found in approximately 2–3% of patients greater than 50 years of age and in 3–5% of persons older than 70 years.[172] It is defined by the presence of a serum M protein less than 3 g/dL and fewer than 10% plasma cells in the bone marrow in the absence of multiple myeloma, Waldenstrom's macroglobulinemia, primary amyloidosis, cryoglobulinemia, or POEMS syndrome.

The most convincing data for the connection of MGUS and PN was published in the 1980s.[173,174] Kahn and colleagues detected 58 cases of monoclonal gammopathy without evidence of myeloma or Waldenstrom's macroglobulinemia in 14 000 serum samples (0.4%) obtained from patients admitted to a neurologic tertiary care center;[173] 16 of those 58 patients (28%) had PN. The second published study of import establishing a relationship between MGUS and PN was by Kelly *et al.* This study was conducted over a one-year period in 692 patients with a clinically apparent PN who were identified in the electromyography laboratory at the Mayo Clinic.[174] Three hundred and fifty-eight patients had an identifiable systemic disease known to cause PN such as diabetes mellitus, or alcoholism (secondary neuropathy group); 334 were apparently idiopathic. Approximately 80% of patients in each group had serum protein electrophoretic studies. In the secondary group 2.5% of the patients had an M protein, while in the idiopathic group, 10% had an M protein: MGUS (16 patients); primary systemic amyloidosis (7 patients); Waldenstrom's macroglobulinemia (1 patient); and gamma heavy chain disease (1 patient). The age-matched rate of monoclonal gammopathy was statistically significantly higher in patients with PN as compared to normal populations in Minnesota and Sweden. Not all studies support the association.[175]

The pathogenesis of MGUS neuropathy (especially IgM) is sometimes related to the reactivity of the monoclonal immunoglobulins to specific antigens expressed on peripheral nerves such as myelin-associated glycoprotein (MAG), gangliosides, chondroitin sulfate, and sulfatide.[176] The most convincing pathogenic relationship is between IgM MGUS neuropathy and MAG antibodies, although there is still some controversy. Quarles and Weiss provide a comprehensive review of autoantibodies associated with PN.[177]

Typically MGUS-associated neuropathy has the following features: (1) there is an M protein in the serum, most commonly IgM, followed in frequency by IgG and then IgA; (2) there is a symmetric sensorimotor polyradiculopathy or neuropathy which begins insidiously and is usually slowly progressive; (3) cranial nerves are not involved; (4) it occurs more often in the sixth to the seventh decade of life; (5) it affects males more frequently than females; (6) POEMS syndrome is not present. Paresthesias, ataxia, and pain may be predominant features, but predisposition for these symptoms depends on the type of monoclonal protein present and whether there are anti-MAG antibodies present. Symptoms usually begin with paresthesias and numbness distally in the feet or hands, and early motor symptoms are rare or minor. The neuropathy then progresses proximally in stocking/glove distribution and may involve motor as well as sensory functions. Ataxia and tremor may be present and sometimes predominate. There is no correlation between the size of the monoclonal protein and the severity of the neuropathy.

Table 11.8. Randomized trials to treat MGUS-associated peripheral neuropathy

Ref	n	Treatment	
179	39	Double-blind plasma exchange vs. sham	Improvement in NDS with PE; especially in IgA and IgG patients
180	24	Chlorambucil vs. chlorambucil and plasma exchange	Sensory component of NDS improved slightly in both arms. No difference between treatments
181	20	Open randomized IFN-α vs. IV Ig	8/10 vs. 1/10 improved NDS at 6 months; persistent at 12 months. Sensory improvement only. Decreased IgM in 2 IFN-α patients. MAG Ab persist
182	22	IV Ig vs. placebo	Improved hand grip, 10 meter walking time, and sensory symptom score in IV Ig group as compared to baseline. Only difference at 4 weeks was hand grip
183	24	Double-blind randomized IFN-α vs. placebo	3/12 patients in each arm improved clinically. No benefit to IFN-α

Note: NDS: neuropathy disability score.
Source: Modified from Dispenzieri and Kyle.[175]

Treatment and prognosis

Initiation of treatment is largely based on comparing the potential risk of therapy to its potential benefit. In one study of 25 patients, after a mean follow-up of 8.5 years (range 2–13 years) and a mean duration of neuropathy symptoms of 11.8 years (range 3–18, > 10 years in 16), 17 patients (68%) were alive.[178] The eight (32%) who died did so 3–15 years (mean 10.6) after neuropathy onset; in none of them was death caused by the neuropathy, although in three it was possibly related to the therapy for the neuropathy. The authors also found that at last follow-up or prior to death, 11 patients (44%) were disabled by severe hand tremor, gait ataxia, or both, with disability rates at 5, 10, and 15 years from neuropathy onset of 16%, 24%, and 50%, respectively.

To date, treatment strategies have been directed toward reducing the IgM paraprotein level either by removing the antibody or targeting the presumed monoclonal B-cell clone, or toward interfering with the presumed effector mechanisms such as complement activation or macrophage recruitment. There are limited published data regarding efficacy of the various immunosuppressive regimens in IgM paraproteinemic neuropathies and only six randomized controlled trials (Table 11.8).[179,180,182–184] Most case series are small, include diverse groups of patients and measurements of efficacy differ between trials.

The first of these randomized trials in patients with MGUS-associated PN was a comparison of plasma exchange to sham exchange in 39 patients, 21 of whom had an IgM paraprotein.[179] Patients received either plasma exchange twice weekly or sham-plasma exchange in a double-blind trial. Sham-plasma exchange patients subsequently underwent plasma exchange in an open trial. The average neuropathy disability score improved significantly in the plasma exchange group. In both the double-blind and open trials IgG or IgA gammopathy had a better response to plasma exchange than those with IgM gammopathy.[179] In multiple small studies of plasma exchange used as monotherapy, improvement has been reported in more than 50% of cases of MGUS-associated neuropathy.[178,185,186] Improvement with plasma exchange in combination with other drugs has been described. However, in a prospective study of 44 patients with an IgM MGUS and PN, patients were randomized to receive either chlorambucil orally or chlorambucil plus 15 courses of plasma exchange during the first four months of therapy. There was no difference in the two treatment groups.[180]

Alkylators may be used, with the knowledge that secondary myelodysplastic syndrome or acute leukemia are possible complications. Small studies indicate response rates of ~33%. Corticosteroids are not usually effective in patients with neuropathy and IgM MGUS.[185]

Based on the results of a small open-label randomized study in which patients were randomized to either IFN-α or intravenous (IV) Ig, it was thought that IFN-α was an effective therapy in patients with IgM MAG-associated PN. A successor study, which was a blinded comparison of IFN-α and placebo, however, was negative.[183]

Intravenous gammaglobulin produces benefit in some patients with CIDP and may be used for patients with sensorimotor PN and MGUS. IV immunoglobulin is beneficial in 25–50% of patients.[182,184] Dalakas *et al.* randomized 11 patients with IgM MAG-associated PN to either IV gammaglobulin or placebo; at 3 months patients crossed over to the other therapy. There was improvement in 27% (improved strength in two patients and improved sensory symptoms in another), without any change in MAG or sulfoglucuronyl paragloboside (SGPG) titers.[184] Comi *et al.* treated 22 patients with IgM MAG-associated PN with either IV gammaglobulin or placebo, and found short-term intrapatient improvement.[182]

Novel therapies such as purine nucleoside analogs[187,188] and rituximab[189–191] may be useful. Fludarabine, a purine analog, produced benefit in three of four patients with an IgM MGUS.[188] Thirty-five patients have been treated with anti-CD20 antibodies in three open studies with response rates of 66–100%.[189–191] Lowering of both IgM levels and anti-MAG antibody titers is observed.[190] Pestronk *et al.* treated 21 patients with IgM MAG-(7 patients) or IgM ganglioside-(14 patients) associated neuropathy with rituximab, with an option to retreat, followed by a maintenance course of a dose every 10 weeks for 2 years. Eighty-one percent had improvement in the functional scores over baseline at the conclusion of the study.[191]

Scleromyxedema

Scleromyxedema is a cutaneous mucinosis characterized by a generalized papular and sclerodermoid eruption, mucin deposition, increased fibroblast proliferation, fibrosis, and monoclonal gammopathy in the absence of thyroid disease. Extracutaneous manifestations may involve the cardiovascular, gastrointestinal, pulmonary, rheumatologic, and central nervous systems. (See recent review by Cokonis Georgakis *et al.*[192]) The disorder was previously described by Dubruilh in 1906 under the alternate name of lichen myxedematosus and distinguished from sclerederma and generalized myxedema by Montgomery and Underwood in 1953. More recently, scleromyxedema has been used as the generalized form of lichen myxedematosus while papular mucinosis is thought to be the localized form of the disease.[192]

The pathogenesis of the disorder is not understood. In vitro serum from patients with scleromyxedema stimulates dermal fibroblast proliferation with resultant hyaluronic acid and protaglandin E production.[193] Isolated serum IgG does not stimulate this effect despite the fact that 83% of patients with the disorder have an IgG monoclonal protein.[192]

Diagnosis of scleromyxedema should fulfill the following criteria: (1) generalized papular and sclerodermoid eruption; (2) mucin deposition, fibroblast proliferation, and fibrosis; (3) monoclonal gammopathy; and (4) the absence of thyroid disease.[194] The connective tissue diseases that are in the differential diagnosis are systemic sclerosis, dermatomyositis, and rheumatoid arthritis. Nephrogenic fibrosing dermopathy shares dermatologic features with scleromyxedema.[193]

This rare disorder appears to affect men at a slightly higher rate than women, with a mean age of the sixth decade.[195] The hallmark of the disorder is the rash, which consists of small (2–3 mm), waxy, firm papules that are closely spaced and often arranged linearly. They may be dome shaped or flat topped, and they most commonly affect the face, neck, distal forearms, and hands. The skin may exhibit diffuse erythema, edema, and a brownish discoloration and there is often loss of skin appendages. In those patients with diffuse mucin deposition within the glabella, there is a leonine facies appearance. Pruritis may or may not be present. The mucin infiltration in the skin results in stiffening of the skin and decreased range of motion in the hands, lips, and extremities. The infiltration is not limited to skin, however, and mucin deposition in adventitia around vessels in many organ systems can cause life-threatening extracutaneous complications.

The majority of patients have extracutaneous manifestations, the most common of which is gastrointestinal, especially dysphagia.[195] Patients not infrequently have esophageal dysmotility, aspiration, and vocal hoarseness. Approximately 25% of patients develop proximal weakness and myopathy. Histologically, the most common muscle feature is vascular myopathy. Mucin deposits in the muscle are rare, and occasionally there are interstitial inflammatory infiltrates. Very rarely, patients may have an inflammatory arthritis. Carpal tunnel has been reported in association with the disease as well. Neurologic and psychiatric disorders have been described with scleromyxedema.[196] Central nervous system findings including seizures, stroke, encephalopathy, and psychosis have been reported. Reported peripheral nervous system associations include PN and mononeuritis multiplex. Myopathy, myositis, and rhabdomyolysis have also been reported. Dyspnea is not unusual, and upon testing obstructive and/or restrictive pulmonary disease can be seen in about one-fourth of patients.[195] In one study 10% of patients had cardiac manifestations.[197]

Treatment and prognosis

The most commonly used upfront therapies have included systemic corticosteroids, melphalan, and plasmapheresis. More recently, novel treatments like high-dose chemotherapy with peripheral blood SCT and thalidomide have shown to be effective, at least in the short term.[198,199] Other agents with variable utility include isotretinonin, etretinate, intralesional corticosteroids, intravenous gammaglobulin, purine nucleoside analogs, IFN-α, PUVA (psoralen and ultraviolet radiation), radiation, surgery, and methotexate.[192] Although it may improve the skin manifestations, low-dose alkylator therapy should be used with caution since secondary acute leukemia has been reported.[195] In one series, more than half of the patients treated with oral melphalan died of treatment-related causes.

Necrobiotic xanthogranuloma

Necrobiotic xanthogranuloma (NXG) is a rare chronic granulomatous disease of the skin and extracutaneous tissues. It was originally described in 1980 by Kossard and Winkelmann as a distinctive disorder consisting of cutaneous and subcutaneous xanthomatous plaques, which frequently were associated with monoclonal protein and/or lymphoproliferative diseases. (See recent review.[200])

The pathogenesis of the disorder is poorly understood. Approximately 80–90% of cases have a monoclonal gammopathy, IgG kappa in approximately 60% and IgG lambda in nearly 30%.[201] One theory is that the monoclonal protein has functional features of a lipoprotein, binding to lipoprotein receptors of monocytes, thereby inducing xanthoma formation.[202] The activation of monocytes may contribute to an intracellular accumulation of lipoprotein-derived lipids in the skin.[200] Matsuura *et al.* observed one patient who had increased serum levels of macrophage colony-stimulating factor.[203] On light microscopy, changes are seen in the deep dermis and subcutaneous tissue. The superficial dermis and epidermis are typically spared. There are large areas of hyaline necrobiosis with degenerated collagen bundles, nuclear debris, and granulomatous inflammation. The granulomas are comprised of sheets of xanthomatized histiocytes, multinucleate giant cells, and a few lymphocytes. Cholesterol clefts may also be seen. Vasculitis is not usually present.

Besides MGUS, other hematologic disorders seen with NXG include multiple myeloma, amyloidosis, Waldenstrom's macroglobulinemia, cryoglobulinemia, chronic lymphocytic leukemia, Hodgkin lymphoma, non-Hodgkin lymphoma, and myelodysplastic syndrome.[200]

It is a progressive multiple organ disease with an indolent course for most patients. NXG is a progressive, histiocytic disease characterized by destructive cutaneous lesions, a monoclonal protein, and extracutaneous manifestations. It tends to occur in the sixth decade and is without sex predilection.[200] The skin manifestations consist of multiple indurated yellow–red plaques or nodules, most commonly collecting around the periorbital region. The symmetric involvement around the eyes may produce a variety of symptoms including pain and blurred vision. There can be conjunctival involvement, keratitis, scleritis, episcleritis, corneal perforation, and uveitis.[200]

The lesions start as papules, but become confluent, as indurated plaques. The plaques often have a yellowish hue and may have telangiectasia; they can become atrophied and ulcerate. Nearly half of the cases ulcerate. Extracutaneous sites of involvement include the spleen, heart, lung, kidney, intestine, larynx, pharynx, skeletal muscle, and central nervous system.[201] Most of the visceral lesions are asymptomatic and only discovered post-mortem.

Treatment and prognosis

There are no standardized treatments for NXG. Alkylator-based therapies like low-dose melphalan, cyclophosphamide, or chlorambucil with or without prednisone have been used[201] as has IFN-α with some response.[204] Other agents like azathioprine and methotrexate have not been useful.[201] We recently reported a case of a patient treated with high-dose chemotherapy with peripheral blood SCT who had an excellent response.[205] He had a transient response to splenectomy predating his transplant. Intralesional corticosteroid injections, radiation therapy, plasmapheresis, and surgical removal have all been tried with limited efficacy.[200] The course tends to be indolent, but progressive. The prognosis is dependent on extracutaneous involvement and whether the disease is associated with a hematologic malignancy or not.

Schnitzler's syndrome

Schnitzler's syndrome is a poorly defined syndrome characterized by chronic urticaria, IgM monoclonal gammopathy, bone pain, elevated erythrocyte sedimentation rate (ESR), lymphadenopathy, and recurrent fever.[206] (See two excellent reviews by Lipsker *et al.*[207] and by de Koning *et al.*[208]) A variant with a similar phenotype but an IgG monoclonal protein has also been described, and is now recognized as a variant of the syndrome.[208]

The pathophysiology of this disorder is not well understood. It has been postulated that the monoclonal protein serves as an autoantibody that deposits triggering a local inflammatory response that could induce the skin lesions. The typical histologic appearance of a skin lesion is that of neutrophilic urticaria.[209] Cytokine aberrations have been implicated including elevations in interleukin-6 and antibodies against interleukin-1.[208,210,211]

Because it is a rare disorder, it is under-recognized and the time from symptoms to diagnosis is usually more than 5 years.[207] De Koning *et al.* have recently published a review of 94 cases of Schnitzler's syndrome. The mean age of onset was 51 years.[208] The rash is pale rose, slightly elevated papules and plaques. Individual lesions measure 0.5–3 cm in diameter. New lesions appear daily and disappear in 12–24 hours. It can be chronic and unrelenting, but patients can go 1–2 weeks without eruptions. Head and neck are usually spared, and the trunk and extremities are most commonly affected. Approximately 45% of patients experience pruritus, but this tends to be a later finding. Angioedema is rare. Extra-dermatologic manifestations include: fever (88%), arthralgia/arthritis (82%), bone pain (72%), weight loss (64%), lymphadenopathy (44%), hepatomegaly (29%), and splenomegaly (12%).[208]

Typical laboratory findings include a moderately increased ESR, leukocytosis, mild anemia, and an elevated C-reactive protein. On immunofixation, an IgM monoclonal protein will be found. Since the monoclonal protein is typically small, it can be missed by merely measuring quantitative immunoglobulins by nephelometry or by screening with a serum

Table 11.9. Diagnostic criteria of the Schnitzler's syndrome

Criteria
Major
Chronic urticarial rash
Monoclonal IgM (or IgG: variant type)
Minor
Intermittent fever
Arthralgia or arthritis
Bone pain
Lymphadenopathy
Hepato- and/or splenomegaly
Elevated ESR and/or leukocytosis
Bone abnormalities (radiologic or histologic)

Note: To meet criteria, patient must have both major criteria and at least two minor criteria after exclusion of other causes.
Sources: de Koning *et al.*[208] and Lipsker *et al.*[212]

protein electrophoresis. Occasionally, there will be an IgG monoclonal protein instead. Complement levels are normal. The bone marrow biopsy may be "negative" and lymph nodes tend to show only reactive hyperplasia. Bone radiographs are most commonly normal, but increased bone density, lytic lesions, and periosteal apposition have been described.[207,208]

Table 11.9 contains the criteria for Schnitzler's syndrome as published by de Koning *et al.*,[208] which were based on cumulative data and criteria presented by Lipsker *et al.*[207,212] The differential diagnosis includes idiopathic chronic urticaria, cryoglobulinemia, mastocytosis, hypocomplementemic urticarial vasculitis, acquired C1 inhibitor deficiency, hyper IgD syndrome, adult-onset Still disease, systemic lupus erythematosus, Behcet's disease, and hereditary auto-inflammatory syndromes (e.g., cryopyrin-associated syndrome, familial cold urticaria, Muckle–Wells syndrome, and chronic infantile neurologic cutaneous and articular syndrome).[207,208]

Treatment and prognosis

Treatments that have provided varying degrees of relief include anakinra (an interleukin-receptor antagonist), oral corticosteroids, thalidomide, PUVA, antihistamines, nonsteroidal anti-inflammatory drugs, interferon, rituximab, intravenous gammaglobulin, colchicine, dapsone, ciclosporin, alkylating agents, purine nucleoside analogs, methotrexate, and plasma exchange.[207,208] The demonstrated clinical efficacy of the interleukin-1β inhibitor anakinra against this disorder would suggest that interleukin-1β plays an important role in the pathophysiology.[209–212]

Patients are at risk for both progression to Waldenstrom's macroglobulinemia and amyloid A amyloidosis. AL amyloidosis has not been reported. In a recent study of 94 patients, the 15-year survival rate was 91%.[213] In this same series, 11 patients developed Waldenstrom's macroglobulinemia.

References

1. Kyle RA, Linos A, Beard CM, *et al.* Incidence and natural history of primary systemic amyloidosis in Olmsted County, Minnesota, 1950 through 1989. *Blood* 1992;**79**:1817–22.
2. Rajkumar SV, Dispenzieri A, Kyle RA. Monoclonal gammopathy of undetermined significance, Waldenstrom macroglobulinemia, AL amyloidosis, and related plasma cell disorders: diagnosis and treatment. *Mayo Clin Proc* 2006;**81**:693–703.
3. Palladini G, Kyle RA, Larson DR, *et al.* Multicentre versus single centre approach to rare diseases: the model of systemic light chain amyloidosis. *Amyloid* 2005;**12**:120–6.
4. Lachmann HJ, Booth DR, Booth SE, *et al.* Misdiagnosis of hereditary amyloidosis as AL (primary) amyloidosis. *N Engl J Med* 2002;**346**:1786–91.
5. Comenzo RL, Zhou P, Fleisher M, *et al.* Seeking confidence in the diagnosis of systemic AL (Ig light-chain) amyloidosis: patients can have both monoclonal gammopathies and hereditary amyloid proteins. *Blood* 2006;**107**:3489–91.
6. Gertz MA, Lacy MQ, Dispenzieri A, *et al.* Amyloidosis: diagnosis and management. *Clin Lymphoma Myeloma* 2005;**6**:208–19.
7. Hamidi Asl K, Liepnieks JJ, Nakamura M, *et al.* Organ-specific (localized) synthesis of Ig light chain amyloid. *J Immunol* 1999;**162**:5556–60.
8. Gertz MA, Comenzo R, Falk RH, *et al.* Definition of organ involvement and treatment response in immunoglobulin light chain amyloidosis (AL): a consensus opinion from the 10th International Symposium on Amyloid and Amyloidosis, Tours, France, 18–22 April 2004. *Am J Hematol* 2005; **79**:319–28.
9. Trinkaus-Randall V, Walsh MT, Steeves S, *et al.* Cellular response of cardiac fibroblasts to amyloidogenic light chains. *Am J Pathol* 2005;**166**:197–208.
10. Gertz MA, Lacy MQ, Dispenzieri A, *et al.* Effect of hematologic response on outcome of patients undergoing transplantation for primary amyloidosis: importance of achieving a complete response. *Haematologica* 2007;**92**:1415–18.
11. Gertz MA, Lacy MQ, Dispenzieri A, *et al.* Risk-adjusted manipulation of melphalan dose before stem cell transplantation in patients with amyloidosis is associated with a lower response rate. *Bone Marrow Transplant* 2004;**34**:1025–31.
12. Dispenzieri A, Gertz MA, Kyle RA, *et al.* Prognostication of survival using cardiac troponins and N-terminal pro-brain natriuretic peptide in patients with primary systemic amyloidosis undergoing peripheral blood stem cell transplantation. *Blood* 2004;**104**:1881–7.
13. Gertz MA, Lacy MQ, Dispenzieri A, *et al.* Transplantation for amyloidosis. *Curr Opin Oncol* 2007;**19**:136–41.
14. Moreau P, Milpied N, de Faucal P, *et al.* High-dose melphalan and autologous

bone marrow transplantation for systemic AL amyloidosis with cardiac involvement. *Blood* 1996;**87**:3063–4.

15. Comenzo RL, Vosburgh E, Falk RH, *et al.* Dose-intensive melphalan with blood stem-cell support for the treatment of AL (amyloid light-chain) amyloidosis: survival and responses in 25 patients. *Blood* 1998;**91**:3662–70.
16. Skinner M, Sanchorawala V, Seldin DC, *et al.* High-dose melphalan and autologous stem-cell transplantation in patients with AL amyloidosis: an 8-year study. *Ann Intern Med* 2004;**140**:85–93.
17. Jaccard A, Moreau P, Leblond V, *et al.* High-dose melphalan versus melphalan plus dexamethasone for AL amyloidosis. *N Engl J Med* 2007;**357**:1083–93.
18. Vesole DH, Perez WS, Akasheh M, *et al.* High-dose therapy and autologous hematopoietic stem cell transplantation for patients with primary systemic amyloidosis: a Center for International Blood and Marrow Transplant Research Study. *Mayo Clin Proc* 2006;**81**:880–8.
19. Dispenzieri A, Kyle RA, Lacy MQ, *et al.* Superior survival in primary systemic amyloidosis patients undergoing peripheral blood stem cell transplantation: a case-control study. *Blood* 2004;**103**:3960–3.
20. Schonland SO, Lokhorst H, Buzyn A, *et al.* Allogeneic and syngeneic hematopoietic cell transplantation in patients with amyloid light-chain amyloidosis: a report from the European Group for Blood and Marrow Transplantation. *Blood* 2006;**107**:2578–84.
21. Jones NF, Hilton PJ, Tighe JR, *et al.* Treatment of "primary" renal amyloidosis with melphalan. *Lancet* 1972;**2**:616–19.
22. Cohen HJ, Lessin LS, Hallal J, *et al.* Resolution of primary amyloidosis during chemotherapy. Studies in a patient with nephrotic syndrome. *Ann Intern Med* 1975;**82**:466–73.
23. Kyle RA, Greipp PR, Garton JP, *et al.* Primary systemic amyloidosis. Comparison of melphalan/prednisone versus colchicine. *Am J Med* 1985;**79**:708–16.
24. Kyle RA, Greipp PR. Primary systemic amyloidosis: comparison of melphalan and prednisone versus placebo. *Blood* 1978;**52**:818–27.
25. Kyle RA, Gertz MA, Greipp PR, *et al.* A trial of three regimens for primary amyloidosis: colchicine alone, melphalan and prednisone, and melphalan, prednisone, and colchicine. *N Engl J Med* 1997;**336**:1202–7.
26. Skinner M, Anderson J, Simms R, *et al.* Treatment of 100 patients with primary amyloidosis: a randomized trial of melphalan, prednisone, and colchicine versus colchicine only. *Am J Med* 1996;**100**:290–8.
27. Gertz MA, Lacy MQ, Lust JA, *et al.* Prospective randomized trial of melphalan and prednisone versus vincristine, carmustine, melphalan, cyclophosphamide, and prednisone in the treatment of primary systemic amyloidosis. *J Clin Oncol* 1999;**17**:262–7.
28. Lachmann HJ, Gallimore R, Gillmore JD, *et al.* Outcome in systemic AL amyloidosis in relation to changes in concentration of circulating free immunoglobulin light chains following chemotherapy. *Br J Haematol* 2003;**122**:78–84.
29. Palladini G, Perfetti V, Obici L, *et al.* Association of melphalan and high-dose dexamethasone is effective and well tolerated in patients with AL (primary) amyloidosis who are ineligible for stem cell transplantation. *Blood* 2004;**103**:2936–8.
30. Gertz MA, Lacy MQ, Lust JA, *et al.* Phase II trial of high-dose dexamethasone for previously treated immunoglobulin light-chain amyloidosis. *Am J Hematol* 1999;**61**:115–19.
31. Gertz MA, Lacy MQ, Lust JA, *et al.* Phase II trial of high-dose dexamethasone for untreated patients with primary systemic amyloidosis. *Med Oncol* 1999;**16**:104–9.
32. Dhodapkar MV, Hussein MA, Rasmussen E, *et al.* Clinical efficacy of high-dose dexamethasone with maintenance dexamethasone/alpha interferon in patients with primary systemic amyloidosis: results of United States Intergroup Trial Southwest Oncology Group (SWOG) S9628. *Blood* 2004;**104**:3520–6.
33. Levy Y, Belghiti-Deprez D, Sobel A. Treatment of AL amyloidosis without myeloma. *Ann Med Interne (Paris)* 1988;**139**:190–3.
34. Wardley AM, Jayson GC, Goldsmith DJ, *et al.* The treatment of nephrotic syndrome caused by primary (light chain) amyloid with vincristine, doxorubicin and dexamethasone. *Br J Cancer* 1998;**78**:774–6.
35. van Gameren I, Hazenberg BP, Jager PL, *et al.* AL amyloidosis treated with induction chemotherapy with VAD followed by high dose melphalan and autologous stem cell transplantation. *Amyloid* 2002;**9**:165–74.
36. Ichida M, Imagawa S, Ohmine K, *et al.* Successful treatment of multiple myeloma-associated amyloidosis by interferon-alpha, dimethyl sulfoxide, and VAD (vincristine, adriamycin, and dexamethasone). *Int J Hematol* 2000;**72**:491–3.
37. Gono T, Matsuda M, Shimojima Y, *et al.* VAD with or without subsequent high-dose melphalan followed by autologous stem cell support in AL amyloidosis: Japanese experience and criteria for patient selection. *Amyloid* 2004;**11**:245–56.
38. Gertz MA, Kyle RA, Greipp PR. Response rates and survival in primary systemic amyloidosis. *Blood* 1991;**77**:257–62.
39. Palladini G, Russo P, Nuvolone M, *et al.* Treatment with oral melphalan plus dexamethasone produces long-term remissions in AL amyloidosis. *Blood* 2007;**110**:787–8.
40. Gertz MA, Kyle RA. Acute leukemia and cytogenetic abnormalities complicating melphalan treatment of primary systemic amyloidosis. *Arch Intern Med* 1990;**150**:629–33.
41. Seldin DC, Choufani EB, Dember LM, *et al.* Tolerability and efficacy of thalidomide for the treatment of patients with light chain-associated (AL) amyloidosis. *Clin Lymphoma* 2003;**3**:241–6.
42. Palladini G, Perfetti V, Perlini S, *et al.* The combination of thalidomide and intermediate-dose dexamethasone is an effective but toxic treatment for patients with primary amyloidosis (AL). *Blood* 2005;**105**:2949–51.
43. Dispenzieri A, Lacy MQ, Rajkumar SV, *et al.* Poor tolerance to high doses of thalidomide in patients with primary systemic amyloidosis. *Amyloid* 2003;**10**:257–61.
44. Dispenzieri A, Lacy MQ, Geyer SM, *et al.* Low dose single agent thalidomide is tolerated in patients with primary systemic amyloidosis, but responses are limited. *ASH Annual Meeting Abstracts* 2004;**104**:4920.

45. Wechalekar AD, Goodman HJ, Lachmann HJ, *et al.* Safety and efficacy of risk-adapted cyclophosphamide, thalidomide, and dexamethasone in systemic AL amyloidosis. *Blood* 2007;**109**:457–64.

46. Dispenzieri A, Lacy MQ, Zeldenrust SR, *et al.* The activity of lenalidomide with or without dexamethasone in patients with primary systemic amyloidosis. *Blood* 2007;**109**:465–70.

47. Sanchorawala V, Wright DG, Rosenzweig M, *et al.* Lenalidomide and dexamethasone in the treatment of AL amyloidosis: results of a phase 2 trial. *Blood* 2007;**109**:492–6.

48. Kastritis E, Anagnostopoulos A, Roussou M, *et al.* Treatment of light chain (AL) amyloidosis with the combination of bortezomib and dexamethasone. *Haematologica* 2007;**92**:1351–8.

49. Wechalekar AD, Lachmann HJ, Offer M, *et al.* Efficacy of bortezomib in systemic AL amyloidosis with relapsed/refractory clonal disease. *Haematologica* 2008;**93**:295–8.

50. Reece DE, Sanchorawala V, Hegenbart U, *et al.* Weekly and twice-weekly bortezomib in patients with systemic AL amyloidosis: results of a phase 1 dose-escalation study. *Blood* 2009;**114** (8):1489–97.

51. Dispenzieri A, Kyle RA, Lacy MQ, *et al.* POEMS syndrome: definitions and long-term outcome. *Blood* 2003;**101**:2496–506.

52. Gertz MA, Kyle RA, Greipp PR, *et al.* Beta 2-microglobulin predicts survival in primary systemic amyloidosis. *Am J Med* 1990;**89**:609–14.

53. Dispenzieri A, Lacy MQ, Katzmann JA, *et al.* Absolute values of immunoglobulin free light chains are prognostic in patients with primary systemic amyloidosis undergoing peripheral blood stem cell transplantation. *Blood* 2006;**107**:3378–83.

54. Moreau P, Leblond V, Bourquelot P, *et al.* Prognostic factors for survival and response after high-dose therapy and autologous stem cell transplantation in systemic AL amyloidosis: a report on 21 patients. *Br J Haematol* 1998;**101**:766–9.

55. Gertz MA, Lacy MQ, Dispenzieri A, *et al.* Amyloidosis. *Best Pract Res Clin Haematol* 2005;**18**:709–27.

56. Cueto-Garcia L, Reeder GS, Kyle RA, *et al.* Echocardiographic findings in systemic amyloidosis: spectrum of cardiac involvement and relation to survival. *J Am Coll Cardiol* 1985;**6**:737–43.

57. Dispenzieri A, Kyle RA, Gertz MA, *et al.* Survival in patients with primary systemic amyloidosis and raised serum cardiac troponins. *Lancet* 2003;**361**:1787–9.

58. Dispenzieri A, Gertz MA, Kyle RA, *et al.* Serum cardiac troponins and N-terminal pro-brain natriuretic peptide: a staging system for primary systemic amyloidosis. *J Clin Oncol* 2004; **22**:3751–7.

59. Palladini G, Campana C, Klersy C, *et al.* Serum N-terminal pro-brain natriuretic peptide is a sensitive marker of myocardial dysfunction in AL amyloidosis. *Circulation* 2003;**107**:2440–5.

60. Gertz M, Lacy M, Dispenzieri A, *et al.* Troponin T level as an exclusion criterion for stem cell transplantation in light-chain amyloidosis. *Leuk Lymphoma* 2008;**49**:36–41.

61. Sanchorawala V, Seldin DC, Magnani B, *et al.* Serum free light-chain responses after high-dose intravenous melphalan and autologous stem cell transplantation for AL (primary) amyloidosis. *Bone Marrow Transplant* 2005;**36**:597–600.

62. Cohen AD, Zhou P, Chou J, *et al.* Risk-adapted autologous stem cell transplantation with adjuvant dexamethasone +/— thalidomide for systemic light-chain amyloidosis: results of a phase II trial. *Br J Haematol* 2007;**139**:224–33.

63. Biewend ML, Menke DM, Calamia KT. The spectrum of localized amyloidosis: a case series of 20 patients and review of the literature. *Amyloid* 2006; **13**:135–42.

64. Utz JP, Gertz MA, Kalra S. External-beam radiation therapy in the treatment of diffuse tracheobronchial amyloidosis. *Chest* 2001;**120**:1735–8.

65. Pitz MW, Gibson IW, Johnston JB. Isolated pulmonary amyloidosis: case report and review of the literature. *Am J Hematol* 2006;**81**:212–13.

66. Dundore PA, Aisner SC, Templeton PA, *et al.* Nodular pulmonary amyloidosis: diagnosis by fine-needle aspiration cytology and a review of the literature. *Diagn Cytopathol* 1993;**9**:562–4.

67. Neben-Wittich MA, Foote RL, Kalra S. Electron beam radiation therapy for tracheobronchial amyloidosis. *Chest* 2007;**132**:262–7.

68. Mariani AJ, Barrett DM, Kurtz SB, *et al.* Bilateral localized amyloidosis of the ureter presenting with anuria. *J Urol* 1978;**120**:757–9.

69. Shittu OB, Weston PM. Localised amyloidosis of the urinary bladder: a case report and review of treatment. *West Afr J Med* 1994;**13**:252–3.

70. Malek RS, Wahner-Roedler DL, *et al.* Primary localized amyloidosis of the bladder: experience with dimethyl sulfoxide therapy. *J Urol* 2002;**168**:1018–20.

71. Bardwick PA, Zvaifler NJ, Gill GN, *et al.* Plasma cell dyscrasia with polyneuropathy, organomegaly, endocrinopathy, M protein, and skin changes: the POEMS syndrome. Report on two cases and a review of the literature. *Medicine* 1980;**59**:311–22.

72. Dispenzieri A, Kyle RA, Lacy MQ, *et al.* POEMS syndrome: definitions and long-term outcome. *Blood* 2003;**101**:2496–506.

73. Takatsuki K, Sanada I. Plasma cell dyscrasia with polyneuropathy and endocrine disorder: clinical and laboratory features of 109 reported cases. *Jpn J Clin Oncol* 1983;**13**:543–55.

74. Nakanishi T, Sobue I, Toyokura Y, *et al.* The Crow-Fukase syndrome: a study of 102 cases in Japan. *Neurology* 1984;**34**:712–20.

75. Dispenzieri A. POEMS syndrome. *Blood Reviews* 2007;**21**:285–99.

76. Watanabe O, Arimura K, Kitajima I, *et al.* Greatly raised vascular endothelial growth factor (VEGF) in POEMS syndrome [letter]. *Lancet* 1996;**347**:702.

77. Soubrier M, Dubost JJ, Serre AF, *et al.* Growth factors in POEMS syndrome: evidence for a marked increase in circulating vascular endothelial growth factor. *Arthritis Rheum* 1997;**40**:786–7.

78. Hashiguchi T, Arimura K, Matsumuro K, *et al.* Highly concentrated vascular endothelial growth factor in platelets in Crow-Fukase syndrome. *Muscle Nerve* 2000;**23**:1051–6.

79. Watanabe O, Maruyama I, Arimura K, *et al.* Overproduction of vascular endothelial growth factor/vascular

permeability factor is causative in Crow-Fukase (POEMS) syndrome. *Muscle Nerve* 1998;**21**:1390–7.

80. Scarlato M, Previtali SC, Carpo M, *et al.* Polyneuropathy in POEMS syndrome: role of angiogenic factors in the pathogenesis. *Brain* 2005;**128**:1911–20.
81. Kelly JJ Jr, Kyle RA, Miles JM, *et al.* Osteosclerotic myeloma and peripheral neuropathy. *Neurology* 1983;**33**:202–10.
82. Ghandi GY, Basu R, Dispenzieri A, *et al.* Endocrinopathy in POEMS syndrome: the Mayo Clinic experience. *Mayo Clin Proc* 2007;**82**:836–42.
83. Sanada S, Ookawara S, Karube H, *et al.* Marked recovery of severe renal lesions in POEMS syndrome with high-dose melphalan therapy supported by autologous blood stem cell transplantation. *Am J Kidney Dis* 2006;**47**:672–9.
84. Soubrier MJ, Dubost JJ, Sauvezie BJ. POEMS syndrome: a study of 25 cases and a review of the literature. French Study Group on POEMS Syndrome. *Am J Med* 1994;**97**:543–53.
85. Lesprit P, Authier FJ, Gherardi R, *et al.* Acute arterial obliteration: a new feature of the POEMS syndrome? *Medicine* 1996;**75**:226–32.
86. Zenone T, Bastion Y, Salles G, *et al.* POEMS syndrome, arterial thrombosis and thrombocythaemia. *J Intern Med* 1996;**240**:107–9.
87. Soubrier M, Guillon R, Dubost JJ, *et al.* Arterial obliteration in POEMS syndrome: possible role of vascular endothelial growth factor. *J Rheumatol* 1998;**25**:813–15.
88. Bova G, Pasqui AL, Saletti M, *et al.* POEMS syndrome with vascular lesions: a role for interleukin-1beta and interleukin-6 increase–a case report. *Angiology* 1998;**49**:937–40.
89. Kang K, Chu K, Kim DE, *et al.* POEMS syndrome associated with ischemic stroke. *Arch Neurol* 2003;**60**:745–9.
90. Mufti GJ, Hamblin TJ, Gordon J. Melphalan-induced pulmonary fibrosis in osteosclerotic myeloma [letter]. *Acta Haematologica* 1983;**69**:140–1.
91. Iwasaki H, Ogawa K, Yoshida H, *et al.* Crow-Fukase syndrome associated with pulmonary hypertension. *Intern Med* 1993;**32**:556–60.
92. Lesprit P, Godeau B, Authier FJ, *et al.* Pulmonary hypertension in POEMS syndrome: a new feature mediated by cytokines. *Am J Respir Crit Care Med* 1998;**157**:907–11.
93. Dispenzieri A, Moreno-Aspitia A, Suarez GA, *et al.* Peripheral blood stem cell transplantation in 16 patients with POEMS syndrome, and a review of the literature. *Blood* 2004;**104**:3400–7.
94. Allam JS, Kennedy CC, Aksamit TR, *et al.* Pulmonary manifestations in patients with POEMS syndrome: a retrospective review of 137 patients. *Chest* 2008;**133**:969–74.
95. Barrier JH, Le Noan H, Mussini JM, *et al.* Stabilisation of a severe case of P.O.E.M.S. syndrome after tamoxifen administration [letter]. *J Neurol Neurosurg Psychiatry* 1989;**52**:286.
96. Matsui H, Udaka F, Kubori T, *et al.* POEMS syndrome demonstrating VEGF decrease by ticlopidine. *Intern Med* 2004;**43**:1082–3.
97. Tokashiki T, Hashiguchi T, Arimura K, *et al.* Predictive value of serial platelet count and VEGF determination for the management of DIC in the Crow-Fukase (POEMS) syndrome. *Intern Med* 2003;**42**:1240–3.
98. Saida K, Kawakami H, Ohta M, *et al.* Coagulation and vascular abnormalities in Crow-Fukase syndrome. *Muscle Nerve* 1997;**20**:486–92.
99. Coto V, Auletta M, Oliviero U, *et al.* POEMS syndrome: an Italian case with diagnostic and therapeutic implications. *Ann Ital Med Int* 1991;**6**:416–19.
100. Authier FJ, Belec L, Levy Y, *et al.* All-trans-retinoic acid in POEMS syndrome. Therapeutic effect associated with decreased circulating levels of proinflammatory cytokines. *Arthritis Rheum* 1996;**39**:1423–6.
101. Sternberg AJ, Davies P, Macmillan C, *et al.* Strontium-89: a novel treatment for a case of osteosclerotic myeloma associated with life-threatening neuropathy. *Br J Haematol* 2002;**118**:821–4.
102. Kim SY, Lee SA, Ryoo HM, *et al.* Thalidomide for POEMS syndrome. *Ann Hematol* 2006;**85**:545–6.
103. Sinisalo M, Hietaharju A, Sauranen J, *et al.* Thalidomide in POEMS syndrome: case report. *Am J Hematol* 2004;**76**:66–8.
104. Badros A, Porter N, Zimrin A. Bevacizumab therapy for POEMS syndrome. *Blood* 2005;**106**:1135.
105. Straume O, Bergheim J, Ernst P. Bevacizumab therapy for POEMS syndrome. *Blood* 2006;**107**:4972–3; author reply 4973–4.
106. Dispenzieri A, Klein CJ, Mauermann ML. Lenalidomide therapy in a patient with POEMS syndrome. *Blood* 2007;**110**:1075–6.
107. Dispenzieri A, Lacy MQ, Hayman SR, *et al.* Peripheral blood stem cell transplant for POEMS syndrome is associated with high rates of engraftment syndrome. *Eur J Haematol* 2008;**80**:397–406.
108. Nakano A, Mitsui T, Endo I, *et al.* Solitary plasmacytoma with VEGF overproduction: report of a patient with polyneuropathy. *Neurology* 2001;**56**:818–19.
109. Mineta M, Hatori M, Sano H, *et al.* Recurrent Crow-Fukase syndrome associated with increased serum levels of vascular endothelial growth factor: a case report and review of the literature. *Tohoku J Exp Med* 2006;**210**:269–77.
110. Soubrier M, Ruivard M, Dubost JJ, *et al.* Successful use of autologous bone marrow transplantation in treating a patient with POEMS syndrome. *Bone Marrow Transplant* 2002;**30**:61–2.
111. Jaccard A, Royer B, Bordessoule D, *et al.* High-dose therapy and autologous blood stem cell transplantation in POEMS syndrome. *Blood* 2002;**99**:3057–9.
112. Singhal S, Mehta J, Desikan R, *et al.* Antitumor activity of thalidomide in refractory multiple myeloma. *N Engl J Med* 1999;**341**:1565–71.
113. Dispenzieri A, Gorevic PD. Cryoglobulinemia. *Hematol Oncol Clin North Am* 1999;**13**:1315–49.
114. Meltzer M, Franklin EC, Elias K, *et al.* Cryoglobulinemia–a clinical and laboratory study. II. Cryoglobulins with rheumatoid factor activity. *Am J Med* 1966;**40**:837–56.
115. Brouet J, Clauvel J, Danon F, *et al.* Biological and clinical significance of cryoglobulins. A report of 86 cases. *Am J Med* 1974;**57**:775–88.
116. Gorevic PD, Kassab HJ, Levo Y, *et al.* Mixed cryoglobulinemia: clinical aspects and long-term follow-up of 40 patients. *Am J Med* 1980;**69**:287–308.
117. Monti G, Galli M, Invernizzi F, *et al.* Cryoglobulinaemias: a multi-centre

study of the early clinical and laboratory manifestations of primary and secondary disease. GISC. Italian Group for the Study of Cryoglobulinaemias. *QJM* 1995;**88**:115–26.

118. Pascual M, Perrin L, Giostra E, *et al.* Hepatitis C virus in patients with cryoglobulinemia type II. *J Infect Dis* 1990;**162**:569–70.
119. Ferri C, Greco F, Longombardo G, *et al.* Antibodies to hepatitis C virus in patients with mixed cryoglobulinemia. *Arthritis Rheum* 1991;**34**:1606–10.
120. Mendez P, Saeian K, Reddy KR, *et al.* Hepatitis C, cryoglobulinemia, and cutaneous vasculitis associated with unusual and serious manifestations. *Am J Gastroenterol* 2001;**96**:2489–93.
121. Donada C, Crucitti A, Donadon V, *et al.* Systemic manifestations and liver disease in patients with chronic hepatitis C and type II or III mixed cryoglobulinaemia. *J Viral Hepat* 1998;**5**:179–85.
122. Montagnino G. Reappraisal of the clinical expression of mixed cryoglobulinemia. *Springer Semin Immunopathol* 1988;**10**:1–19.
123. Cohen SJ, Pittelkow MR, Su WP. Cutaneous manifestations of cryoglobulinemia: clinical and histopathologic study of seventy-two patients. *J Am Acad Dermatol* 1991;**25**:21–7.
124. Ferri C, La Civita L, Longombardo G, *et al.* Mixed cryoglobulinaemia: a cross-road between autoimmune and lymphoproliferative disorders. *Lupus* 1998;**7**:275–9.
125. Trejo O, Ramos-Casals M, Garcia-Carrasco M, *et al.* Cryoglobulinemia: study of etiologic factors and clinical and immunologic features in 443 patients from a single center. *Medicine (Baltimore)* 2001;**80**:252–62.
126. Cordonnier D, Vialtel P, Renversez JC, *et al.* Renal diseases in 18 patients with mixed type II IgM-IgG cryoglobulinemia: monoclonal lymphoid infiltration (2 cases) and membranoproliferative glomerulonephritis (14 cases). *Adv Nephrol Necker Hosp* 1983; **12**:177–204.
127. Invernizzi F, Galli M, Serino G, *et al.* Secondary and essential cryoglobulinemias. Frequency, nosological classification, and long-term follow-up. *Acta Haematol* 1983;**70**:73–82.
128. Tarantino A, Campise M, Banfi G, *et al.* Long-term predictors of survival in essential mixed cryoglobulinemic glomerulonephritis. *Kidney Int* 1995;**47**:618–23.
129. Gorevic PD, Frangione B. Mixed cryoglobulinemia cross-reactive idiotypes: implications for the relationship of MC to rheumatic and lymphoproliferative diseases. *Semin Hematol* 1991;**28**:79–94.
130. Singer DR, Venning MC, Lockwood CM, *et al.* Cryoglobulinaemia: clinical features and response to treatment. *Ann Med Interne (Paris)* 1986;**137**:251–3.
131. Gemignani F, Brindani F, Alfieri S, *et al.* Clinical spectrum of cryoglobulinaemic neuropathy. *J Neurol Neurosurg Psychiatry* 2005;**76**:1410–14.
132. Chad D, Pariser K, Bradley WG, *et al.* The pathogenesis of cryoglobulinemic neuropathy. *Neurology* 1982;**32**:725–9.
133. Nemni R, Corbo M, Fazio R, *et al.* Cryoglobulinaemic neuropathy. A clinical, morphological and immunocytochemical study of 8 cases. *Brain* 1988;**111**:541–52.
134. Cavaletti G, Petruccioli MG, Crespi V, *et al.* A clinico-pathological and follow up study of 10 cases of essential type II cryoglobulinaemic neuropathy. *J Neurol Neurosurg Psychiatry* 1990;**53**:886–9.
135. Ammendola A, Sampaolo S, Ambrosone L, *et al.* Peripheral neuropathy in hepatitis-related mixed cryoglobulinemia: electrophysiologic follow-up study. *Muscle Nerve* 2005;**31**:382–5.
136. Bryce AH, Kyle RA, Dispenzieri A, *et al.* Natural history and therapy of 66 patients with mixed cryoglobulinemia. *Am J Hematol* 2006;**81**:511–18.
137. Tarantino A, Anelli A, Costantino A, *et al.* Serum complement pattern in essential mixed cryoglobulinaemia. *Clin Exp Immunol* 1978;**32**:77–85.
138. Ferri C, Moriconi L, Gremignai G, *et al.* Treatment of the renal involvement in mixed cryoglobulinemia with prolonged plasma exchange. *Nephron* 1986;**43**:246–53.
139. Frankel AH, Singer DR, Winearls CG, *et al.* Type II essential mixed cryoglobulinaemia: presentation, treatment and outcome in 13 patients. *Q J Med* 1992;**82**:101–24.
140. Monti G, Saccardo F, Pioltelli P, *et al.* The natural history of cryoglobulinemia: symptoms at onset and during follow-up. A report by the Italian Group for the Study of Cryoglobulinemias (GISC). *Clin Exp Rheumatol* 1995;**13**:S129–33.
141. Ferri C, Marzo E, Longombardo G, *et al.* Interferon-alpha in mixed cryoglobulinemia patients: a randomized, crossover-controlled trial. *Blood* 1993;**81**:1132–6.
142. Ferri C, Sebastiani M, Giuggioli D, *et al.* Mixed cryoglobulinemia: demographic, clinical, and serologic features and survival in 231 patients. *Semin Arthritis Rheum* 2004;**33**:355–74.
143. Rieu V, Cohen P, Andre MH, *et al.* Characteristics and outcome of 49 patients with symptomatic cryoglobulinaemia. *Rheumatology (Oxford)* 2002;**41**:290–300.
144. Ferri C, Marzo E, Longombardo G, *et al.* Interferon alfa-2b in mixed cryoglobulinaemia: a controlled crossover trial. *Gut* 1993;**34**: S144–5.
145. Misiani R, Bellavita P, Fenili D, *et al.* Interferon alfa-2a therapy in cryoglobulinemia associated with hepatitis C virus. *N Engl J Med* 1994;**330**:751–6.
146. Dammacco F, Sansonno D, Han JH, *et al.* Natural interferon-alpha versus its combination with 6-methyl-prednisolone in the therapy of type II mixed cryoglobulinemia: a long-term, randomized, controlled study. *Blood* 1994;**84**:3336–43.
147. Lauta VM, De Sangro MA. Long-term results regarding the use of recombinant interferon alpha-2b in the treatment of II type mixed essential cryoglobulinemia. *Med Oncol* 1995;**12**:223–30.
148. Mazzaro C, Lacchin T, Moretti M, *et al.* Effects of two different alpha-interferon regimens on clinical and virological findings in mixed cryoglobulinemia. *Clin Exp Rheumatol* 1995;**13**:S181–5.
149. Ferri C, Pietrogrande M, Cecchetti R, *et al.* Low-antigen-content diet in the treatment of patients with mixed cryoglobulinemia. *Am J Med* 1989;**87**:519–24.
150. D'Amico G. Renal involvement in hepatitis C infection: cryoglobulinemic glomerulonephritis. *Kidney Int* 1998;**54**:650–71.

151. Alric L, Plaisier E, Thebault S, *et al.* Influence of antiviral therapy in hepatitis C virus-associated cryoglobulinemic MPGN. *Am J Kidney Dis* 2004;**43**:617–23.
152. Zignego AL, Ferri C, Pileri SA, *et al.* Extrahepatic manifestations of Hepatitis C Virus infection: a general overview and guidelines for a clinical approach. *Dig Liver Dis* 2007;**39**:2–17.
153. Geltner D, Kohn RW, Gorevic P, *et al.* The effect of combination therapy (steroids, immunosuppressives, and plasmapheresis) on 5 mixed cryoglobulinemia patients with renal, neurologic, and vascular involvement. *Arthritis Rheum* 1981;**24**:1121–7.
154. Valbonesi M, Montani F, Mosconi L, *et al.* Plasmapheresis and cytotoxic drugs for mixed cryoglobulinemia. *Haematologia* 1984;**17**:341–51.
155. Sinico RA, Fornasieri A, Fiorini G, *et al.* Plasma exchange in the treatment of essential mixed cryoglobulinemia nephropathy. Long-term follow up. *Int J Artif Organs* 1985;**2**:15–18.
156. Migliaresi S, Tirri G. Interferon in the treatment of mixed cryoglobulinemia. *Clin Exp Rheumatol* 1995;**13**:S175–80.
157. Bruchfeld A, Lindahl K, Stahle L, *et al.* Interferon and ribavirin treatment in patients with hepatitis C-associated renal disease and renal insufficiency. *Nephrol Dial Transplant* 2003;**18**:1573–80.
158. Casato M, Lagana B, Antonelli G, *et al.* Long-term results of therapy with interferon-alpha for type II essential mixed cryoglobulinemia. *Blood* 1991;**78**:3142–7.
159. Ohta S, Yokoyama H, Wada T, *et al.* Exacerbation of glomerulonephritis in subjects with chronic hepatitis C virus infection after interferon therapy. *Am J Kidney Dis* 1999;**33**:1040–8.
160. Beuthien W, Mellinghoff HU, Kempis J. Vasculitic complications of interferon-alpha treatment for chronic hepatitis C virus infection: case report and review of the literature. *Clin Rheumatol* 2005;**24**:507–15.
161. Cid MC, Hernandez-Rodriguez J, Robert J, *et al.* Interferon-alpha may exacerbate cryoglobulinemia-related ischemic manifestations: an adverse effect potentially related to its anti-angiogenic activity. *Arthritis Rheum* 1999;**42**:1051–5.
162. Zaja F, De Vita S, Mazzaro C, *et al.* Efficacy and safety of rituximab in type II mixed cryoglobulinemia. *Blood* 2003;**101**:3827–34.
163. Sansonno D, De Re V, Lauletta G, *et al.* Monoclonal antibody treatment of mixed cryoglobulinemia resistant to interferon alpha with an anti-CD20. *Blood* 2003;**101**:3818–26.
164. Bryce AH, Dispenzieri A, Kyle RA, *et al.* Response to rituximab in patients with type II cryoglobulinemia. *Clin Lymphoma Myeloma* 2006;**7**:140–4.
165. Roccatello D, Baldovino S, Rossi D, *et al.* Long-term effects of anti-CD20 monoclonal antibody treatment of cryoglobulinaemic glomerulonephritis. *Nephrol Dial Transplant* 2004; **19**:3054–61.
166. Basse G, Ribes D, Kamar N, *et al.* Rituximab therapy for mixed cryoglobulinemia in seven renal transplant patients. *Transplant Proc* 2006;**38**:2308–10.
167. Ghobrial IM, Uslan DZ, Call TG, *et al.* Initial increase in the cryoglobulin level after rituximab therapy for type II cryoglobulinemia secondary to Waldenstrom macroglobulinemia does not indicate failure of response. *Am J Hematol* 2004;**77**:329–30.
168. Frickhofen N, Wiesneth M, Jainta C, *et al.* Hepatitis C virus infection is a risk factor for liver failure from veno-occlusive disease after bone marrow transplantation. *Blood* 1994;**83**:1998–2004.
169. Mathison DA, Condemi JJ, Leddy JP, *et al.* Purpura, arthralgia, and IgM-IgM cryoglobulinemia with rheumatoid factor activity. Response to cyclophosphamide and splenectomy. *Ann Intern Med* 1971;**74**:383–90.
170. Ubara Y, Hara S, Katori H, *et al.* Splenectomy may improve the glomerulopathy of type II mixed cryoglobulinemia. *Am J Kidney Dis* 2000;**35**:1186–92.
171. Meltzer M, Franklin EC. Cryoglobulinemia–a study of twenty-nine patients. I. IgG and IgM cryoglobulins and factors affecting cryoprecipitability. *Am J Med* 1966;**40**:828–56.
172. Kyle RA, Therneau TM, Rajkumar SV, *et al.* A long-term study of prognosis in monoclonal gammopathy of undetermined significance. *N Engl J Med* 2002;**346**:564–9.
173. Kahn SN, Riches PG, Kohn J. Paraproteinaemia in neurological disease: incidence, associations, and classification of monoclonal immunoglobulins. *J Clin Pathol* 1980;**33**:617–21.
174. Kelly JJ Jr, Kyle RA, O'Brien PC, *et al.* Prevalence of monoclonal protein in peripheral neuropathy. *Neurology* 1981;**31**:1480–3.
175. Dispenzieri A, Kyle RA. Neurological aspects of multiple myeloma and related disorders. *Best Pract Res Clin Haematol* 2005;**18**:673–88.
176. Latov N, Sherman WH, Nemni R, *et al.* Plasma-cell dyscrasia and peripheral neuropathy with a monoclonal antibody to peripheral-nerve myelin. *N Engl J Med* 1980;**303**:618–21.
177. Quarles RH, Weiss MD. Autoantibodies associated with peripheral neuropathy. *Muscle Nerve* 1999;**22**:800–22.
178. Nobile-Orazio E, Meucci N, Baldini L, *et al.* Long-term prognosis of neuropathy associated with anti-MAG IgM M-proteins and its relationship to immune therapies. *Brain* 2000;**123**:710–17.
179. Dyck PJ, Low PA, Windebank AJ, *et al.* Plasma exchange in polyneuropathy associated with monoclonal gammopathy of undetermined significance. *N Engl J Med* 1991;**325**:1482–6.
180. Oksenhendler E, Chevret S, Leger JM, *et al.* Plasma exchange and chlorambucil in polyneuropathy associated with monoclonal IgM gammopathy. IgM-associated Polyneuropathy Study Group. *J Neurol Neurosurg Psychiatry* 1995;**59**:243–7.
181. Mariette X, Chastang C, Clavelou P, *et al.* A randomised clinical trial comparing interferon-alpha and intravenous immunoglobulin in polyneuropathy associated with monoclonal IgM. The IgM-associated Polyneuropathy Study Group. *J Neurol Neurosurg Psychiatry* 1997;**63**:28–34.
182. Comi G, Roveri L, Swan A, *et al.* A randomised controlled trial of intravenous immunoglobulin in IgM paraprotein associated demyelinating neuropathy. *J Neurol* 2002;**249**:1370–7.
183. Mariette X, Brouet JC, Chevret S, *et al.* A randomised double blind trial versus placebo does not confirm the benefit of alpha-interferon in polyneuropathy associated with monoclonal IgM [letter]. *J Neurol Neurosurg Psychiatry* 2000;**69**:279–80.

184. Dalakas MC, Quarles RH, Farrer RG, *et al.* A controlled study of intravenous immunoglobulin in demyelinating neuropathy with IgM gammopathy. *Ann Neurol* 1996;**40**:792–5.

185. Gorson KC, Allam G, Ropper AH. Chronic inflammatory demyelinating polyneuropathy: clinical features and response to treatment in 67 consecutive patients with and without a monoclonal gammopathy. *Neurology* 1997;**48**:321–8.

186. Sherman WH, Olarte MR, McKiernan G, *et al.* Plasma exchange treatment of peripheral neuropathy associated with plasma cell dyscrasia. *J Neurol Neurosurg Psychiatry* 1984;**47**:813–19.

187. Yeung KB, Thomas PK, King RH, *et al.* The clinical spectrum of peripheral neuropathies associated with benign monoclonal IgM, IgG and IgA paraproteinaemia. Comparative clinical, immunological and nerve biopsy findings. *J Neurol* 1991;**238**:383–91.

188. Wilson HC, Lunn MP, Schey S, *et al.* Successful treatment of IgM paraproteinaemic neuropathy with fludarabine. *J Neurol, Neurosurg Psychiatry* 1999;**66**:575–80.

189. Levine TD, Pestronk A. IgM antibody-related polyneuropathies: B-cell depletion chemotherapy using Rituximab. *Neurology* 1999;**52**:1701–4.

190. Renaud S, Gregor M, Fuhr P, *et al.* Rituximab in the treatment of polyneuropathy associated with anti-MAG antibodies. *Muscle Nerve* 2003;**27**:611–15.

191. Pestronk A, Florence J, Miller T, *et al.* Treatment of IgM antibody associated polyneuropathies using rituximab. *J Neurol Neurosurg Psychiatry* 2003;**74**:485–9.

192. Cokonis Georgakis CD, Falasca G, Georgakis A, *et al.* Scleromyxedema. *Clin Dermatol* 2006;**24**:493–7.

193. Kucher C, Xu X, Pasha T, *et al.* Histopathologic comparison of nephrogenic fibrosing dermopathy and scleromyxedema. *J Cutan Pathol* 2005;**32**:484–90.

194. Rongioletti F, Rebora A. Updated classification of papular mucinosis, lichen myxedematosus, and scleromyxedema. *J Am Acad Dermatol* 2001;**44**:273–81.

195. Dinneen AM, Dicken CH. Scleromyxedema. *J Am Acad Dermatol* 1995;**33**:37–43.

196. Berger JR, Dobbs MR, Terhune MH, *et al.* The neurologic complications of scleromyxedema. *Medicine (Baltimore)* 2001;**80**:313–19.

197. Pomann JJ, Rudner EJ. Scleromyxedema revisited. *Int J Dermatol* 2003;**42**:31–5.

198. Lacy MQ, Hogan WJ, Gertz MA, *et al.* Successful treatment of scleromyxedema with autologous peripheral blood stem cell transplantation. *Arch Dermatol* 2005;**141**:1277–82.

199. Sansbury JC, Cocuroccia B, Jorizzo JL, *et al.* Treatment of recalcitrant scleromyxedema with thalidomide in 3 patients. *J Am Acad Dermatol* 2004;**51**:126–31.

200. Fernandez-Herrera J, Pedraz J. Necrobiotic xanthogranuloma. *Semin Cutan Med Surg* 2007;**26**:108–13.

201. Finan MC, Winkelmann RK. Necrobiotic xanthogranuloma with paraproteinemia. A review of 22 cases. *Medicine (Baltimore)* 1986;**65**:376–88.

202. Bullock JD, Bartley GB, Campbell RJ, *et al.* Necrobiotic xanthogranuloma with paraproteinemia: case report and a pathogenetic theory. *Trans Am Ophthalmol Soc* 1986;**84**:342–54.

203. Matsuura F, Yamashita S, Hirano K, *et al.* Activation of monocytes in vivo causes intracellular accumulation of lipoprotein-derived lipids and marked hypocholesterolemia–a possible pathogenesis of necrobiotic xanthogranuloma. *Atherosclerosis* 1999;**142**:355–65.

204. Venencie PY, Le Bras P, Toan ND, *et al.* Recombinant interferon alfa-2b treatment of necrobiotic xanthogranuloma with paraproteinemia. *J Am Acad Dermatol* 1995;**32**:666–7.

205. Goede JS, Misselwitz B, Taverna C, *et al.* Necrobiotic xanthogranuloma successfully treated with autologous stem cell transplantation. *Ann Hematol* 2007;**86**:303–6.

206. Schnitzler L, Schubert B, Boasson M, *et al.* Urticaire chronique, lesions osseuses, macroglobulinemie IgM: maladie de Waldenstrom-IIe presentation. *Bull Soc Fr Dermatol Syphiligr* 1974;**81**:363.

207. Lipsker D, Veran Y, Grunenberger F, *et al.* The Schnitzler syndrome. Four new cases and review of the literature. *Medicine (Baltimore)* 2001; **80**:37–44.

208. de Koning HD, Bodar EJ, van der Meer JW, *et al.* Schnitzler syndrome: beyond the case reports: review and follow-up of 94 patients with an emphasis on prognosis and treatment. *Semin Arthritis Rheum* 2007;**37**:137–48.

209. de Castro FR, Masouye I, Winkelmann RK, *et al.* Urticarial pathology in Schnitzler's (hyper-IgM) syndrome. *Dermatology* 1996;**193**:94–9.

210. Schneider SW, Gaubitz M, Luger TA, *et al.* Prompt response of refractory Schnitzler syndrome to treatment with anakinra. *J Am Acad Dermatol* 2007;**56**: S120–2.

211. Eiling E, Moller M, Kreiselmaier I, *et al.* Schnitzler syndrome: treatment failure to rituximab but response to anakinra. *J Am Acad Dermatol* 2007;**57**:361–4.

212. Lipsker D, Imrie K, Simon A, *et al.* Hot and hobbling with hives: Schnitzler syndrome. *Clin Immunol* 2006; **119**:131–4.

213. Martinez-Taboada VM, Fontalba A, Blanco R, *et al.* Successful treatment of refractory Schnitzler's syndrome with anakinra: comment on the article by Hawkins *et al.* *Arthritis Rheum* 2005;**52**:2226–7.

Chapter 12

Waldenstrom's macroglobulinemia/lymphoplasmacytic lymphoma

Steven P. Treon and Giampaolo Merlini

Introduction

Waldenstrom's macroglobulinemia (WM) is a distinct clinicopathologic entity resulting from the accumulation, predominantly in the bone marrow, of clonally related lymphocytes, lymphoplasmacytic cells, and plasma cells which secrete a monoclonal IgM protein (Figure 12.1).[1] This condition is considered to correspond to the lymphoplasmacytic lymphoma (LPL) as defined by the Revised European–American Lymphoma (REAL) and World Health Organization (WHO) classification systems.[2,3] Most cases of LPL are WM, with less than 5% of cases made up of IgA, IgG, and non-secreting LPL.

Epidemiology and etiology

WM is an uncommon disease, with a reported age-adjusted incidence rate of 3.4 per million among males and 1.7 per million among females in the USA, and a geometrical increase with age.[4,5] The incidence rate for WM is higher among Caucasians, with African descendants representing only 5% of all patients. Genetic factors appear to be an important factor to the pathogenesis of WM. Approximately 20% of WM patients have an Ashkenazi (Eastern European) Jewish ethnic background, and there have been numerous reports of familiar disease, including multigenerational clustering of WM and other B-cell lymphoproliferative diseases.[6–10] In a recent study, approximately 20% of 257 serial WM patients presenting to a tertiary referral had a first-degree relative with either WM or another B-cell disorder.[7] Frequent familiar association with other immunologic disorders in healthy relatives, including hypogammaglobulinemia and hypergammaglobulinemia (particularly polyclonal IgM), autoantibody (particularly to thyroid) production, and manifestation of hyperactive B cells have also been reported.[9,10] Increased expression of the *BCL2* gene with enhanced B-cell survival may underlie the increased immunoglobulin synthesis in familial WM.[9]

The role of environmental factors in WM remains to be clarified, but chronic antigenic stimulation from infections and certain drug and agent orange exposures remain suspect. An etiologic role for hepatitis C virus (HCV) infection has been suggested, though in a recent study examining 100 consecutive patients with WM, no association could be established using both serologic and molecular diagnostic studies for HCV infection.[11–13]

Biology

Cytogenetic findings

Several studies, usually performed on limited series of patients, have been published on cytogenetic findings in WM demonstrating a great variety of numerical and structural chromosome abnormalities. Numerical losses involving chromosomes 17, 18, 19, 20, 21, 22, X, and Y have been commonly observed, though gains in chromosomes 3, 4, and 12 have also been reported.[7,14–19] Chromosome 6q deletions encompassing 6q21-q22 have been observed in up to half of WM patients, and at a comparable frequency amongst patients with and without a familial history.[7,19] The presence of 6q deletions has been suggested in one study to discern patients with WM from those with IgM monoclonal gammopathy of unknown significance (MGUS), and to have potential prognostic significance, though others have reported no prognostic significance to the presence of 6q deletions in WM.[20,21] While 6q deletions have been reported in other B-cell malignancies, several candidate tumor suppressor genes in this region are under investigation in WM patients including *BLIMP-1*,[22] a master regulatory gene implicated in lymphoplasmacytic differentiation. Notable, however, is the absence of IGH switch region rearrangements in WM, a finding which may be used to discern cases of IgM myeloma where IGH switch region rearrangements are a predominant feature.[23]

Nature of the clonal cell

The WM bone marrow B-cell clone shows intraclonal differentiation from small lymphocytes with large focal deposits of surface immunoglobulins, to lymphoplasmacytic cells, to mature plasma cells that contain intracytoplasmic

Management of Hematologic Malignancies, ed. Susan M. O'Brien, Julie M. Vose, and Hagop M. Kantarjian. Published by Cambridge University Press.

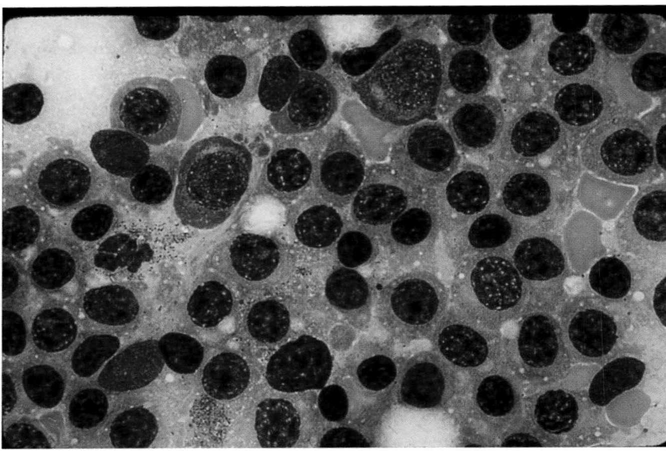

Figure 12.1 Aspirate from a patient with Waldenstrom's macroglobulinemia demonstrating excess mature lymphocytes, lymphoplasmacytic cells, and plasma cells (original magnification × 200). Courtesy of Marvin Stone MD.

immunoglobulins.[24] Clonal B cells are detectable among blood B lymphocytes, and their number increases in patients who fail to respond to therapy or who progress.[25] These clonal blood cells present the peculiar capacity to differentiate spontaneously, in in vitro culture, to plasma cells. This is through an interleukin-6 (IL-6)-dependent process in IgM MGUS and mostly an IL-6-independent process in WM patients.[26] All these cells express the monoclonal IgM present in the blood and a variable percentage of them also express surface IgD. The characteristic immunophenotypic profile of the lymphoplasmacytic cells in WM includes the expression of the pan-B-cell markers CD19, CD20, CD22, CD79, and FMC7.2.[27–29] Expression of CD5, CD10, and CD23 may be found in 10–20% of cases, and does not exclude the diagnosis of WM.[30]

The phenotype of lymphoplasmacytic cells in WM suggests that the clone is a post-germinal center B cell. This indication is further strengthened by the results of the analysis of the nature (silent or amino-acid replacing) and distribution (in framework or CDR regions) of somatic mutations in immunoglobulin (Ig) heavy- and light-chain variable regions performed in patients with WM.[31,32] This analysis showed a high rate of replacement mutations, compared with the closest germline genes, clustering in the CDR regions and without intraclonal variation. Subsequent studies showed a strong preferential usage of VH3/JH4 gene families, no intraclonal variation, and no evidence for any isotype-switched transcripts.[33,34] These data indicate that WM may originate from an IgM+ and/or IgM+ IgD+ memory B cell. Normal IgM+ memory B cells localize in bone marrow, where they mature to IgM-secreting cells.[35]

Bone marrow microenvironment

Increased numbers of mast cells are found in the bone marrow of WM patients, wherein they are usually admixed with tumor aggregates.[29,36] Recent studies have helped clarify the role of mast cells in WM. Co-culture of primary autologous or mast cell lines with WM lymphoplasmacytic cells (LPC) resulted in dose-dependent WM cell proliferation and/or tumor colony formation, primarily through CD40 ligand (CD40L) signaling. Furthermore, WM cells through elaboration of soluble CD27 (sCD27) induced the upregulation of CD40L on mast cells derived from WM patients and mast cell lines.[37]

Clinical features

The clinical and laboratory findings at time of diagnosis of WM in one large institutional study[7] are presented in Table 12.1. Unlike most indolent lymphomas, splenomegaly and lymphadenopathy are prominent in only a minority of patients (~15%). Purpura is frequently associated with cryoglobulinemia and more rarely with amyloid light chain (AL) amyloidosis, while hemorrhagic manifestations and neuropathies are multifactorial (see later). The morbidity associated with WM is caused by the concurrence of two main components: tissue infiltration by neoplastic cells and, more importantly, the physicochemical and immunologic properties of the monoclonal IgM. As shown in Table 12.2, the monoclonal IgM can produce clinical manifestations through several different mechanisms related to its physicochemical properties, non-specific interactions with other proteins, antibody activity, and tendency to deposit in tissues.[38–40]

Morbidity mediated by the effects of IgM

Hyperviscosity syndrome

Blood hyperviscosity is effected by increased serum IgM levels leading to hyperviscosity-related complications.[41] The mechanisms behind the marked increase in the resistance to blood flow and the resulting impaired transit through the microcirculatory system are rather complex.[41–43] The main determinants are: (1) a high concentration of monoclonal IgMs, which may form aggregates and may bind water through their carbohydrate component; and (2) their interaction with blood cells. Monoclonal IgMs increase red cell aggregation (*rouleaux* formation) and red cell internal viscosity while also reducing deformability. The possible presence of cryoglobulins can contribute to increasing blood viscosity as well as to the tendency to induce erythrocyte aggregation. Serum viscosity is proportional to IgM concentration up to 30 g/L, then increases sharply at higher levels. Plasma viscosity and hematocrit are directly regulated by the body. Increased plasma viscosity may also contribute to inappropriately low erythropoietin production, which is the major reason for anemia in these patients.[44] Clinical manifestations are related to circulatory disturbances that can be best appreciated by ophthalmoscopy, which shows distended and tortuous retinal veins, hemorrhages, and papilledema[45]

Table 12.1. Clinical and laboratory findings for 149 consecutive newly diagnosed patients with the consensus panel diagnosis of WM presenting to the Dana Farber Cancer Institute

	Median	Range	Institutional normal reference range
Age (yr)	59	34–84	NA
Gender (male/female)	85/64		NA
Bone marrow involvement	30%	5–95%	NA
Adenopathy	16%		NA
Splenomegaly	10%		NA
IgM (mg/dL)	2870	267–12 400	40–230
IgG (mg/dL)	587	47–2770	700–1600
IgA (mg/dL)	47	8–509	70–400
Serum viscosity (cp)	2.0	1.4–6.6	1.4–1.9
Hct (%)	35.0	17.2–45.4	34.8–43.6
Plt ($\times 10^9$/L)	253	24–649	155–410
WBC ($\times 10^9$/L)	6.0	0.3–13	3.8–9.2
β_2M (mg/dL)	3.0	1.3–13.7	0–2.7
LDH	395	122–1131	313–618

Notes: Hct: hematocrit; Plt: platelets; WBC: white blood cells; β_2M: β_2-microglobulin; LDH: lactate dehydrogenase; NA: not applicable.

Table 12.2. Physicochemical and immunologic properties of the monoclonal IgM protein in Waldenstrom's macroglobulinemia

Properties of IgM monoclonal protein	Diagnostic condition	Clinical manifestations
Pentameric structure	Hyperviscosity	Headaches, blurred vision, epistaxis, retinal hemorrhages, leg cramps, impaired mentation, intracranial hemorrhage
Precipitation on cooling	Cryoglobulinemia (type I)	Raynaud's phenomenon, acrocyanosis, ulcers, purpura, cold urticaria
Auto antibody activity to myelin-associated glycoprotein (MAG), ganglioside M1 (GM1), sulfatide moieties on peripheral nerve sheaths	Peripheral neuropathies	Sensorimotor neuropathies, painful neuropathies, ataxic gait, bilateral foot drop
Auto antibody activity to IgG	Cryoglobulinemia (type II)	Purpura, arthralgias, renal failure, sensorimotor neuropathies
Auto antibody activity to red blood cell antigens	Cold agglutinins	Hemolytic anemia, Raynaud's phenomenon, acrocyanosis, livedo reticularis
Tissue deposition as amorphous aggregates	Organ dysfunction	Skin: bullous skin disease, papules, Schnitzler's syndrome Gastrointestinal: diarrhea, malabsorption, bleeding Kidney: proteinuria, renal failure (light chain component)
Tissue deposition as amyloid fibrils (light chain component most commonly)	Organ dysfunction	Fatigue, weight loss, edema, hepatomegaly, macroglossia, organ dysfunction of involved organs: heart, kidney, liver, peripheral sensory and autonomic nerves

(Figure 12.2). Symptoms usually occur when the monoclonal IgM concentration exceeds 50 g/L or when serum viscosity is $>$ 4.0 centipoises (cp), but there is a great individual variability, with some patients showing no evidence of hyperviscosity even at 10 cp.[41] The most common symptoms are oronasal bleeding, visual disturbances due to retinal bleeding, and dizziness that may rarely lead to coma. Heart failure can be aggravated, particularly in the elderly, owing to increased

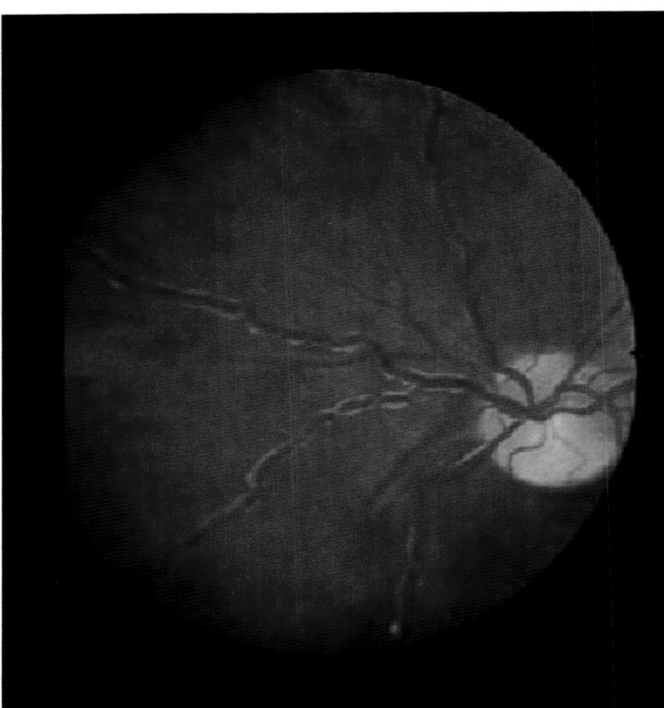

Figure 12.2 Funduscopic examination of a patient with Waldenstrom's macroglobulinemia demonstrating hyperviscosity-related changes including dilated retinal vessels, peripheral hemorrhages, and "venous sausaging" (original magnification × 16). Courtesy of Marvin Stone MD.

blood viscosity, expanded plasma volume, and anemia. Inappropriate transfusion can exacerbate hyperviscosity and may precipitate cardiac failure.

Cryoglobulinemia

In up to 20% of WM patients, the monoclonal IgM can behave as a cryoglobulin (type I), but it is symptomatic in 5% or less of the cases.[46] Cryoprecipitation is mainly dependent on the concentration of monoclonal IgM; for this reason plasmapheresis or plasma exchange are commonly effective in this condition. Symptoms result from impaired blood flow in small vessels and include Raynaud's phenomenon, acrocyanosis, and necrosis of the regions most exposed to cold such as the tip of the nose, ears, fingers, and toes (Figure 12.3), malleolar ulcers, purpura, and cold urticaria. Renal manifestations may occur but are infrequent.

IgM-related neuropathy

Monoclonal IgM may exert its pathogenic effects through specific recognition of autologous antigens, the most notable being components of myelin sheaths leading to peripheral neuropathy.

In a series of 215 patients with WM, Merlini *et al.* reported the clinical presence of peripheral neuropathy in 24% of WM patients,[46] although prevalence rates ranging from 5% to 38% have been reported in other series.[47,48] An estimated 6.5–10% of idiopathic neuropathies are associated with a monoclonal gammopathy, with a preponderance of IgM (60%) followed by IgG (30%) and IgA (10%) (reviewed in Nemni *et al.*[49] and Ropper and Gorson[50]). In WM patients, the nerve damage is mediated by diverse pathogenetic mechanisms: IgM antibody activity toward nerve constituents causing demyelinating polyneuropathies; endoneurial granulofibrillar deposits of IgM without antibody activity, associated with axonal polyneuropathy; occasionally by tubular deposits in the endoneurium associated with IgM cryoglobulin; and, rarely, by amyloid deposits or by neoplastic cell infiltration of nerve structures.[51] Half of the patients with IgM neuropathy have a distinctive clinical syndrome that is associated with antibodies against a minor 100-kDa glycoprotein component of nerve, myelin-associated glycoprotein (MAG). Anti-MAG antibodies are generally monoclonal IgMκ, and usually also exhibit reactivity with other glycoproteins or glycolipids that share antigenic determinants with MAG.[52–54]

The anti-MAG-related neuropathy is typically distal and symmetrical, affecting both motor and sensory functions; it is slowly progressive with a long period of stability.[48,55] Most patients present with sensory complaints (paresthesias, aching discomfort, dysesthesias, or lancinating pains), imbalance and gait ataxia, owing to lack of proprioception, and leg muscles atrophy in advanced stage. Patients with predominantly demyelinating sensory neuropathy in association with monoclonal IgM to gangliosides with disialosyl moieties, such as GD1b, GD3, GD2, GT1b, and GQ1b, have also been reported.[56,57] Anti-GD1b and anti-GQ1b antibodies were significantly associated with predominantly sensory ataxic neuropathy.[58] These antiganglioside monoclonal IgMs present core clinical features of chronic ataxic neuropathy with variably present ophthalmoplegia and/or red blood cell cold agglutinating activity. The disialosyl epitope is also present on red blood cell glycophorins, thereby accounting for the red cell cold agglutinin activity of anti-Pr2 specificity.[59,60] Monoclonal IgM proteins that bind to gangliosides with a terminal trisaccharide moiety, including GM2 and GalNac-GD1A, are associated with chronic demyelinating neuropathy and severe sensory ataxia, unresponsive to corticosteroids.[61]

Antiganglioside IgM proteins may also cross-react with lipopolysaccharides of *Campylobacter jejuni*, whose infection is known to precipitate the Miller Fisher syndrome, a variant of the Guillain–Barré syndrome.[58] This finding indicates that molecular mimicry may play a role in this condition. Antisulfatide monoclonal IgM proteins, associated with sensory/sensorimotor neuropathy, have been detected in 5% of patients with IgM monoclonal gammopathy and neuropathy.[62] Motor neuron disease has been reported in patients with WM, and monoclonal IgM with anti-GM1 and sulfoglucuronyl paragloboside activity.[63] POEMS (polyradiculoneuropathy, organomegaly, endocrinopathy, M protein, and skin changes) syndrome is rarely associated with WM.[64]

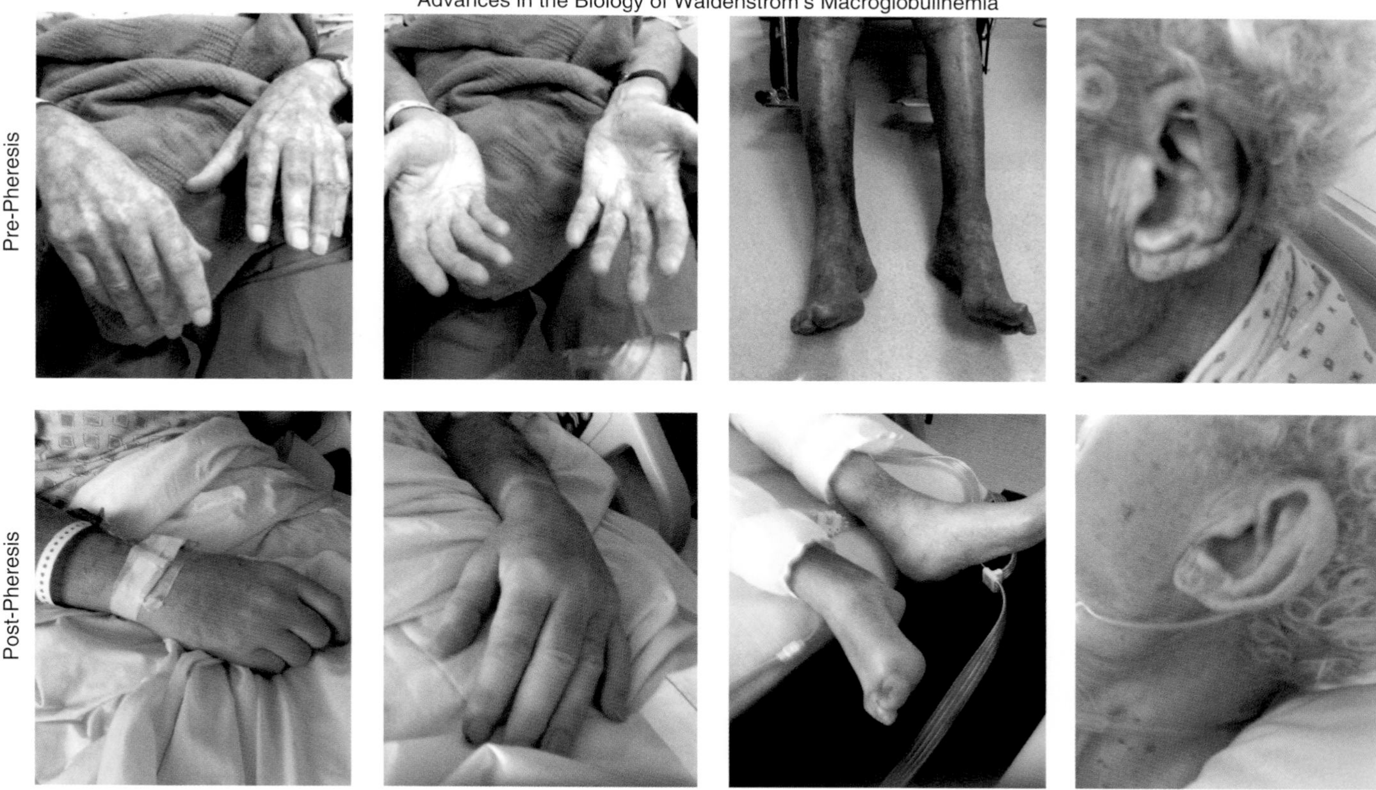

Figure 12.3 Cryoglobulinemia manifesting with severe acrocyanosis in a patient with Waldenstrom's macroglobulinemia before (pre-pheresis) and following warming and plasmapheresis (post-pheresis).

Cold agglutinin hemolytic anemia

Monoclonal IgM may present with cold agglutinin activity, i.e., it can recognize specific red cell antigens at temperatures below physiologic, producing chronic hemolytic anemia. This disorder occurs in $< 10\%$ of WM patients[65] and is associated with cold agglutinin titers $> 1{:}1000$ in most cases. The monoclonal component is usually an IgMκ and reacts most commonly with I/i antigens, with complement fixation and activation.[66,67] Mild chronic hemolytic anemia can be exacerbated after cold exposure but rarely does hemoglobin drop below 70 g/L. The hemolysis is usually extravascular (removal of C3b opsonized cells by the reticuloendothelial system, primarily in the liver) and rarely intravascular from complement destruction of red blood cell membrane. The agglutination of red blood cells in the cooler peripheral circulation also causes Raynaud's syndrome, acrocyanosis, and livedo reticularis. Macroglobulins with the properties of both cryoglobulins and cold agglutinins with anti-Pr specificity have been reported. These properties may have as a common basis the immune binding of the sialic acid-containing carbohydrate present on red blood cell glycophorins and on Ig molecules. Several other macroglobulins with various antibody activity toward autologous antigens (i.e., phospholipids, tissue and plasma proteins, etc.) and foreign ligands have also been reported.

IgM tissue deposition

The monoclonal protein can deposit in several tissues as amorphous aggregates. Linear deposition of monoclonal IgM along the skin basement membrane is associated with bullous skin disease.[68] Amorphous IgM deposits in the dermis determine the so-called IgM storage papules on the extensor surface of the extremities – macroglobulinemia cutis.[69] Deposition of monoclonal IgM in the lamina propria and/or submucosa of the intestine may be associated with diarrhea, malabsorption, and gastrointestinal bleeding.[70,71] It is well known that kidney involvement is less common and less severe in WM than in multiple myeloma, probably because the amount of light chain excreted in the urine is generally lower in WM than in myeloma and because of the absence of contributing factors, such as hypercalcemia, although cast nephropathy has also been described in WM.[72] On the other hand, the IgM macromolecule is more susceptible to being trapped in the glomerular loops where ultrafiltration presumably contributes to its precipitation, forming subendothelial deposits of aggregated IgM proteins that occlude the glomerular capillaries.[73] Mild and reversible proteinuria may result and most patients are asymptomatic. The deposition of monoclonal light chain as fibrillar amyloid deposits (AL amyloidosis) is uncommon in patients with WM.[74] Clinical expression and prognosis are similar to those of other AL patients with involvement of heart (44%), kidneys (32%), liver (14%), lungs (10%), peripheral/autonomic nerves (38%), and soft tissues (18%). However, the incidence of cardiac and pulmonary involvement is higher in patients with monoclonal IgM than with other immunoglobulin isotypes. The association of WM with reactive amyloidosis (AA) has been documented rarely.[75,76] Simultaneous occurrence of fibrillary glomerulopathy, characterized by glomerular deposits of wide non-congophilic fibrils and amyloid deposits, has been reported in WM.[77]

Manifestations related to tissue infiltration by neoplastic cells

Tissue infiltration by neoplastic cells is rare and can involve various organs and tissues, from the bone marrow (described later) to the liver, spleen, lymph nodes, and possibly the lungs, gastrointestinal tract, kidneys, skin, eyes, and central nervous system. Pulmonary involvement in the form of masses, nodules, diffuse infiltrate, or pleural effusions is relatively rare, since the overall incidence of pulmonary and pleural findings reported for WM is only 3–5%.[78–80] Cough is the most common presenting symptom, followed by dyspnea and chest pain. Chest radiographic findings include parenchymal infiltrates, confluent masses, and effusions. Malabsorption, diarrhea, bleeding, or obstruction may indicate involvement of the gastrointestinal tract at the level of the stomach, duodenum, or small intestine.[81–84] In contrast to multiple myeloma, infiltration of the kidney interstitium with lymphoplasmacytoid cell has been reported in WM,[85] while renal or perirenal masses are not uncommon.[86] The skin can be the site of dense lymphoplasmacytic infiltrates, similar to that seen in the liver, spleen, and lymph nodes, forming cutaneous plaques and, rarely, nodules.[87] Chronic urticaria and IgM gammopathy are the two cardinal features of Schnitzler's syndrome, which is not usually associated initially with clinical features of WM,[88] although evolution to WM is not uncommon. Thus, close follow-up of these patients is warranted. Invasion of articular and periarticular structures by WM malignant cells is rarely reported.[89] The neoplastic cells can infiltrate the periorbital structures, lacrimal gland, and retro-orbital lymphoid tissues, resulting in ocular nerve palsies.[90,91] Direct infiltration of the central nervous system by monoclonal lymphoplasmacytic cells as infiltrates or as tumors constitutes the rarely observed Bing–Neel syndrome, characterized clinically by confusion, memory loss, disorientation, and motor dysfunction (reviewed in Civit *et al.*[92]).

Laboratory investigations and findings

Hematological abnormalities

Anemia is the most common finding in patients with symptomatic WM and is caused by a combination of factors: mild decrease in red cell survival, impaired erythropoiesis, hemolysis, moderate plasma volume expansion, and blood loss from the gastrointestinal tract. Blood smears are usually normocytic and normochromic, and rouleaux formation is often pronounced. Electronically measured mean corpuscular volume may be elevated spuriously owing to erythrocyte aggregation. In addition, the hemoglobin estimate can be inaccurate, i.e., falsely high, because of interaction between the monoclonal protein and the diluent used in some automated analyzers.[93] Leukocyte and platelet counts are usually within the reference range at presentation, although patients may occasionally present with severe thrombocytopenia. As reported above, monoclonal B lymphocytes expressing surface IgM and late-differentiation B-cell markers are uncommonly detected in blood by flow cytometry. A raised erythrocyte sedimentation rate is almost constantly observed in WM and may be the first clue to the presence of the macroglobulin. The clotting abnormality detected most frequently is prolongation of thrombin time. AL amyloidosis should be suspected in all patients with nephrotic syndrome, cardiomyopathy, hepatomegaly, or peripheral neuropathy. Diagnosis requires the demonstration of green birefringence under polarized light of amyloid deposits stained with Congo red.

Biochemical investigations

High-resolution electrophoresis combined with immunofixation of serum and urine are recommended for identification and characterization of the IgM monoclonal protein. The light chain of the monoclonal IgM is κ in 75–80% of patients. A few WM patients have more than one M-component. The concentration of the serum monoclonal protein is very variable but in most cases lies within the range of 15–45 g/L. Densitometry should be adopted to determine IgM levels for serial evaluations because nephelometry is unreliable and shows large intralaboratory as well as interlaboratory variation. The presence of cold agglutinins or cryoglobulins may affect determination of IgM levels and, therefore, testing for cold agglutinins and cryoglobulins should be performed at diagnosis. If present, subsequent serum samples should be analyzed under warm conditions for determination of serum monoclonal IgM level. Although Bence Jones proteinuria is frequently present, it exceeds 1 g/24 hours in only 3% of cases. While IgM levels are elevated in WM patients, IgA and IgG levels are most often depressed and do not demonstrate recovery even after successful treatment suggesting that patients with WM harbor a defect which prevents normal plasma cell development and/or Ig heavy chain rearrangements.[94,95]

Serum viscosity

Because of their large size (almost 1 000 000 daltons), most IgM molecules are retained within the intravascular compartment and can exert an undue effect on serum viscosity. Therefore, serum viscosity should be measured if the patient has signs or symptoms of hyperviscosity syndrome. Funduscopic examination remains an excellent indicator of clinically relevant hyperviscosity. Among the first clinical signs of hyperviscosity are the appearance of peripheral and mid-peripheral dot and blot-like hemorrhages in the retina, which are best appreciated with indirect ophthalmoscopy and scleral depression.[45] In more severe cases of hyperviscosity, dot, blot, and flame-shaped hemorrhages can appear in the macular area along with markedly dilated and tortuous veins with focal constrictions resulting in "venous sausaging," as well as papilledema.

Bone marrow findings

The bone marrow is always involved in WM. Central to the diagnosis of WM is the demonstration, by trephine biopsy, of bone marrow infiltration by a lymphoplasmacytic cell population constituted by small lymphocytes with evidence of plasmacytoid/plasma cell differentiation (Figure 12.1). The pattern of bone marrow infiltration may be diffuse, interstitial, or nodular, showing usually an intertrabecular pattern of infiltration. A solely paratrabecular pattern of infiltration is unusual and should raise the possibility of follicular lymphoma.[1] The bone marrow infiltration should routinely be confirmed by immunophenotypic studies (flow cytometry and/or immunohistochemistry) showing the following profile: sIgM+CD19+CD20+CD22+CD79+.[27–29] Up to 20% of cases may express either CD5, CD10, or CD23.[30] In these cases, care should be taken to satisfactorily exclude chronic lymphocytic leukemia and mantle cell lymphoma.[1] "Intranuclear" periodic acid-Schiff (PAS)-positive inclusions (Dutcher–Fahey bodies)[96] consisting of IgM deposits in the perinuclear space, and sometimes in intranuclear vacuoles, may be seen occasionally in lymphoid cells in WM. An increased number of mast cells, usually in association with the lymphoid aggregates, is commonly found in WM, and their presence may help in differentiating WM from other B-cell lymphomas.[2,3]

Other investigations

Magnetic resonance imaging (MRI) of the spine in conjunction with computed tomography (CT) of the abdomen and pelvis are useful in evaluating the disease status in WM.[97] Bone marrow involvement can be documented by MRI studies of the spine in over 90% of patients, while CT of the abdomen and pelvis demonstrated enlarged nodes in 43% of WM patients.[97] Lymph node biopsy may show preserved architecture or replacement by infiltration of neoplastic cells with lymphoplasmacytoid, lymphoplasmacytic, or polymorphous cytologic patterns. The residual disease after high-dose chemotherapy with allogeneic or autologous stem cell rescue can be monitored by polymerase chain reaction (PCR)-based methods using primers specific for the monoclonal Ig variable regions.

Prognosis

Waldenstrom's macroglobulinemia typically presents as an indolent disease though considerable variability in prognosis can be seen. The median survival reported in several large series has ranged from 5 to 10 years,[98–104] though in a recent follow-up of 436 consecutive patients diagnosed with WM, the median overall survival from time of diagnosis was in excess of 10 years.[105] The presence of 6q deletions have been suggested to have prognostic significance in one study, though others have reported no such association in WM.[20,21] Age is consistently an important prognostic factor (> 60–70 years),[98,99,101,104] but this factor is often impacted by unrelated morbidities. Anemia, which reflects both marrow involvement and the serum level of the IgM monoclonal protein due to the impact of IgM on intravascular fluid retention, has emerged as a strong adverse prognostic factor with hemoglobin levels of < 9–12 g/dL associated with decreased survival in several series.[98–101,104] Cytopenias have also been regularly identified as a significant predictor of survival.[99] However, the precise level of cytopenias with prognostic significance remains to be determined.[101] Some series have identified a platelet count of $< 100–150 \times 10^9$/L and a granulocyte count of $< 1.5 \times 10^9$/L as independent prognostic factors.[98,99,101,104] The number of cytopenias in a given patient has been proposed as a strong prognostic factor.[99] Serum albumin levels have also correlated with survival in WM patients in certain but not all studies using multivariate analyses.[99,101,102] High beta-2 microglobulin levels (> 3–3.5 g/dL) were shown in several studies,[100–104] along with a high serum IgM M-protein (> 7 g/dL)[104] as well as a low serum IgM M-protein (< 4 g/dL)[102] and the presence of cryoglobulins,[98] to be adverse factors. A few scoring systems have been proposed based on these analyses (Table 12.3).

Treatment of Waldenstrom's macroglobulinemia

As part of the Second International Workshop on Waldenstrom's Macroglobulinemia, a consensus panel was organized to recommend criteria for the initiation of therapy in patients with WM.[101] The panel recommended that initiation of therapy should not be based on the IgM level per se, since this may not correlate with the clinical manifestations of WM. The consensus panel, however, agreed that initiation of therapy was appropriate for patients with constitutional symptoms, such as recurrent fever, night sweats, fatigue due to anemia, or weight loss. The presence of progressive symptomatic lymphadenopathy or splenomegaly provides additional reasons to begin therapy. The presence of anemia with a hemoglobin value of ≤ 10 g/dL or a platelet count $\leq 100 \times 10^9$/L owing to marrow infiltration also justifies treatment. Certain complications, such as hyperviscosity syndrome, symptomatic sensorimotor peripheral neuropathy, systemic amyloidosis, renal insufficiency, or symptomatic cryoglobulinemia, may also be indications for therapy.[101]

Table 12.3. Prognostic scoring systems in Waldenstrom's macroglobulinemia

Study	Adverse prognostic factors	Number of groups	Survival
Gobbi *et al.* [98]	Hb $<$ 9 g/dL	0–1 prognostic factors	Median: 48 mo
	Age $>$ 70 yr	2–4 prognostic factors	Median: 80 mo
	Weight loss		
	Cryoglobulinemia		
Morel *et al.* [99]	Age $\geq$ 65 yr	0–1 prognostic factors	5 yr: 87%
	Albumin $<$ 4 g/dL	2 prognostic factors	5 yr: 62%
	Number of cytopenias:	3–4 prognostic factors	5 yr: 25%
	Hb $<$ 12 g/dL		
	Platelets $< 150 \times 10^9$/L		
	WBC $< 4 \times 10^9$/L		
Dhodapkar *et al.* [100]	β_2M $\geq$ 3 g/dL	β_2M $<$ 3 mg/dL + Hb $\geq$ 12 g/dL	5 yr: 87%
	Hb $<$ 12 g/dL		
	IgM $<$ 4 g/dL	β_2M $<$ 3 mg/dL + Hb $<$ 12 g/dL	5 yr: 63%
		β_2M $\geq$ 3 mg/dL + IgM $\geq$ 4 g/dL	5 yr: 53%
		β_2M $\geq$ 3 mg/dL + IgM $<$ 4 g/dL	5 yr: 21%
Application of International Staging System Criteria for Myeloma to WM	Albumin $\leq$ 3.5 g/dL	Albumin $\geq$ 3.5 g/dL + β_2M $<$ 3.5 mg/dL	Median: NR
	β_2M $\geq$ 3.5 mg/L		
		Albumin $\leq$ 3.5 g/dL + β_2M $<$ 3.5 or β_2M 3.5–5.5 mg/dL	Median: 116 mo
		β_2M $>$ 5.5 mg/dL	Median: 54 mo
Dimopoulos *et al.* [102]			
International Prognostic Scoring System for WM	Age $>$ 65 yr	0–1 prognostic factors[a]	5 yr: 87%
Morel *et al.* [104]	Hb $<$ 11.5 g/dL	2 prognostic factors[b]	5 yr: 68%
	Platelets $< 100 \times 10^9$/L	3–5 prognostic factors	5 yr: 36%
	β_2M $>$ 3 mg/L		
	IgM $>$ 7 g/dL		

Notes: [a]excluding age.
[b]or age $>$ 65.
Hb: hemoglobin.

Frontline therapy

While a precise therapeutic algorithm for therapy of WM remains to be defined given the paucity of randomized clinical trials, consensus panels composed of experts who treat WM were organized as part of the International Workshops on Waldenstrom's macroglobulinemia and have formulated recommendations for both frontline and salvage therapy of WM based on the best available clinical trials evidence. Among frontline options, the panels considered alkylator agents (e.g., chlorambucil), nucleoside analogs (cladribine or fludarabine), the monoclonal antibody rituximab as well as combinations thereof as reasonable choices for the upfront therapy of WM.[106–108] Importantly, the panel felt that individual patient considerations, including the presence of cytopenias, need for more rapid disease control, age, and candidacy for autologous transplant therapy, should be taken into account in making the choice of a first-line agent. For patients who are candidates for autologous transplant therapy, which typically is reserved for those patients < 70 years of age, the panel recommended that exposure to alkylator or nucleoside analog therapy should be limited. The use of nucleoside analogs should be approached cautiously in patients with WM since there appears to be an increased risk for the development of disease transformation as well as myelodysplasia and acute myelogenous leukemia.

Alkylator-based therapy

Oral alkylating drugs, alone and in combination therapy with corticosteroids, have been extensively evaluated in the upfront treatment of WM. The greatest experience with oral alkylator therapy has been with chlorambucil, which has been administered on both a continuous (i.e., daily dose schedule) as well as an intermittent schedule. Patients receiving chlorambucil on a continuous schedule typically receive 0.1 mg/kg per day, whilst on the intermittent schedule patients will typically receive 0.3 mg/kg for 7 days, every 6 weeks. In a prospective randomized study, Kyle *et al.* reported no significant difference in the overall response rate between these schedules, although interestingly the median response duration was greater for patients receiving intermittent versus continuously dosed chlorambucil (46 vs. 26 months).[109] Despite the favorable median response duration in this study for use of the intermittent schedule, no difference in the median overall survival was observed. Moreover, an increased incidence for development of myelodysplasia and acute myelogenous leukemia with the intermittent (3 of 22 patients) versus the continuous (0 of 24 patients) chlorambucil schedule prompted the authors of this study to express preference for use of continuous chlorambucil dosing. The use of corticosteroids in combination with alkylator therapy has also been explored. Dimopoulos and Alexanian evaluated chlorambucil (8 mg/m^2) along with prednisone (40 mg/m^2) given orally for 10 days, every 6 weeks, and reported a major response (i.e., reduction of IgM by greater than 50%) in 72% of patients.[110] Non-chlorambucil-based alkylator regimens employing melphalan and cyclophosphamide in combination with corticosteroids have also been examined by Petrucci *et al.*[111] and Case *et al.*[112] producing slightly higher overall response rates and response durations, although the benefit of these more complex regimens over chlorambucil remains to be demonstrated. Facon *et al.* have evaluated parameters predicting for response to alkylator therapy.[113] Their studies in patients receiving single-agent chlorambucil demonstrated that age 60, male sex, symptomatic status, and cytopenias (but, interestingly, not high tumor burden and serum IgM levels) were associated with poor response to alkylator therapy. Additional factors to be taken into account in considering alkylator therapy for patients with WM include necessity for more rapid disease control given the slow nature of response to alkylator therapy, as well as consideration for preserving stem cells in patients who are candidates for autologous transplant therapy.

Nucleoside analog therapy

Both cladribine and fludarabine have been extensively evaluated in untreated as well as previously treated WM patients. Cladribine administered as a single agent by continuous intravenous (IV) infusion, by 2-hour daily infusion, or by subcutaneous bolus injections for 5–7 days has resulted in major responses in 40–90% of patients who received primary therapy, whilst in the salvage setting responses have ranged from 38% to 54%.[113–120] Median time to achievement of response in responding patients following cladribine ranged from 1.2 to 5 months. The overall response rate with daily infusional fludarabine therapy administered mainly on 5-day schedules in previously untreated and treated WM patients has ranged from 38% to 100% and 30% to 40%, respectively,[121–126] which are on par with the response data for cladribine. Median time to achievement of response for fludarabine was also on par with cladribine at 3–6 months. In general, response rates and durations of responses have been greater for patients receiving nucleoside analogs as first-line agents, although in several of the above studies wherein both untreated and previously treated patients were enrolled, no substantial difference in the overall response rate was reported.

Myelosuppression commonly occurred following prolonged exposure to either of the nucleoside analogs, as did lymphopenia with sustained depletion of both CD4+ and CD8+ T lymphocytes observed in WM patients 1 year following initiation of therapy.[113,115] Treatment-related mortality due to myelosuppression and/or opportunistic infections attributable to immunosuppression occurred in up to 5% of all treated patients in some series with either nucleoside analog. Factors predicting for response to nucleoside analogs in WM included age at start of treatment (< 70 years), pretreatment hemoglobin > 95 g/L, platelets $> 75\,000$/ml^3, disease relapsing off therapy, patients with resistant disease within the first year of diagnosis, and a long interval between first-line therapy and initiation of a nucleoside analog in relapsing patients.[113,119,125] There are limited data on the use of an alternate nucleoside analog to salvage patients whose disease relapsed or demonstrated resistance to cladribine or fludarabine therapy.[127,128] Three of four (75%) patients responded to cladribine to salvage patients who progressed following an unmaintained remission to fludarabine, whereas only one of ten (10%) with disease resistant to fludarabine responded to cladribine.[127] However, Lewandowski *et al.*[128] reported a response in two of six patients (33%) and disease stabilization in the remaining patients to fludarabine, in spite of an inadequate response or progressive disease following cladribine therapy.

The safety of nucleoside analogs has been the subject of investigation in several recent studies. Thomas *et al.* recently reported their experiences in harvesting stem cells in 21 patients with symptomatic WM in whom autologous peripheral blood stem cell collection was attempted. Autologous stem cell collection (ASCC) succeeded on first attempt in 14/15 patients who received non-nucleoside analog based therapy versus 2/6 patients who received a nucleoside analog.[129] The long-term safety of nucleoside analogs in WM was recently examined by Leleu *et al.* in a large series of WM patients.[105] A sevenfold increase in transformation to an aggressive lymphoma and a threefold increase in the development of acute myelogenous leukemia/myelodysplasia were observed amongst patients who received a nucleoside analog versus other therapies for their WM. A recent meta-analysis by Leleu *et al.*[130] of several trials utilizing nucleoside analogs in WM patients, which included patients who had previously received an alkylator agent, showed a crude incidence of 6.6–10% for development of disease transformation, and 1.4–8.9% for development of myelodysplasia or acute myeloid leukemia (AML). None of the studied risk factors, i.e., gender, age, family history of WM or B-cell malignancies, typical markers of tumor burden and prognosis, type of nucleoside analog therapy (cladribine vs. fludarabine), time from diagnosis to nucleoside analog use, nucleoside analog treatment as primary or salvage therapy, as well as treatment with an oral alkylator (i.e., chlorambucil), predicted for the occurrence of transformation or development of myelodysplasia/acute myelogenous leukemia for WM patients treated with a nucleoside analog.[130]

CD20-directed antibody therapy

Rituximab is a chimeric monoclonal antibody which targets CD20, a widely expressed antigen on lymphoplasmacytic cells in WM.[131] Several retrospective and prospective studies have indicated that rituximab, when used at standard dosimetry (i.e., four weekly infusions at 375 mg/m^2), induced major responses in approximately 27–35% of previously treated and untreated patients.[132–138] Furthermore, it was shown in some of these studies that patients who achieved minor responses or even stable disease benefited from rituximab as evidenced by improved hemoglobin and platelet counts, and reduction of lymphadenopathy and/or splenomegaly. The median time to treatment failure in these studies was found to range from 8 to 27+ months. Studies evaluating an extended rituximab schedule consisting of four weekly courses at 375 mg/m^2 per week, repeated 3 months later by another 4-week course, have demonstrated major response rates of 44–48%, with time to progression estimates of 16+ to 29+ months.[138,139]

In many WM patients, a transient increase of serum IgM may be noted immediately following initiation of treatment.[138,140–142] Such an increase does not herald treatment failure, and while most patients will return to their baseline serum IgM level by 12 weeks, some continue to show prolonged spiking despite demonstrating a reduction in their bone marrow tumor load. However, patients with baseline serum IgM levels of > 50 g/dL or serum viscosity of > 3.5 cp may be particularly at risk for a hyperviscosity-related event and in such patients plasmapheresis should be considered in advance of rituximab therapy.[141] Because of the decreased likelihood of response in patients with higher IgM levels, as well as the possibility that serum IgM and viscosity levels may abruptly rise, rituximab monotherapy should not be used as sole therapy for the treatment of patients at risk for hyperviscosity symptoms.

Time to response after rituximab is slow and exceeds 3 months on average. The time to best response in one study was 18 months.[139] Patients with baseline serum IgM levels of < 60 g/dL are more likely to respond, irrespective of the underlying bone marrow involvement by tumor cells.[138,139] A recent analysis of 52 patients who were treated with single-agent rituximab has indicated that the objective response rate was significantly lower in patients who had either low serum albumin (< 35 g/L) or elevated serum monoclonal protein (> 40 g/L M-spike). Furthermore, the presence of both adverse prognostic factors was related with a short time to progression (3.6 months). Moreover, patients who had normal serum albumin and relatively low serum monoclonal protein levels derived a substantial benefit from rituximab with a time to progression exceeding 40 months.[143]

The genetic background of patients may also be important for determining response to rituximab. In particular, a correlation between polymorphisms at position 158 in the FcγRIIIa receptor (CD16), an activating Fc receptor on important effector cells that mediate antibody-dependent cell-mediated cytotoxicity (ADCC), and rituximab response was observed in WM patients. Individuals may encode either the amino acid valine or phenylalanine at position 158 in the FcγRIIIa receptor. WM patients who carried the valine amino acid (either in a homozygous or heterozygous pattern) had a fourfold higher major response rate (i.e., 50% decline in serum IgM levels) to rituximab versus those patients who expressed phenylalanine in a homozygous pattern.[144]

Combination therapies

Because rituximab is an active and a non-myelosuppressive agent, its combination with chemotherapy has been explored in WM patients. Weber *et al.* administered rituximab along with cladribine and cyclophosphamide to 17 previously untreated patients with WM.[145] At least a partial response was documented in 94% of WM patients including a complete response in 18%. With a median follow-up of 21 months no patient has relapsed. In a study by the Waldenstrom's Macroglobulinemia Clinical Trials Group (WMCTG), the combination of rituximab and fludarabine was evaluated in 43 WM patients, 32 (74%) of whom were previously untreated.[146] The overall response rate was 95.3%, with 83% of patients achieving a major response (i.e., 50% reduction in disease burden). The median time to progression was 51.2 months in this series, and was longer for those patients who were previously untreated and for those achieving a very good partial response (VGPR) (i.e., 90% reduction in disease) or better. Hematological toxicity was common with grade 3 neutropenia and thrombocytopenia observed in 27 and 4 patients, respectively. Two deaths occurred in this study due to non-*Pneumocystis carinii* pneumonia. Secondary malignancies including transformation to aggressive lymphoma and development of myelodysplasia or AML were observed in six patients in this series. The addition of rituximab to fludarabine and cyclophosphamide has also been explored in the salvage setting by Tam *et al.*, wherein four of five patients demonstrated a response.[147] In another combination study with rituximab, Hensel *et al.* administered rituximab along with pentostatin and cyclophosphamide to 13 patients with untreated and previously treated WM or lymphoplasmacytic lymphoma.[148] A major response was observed in 77% of patients. In a study by Dimopoulos *et al.* the combination of rituximab, dexamethasone, and cyclophosphamide was used as primary therapy to treat 72 patients with WM.[149] At least a major response was observed in 74% of patients in this study, and the 2-year progression-free survival was 67%. Therapy was well tolerated, though one patient died of interstitial pneumonia.

In addition to nucleoside analog-based trials with rituximab, two studies have examined CHOP (cyclophosphamide, doxorubicin, vincristine, prednisone) in combination with rituximab (CHOP-R). In a randomized frontline study by the German Low Grade Lymphoma Study Group (GLSG) involving 69 patients, most of whom had WM, the addition of rituximab to CHOP resulted in a higher overall response rate (94% vs. 67%) and median time to progression (63 vs. 22 months) in comparison to patients treated with CHOP alone.[150] Treon *et al.* have also evaluated CHOP-R in 13 WM patients, 8 and 5 of whom were relapsed or refractory to nucleoside analogs and single-agent rituximab, respectively.[151] Among 13 evaluable patients, 10 patients achieved a major response (77%) including 3 complete responses (CRs) and 7 partial responses (PRs), and 2 patients achieved a minor response. In a retrospective study, Ioakimidis *et al.* examined the outcomes of symptomatic WM patients who received CHOP-R, CVP-R (cyclophosphamide, vincristine, prednisone, and rituximab), or CP-R.[152] Baseline characteristics for all three cohorts were similar for age, prior therapies, bone marrow involvement, hematocrit, platelet count, and serum β2-microglobulin, though serum IgM levels were higher in patients treated with CHOP-R. The overall response rates to therapy were comparable among all three treatment groups: CHOP-R (96%), CVP-R (88%), and CP-R (95%), though there was a trend for more CRs among patients treated with CVP-R and CHOP-R. Adverse events attributed to therapy showed a higher incidence for neutropenic fever and treatment-related neuropathy for CHOP-R and CVP-R versus CP-R. The results of this study suggest that in WM, the use of CP-R may provide analogous treatment responses to more intense cyclophosphamide-based regimens, while minimizing treatment-related complications.

The addition of alkylating agents to nucleoside analogs has also been explored in WM. Weber *et al.* administered two cycles of oral cyclophosphamide along with subcutaneous cladribine to 37 patients with previously untreated WM.[145] At least a PR was observed in 84% of patients and the median duration of response was 36 months. Dimopoulos *et al.* examined fludarabine in combination with intravenous cyclophosphamide and observed partial responses in 6 of 11 (55%) WM patients either with primary refractory disease or who had relapsed on treatment.[153] The combination of fludarabine plus cyclophosphamide was also evaluated in a recent study by Tamburini *et al.* involving 49 patients, 35 of whom were previously treated.[154] Seventy-eight percent of the patients in this study achieved a response and median time to treatment failure was 27 months. Hematological toxicity was commonly observed and three patients died of treatment-related toxicities. Interesting findings in this study were the development of acute leukemia in two patients, histologic transformation to diffuse large cell lymphoma in one patient, and two cases of solid malignancies (prostate and melanoma), as well as failure to mobilize stem cells in four of six patients.

In view of the above data, the consensus panel on therapeutics amended its original recommendations for the therapy of WM to include the use of combination therapy with either nucleoside analogs and alkylator agents, or rituximab in combination with nucleoside analog, nucleoside analogs plus alkylator agents, or cyclophosphamide-based therapy as reasonable therapeutics options for the treatment of WM.[107,108]

Salvage therapy including novel agents

For patients in relapse or who have refractory disease, the consensus panels recommended the use of an alternative first-line agent as defined above, with the caveat that for those patients for whom autologous transplantation was being seriously considered, further exposure to stem cell-damaging agents (i.e., many alkylator agents and nucleoside analog drugs) should be avoided, and a non-stem-cell toxic agent should be considered if stem cells had not previously been harvested.[107,108] Recent studies have also demonstrated activity for several novel agents including bortezomib, thalidomide alone or in combination, and alemtuzumab which can be considered in the treatment of relapsed/refractory WM. Lastly, autologous stem cell transplant remains an option for the salvage therapy of WM particularly among younger patients who have had multiple relapses, or have primary refractory disease.

Proteasome inhibitor

Bortezomib, a stem cell-sparing agent,[155–157] is a proteasome inhibitor which induces apoptosis of primary WM lymphoplasmacytic cells, as well as the WM-WSU WM cell line at pharmacologically achievable levels.[158] Moreover, bortezomib may also impact on bone marrow microenvironmental support for lymphoplasmacytic cells. In a multicenter study of the

WMCTG,[159] 27 patients received up to eight cycles of bortezomib at 1.3 mg/m^2 on days 1, 4, 8, and 11. All but one patient had relapsed or refractory disease. Following therapy, median serum IgM levels declined from 4660 mg/dL to 2092 mg/dL ($p < 0.0001$). The overall response rate was 85%, with 10 and 13 patients achieving a minor (< 25% decrease in IgM) and major (< 50% decrease in IgM) response. Responses were prompt, and occurred at a median of 1.4 months. The median time to progression for all responding patients in this study was 7.9 (range 3–21.4+) months, and the most common grade 3/4 toxicities occurring in ≥ 5% of patients were sensory neuropathies (22.2%); leukopenia (18.5%); neutropenia (14.8%); dizziness (11.1%); and thrombocytopenia (7.4%). Importantly, sensory neuropathies resolved or improved in nearly all patients following cessation of therapy. As part of a National Cancer Institute of Canada study, Chen *et al.* treated 27 patients with both untreated (44%) and previously treated (56%) disease.[160] Patients in this study received bortezomib utilizing the standard schedule until they either demonstrated progressive disease, or two cycles beyond a CR or stable disease. The overall response rate in this study was 78%, with major responses observed in 44% of patients. Sensory neuropathy occurred in 20 patients, 5 with grade > 3, and occurred following two to four cycles of therapy. Among the 20 patients developing a neuropathy, 14 patients resolved and 1 patient demonstrated a one-grade improvement at 2–13 months. In addition to the above experiences with bortezomib monotherapy in WM, Dimopoulos *et al.*[161] observed major responses in six of ten (60%) previously treated WM patients, while Goy *et al.*[162] observed a major response in one of two WM patients who were included in a series of relapsed or refractory patients with non-Hodgkin lymphoma (NHL). In view of the single-agent activity of bortezomib in WM, Treon *et al.* have examined the combination of bortezomib, dexamethasone, and rituximab (BDR) as primary therapy in patients with WM.[163] An overall response rate of 96% and a major response rate of 83% were observed with the BDR combination. The incidence of grade 3 neuropathy was about 30% in this study, but was reversible in most patients following discontinuation of therapy. An increased incidence of herpes zoster was also observed prompting the prophylactic use of antiviral therapy with BDR. Alternative schedules for administration of bortezomib (i.e., once weekly at higher doses) in combination with rituximab are also being examined by Ghobrial *et al.*[164] and Agathocleous *et al.*[165] in patients with WM with overall response rates of 80–90%. The impact of these schedules on the development of bortezomib-related peripheral neuropathy remains to be clarified, though in one study it appeared to be diminished.[164]

CD52-directed antibody therapy

Alemtuzumab is a humanized monoclonal antibody which targets CD52, an antigen widely expressed on bone marrow leukemic progenitor cells (LPC) in WM patients, as well as on mast cells which are increased in the BM of patients with WM and provide growth and survival signals to WM LPC through several tumor necrosis factor family ligands (CD40L, APRIL, BLYS).[166] As part of a WMCTG effort,[167] 28 subjects with the REAL/WHO clinicopathologic diagnosis of LPL, including 27 patients with IgM (WM) and 1 with IgA monoclonal gammopathy, were enrolled in this prospective, multicenter study. Five patients were untreated and 23 were previously treated, all of whom had previously received rituximab. Patients received three daily test doses of alemtuzumab (3, 10, and 30 mg IV) followed by 30 mg alemtuzumab IV three times a week for up to 12 weeks. All patients received aciclovir and bactrim or equivalent prophylaxis for the duration of therapy plus 8 weeks following the last infusion of alemtuzumab. Among 25 patients evaluable for response, the overall response rate was 76%, which included 8 (32%) major responders, and 11 (44%) minor responders. Hematological toxicities were common among previously treated (but not untreated) patients and included grade 3/4 neutropenia 39%; thrombocytopenia 18%; and anemia 7%. Grade 3/4 non-hematological toxicity for all patients included dermatitis 11%; fatigue 7%; and infection 7%. Cytomegalovirus (CMV) reactivation and infection was commonly seen among previously treated patients and may have been etiologic for one death on study. With a median follow-up of 8.5+ months, 11/19 responding patients remain free of progression. High rates of response with the use of alemtuzumab as salvage therapy have also been reported by Owen *et al.*[168] in a small series of heavily pretreated WM patients (with a median number prior therapies of four) who received up to 12 weeks of therapy (at 30 mg IV thrice weekly) following initial dose escalation. Among the seven patients receiving alemtuzumab, five patients achieved a partial response and one patient a complete response. Infectious complications were common, with CMV reactivation occurring in three patients requiring ganciclovir therapy, and hospitalization for three patients for bacterial infections. Opportunistic infection occurred in two patients, and was responsible for their deaths.

Thalidomide and lenalidomide

Thalidomide as a single agent, and in combination with dexamethasone and clarithromycin, has also been examined in patients with WM, in view of the success of these regimens in patients with advanced multiple myeloma. Dimopoulos *et al.* demonstrated a major response in 5 of 20 (25%) previously untreated and treated patients who received single-agent thalidomide.[169] Dose escalation from the thalidomide start dose of 200 mg daily was hindered by development of side effects, including the development of peripheral neuropathy in five patients obligating discontinuation or dose reduction. Low doses of thalidomide (50 mg orally daily) in combination with dexamethasone (40 mg orally once a week) and clarithromycin (250 mg orally twice a day) have also been examined, with 10 of 12 (83%) previously treated patients demonstrating at least a major response.[170] However, in a follow-up study by Dimopoulos *et al.* using a higher thalidomide dose (200 mg orally daily) along with dexamethasone (40 g orally once a week) and clarithromycin (500 mg orally twice a day), only two of ten (20%) previously treated patients responded.[171] In a previous study, the immunomodulators thalidomide and its analog lenalidomide significantly augmented rituximab-mediated ADCC against lymphoplasmacytic cells.[172] Moreover, an expansion of natural killer cells has been observed with thalidomide, which in previous studies has been shown to be associated with rituximab response.[173,174] In view of these data, the WMCTG conducted two phase II clinical trials in symptomatic patients with WM combining thalidomide or lenalidomide with rituximab.[175,176] Intended therapy for those patients treated on the thalidomide plus rituximab study consisted of thalidomide administered at 200 mg daily for 2 weeks, followed by 400 mg daily thereafter for one year. Patients received four weekly infusions of rituximab at 375 mg/m^2 beginning one week after initiation of thalidomide, followed by four additional weekly infusions of rituximab at 375 mg/m^2 beginning at week 13. The overall and major response rates (i.e., $\geq$ 50% decrease in IgM) were 72% and 64%, respectively. Median serum IgM levels decreased from 3670 to 1590 mg/dL, while the median hematocrit rose from 33.0% to 37.6% at best response. The median time to progression for responders was 38 months in these series. Dose reduction of thalidomide occurred in all patients and led to discontinuation in 11 patients. Among 11 patients experiencing grade $\geq$ 2 neuroparesthesias, 10 demonstrated resolution to grade 1 or less at a median of 6.7 months. Given the high incidence of treatment-related neuropathy, the investigators recommended that lower doses of thalidomide (i.e., $\leq$ 200 mg/day) should be considered in this patient population.

In a phase II study of lenalidomide and rituximab in WM,[176] patients were initiated on lenalidomide at 25 mg daily on a syncopated schedule wherein therapy was administered for 3 weeks, followed by a 1 week pause for an intended duration of 48 weeks. Patients received 1 week of therapy with lenalidomide, after which rituximab (375 mg/m^2) was administered weekly on weeks 2–5, then 13–16. The overall and major response rates in this study were 50% and 25%, respectively, and a median time to progression for responders was 18.9 months. In two patients with bulky disease, significant reduction in extramedullary disease was observed. However, an acute decrease in hematocrit was observed during the first 2 weeks of lenalidomide therapy in 13/16 (81%) patients with a median absolute decrease in hematocrit of 4.8%, resulting in anemia-related complications and hospitalizations in four patients. Despite dose reduction, most patients in this study continued to demonstrate aggravated anemia with lenalidomide. There was no evidence of hemolysis or more general myelosuppression with lenalidomide in this study. Therefore, the mechanism for lenalidomide-related anemia in WM patients remains to be determined, and the use of this agent among WM patients should be avoided.

High-dose therapy and stem cell transplantation

The use of stem cell transplantation (SCT) therapy has also been explored in patients with WM. Desikan *et al.* reported their initial experience of high-dose chemotherapy and autologous SCT (ASCT),[177] which has more recently been updated by Munshi *et al.*[178] Their studies involved eight previously treated WM patients between the ages of 45 and 69 years, who received either melphalan at 200 mg/m^2 (n = 7) or melphalan at 140 mg/m^2 along with total body irradiation. Stem cells were successfully collected in all eight patients, although a second collection procedure was required for two patients who had extensive previous nucleoside analog exposure. There were no transplant-related mortalities and toxicities were manageable. All eight patients responded, with seven of eight patients achieving a major response, and one patient achieving a complete response with durations of response ranging from 5+ to 77+ months. Dreger *et al.* investigated the use of the DEXA-BEAM (dexamethasone, carmustine [BCNU], etoposide, cytarabine, melphalan) regimen followed by myeloablative therapy with cyclophosphamide, and total body irradiation and ASCT in seven WM patients, which included four untreated patients.[179] Serum IgM levels declined by > 50% following DEXA-BEAM and myeloablative therapy for six of seven patients, with progression-free survival ranging from 4+ to 30+ months. All three evaluable patients, who were previously treated, also attained a major response in a study by Anagnostopoulos *et al.* in which WM patients received various preparative regimens and showed event-free survivals of 26+, 31+, and 108+ months.[180] Tournilhac *et al.* recently reported the outcome of 18 WM patients in France who received high-dose chemotherapy followed by ASCT.[181] All patients were previously treated with a median of three (range 1–5) prior regimens. Therapy was well tolerated with an improvement in response status observed for seven patients (six PRs to CRs; one stable disease [SD] to PR), while only one patient demonstrated progressive disease. The median event-free survival for all non-progressing patients was 12 months. Tournilhac *et al.* have also reported the outcome of allogeneic transplantation in ten previously treated WM patients (ages 35–46) who received a median of three prior therapies, including three patients with progressive disease despite therapy.[181] Two of three patients with progressive disease responded, and an improvement in response status was observed in five patients. The median event-free survival for non-progressing, evaluable patients was 31 months. Concerning in this series was the death of three patients owing to transplantation-related toxicity. Anagnostopoulos *et al.*[182] have also reported on a retrospective review of WM patients who underwent either autologous or allogeneic transplantation, and whose outcomes were reported to the International Blood and Marrow Transplant Registry. Seventy-eight percent of patients in this cohort had two or more previous therapies, and 58% of them were resistant to their previous therapy. The relapse rate

Table 12.4. Summary of updated response criteria from the Third International Workshop on Waldenstrom's Macroglobulinemia

Complete response	CR	Disappearance of monoclonal protein by immunofixation; no histologic evidence of bone marrow involvement, and resolution of any adenopathy/organomegaly (confirmed by CT scan), along with no signs or symptoms attributable to WM. Reconfirmation of the CR status is required at least 6 weeks apart with a second immunofixation
Partial response	PR	A ≥ 50% reduction of serum monoclonal IgM concentration on protein electrophoresis and ≥ 50% decrease in adenopathy/organomegaly on physical examination or on CT scan. No new symptoms or signs of active disease
Minor response	MR	A ≥ 25% but < 50% reduction of serum monoclonal IgM by protein electrophoresis. No new symptoms or signs of active disease
Stable disease	SD	A < 25% reduction and < 25% increase of serum monoclonal IgM by electrophoresis without progression of adenopathy/ organomegaly, cytopenias or clinically significant symptoms due to disease and/ or signs of WM
Progressive disease	PD	A ≥ 25% increase in serum monoclonal IgM by protein electrophoresis confirmed by a second measurement or progression of clinically significant findings due to disease (i.e., anemia, thrombocytopenia, leukopenia, bulky adenopathy/ organomegaly) or symptoms (unexplained recurrent fever ≥ 38.4 °C, drenching night sweats, ≥ 10% body weight loss, or hyperviscosity, neuropathy, symptomatic cryoglobulinemia or amyloidosis) attributable to WM

Source: Kimby *et al.*[186]

at 3 years was 29% in the allogeneic group, and 24% in the autologous group. Non-relapse mortality, however, was 40% in the allogeneic group, and 11% in the autologous group in this series.

Kyriakou *et al.* recently provided an update of data from the European Bone Marrow Transplant (EBMT) registry on the outcome of WM patients who received either an autologous or allogeneic SCT.[183] Among 202 WM patients receiving an ASCT, which included primarily relapsed or refractory patients, the 5-year progression-free and overall survival rates were 61% and 33%, respectively. Chemosensitive disease at time of the ASCT was the most important prognostic factor for non-relapse mortality, response rate, and progression-free and overall survival. The EBMT registry experience with 106 allogeneic transplantations, which included 44 patients who received a conventional myeloablative allogeneic SCT and 62 patients who received a reduced intensity conditioning (RIC) allogeneic SCT was also presented by Kyriakou *et al.*,[183] which included predominately more advanced WM patients and was notable for a 3-year non-relapse mortality rate of 33%. The 5-year progression-free and overall survival rates in this series were 48% and 63%, respectively. Among the 106 patients who underwent an allogeneic SCT, 48 developed acute and 16 and 11 patients developed limited and extensive chronic graft-versus-host disease, respectively. The potential role for RIC allogeneic SCT to induce responses, including CRs, among patients with very advanced WM was reported by Maloney who observed 6 CRs, 1 near CR, and 4 PRs among 12 evaluable patients.[184] In consensus statements adopted at the fifth International Workshop, the use of autologous as well as RIC allogeneic SCT were deemed appropriate modalities for the treatment of relapsed/refractory WM patients, though the risks and benefits of these modalities should be carefully weighed against other available treatment options.

Response criteria in Waldenstrom's macroglobulinemia

Assessment of response to treatment in WM has been widely heterogeneous. As a consequence studies using the same regimen have reported significantly different response rates. As part of the Second and Third International Workshops on Waldenstrom's Macroglobulinemia, consensus panels developed guidelines for uniform response criteria in WM.[185,186] The category of minor response was adopted at the Third International Workshop on Waldenstrom's Macroglobulinemia, given that clinically meaningful responses were observed with newer biologic agents, and is based on ≥ 25% to < 50% decrease in serum IgM level, which is used as a surrogate marker of disease in WM. In distinction, the term major response is used to denote a response of ≥ 50% decrease in serum IgM levels, and includes PRs and CRs.[186] Response categories and criteria for progressive disease in WM based on consensus recommendations are summarized in Table 12.4. An important concern with the use of IgM as a surrogate marker of disease is that it can fluctuate, independent of tumor cell killing, particularly with newer biologically targeted agents such as rituximab and bortezomib.[134–136,152,178] Rituximab induces a spike or flare in serum IgM levels which can occur when used as monotherapy and in combination with other agents including cyclophosphamide, nucleoside analog, thalidomide, and lenalidomide, and last for several weeks to months,[138,141,142,152,159,175,176,187] whereas bortezomib can suppress IgM levels independent of tumor cell killing in certain patients.[159,188] Moreover, Owen[189] showed that in patients treated with selective B-cell-depleting agents, such as rituximab and alemtuzumab, residual IgM-producing plasma cells are spared and continue to persist, thus potentially skewing the relative response and assessment to treatment. Therefore, in circumstances where the serum IgM levels appear out of context with the clinical progress of the patient, a bone marrow biopsy should be considered in order to clarify the patient's underlying disease burden. A recent study by Ho *et al.*[37] suggests that soluble CD27 may serve as an alternative surrogate marker in WM, and may remain a faithful marker of disease in patients experiencing a rituximab-related IgM flare, as well as plasmapheresis.[190]

References

1. Owen RG, Treon SP, Al-Katib A, *et al.* Clinicopathologic definition of Waldenström's macroglobulinemia: Consensus Panel Recommendations from the Second International Workshop on Waldenström's macroglobulinemia. *Semin Oncol* 2003;**30**:110–15.
2. Harris NL, Jaffe ES, Stein H, *et al.* A revised European-American classification of lymphoid neoplasms: a proposal from the International Lymphoma Study Group. *Blood* 1994;**84**:1361–92.
3. Harris NL, Jaffe ES, Diebold J, *et al.* The World Health Organization classification of neoplastic diseases of the hematopoietic and lymphoid tissues. Report of the Clinical Advisory Committee meeting, Airlie House, Virginia, November, 1997. *Ann Oncol* 1999;**10**:1419–32.
4. Groves FD, Travis LB, Devesa SS, *et al.* Waldenström's macroglobulinemia: incidence patterns in the United States, 1988–1994. *Cancer* 1998;**82**:1078–81.
5. Herrinton LJ, Weiss NS. Incidence of Waldenström's macroglobulinemia. *Blood* 1993;**82**:3148–50.
6. Bjornsson OG, Arnason A, Gudmunosson S, *et al.* Macroglobulinaemia in an Icelandic family. *Acta Med Scand* 1978;**203**:283–8.
7. Treon SP, Hunter ZR, Aggarwal A, *et al.* Characterization of familial Waldenstrom's macroglobulinemia. *Ann Oncol* 2006;**17**:488–94.
8. Renier G, Ifrah N, Chevailler A, *et al.* Four brothers with Waldenström's macroglobulinemia. *Cancer* 1989;**64**:1554–9.
9. Ogmundsdottir HM, Sveinsdottir S, Sigfusson A, *et al.* Enhanced B cell survival in familial macroglobulinaemia is associated with increased expression of Bcl-2. *Clin Exp Immunol* 1999;**117**:252–60.
10. Linet MS, Humphrey RL, Mehl ES, *et al.* A case-control and family study of Waldenström's macroglobulinemia. *Leukemia* 1993;**7**:1363–9.
11. Santini GF, Crovatto M, Modolo ML, *et al.* Waldenström macroglobulinemia: a role of HCV infection? *Blood* 1993;**82**:2932.
12. Silvestri F, Barillari G, Fanin R, *et al.* Risk of hepatitis C virus infection, Waldenström's macroglobulinemia, and monoclonal gammopathies. *Blood* 1996;**88**:1125–6.
13. Leleu X, O'Connor K, Ho A, *et al.* Hepatitis C viral infection is not associated with Waldenström's macroglobulinemia. *Am J Hematol* 2007;**82**:83–4.
14. Carbone P, Caradonna F, Granata G, *et al.* Chromosomal abnormalities in Waldenstrom's macroglobulinemia. *Cancer Genet Cytogenet* 1992; **61**:147–51.
15. Mansoor A, Medeiros LJ, Weber DM, *et al.* Cytogenetic findings in lymphoplasmacytic lymphoma/ Waldenström macroglobulinemia. Chromosomal abnormalities are associated with the polymorphous subtype and an aggressive clinical course. *Am J Clin Pathol* 2001;**116**:543–9.
16. Han T, Sadamori N, Takeuchi J, *et al.* Clonal chromosome abnormalities in patients with Waldenstrom's and CLL-associated macroglobulinemia: significance of trisomy 12. *Blood* 1983;**62**:525–31.
17. Rivera AI, Li MM, Beltran G, *et al.* Trisomy 4 as the sole cytogenetic abnormality in a Waldenstrom macroglobulinemia. *Cancer Genet Cytogenet* 2002;**133**:172–3.
18. Wong KF, So CC, Chan JC, *et al.* Gain of chromosome 3/3q in B-cell chronic lymphoproliferative disorder is associated with plasmacytoid differentiation with or without IgM overproduction. *Cancer Genet Cytogenet* 2002;**136**:82–5.
19. Schop RF, Kuehl WM, Van Wier SA, *et al.* Waldenström macroglobulinemia neoplastic cells lack immunoglobulin heavy chain locus translocations but have frequent 6q deletions. *Blood* 2002;**100**:2996–3001.
20. Ocio EM, Schop RF, Gonzalez B, *et al.* 6q deletion in Waldenstrom's macroglobulinemia is associated with features of adverse prognosis. *Br J Haematol* 2007;**136**:80–6.
21. Chang H, Qi C, Trieu Y, *et al.* Prognostic relevance of 6q deletion in Waldenstrom's macroglobulinemia. *Proceedings of the Fifth International Workshop on Waldenstrom's Macroglobulinemia*, Stockholm, Sweden 2008 (Abstract 125).
22. Leleu X, Hunter ZR, Xu L, *et al.* Expression of regulatory genes for lymphoplasmacytic cell differentiation in Waldenstrom macroglobulinemia. *Br J Haematol* 2009;**145**:59–63.
23. Avet-Loiseau H, Garand R, Lode L, *et al.* 14q32 translocations discriminate IgM multiple myeloma from Waldenstrom's macroglobulinemia. *Semin Oncol* 2003;**30**:153–5.
24. Preud'homme JL, Seligmann M. Immunoglobulins on the surface of lymphoid cells in Waldenström's macroglobulinemia. *J Clin Invest* 1972;**51**:701–5.
25. Smith BR, Robert NJ, Ault KA. In Waldenstrom's macroglobulinemia the quantity of detectable circulating monoclonal B lymphocytes correlates with clinical course. *Blood* 1983; **61**:911–14.
26. Levy Y, Fermand JP, Navarro S, *et al.* Interleukin 6 dependence of spontaneous in vitro differentiation of B cells from patients with IgM gammopathy. *Proc Natl Acad Sci USA* 1990;**87**:3309–13.
27. Owen RG, Barrans SL, Richards SJ, *et al.* Waldenström macroglobulinemia. Development of diagnostic criteria and identification of prognostic factors. *Am J Clin Pathol* 2001; **116**:420–8.
28. Feiner HD, Rizk CC, Finfer MD, *et al.* IgM monoclonal gammopathy/ Waldenström's macroglobulinemia: a morphological and immunophenotypic study of the bone marrow. *Mod Pathol* 1990;**3**:348–56.
29. San Miguel JF, Vidriales MB, Ocio E, *et al.* Immunophenotypic analysis of Waldenstrom's macroglobulinemia. *Semin Oncol* 2003;**30**:187–95.

30. Hunter ZR, Branagan AR, Manning R, *et al.* CD5, CD10, CD23 expression in Waldenstrom's macroglobulinemia. *Clin Lymphoma* 2005;**5**:246–9.
31. Wagner SD, Martinelli V, Luzzatto L. Similar patterns of V kappa gene usage but different degrees of somatic mutation in hairy cell leukemia, prolymphocytic leukemia, Waldenström's macroglobulinemia, and myeloma. *Blood* 1994;**83**:3647–53.
32. Aoki H, Takishita M, Kosaka M, *et al.* Frequent somatic mutations in D and/or JH segments of Ig gene in Waldenström's macroglobulinemia and chronic lymphocytic leukemia (CLL) with Richter's syndrome but not in common CLL. *Blood* 1995;**85**:1913–19.
33. Shiokawa S, Suehiro Y, Uike N, *et al.* Sequence and expression analyses of mu and delta transcripts in patients with Waldenström's macroglobulinemia. *Am J Hematol* 2001;**68**:139–43.
34. Sahota SS, Forconi F, Ottensmeier CH, *et al.* Typical Waldenström macroglobulinemia is derived from a B-cell arrested after cessation of somatic mutation but prior to isotype switch events. *Blood* 2002; **100**:1505–7.
35. Paramithiotis E, Cooper MD. Memory B lymphocytes migrate to bone marrow in humans. *Proc Natl Acad Sci U S A* 1997;**94**:208–12.
36. Tournilhac O, Santos DD, Xu L, *et al.* Mast cells in Waldenstrom's macroglobulinemia support lymphoplasmacytic cell growth through CD154/CD40 signaling. *Ann Oncol* 2006;**17**:1275–82.
37. Ho A, Leleu X, Hatjiharissi E, *et al.* CD27-CD70 interactions in the pathogenesis of Waldenstrom's macroglobulinemia. *Blood* 2008;**112**:4683–9.
38. Merlini G, Farhangi M, Osserman EF. Monoclonal immunoglobulins with antibody activity in myeloma, macroglobulinemia and related plasma cell dyscrasias. *Semin Oncol* 1986;**13**:350–65.
39. Farhangi M, Merlini G. The clinical implications of monoclonal immunoglobulins. *Semin Oncol* 1986;**13**:366–79.
40. Marmont AM, Merlini G. Monoclonal autoimmunity in hematology. *Haematologica* 1991;**76**:449–59.
41. Mackenzie MR, Babcock J. Studies of the hyperviscosity syndrome. II. Macroglobulinemia. *J Lab Clin Med* 1975;**85**:227–34.
42. Gertz MA, Kyle RA. Hyperviscosity syndrome. *J Intensive Care Med* 1995;**10**:128–41.
43. Kwaan HC, Bongu A. The hyperviscosity syndromes. *Semin Thromb Hemost* 1999;**25**:199–208.
44. Singh A, Eckardt KU, Zimmermann A, *et al.* Increased plasma viscosity as a reason for inappropriate erythropoietin formation. *J Clin Invest* 1993;**91**:251–6.
45. Menke MN, Feke GT, McMeel JW, *et al.* Hyperviscosity-related retinopathy in Waldenstrom's macroglobulinemia. *Arch Ophthalmol* 2006;**124**:1601–6.
46. Merlini G, Baldini L, Broglia C, *et al.* Prognostic factors in symptomatic Waldenström's macroglobulinemia. *Semin Oncol* 2003;**30**:211–15.
47. Dellagi K, Dupouey P, Brouet JC, *et al.* Waldenström's macroglobulinemia and peripheral neuropathy: a clinical and immunologic study of 25 patients. *Blood* 1983;**62**:280–5.
48. Nobile-Orazio E, Marmiroli P, Baldini L, *et al.* Peripheral neuropathy in macroglobulinemia: incidence and antigen-specificity of M proteins. *Neurology* 1987;**37**:1506–14.
49. Nemni R, Gerosa E, Piccolo G, *et al.* Neuropathies associated with monoclonal gammopathies. *Haematologica* 1994;**79**:557–66.
50. Ropper AH, Gorson KC. Neuropathies associated with paraproteinemia. *N Engl J Med* 1998;**338**:1601–7.
51. Vital A. Paraproteinemic neuropathies. *Brain Pathol* 2001;**11**:399–407.
52. Latov N, Braun PE, Gross RB, *et al.* Plasma cell dyscrasia and peripheral neuropathy: identification of the myelin antigens that react with human paraproteins. *Proc Natl Acad Sci U S A* 1981;**78**:7139–42.
53. Chassande B, Leger JM, Younes-Chennoufi AB, *et al.* Peripheral neuropathy associated with IgM monoclonal gammopathy: correlations between M-protein antibody activity and clinical/electrophysiological features in 40 cases. *Muscle Nerve* 1998;**21**:55–62.
54. Weiss MD, Dalakas MC, Lauter CJ, *et al.* Variability in the binding of anti-MAG and anti-SGPG antibodies to target antigens in demyelinating neuropathy and IgM paraproteinemia. *J Neuroimmunol* 1999;**95**:174–84.
55. Latov N, Hays AP, Sherman WH. Peripheral neuropathy and anti-MAG antibodies. *Crit Rev Neurobiol* 1988;**3**:301–32.
56. Dalakas MC, Quarles RH. Autoimmune ataxic neuropathies (sensory ganglionopathies): are glycolipids the responsible autoantigens? *Ann Neurol* 1996;**39**:419–22.
57. Eurelings M, Ang CW, Notermans NC, *et al.* Antiganglioside antibodies in polyneuropathy associated with monoclonal gammopathy. *Neurology* 2001;**57**:1909–12.
58. Jacobs BC, O'Hanlon GM, Breedland EG, *et al.* Human IgM paraproteins demonstrate shared reactivity between *Campylobacter jejuni* lipopolysaccharides and human peripheral nerve disialylated gangliosides. *J Neuroimmunol* 1997;**80**:23–30.
59. Ilyas AA, Quarles RH, Dalakas MC, *et al.* Monoclonal IgM in a patient with paraproteinemic polyneuropathy binds to gangliosides containing disialosyl groups. *Ann Neurol* 1985;**18**:655–9.
60. Willison HJ, O'Leary CP, Veitch J, *et al.* The clinical and laboratory features of chronic sensory ataxic neuropathy with anti-disialosyl IgM antibodies. *Brain* 2001;**124**:1968–77.
61. Lopate G, Choksi R, Pestronk A. Severe sensory ataxia and demyelinating polyneuropathy with IgM anti-GM2 and GalNAc-GD1A antibodies. *Muscle Nerve* 2002;**25**:828–36.
62. Nobile-Orazio E, Manfredini E, Carpo M, *et al.* Frequency and clinical correlates of antineural IgM antibodies in neuropathy associated with IgM monoclonal gammopathy. *Ann Neurol* 1994;**36**:416–24.
63. Gordon PH, Rowland LP, Younger DS, *et al.* Lymphoproliferative disorders and motor neuron disease: an update. *Neurology* 1997;**48**:1671–8.
64. Pavord SR, Murphy PT, Mitchell VE. POEMS syndrome and Waldenström's macroglobulinaemia. *J Clin Pathol* 1996;**49**:181–2.
65. Crisp D, Pruzanski W. B-cell neoplasms with homogeneous cold-reacting antibodies (cold agglutinins). *Am J Med* 1982;**72**:915–22.

66. Pruzanski W, Shumak KH. Biologic activity of cold-reacting autoantibodies (first of two parts). *N Engl J Med* 1977;**297**:538–42.

67. Pruzanski W, Shumak KH. Biologic activity of cold-reacting autoantibodies (second of two parts). *N Engl J Med* 1977;**297**:583–9.

68. Whittaker SJ, Bhogal BS, Black MM. Acquired immunobullous disease: a cutaneous manifestation of IgM macroglobulinaemia. *Br J Dermatol* 1996;**135**:283–6.

69. Daoud MS, Lust JA, Kyle RA, *et al.* Monoclonal gammopathies and associated skin disorders. *J Am Acad Dermatol* 1999;**40**:507–35.

70. Gad A, Willen R, Carlen B, *et al.* Duodenal involvement in Waldenström's macroglobulinemia. *J Clin Gastroenterol* 1995;**20**:174–6.

71. Case records of the Massachusetts General Hospital. Weekly clinicopathological exercises. Case 3-1990. A 66-year-old woman with Waldenström's macroglobulinemia, diarrhea, anemia, and persistent gastrointestinal bleeding. *N Engl J Med* 1990;**322**:183–92.

72. Isaac J, Herrera GA. Cast nephropathy in a case of Waldenström's macroglobulinemia. *Nephron* 2002;**91**:512–15.

73. Morel-Maroger L, Basch A, Danon F, *et al.* Pathology of the kidney in Waldenström's macroglobulinemia. Study of sixteen cases. *N Engl J Med* 1970;**283**:123–9.

74. Gertz MA, Kyle RA, Noel P. Primary systemic amyloidosis: a rare complication of immunoglobulin M monoclonal gammopathies and Waldenström's macroglobulinemia. *J Clin Oncol* 1993;**11**:914–20.

75. Moyner K, Sletten K, Husby G, *et al.* An unusually large (83 amino acid residues) amyloid fibril protein AA from a patient with Waldenström's macroglobulinaemia and amyloidosis. *Scand J Immunol* 1980;**11**:549–54.

76. Gardyn J, Schwartz A, Gal R, *et al.* Waldenström's macroglobulinemia associated with AA amyloidosis. *Int J Hematol* 2001;**74**:76–8.

77. Dussol B, Kaplanski G, Daniel L, *et al.* Simultaneous occurrence of fibrillary glomerulopathy and AL amyloid. *Nephrol Dial Transplant* 1998;**13**:2630–2.

78. Rausch PG, Herion JC. Pulmonary manifestations of Waldenström macroglobulinemia. *Am J Hematol* 1980;**9**:201–9.

79. Fadil A, Taylor DE. The lung and Waldenström's macroglobulinemia. *South Med J* 1998;**91**:681–5.

80. Kyrtsonis MC, Angelopoulou MK, Kontopidou FN, *et al.* Primary lung involvement in Waldenström's macroglobulinaemia: report of two cases and review of the literature. *Acta Haematol* 2001;**105**:92–6.

81. Kaila VL, el Newihi HM, Dreiling BJ, *et al.* Waldenström's macroglobulinemia of the stomach presenting with upper gastrointestinal hemorrhage. *Gastrointest Endosc* 1996;**44**:73–5.

82. Yasui O, Tukamoto F, Sasaki N, *et al.* Malignant lymphoma of the transverse colon associated with macroglobulinemia. *Am J Gastroenterol* 1997;**92**:2299–301.

83. Rosenthal JA, Curran WJ Jr, Schuster SJ. Waldenström's macroglobulinemia resulting from localized gastric lymphoplasmacytoid lymphoma. *Am J Hematol* 1998;**58**:244–5.

84. Recine MA, Perez MT, Cabello-Inchausti B, *et al.* Extranodal lymphoplasmacytoid lymphoma (immunocytoma) presenting as small intestinal obstruction. *Arch Pathol Lab Med* 2001;**125**:677–9.

85. Veltman GA, van Veen S, Kluin-Nelemans JC, *et al.* Renal disease in Waldenström's macroglobulinaemia. *Nephrol Dial Transplant* 1997;**12**:1256–9.

86. Moore DF Jr, Moulopoulos LA, Dimopoulos MA. Waldenström macroglobulinemia presenting as a renal or perirenal mass: clinical and radiographic features. *Leuk Lymphoma* 1995;**17**:331–4.

87. Mascaro JM, Montserrat E, Estrach T, *et al.* Specific cutaneous manifestations of Waldenström's macroglobulinaemia. A report of two cases. *Br J Dermatol* 1982;**106**:17–22.

88. Schnitzler L, Schubert B, Boasson M, *et al.* Urticaire chronique, lésions osseuses, macroglobulinémie IgM: Maladie de Waldenström? *Bull Soc Fr Dermatol Syphiligr* 1974;**81**:363–8.

89. Roux S, Fermand JP, Brechignac S, *et al.* Tumoral joint involvement in multiple myeloma and Waldenström's macroglobulinemia – report of 4 cases. *J Rheumatol* 1996;**23**:2175–8.

90. Orellana J, Friedman AH. Ocular manifestations of multiple myeloma, Waldenström's macroglobulinemia and benign monoclonal gammopathy. *Surv Ophthalmol* 1981;**26**:157–69.

91. Ettl AR, Birbamer GG, Philipp W. Orbital involvement in Waldenström's macroglobulinemia: ultrasound, computed tomography and magnetic resonance findings. *Ophthalmologica* 1992;**205**:40–5.

92. Civit T, Coulbois S, Baylac F, *et al.* Waldenström's macroglobulinemia and cerebral lymphoplasmocytic proliferation: Bing and Neel syndrome. Apropos of a new case. *Neurochirurgie* 1997;**43**:245–9.

93. McMullin MF, Wilkin HJ, Elder E. Inaccurate haemoglobin estimation in Waldenström's macroglobulinaemia. *J Clin Pathol* 1995;**48**:787.

94. Treon SP, Branagan AR, Hunter Z, *et al.* IgA and IgG hypogammaglobulinemia persists in most patients with Waldenstrom's macroglobulinemia despite therapeutic responses, including complete remissions. *Blood* 2004;**104**:306b.

95. Treon SP, Hunter Z, Ciccarelli BT, *et al.* IgA and IgG hypogammaglobulinemia is a constitutive feature in most Waldenstrom's macroglobulinemia patients and may be related to mutations associated with common variable immunodeficiency disorder (CVID). *Blood* 2008;**112**:3749.

96. Dutcher TF, Fahey JL. The histopathology of macroglobulinemia of Waldenström. *J Natl Cancer Inst* 1959;**22**:887–917.

97. Moulopoulos LA, Dimopoulos MA, Varma DG, *et al.* Waldenström macroglobulinemia: MR imaging of the spine and CT of the abdomen and pelvis. *Radiology* 1993;**188**:669–73.

98. Gobbi PG, Bettini R, Montecucco C, *et al.* Study of prognosis in Waldenström's macroglobulinemia: a proposal for a simple binary classification with clinical and investigational utility. *Blood* 1994;**83**:2939–45.

99. Morel P, Monconduit M, Jacomy D, *et al.* Prognostic factors in Waldenström macroglobulinemia: a report on 232 patients with the description of a new scoring system and

its validation on 253 other patients. *Blood* 2000;**96**:852–8.

100. Dhodapkar MV, Jacobson JL, Gertz MA, *et al.* Prognostic factors and response to fludarabine therapy in patients with Waldenström macroglobulinemia: results of United States intergroup trial (Southwest Oncology Group S9003). *Blood* 2001;**98**:41–8.

101. Kyle RA, Treon SP, Alexanian R, *et al.* Prognostic markers and criteria to initiate therapy in Waldenström's macroglobulinemia: Consensus Panel Recommendations from the Second International Workshop on Waldenström's macroglobulinemia. *Semin Oncol* 2003;**30**:116–20.

102. Dimopoulos M, Gika D, Zervas K, *et al.* The international staging system for multiple myeloma is applicable in symptomatic Waldenstrom's macroglobulinemia. *Leuk Lymphoma* 2004;**45**:1809–13.

103. Anagnostopoulos A, Zervas K, Kyrtsonis M, *et al.* Prognostic value of serum beta 2-microglobulin in patients with Waldenstrom's macroglobulinemia requiring therapy. *Clin Lymphoma Myeloma* 2006;7:205–9.

104. Morel P, Duhamel A, Gobbi P, *et al.* International prognostic scoring system for Waldenstrom's macroglobulinemia. *Blood* 2009;**113**:4163–70.

105. Leleu XP, Manning R, Soumerai JD, *et al.* Increased incidence of transformation and myelodysplasia/acute leukemia in patients with Waldenström macroglobulinemia treated with nucleoside analogs. *J Clin Oncol* 2009;**27**:250–5.

106. Gertz M, Anagnostopoulos A, Anderson KC, *et al.* Treatment recommendations in Waldenström's macroglobulinemia: Consensus Panel Recommendations from the Second International Workshop on Waldenström's Macroglobulinemia. *Semin Oncol* 2003;**30**:121–6.

107. Treon SP, Gertz MA, Dimopoulos MA, *et al.* Update on treatment recommendations from the Third International Workshop on Waldenstrom's Macroglobulinemia. *Blood* 2006;**107**:3442–6.

108. Dimopoulos MA, Gertz MA, Kastritis E, *et al.* Update on treatment recommendations from the Fourth International Workshop on Waldenstrom's Macroglobulinemia. *J Clin Oncol* 2009;**27**:120–6.

109. Kyle RA, Greipp PR, Gertz MA, *et al.* Waldenström's macroglobulinaemia: a prospective study comparing daily with intermittent oral chlorambucil. *Br J Haematol* 2000;**108**:737–42.

110. Dimopoulos MA, Alexanian R. Waldenstrom's macroglobulinemia. *Blood* 1994;**83**:1452–9.

111. Petrucci MT, Avvisati G, Tribalto M, *et al.* Waldenström's macroglobulinaemia: results of a combined oral treatment in 34 newly diagnosed patients. *J Intern Med* 1989;**226**:443–7.

112. Case DC Jr, Ervin TJ, Boyd MA, *et al.* Waldenström's macroglobulinemia: long-term results with the M-2 protocol. *Cancer Invest* 1991;**9**:1–7.

113. Facon T, Brouillard M, Duhamel A, *et al.* Prognostic factors in Waldenström's macroglobulinemia: a report of 167 cases. *J Clin Oncol* 1993;**11**:1553–8.

114. Dimopoulos MA, Kantarjian H, Weber D, *et al.* Primary therapy of Waldenström's macroglobulinemia with 2-chlorodeoxyadenosine. *J Clin Oncol* 1994;**12**:2694–8.

115. Delannoy A, Ferrant A, Martiat P, *et al.* 2-Chlorodeoxyadenosine therapy in Waldenström's macroglobulinaemia. *Nouv Rev Fr Hematol* 1994;**36**:317–20.

116. Fridrik MA, Jager G, Baldinger C, *et al.* First-line treatment of Waldenström's disease with cladribine. Arbeitsgemeinschaft Medikamentöse Tumortherapie. *Ann Hematol* 1997;**74**:7–10.

117. Liu ES, Burian C, Miller WE, *et al.* Bolus administration of cladribine in the treatment of Waldenström macroglobulinaemia. *Br J Haematol* 1998;**103**:690–5.

118. Hellmann A, Lewandowski K, Zaucha JM, *et al.* Effect of a 2-hour infusion of 2-chlorodeoxyadenosine in the treatment of refractory or previously untreated Waldenström's macroglobulinemia. *Eur J Haematol* 1999;**63**:35–41.

119. Betticher DC, Hsu Schmitz SF, Ratschiller D, *et al.* Cladribine (2-CDA) given as subcutaneous bolus injections is active in pretreated Waldenström's macroglobulinaemia. Swiss Group for Clinical Cancer Research (SAKK). *Br J Haematol* 1997;**99**:358–63.

120. Dimopoulos MA, Weber D, Delasalle KB, *et al.* Treatment of Waldenström's macroglobulinemia resistant to standard therapy with 2-chlorodeoxyadenosine: identification of prognostic factors. *Ann Oncol* 1995;**6**:49–52.

121. Dimopoulos MA, O'Brien S, Kantarjian H, *et al.* Fludarabine therapy in Waldenström's macroglobulinemia. *Am J Med* 1993;**95**:49–52.

122. Foran JM, Rohatiner AZ, Coiffier B, *et al.* Multicenter phase II study of fludarabine phosphate for patients with newly diagnosed lymphoplasmacytoid lymphoma, Waldenström's macroglobulinemia, and mantle-cell lymphoma. *J Clin Oncol* 1999; **17**:546–53.

123. Thalhammer-Scherrer R, Geissler K, Schwarzinger I, *et al.* Fludarabine therapy in Waldenström's macroglobulinemia. *Ann Hematol* 2000;**79**:556–9.

124. Dhodapkar MV, Jacobson JL, Gertz MA, *et al.* Prognostic factors and response to fludarabine therapy in patients with Waldenström macroglobulinemia: results of United States intergroup trial (Southwest Oncology Group S9003). *Blood* 2001;**98**:41–8.

125. Zinzani PL, Gherlinzoni F, Bendandi M, *et al.* Fludarabine treatment in resistant Waldenström's macroglobulinemia. *Eur J Haematol* 1995;**54**:120–3.

126. Leblond V, Ben Othman T, Deconinck E, *et al.* Activity of fludarabine in previously treated Waldenström's macroglobulinemia: a report of 71 cases. Groupe Cooperatif Macroglobulinemie. *J Clin Oncol* 1998;**16**:2060–4.

127. Dimopoulos MA, Weber DM, Kantarjian H, *et al.* 2-Chlorodeoxyadenosine therapy of patients with Waldenström macroglobulinemia previously treated with fludarabine. *Ann Oncol* 1994;**5**:288–9.

128. Lewandowski K, Halaburda K, Hellmann A. Fludarabine therapy in Waldenström's macroglobulinemia patients treated previously with 2-chlorodeoxyadenosine. *Leuk Lymphoma* 2002;**43**:361–3.

129. Thomas S, Hosing C, Delasalle KB, *et al.* Success rates of autologous stem cell collection in patients with Waldenstrom's macroglobulinemia. Proceedings of the Fifth International Workshop on Waldenstrom's Macroglobulinemia 2008 (Supplemental Abstract).

130. Leleu X, Tamburini J, Roccaro A, *et al.* Balancing risk versus benefit in the treatment of Waldenstrom's macroglobulinemia patients with nucleoside analogue-based therapy. *Clin Lymphoma Myeloma* 2009;**9**:71–3.

131. Treon SP, Kelliher A, Keele B, *et al.* Expression of serotherapy target antigens in Waldenstrom's macroglobulinemia: therapeutic applications and considerations. *Semin Oncol* 2003;**30**:248–52.

132. Treon SP, Shima Y, Preffer FI, *et al.* Treatment of plasma cell dyscrasias with antibody-mediated immunotherapy. *Semin Oncol* 1999;**26** Suppl 14:97–106.

133. Byrd JC, White CA, Link B, *et al.* Rituximab therapy in Waldenstrom's macroglobulinemia: preliminary evidence of clinical activity. *Ann Oncol* 1999;**10**:1525–7.

134. Weber DM, Gavino M, Huh Y, *et al.* Phenotypic and clinical evidence supports rituximab for Waldenstrom's macroglobulinemia. *Blood* 1999;**94**:125a.

135. Foran JM, Rohatiner AZ, Cunningham D, *et al.* European phase II study of rituximab (chimeric anti-CD20 monoclonal antibody) for patients with newly diagnosed mantle-cell lymphoma and previously treated mantle-cell lymphoma, immunocytoma, and small B-cell lymphocytic lymphoma. *J Clin Oncol* 2000;**18**:317–24.

136. Treon SP, Agus DB, Link B, *et al.* CD20-Directed antibody-mediated immunotherapy induces responses and facilitates hematologic recovery in patients with Waldenstrom's macroglobulinemia. *J Immunother* 2001;**24**:272–9.

137. Gertz MA, Rue M, Blood E, *et al.* Multicenter phase 2 trial of rituximab for Waldenstrom macroglobulinemia (WM): An Eastern Cooperative Oncology Group Study (E3A98). *Leuk Lymphoma* 2004;**45**:2047–55.

138. Dimopoulos MA, Zervas C, Zomas A, *et al.* Treatment of Waldenstrom's macroglobulinemia with rituximab. *J Clin Oncol* 2002;**20**:2327–33.

139. Treon SP, Emmanouilides C, Kimby E, *et al.* Extended rituximab therapy in Waldenström's macroglobulinemia. *Ann Oncol* 2005;**16**:132–8.

140. Donnelly GB, Bober-Sorcinelli K, Jacobson R, *et al.* Abrupt IgM rise following treatment with rituximab in patients with Waldenstrom's macroglobulinemia. *Blood* 2001;**98**:240b.

141. Treon SP, Branagan AR, Hunter Z, *et al.* Paradoxical increases in serum IgM and viscosity levels following rituximab therapy in Waldenstrom's Macroglobulinemia. *Ann Oncol* 2004;**15**:1481–3.

142. Ghobrial IM, Fonseca R, Greipp PR, *et al.* Initial immunoglobulin M "flare" after rituximab therapy in patients with Waldenstrom Macroglobulinemia: An Eastern Cooperative Oncology Group Study. *Cancer* 2004;**101**:2593–8.

143. Dimopoulos MA, Anagnostopoulos A, Zervas C, *et al.* Predictive factors for response to rituximab in Waldenstrom's macroglobulinemia. *Clin Lymphoma* 2005;**5**:270–2.

144. Treon SP, Hansen M, Branagan AR, *et al.* Polymorphisms in FcgammaRIIIA (CD16) receptor expression are associated with clinical responses to rituximab in Waldenstrom's macroglobulinemia. *J Clin Oncol* 2005;**23**:474–81.

145. Weber DM, Dimopoulos MA, Delasalle K, *et al.* 2-chlorodeoxyadenosine alone and in combination for previously untreated Waldenstrom's macroglobulinemia. *Semin Oncol* 2003;**30**:243–7.

146. Treon SP, Branagan AR, Ioakimidis L, *et al.* Long-term outcomes to fludarabine and rituximab in Waldenstrom's macroglobulinemia. *Blood* 2009;**113**:3673–8.

147. Tam CS, Wolf MM, Westerman D, *et al.* Fludarabine combination therapy is highly effective in first-line and salvage treatment of patients with Waldenstrom's macroglobulinemia. *Clin Lymphoma Myeloma* 2005; **6**:136–9.

148. Hensel M, Villalobos M, Kornacker M, *et al.* Pentostatin/cyclophosphamide with or without rituximab: an effective regimen for patients with Waldenstrom's macroglobulinemia/ lymphoplasmacytic lymphoma. *Clin Lymphoma Myeloma* 2005;**6**:131–5.

149. Dimopoulos MA, Anagnostopoulos A, Kyrtsonis MC, *et al.* Primary treatment of Waldenstrom's macroglobulinemia with dexamethasone, rituximab and cyclophosphamide. *J Clin Oncol* 2007;**25**:3344–9.

150. Buske C, Hoster E, Dreyling MH, *et al.* The addition of rituximab to front-line therapy with CHOP (R-CHOP) results in a higher response rate and longer time to treatment failure in patients with lymphoplasmacytic lymphoma: results of a randomized trial of the German Low-Grade Lymphoma Study Group (GLSG). *Leukemia* 2009;**23**:153–61.

151. Treon SP, Hunter Z, Branagan A. CHOP plus rituximab therapy in Waldenström's macroglobulinemia. *Clin Lymphoma Myeloma* 2005;**5**: 273–7.

152. Ioakimidis L, Patterson CJ, Hunter ZR, *et al.* Comparative outcomes following CP-R, CVP-R and CHOP-R in Waldenström's macroglobulinemia. *Clin Lymphoma Myeloma* 2009;**9**:62–6.

153. Dimopoulos MA, Hamilos G, Efstathiou E, *et al.* Treatment of Waldenstrom's macroglobulinemia with the combination of fludarabine and cyclophosphamide. *Leuk Lymphoma* 2003;**44**:993–6.

154. Tamburini J, Levy V, Chateilex C, *et al.* Fludarabine plus cyclophosphamide in Waldenstrom's macroglobulinemia: results in 49 patients. *Leukemia* 2005;**19**:1831–4.

155. Jagannath S, Durie BG, Wolf J, *et al.* Bortezomib therapy alone and in combination with dexamethasone for previously untreated symptomatic multiple myeloma. *Br J Haematol* 2005;**129**:776–83.

156. Oakervee HE, Popat R, Curry N, *et al.* PAD combination therapy (PS-341/ bortezomib, doxorubicin and dexamethasone) for previously untreated patients with multiple myeloma. *Br J Haematol* 2005;**129**:755–62.

157. Harousseau JL, Attal M, Leleu X, *et al.* Bortezomib plus dexamethasone as induction treatment prior to autologous stem cell transplantation in patients with newly diagnosed multiple myeloma. Preliminary results of an IFM phase II study. *Blood* 2004;**104**:416a.

158. Mitsiades CS, Mitsiades N, McMullan CJ, *et al.* The proteasome inhibitor

bortezomib (PS-341) is active against Waldenstrom's macroglobulinemia. *Blood* 2003;**102**:181a.

159. Treon SP, Hunter ZR, Matous J, *et al.* Multicenter clinical trial of bortezomib in relapsed/refractory Waldenstrom's macroglobulinemia: results of WMCTG Trial 03-248. *Clin Cancer Res* 2007;**13**:3320–5.

160. Chen CI, Kouroukis CT, White D, *et al.* Bortezomib is active in patients with untreated or relapsed Waldenstrom's macroglobulinemia: a phase II study of the National Cancer Institute of Canada Clinical Trials Group. *J Clin Oncol* 2007;**25**:1570–5.

161. Dimopoulos MA, Anagnostopoulos A, Kyrtsonis MC, *et al.* Treatment of relapsed or refractory Waldenstrom's macroglobulinemia with bortezomib. *Haematologica* 2005;**90**:1655–7.

162. Goy A, Younes A, McLaughlin P, *et al.* Phase II study of proteasome inhibitor bortezomib in relapsed or refractory B-cell non-Hodgkin's lymphoma. *J Clin Oncol* 2005; **23**:667–75.

163. Treon SP, Ioakimidis L, Soumerai JD, *et al.* Primary therapy of Waldenstrom's macroglobulinemia with bortezomib, dexamethasone and rituximab: WMCTG clinical trial 05-180. *J Clin Oncol* 2009;**27**:3830–5.

164. Ghobrial IM, Hong F, Padmanabhan S, *et al.* Phase II of weekly bortezomib in combination with rituximab in relapsed or relapsed/refractory Waldenstrom's Macroglobulinemia. *J Clin Oncol* 2010;**28**(8):1422–8.

165. Agathocleous A, Rule S, Johson P. Preliminary results of a phase I/II study of weekly or twice weekly bortezomib in combination with rituximab in patients with follicular lymphoma, mantle cell lymphoma, and Waldenstrom's macroglobulinemia. *Blood* 2007;**110**:754a.

166. Santos DD, Hatjiharissi E, Tournilhac O, *et al.* CD52 is expressed on human mast cells and is a potential therapeutic target in Waldenstrom's macroglobulinemia and mast cell disorders. *Clin Lymphoma Myeloma* 2006;**6**:478–83.

167. Hunter ZR, Boxer M, Kahl B, *et al.* Phase II study of alemtuzumab in lymphoplasmacytic lymphoma: results of WMCTG trial 02–079. *Proc Am Soc Clin Oncol* 2006;**24**:427s.

168. Owen RG, Rawstron AC, Osterborg A, *et al.* Activity of alemtuzumab in relapsed/refractory Waldenstrom's macroglobulinemia. *Blood* 2003;**102**:644a.

169. Dimopoulos MA, Zomas A, Viniou NA, *et al.* Treatment of Waldenström's macroglobulinemia with thalidomide. *J Clin Oncol* 2001;**19**:3596–601.

170. Coleman M, Leonard J, Lyons L, *et al.* Treatment of Waldenström's macroglobulinemia with clarithromycin, low-dose thalidomide and dexamethasone. *Semin Oncol* 2003;**30**:270–4.

171. Dimopoulos MA, Zomas K, Tsatalas K, *et al.* Treatment of Waldenström's macroglobulinemia with single agent thalidomide or with combination of clarithromycin, thalidomide and dexamethasone. *Semin Oncol* 2003;**30**:265–9.

172. Hayashi T, Hideshima T, Akiyama M, *et al.* Molecular mechanisms whereby immunomodulatory drugs activate natural killer cells: clinical application. *Br J Haematol* 2005;**128**:192–203.

173. Davies FE, Raje N, Hideshima T, *et al.* Thalidomide and immunomodulatory derivatives augment natural killer cell cytotoxicity in multiple myeloma. *Blood* 2001;**98**:210–16.

174. Janakiraman N, McLaughlin P, White CA, *et al.* Rituximab: correlation between effector cells and clinical activity in NHL. *Blood* 1998;**92**:337a.

175. Treon SP, Soumerai JD, Branagan AR, *et al.* Thalidomide and rituximab in Waldenstrom's macroglobulinemia. *Blood* 2008;**112**:4452–7.

176. Treon SP, Soumerai JD, Branagan AR, *et al.* Lenalidomide and rituximab in Waldenström's macroglobulinemia. *Clin Cancer Res* 2008;**15**:355–60.

177. Desikan R, Dhodapkar M, Siegel D, *et al.* High-dose therapy with autologous haemopoietic stem cell support for Waldenström's macroglobulinaemia. *Br J Haematol* 1999;**105**:993–6.

178. Munshi NC, Barlogie B. Role for high dose therapy with autologous hematopoietic stem cell support in Waldenström's macroglobulinemia. *Semin Oncol* 2003;**30**:282–5.

179. Dreger P, Glass B, Kuse R, *et al.* Myeloablative radiochemotherapy followed by reinfusion of purged autologous stem cells for Waldenström's macroglobulinaemia. *Br J Haematol* 1999;**106**:115–18.

180. Anagnostopoulos A, Dimopoulos MA, Aleman A, *et al.* High-dose chemotherapy followed by stem cell transplantation in patients with resistant Waldenström's macroglobulinemia. *Bone Marrow Transplant* 2001;**27**:1027–9.

181. Tournilhac O, Leblond V, Tabrizi R, *et al.* Transplantation in Waldenström's macroglobulinemia – the French Experience. *Semin Oncol* 2003; **30**:291–6.

182. Anagnostopoulos A, Hari PN, Perez WS, *et al.* Autologous or allogeneic stem cell transplantation in patients with Waldenstrom's macroglobulinemia. *Biol Blood Marrow Transplant* 2006;**12**:845–54.

183. Kyriakou H, on behalf of the Lymphoma Working Party of the European Group for Blood and Bone Marrow Transplantation. Haematopoietic stem cell transplantation for Waldenstrom's macroglobulinemia. Proceedings of the Fifth International Workshop on Waldenstrom's Macroglobulinemia, Stockholm, Sweden 2008 (Abstract 146).

184. Maloney D. Evidence for GVWM following mini-allo in Waldenstrom's macroglobulinemia. Proceedings of the Fifth International Workshop on Waldenstrom's Macroglobulinemia, Stockholm, Sweden 2008 (Abstract 147).

185. Weber D, Treon SP, Emmanouilides C, *et al.* Uniform response criteria in Waldenstrom's macroglobulinemia: consensus panel recommendations from the Second International Workshop on Waldenstrom's Macroglobulinemia. *Semin Oncol* 2003;**30**:127–31.

186. Kimby E, Treon SP, Anagnostopoulos A, *et al.* Update on recommendations for assessing response from the Third International Workshop on Waldenstrom's Macroglobulinemia. *Clin Lymphoma Myeloma* 2006; **6**:380–3.

187. Nichols GL, Savage DG. Timing of rituximab/fludarabine in Waldenstrom's macroglobulinemia may avert hyperviscosity. *Blood* 2004;**104**:237b.

188. Strauss SJ, Maharaj L, Hoare S, *et al.* Bortezomib therapy in patients with relapsed or refractory lymphoma: potential correlation of in vitro sensitivity and tumor necrosis factor alpha response with clinical activity. *J Clin Oncol* 2006;**24**:2105–12.

189. Owen R. Complexities of assessing response in Waldenstrom's macroglobulinemia. Proceedings of the Fifth International Workshop on Waldenstrom's Macroglobulinemia, Stockholm, Sweden 2008 (Abstract 128).

190. Ciccarelli BT, Yang G, Hatjiharissi E, *et al.* Soluble CD27 is a faithful marker of disease burden and is unaffected by the rituximab-induced IgM flare, as well as plasmapheresis, in patients with Waldenström's macroglobulinemia. *Clin Lymphoma Myeloma* 2009;**9**:56–8.

Chapter 13

WHO classification of lymphomas

William W. L. Choi and Wing C. Chan

Introduction

The latest fourth edition of the World Health Organization (WHO) classification of tumors of hematopoietic and lymphoid tissues (WHO classification) was published in 2008.[1] The current and the previous (2001) editions of the WHO classification adopt the guiding principles of the widely accepted Revised European–American Classification of Lymphoid Neoplasms (REAL) classification published in 1994.[2] Both the REAL and the WHO classifications aim at defining distinct disease entities that are both recognizable by pathologists and are meaningful to the clinicians. All available information from morphologic, immunophenotypic, genetic, and clinical assessments was utilized to define non-overlapping disease entities. Additionally, the complexity of the field necessitated the recruitment of a larger number of expert pathologists from around the world, and the inclusion of input from the clinicians in the development of the WHO classification. Broad agreement among the pathologists was required, even at the expense of compromise, which was considered vital for wide acceptance of the WHO classification.[1]

Essential elements of the WHO classification

The WHO classification takes into account a combination of clinical, morphologic, immunophenotypic, and genetic information in recognizing distinct lymphoma entities, although the weight of each of these four parameters varies. Indeed, there is no 'gold standard' among these four features when defining individual entities.[1]

Morphology

Morphologic features remain the foundation in the WHO classification and in day-to-day lymphoma diagnosis. Some disease entities, like the various subtypes of Hodgkin lymphomas (HLs), are still defined and diagnosed on morphologic grounds, with support from immunophenotypic results. For the non-Hodgkin lymphomas (NHLs), histologic and cytologic features are often needed to guide the more sophisticated and expensive tests (e.g., panels of immunostains). The interpretation of other ancillary tests should also be considered in the context of morphology. For instance, flow cytometric immunophenotyping of a thymoma could yield a lot of CD4+CD8+ T cells with nuclear expression of terminal deoxynucleotidyl transferase (TdT), which may lead to an erroneous diagnosis of T lymphoblastic lymphoma (T-LBL) if morphologic features were overlooked.[3] Therefore, the importance of maintaining the highest standard in obtaining and processing a specimen for the interpretation of morphologic features cannot be overemphasized.

Immunophenotype

The advent of immunohistochemistry and flow cytometry during the 1980s greatly facilitated the understanding of marker expression on immune cells and enhanced the classification and diagnosis of lymphomas. However, only a handful of lymphoid malignancies have characteristic immunophenotypic patterns that are virtually diagnostic of those entities. A prominent example is the coexpression of surface CD11c, CD25, and CD103 on hairy cell leukemia (HCL) cells.[4] Nevertheless, most immunophenotypic markers or marker patterns are neither sensitive nor specific enough for a definitive diagnosis.

Genetic aberrations

One of the important characteristics of the WHO classification is the incorporation of unique genetic abnormalities in the definition of certain disease entities. The vast majority of genetic changes thus far included in the WHO classification are chromosomal translocations. However, it is possible that novel discoveries may allow subtle genetic changes (e.g., microdeletions, point mutations, etc.), or changes involving other mechanisms of gene activation or silencing, to become a component of future lymphoma classifications. New genetic and molecular techniques, such as array comparative genomic hybridization (aCGH), gene expression profiling (GEP), and mutation analysis may play an increasingly important role in future lymphoma classifications.

Management of Hematologic Malignancies, ed. Susan M. O'Brien, Julie M. Vose, and Hagop M. Kantarjian. Published by Cambridge University Press.

Clinical features

Clinical features are an integral part of some entities in the WHO classification. Post-transplant lymphoproliferative disorders (PTLDs), as the name implies, defines lymphoproliferative disorders (LPDs) developing after allogeneic stem cell or solid organ transplantation. Certain primary cutaneous lymphomas require clinical input to differentiate from their systemic counterparts, which share identical morphologic, cytologic, and immunophenotypic features, but very different prognosis.

Clinical implications

The requirement to have comprehensive clinical, morphologic, immunophenotypic, and genetic information in lymphoma diagnosis has several implications to the clinicians. First, providing the diagnostic pathologists with accurate and relevant clinical information is a prerequisite for making an accurate pathologic diagnosis. Second, excisional biopsies are usually significantly superior to small incisional biopsies or needle core biopsies for making the correct and complete diagnosis. Small biopsies tend to have limited areas for assessing morphologic features and architecture of the lymphoid tissue, and may not be representative of the whole lesion. The morphology of these small biopsies is often distorted secondary to traction forces during the biopsy process. Even more importantly, the limited amount of tissue may preclude immunophenotypic and genetic tests, which could provide essential information for diagnosis. Therefore, an excisional biopsy of a lymph node is recommended if a superficial and easily accessible site is involved. Needle core biopsies of a lymph node should be reserved for less accessible sites (e.g., retroperitoneal lymph nodes). Third, the entire specimen or a portion of the specimen should be sent fresh and sterile, or put in special transport media in anticipation of possible ancillary tests, which include flow cytometry, cytogenetic karyotyping, and molecular analyses. If there is enough tissue, a portion may also be snap frozen and stored at −80 °C for possible special immunohistochemical or molecular tests. To facilitate these arrangements, a standard protocol should be developed for handling specimens suspicious for lymphoma involvement. Fourth, the need for additional laboratory tests in lymphoma diagnosis may translate into a longer turn-around-time for issuing a final report.

Lymphoma entities in the WHO classification

The WHO classification segregates lymphoid neoplasms into five major categories: precursor lymphoid neoplasms, mature B-cell neoplasms, mature T- and natural killer (NK)-cell neoplasms, HL, and immunodeficiency-associated LPDs. Table 13.1 summarizes the various entities recognized by the WHO classification.

It is noteworthy that both lymphomas and lymphoid leukemias are included in the classification. These two phases may

Table 13.1. Summary of the 2008 World Health Organization classification of lymphoid neoplasms

PRECURSOR LYMPHOID NEOPLASMS
B lymphoblastic leukemia/lymphoma, NOS
B lymphoblastic leukemia/lymphoma with recurrent genetic abnormalities
• B lymphoblastic leukemia/lymphoma with t(9;22)(q34; q11.2); *BCR-ABL1*
• B lymphoblastic leukemia/lymphoma with t(v;11q23); *MLL* rearranged
• B lymphoblastic leukemia/lymphoma with t(12;21)(p13;q22); *TEL-AML1 (ETV6-RUNX1)*
• B lymphoblastic leukemia/lymphoma with hyperdiploidy
• B lymphoblastic leukemia/lymphoma with hypodiploidy (hypodiploid ALL)
• B lymphoblastic leukemia/lymphoma with t(5;14)(q31;q32); *IL3-IGH*
• B lymphoblastic leukemia/lymphoma with t(1;19)(q23; q13.3); *E2A-PBX1(TCF3-PBX1)*
T lymphoblastic leukemia/lymphoma
MATURE B-CELL NEOPLASMS
Chronic lymphocytic leukemia/small lymphocytic lymphoma
B-cell prolymphocytic leukemia
Splenic B-cell marginal zone lymphoma
Hairy cell leukemia
Splenic B-cell lymphoma/leukemia, unclassifiable
• Splenic diffuse red pulp small B-cell lymphoma
• Hairy cell leukemia-variant
Lymphoplasmacytic lymphoma
Heavy chain diseases
• Gamma heavy chain disease
• Mu heavy chain disease
• Alpha heavy chain disease
Plasma cell neoplasms
• Monoclonal gammopathy of undetermined significance (MGUS)
• Plasma cell myeloma
• Solitary plasmacytoma of bone
• Extraosseous plasmacytoma
• Monoclonal immunoglobulin deposition diseases
Extranodal marginal zone lymphoma of mucosa-associated lymphoid tissue (MALT lymphoma)
Nodal marginal zone lymphoma
Follicular lymphoma

Table 13.1. *(cont.)*

Primary cutaneous follicle center lymphoma
Mantle cell lymphoma
Diffuse large B-cell lymphoma (DLBCL), NOS
DLBCL subtypes
• T-cell/histiocyte-rich large B-cell lymphoma
• Primary DLBCL of the CNS
• Primary cutaneous DLBCL, leg type
• Epstein–Barr virus (EBV)-positive DLBCL of the elderly
Other lymphomas of large B cells
• DLBCL associated with chronic inflammation
• Lymphomatoid granulomatosis
• Primary mediastinal (thymic) large B-cell lymphoma
• Intravascular large B-cell lymphoma
• ALK-positive large B-cell lymphoma
• Plasmablastic lymphoma
• Large B-cell lymphoma arising in HHV-8-associated multicentric Castleman's disease
• Primary effusion lymphoma
Borderline cases
• B-cell lymphoma, unclassifiable, with features intermediate between DLBCL and Burkitt lymphoma
• B-cell lymphoma, unclassifiable, with features intermediate between DLBCL and classical Hodgkin lymphoma
MATURE T-CELL AND NK-CELL NEOPLASMS
T-cell prolymphocytic leukemia
T-cell large granular lymphocytic leukemia
Chronic lymphoproliferative disorder of NK cells
Aggressive NK-cell leukemia
EBV-positive T-cell lymphoproliferative diseases of childhood
• Systemic EBV+ T-cell lymphoproliferative disease of childhood
• Hydroa vacciniforme-like lymphoma[a]
Adult T-cell leukemia/lymphoma
Extranodal NK/T-cell lymphoma, nasal type
Enteropathy-associated T-cell lymphoma
Hepatosplenic T-cell lymphoma
Subcutaneous panniculitis-like T-cell lymphoma
Mycosis fungoides
Sézary syndrome
Primary cutaneous CD30-positive T-cell lymphoproliferative disorders
Primary cutaneous peripheral T-cell lymphomas, rare subtypes
• Primary cutaneous gamma-delta T-cell lymphoma
• Primary cutaneous CD8-positive aggressive epidermotropic cytotoxic T-cell lymphoma
• Primary cutaneous CD4-positive small/medium T-cell lymphoma
Peripheral T-cell lymphoma, NOS
Angioimmunoblastic T-cell lymphoma
Anaplastic large cell lymphoma, ALK positive
Anaplastic large cell lymphoma, ALK negative
HODGKIN LYMPHOMA
Nodular lymphocyte predominant Hodgkin lymphoma
Classical Hodgkin lymphoma
Nodular sclerosis classical Hodgkin lymphoma
Mixed cellularity classical Hodgkin lymphoma
Lymphocyte-rich classical Hodgkin lymphoma
Lymphocyte-depleted classical Hodgkin lymphoma
IMMUNODEFICIENCY-ASSOCIATED LYMPHOPROLIFERATIVE DISORDERS
Lymphoproliferative diseases associated with primary immune disorders
Lymphomas associated with HIV infection
Post-transplant lymphoproliferative disorders (PTLD)
• Plasmacytic hyperplasia and infectious-mononucleosis-like PTLD
• Polymorphic PTLD
• Monomorphic PTLD
• Classical Hodgkin lymphoma-type PTLD
Other iatrogenic immunodeficiency-associated lymphoproliferative disorders

Note: [a]Derived from cytotoxic T-cells or NK-cells.
NOS: not otherwise specified; ALK: anaplastic large cell lymphoma kinase; CNS: central nervous system; HHV-8: human herpesvirus 8.
Source: Swerdlow *et al.*[1]

represent two facets of the same lymphoid neoplasm if they share similar clinical, morphologic, immunophenotypic, and genetic characteristics. Moreover, both phases may co-exist in the same patient. An example is chronic lymphocytic leukemia/small lymphocytic lymphoma (CLL/SLL), where both the solid and leukemic phases are common and may be found concomitantly or sequentially in a given patient.

A detailed account of every single entity is beyond the scope of this chapter. In the following sections, a brief account of the entities recognized by the WHO classification is given, with an emphasis on recent genetic and molecular findings. The entities discussed are grouped according to the lineage of the cell of origin and the major patterns of clinical presentation.

Precursor lymphoid neoplasms

B and T lymphoblastic leukemia/lymphoma (B- and T-ALL/LBL)

B- and T-ALL/LBL arise from lymphoblasts that are committed to either the B- or T-cell lineage, respectively. The use of the terms leukemia or lymphoma is arbitrary and depends on whether the disease process is restricted to a mass lesion with no or little evidence of blood and bone marrow involvement (lymphoma), or there is predominantly bone marrow and blood involvement (leukemia). If the presentation is a mass lesion and there are 25% or fewer lymphoblasts in the bone marrow, the designation of lymphoma is preferred.[1]

T-LBL is much more common than B-LBL, with the former representing 85–90% of all LBLs.[5] T-LBL has a predilection for the mediastinum, with approximately 50% of the cases presenting as a mediastinal mass.[1] In contrast, only about 15% of pediatric ALL and 25% of adult ALL are T-ALL.[5]

Lymphoblastic neoplasms of both B and T lineages are more common in children and adolescents. Adult B-ALL tends to have worse prognosis than pediatric B-ALL, with a 5-year complete remission rate of 60–85% for the former and 95% for the latter.[1]

The expert panel of the WHO classification has borrowed the concept in classifying acute myeloid leukemia to classify B-ALL/LBL by recognizing certain B-ALL/LBL cases with recurrent genetic abnormalities as distinct entities (Table 13.1). These entities are associated with characteristic clinical, phenotypic, prognostic, and biologic features and are mutually exclusive to each other. For instance, patients with the t(12;21)/*TEL-AML1* fusion, the t(1;19)/*E2A-PBX1* fusion, and hyperdiploidy (> 50 chromosomes) have the best prognosis, with long-term event-free survival of these patients reaching 85–90%. In contrast, patients with the Philadelphia chromosome or the t(4;11)/*MLL-AF4* fusion are associated with a long-term event-free survival of only 25–30%.[6]

It has been noted that about 56% of pediatric and adolescent T-ALL harbor at least one activating *NOTCH1* mutation.[7] This finding may have therapeutic implications because γ-secretase is required for the signaling of these activated NOTCH1 receptors and γ-secretase inhibitors have been developed for Alzheimer's disease and are currently being tested in clinical trials.[5,6,8] In addition to mutations, common cytogenetic abnormalities seen in T-ALL include del(6q) (15–18%), abnormalities of 9p21 (loss of *p16INK4α* gene) (about 15%), t(10;14)(q24;q11)/*HOX11-TCR-α* (5–10%), other translocations involving the *TCR-α* locus, and amplification of the *ABL* gene.[5] Rare cases of T-ALL/LBL harbor cytogenetic abnormalities involving the *MLL* gene at 11q23. One such example, the t(11;19)(q23;q13.3), which can be seen in both T-ALL/LBL and B-ALL, fuses the *MLL* with the *ENL*. In T-ALL/LBL, this translocation is associated with the γδ T-cell phenotype and a dismal prognosis. Several other translocations have also been linked to specific stages of developmental arrest of T lymphoblasts.[5]

Mature B-cell neoplasms

Diffuse large B-cell lymphoma (DLBCL) and its subtypes, other large B-cell lymphomas, and Burkitt lymphoma (BL)

DLBCL is the most common lymphoma category among all the NHLs.[9] The latest WHO classification identifies the following DLBCL subtypes: DLBCL, not otherwise specified (NOS), T-cell/histiocyte-rich large B-cell lymphoma (THRLBCL), primary DLBCL of the central nervous system (CNS), primary cutaneous DLBCL (PCDLBCL), leg type, and Epstein–Barr virus (EBV)-positive DLBCL of the elderly.[1] Additional large B-cell lymphomas recognized by the WHO classification as distinct entities also include: primary mediastinal (thymic) large B-cell lymphoma (PMLBCL), intravascular large B-cell lymphoma (IVLBCL), DLBCL associated with chronic inflammation, lymphomatoid granulomatosis (LYG), anaplastic lymphoma kinase (ALK)-positive LBCL, plasmablastic lymphoma, large B-cell lymphoma arising in human herpesvirus 8 (HHV-8)-associated multicentric Castleman disease (MCD), and primary effusion lymphoma (PEL) (Table 13.1).[1]

DLBCL, NOS is by far the most common entity among all the DLBCL subtypes and large B-cell lymphomas. It may be de novo or may represent a transformation from a low-grade B-cell NHL. Nodular lymphocyte predominant HL (NLPHL) can also transform into DLBCL, NOS, or THRLBCL (Figure 13.1a).[10,11] DLBCL, NOS may present as nodal or extranodal disease, and up to 40% of cases confine initially to an extranodal site.[1] Rare cases may show prominent sinusoidal involvement only, prompting the differential diagnosis of metastatic carcinoma (Figure 13.1d). Previous studies have shown that 11–48% of DLBCL, NOS patients had bone marrow involvement by a B-cell NHL upon presentation,[12–15] and a concordant histology signified worse prognosis compared to a discordant histology.[12–16] A proportion of large cells (Figure 13.2a) of at least 50%, or at least 70% bone marrow involvement also predicted for a worse overall survival.[17]

In addition to morphology, GEP also defines distinct subgroups of DLBCL, NOS: the germinal center-B-cell-like (GCB), the activated B-cell-like (ABC), and a small subgroup that cannot be classified as such, the GEP-unclassified subgroup. The GCB subgroup has a better prognosis than the other two even when rituximab is added to the chemotherapy regimen.[18,19] These GEP-defined subgroups are also associated with different patterns of cytogenetic abnormalities, with the t(14;18) and gains of 12q12 more commonly seen in the GCB subtype,[20,21] whereas 3q27 (*BCL6*) translocations are more commonly seen in PMBL and the ABC subtype of DLBCL.[22] Trisomy 3, gains of 3q and 18q21-q22, and losses of 6q21-q22 are abnormalities often associated with the ABC subtype. GEP is not currently used in routine clinical practice

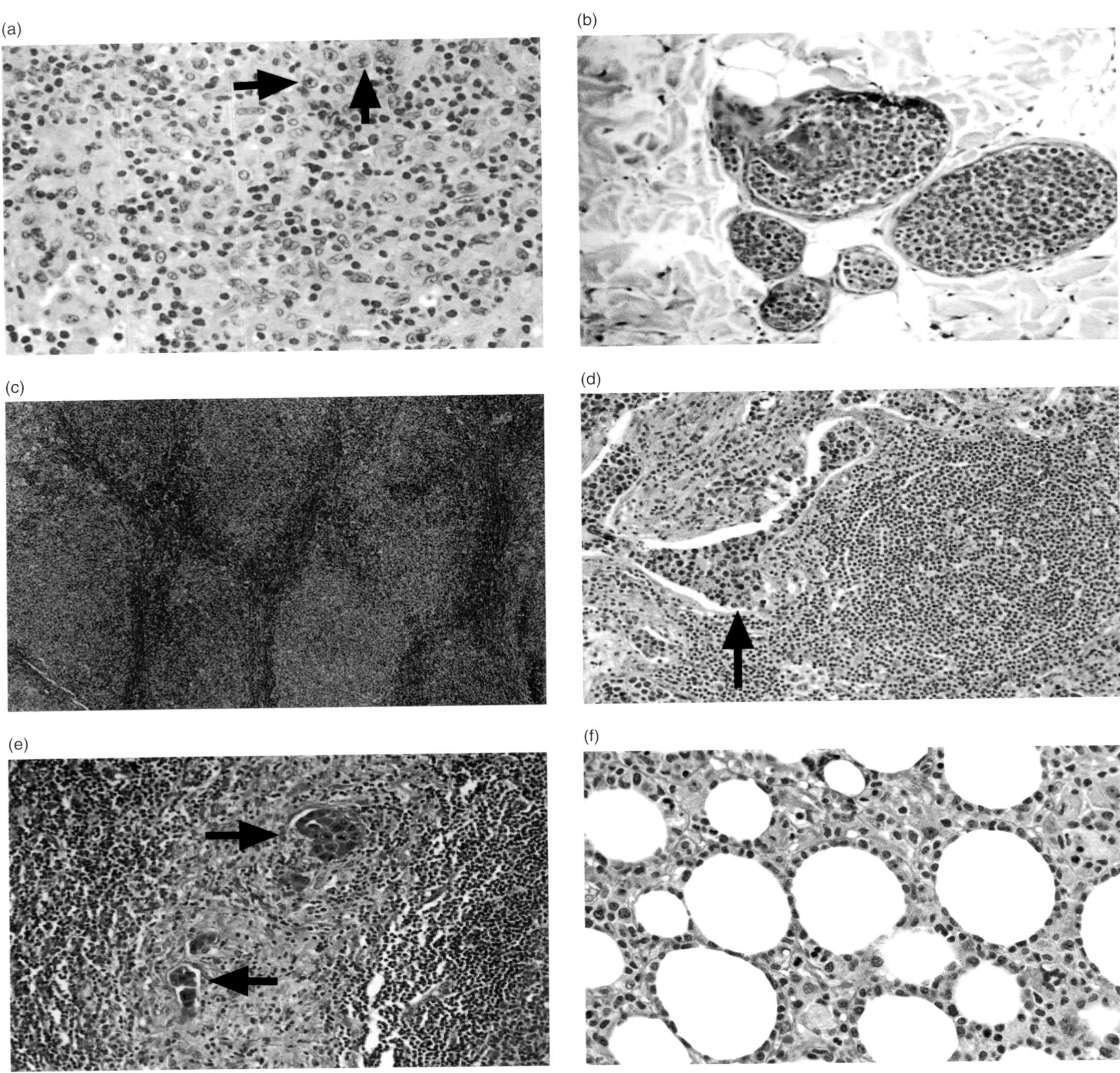

Figure 13.1 Morphologic patterns of lymphoma are diverse. The lymphoma cells can at times constitute the minor population of the cellular infiltrate, as illustrated in this case of T-cell/histiocyte-rich large B-cell lymphoma, where the large neoplastic B cells with prominent nucleoli (arrows) are scant and far outnumbered by the infiltrating histiocytes and small lymphocytes in the involved tissue (a, original magnification × 400). Intravascular large B-cell lymphoma is a distinct entity with the lymphoma cells restricted in vessel lumens (b, original magnification × 100). Numerous back-to-back follicles are seen in follicular lymphoma (c, original magnification × 20). Prominent sinusoidal involvement (arrow) in a rare case of diffuse large B-cell lymphoma (d, original magnification × 100) or cohesive clusters of lymphoma cells (arrows) in anaplastic large T-cell lymphoma (e, original magnification × 200) may simulate metastatic carcinoma. Lymphomatous T cells rim adipocytes in subcutaneous panniculitis-like T-cell lymphoma (f, original magnification × 200) (hematoxylin and eosin [H&E] stain for all panels).

but there have been attempts in simulating the GEP classification using immunohistochemical assays.[23,24] GEP has also been performed on CD5+ DLBCL and a series of genes were identified to distinguish CD5+ DLBCL from CD5− DLBCL and mantle cell lymphomas (MCL).[25] Because of the large number of DLBCL entities, we attempt to group them under certain headings to facilitate further discussion and the conceptualization of this classification.

(a)

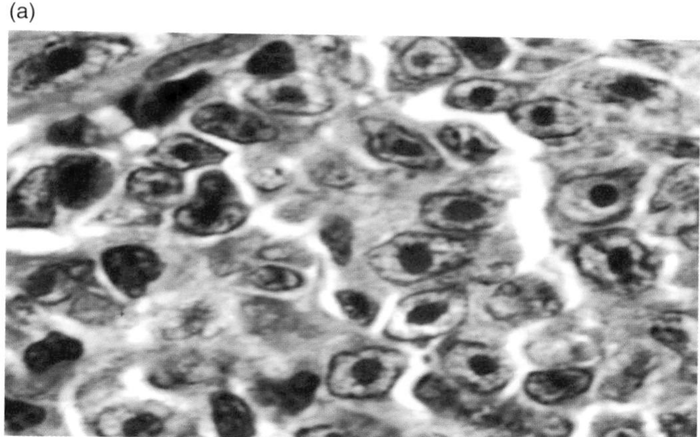

(b)

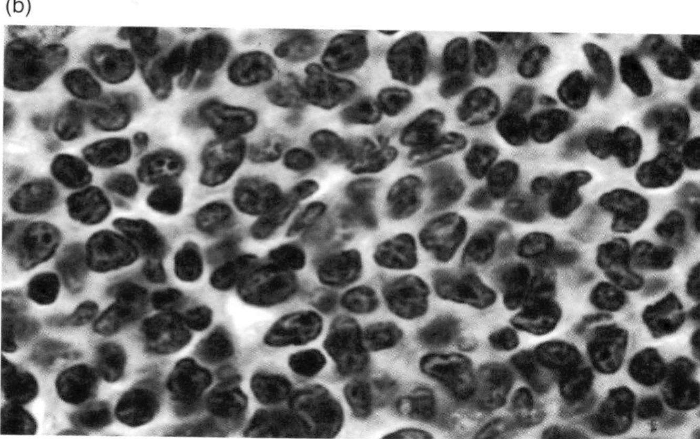

Figure 13.2 The nuclear size, chromatin pattern, and nucleolus of high-grade and low-grade B-cell non-Hodgkin lymphomas are in general distinctly different. High-grade B-cell non-Hodgkin lymphoma cells usually have large nuclei with dispersed nuclear chromatin and prominent nucleoli, as illustrated in a case of diffuse large B-cell lymphoma (a, H&E stain and original magnification × 400). In contrast, low-grade B-cell non-Hodgkin lymphoma cells, as demonstrated in a grade 1 follicular lymphoma in panel b, are usually small with condensed chromatin and no visible or small nucleolus (b H&E stain and original magnification × 1000).

Large B-cell lymphomas associated with EBV in the setting of immunodeficiency

These include the rare entities of plasmablastic lymphoma, DLBCL arising in HHV-8-associated MCD, and PEL. All of them are most commonly found in human immunodeficiency virus (HIV)-infected individuals. The latter two entities are additionally associated with HHV-8.

Plasmablastic lymphoma is mostly seen in HIV-positive individuals but it can also be seen in other immunodeficiency states, and in the elderly. It most frequently occurs as a mass lesion in the oral cavity, but other extranodal mucosal sites may also be involved. The lymphoma cells typically show plasmacytic differentiation with expression of CD38, CD79a (majority), CD138, VS38, interferon regulatory factor 4/multiple myeloma oncogene 1 (IRF4/MUM-1), and cytoplasmic immunoglobulin G (IgG) with light chain restriction, but not leukocyte common antigen (CD45) and the B-cell markers CD20 and paired box gene 5 (PAX5). The lymphoma cells also express epithelial membrane antigen (EMA) and CD30, and the majority of the cases are positive for EBV. HHV-8 is, however, not associated with this lymphoma.[26–28]

DLBCL arising in HHV-8-associated MCD is a lymphoma that arises in a setting of MCD most commonly seen in HIV-infected individuals. In contrast to plasmablastic lymphoma described above, this entity usually affects lymph nodes and the spleen. HHV-8 latency-associated nuclear antigen-1 (LANA-1) is found in the neoplastic cells of this entity. However, large B-cell lymphoma arising in HHV-8-associated MCD is negative for EBV-encoded RNAs (EBER) and CD79a, but is positive for CD20. This expression pattern is reciprocal to that of plasmablastic lymphoma for these antigens. Finally, the lymphoma cells in this disease consistently express cytoplasmic IgM that has not undergone somatic hypermutation. In contrast, plasmablastic lymphoma cells are usually class-switched with hypermutated Ig genes.[1,29]

PEL usually arises in the setting of HIV infection. Immunostaining for LANA-1 and *in situ* hybridization for EBER demonstrate universal presence of HHV-8 and frequent presence of EBV in the lymphoma cells. Rare cases associated with MCD have also been reported. Patients typically present with lymphomatous effusions of one body cavity (pleural, pericardial, and peritoneal) with no mass lesion. The prognosis is guarded. The lymphoma cells exhibit a highly abnormal immunophenotype with frequent loss of expression of pan-B-cell antigens including CD19, CD20, CD22, and CD79a.[30] There is expression of CD45, IRF4/MUM-1, and CD138.[31] PEL demonstrated a plasmablastic gene expression profile.[32]

DLBCL associated with EBV in patients without overt immunodeficiency

These include EBV-positive DLBCL of the elderly, LYG, and DLBCL associated with chronic inflammation.

EBV-positive DLBCL of the elderly is defined as an EBV-positive DLBCL demonstrable by *in situ* hybridization targeting EBER, in patients older than 50 years of age and without any known immunodeficiency or prior lymphoma, that cannot be classified as other specific EBV-positive lymphomas, such as plasmablastic lymphoma.[1] These cases represent 8–10% of DLBCL in Asian patients without known immunodeficiency, and appear to be an aggressive disease with a median survival of about 2 years.[33,34]

LYG is an EBV-driven, extranodal LPD. The most common sites of involvement are the lungs, kidneys, liver, skin, and brain. The disease is divided into three grades with progressively increased number of large pleomorphic B cells. Grade 1 and 2 lesions have a large number of reactive T cells admixed with EBV-transformed B cells. Grade 3 LYG is equivalent to an EBV-positive DLBCL. The natural history of LYG is variable, with a small proportion of patients undergoing spontaneous regression. Approximately 30–40% of patients succumb to the disease.[35,36] Interestingly, low-grade disease may respond well to interferon alpha therapy.

Pyothorax-associated lymphoma is the prototype of DLBCL associated with chronic inflammation. Other cases are found in association with chronic suppuration or chronic inflammation, such as chronic osteomyelitis, chronic skin ulcer, and in areas around metallic implants. While most cases are EBV-associated and are found in body cavities or narrow spaces (e.g., joint), they should be distinguished from PEL because they usually express B-lineage markers CD20 and CD79a, and are not associated with HHV-8. GEP of pyothorax-associated lymphoma showed a distinctive pattern from nodal DLBCL.[37]

DLBCL and large B-cell lymphoma specific to an anatomic site

DLBCL associated with certain anatomic sites may have unique biologic, clinical, and prognostic characteristics and they are therefore separated in the classification. These include the DLBCL subtypes: primary DLBCL of the CNS; PCDLBCL, leg type; and the large B-cell lymphomas: PMBL and IVBCL. These entities are not generally associated with EBV.

Primary DLBCL of the CNS are the intracerebral or intraocular DLBCL that are not associated with systemic disease or an immunodeficiency state.[1] Translocations involving the *BCL6* gene are at 30–40%, while the t(14;18)(q32;q21) and the t(8;14)(q24;q32) are rare.[38]

PCDLBCL, leg type, will be discussed in the section on WHO-European Organization for Research and Treatment of Cancer (EORTC) classification of cutaneous lymphomas.

PMBL is a lymphoma associated with a favorable prognosis. It is postulated to arise from thymic B cells and typically presents in the mediastinum of young females.[1,39] It can share some of the clinical, histologic, and immunophenotypic features with nodular sclerosis classical Hodgkin lymphoma (CHL).[39] A unique gene expression signature has been identified for PMBL,[40,41] and there are suggestions that PMBL and nodular sclerosis CHL share some characteristics in survival pathways.[41] PMBL frequently contains gains of 9p21-pter and 2p14-p16,[21] and these abnormalities are also common in CHL.[42] Indeed, some cases are difficult to put into either category because of intermediate morphologic and immunophenotypic features. The latest WHO classification establishes a new category termed “B-cell lymphoma, unclassifiable, with features intermediate between diffuse large B-cell lymphoma and classical Hodgkin lymphoma” to accommodate these cases.[1]

IVLBCL is rare and is confined to vascular lumens (Figure 13.1b). Clinical presentation is protean and is secondary to the occlusion of small blood vessels of various organs by the lymphoma cells. Recently, it has been observed that IVLBCL comes in two subtypes: a classical subtype with frequent skin and CNS involvement, and a second subtype associated with hemophagocytic syndrome, high incidence of hepatosplenic and bone marrow infiltration, cytopenias, and absence of skin involvement. The second subtype is reported mostly from Asia.[43] While skin lesions are common for the classical form, a recent study showed that even random skin biopsies have a high yield of observing lymphoma cells.[44]

Other DLBCL subtypes and large B-cell lymphomas

These include THRLBCL and ALK-positive large B-cell lymphoma.

THRLBCL is characterized by the scarcity of large, atypical neoplastic B cells among a background of numerous T cells and frequent histiocytes. It is considered an aggressive lymphoma, usually presented at a high stage and often refractory to chemotherapeutic agents commonly in use.[1] It seems that those cases with abundant histiocytes represent a more homogeneous group demonstrating more aggressive behavior.[45,46]

ALK-positive large B-cell lymphoma is a rare B-cell lymphoma with large cells that strongly express the ALK protein. This tumor shows a peculiar immunophenotype with expression of EMA, plasma cell markers CD138 and VS38, cytoplasmic IgA with light chain restriction, and weak to negative expression of CD45, but no expression of CD3, CD20, CD79a, and CD30.[47] This entity harbors a translocation involving the *ALK* gene, with the most frequent one being the t(2;17)(p23;q23) leading to a clathrin-ALK fusion protein.[48]

BL is a highly aggressive lymphoma often presenting in extranodal sites or less commonly as Burkitt leukemia (Figure 13.3a). It encompasses three clinical variants: endemic, sporadic, and immunodeficiency-associated BL, which are different in terms of geographic distribution, EBV association, pattern of c-Myc translocation, typical age distribution, and the anatomic sites of involvement.[49] Cases of BL typically express CD20, CD10, and BCL6, but not BCL2. Immunostaining for Ki-67 is classically close to 100%.

Although DLBCL and BL are both aggressive NHLs, the prognosis of BL has traditionally been better, with about 90% of pediatric patients and 50–70% of adult patients achieving long-term survival after high-intensity chemotherapy.[49,50] These figures are in contrast to the 40% long-term survival of DLBCL patients treated with anthracycline-based chemotherapy regimens. However, this prognostic gap has been narrowed significantly in recent years with the introduction of rituximab to DLBCL regimens. A recent study showed that the 5-year overall survival rate for DLBCL patients treated with rituximab plus a traditional anthracycline-based chemotherapeutic protocol may reach around 75–80%.[51]

While differentiating DLBCL from BL has therapeutic and possibly prognostic significance, this can be difficult at times due to morphologic and immunophenotypic overlap of these two groups of diseases. Recently, studies using GEP and cytogenetic techniques have shown that DLBCL and BL have distinct gene expression patterns[52,53] and cytogenetic abnormalities,[53] which may impact future classification systems and clinical trials.

The latest WHO classification adds a new category, “B-cell lymphoma, unclassifiable with features intermediate between DLBCL and BL,” to recognize those aggressive B-cell

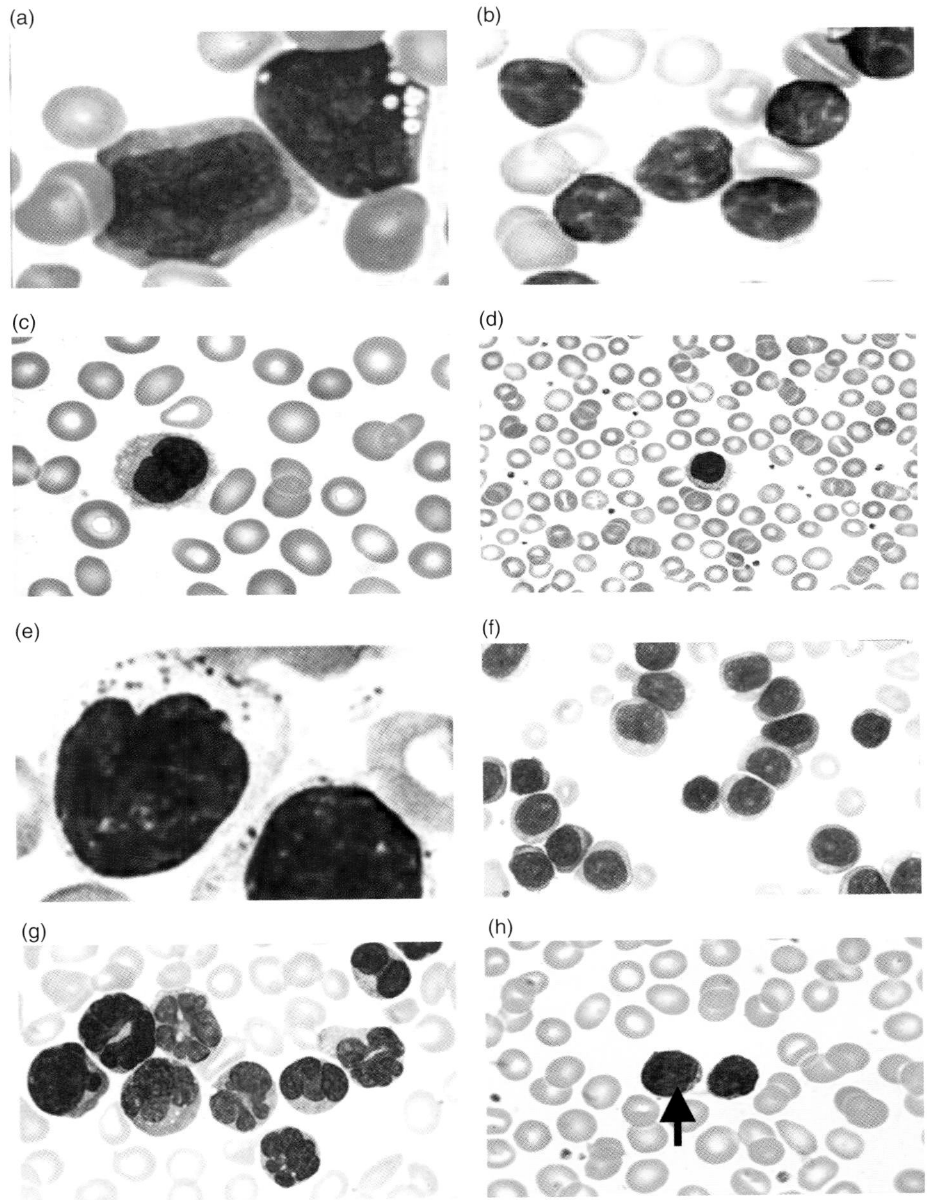

Figure 13.3 Some mature lymphoid malignancies consist of a prominent leukemic component. Burkitt leukemia cells have moderately high nuclear-to-cytoplasmic ratio, prominent multiple nucleoli, dark-blue cytoplasm, and cytoplasmic vacuoles (a). Chronic lymphocytic leukemia cells are small with round nuclei, clumped chromatin, and minimal cytoplasm (b). Circulating hairy cell leukemia cells show 'hairy' cytoplasmic projections, abundant cytoplasm, and indented nuclei without prominent nucleoli (c). In contrast, cells in hairy cell leukemia variant contain round nuclei with a prominent, central nucleolus, in addition to the hairy cytoplasmic projections (d). T-cell large granular cell leukemia cells contain abundant pale cytoplasm with cytoplasmic azurophilic granules (e). T-cell prolymphocytic leukemia is characterized by rapidly progressive lymphocytosis. The leukemic cells show nuclei with a prominent central nucleolus and fair amount of cytoplasm (f). Bizarre circulating lymphoma cells exhibiting highly convoluted nuclear contours are seen in a case of adult T-cell leukemia/lymphoma. These cells are called flower cells because of this flower-like morphology of the nucleus (g). Two circulating Sézary cells are seen in the peripheral blood smear of a patient with Sézary syndrome. Note the deep nuclear groove (h, arrow) (Wright–Giemsa stain for all panels, original magnification × 400 for panel D and × 1000 for all other panels).

lymphomas that fall into the gray zone between DLBCL and BL. The creation of this new category also helps to keep the distinct DLBCL subtypes and BL non-overlapping. The cases in this category more commonly resemble BL morphologically, but cannot be diagnosed as BL or DLBCL because of one or more morphologic or immunophenotypic features. Some of these cases were previously labeled as Burkitt-like lymphoma. There is a lack of predilection to the ileocecal region or jaws like the BL, and cases in this category more commonly show a complex karyotype as compared to the usually low genetic complexity seen in typical BL.[54] Most of the 'double-hit' aggressive B-cell lymphomas containing a *c-MYC*/8q24 break and a *BCL2*/18q21 break with or without a *BCL6*/3q27 break would be put into this category. Cases of otherwise typical DLBCL with high proliferative index, or with a *c-MYC* rearrangement, or cases of otherwise typical BL without a demonstrable *c-MYC* rearrangement should not be placed in this category.[1,55]

Follicular lymphoma (FL)

FL is the second most common NHL and is more common in the United States than in other parts of the world. It exemplifies the concept that a distinct entity in the WHO classification can span a spectrum of histologic grades. It is primarily a nodal disease at presentation. Spleen and bone marrow involvement is also common, especially for the low-grade (grades 1 and 2) lesions. Dissemination to extranodal sites usually occurs later in the disease course. FL usually affects older adults, but pediatric FL can rarely occur, and pediatric FL is recognized as a provisional entity in the latest WHO classification.

An individual case of FL may consist of an admixture of both follicular and diffuse areas, and the WHO classification advocates reporting the proportion of follicular areas. To this end, the pattern can be reported as follicular (> 75% follicular) (Figure 13.1c), follicular and diffuse (25–75% follicular), focally follicular (< 25% follicular), or diffuse (0% follicular).[1] For grade 1 and grade 2 FL (Figure 13.2b), it is unclear as to whether the presence and extent of diffuse areas affect the prognosis. Since both grade 1 and grade 2 diseases are indolent, the WHO classification does not encourage distinguishing between these two grades.[1] For grade 3 FL, it has recently been shown that the presence of diffuse areas greater than 50% of the entire lesion confers a worse prognosis.[23] The WHO classification further states that any diffuse areas containing more than 15 centroblasts per high-power field should be reported as DLBCL and the approximate percentage of the areas indicated.[1] Grade 3 FL can be subdivided into grade 3A (centroblasts plus centrocytes) and grade 3B (centroblasts only) FL. The t(14;18) or CD10 expression are uncommon in grade 3B FLs, which more often contain 3q27 translocations.[56–59] Grade 3B FLs frequently have extensive diffuse areas and are better considered to behave more aggressively like a DLBCL rather than a FL.

Pediatric FLs are more likely to be indolent (despite a grade 3 morphology), localized, and negative for both BCL2 expression and translocations involving the *BCL2* gene.[60] Additionally, the neoplastic follicles tend to be large. Extranodal involvement of the testicles is well described.[60]

Mantle cell lymphoma (MCL)

MCL is a B-cell NHL that exhibits the unfavorable characteristics of both the indolent (incurability) and aggressive lymphomas (aggressive clinical course). It is a predominantly nodal disease, with frequent gastrointestinal, bone marrow, and Waldeyer's ring involvement. While earlier studies indicated that up to 30% of MCL patients have gastrointestinal disease, more recent studies showed microscopic involvement along the gastrointestinal tract in the vast majority of patients.[61,62] Most MCL cases express CD5 and have the characteristic t(11;14), juxtaposing the *CCND1* gene on chromosome 11 to the Ig heavy chain (*IGH*) locus on chromosome 14. This translocation leads to an overexpression of cyclin D1 that can readily be detected by immunohistochemistry on tissue sections. The t(11;14) can also be detected by conventional cytogenetic karyotyping but fluorescence *in situ* hybridization (FISH) for the t(11;14) can additionally be performed on formalin-fixed, paraffin-embedded tissue. These cytogenetic tests can serve as an adjunct or confirmation to immunohistochemical studies. Due to the widely scattered breakpoints on the *CCND1* locus, polymerase chain reaction (PCR) and Southern blot are not very useful in the diagnosis of MCL. Quantitating the *CCND1* transcript by quantitative reverse transcriptase-PCR (qRT-PCR) has been shown to be useful as a diagnostic test, but it has not been widely accepted in practice.[63–72] Cyclin D1 can sometimes be expressed weakly and focally in the proliferation centers of CLL/SLL,[73] in a proportion of HCL (usually weak, partial)[74,75] and plasma cell myeloma (PCM).[76] However, the t(11;14) is only commonly seen in MCL and PCM. Rare cases of MCL lacking the t(11;14) have been identified by GEP studies and are difficult to diagnose.[77] These cases may overexpress cyclin D2 or cyclin D3, but the mechanism is unclear except for rare cases with chromosomal translocations involving the *CCND2* and *CCND3* genes.[78,79] Most recently, SOX11 protein expression was demonstrated by immunohistochemistry in cyclin D1-negative MCL, which may facilitate the diagnosis of cyclin D1-negative MCL using formalin-fixed paraffin-embedded materials.[80,81]

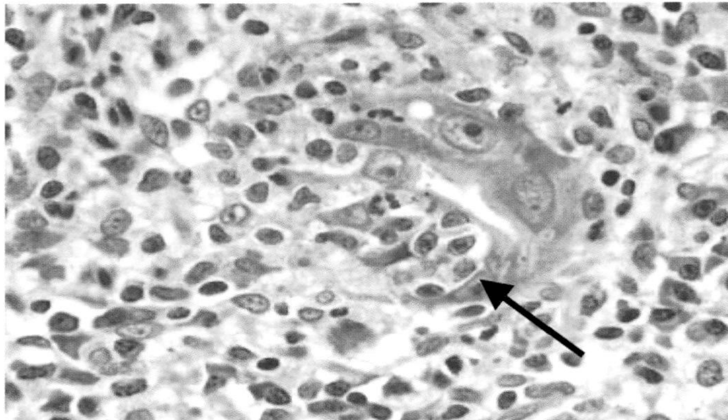

Figure 13.4 Lymphoma cells in extranodal marginal zone lymphoma of mucosa-associated lymphoid tissue (MALT lymphoma) invade into epithelial crypts (arrow), forming lymphoepithelial lesions (original magnification × 400).

Nodal marginal zone lymphoma (NMZL), extranodal marginal zone lymphoma of mucosa-associated lymphoid tissue (MALT lymphoma) and splenic B-cell marginal zone lymphoma (SMZL)

NMZL and MALT lymphoma consist of small B cells that resemble the marginal zone B cells or monocytoid B cells. In MALT lymphomas, the neoplastic cells invade into epithelial structures forming lymphoepithelial lesions (Figure 13.4). MALT lymphoma most commonly affects the stomach. Other epithelial tissues, including other parts of the aerodigestive tract, thyroid gland, salivary gland, lacrimal gland, and skin, can also be the primary sites of the disease. Rare cases may also arise in the thymus, dura mater, or skeletal muscle. MALT lymphomas are usually associated with a history of chronic inflammation and are linked to various infectious agents and autoimmune diseases. Most notably, *Helicobacter pylori* is associated with gastric MALT lymphomas and eradication of the bacteria may lead to regression of the lymphoma in some cases. *Campylobacter jejuni*, *Borrelia burgdorferi*, and *Chlamydia psittaci* have also been associated with immunoproliferative small intestinal disease, primary cutaneous marginal zone lymphoma, and ocular marginal zone lymphoma, respectively.[82]

NMZL is a lymphoma having similar cytologic features to MALT lymphomas. Therefore, it is often difficult to differentiate primary nodal disease from involvement by the latter. Clinical information is crucial in this situation.

SMZL is a small B-cell lymphoma involving the spleen, splenic hilar lymph nodes, bone marrow, and the peripheral blood. Patients typically present with splenomegaly, with or without autoimmune thrombocytopenia or anemia. Circulating lymphoma cells are variable in number, and some may have villous projections on smears. In the spleen, the neoplastic cells typically surround the white pulps in the marginal zone. The white pulps are totally obliterated by neoplastic cells when the disease progresses. The red pulp is also frequently infiltrated.

The most common abnormalities found in MALT lymphomas include trisomy 3, the t(11;18)(q21;q21) involving the *API2* and *MALT1* genes on chromosomes 11 and 18, respectively, the t(14;18)(q32;q21) involving the *IGH* locus, and the *MALT1* gene. Uncommon translocations involving other genes such as *BCL10* on 1p22 and *FOXP1* on 3p14.1 have been reported.[83,84] Certain cytogenetic abnormalities are associated with the anatomic sites of the MALT lymphoma.[85] The t(11;18)-positive gastric MALT lymphomas are more commonly negative for *H. pylori* or resistant to *H. pylori* eradication therapy.[86] For SMZL, the most common cytogenetic abnormalities are del(7)(q22-q32) and trisomy 3/3q.[87] Studies on the genetic abnormalities of NMZL are scarce. Trisomy 3 is the most common abnormality, but the t(11;18) seen in MALT lymphoma is absent.[88] A common theme of MZL lymphomagenesis is the over-expression of *BCL10*, *MALT1*, and *FOXP1* leading to activation of the nuclear factor-kappa B (NF-κB) pathway.[89]

Lymphoplasmacytic lymphoma (LPL) and the heavy chain diseases (HCD)

LPL is a B-cell NHL consisting of an admixture of neoplastic small lymphocytes, plasmacytoid lymphocytes, and plasma cells. Lymph nodes can be affected and there is a high frequency of bone marrow involvement upon presentation. It is a diagnosis of exclusion because many B-cell NHLs, most commonly MZL, can also have prominent plasmacytic differentiation. Given the overlapping morphologic features of LPL and MZL, and the lack of defining immunophenotypic and genetic abnormalities for both LPL and MZL, it can prove challenging to make a definite distinction. Some cases are difficult to classify and may need to be called small B-cell lymphoma with plasmacytic differentiation with a differential diagnosis listed.[1] The majority of patients with LPL have accompanying Waldenstrom's macroglobulinemia (WM), which is now defined as LPL with bone marrow involvement and an IgM monoclonal gammopathy of any concentration.[90] The t(9;14)(p13;q32) juxtaposing the *PAX5* gene to the *IGH* locus was previously reported to be common in older studies,[91,92] but this finding has not been substantiated by more recent data, which only showed chromosome 6q deletions[93–96] and trisomy 4[97] as common recurrent cytogenetic abnormalities. GEP studies showed upregulation of the *interleukin 6* (*IL6*) gene in WM,[98,99] and WM clustered with CLL and normal B cells, but not PCM, by unsupervised hierarchical clustering in GEP studies.[98]

The HCD consist of three rare B-cell neoplasms that produce and secrete monoclonal IgG (gamma HCD), IgA (alpha HCD), and IgM (mu HCD). The three HCD resemble LPL, MALT lymphoma, and CLL, respectively, on a morphologic basis. The corresponding heavy chain gene is usually affected by partial deletions and incapable of full assembly. The defective Ig heavy chain thus produced may not be captured by serum protein electrophoresis and requires immunofixation to detect. The most common of these three is alpha HCD, which was also called immunoproliferative small intestinal disease (IPSID) in earlier editions of the WHO classification. Alpha HCD or IPSID involves mainly the small intestine and mesenteric lymph nodes and is believed to associate with chronic *Campylobacter jejuni* infection. Both gamma HCD and alpha HCD may transform into DLBCL, and mu HCD is usually slowly progressive.[1]

Plasma cell myeloma (PCM) and related disorders

Plasma cell disorders are included under the section of mature B-cell neoplasms in the WHO classification because plasma cells represent the end stage of mature B-cell differentiation.

There are specific diagnostic criteria for PCM, and monoclonal gammopathy of undetermined significance.[1] PCM is now classified into symptomatic PCM and asymptomatic (smoldering) PCM. Symptomatic PCM cases have M proteins in the serum or urine, clonal plasma cells in the bone marrow or plasmacytomas, and related organ or tissue impairment. Asymptomatic PCM has an M protein in serum > 30 g/L, and/or 10% or more clonal plasma cells in the bone marrow, and no related organ or tissue impairment. In the majority of PCM, the M protein is an IgG (50%), an IgA (20%), or a serum free light chain (Bence-Jones protein) (15%). IgD-secreting PCM, PCM with biclonal gammopathies, or non-secretory PCM make up the rest of the cases. IgM- and IgE-secreting PCM are very rare.

Apart from PCM, the WHO classification also includes solitary plasmacytoma of bone (SPB) and extraosseous plasmacytoma (EP) as distinct entities. SPB and EP represent clonal proliferation of plasma cells in either a bone or an extraosseous site, respectively, with no signs of widespread bone marrow involvement. Histologically, SPB and EP have to be differentiated from MZL with prominent plasmacytic differentiation. It is important to recognize SPB and EP because the initial treatment involves radiation or surgery, rather than systemic chemotherapy.[100,101] One study showed

53% of SPB and 36% of EP converted to PCM, and the median survival after this conversion was 14.5 months.[102]

PCM cells almost universally harbor multiple cytogenetic abnormalities. Aneuploidy with trisomies of chromosomes 3, 5, 7, 9, 11, 15, 19, and 21, and monosomies of chromosomes 13, 14, 16, and 22 are frequently seen.[103] Other frequently encountered chromosomal abnormalities include del(13)(q14),[104] and balanced translocations involving the *IGH* locus on chromosome 14q32 and the *CCND1* gene on 11q13, *FGFR3* on 4p16, *c-MAF* on 16q23, and *CCND3* on 6p21.[105] Other common genetic abnormalities include chromosome 1 abnormalities,[103] activating *RAS* mutations,[105] and deletions or mutations involving the *TP53* gene.[106] Constitutive activation of the NF-κB pathway has also been observed in PCM, but the underlying mechanism is poorly understood.[107] A GEP study classified PCM into low- and high-risk subgroups that are associated with the aforementioned chromosomal and genetic alterations.[108]

Other clonal plasma cell disorders that are more defined by the consequence of tissue monoclonal Ig deposition include primary amyloidosis, the monoclonal light chain and heavy chain deposition diseases, and osteosclerotic myeloma (polyradiculoneuropathy, organomegaly, endocrinopathy, monoclonal gammopathy, and skin changes [POEMS syndrome]).

Chronic lymphocytic leukemia/small lymphocytic lymphoma (CLL/SLL)

CLL/SLL is a small B-cell neoplasm that commonly shows variable extent of peripheral blood, bone marrow (Figure 13.3b), spleen, and lymph node involvement. The term SLL is restricted to patients with a mass lesion but no leukemia. Bone marrow involvement in these cases is regarded as "bone marrow involvement by SLL."

The latest WHO classification requires at least 5×10^9/L monoclonal lymphocytes with a CLL immunophenotype in the peripheral blood to diagnose CLL.[1] The typical CLL coexpresses CD5, weak CD11c, CD19, dim CD20, CD22, CD23, CD43, CD79a, dim surface IgM, or IgD, but is negative for CD10, CD79b, and FMC-7.[1] Flow cytometric analysis is highly sensitive and can detect clonal populations down to levels less than 1% of all nucleated cells in the specimen. It is not surprising, therefore, that B-cell clones with a CLL phenotype could be detected in the peripheral blood in up to 3.5% of healthy individuals.[109] In 2005, the Familial CLL Consortium defined monoclonal B-cell lymphocytosis (MBL) as the presence of a persistent monoclonal B-cell population in the peripheral blood for at least 3 months. The absolute B-lymphocyte count has to be less than 5.0×10^9/L, and there should be no concomitant lymphadenopathy, organomegaly, or autoimmune/infectious disease.[110] Progression of MBL to CLL or other B-cell NHL ranges from 0% in 30 months to 18% in 12 years.[111–113] Further longitudinal studies are required to give a more accurate estimate of the prognosis of this condition.

Although most patients with CLL/SLL experience an indolent clinical course, a subset of cases is more aggressive and is associated with certain immunophenotypic and genetic markers (Table 13.2). Some cases may transform into a more aggressive leukemia or lymphoma during the disease course, such as prolymphocytic leukemia, DLBCL (Richter syndrome), and CHL.

Table 13.2. Adverse immunophenotypic, cytogenetic, and molecular prognostic markers of chronic lymphocytic leukemia/small lymphocytic lymphoma

Protein markers detected by immunophenotyping
ZAP-70 expression
CD38 expression
Cytogenetic aberrations
del(11q)
del(17p)
Molecular markers
Unmutated immunoglobulin heavy chain variable region (*VH*) gene
Rearrangement of the VH using the *V3–21* gene

Note: ZAP: zeta-chain-associated protein kinase.

Mature B-cell neoplasms that manifest predominantly as lymphoid leukemias

These include B-cell prolymphocytic leukemia (B-PLL), SMZL (also see above discussion of MZLs), and HCL (Figure 13.3c). Two provisional entities are recognized under the newly created category "splenic B-cell lymphoma/leukemia, unclassifiable," namely, hairy cell leukemia variant (HCL-V) (Figure 13.3d), and splenic diffuse red pulp small B-cell lymphoma. These two entities are also commonly included as differential diagnosis of predominantly leukemic B-cell lymphoid neoplasms. The features of these five entities are compared in Table 13.3.

Mature T-cell and NK-cell neoplasms

Mature T-cell and NK-cell leukemias

Mature NK-cell and T-cell leukemias are clonal proliferations of NK cells and post-thymic T cells. The distinct entities recognized by the WHO classification include T-cell large granular lymphocytic leukemia (T-LGLL), chronic LPD of NK cells, T-cell prolymphocytic leukemia (T-PLL), aggressive NK-cell leukemia, adult T-cell leukemia/lymphoma (ATLL), and Sézary syndrome (SS).

T-LGLL is an indolent T-cell LPD of CD8+ T cells that is frequently associated with neutropenia and anemia (50%), certain autoantibodies (e.g., rheumatoid factor), and serologic abnormalities (e.g., elevated β2-microglobulin).[127] T-LGLL cells have abundant pale cytoplasm, with variable number of cytoplasmic azurophilic granules (Figure 13.3e). The peripheral blood large granular lymphocytosis is persistent (more than 6 months) and the level is usually between 2 and

Table 13.3. Comparison of the clinical, hematologic, cytologic, and immunophenotypic features of mature B-cell neoplasms manifesting predominantly as lymphoid leukemias

	HCL	HCL-V	SDRPSBCL	SMZL	B-PLL
M:F[1,114,115]	5:1	4:1	1.6:1	1:1	1.6:1
Median age[1,114,115]	55	78	77	68	70
Complete blood count[1,115]	Monocytopenia, pancytopenia, few circulating hairy cell leukemia cells	Lymphocytosis with lymphocytes having central nucleoli, normal monocyte count, and occasional cytopenia	Lymphocytosis in the majority (76%) of cases, usually of relatively low level; small or invisible nucleoli	Circulating lymphoma cells present, nucleoli uncommon and associated with progression	Rapidly progressive, marked lymphocytosis with most of the cells being prolymphocytes
Bone marrow aspiration[1]	Dry tap	Bone marrow easily aspirated	Bone marrow easily aspirated	Bone marrow easily aspirated	Bone marrow easily aspirated
'Hairy' cytoplasmic projections[1,115]	Circumferential	Circumferential	Polar	Polar	None
TRAP[1,116–118]	+ (> 90%, strong, diffuse)	+ (10–30%, weak)	–	–	–
CD11c[1,114,115,118,119]	+ (> 60%, bright)	+ (> 60%)	+ (97%)	+ (31–60%)	+ (10–30%)
CD25[1,114,115,118,119]	+ (> 60%)	–	–	+ (10–30%)	+ (10–30%)
CD103[1,114,115,118,119]	+ (> 60%, bright)	+ (31–60%, usually dim)	+ (38%)	–	–
CD123[115,120,121]	+ (> 60%)	–	+ (16%)	–	–
DBA.44[116,117,122–124]	+ (> 60%)	+ (31–60%)	unknown	+ (10–30%)	uncertain
Surface imunoglobulin[1,114,115,124–126]	IgG, or mixed pre- and post-isotype switch immunoglobulin isotypes	IgG, or mixed pre- and post-isotype switch immunoglobulin isotypes	IgM and IgD (31%), IgM and IgG (19%), IgM only (19%), or IgG only (19%)	IgM +/– IgD	IgM +/– IgD

Notes: HCL: hairy cell leukemia; HCL-V: hairy cell leukemia variant; SDRPSBCL: splenic diffuse red pulp small B-cell lymphoma; SMZL: splenic B-cell marginal zone lymphoma; B-PLL: B-cell prolymphocytic leukemia; TRAP: tartrate-resistant acid phosphatase.

20×10^6/L. Most patients run an indolent course, and morbidity is usually secondary to the accompanying neutropenia. A diagnosis of T-LGLL can be made with a large granular lymphocyte (LGL) count less than 2×10^6/L, provided all typical clinicopathologic features, including clonality, can be demonstrated. Establishing clonality is important to distinguish T-LGLL from reactive increase of T-LGL in conditions such as neoplastic diseases and infections. Apart from PCR and Southern blot techniques for clonal T-cell receptor (TCR) gene rearrangements, flow cytometry can be used to demonstrate T-cell clonality by showing a restricted expression of the TCR β-chain variable region family members.[128,129] An abnormal killer cell Ig-like receptor (KIR) expression profile by flow cytometry can also provide additional evidence of clonality of the T-LGL expansion.[130,131] Flow cytometry may also detect immunophenotypic abnormalities of pan-T-cell antigen expression in these T-LGL cells.[132–134] There is a high incidence of expression of CD16, CD57, and cytotoxic molecules (e.g., granzyme B) in T-LGLL. CD5 expression is typically dim.[135,136] Rarely, T-LGLL can be CD4+ or express γδ TCR rather than the typical αβ TCR. Cytogenetic abnormalities are rarely detected in T-LGLL.[137,138]

Chronic LPD of NK cells are the NK-cell counterpart of T-LGLL. This entity is defined similarly to T-LGLL as a persistent (more than 6 months) increase in peripheral blood NK cells greater than 2×10^9/L without a clearly identified cause. The clinical presentation is also similar to T-LGLL, with most patients being asymptomatic or having symptoms attributable to cytopenias. Immunophenotypically, these cells express cytotoxic molecules (T-cell intracellular antigen 1 [TIA-1], granzyme B, and granzyme M). In contrast to T-LGLL, the NK cells in this entity express CD16 and CD56 but not surface CD3, and do not rearrange the TCR genes. Expression of the KIR family of NK-cell receptors either shows restricted KIR isoform expression or a complete lack of detectable KIR using currently available antibodies.[131,132,139–141]

T-PLL is the most common subtype of mature T-cell leukemia, accounting for about 2% of small lymphocytic leukemias in adults.[1] The disease is aggressive and resistant to conventional chemotherapy, but 60% of patients may achieve a complete response with alemtuzumab treatment.[142] Patients usually present with a high lymphocyte count (usually over 100×10^6/L, but may be greater than 900×10^6/L)[1,143] that may rise rapidly with a doubling time in the range of weeks to months.[144] The leukemia cells are medium in size, and contain central nucleoli on peripheral blood smear (Figure 13.3f). The most common clinical signs include marked hepatosplenomegaly, generalized lymphadenopathy, and skin rash. Accompanying anemia and thrombocytopenia are frequently seen.[1,143] However, occasional cases of "indolent T-PLL" have been described,[145–147] which can become more aggressive over several years.[148] Unlike the B-cell leukemias where both B-CLL and B-PLL are recognized, T-CLL is not currently recognized as a distinct entity. Most T-PLL cases show a CD4+/CD8- helper T-cell phenotype, but approximately one-third of the cases are double positive for CD4 and CD8, while 15% of the cases are CD4-/CD8+.[1] Expression of the TCL1 protein is helpful in the diagnosis of T-PLL because TCL1 is expressed in approximately 70% of T-PLL but not in other mature T-cell leukemias.[144] The upregulation of TCL1 in T-PLL is secondary to recurrent chromosomal rearrangements including inv(14)(q11q32), t(14;14)(q11;q32), and t(7;14)(q35; q32) that involve the *TCL1* locus on 14q32, the *TCR-αδ* on 14q11, and the *TCRβ* on 7q35.[143,147] Other genetic abnormalities include translocations involving the *MTCP-1* gene on Xq28, abnormalities of the *ATM* gene on 11q23, deletions of 12p13, and abnormalities of chromosome 8.[147]

Aggressive NK-cell leukemia is a rare, aggressive NK-cell neoplasm that is more prevalent in Asians. It commonly involves the peripheral blood and bone marrow and infiltrates the liver and spleen. In some patients, the disease is associated with cytopenias, hemophagocytic syndrome, coagulopathy, and multiorgan failure.[1,149] Since it is strongly associated with EBV and shares a similar immunophenotype with extranodal NK/T-cell lymphoma, nasal type, some believe that this entity may represent the leukemic counterpart or the leukemic presentation of the latter.[150] However, a recent array CGH study cast doubt on this speculation by showing that these entities display non-overlapping chromosomal changes in many regions.[151]

ATLL is a peripheral T-cell leukemia/lymphoma caused by the human T-cell leukemia virus type 1 (HTLV-1).[152,153] Anecdotal reports of ATLLs that are negative for HTLV-1 but positive for HTLV-2 have also been described,[143] but the etiologic link between HTLV-2 and ATLL is not as well-established. ATLL is endemic in Southwestern Japan, the Caribbean, and parts of central Africa. There are four clinical variants: acute, lymphomatous, chronic, and smoldering.[154] The acute and lymphomatous variants are associated with poor overall survival that ranges from 2 weeks to a year for most patients. In contrast, about 50% and 65% of patients with chronic and smoldering variants, respectively, survive at 2 years.[1] The morphologic features are variable, but there is no consistent correlation of the clinical variants with specific morphologic features. The lymphoma or leukemia cells are medium to large with nuclear pleomorphism in the acute and lymphomatous variants. The circulating neoplastic cells have deeply basophilic cytoplasm, condensed chromatin, and a highly convoluted or polylobated nucleus, which are termed 'flower cells' (Figure 13.3g). The neoplastic T cells do not express CD7 or CD8,[143] and CD3 and TCR β-chain expression may be weak or negative on the cell membrane but positive in the cytoplasm. CD25 is typically highly expressed[155] and the CD4+CD25+ immunophenotype is reminiscent of regulatory T cells. Additionally, many patients have opportunistic infections secondary to a T-cell immunodeficiency. These observations lead to the speculation that the cells of origin of ATLL may be regulatory T cells. Forkhead/winged helix transcription factor 3 (FOXP3), a key protein for differentiation and function of regulatory T cells, is expressed in a subset (36–68%) of ATLL,[156–158] and the expression of FOXP3 is clinically associated with immunosuppression (severe infections and increased number of EBV+ cells).[159] No distinct karyotypic or molecular abnormalities are associated with ATLL, but most ATLL cases have a complex karyotype.[160] Mutations of the tumor suppressor genes *CDKN2A*, *CDKN2B*, and *TP53* were also observed.[155] *TP53* mutations are predictive for resistance to zidovudine treatment,[161] which, when combined with interferon alpha, has achieved 65–92% complete response rates in two prospective trials.[162,163] Most ATLL cases have clonally integrated HTLV-1,[164] but demonstration of this is not required for diagnosis. Rather, serologic confirmation of HTLV-1 (or rarely HTLV-2) infection is sufficient.[143]

SS will be discussed in detail with mycosis fungoides (MF) in a subsequent section "Predominantly extranodal mature T-cell and NK-cell neoplasms."

Anaplastic large cell lymphoma (ALCL) and primary cutaneous CD30-positive T-cell LPDs

ALCL is a lymphoma of possible cytotoxic T-cell origin. It usually affects both lymph nodes and extranodal sites, such as skin, bone, soft tissue, lungs, and liver. Bone marrow involvement is also commonly seen, but it can be subtle and requires immunohistochemical stains to confirm.

The majority of ALCL (60–85%) expresses ALK, but this figure can vary considerably due to different patient demographics (proportion of young patients) and variable thresholds of diagnosing ALK-negative ALCL in different institutions (see below).[165] ALK is a receptor tyrosine kinase not normally expressed in postnatal human tissues, except in a small subset of central and peripheral nervous system cells.[165,166] The latest WHO classification segregates ALK-positive ALCL and ALK-negative ALCL into separate entities.[1]

In ALK-positive ALCL, the aberrant expression of ALK is secondary to a translocation of the *ALK* gene to a ubiquitously expressed partner gene. These translocations result in a fusion protein retaining the tyrosine kinase domain of ALK and constitutive activation of its function. There are nine partners

Table 13.4. Translocations involving the *ALK* gene in ALK-positive anaplastic large cell lymphoma

Translocations	Partner genes	Staining patterns	Frequency
t(2;5)(p23; q35)[167]	*NPM*	Diffuse cytoplasmic, nuclear, and nucleolar	70–80%
t(1;2)(q25;p23)[a]	*TPM3*	Diffuse cytoplasmic with peripheral intensification	10–20%
inv(2) (p23q35)[168]	*ATIC*[169–171]	Diffuse cytoplasmic	2–5%
t(2;3)(p23;q21)[b]	*TFG*[172]	Diffuse cytoplasmic[172,173]	Uncommon
t(2;17)(p23; q23)[c]	*CLTC*	Granular cytoplasmic	Uncommon
t(2;19)(p23; p13.1)[174]	*TPM4*	Diffuse cytoplasmic	Uncommon
t(2;X)(p23; q11-q12)[175]	*MSN*	Membranous	Uncommon
t(2;17)(p23; q25)[176]	*ALO17*	Diffuse cytoplasmic	Uncommon
t(2;22)(p23; q11.2)[177]	*MYH9*	Diffuse cytoplasmic	Uncommon

Notes: [a]In the original reports of the t(1;2)(q25;p23), the breakpoint on chromosome 1 was reported at 1q25.[166,178,179] The *TPM3* gene is mapped to 1q22-q23.[180]
[b]One of the two cases originally reported by Hernandez *et al.*[172] had been karyotyped as t(2;3)(p23;q21).[173] The *TFG* gene is mapped to 3q11-q12.[181]
[c]The initial report of this variant translocation had identified the clathrin heavy polypeptide-like (*CLTCL*) gene at 22q11.2 as the translocation partner,[182] but it was later noted that the clathrin heavy polypeptide-like sequence had in fact been clathrin heavy chain due to an error in GenBank.[183] The clathrin heavy chain gene, *CLTC*, is mapped to 17q23.

of *ALK* fusion recognized so far (Table 13.4). While ALK is normally expressed in the cytoplasmic membrane, most of these fusion products are aberrantly expressed in other subcellular compartments as directed by the fusion partner (Table 13.4).

ALCL demonstrates several peculiar histologic features that are unusual for lymphomas and may be challenging for the pathologists. Lymph node involvement can be subtle in the paracortical or perifollicular areas in some cases. ALCL cells characteristically infiltrate lymph node sinuses prominently or exclusively, and the lymphoma cells can appear cohesive (Figure 13.1e), thereby mimicking metastatic carcinoma. There are several histologic variants of ALCL: classical, lymphohistiocytic, small cell, hypocellular, sarcomatoid, monomorphic, mixed cell, and giant cell.[1,3] The lymphohistiocytic, small cell, hypocellular, and sarcomatoid variants are notoriously

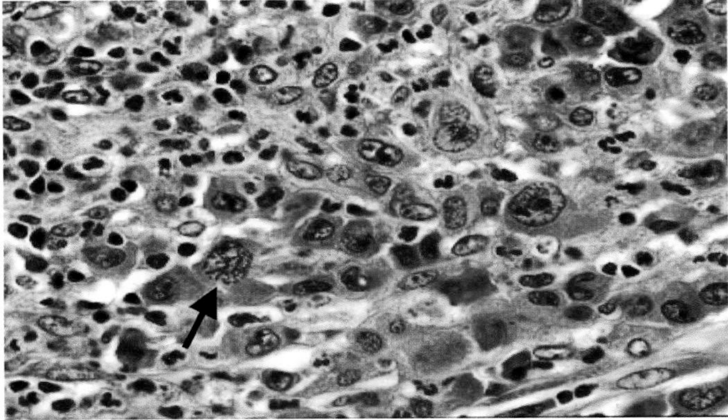

Figure 13.5 A hallmark cell in anaplastic large T-cell lymphoma is a large cell with abundant cytoplasm and a C-shaped nucleus. A donut cell is a similar cell with a complete ring of nucleus (arrow). Note the polymorphic background with numerous admixed small lymphocytes and eosinophils (H&E stain, original magnification × 400).

deceptive and require a high index of suspicion for a correct diagnosis. Common to all these variants are the presence of the hallmark cell, which is a large cell with an eccentric, C-shaped or reniform nucleus, a distinct eosinophilic Golgi zone, and voluminous cytoplasm. Lymphoma cells with their nuclei forming a 'closed-loop' are called donut cells (Figure 13.5). However, these characteristic cells can be scanty in those deceptive variants aforementioned, and demonstration of ALK and CD30 expression would be pivotal in pinpointing the diagnosis. A significant proportion of ALCL may lack expression of CD45 and many T-cell markers (e.g., CD3). The term ALCL of null cell type may be used if no immunophenotypic and/or genetic evidence of T-cell lineage is demonstrable. ALCL expresses cytotoxic molecules (e.g., granzyme B), despite a CD4+CD8- phenotype. Clusterin and EMA are also commonly expressed. Rearrangement of TCR genes is positive in the vast majority of cases.[184]

ALK-negative ALCL is now considered a provisional entity. The strictest definition only includes those cases sharing most of the histologic and immunophenotypic features of the classical variant of ALK-positive ALCL, except for the lack of ALK expression. Most ALK-negative ALCL are morphologically similar to the classical variant, since it is extremely difficult to identify the non-classical variants as an ALCL without the ALK expression.[165] Despite the rather unique features of ALK-negative ALCL, it is still controversial whether ALK-negative ALCL should be classified as ALCL. CGH studies showed that ALK-positive and ALK-negative ALCL have different chromosomal gains and losses.[185,186] Some investigators proposed that ALK-negative ALCL should be grouped with the rest of the peripheral T-cell lymphomas, not otherwise specified (PTCL, NOS), because there are no distinct cytogenetic and molecular changes to characterize ALK-negative ALCL. However, ALK-negative ALCL has significantly better prognosis than PTCL, NOS.[187]

The segregation of ALCL into ALK-positive and ALK-negative subgroups is of prognostic significance. ALK-positive ALCL is predominantly seen in the first three decades and shows a male predominance. It is associated with a better prognosis, with a 5-year overall survival of 70%, compared with the corresponding figure of 49% for ALK-negative ALCL.[187–190] ALK-negative ALCL tends to affect older adults with an equal sex incidence and a better overall survival than PTCL, NOS (5-year overall survival 32%).[187]

When the skin is the only affected site, systemic ALCL has to be differentiated from primary cutaneous ALCL, since the latter has excellent prognosis and requires different treatment. Clinical history and staging play an important role in this setting. Besides, primary cutaneous ALCL rarely expresses ALK and EMA,[191–193] and has a lower incidence of CD3 expression.[194] Zeta-chain-associated protein 70 (ZAP-70) is expressed in about 30–60% of primary cutaneous lesions but in only 10% of systemic ALCL.[194,195]

Under the umbrella term primary cutaneous CD30-positive T-cell LPDs, three subtypes of disorders are recognized: primary cutaneous anaplastic large cell lymphoma (C-ALCL), lymphomatoid papulosis (LyP), and borderline lesions. Clinical features play an important role in differentiating C-ALCL from LyP. The features suggestive of C-ALCL include solitary growth, large nodules greater than 2 cm, and progressive enlargement of the lesions with no regression. In contrast, classical LyP are small (less than 1 cm) papules growing in crops or clusters, with a waxing and waning history. The lesions heal with a scar after regression.[196] Histologically, the lymphoma cells are arranged in sheets and may invade the subcutis in C-ALCL. For LyP, three histologic variants (Types A-C) are described. Type A LyP infiltrates the dermis in a wedge-shaped and perivascular pattern. The infiltrates contain a small number of Reed–Sternberg (RS)-like large cells (medium to large, some multinucleated) in a background of small lymphocytes, neutrophils, and eosinophils. Type B LyP lesions show a band of lymphoid infiltrate in the reticular dermis. Epidermotropism is common and the atypical cells are usually small to medium in size. Some cases may have admixed neutrophils and eosinophils. Type C LyP lesions resemble C-ALCL and contain many large CD30-positive atypical cells in both the superficial and deep dermis, but not the subcutis.[197,198] Finally, the borderline lesions are the ones where the clinical and histologic features are contradictory (e.g., clinical features of C-ALCL but histologic features of LyP or vice versa).[193] TCR genes are clonally rearranged in most of the C-ALCL[193,199] and in about 60–80% of LyP.[200,201] The ALK translocations that characterize systemic ALK-positive ALCL are absent in C-ALCL.[202]

Predominantly nodal mature T-cell neoplasms

Angioimmunoblastic T-cell lymphoma (AITL) and PTCL, NOS present primarily as nodal disease. Extranodal involvement is possible but usually in the context of widespread disease.

AITL is a peripheral T-cell lymphoma with a prominent arborizing proliferation of post-capillary venules amid the neoplastic T-cell proliferation. Patients commonly show some immunologic abnormalities, including hypergammaglobulinemia, drug hypersensitivity, circulating immune complexes, cold agglutinins with hemolytic anemia, positive rheumatoid factor, and other autoimmune antibodies. The dysregulation of immunologic function is also present in the lymphoma milieu, leading to the presence of EBV-positive B cells in the affected lymph nodes. Some of these B cells may at times proliferate and develop into a clonal, EBV-driven B-cell LPD. The neoplastic T cells are CD4+CD8- helper T cells. Recent studies showed coexpression of CD10 and BCL6 in the lymphoma cells, suggesting a T-follicular helper (T_{FH}) origin.[203–206] Additional support of this notion came from studies showing CXCL13 expression, a cytokine produced by T_{FH} cells, in most AITL cases. In contrast, only a small proportion of PTCL, NOS expresses this marker, and other specific T-cell lymphomas have not been shown to express CXCL13.[205,206] Most recently, GEP studies further confirmed this hypothesis by demonstrating enriched expression of the molecular signature of T_{FH} cells by AITL.[207,208]

PTCL, NOS is used for all the PTCL that cannot be otherwise assigned to other specific T-cell NHL categories. They constitute the largest proportion of mature T-cell lymphomas. It is understandable that this is a heterogeneous group and may represent multiple as yet undiscovered disease subtypes. Various morphologic variants have been described, such as Lennert (lymphoepithelioid) lymphoma, T-zone lymphoma, and follicular T-cell lymphoma.[1,3] Whether some of these morphologic variants represent distinct disease entities remains to be determined. In particular, the follicular T-cell lymphoma has been reported to express CD10 and BCL 6 and associate with germinal centers leading to the speculation that it might be related to AITL.[209] A group of cytotoxic PTCL may also be identified and separated from PTCL, NOS.[210] Most of the PTCL, NOS cases are aggressive tumors with poor response to chemotherapeutic treatment irrespective of the morphology.

Predominantly extranodal mature T-cell and NK-cell neoplasms

These include extranodal NK/T-cell lymphoma, nasal type, enteropathy-type T-cell lymphoma, hepatosplenic T-cell lymphoma, subcutaneous panniculitis-like T-cell lymphoma, MF/SS, and EBV-positive T-cell lymphoproliferative disorders of childhood.

Extranodal NK/T-cell lymphoma, nasal type, is an aggressive, angiocentric, and angiodestructive lymphoma affecting primarily extranodal sites. Most of the cases demonstrate evidence of an NK-cell origin, but rare cases show a cytotoxic T-cell phenotype. The size of the neoplastic cells can be variable, ranging from small, to intermediate, to large. Giemsa stain on touch preparations of the tumorous tissue highlights azurophilic granules in the cytoplasm of neoplastic cells. These granules contain cytotoxic molecules including TIA-1, granzyme B, and perforin, a reflection of the NK or cytotoxic T-cell nature of the neoplastic cells. Irrespective of the cell lineage, EBV is present in all the cases. The qualifier 'nasal type' signifies that the nasal cavity is the most common site of involvement, and the prototypic disease in this anatomic site is called nasal NK/T-cell lymphoma. Extranodal NK/T-cell lymphoma, nasal type is sensitive to radiotherapy, which is the primary modality of treatment for localized disease.

Enteropathy-associated T-cell lymphoma (ETL) is the most frequent T-cell NHL arising primarily in the intestine. It occurs most commonly in the proximal jejunum, and less frequently in other parts of the small intestine, colon, or stomach.[211] The presenting symptoms are abdominal pain and intestinal obstruction secondary to a single or multiple intestinal mass(es) or ulcerated lesions. Recently, Deleeuw *et al.*[212] suggested that ETL can be further subdivided into two distinct subgroups. Type 1 ETL comprises 80% of all ETL and is characterized by pleomorphic lymphoma cells, a prior history of celiac disease (about 30%) and mucosal changes of celiac disease near the lymphoma (about 85%), HLA-DQB1 genotype pattern of celiac disease, a CD3+CD5-CD7+CD4-CD8-CD56- immunophenotype, and gains of chromosome 1q and 5q.[212] In contrast, type 2 ETL shows monomorphic small- to medium-sized cells, infrequent association with celiac disease, HLA-DQB1 genotype pattern similar to the normal white population, frequent expression of CD8 and CD56, *c-MYC* gene locus gains, and rare gains of 1q and 5q.[212] CGH studies showed that complex gains of chromosome 9q31.3-qter are frequent in both types (overall 70%), with the vast majority of these gains clustering in 9q33.2-q33.3.[212,213] Since 9q gain is rarely found in other subtypes of PTCL,[186,214–216] FISH using a probe targeting this region may be useful in the diagnosis of ETL.[211] Type 1 ETL cells resemble the majority of intraepithelial αβ T cells immunophenotypically, while type 2 ETL may derive from activated intraepithelial αβ T cells.[212] Rare gastrointestinal mucosal γδ T-cell lymphoma have been reported and most of them seem to be aggressive and carry a bad prognosis.[217,218]

Hepatosplenic T-cell lymphoma involves the liver, spleen, and bone marrow with a characteristic sinusoidal distribution of medium-sized pleomorphic lymphoma cells. Most cases derive from γδ T cells, but a minority of hepatosplenic αβ T-cell lymphomas has also been reported.[219] Approximately 70% of cases harbor a characteristic isochromosome 7, and about 50% of cases additionally show trisomy 8.[220,221] There are suggestions that hepatosplenic γδ T-cell lymphoma is more common among immunosuppressed patients after solid organ transplantation. This lymphoma is aggressive and is associated with a poor prognosis.[1]

Subcutaneous panniculitis-like T-cell lymphoma (SPTL) is a NHL of mature cytotoxic T cells. The usual presentation is multiple subcutaneous nodules affecting both the trunk and extremities (most commonly in the lower limbs). Hemophagocytic syndrome may be seen in some of the cases. The lymphoma cells are usually of small to medium size and involve the subcutaneous adipose tissue, sparing the dermis and epidermis. The adipose cells are characteristically rimmed by the lymphoma cells (Figure 13.1f). There are usually many intermixed histiocytes, with necrosis and karyorrhexis often present. Expression of the cytotoxic molecules TIA-1, granzyme B, and perforin can be demonstrated by immunohistochemistry. The designation SPTL is now restricted to tumors expressing the αβ T-cell receptors. These cases show the classical histologic features described above, and the lymphoma cells are usually CD4-CD8+CD56-. The disease course in a significant percentage of patients is relatively indolent. In contrast, cases derived from γδ T cells tend to involve the dermis and epidermis in addition to the subcutis. These tumors frequently demonstrate a CD4-CD8-CD56+ immunophenotype, and invariably associate with a very poor prognosis.[222–225] Therefore, a provisional category 'cutaneous γδ T-cell lymphoma' was proposed in the WHO–EORTC classification for these cases (see below).[199]

MF is the most common type of primary cutaneous T-cell lymphoma, accounting for approximately 50% of such cases.[199] It is recommended that this diagnostic label be used only in cases that show a typical clinical course,[199] which is protracted and limited to the skin for a long period of time before systemic dissemination. In the early patch stage, the lymphoma cells are arranged in a band beneath the dermo-epidermal junction. There is also epidermotropism, with collections of lymphoma cells in the epidermis (Pautrier microabscesses) sometimes observed. The lymphoma cells are small- to medium-sized and have highly convoluted nuclei (cerebriform cells), typically showing a CD3+CD4+CD8-CD45RO+ memory T-cell phenotype, and demonstrate variable loss of the pan-T-cell antigens CD2, CD5, and CD7. Expression of CD30 is not common, and is usually associated with large cell transformation. Demonstration by flow cytometry of restricted TCR β-chain variable region family usage,[226] and molecular studies demonstrating a clonal TCR rearrangement, are important adjuncts for differentiating MF from reactive dermatoses.[227]

SS is conventionally defined by the triad of erythroderma, generalized lymphadenopathy, and the presence of Sézary cells in skin, lymph nodes, and peripheral blood (Figure 13.3h).[228] In 2002, the International Society for Cutaneous Lymphomas (ISCL) proposed one or more of the following features for the diagnosis of SS: an absolute peripheral blood Sézary cell count of at least 1000 cells/mm^3, demonstration of immunophenotypic abnormalities (CD4/CD8 ratio greater than 10, loss of pan-T-cell antigens, or both), or demonstration of T-cell clonality in the peripheral blood by molecular or cytogenetic methods.[229] The WHO–EORTC classification recommended the presence of at least one of the cytomorphologic or immunophenotypic features proposed by the ISCL, plus the demonstration of T-cell clonality (preferably the same clone in blood and skin) as the minimal diagnostic criteria of SS.[199] Demonstration of T-cell clonality serves to avoid over-diagnosing benign conditions as SS.[199] Clinically, SS can be divided into primary SS, which presents as a primary leukemic disorder, and secondary SS, which develops after a long history of MF. It is noted that patients with primary SS have a much worse clinical outcome.[229] The circulating Sézary cells exhibit cerebriform nuclear outlines, and the immunophenotype is also similar to the neoplastic cells seen in MF with coexpression of

CD4 and CD25. Patients with late-stage MF and SS are immunosuppressed, which is postulated to be due to T-helper 2 (Th-2)-skewing of the helper T cells.[230–232]

A GEP study using cDNA microarrays identified a signature of 27 genes implicated in the pathogenesis of MF.[233] This study also derived and validated a six-gene classifier for MF and gene expression signatures associated with more aggressive disease, aberrant immunophenotype, and tumor stage.[233] Another GEP study on SS has identified highly expressed genes that include Th-2-specific transcription factors Gata-3 and Jun B, which coincides with the Th-2-skewing aforementioned. A diagnostic signature and prognostic model have also been established in SS patients.[234]

Two types of EBV-associated T-cell LPDs of childhood are recognized by the WHO classification. They include systemic EBV-positive T-cell LPD of childhood and hydroa vacciniforme-like lymphoma. Both of them occur more often in East Asians and in Native Americans from Mexico and Central and South America. Systemic EBV-positive T-cell LPD of childhood is a life-threatening disease with a clonal proliferation of EBV-infected cytotoxic T cells. It may occur shortly after primary acute EBV infection or in the setting of chronic active EBV infection.[235,236] Patients usually present with abrupt onset of fever, with hepatosplenomegaly, hepatic failure, and sometimes lymphadenopathy. Hemophagocytic syndrome and multiorgan failure are common and most patients run a fulminant, fatal, acute clinical course.[237] Hydroa vacciniforme-like lymphoma is a cutaneous cytotoxic T-cell or NK-cell lymphoma affecting sun-exposed skin, and is associated with insect bite sensitivity. The patients usually have papulovesicular eruptions, which proceed to ulceration and scarring over time. The clinical course is variable, ranging from an indolent disease for over 10 years to aggressive systemic involvement.

Hodgkin lymphoma

HLs are divided into two main categories: NLPHL and CHL. NLPHL and the vast majority of CHL are derived from germinal and post-germinal center B cells, respectively.[238–240] Very rare cases of CHL of T-cell origin have also been described.[210,211] In developed nations, NLPHL and CHL peak in late adolescence and early adulthood, and CHL has a second peak in late adulthood. Both NLPHL and CHL typically display relatively few neoplastic cells in a polymorphic background.

The prototypic neoplastic cells in CHL are the RS cells, which are large cells with abundant cytoplasm, bilobed nuclei, and a macronucleolus in each nucleus or nuclear lobe. The nucleoli are at least as large as the nuclei of small lymphocytes, and there are halos around the nucleoli (Figure 13.6a). Variant forms of RS cells called RS variants or Hodgkin cells that do not fit the description of classical RS cells can also be seen (Figure 13.6b). The Hodgkin and RS (HRS) cells secrete an array of cytokines that attract the background cellular components of polymorphonuclear cells, T lymphocytes, and histiocytes.[243] For the B-cell-derived CHL, the HRS cells are post-germinal center B cells often showing deleterious mutations of the Ig genes.[239] Additionally, suppression of several transcription factors important for Ig transcription, including PU.1, BOB1, and OCT2, plays an even more important role in the lack of expression of Ig transcripts in the HRS cells.[240,244–247] Downregulation of genes encoding essential B-cell signaling pathway proteins has also been observed in HRS cells.[248] Although many of the markers of B-cell differentiation are lost in HRS cells, a B-cell origin can be established because of the retained PAX5 (a B-lineage-specific transcription factor) expression,[249] and Ig heavy and light chain gene rearrangements.[239,240,242] CHL is further subdivided into four histologic variants: nodular sclerosis, mixed cellularity, lymphocyte rich, and lymphocyte depleted. These morphologic variants have different demographics, incidence of EBV positivity, and clinical features.[1]

Nodular sclerosis CHL is the most common morphologic subtype of CHL and frequently presents as a mediastinal mass. It affects both sexes equally, in contrast with the male predominance in the other morphologic subtypes. Most patients present at an early stage. The affected lymph nodes show a nodular architecture with the nodules surrounded by fibrous collagen bands. The RS cell variant in this subtype is called a lacunar cell (Figure 13.6c), due to a rim of empty space around the neoplastic cell nucleus if the tissue is fixed in formalin. There is a low incidence of EBV (approximately 10%).

Mixed cellularity CHL is the second most common morphologic subtype and has a higher EBV association (overall 75%). Patients usually present at an advanced stage. The histologic pattern is usually diffuse or vaguely nodular. The RS cells are present in a mixed inflammatory background represented by classical RS cells and mononuclear variants. This is the morphologic subtype most commonly seen in patients with HIV infection and in developing countries. The cases associated with HIV are 100% EBV positive.[250] Although the advent of highly active antiretroviral therapy has led to the decline of NHL in AIDS patients, the incidence of HL remains steady[251] or even increases.[252–254]

Lymphocyte-rich CHL is a rare subtype of CHL typically showing peripheral lymph nodes and mediastinal involvement. It usually has a nodular pattern but rarely a diffuse pattern can also be observed. The background cells are usually small B cells with IgM and IgD expression. Rosetting of the neoplastic large cells by CD3-positive T-cells can be seen, but these cells are not CD57-positive, in contrast with NLPHL.[255] This feature, together with the difference in the cytology and immunophenotype between the HRS cells in lymphocyte-rich CHL and the lymphocytic and histiocytic (L&H) cells in NLPHL, serves to differentiate these two entities with very similar histologic patterns. Most patients present with early-stage disease.

Lymphocyte-depleted CHL is the rarest of all CHL subtypes. It has to be distinguished from nodular sclerosis CHL with lymphocyte depletion, which has abundant lacunar cells. The syncytial variant of nodular sclerosis CHL should, in addition,

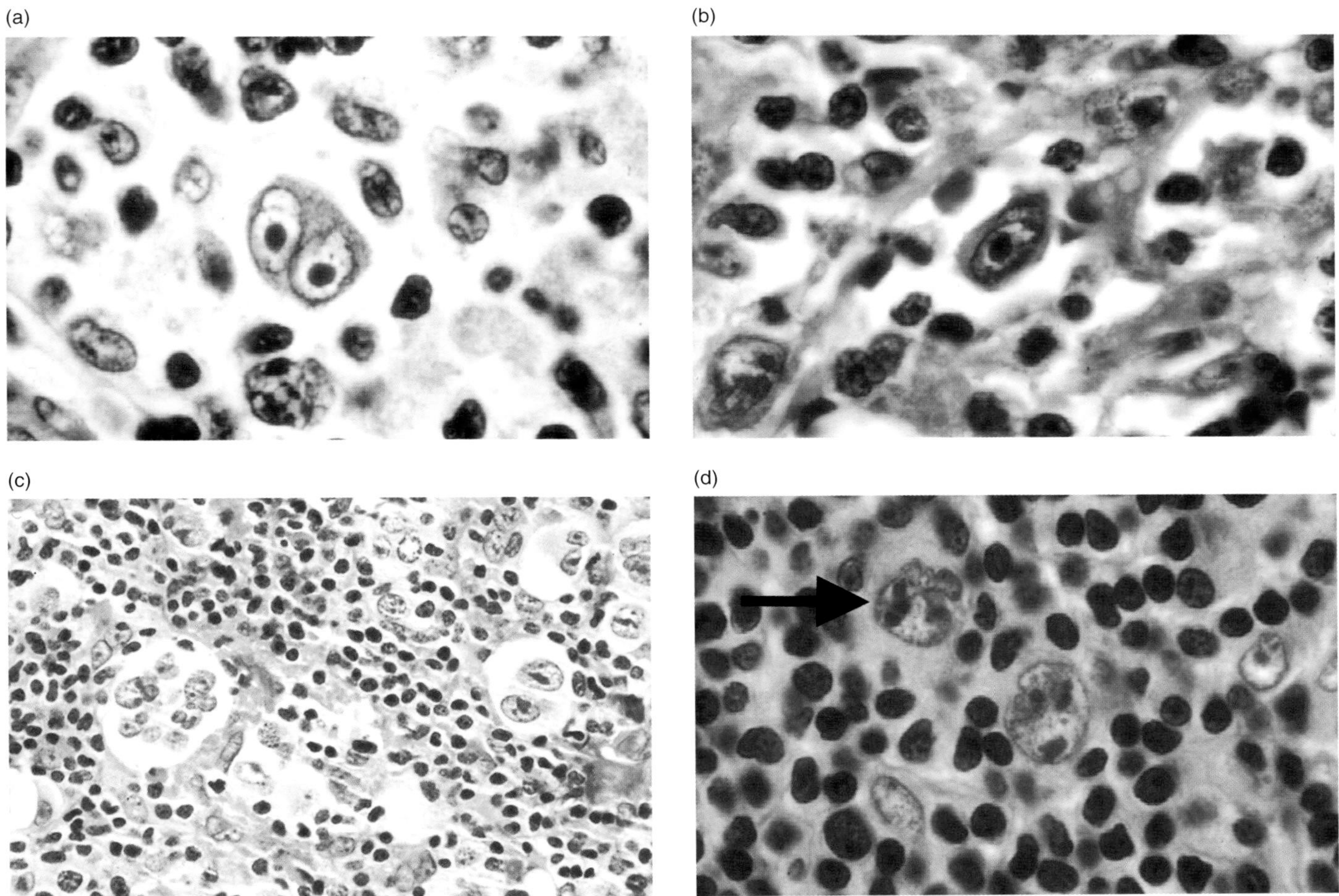

Figure 13.6 The neoplastic cells in Hodgkin lymphomas demonstrate various morphologic features. Panel a demonstrates a classical Reed–Sternberg cell with large, bilobar nuclei with macronucleoli (the owl's eyes appearance), and perinucleolar halo. The mononuclear variant is typically seen in mixed cellularity Hodgkin lymphoma (b). The lacunar cell is a variant Reed–Sternberg cell seen in nodular sclerosis classical Hodgkin lymphoma. The lacuna where the cell resides is a result of cytoplasmic retraction secondary to formalin fixation (c). The lymphocytic and histiocytic cell of nodular lymphocyte predominant Hodgkin lymphoma is a large cell with multilobated nuclei, which leads to its descriptive name popcorn cell (arrow). The background small lymphocytes are predominantly B cells (d) (H&E stain for all panels, original magnification × 400 for panel c and × 1000 for all other panels).

display a syncytial pattern (sheets of neoplastic cells with no distinct borders) of the neoplastic cells as its name implies. Lymphocyte-depleted CHL and the syncytial variant of nodular sclerosis CHL should also be distinguished from ALCL and the morphologic variant of anaplastic DLBCL by immunohistochemical, cytogenetic, or molecular diagnostic studies.

CGH studies performed on RS cells obtained by laser capture microdissection revealed recurrent chromosome gains of 2p, 12q, and 17p, and loss of 13q.[256,257] A GEP study of classical CHL cell lines showed global silencing of the B-cell-specific gene expression program, including genes involved in B-cell receptor signaling.[248] Another GEP study using cDNA arrays targeting the mRNA of approximately 1000 selected genes on 21 patient samples of nodular sclerosis and mixed cellularity CHL demonstrated three gene expression signatures that corresponded to mixed cellularity CHL, nodular sclerosis CHL with good prognosis, and nodular sclerosis CHL with bad prognosis.[258]

NLPHL is characterized by a nodular or mixed nodular and diffuse proliferation of mostly small lymphocytes with a variable admixture of histiocytes and a variant of RS cells, the L&H cells (Figure 13.6d), which are large neoplastic centroblasts with multilobated nuclei and high nuclear-to-cytoplasmic ratio. Patients usually present with localized peripheral lymphadenopathy. Involvement of deep-seated lymph nodes, spleen, and bone marrow is uncommon. Some cases are associated with concomitant progressive transformation of germinal centers (PTGC), which are enlarged follicles with a predominance of mantle zone B cells and fragmented germinal centers. It is postulated that PTGC could represent the precursor lesions of NLPHL. However, PTGC may occur without the development of HL even in patients with previously diagnosed NLPHL. Despite the possibility of multiple relapses, most patients have long survival. On the other hand, NLPHL can transform into DLBCL that may occasionally resemble a THRLBCL, which is associated with a worse survival.

Immunodeficiency-associated LPDs

Four immunodeficiency states associated with an increased risk of LPD are recognized by the WHO classification. They include primary immune disorders, HIV infection, iatrogenic immunosuppression in allogeneic transplant recipients, and other iatrogenic immunodeficiency states caused by immunosuppressive drugs. A proportion of these LPDs resemble polymorphic lymphoid proliferations that are seen in infectious mononucleosis (IM). An example is polymorphic post-transplant lymphoproliferative disorder (PTLD), which is classified as a B-cell proliferation of uncertain malignant potential because reducing immunosuppression may lead to disease regression in some cases. These IM-like, polymorphic LPDs are usually positive for EBV. Other immunodeficiency-associated LPDs may manifest as a predominantly plasmacytic proliferation, or they may resemble one of the recognized sporadic HL or NHL subtypes discussed above. The incidence of EBV positivity is variable depending on the predisposing conditions and the time elapsed after the start of the immunosuppression. These LPDs should be classified as the corresponding HL or NHL subtypes if the diagnostic criteria are met.

WHO–EORTC classification of cutaneous lymphomas

The skin is the second most common site for primary extranodal lymphomas, and it is also commonly involved by systemic lymphomas. Certain primary cutaneous lymphomas are unique to the skin, such as MF. Other cutaneous lymphomas share similar histologic features with some nodal lymphoma subtypes, but may differ in terms of immunophenotype, molecular abnormalities, clinical behavior, and prognosis. Therefore, distinguishing a primary cutaneous lymphoma and cutaneous involvement by a systemic lymphoma is crucial for patient management. For example, primary cutaneous follicle center lymphoma (PCFCL) is frequently negative for BCL2 expression, is negative for the t(14;18), and has a much better prognosis than systemic FL.

The WHO and the EORTC had previously proposed separate classification systems for cutaneous lymphomas.[1,193] To minimize the confusion to pathologists and clinicians, the representatives of the WHO and the EORTC cutaneous lymphoma classification systems jointly developed a unified consensus WHO–EORTC classification of cutaneous lymphomas that was published in 2005.[168] The lymphoma entities are classified into categories of T-cell and NK-cell lymphomas, B-cell lymphomas, and precursor hematologic neoplasms (Table 13.5).

The 2005 WHO–EORTC classification recognizes PCFCL and PCDLBCL as distinct entities from their systemic counterparts. Patients with the PCFCL have an excellent prognosis (5-year survival rate of over 95%) and grading appears to have minimal effect on prognosis. The PCDLBCL are further subclassified into PCDLBCL, leg type; PCDLBCL, other; and intravascular large B-cell lymphoma. The PCDLBCL, leg type appears to have an ABC gene expression profile and has a 5-year disease-specific survival of about 50%. It appears that this disease should be treated with systemic, anthracycline-based chemotherapy like its systemic counterpart. The other category, PCDLBCL, other, essentially includes all the other PCDLBCL that do not fit into the leg type or the entity IVLBCL.[199]

For the primary cutaneous T-cell lymphomas, the WHO-EORTC classification recognizes three MF variants (folliculotropic MF, pagetoid reticulosis, and granulomatous slack skin) in addition to MF, SS, and primary cutaneous CD30-positive T-cell LPD. Several provisional entities within the primary cutaneous peripheral T-cell lymphoma, unspecified, are also included (Table 13.5), which await additional studies for further characterization.

Table 13.5. Summary of the 2005 World Health Organization–European Organization for Research and Treatment of Cancer classification of lymphomas with primary cutaneous involvement and presentation

Cutaneous T-cell and NK-cell lymphomas
Mycosis fungoides
Mycosis fungoides variants and subtypes
Folliculotropic mycosis fungoides
Pagetoid reticulosis
Granulomatous slack skin
Sézary syndrome
Adult T-cell leukemia/lymphoma
Primary cutaneous CD30+ lymphoproliferative disorders
Primary cutaneous anaplastic large cell lymphoma
Lymphomatoid papulosis
Subcutaneous panniculitis-like T-cell lymphoma
Extranodal NK/T-cell lymphoma, nasal type
Primary cutaneous T-cell lymphoma, unspecified
Primary cutaneous aggressive epidermotropic CD8+ T-cell lymphoma (provisional)
Cutaneous γ/δ T-cell lymphoma (provisional)
Primary cutaneous CD4+ small/medium-sized pleomorphic T-cell lymphoma (provisional)
Cutaneous B-cell lymphomas
Primary cutaneous marginal zone B-cell lymphoma
Primary cutaneous follicle center lymphoma
Primary cutaneous diffuse large B-cell lymphoma, leg type
Primary cutaneous diffuse large B-cell lymphoma, other
Intravascular large B-cell lymphoma
Precursor hematologic neoplasm
CD4+/CD56+ hematodermic neoplasm (blastic NK-cell lymphoma)

Source: Produced from Willemze *et al.*[199]

Blastic plasmacytoid dendritic cell neoplasm (also called CD4+/CD56+ hematodermic neoplasm) was previously called blastic NK-cell lymphoma. It was classified as a putative NK-cell tumor in the 2001 WHO classification of tumors of the hematopoietic and lymphoid tissues, because the neoplastic cells resemble blasts and frequently express CD56. Evidence accumulated from recent studies indicated a probable plasmacytoid dendritic cell origin of these tumors.[259–263] Petrella *et al.* first proposed the term "agranular CD4+CD56+ hematodermic neoplasms."[260,264] The 2005 WHO-EORTC classification of cutaneous lymphomas thus adopted and slightly modified this proposed nomenclature to CD4+/CD56+ hematodermic neoplasm (blastic NK-cell lymphoma) under the category of precursor hematologic neoplasm (Table 13.5).[199] In the latest WHO classification of tumors of hematopoietic and lymphoid tissues, this entity is further renamed as blastic plasmacytoid dendritic cell neoplasm to highlight the current concept of its cell of origin.[1] The frequent CD4 expression and the blastic appearance of the tumor cells necessitate the inclusion of cutaneous acute myelomonocytic and acute monoblast/monocytic leukemia as the major differential diagnosis. However, the tumor cells do not resemble monocytic cells and most myeloid markers are usually absent.[262,264] Expression of CD123 and T-cell leukemia 1 (TCL1) antigens supports the diagnosis of this entity.[265] A recent study further showed that blastic plasmacytoid dendritic cell neoplasm and cutaneous myelomonocytic leukemias are different by GEP and in terms of chromosomal aberrations.[266] Most cases of blastic plasmacytoid dendritic cell neoplasm harbor complex cytogenetic abnormalities, and the most common ones include deletions or translocations involving 5q (72%), deletions of 12p (64%), and deletions of 13q (64%).[267]

Conclusions

The latest WHO classification of tumors of hematopoietic and lymphoid tissues has been developed by a large panel of pathologists and clinicians around the world. The extensive international collaboration ensures the integration of as much expert opinion as possible, and allows the adoption of this classification system as the common language among clinicians, pathologists, and scientists working in this field. As new information, including contributions from many genome-wide investigations, is accumulating rapidly, novel entities and/or critical changes to the current WHO classification system may be anticipated in the foreseeable future.

References

1. Swerdlow SH, Campo E, Harris NL, *et al.* (eds.). *WHO Classification of Tumours of the Haematopoietic and Lymphoid Tissues*. Lyon, IARC Press, 2008.
2. Harris NL, Jaffe ES, Stein H, *et al.* A revised European-American classification of lymphoid neoplasms: a proposal from the International Lymphoma Study Group. *Blood* 1994;**84**:1361–92.
3. Chan JKC. Tumors of the lymphoreticular system. In: Fletcher CDM, ed. *Diagnostic Histopathology of Tumors*, 3rd edn. Edinburgh, Churchill Livingstone. 2007; 1139–288.
4. Matutes E, Catovsky D. The value of scoring systems for the diagnosis of biphenotypic leukemia and mature B-cell disorders. *Leuk Lymphoma* 1994;**13** Suppl 1:11–14.
5. Han X, Bueso-Ramos CE. Precursor T-cell acute lymphoblastic leukemia/lymphoblastic lymphoma and acute biphenotypic leukemias. *Am J Clin Pathol* 2007;**127**:528–44.
6. Pui CH, Robison LL, Look AT. Acute lymphoblastic leukemia. *Lancet* 2008;**371**:1030–43.
7. Weng AP, Ferrando AA, Lee W, *et al.* Activating mutations of NOTCH1 in human T cell acute lymphoblastic leukemia. *Science* 2004;**306**:269–71.
8. Wolfe MS. Gamma-Secretase inhibition and modulation for Alzheimer's disease. *Curr Alzheimer Res* 2008;**5**:158–64.
9. The Non-Hodgkin's Lymphoma Classification Project. A clinical evaluation of the International Lymphoma Study Group classification of non-Hodgkin's lymphoma. *Blood* 1997;**89**:3909–18.
10. Shimodaira S, Hidaka E, Katsuyama T. Clonal identity of nodular lymphocyte-predominant Hodgkin's disease and T-cell-rich B-cell lymphoma. *N Engl J Med* 2000;**343**:1124–5.
11. Chan WC. Cellular origin of nodular lymphocyte-predominant Hodgkin's lymphoma: immunophenotypic and molecular studies. *Semin Hematol* 1999;**36**:242–52.
12. Campbell J, Seymour JF, Matthews J, *et al.* The prognostic impact of bone marrow involvement in patients with diffuse large cell lymphoma varies according to the degree of infiltration and presence of discordant marrow involvement. *Eur J Haematol* 2006;**76**:473–80.
13. Chung R, Lai R, Wei P, *et al.* Concordant but not discordant bone marrow involvement in diffuse large B-cell lymphoma predicts a poor clinical outcome independent of the International Prognostic Index. *Blood* 2007;**110**:1278–82.
14. Hodges GF, Lenhardt TM, Cotelingam JD. Bone marrow involvement in large-cell lymphoma. Prognostic implications of discordant disease. *Am J Clin Pathol* 1994;**101**:305–11.
15. Robertson LE, Redman JR, Butler JJ, *et al.* Discordant bone marrow involvement in diffuse large-cell lymphoma: a distinct clinical-pathologic entity associated with a continuous risk of relapse. *J Clin Oncol* 1991;**9**:236–42.
16. Fisher DE, Jacobson JO, Ault KA, *et al.* Diffuse large cell lymphoma with discordant bone marrow histology. Clinical features and biological implications. *Cancer* 1989;**64**: 1879–87.
17. Yan Y, Chan WC, Weisenburger DD, *et al.* Clinical and prognostic significance of bone marrow involvement in patients with diffuse aggressive B-cell lymphoma. *J Clin Oncol* 1995;**13**:1336–42.
18. Rosenwald A, Wright G, Chan WC, *et al.* The use of molecular profiling to predict survival after chemotherapy for diffuse large-B-cell lymphoma. *N Engl J Med* 2002;**346**:1937–47.

19. Shipp MA, Ross KN, Tamayo P, *et al.* Diffuse large B-cell lymphoma outcome prediction by gene-expression profiling and supervised machine learning. *Nat Med* 2002;**8**:68–74.

20. Iqbal J, Sanger WG, Horsman DE, *et al.* BCL2 translocation defines a unique tumor subset within the germinal center B-cell-like diffuse large B-cell lymphoma. *Am J Pathol* 2004;**165**:159–66.

21. Bea S, Zettl A, Wright G, *et al.* Diffuse large B-cell lymphoma subgroups have distinct genetic profiles that influence tumor biology and improve gene-expression-based survival prediction. *Blood* 2005;**106**:3183–90.

22. Iqbal J, Greiner TC, Patel K, *et al.* Distinctive patterns of BCL6 molecular alterations and their functional consequences in different subgroups of diffuse large B-cell lymphoma. *Leukemia* 2007;**21**:2332–43.

23. Hans CP, Weisenburger DD, Vose JM, *et al.* A significant diffuse component predicts for inferior survival in grade 3 follicular lymphoma, but cytologic subtypes do not predict survival. *Blood* 2003;**101**:2363–7.

24. Choi WW, Weisenburger DD, Greiner TC, *et al.* A new immunostain algorithm classifies diffuse large B-cell lymphoma into molecular subtypes with high accuracy. *Clin Cancer Res* 2009;**15**:5494–502.

25. Kobayashi T, Yamaguchi M, Kim S, *et al.* Microarray reveals differences in both tumors and vascular specific gene expression in de novo CD5+ and CD5- diffuse large B-cell lymphomas. *Cancer Res* 2003;**63**:60–6.

26. Colomo L, Loong F, Rives S, *et al.* Diffuse large B-cell lymphomas with plasmablastic differentiation represent a heterogeneous group of disease entities. *Am J Surg Pathol* 2004;**28**:736–47.

27. Delecluse HJ, Anagnostopoulos I, Dallenbach F, *et al.* Plasmablastic lymphomas of the oral cavity: a new entity associated with the human immunodeficiency virus infection. *Blood* 1997;**89**:1413–20.

28. Dong HY, Scadden DT, de Leval L, *et al.* Plasmablastic lymphoma in HIV-positive patients: an aggressive Epstein-Barr virus-associated extramedullary plasmacytic neoplasm. *Am J Surg Pathol* 2005;**29**:1633–41.

29. Oksenhendler E, Boulanger E, Galicier L, *et al.* High incidence of Kaposi sarcoma-associated herpesvirus-related non-Hodgkin lymphoma in patients with HIV infection and multicentric Castleman disease. *Blood* 2002;**99**:2331–6.

30. Nador RG, Cesarman E, Chadburn A, *et al.* Primary effusion lymphoma: a distinct clinicopathologic entity associated with the Kaposi's sarcoma-associated herpes virus. *Blood* 1996;**88**:645–56.

31. Carbone A, Gloghini A, Cozzi MR, *et al.* Expression of MUM-1/IRF4 selectively clusters with primary effusion lymphoma among lymphomatous effusions: implications for disease histogenesis and pathogenesis. *Br J Haematol* 2000;**111**:247–57.

32. Klein U, Gloghini A, Gaidano G, *et al.* Gene expression profile analysis of AIDS-related primary effusion lymphoma (PEL) suggests a plasmablastic derivation and identifies PEL-specific transcripts. *Blood* 2003;**101**:4115–21.

33. Oyama T, Yamamoto K, Asano N, *et al.* Age-related EBV-associated B-cell lymphoproliferative disorders constitute a distinct clinicopathologic group: a study of 96 patients. *Clin Cancer Res* 2007;**13**:5124–32.

34. Park S, Lee J, Ko YH, *et al.* The impact of Epstein-Barr virus status on clinical outcome in diffuse large B-cell lymphoma. *Blood* 2007;**110**:972–8.

35. Guinee DG Jr, Perkins SL, Travis WD, *et al.* Proliferation and cellular phenotype in lymphomatoid granulomatosis: implications of a higher proliferation index in B cells. *Am J Surg Pathol* 1998;**22**:1093–100.

36. Koss MN, Hochholzer L, Langloss JM, *et al.* Lymphomatoid granulomatosis: a clinicopathologic study of 42 patients. *Pathology* 1986;**18**:283–8.

37. Nishiu M, Tomita Y, Nakatsuka S, *et al.* Distinct pattern of gene expression in pyothorax-associated lymphoma (PAL), a lymphoma developing in long-standing inflammation. *Cancer Sci* 2004;**95**:828–34.

38. Cobbers JM, Wolter M, Reifenberger J, *et al.* Frequent inactivation of CDKN2A and rare mutation of TP53 in PCNSL. *Brain Pathol* 1998;**8**:263–76.

39. Boleti E, Johnson PW. Primary mediastinal B-cell lymphoma. *Hematol Oncol* 2007;**25**:157–63.

40. Rosenwald A, Wright G, Leroy K, *et al.* Molecular diagnosis of primary mediastinal B cell lymphoma identifies a clinically favorable subgroup of diffuse large B cell lymphoma related to Hodgkin lymphoma. *J Exp Med* 2003;**198**:851–62.

41. Savage KJ, Monti S, Kutok JL, *et al.* The molecular signature of mediastinal large B-cell lymphoma differs from that of other diffuse large B-cell lymphomas and shares features with classical Hodgkin lymphoma. *Blood* 2003;**102**:3871–9.

42. Joos S, Kupper M, Ohl S, *et al.* Genomic imbalances including amplification of the tyrosine kinase gene JAK2 in CD30+ Hodgkin cells. *Cancer Res* 2000;**60**:549–52.

43. Ferreri AJ, Dognini GP, Campo E, *et al.* Variations in clinical presentation, frequency of hemophagocytosis and clinical behavior of intravascular lymphoma diagnosed in different geographical regions. *Haematologica* 2007;**92**:486–92.

44. Matsue K, Asada N, Takeuchi M, *et al.* A clinicopathological study of 13 cases of intravascular lymphoma: experience in a single institution over a 9-yr period. *Eur J Haematol* 2008;**80**:236–44.

45. Achten R, Verhoef G, Vanuytsel L, *et al.* T-cell/histiocyte-rich large B-cell lymphoma: a distinct clinicopathologic entity. *J Clin Oncol* 2002;**20**:1269–77.

46. Bouabdallah R, Mounier N, Guettier C, *et al.* T-cell/histiocyte-rich large B-cell lymphomas and classical diffuse large B-cell lymphomas have similar outcome after chemotherapy: a matched-control analysis. *J Clin Oncol* 2003;**21**:1271–7.

47. Delsol G, Lamant L, Mariame B, *et al.* A new subtype of large B-cell lymphoma expressing the ALK kinase and lacking the 2; 5 translocation. *Blood* 1997;**89**:1483–90.

48. Chikatsu N, Kojima H, Suzukawa K, *et al.* ALK+, CD30-, CD20- large B-cell lymphoma containing anaplastic lymphoma kinase (ALK) fused to clathrin heavy chain gene (CLTC). *Mod Pathol* 2003;**16**:828–32.

49. Blum KA, Lozanski G, Byrd JC. Adult Burkitt leukemia and lymphoma. *Blood* 2004;**104**:3009–20.

50. Patte C, Auperin A, Michon J, *et al.* The Societe Francaise d'Oncologie Pediatrique LMB89 protocol: highly

effective multiagent chemotherapy tailored to the tumor burden and initial response in 561 unselected children with B-cell lymphomas and L3 leukemia. *Blood* 2001;**97**:3370–9.

51. Nyman H, Adde M, Karjalainen-Lindsberg ML, *et al.* Prognostic impact of immunohistochemically defined germinal center phenotype in diffuse large B-cell lymphoma patients treated with immunochemotherapy. *Blood* 2007;**109**:4930–5.

52. Dave SS, Fu K, Wright GW, *et al.* Molecular diagnosis of Burkitt's lymphoma. *N Engl J Med* 2006;**354**:2431–42.

53. Hummel M, Bentink S, Berger H, *et al.* A biologic definition of Burkitt's lymphoma from transcriptional and genomic profiling. *N Engl J Med* 2006;**354**:2419–30.

54. Le Gouill S, Talmant P, Touzeau C, *et al.* The clinical presentation and prognosis of diffuse large B-cell lymphoma with t(14;18) and 8q24/c-MYC rearrangement. *Haematologica* 2007;**92**:1335–42.

55. Chuang SS, Ye H, Du MQ, *et al.* Histopathology and immunohistochemistry in distinguishing Burkitt lymphoma from diffuse large B-cell lymphoma with very high proliferation index and with or without a starry-sky pattern: a comparative study with EBER and FISH. *Am J Clin Pathol* 2007;**128**:558–64.

56. Ott G, Katzenberger T, Lohr A, *et al.* Cytomorphologic, immunohistochemical, and cytogenetic profiles of follicular lymphoma: 2 types of follicular lymphoma grade 3. *Blood* 2002;**99**:3806–12.

57. Bosga-Bouwer AG, van Imhoff GW, Boonstra R, *et al.* Follicular lymphoma grade 3B includes 3 cytogenetically defined subgroups with primary t(14;18), 3q27, or other translocations: t(14;18) and 3q27 are mutually exclusive. *Blood* 2003;**101**:1149–54.

58. Bosga-Bouwer AG, van den Berg A, Haralambieva E, *et al.* Molecular, cytogenetic, and immunophenotypic characterization of follicular lymphoma grade 3B; a separate entity or part of the spectrum of diffuse large B-cell lymphoma or follicular lymphoma? *Hum Pathol* 2006;**37**:528–33.

59. Katzenberger T, Ott G, Klein T, *et al.* Cytogenetic alterations affecting BCL6 are predominantly found in follicular lymphomas grade 3B with a diffuse large B-cell component. *Am J Pathol* 2004;**165**:481–90.

60. Swerdlow SH. Pediatric follicular lymphomas, marginal zone lymphomas, and marginal zone hyperplasia. *Am J Clin Pathol* 2004;**122** Suppl:S98–109.

61. Salar A, Juanpere N, Bellosillo B, *et al.* Gastrointestinal involvement in mantle cell lymphoma: a prospective clinic, endoscopic, and pathologic study. *Am J Surg Pathol* 2006;**30**:1274–80.

62. Romaguera JE, Medeiros LJ, Hagemeister FB, *et al.* Frequency of gastrointestinal involvement and its clinical significance in mantle cell lymphoma. *Cancer* 2003;**97**:586–91.

63. Suzuki R, Takemura K, Tsutsumi M, *et al.* Detection of cyclin D1 overexpression by real-time reverse-transcriptase-mediated quantitative polymerase chain reaction for the diagnosis of mantle cell lymphoma. *Am J Pathol* 2001;**159**:425–9.

64. Hui P, Howe JG, Crouch J, *et al.* Real-time quantitative RT-PCR of cyclin D1 mRNA in mantle cell lymphoma: comparison with FISH and immunohistochemistry. *Leuk Lymphoma* 2003;**44**:1385–94.

65. Belaud-Rotureau MA, Parrens M, Dubus P, *et al.* A comparative analysis of FISH, RT-PCR, PCR, and immunohistochemistry for the diagnosis of mantle cell lymphomas. *Mod Pathol* 2002;**15**:517–25.

66. Specht K, Kremer M, Muller U, *et al.* Identification of cyclin D1 mRNA overexpression in B-cell neoplasias by real-time reverse transcription-PCR of microdissected paraffin sections. *Clin Cancer Res* 2002;**8**:2902–11.

67. Howe JG, Crouch J, Cooper D, *et al.* Real-time quantitative reverse transcription-PCR for cyclin D1 mRNA in blood, marrow, and tissue specimens for diagnosis of mantle cell lymphoma. *Clin Chem* 2004;**50**:80–7.

68. Thomazy VA, Luthra R, Uthman MO, *et al.* Determination of cyclin D1 and CD20 mRNA levels by real-time quantitative RT-PCR from archival tissue sections of mantle cell lymphoma and other non-Hodgkin's lymphomas. *J Mol Diagn* 2002;**4**:201–8.

69. Medeiros LJ, Hai S, Thomazy VA, *et al.* Real-time RT-PCR assay for quantifying cyclin D1 mRNA in B-cell non-Hodgkin's lymphomas. *Mod Pathol* 2002;**15**:556–64.

70. Bijwaard KE, Aguilera NS, Monczak Y, *et al.* Quantitative real-time reverse transcription-PCR assay for cyclin D1 expression: utility in the diagnosis of mantle cell lymphoma. *Clin Chem* 2001;**47**:195–201.

71. Peghini PE, Fehr J. Analysis of cyclin D1 expression by quantitative real-time reverse transcription-polymerase chain reaction in the diagnosis of mantle cell lymphoma. *Am J Clin Pathol* 2002;**117**:237–45.

72. Brizova H, Kalinova M, Krskova L, *et al.* Quantitative measurement of cyclin D1 mRNA, a potent diagnostic tool to separate mantle cell lymphoma from other B-cell lymphoproliferative disorders. *Diagn Mol Pathol* 2008;**17**:39–50.

73. O'Malley DP, Vance GH, Orazi A. Chronic lymphocytic leukemia/small lymphocytic lymphoma with trisomy 12 and focal cyclin d1 expression: a potential diagnostic pitfall. *Arch Pathol Lab Med* 2005;**129**:92–5.

74. Zukerberg LR, Yang WI, Arnold A, *et al.* Cyclin D1 expression in non-Hodgkin's lymphomas. Detection by immunohistochemistry. *Am J Clin Pathol* 1995;**103**:756–60.

75. Miranda RN, Briggs RC, Kinney MC, *et al.* Immunohistochemical detection of cyclin D1 using optimized conditions is highly specific for mantle cell lymphoma and hairy cell leukemia. *Mod Pathol* 2000;**13**:1308–14.

76. Fonseca R, Blood EA, Oken MM, *et al.* Myeloma and the t(11;14)(q13;q32); evidence for a biologically defined unique subset of patients. *Blood* 2002;**99**:3735–41.

77. Fu K, Weisenburger DD, Greiner TC, *et al.* Cyclin D1-negative mantle cell lymphoma: a clinicopathologic study based on gene expression profiling. *Blood* 2005;**106**:4315–21.

78. Gesk S, Klapper W, Martin-Subero JI, *et al.* A chromosomal translocation in cyclin D1-negative/cyclin D2-positive mantle cell lymphoma fuses the CCND2 gene to the IGK locus. *Blood* 2006;**108**:1109–10.

79. Wlodarska I, Dierickx D, Vanhentenrijk V, *et al.* Translocations targeting CCND2, CCND3, and MYCN do occur in t(11;14)-negative mantle

cell lymphomas. *Blood* 2008;**111**: 5683–90.

80. Ek S, Dictor M, Jerkeman M, *et al.* Nuclear expression of the non B-cell lineage Sox11 transcription factor identifies mantle cell lymphoma. *Blood* 2008;**111**:800–5.
81. Mozos A, Royo C, Hartmann E, *et al.* SOX11 expression is highly specific for mantle cell lymphoma and identifies the cyclin D1-negative subtype. *Haematologica* 2009;**94**:1555–62.
82. Suarez F, Lortholary O, Hermine O, *et al.* Infection-associated lymphomas derived from marginal zone B cells: a model of antigen-driven lymphoproliferation. *Blood* 2006;**107**:3034–44.
83. Dierlamm J. Genetic abnormalities in marginal zone B-cell lymphoma. *Haematologica* 2003;**88**:8–12.
84. Streubel B, Vinatzer U, Lamprecht A, *et al.* T(3;14)(p14.1;q32) involving IGH and FOXP1 is a novel recurrent chromosomal aberration in MALT lymphoma. *Leukemia* 2005;**19**:652–8.
85. Remstein ED, Dogan A, Einerson RR, *et al.* The incidence and anatomic site specificity of chromosomal translocations in primary extranodal marginal zone B-cell lymphoma of mucosa-associated lymphoid tissue (MALT lymphoma) in North America. *Am J Surg Pathol* 2006;**30**:1546–53.
86. Nakamura S, Ye H, Bacon CM, *et al.* Clinical impact of genetic aberrations in gastric MALT lymphoma: a comprehensive analysis using interphase fluorescence in situ hybridisation. *Gut* 2007;**56**:1358–63.
87. Baro C, Salido M, Espinet B, *et al.* New chromosomal alterations in a series of 23 splenic marginal zone lymphoma patients revealed by Spectral Karyotyping (SKY). *Leuk Res* 2008;**32**:727–36.
88. Remstein ED, James CD, Kurtin PJ. Incidence and subtype specificity of API2-MALT1 fusion translocations in extranodal, nodal, and splenic marginal zone lymphomas. *Am J Pathol* 2000;**156**:1183–8.
89. Sagaert X, De Wolf-Peeters C, Noels H, *et al.* The pathogenesis of MALT lymphomas: where do we stand? *Leukemia* 2007;**21**:389–96.
90. Owen RG, Treon SP, Al-Katib A, *et al.* Clinicopathological definition of Waldenstrom's macroglobulinemia: consensus panel recommendations from the Second International Workshop on Waldenstrom's Macroglobulinemia. *Semin Oncol* 2003;**30**:110–15.
91. Offit K, Parsa NZ, Filippa D, *et al.* t(9;14)(p13;q32) denotes a subset of low-grade non-Hodgkin's lymphoma with plasmacytoid differentiation. *Blood* 1992;**80**:2594–9.
92. Iida S, Rao PH, Nallasivam P, *et al.* The t(9;14)(p13;q32) chromosomal translocation associated with lymphoplasmacytoid lymphoma involves the PAX-5 gene. *Blood* 1996;**88**:4110–17.
93. Schop RF, Kuehl WM, Van Wier SA, *et al.* Waldenstrom macroglobulinemia neoplastic cells lack immunoglobulin heavy chain locus translocations but have frequent 6q deletions. *Blood* 2002;**100**:2996–3001.
94. Jankovic GM, Colovic MD, Wiernik PH, *et al.* Multiple karyotypic aberrations in a polymorphous variant of Waldenstrom macroglobulinemia. *Cancer Genet Cytogenet* 1999; **111**:77–80.
95. Mansoor A, Medeiros LJ, Weber DM, *et al.* Cytogenetic findings in lymphoplasmacytic lymphoma/ Waldenstrom macroglobulinemia. Chromosomal abnormalities are associated with the polymorphous subtype and an aggressive clinical course. *Am J Clin Pathol* 2001; **116**:543–9.
96. Wong KF, So CC. Waldenstrom macroglobulinemia with karyotypic aberrations involving both homologous 6q. *Cancer Genet Cytogenet* 2001;**124**:137–9.
97. Terre C, Nguyen-Khac F, Barin C, *et al.* Trisomy 4, a new chromosomal abnormality in Waldenstrom's macroglobulinemia: a study of 39 cases. *Leukemia* 2006;**20**:1634–6.
98. Chng WJ, Schop RF, Price-Troska T, *et al.* Gene-expression profiling of Waldenstrom macroglobulinemia reveals a phenotype more similar to chronic lymphocytic leukemia than multiple myeloma. *Blood* 2006;**108**:2755–63.
99. Gutierrez NC, Ocio EM, de Las Rivas J, *et al.* Gene expression profiling of B lymphocytes and plasma cells from Waldenstrom's macroglobulinemia: comparison with expression patterns of the same cell counterparts from chronic lymphocytic leukemia, multiple myeloma and normal individuals. *Leukemia* 2007;**21**:541–9.
100. Barosi G, Boccadoro M, Cavo M, *et al.* Management of multiple myeloma and related-disorders: guidelines from the Italian Society of Hematology (SIE), Italian Society of Experimental Hematology (SIES) and Italian Group for Bone Marrow Transplantation (GITMO). *Haematologica* 2004; **89**:717–41.
101. Dimopoulos MA, Hamilos G. Solitary bone plasmacytoma and extramedullary plasmacytoma. *Curr Treat Options Oncol* 2002;**3**:255–9.
102. Holland J, Trenkner DA, Wasserman TH, *et al.* Plasmacytoma. Treatment results and conversion to myeloma. *Cancer* 1992;**69**:1513–17.
103. Debes-Marun CS, Dewald GW, Bryant S, *et al.* Chromosome abnormalities clustering and its implications for pathogenesis and prognosis in myeloma. *Leukemia* 2003;**17**:427–36.
104. Fonseca R, Oken MM, Harrington D, *et al.* Deletions of chromosome 13 in multiple myeloma identified by interphase FISH usually denote large deletions of the q arm or monosomy. *Leukemia* 2001;**15**:981–6.
105. Fonseca R, Barlogie B, Bataille R, *et al.* Genetics and cytogenetics of multiple myeloma: a workshop report. *Cancer Res* 2004;**64**:1546–58.
106. Chng WJ, Price-Troska T, Gonzalez-Paz N, *et al.* Clinical significance of TP53 mutation in myeloma. *Leukemia* 2007;**21**:582–4.
107. Romagnoli M, Desplanques G, Maiga S, *et al.* Canonical nuclear factor kappaB pathway inhibition blocks myeloma cell growth and induces apoptosis in strong synergy with TRAIL. *Clin Cancer Res* 2007;**13**:6010–18.
108. Zhan F, Huang Y, Colla S, *et al.* The molecular classification of multiple myeloma. *Blood* 2006;**108**:2020–8.
109. Rawstron AC, Green MJ, Kuzmicki A, *et al.* Monoclonal B lymphocytes with the characteristics of "indolent" chronic lymphocytic leukemia are present in 3.5% of adults with normal blood counts. *Blood* 2002;**100**:635–9.
110. Marti GE, Rawstron AC, Ghia P, *et al.* Diagnostic criteria for monoclonal B-cell lymphocytosis. *Br J Haematol* 2005;**130**:325–32.

111. Fung SS, Hillier KL, Leger CS, *et al.* Clinical progression and outcome of patients with monoclonal B-cell lymphocytosis. *Leuk Lymphoma* 2007;**48**:1087–91.

112. Shim YK, Vogt RF, Middleton D, *et al.* Prevalence and natural history of monoclonal and polyclonal B-cell lymphocytosis in a residential adult population. *Cytometry B Clin Cytom* 2007;**72**:344–53.

113. Rawstron AC. Monoclonal B-cell lymphocytosis: good news for patients and CLL investigators. *Leuk Lymphoma* 2007;**48**:1057–8.

114. Cessna MH, Hartung L, Tripp S, *et al.* Hairy cell leukemia variant: fact or fiction? *Am J Clin Pathol* 2005;**123**: 132–8.

115. Traverse-Glehen A, Baseggio L, Bauchu EC, *et al.* Splenic red pulp lymphoma with numerous basophilic villous lymphocytes: a distinct clinicopathologic and molecular entity? *Blood* 2008;**111**:2253–60.

116. Went PT, Zimpfer A, Pehrs AC, *et al.* High specificity of combined TRAP and DBA.44 expression for hairy cell leukemia. *Am J Surg Pathol* 2005;**29**:474–8.

117. Dunphy CH. Reaction patterns of TRAP and DBA.44 in hairy cell leukemia, hairy cell variant, and nodal and extranodal marginal zone B-cell lymphomas. *Appl Immunohistochem Mol Morphol* 2008;**16**:135–9.

118. Matutes E. Immunophenotyping and differential diagnosis of hairy cell leukemia. *Hematol Oncol Clin North Am* 2006;**20**:1051–63.

119. Matutes E, Morilla R, Owusu-Ankomah K, *et al.* The immunophenotype of hairy cell leukemia (HCL). Proposal for a scoring system to distinguish HCL from B-cell disorders with hairy or villous lymphocytes. *Leuk Lymphoma* 1994;**14** Suppl 1:57–61.

120. Del Giudice I, Matutes E, Morilla R, *et al.* The diagnostic value of CD123 in B-cell disorders with hairy or villous lymphocytes. *Haematologica* 2004;**89**:303–8.

121. Munoz L, Nomdedeu JF, Lopez O, *et al.* Interleukin-3 receptor alpha chain (CD123) is widely expressed in hematologic malignancies. *Haematologica* 2001;**86**: 1261–9.

122. Salomon-Nguyen F, Valensi F, Troussard X, *et al.* The value of the monoclonal antibody, DBA44, in the diagnosis of B-lymphoid disorders. *Leuk Res* 1996;**20**:909–13.

123. Papadaki T, Stamatopoulos K, Belessi C, *et al.* Splenic marginal-zone lymphoma: one or more entities? A histologic, immunohistochemical, and molecular study of 42 cases. *Am J Surg Pathol* 2007;**31**: 438–46.

124. Hammer RD, Glick AD, Greer JP, *et al.* Splenic marginal zone lymphoma. A distinct B-cell neoplasm. *Am J Surg Pathol* 1996;**20**:613–26.

125. Kluin-Nelemans HC, Krouwels MM, Jansen JH, *et al.* Hairy cell leukemia preferentially expresses the IgG3-subclass. *Blood* 1990;**75**:972–5.

126. Forconi F, Sahota SS, Raspadori D, *et al.* Hairy cell leukemia: at the crossroad of somatic mutation and isotype switch. *Blood* 2004;**104**: 3312–17.

127. Lamy T, Loughran TP Jr. Current concepts: large granular lymphocyte leukemia. *Blood Rev* 1999;**13**:230–40.

128. Lima M, Almeida J, Santos AH, *et al.* Immunophenotypic analysis of the TCR-Vbeta repertoire in 98 persistent expansions of CD3(+)/TCR-alphabeta (+) large granular lymphocytes: utility in assessing clonality and insights into the pathogenesis of the disease. *Am J Pathol* 2001;**159**:1861–8.

129. Langerak AW, van Den Beemd R, Wolvers-Tettero IL, *et al.* Molecular and flow cytometric analysis of the Vbeta repertoire for clonality assessment in mature TCRalphabeta T-cell proliferations. *Blood* 2001;**98**: 165–73.

130. O'Malley DP. T-cell large granular leukemia and related proliferations. *Am J Clin Pathol* 2007;**127**:850–9.

131. Hoffmann T, De Libero G, Colonna M, *et al.* Natural killer-type receptors for HLA class I antigens are clonally expressed in lymphoproliferative disorders of natural killer and T-cell type. *Br J Haematol* 2000;**110**: 525–36.

132. Morice WG, Kurtin PJ, Leibson PJ, *et al.* Demonstration of aberrant T-cell and natural killer-cell antigen expression in all cases of granular lymphocytic leukemia. *Br J Haematol* 2003;**120**:1026–36.

133. Lundell R, Hartung L, Hill S, *et al.* T-cell large granular lymphocyte leukemias have multiple phenotypic abnormalities involving pan-T-cell antigens and receptors for MHC molecules. *Am J Clin Pathol* 2005;**124**:937–46.

134. Gorczyca W, Weisberger J, Liu Z, *et al.* An approach to diagnosis of T-cell lymphoproliferative disorders by flow cytometry. *Cytometry* 2002;**50**:177–90.

135. Melenhorst JJ, Sorbara L, Kirby M, *et al.* Large granular lymphocyte leukemia is characterized by a clonal T-cell receptor rearrangement in both memory and effector CD8(+) lymphocyte populations. *Br J Haematol* 2001;**112**:189–94.

136. Melenhorst JJ, Eniafe R, Follmann D, *et al.* T-cell large granular lymphocyte leukemia is characterized by massive TCRBV-restricted clonal CD8 expansion and a generalized overexpression of the effector cell marker CD57. *Hematol J* 2003;**4**:18–25.

137. Wong KF, Chan JC, Liu HS, *et al.* Chromosomal abnormalities in T-cell large granular lymphocyte leukemia: report of two cases and review of the literature. *Br J Haematol* 2002;**116**: 598–600.

138. Man C, Au WY, Pang A, *et al.* Deletion 6q as a recurrent chromosomal aberration in T-cell large granular lymphocyte leukemia. *Cancer Genet Cytogenet* 2002;**139**:71–4.

139. Epling-Burnette PK, Painter JS, Chaurasia P, *et al.* Dysregulated NK receptor expression in patients with lymphoproliferative disease of granular lymphocytes. *Blood* 2004;**103**:3431–9.

140. Pascal V, Schleinitz N, Brunet C, *et al.* Comparative analysis of NK cell subset distribution in normal and lymphoproliferative disease of granular lymphocyte conditions. *Eur J Immunol* 2004;**34**:2930–40.

141. Zambello R, Falco M, Della Chiesa M, *et al.* Expression and function of KIR and natural cytotoxicity receptors in NK-type lymphoproliferative diseases of granular lymphocytes. *Blood* 2003;**102**:1797–805.

142. Dearden CE, Matutes E, Cazin B, *et al.* High remission rate in T-cell prolymphocytic leukemia with CAMPATH-1H. *Blood* 2001;**98**:1721–6.

143. Foucar K. Mature T-cell leukemias including T-prolymphocytic leukemia,

adult T-cell leukemia/lymphoma, and Sezary syndrome. *Am J Clin Pathol* 2007;**127**:496–510.

144. Herling M, Khoury JD, Washington LT, *et al.* A systematic approach to diagnosis of mature T-cell leukemias reveals heterogeneity among WHO categories. *Blood* 2004;**104**:328–35.

145. Moid F, Day E, Schneider MA, *et al.* An indolent case of T-prolymphocytic leukemia with t(3;22)(q21;q11.2) and elevated serum beta2-microglobulin. *Arch Pathol Lab Med* 2005;**129**:1164–7.

146. Soma L, Cornfield DB, Prager D, *et al.* Unusually indolent T-cell prolymphocytic leukemia associated with a complex karyotype: is this T-cell chronic lymphocytic leukemia? *Am J Hematol* 2002;**71**:224–6.

147. Chan WC, Hans CP. Genetic and molecular genetic studies in the diagnosis of T and NK cell neoplasia. *Hum Pathol* 2003;**34**:314–21.

148. Garand R, Goasguen J, Brizard A, *et al.* Indolent course as a relatively frequent presentation in T-prolymphocytic leukemia. Groupe Francais d'Hematologie Cellulaire. *Br J Haematol* 1998;**103**:488–94.

149. Hasserjian RP, Harris NL. NK-cell lymphomas and leukemias: a spectrum of tumors with variable manifestations and immunophenotype. *Am J Clin Pathol* 2007;**127**:860–8.

150. Chan JK. Natural killer cell neoplasms. *Anat Pathol* 1998;**3**:77–145.

151. Nakashima Y, Tagawa H, Suzuki R, *et al.* Genome-wide array-based comparative genomic hybridization of natural killer cell lymphoma/leukemia: different genomic alteration patterns of aggressive NK-cell leukemia and extranodal Nk/T-cell lymphoma, nasal type. *Genes Chromosomes Cancer* 2005;**44**: 247–55.

152. Uchiyama T, Yodoi J, Sagawa K, *et al.* Adult T-cell leukemia: clinical and hematologic features of 16 cases. *Blood* 1977;**50**:481–92.

153. Hinuma Y, Nagata K, Hanaoka M, *et al.* Adult T-cell leukemia: antigen in an ATL cell line and detection of antibodies to the antigen in human sera. *Proc Natl Acad Sci U S A* 1981;**78**: 6476–80.

154. Shimoyama M. Diagnostic criteria and classification of clinical subtypes of adult T-cell leukemia-lymphoma. A report from the Lymphoma Study Group (1984–87). *Br J Haematol* 1991;**79**:428–37.

155. Matutes E. Adult T-cell leukaemia/ lymphoma. *J Clin Pathol* 2007;**60**: 1373–7.

156. Karube K, Ohshima K, Tsuchiya T, *et al.* Expression of FoxP3, a key molecule in CD4CD25 regulatory T cells, in adult T-cell leukemia/ lymphoma cells. *Br J Haematol* 2004;**126**:81–4.

157. Matsubara Y, Hori T, Morita R, *et al.* Phenotypic and functional relationship between adult T-cell leukemia cells and regulatory T cells. *Leukemia* 2005;**19**:482–3.

158. Roncador G, Garcia JF, Garcia JF, *et al.* FOXP3, a selective marker for a subset of adult T-cell leukemia/ lymphoma. *Leukemia* 2005;**19**: 2247–53.

159. Karube K, Aoki R, Sugita Y, *et al.* The relationship of FOXP3 expression and clinicopathological characteristics in adult T-cell leukemia/lymphoma. *Mod Pathol* 2008;**21**:617–25.

160. Correlation of chromosome abnormalities with histologic and immunologic characteristics in non-Hodgkin's lymphoma and adult T cell leukemia-lymphoma. Fifth International Workshop on Chromosomes in Leukemia-Lymphoma. *Blood* 1987;**70**: 1554–64.

161. Datta A, Bellon M, Sinha-Datta U, *et al.* Persistent inhibition of telomerase reprograms adult T-cell leukemia to p53-dependent senescence. *Blood* 2006;**108**:1021–9.

162. Matutes E, Taylor GP, Cavenagh J, *et al.* Interferon alpha and zidovudine therapy in adult T-cell leukemia lymphoma: response and outcome in 15 patients. *Br J Haematol* 2001;**113**: 779–84.

163. Hermine O, Allard I, Levy V, *et al.* A prospective phase II clinical trial with the use of zidovudine and interferon-alpha in the acute and lymphoma forms of adult T-cell leukemia/lymphoma. *Hematol J* 2002;**3**:276–82.

164. Tsukasaki K, Tsushima H, Yamamura M, *et al.* Integration patterns of HTLV-I provirus in relation to the clinical course of ATL: frequent clonal change at crisis from indolent disease. *Blood* 1997;**89**:948–56.

165. Medeiros LJ, Elenitoba-Johnson KS. Anaplastic large cell lymphoma. *Am J Clin Pathol* 2007;**127**:707–22.

166. Pulford K, Lamant L, Morris SW, *et al.* Detection of anaplastic lymphoma kinase (ALK) and nucleolar protein nucleophosmin (NPM)-ALK proteins in normal and neoplastic cells with the monoclonal antibody ALK1. *Blood* 1997;**89**:1394–404.

167. Morris SW, Kirstein MN, Valentine MB, *et al.* Fusion of a kinase gene, ALK, to a nucleolar protein gene, NPM, in non-Hodgkin's lymphoma. *Science* 1994;**263**:1281–4.

168. Wlodarska I, De Wolf-Peeters C, Falini B, *et al.* The cryptic inv(2)(p23q35) defines a new molecular genetic subtype of ALK-positive anaplastic large-cell lymphoma. *Blood* 1998;**92**:2688–95.

169. Ma Z, Cools J, Marynen P, *et al.* Inv(2) (p23q35) in anaplastic large-cell lymphoma induces constitutive anaplastic lymphoma kinase (ALK) tyrosine kinase activation by fusion to ATIC, an enzyme involved in purine nucleotide biosynthesis. *Blood* 2000; **95**:2144–9.

170. Colleoni GW, Bridge JA, Garicochea B, *et al.* ATIC-ALK: a novel variant ALK gene fusion in anaplastic large cell lymphoma resulting from the recurrent cryptic chromosomal inversion, inv(2) (p23q35). *Am J Pathol* 2000;**156**:781–9.

171. Trinei M, Lanfrancone L, Campo E, *et al.* A new variant anaplastic lymphoma kinase (ALK)-fusion protein (ATIC-ALK) in a case of ALK-positive anaplastic large cell lymphoma. *Cancer Res* 2000;**60**:793–8.

172. Hernandez L, Pinyol M, Hernandez S, *et al.* TRK-fused gene (TFG) is a new partner of ALK in anaplastic large cell lymphoma producing two structurally different TFG-ALK translocations. *Blood* 1999;**94**:3265–8.

173. Rosenwald A, Ott G, Pulford K, *et al.* t(1;2)(q21;p23) and t(2;3)(p23;q21): two novel variant translocations of the t(2;5)(p23;q35) in anaplastic large cell lymphoma. *Blood* 1999; **94**:362–4.

174. Meech SJ, McGavran L, Odom LF, *et al.* Unusual childhood extramedullary hematologic malignancy with natural killer cell properties that contains tropomyosin 4–anaplastic lymphoma kinase gene fusion. *Blood* 2001;**98**:1209–16.

175. Tort F, Pinyol M, Pulford K, *et al.* Molecular characterization of a new ALK translocation involving moesin (MSN-ALK) in anaplastic large cell lymphoma. *Lab Invest* 2001;**81**:419–26.

176. Cools J, Wlodarska I, Somers R, *et al.* Identification of novel fusion partners of ALK, the anaplastic lymphoma kinase, in anaplastic large-cell lymphoma and inflammatory myofibroblastic tumor. *Genes Chromosomes Cancer* 2002;**34**:354–62.

177. Lamant L, Gascoyne RD, Duplantier MM, *et al.* Non-muscle myosin heavy chain (MYH9): a new partner fused to ALK in anaplastic large cell lymphoma. *Genes Chromosomes Cancer* 2003;**37**:427–32.

178. Lamant L, Meggetto F, al Saati T, *et al.* High incidence of the t(2;5)(p23;q35) translocation in anaplastic large cell lymphoma and its lack of detection in Hodgkin's disease. Comparison of cytogenetic analysis, reverse transcriptase-polymerase chain reaction, and P-80 immunostaining. *Blood* 1996;**87**: 284–91.

179. Lamant L, Dastugue N, Pulford K, *et al.* A new fusion gene TPM3-ALK in anaplastic large cell lymphoma created by a (1;2)(q25;p23) translocation. *Blood* 1999;**93**:3088–95.

180. Wilton SD, Eyre H, Akkari PA, *et al.* Assignment of the human a-tropomyosin gene TPM3 to 1q22–>q23 by fluorescence in situ hybridisation. *Cytogenet Cell Genet* 1995;**68**:122–4.

181. Mencinger M, Panagopoulos I, Andreasson P, *et al.* Characterization and chromosomal mapping of the human TFG gene involved in thyroid carcinoma. *Genomics* 1997;**41**:327–31.

182. Touriol C, Greenland C, Lamant L, *et al.* Further demonstration of the diversity of chromosomal changes involving 2p23 in ALK-positive lymphoma: 2 cases expressing ALK kinase fused to CLTCL (clathrin chain polypeptide-like). *Blood* 2000; **95**:3204–7.

183. Gascoyne RD, Lamant L, Martin-Subero JI, *et al.* ALK-positive diffuse large B-cell lymphoma is associated with Clathrin-ALK rearrangements: report of 6 cases. *Blood* 2003; **102**:2568–73.

184. Foss HD, Anagnostopoulos I, Araujo I, *et al.* Anaplastic large-cell lymphomas of T-cell and null-cell phenotype express cytotoxic molecules. *Blood* 1996;**88**:4005–11.

185. Salaverria I, Bea S, Lopez-Guillermo A, *et al.* Genomic profiling reveals different genetic aberrations in systemic ALK-positive and ALK-negative anaplastic large cell lymphomas. *Br J Haematol* 2008;**140**:516–26.

186. Zettl A, Rudiger T, Konrad MA, *et al.* Genomic profiling of peripheral T-cell lymphoma, unspecified, and anaplastic large T-cell lymphoma delineates novel recurrent chromosomal alterations. *Am J Pathol* 2004;**164**:1837–48.

187. Savage KJ, Harris NL, Vose JM, *et al.* ALK-negative anaplastic large-cell lymphoma (ALCL) is clinically and immunophenotypically different from both ALK-positive ALCL and peripheral T-cell lymphoma, not otherwise specified: report from the International Peripheral T-Cell Lymphoma Project. *Blood* 2008;**111**:5496–504.

188. Falini B, Pileri S, Zinzani PL, *et al.* ALK+ lymphoma: clinico-pathological findings and outcome. *Blood* 1999;**93**:2697–706.

189. Gascoyne RD, Aoun P, Wu D, *et al.* Prognostic significance of anaplastic lymphoma kinase (ALK) protein expression in adults with anaplastic large cell lymphoma. *Blood* 1999;**93**:3913–21.

190. Shiota M, Nakamura S, Ichinohasama R, *et al.* Anaplastic large cell lymphomas expressing the novel chimeric protein p80NPM/ALK: a distinct clinicopathologic entity. *Blood* 1995;**86**:1954–60.

191. ten Berge RL, Oudejans JJ, Ossenkoppele GJ, *et al.* ALK expression in extranodal anaplastic large cell lymphoma favours systemic disease with (primary) nodal involvement and a good prognosis and occurs before dissemination. *J Clin Pathol* 2000;**53**:445–50.

192. Sasaki K, Sugaya M, Fujita H, *et al.* A case of primary cutaneous anaplastic large cell lymphoma with variant anaplastic lymphoma kinase translocation. *Br J Dermatol* 2004;**150**:1202–7.

193. Willemze R, Kerl H, Sterry W, *et al.* EORTC classification for primary cutaneous lymphomas: a proposal from the Cutaneous Lymphoma Study Group of the European Organization for Research and Treatment of Cancer. *Blood* 1997;**90**:354–71.

194. Bonzheim I, Geissinger E, Roth S, *et al.* Anaplastic large cell lymphomas lack the expression of T-cell receptor molecules or molecules of proximal T-cell receptor signaling. *Blood* 2004;**104**:3358–60.

195. Admirand JH, Rassidakis GZ, Abruzzo LV, *et al.* Immunohistochemical detection of ZAP-70 in 341 cases of non-Hodgkin and Hodgkin lymphoma. *Mod Pathol* 2004;**17**:954–61.

196. Kinney MC, Jones D. Cutaneous T-cell and NK-cell lymphomas: the WHO-EORTC classification and the increasing recognition of specialized tumor types. *Am J Clin Pathol* 2007;**127**:670–86.

197. El Shabrawi-Caelen L, Kerl H, Cerroni L. Lymphomatoid papulosis: reappraisal of clinicopathologic presentation and classification into subtypes A, B, and C. *Arch Dermatol* 2004;**140**:441–7.

198. Willemze R, Beljaards RC. Spectrum of primary cutaneous CD30 (Ki-1)-positive lymphoproliferative disorders. A proposal for classification and guidelines for management and treatment. *J Am Acad Dermatol* 1993;**28**:973–80.

199. Willemze R, Jaffe ES, Burg G, *et al.* WHO-EORTC classification for cutaneous lymphomas. *Blood* 2005;**105**:3768–85.

200. Weiss LM, Wood GS, Trela M, *et al.* Clonal T-cell populations in lymphomatoid papulosis. Evidence of a lymphoproliferative origin for a clinically benign disease. *N Engl J Med* 1986;**315**:475–9.

201. Whittaker S, Smith N, Jones RR, *et al.* Analysis of beta, gamma, and delta T-cell receptor genes in lymphomatoid papulosis: cellular basis of two distinct histologic subsets. *J Invest Dermatol* 1991;**96**:786–91.

202. DeCoteau JF, Butmarc JR, Kinney MC, *et al.* The t(2;5) chromosomal translocation is not a common feature of primary cutaneous CD30+ lymphoproliferative disorders: comparison with anaplastic large-cell lymphoma of nodal origin. *Blood* 1996;**87**:3437–41.

203. Attygalle A, Al-Jehani R, Diss TC, *et al.* Neoplastic T cells in

angioimmunoblastic T-cell lymphoma express CD10. *Blood* 2002;**99**:627–33.

204. Grogg KL, Attygalle AD, Macon WR, *et al.* Angioimmunoblastic T-cell lymphoma: a neoplasm of germinal-center T-helper cells? *Blood* 2005;**106**:1501–2.

205. Grogg KL, Attygalle AD, Macon WR, *et al.* Expression of CXCL13, a chemokine highly upregulated in germinal center T-helper cells, distinguishes angioimmunoblastic T-cell lymphoma from peripheral T-cell lymphoma, unspecified. *Mod Pathol* 2006;**19**:1101–7.

206. Dupuis J, Boye K, Martin N, *et al.* Expression of CXCL13 by neoplastic cells in angioimmunoblastic T-cell lymphoma (AITL): a new diagnostic marker providing evidence that AITL derives from follicular helper T cells. *Am J Surg Pathol* 2006;**30**:490–4.

207. Piccaluga PP, Agostinelli C, Califano A, *et al.* Gene expression analysis of angioimmunoblastic lymphoma indicates derivation from T follicular helper cells and vascular endothelial growth factor deregulation. *Cancer Res* 2007;**67**:10 703–10.

208. de Leval L, Rickman DS, Thielen C, *et al.* The gene expression profile of nodal peripheral T-cell lymphoma demonstrates a molecular link between angioimmunoblastic T-cell lymphoma (AITL) and follicular helper T (TFH) cells. *Blood* 2007;**109**:4952–63.

209. de Leval L, Savilo E, Longtine J, *et al.* Peripheral T-cell lymphoma with follicular involvement and a CD4+/BCL6+ phenotype. *Am J Surg Pathol* 2001;**25**:395–400.

210. Iqbal J, Weisenburger DD, Greiner TC, *et al.* Molecular signatures to improve diagnosis in peripheral T-cell lymphoma and prognostication in angioimmunoblastic T-cell lymphoma. *Blood* 2010;**115**:1026–36.

211. Zettl A, deLeeuw R, Haralambieva E, *et al.* Enteropathy-type T-cell lymphoma. *Am J Clin Pathol* 2007;**127**:701–6.

212. Deleeuw RJ, Zettl A, Klinker E, *et al.* Whole-genome analysis and HLA genotyping of enteropathy-type T-cell lymphoma reveals 2 distinct lymphoma subtypes. *Gastroenterology* 2007;**132**:1902–11.

213. Zettl A, Ott G, Makulik A, *et al.* Chromosomal gains at 9q characterize enteropathy-type T-cell lymphoma. *Am J Pathol* 2002;**161**:1635–45.

214. Tsukasaki K, Krebs J, Nagai K, *et al.* Comparative genomic hybridization analysis in adult T-cell leukemia/lymphoma: correlation with clinical course. *Blood* 2001;**97**:3875–81.

215. Soulier J, Pierron G, Vecchione D, *et al.* A complex pattern of recurrent chromosomal losses and gains in T-cell prolymphocytic leukemia. *Genes Chromosomes Cancer* 2001;**31**:248–54.

216. Siu LL, Wong KF, Chan JK, *et al.* Comparative genomic hybridization analysis of natural killer cell lymphoma/leukemia. Recognition of consistent patterns of genetic alterations. *Am J Pathol* 1999;**155**:1419–25.

217. Arnulf B, Copie-Bergman C, Delfau-Larue MH, *et al.* Nonhepatosplenic gammadelta T-cell lymphoma: a subset of cytotoxic lymphomas with mucosal or skin localization. *Blood* 1998;**91**:1723–31.

218. Katoh A, Ohshima K, Kanda M, *et al.* Gastrointestinal T cell lymphoma: predominant cytotoxic phenotypes, including alpha/beta, gamma/delta T cell and natural killer cells. *Leuk Lymphoma* 2000;**39**:97–111.

219. Macon WR, Levy NB, Kurtin PJ, *et al.* Hepatosplenic alphabeta T-cell lymphomas: a report of 14 cases and comparison with hepatosplenic gammadelta T-cell lymphomas. *Am J Surg Pathol* 2001;**25**:285–96.

220. Weidmann E. Hepatosplenic T cell lymphoma. A review on 45 cases since the first report describing the disease as a distinct lymphoma entity in 1990. *Leukemia* 2000;**14**:991–7.

221. Belhadj K, Reyes F, Farcet JP, *et al.* Hepatosplenic gammadelta T-cell lymphoma is a rare clinicopathologic entity with poor outcome: report on a series of 21 patients. *Blood* 2003;**102**:4261–9.

222. Salhany KE, Macon WR, Choi JK, *et al.* Subcutaneous panniculitis-like T-cell lymphoma: clinicopathologic, immunophenotypic, and genotypic analysis of alpha/beta and gamma/delta subtypes. *Am J Surg Pathol* 1998;**22**:881–93.

223. Santucci M, Pimpinelli N, Massi D, *et al.* Cytotoxic/natural killer cell cutaneous lymphomas. Report of EORTC Cutaneous Lymphoma Task Force Workshop. *Cancer* 2003;**97**:610–27.

224. Hoque SR, Child FJ, Whittaker SJ, *et al.* Subcutaneous panniculitis-like T-cell lymphoma: a clinicopathological, immunophenotypic and molecular analysis of six patients. *Br J Dermatol* 2003;**148**:516–25.

225. Takeshita M, Imayama S, Oshiro Y, *et al.* Clinicopathologic analysis of 22 cases of subcutaneous panniculitis-like CD56- or CD56+ lymphoma and review of 44 other reported cases. *Am J Clin Pathol* 2004;**121**:408–16.

226. Sibaud V, Beylot-Barry M, Thiebaut R, *et al.* Bone marrow histopathologic and molecular staging in epidermotropic T-cell lymphomas. *Am J Clin Pathol* 2003;**119**:414–23.

227. Ponti R, Quaglino P, Novelli M, *et al.* T-cell receptor gamma gene rearrangement by multiplex polymerase chain reaction/heteroduplex analysis in patients with cutaneous T-cell lymphoma (mycosis fungoides/Sezary syndrome) and benign inflammatory disease: correlation with clinical, histological and immunophenotypical findings. *Br J Dermatol* 2005;**153**:565–73.

228. Wieselthier JS, Koh HK. Sezary syndrome: diagnosis, prognosis, and critical review of treatment options. *J Am Acad Dermatol* 1990;**22**:381–401.

229. Vonderheid EC, Bernengo MG, Burg G, *et al.* Update on erythrodermic cutaneous T-cell lymphoma: report of the International Society for Cutaneous Lymphomas. *J Am Acad Dermatol* 2002;**46**:95–106.

230. Yamanaka K, Clark R, Dowgiert R, *et al.* Expression of interleukin-18 and caspase-1 in cutaneous T-cell lymphoma. *Clin Cancer Res* 2006;**12**:376–82.

231. Vowels BR, Cassin M, Vonderheid EC, *et al.* Aberrant cytokine production by Sezary syndrome patients: cytokine secretion pattern resembles murine Th-2 cells. *J Invest Dermatol* 1992;**99**:90–4.

232. Vowels BR, Lessin SR, Cassin M, *et al.* Th-2 cytokine mRNA expression in skin in cutaneous T-cell lymphoma. *J Invest Dermatol* 1994;**103**:669–73.

233. Tracey L, Villuendas R, Dotor AM, *et al.* Mycosis fungoides shows concurrent deregulation of multiple genes involved in the TNF signaling

pathway: an expression profile study. *Blood* 2003;**102**:1042–50.

234. Kari L, Loboda A, Nebozhyn M, *et al.* Classification and prediction of survival in patients with the leukemic phase of cutaneous T cell lymphoma. *J Exp Med* 2003;**197**:1477–88.

235. Jones JF, Shurin S, Abramowsky C, *et al.* T-cell lymphomas containing Epstein-Barr viral DNA in patients with chronic Epstein-Barr virus infections. *N Engl J Med* 1988;**318**:733–41.

236. Kanegane H, Bhatia K, Gutierrez M, *et al.* A syndrome of peripheral blood T-cell infection with Epstein-Barr virus (EBV) followed by EBV-positive T-cell lymphoma. *Blood* 1998;**91**: 2085–91.

237. Quintanilla-Martinez L, Kumar S, Fend F, *et al.* Fulminant EBV(+) T-cell lymphoproliferative disorder following acute/chronic EBV infection: a distinct clinicopathologic syndrome. *Blood* 2000;**96**:443–51.

238. Braeuninger A, Kuppers R, Strickler JG, *et al.* Hodgkin and Reed-Sternberg cells in lymphocyte predominant Hodgkin disease represent clonal populations of germinal center-derived tumor B cells. *Proc Natl Acad Sci U S A* 1997;**94**: 9337–42.

239. Kanzler H, Kuppers R, Hansmann ML, *et al.* Hodgkin and Reed-Sternberg cells in Hodgkin's disease represent the outgrowth of a dominant tumor clone derived from (crippled) germinal center B cells. *J Exp Med* 1996;**184**: 1495–505.

240. Marafioti T, Hummel M, Foss HD, *et al.* Hodgkin and reed-sternberg cells represent an expansion of a single clone originating from a germinal center B-cell with functional immunoglobulin gene rearrangements but defective immunoglobulin transcription. *Blood* 2000;**95**:1443–50.

241. Muschen M, Rajewsky K, Brauninger A, *et al.* Rare occurrence of classical Hodgkin's disease as a T cell lymphoma. *J Exp Med* 2000;**191**: 387–94.

242. Seitz V, Hummel M, Marafioti T, *et al.* Detection of clonal T-cell receptor gamma-chain gene rearrangements in Reed-Sternberg cells of classic Hodgkin disease. *Blood* 2000;**95**:3020–4.

243. Skinnider BF, Mak TW. The role of cytokines in classical Hodgkin lymphoma. *Blood* 2002;**99**:4283–97.

244. Stein H, Marafioti T, Foss HD, *et al.* Down-regulation of BOB.1/OBF.1 and Oct2 in classical Hodgkin disease but not in lymphocyte predominant Hodgkin disease correlates with immunoglobulin transcription. *Blood* 2001;**97**:496–501.

245. Jundt F, Kley K, Anagnostopoulos I, *et al.* Loss of PU.1 expression is associated with defective immunoglobulin transcription in Hodgkin and Reed-Sternberg cells of classical Hodgkin disease. *Blood* 2002;**99**:3060–2.

246. Theil J, Laumen H, Marafioti T, *et al.* Defective octamer-dependent transcription is responsible for silenced immunoglobulin transcription in Reed-Sternberg cells. *Blood* 2001;**97**: 3191–6.

247. Re D, Muschen M, Ahmadi T, *et al.* Oct-2 and Bob-1 deficiency in Hodgkin and Reed Sternberg cells. *Cancer Res* 2001;**61**:2080–4.

248. Schwering I, Brauninger A, Klein U, *et al.* Loss of the B-lineage-specific gene expression program in Hodgkin and Reed-Sternberg cells of Hodgkin lymphoma. *Blood* 2003;**101**:1505–12.

249. Torlakovic E, Torlakovic G, Nguyen PL, *et al.* The value of anti-pax-5 immunostaining in routinely fixed and paraffin-embedded sections: a novel pan pre-B and B-cell marker. *Am J Surg Pathol* 2002;**26**:1343–50.

250. Bellas C, Santon A, Manzanal A, *et al.* Pathological, immunological, and molecular features of Hodgkin's disease associated with HIV infection. Comparison with ordinary Hodgkin's disease. *Am J Surg Pathol* 1996;**20**: 1520–4.

251. International collaboration on HIV and cancer. Highly active antiretroviral therapy and incidence of cancer in human immunodeficiency virus-infected adults. *J Natl Cancer Inst* 2000;**92**:1823–30.

252. Engels EA, Pfeiffer RM, Goedert JJ, *et al.* Trends in cancer risk among people with AIDS in the United States 1980–2002. *Aids* 2006;**20**:1645–54.

253. Clifford GM, Polesel J, Rickenbach M, *et al.* Cancer risk in the Swiss HIV Cohort Study: associations with immunodeficiency, smoking, and highly active antiretroviral therapy. *J Natl Cancer Inst* 2005;**97**: 425–32.

254. Engels EA, Biggar RJ, Hall HI, *et al.* Cancer risk in people infected with human immunodeficiency virus in the United States. *Int J Cancer* 2008;**123**:187–94.

255. Kraus MD, Haley J. Lymphocyte predominance Hodgkin's disease: the use of BCL6 and CD57 in diagnosis and differential diagnosis. *Am J Surg Pathol* 2000;**24**:1068–78.

256. Joos S, Menz CK, Wrobel G, *et al.* Classical Hodgkin lymphoma is characterized by recurrent copy number gains of the short arm of chromosome 2. *Blood* 2002;**99**: 1381–7.

257. Chui DT, Hammond D, Baird M, *et al.* Classical Hodgkin lymphoma is associated with frequent gains of 17q. *Genes Chromosomes Cancer* 2003;**38**:126–36.

258. Devilard E, Bertucci F, Trempat P, *et al.* Gene expression profiling defines molecular subtypes of classical Hodgkin's disease. *Oncogene* 2002;**21**:3095–102.

259. Chaperot L, Bendriss N, Manches O, *et al.* Identification of a leukemic counterpart of the plasmacytoid dendritic cells. *Blood* 2001;**97**:3210–17.

260. Petrella T, Comeau MR, Maynadie M, *et al.* 'Agranular CD4+ CD56+ hematodermic neoplasm' (blastic NK-cell lymphoma) originates from a population of CD56+ precursor cells related to plasmacytoid monocytes. *Am J Surg Pathol* 2002;**26**:852–62.

261. Urosevic M, Conrad C, Kamarashev J, *et al.* CD4+CD56+ hematodermic neoplasms bear a plasmacytoid dendritic cell phenotype. *Hum Pathol* 2005;**36**:1020–4.

262. Jacob MC, Chaperot L, Mossuz P, *et al.* CD4+ CD56+ lineage negative malignancies: a new entity developed from malignant early plasmacytoid dendritic cells. *Haematologica* 2003;**88**:941–55.

263. Grouard G, Rissoan MC, Filgueira L, *et al.* The enigmatic plasmacytoid T cells develop into dendritic cells with interleukin (IL)-3 and CD40-ligand. *J Exp Med* 1997;**185**: 1101–11.

264. Petrella T, Bagot M, Willemze R, *et al.* Blastic NK-cell lymphomas (agranular CD4+CD56+ hematodermic neoplasms): a review. *Am J Clin Pathol* 2005;**123**:662–75.

265. Herling M, Jones D. CD4+/CD56+ hematodermic tumor: the features of an evolving entity and its relationship to dendritic cells. *Am J Clin Pathol* 2007;**127**:687–700.

266. Dijkman R, van Doorn R, Szuhai K, *et al*. Gene-expression profiling and array-based CGH classify CD4+CD56+ hematodermic neoplasm and cutaneous myelomonocytic leukemia as distinct disease entities. *Blood* 2007;**109**:1720–7.

267. Leroux D, Mugneret F, Callanan M, *et al*. CD4(+), CD56(+) DC2 acute leukemia is characterized by recurrent clonal chromosomal changes affecting 6 major targets: a study of 21 cases by the Groupe Francais de Cytogenetique Hematologique. *Blood* 2002;**99**:4154–9.

Chapter 14

Molecular pathology of lymphoma

David J. Good and Randy D. Gascoyne

Introduction

The non-Hodgkin lymphomas (NHLs) encompass a wide spectrum of disorders with varying clinical and biologic features. The appropriate diagnosis and classification forms the basis of clinical patient management and the choice of treatment protocol. The diagnosis of lymphoma begins by a thorough evaluation of the histologic and cytologic features. However, this is often inadequate for accurate classification as there is often significant overlap between these entities. Immunophenotyping studies, either by flow cytometry or immunohistochemical staining, are often initially done to determine lineage and possibly clonality. Molecular techniques are of increasing practical importance as they provide an additional level of testing. This is particularly useful in cases where the histologic features or the immunophenotypic findings are not conclusive, or the biopsy is small, hampering an accurate assessment. As well, molecular testing can detect specific lymphomas that have distinctive molecular abnormalities. Figure 14.1 describes an algorithm, outlining how ancillary testing can be utilized in the diagnosis of lymphoma.

This chapter attempts to summarize the basic molecular biology, principles of the molecular techniques, common molecular aberrations, and the application of molecular diagnostics as a key ancillary tool in the diagnosis and classification of lymphoma.

IG and *TCR* gene rearrangements

Human lymphocytes have the ability to specifically recognize millions of different antigens and antigenic epitopes. This is based on the enormous diversity of their antigen-specific receptors, known as immunoglobulin (IG) and T-cell receptor (TCR) molecules.[1,2] Each single B or T lymphocyte has a distinct IG or TCR and expresses approximately 10^5 molecules with identical antigen specificity.

Many genetic mechanisms occur in order to generate the varied set of IG/TCR molecules to cope with a multitude of antigens. Combinatorial diversity, which is the result of different V(D)J combinations, is one of the first mechanisms. For the immunoglobulin heavy chain gene (*IGH*) complex, at least 40 functional variable (V) gene segments, 27 diversity (D) gene segments, and 6 joining (J) gene segments can be combined, resulting in approximately 6000 possible VH-DH-JH combinations.[3] Combining the heavy chain with the numerous V-J combinations of the *IGK* and *IGL* genes, an enormous number of combinations can be achieved. Similar combinatorial diversity can be achieved for the TCR molecules.

Junctional diversity is due to imprecise joining of V, D, and J gene segments. The exact positions at which the genes for the V and J or the V, D, and J segments are joined are not constant and imprecise DNA recombination can lead to changes in the nucleotides and subsequent amino acids at these junction sites. These changes can affect the antigen binding site as they occur in parts of the hypervariable region, where complementarity to the antigen is determined.

Insertional diversity results when small numbers of nucleotides are randomly inserted at the V-D and D-J junctions by the enzyme terminal deoxynucleotidyl transferase (TdT) without the need for a template.[4]

A further method for increasing the repertoire of Ig molecules is through the process of antigen-induced somatic hypermutations in the V(D)J exons of rearranged *IG* genes.[5,6] These are point mutations that occur in the B lymphocytes of secondary follicles and act to fine tune the immune response and increase the affinity of the antibody for its specific antigen.

IG/TCR rearrangements as clonal markers of lymphoid malignancies

Lymphoid malignancies are considered to be the malignant counterparts of normal lymphoid cells.[7] This provides a very beneficial tool for the detection of malignant populations. As with benign lymphoid cells, the majority of lymphoid malignancies also contain rearranged *IG* and/or *TCR* genes. What differs is that they are derived from a single malignantly transformed lymphoid cell and therefore all cells of the malignant population have identically rearranged *IG/TCR* genes. The presence of these clonal *IG/TCR* gene rearrangements

Management of Hematologic Malignancies, ed. Susan M. O'Brien, Julie M. Vose, and Hagop M. Kantarjian. Published by Cambridge University Press.

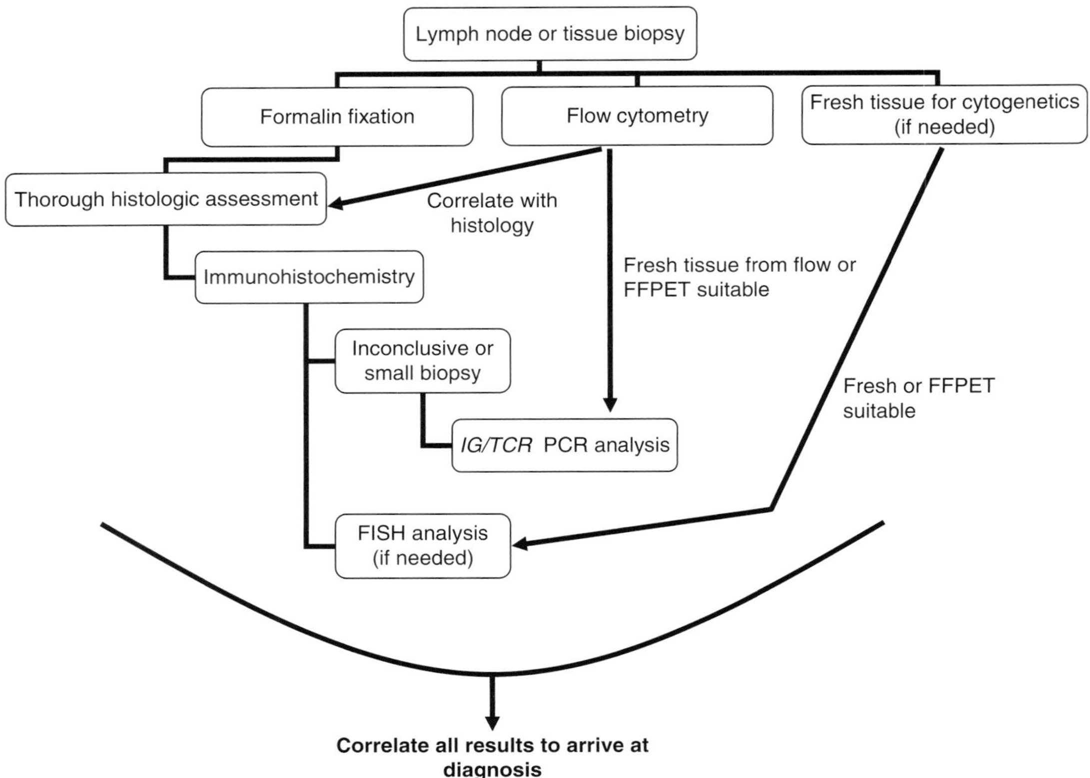

Figure 14.1 Diagnostic algorithm for lymphoma. This algorithm demonstrates the diagnostic pathway for lymphoma from tissue biopsies. There are some caveats to consider. Histologic assessment is still the gold standard so if size of the tissue is limited, the priority is formalin fixation. If sufficient tissue is available, a portion can be sent for flow cytometry and a portion to the cytogenetics laboratory. As well, remaining tissue from flow cytometry can be forwarded to cytogenetics. To save on labor and cost, the cytogenetics laboratory can culture and harvest the metaphases without proceeding to further cytogenetic analysis. The harvested sample can be maintained at 4 °C for months or can be stored indefinitely at −30 °C for analysis at a later date. *IGH/TCR* polymerase chain reaction (PCR) analysis can be performed either on fresh tissue or on formalin-fixed paraffin-embedded tissue (FFPET). If using fresh tissue, one needs to ensure that the tissue is representative as it may differ from what is seen in the paraffin sections, thus yielding a false-negative result. If using FFPET for fluorescence *in situ* hybridization (FISH) analysis, sections can be used and may be suitable for break-apart probes. However, nuclei can overlap and be sectioned through, making scoring difficult. Therefore, it is preferable, especially with colocalization probes, to core the area of interest on the paraffin block. This core can then be disaggregated to make a single cell suspension for FISH analysis. An important point to remember is that none of the ancillary tests should be interpreted in isolation. Correlation of all findings, especially with the histologic appearance, is needed to arrive at the correct diagnosis.

can be used to establish evidence of clonality by methods such as polymerase chain reaction (PCR).[8] (See Figures 14.2 and 14.3.) They also provide an identification target for molecular monitoring of patients during and after therapy.

Previously, detection of lymphoid clonality was largely based on Southern blot analysis of predominantly *IGH* genes. Partial D-J and complete V(D)J rearrangements can be detected and somatic hypermutation does not prevent detection of clonal rearrangements. Chromosomal translocations involving IG/TCR can also be detected. Technical restrictions have led to Southern analysis being replaced by PCR- and/or fluorescent *in situ* hybridization (FISH)-based strategies.

Methods for detection of clonality and chromosomal translocations

Conventional cytogenetics

Cytogenetic analysis has been a valuable tool for the understanding of acquired genetic changes that lead to lymphoma and continues to be a very effective means of surveying the entire genome. Being able to identify chromosomal translocations that are associated with specific subtypes of lymphoma has been the key to understanding how gene dysregulation is involved in the pathogenesis of lymphoma and other malignancies. Conventional cytogenetics was one of the earliest methods of detecting chromosomal changes. Its utility is often forgotten in the molecular era but can provide some very valuable information.

Cytogenetic studies of lymphoma are usually based on analyses of lymph node specimens but lymphoma cells can be cultured from any site, including bone marrow if it is involved.[9] Peripheral blood is generally the most appropriate sample for cytogenetic analysis of the chronic lymphoid leukemias. To achieve optimal results, a portion of lymph node should be transported in sterile tissue culture medium to the cytogenetics laboratory as soon as possible after excision.[9,10] Various methods are used to disaggregate the cells from the node to produce a single cell suspension, which is then added to culture medium. Some of the chronic B- and T-lymphoid

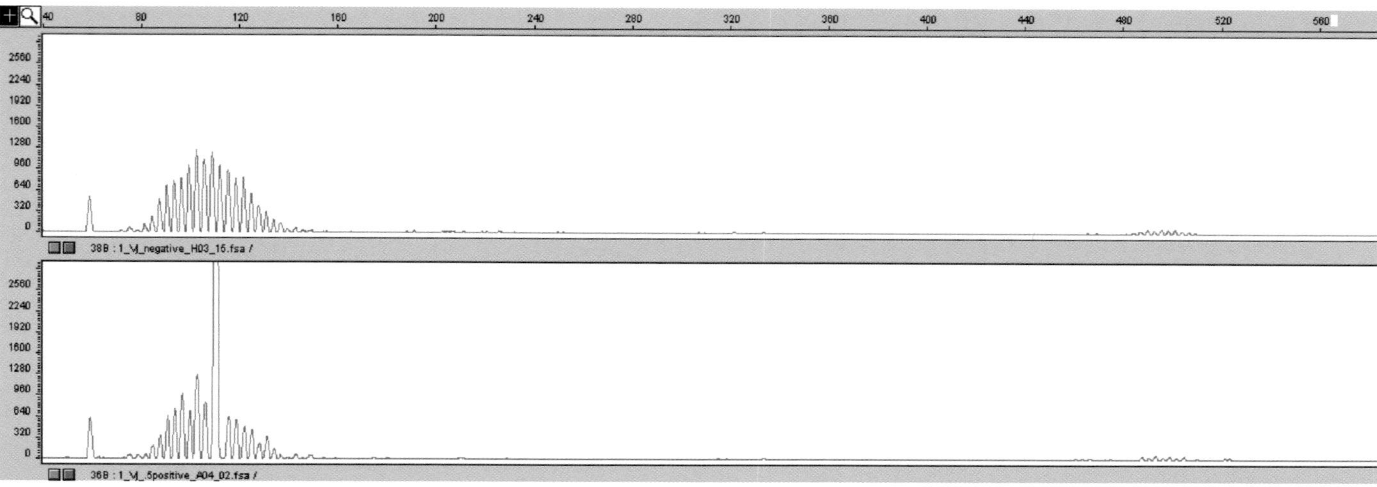

Figure 14.2 These images represent PCR analysis of the *IGH* gene locus. The amplification products are labeled with fluorescent dyes, allowing them to be detected using Genescan analysis. The top image represents a polyclonal population of B cells with *IGH* gene rearrangements of different sizes (vary between 70 and 140 bp), showing a typical bell-shaped distribution. Each spike represents one codon difference in the open reading frame. The bottom image shows a monoclonal peak, arising from a polyclonal background. Internal control DNA with the appropriate fragment size to the gene being analyzed is run with each sample (not shown) to ensure DNA amplification has occurred in order to correctly interpret results.

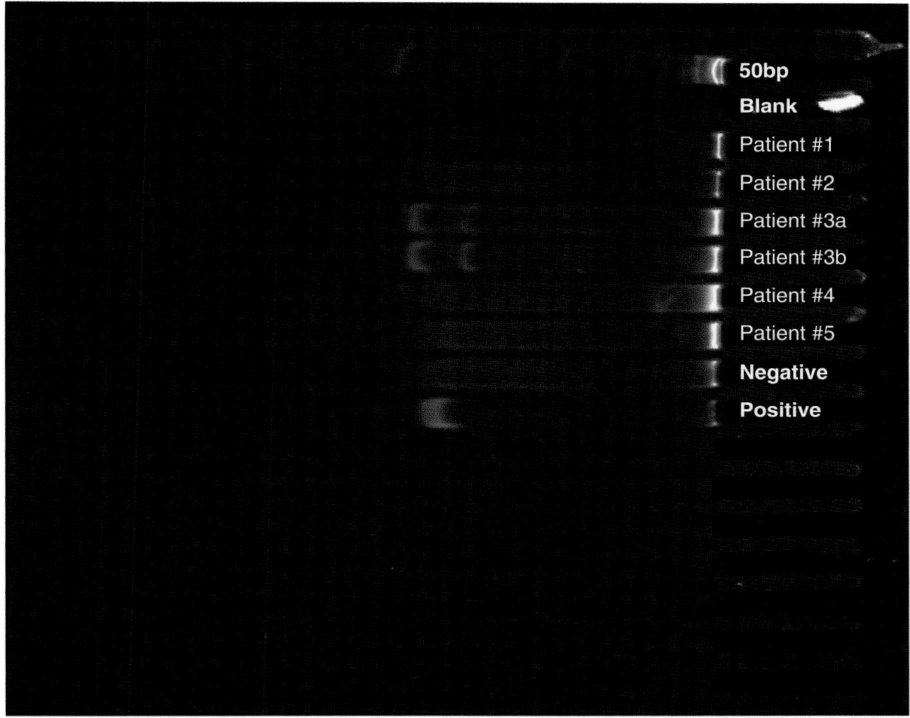

Figure 14.3 This image represents PCR analysis of the *TCR*- gene. The amplification products are subjected to electrophoresis to separate the different sized fragments. On the bottom is the 50 bp size ladder followed by a blank control (no DNA added). Positive and negative controls are seen on the top. Patient samples 3a and 3b represent positive results with distinct bands identified. The remaining patients are negative for monoclonal rearrangements with a smear present in the region of interest.

malignancies can be problematic for conventional cytogenetic analysis as these disorders tend to have low mitotic activity and usually do not respond well to most common mitogens, making it difficult to achieve high-quality metaphases. The development of FISH has allowed detection of numerical and structural abnormalities in the majority of cases, overcoming the inherent difficulties of conventional cytogenetic analysis in this group of disorders. Moreover, FISH techniques can be effectively applied to formalin-fixed paraffin-embedded tissues (FFPET), eliminating the need for fresh tissue.

Most lymphomas will have a dominant clone in which all metaphases will have the same or very similar chromosomal changes. Some metaphases will show additional changes that appear related to the original clone and are referred to as clonal evolution. In some cases, particularly in some forms of lymphoma and especially in clinically progressed disease, cell-to-cell variation may be extreme, making it very difficult to define a distinct clone. However, in most cases, a clonal karyotype can be defined when 20 or more metaphases are examined.

The primary cytogenetic alterations in lymphomas are typically balanced translocations that are closely associated with specific types of lymphoma (i.e., t(14;18) in follicular lymphoma)(see Table 14.1). Often, secondary alterations occur and may be whole chromosomal gains or losses, balanced translocations and inversions or unbalanced derivatives of these changes, and simple or complex deletions and duplications.

Southern blot

The knowledge that the majority of lymphomas contain monoclonal lymphoid populations was established using Southern blot (SB) analysis to detect *IGH* and *TCR* gene rearrangements.[11–13] However, SB has many disadvantages, limiting its utility in a routine clinical laboratory. It requires fresh tissue yielding large amounts of high-quality DNA, which essentially precludes the use of fixed material. SB has a turn-around time of several days and is a relatively expensive and labor-intensive procedure. It also involves the use of radioactive materials, although non-radioactive detection systems are available but are not as widely used. It also has a low analytical sensitivity, limiting its utility in lymphomas that have low numbers of monoclonal cells such as T-cell-rich B-cell lymphoma, and in minimal residual disease (MRD) detection and monitoring.[14] For these reasons, SB has now largely been replaced by polymerase chain reaction (PCR)-based techniques as the primary molecular diagnostic modality, but it still remains the gold standard in clonality testing especially in diagnostically difficult cases.[15,16]

Fluorescent *in situ* hybridization (FISH)

FISH is a valuable technique for the detection of both structural and numerical chromosomal abnormalities, down to the single cell and single gene level.[17] Labeled DNA probes are used that hybridize to chromosome-specific target sequences of interest. The probes employed are highly variable and include whole chromosome paints, centromeric probes, and locus-specific probes. The most common FISH methods used are metaphase and interphase FISH. These are very useful in detecting numerical chromosomal anomalies, by the use of centromeric probes, and for detecting translocations, by using single-, dual-, or triple-color probes.[17–19] They are particularly useful in detecting translocations having widely dispersed breakpoints (such as t(11;14) in mantle cell lymphoma and t(8;14) or variants in Burkitt lymphoma),[20–22] as FISH probes are typically large and can span in excess of 100 Kb of the genome. A disadvantage of metaphase FISH, similar to that of conventional cytogenetic analysis, is that viable cell suspensions are needed and it may be limited in low-grade lymphomas having a low proliferation rate, resulting in a lack of quality metaphases. As well, DNA in metaphase is highly condensed, leading to a relatively low resolution. For these reasons, interphase FISH is more commonly used as it can be used with air-dried smears, paraffin sections, and nuclei isolated from fresh or frozen tissue, or from paraffin sections.[18,21,23] It also has a higher resolution than metaphase FISH.[14] It is the method of choice to detect translocations where no reverse transcriptase-PCR (RT-PCR) assays are

Table 14.1. Molecular aberrations in B-cell and T-cell lymphomas

Lymphoma type	Molecular findings	Detection methods
FL	t(14;18)	- FISH - PCR less sensitive
MCL	t(11;14)	- FISH - Cyclin D1 expression by IHC
CLL/SLL	Trisomy 12 Deletions of 13q14, 11q22-q23, 6q21, 17p13 Rare t(14;19)	- FISH for common translocations - Cytogenetics
SMZL	del 7q31–32	- Cytogenetics and/ or array CGH
MALT	t(11;18), t(14;18), t(1;14), t(3;14), +3, other rare variants	- FISH - Cytogenetics
LPL	Del 6q and 13q	- Cytogenetics and/ or array CGH
Extranodal NK/T-cell lymphoma, nasal type	Gains of 2q, 15q, 17q, and 22q. Losses of 6q, 8p, 11q, 12q, and 13q	- Cytogenetics - Array CGH
PTCL, NOS	Gains of 7q22–31, 1q, 3p, 5p, and 8q2ter, losses of 6q22-q24 and 10p13pter, t(5;9) (q33;q22)	- Cytogenetics - Array CGH - FISH for t(5;9)
AILT	Trisomy 5, 21 and gains of 5q, 3q	- Cytogenetics - Array CGH
Systemic ALCL	t(2;5)(p23;q35) and variants	- ALK expression by IHC - FISH
EATL	Gain of 9q33-q34	- Cytogenetics and/ or array CGH

Notes: FL: follicular lymphoma; MCL: mantle cell lymphoma; CLL/SLL: chronic lymphocytic leukemia/small lymphocytic lymphoma; SMZL: splenic marginal zone lymphoma; MALT: mucosa-associated lymphoid tissue lymphoma; LPL: lymphoplasmacytic lymphoma; PTCL, NOS: peripheral T-cell lymphoma, not otherwise specified; AILT: angioimmunoblastic T-cell lymphoma; ALCL: anaplastic large cell lymphoma; EATL, enteropathy-associated T-cell lymphoma; IHC: immunohistochemistry; CGH: comparative genomic hybridization; ALK: anaplastic lymphoma kinase.

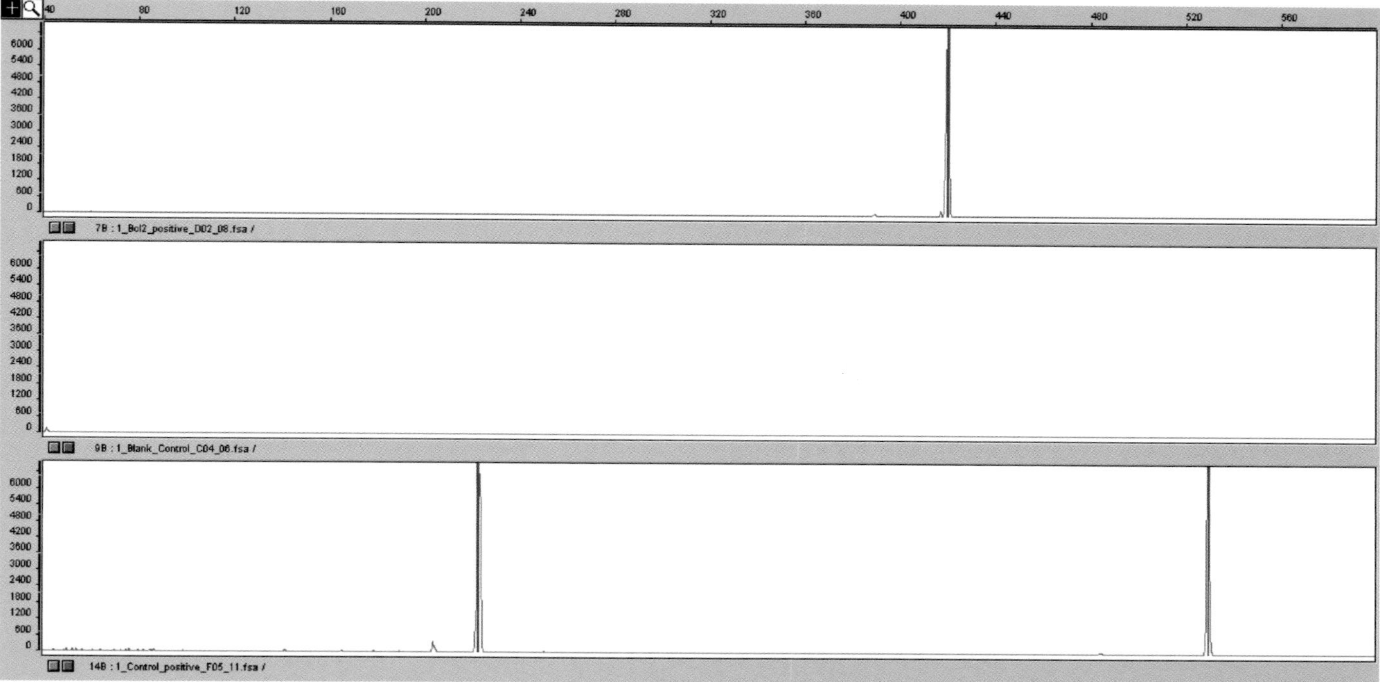

Figure 14.4 The above images represent PCR analysis of the *BCL2* gene. The top image shows a positive result (amplification product approximately 420 bp size) with the middle image showing a blank control. The bottom image shows internal control DNA of housekeeping genes, with the left peak (approximately 220 bp) serving as a control for the *IGH* gene PCR and the right peak (approximately 530 bp) a control for the *BCL2* gene amplification.

available, and where breakpoints are widely dispersed. One disadvantage of interphase FISH, especially in paraffin sections, is the overlapping, and also sectioning, of nuclei which makes it very difficult to accurately score. To circumvent this problem, the areas of interest in the paraffin section can be cored and the cells disaggregated to produce a single cell suspension that can then be spread on a slide. Cytospin and touch preparations can also be used if available. Two basic FISH strategies are used including colocalization and breakapart assays. Co-localization assays are less optimal because of reduced specificity that results from false-positive findings due to overlapping signals. Thus, breakapart assays are preferable. Two probes are used that span the region of interest (e.g., *BCL6*), each being labeled with a different fluorochrome. Any disruption of the genetic locus by a translocation will result in a separation of the fused signals and produces an easily identified split signal. This strategy can also be applied to tissue microarray slides and thus is highly advantageous for studying large numbers of cases.

Polymerase chain reaction (PCR)

As was previously discussed, PCR-based assays are now the preferred approach for the molecular diagnosis of lymphomas.[24–28] PCR is not routinely employed in every case but its utility is seen in cases in which a malignant diagnosis cannot be rendered after morphologic and immunohistochemical assessment. In many cases, PCR analysis enables a diagnosis to be made.[29] PCR assays may not detect all rearrangements demonstrable by SB or FISH,[30] but PCR has many advantages including rapid turn-around time, minimal tissue requirement, and less stringent DNA requirements allowing the use of FFPET. Its relative ease of use allows for automation and it may also be multiplexed, allowing for analysis of more than one chromosomal aberration. It is also much safer as radioactive materials are not required.

DNA-based PCR strategies are employed for the assessment of *IGH/TCR* gene rearrangements and for detecting some chromosomal translocations such as t(14;18), t(11;14), etc. (See Figure 14.4.) RT-PCR is used for detecting chromosome translocations resulting in novel gene fusions and is therefore used mainly in leukemia diagnosis and monitoring. Many different assays are available which vary in design, complexity, cost, and sensitivity. The choice of what type of assay to use depends on the DNA target being tested, and whether it is being used for primary diagnosis or for MRD detection. Each laboratory will need to optimize their assays for their particular needs but also need to be aware of the sensitivity and limitations of each assay being used.[31]

One of the significant advantages of PCR-based assays is the less stringent requirements for large amounts of high-quality DNA. Therefore many different specimens can be suitable for PCR studies. These include small tissue biopsies, fine needle aspiration biopsies, bone marrow aspirates, cells scraped from histologic or cytologic slides, and cells microdissected from tissue specimens.[25,32–37] As well, paraffin-embedded tissue can be used for many PCR assays, often with the sensitivity of clonal detection approaching that of fresh specimens.[38–40] There are many factors that can affect the sensitivity of clonal detection using fixed material. An important factor is the type of fixative with buffered formalin giving the best results.[41,42] Mercury-based fixatives such as B5 are not suitable. The average length of preserved and intact DNA will vary from case to case and institution to institution for FFPET, but on average is typically up to 300 basepairs in length. Thus, PCR strategies where the amplimer is smaller than this are often successfully amplified from paraffin material. Appropriate internal controls (housekeeping genes) are always run with each assay so that false-negative tests secondary to failed amplification of control genes are avoided.

In order to detect rearranged *IG/TCR* genes and chromosome aberrations by PCR, precise knowledge of the rearranged gene segments is needed in order to design appropriate primers. For *IG/TCR* genes, the ability to detect all different V, D, and J gene segments would require a significant number of different primers, which is not practical in routine molecular laboratories. Therefore, consensus primers have been designed, in an attempt to recognize all V and J gene segments of the locus under study. These are generally optimal for portions of the relevant gene segments but other portions show a lower homology. This can lead to false-negative results, particularly in *IG/TCR* genes with many different gene segments.

In the V-region of *IGH* gene segments, three framework regions (FRs) and two complementarity-determining regions (CDRs) are present. The FRs are very homologous among the various *VH* segments, whereas the CDRs are heterogeneous. As well, the CDRs are a site for somatic hypermutation in the germinal center reaction, further increasing the variability within these regions. FRs are usually less affected by somatic mutations but nucleotide substitutions may occur in these regions. Some PCR protocols use single *VH* consensus primers, which are able to bind to one of the three FR regions, mainly FR3. However, these consensus primers are not able to amplify all *VH* segments with the same efficiency. This is partly due to the above mentioned somatic mutations that can occur in FRs, preventing primer annealing and a resultant absence of amplification. Therefore, a significant number of clonal rearrangements cannot be detected by this method, resulting in a false-negative result. This is especially true for follicular lymphoma (FL) and some diffuse large B-cell lymphoma (DLBCL) cases, as these usually contain higher numbers of FR somatic mutations. An attempt to overcome this inherent problem is the addition of further primers to include the FR2 region as well. The European BIOMED-2 project has developed and standardized a multiplex PCR strategy, using multiple primers to detect clonally rearranged *IG* and *TCR* genes and the chromosome aberrations t(11;14) and t(14;18).[28] This has resulted in an extremely high detection rate, even in B-cell malignancies with an increased load of somatic mutations.

Other emerging methodologies

Newer techniques including multicolor FISH (M-FISH)[43] and spectral karyotyping (SKY)[44,45] allow for simultaneous evaluation of multiple targets. These methods rely on color-coded identification of all individual chromosomes within a metaphase spread. (See Figure 14.5.) They vary somewhat in methodology and in the way the signals are analyzed but essentially reveal the same information. M-FISH, and SKY in particular, have some advantages over conventional G-banding.[46] These techniques make it possible to detect otherwise inapparent or complex chromosomal rearrangements and translocations (typically hidden in marker chromosomes). They also have an advantage over conventional FISH in that it is not necessary to know which specific probes to use. M-FISH and SKY, however, do have some shortcomings as they are not sensitive enough to detect small intrachromosomal inversions, duplications, and deletions. As well the need for quality metaphases and the high cost are further drawbacks, making them impractical for routine clinical use at this time.

Comparative genomic hybridization (CGH) is a molecular cytogenetic technique that uses fluorescence-based hybridization to look for genome-wide DNA sequence copy number changes including losses, deletions, gains, and/or amplifications. This information can be gathered in a single hybridization experiment.[47] It cannot be used to detect balanced structural rearrangements such as inversions or translocations common to many lymphomas. However, it is a powerful research tool as it can detect unbalanced genomic alterations which might identify candidate genes involved in lymphoma pathogenesis. Classical CGH uses metaphase chromosomes for analysis but the resolution is limited due to condensation of metaphase DNA. This can now be overcome by hybridization to microarrays of cloned genomic DNA targets or oligonucleotides rather than chromosome metaphases, a technique known as array CGH.[48,49] This results in superior resolution and enables automated analysis.[50–52] The requirement for expensive equipment limits its utility in routine clinical laboratories.

Gene expression profiling or DNA microarray technology is a molecular technique that uses an ordered array of thousands of genes on a solid support. This allows for the simultaneous measurement of mRNA expression levels of each gene on the array, resulting in a profile of gene expression in the particular cell or tumor being analyzed.[53,54] It is beginning to help refine lymphoma subclassification at a molecular level and is able to identify genes of significance involved in pathogenesis and those predictive of clinical behavior. It can also yield valuable information in regards to devising novel targeted therapies.[55] At this point, gene expression profiling is largely a research tool. However, routine pathology laboratories can play an important part in harvesting and storing of fresh lymphoma tissue and normal blood/tissue control samples as these techniques currently require non-degraded mRNA.

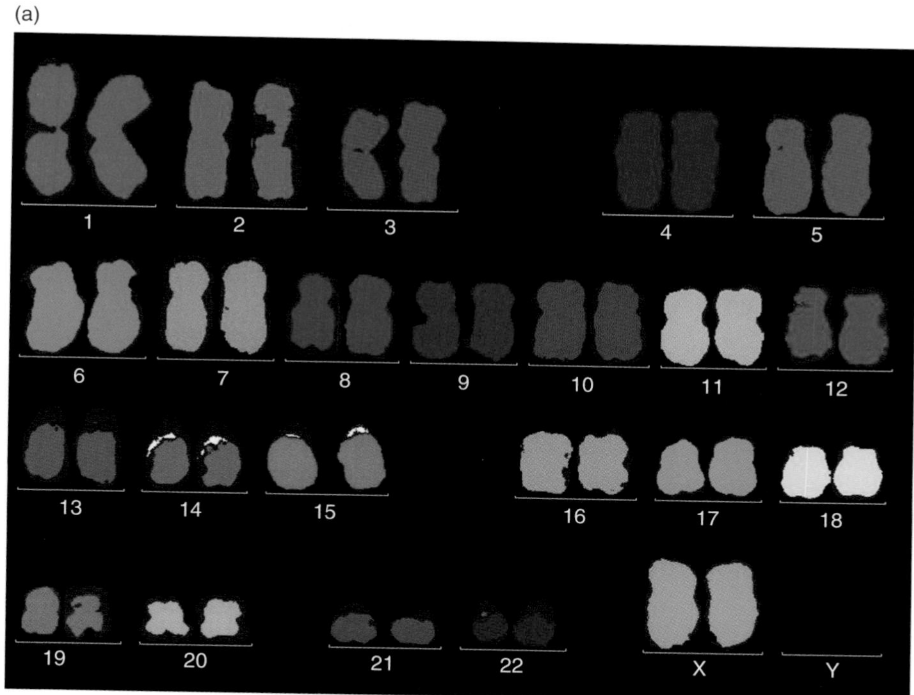

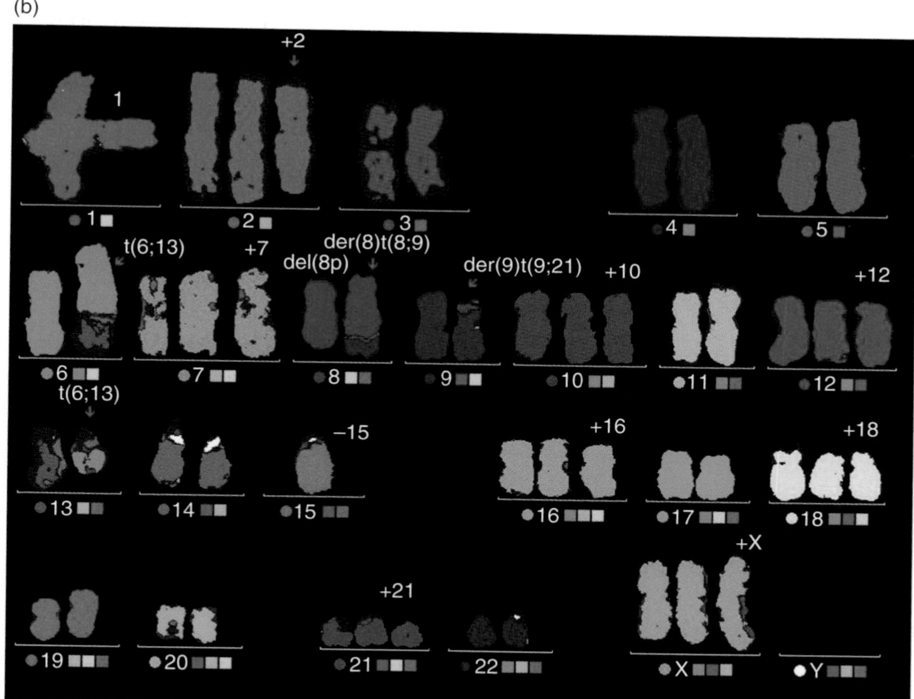

Figure 14.5 Multicolor FISH analysis. (a) A normal female karyotype. (b) A complex karyotype, demonstrating the utility of M-FISH in this situation to sort out the multitude of chromosomal aberrations present.

Molecular genetics of B-cell non-Hodgkin lymphomas

BCL2

The t(14;18)(q32;q21) cytogenetic abnormality was identified in the early 1980s with the translocation partners being cloned and identified by several groups.[56–58] It is a translocation that is present in 80–90% of FLs[59,60] and 10–20% of DLBCLs.[61–65] The translocation brings the *BCL2* gene on chromosome 18 under the control of the *IGH* gene enhancer element on chromosome 14. This results in expression of the BCL2 protein, which should normally be turned off in the majority of

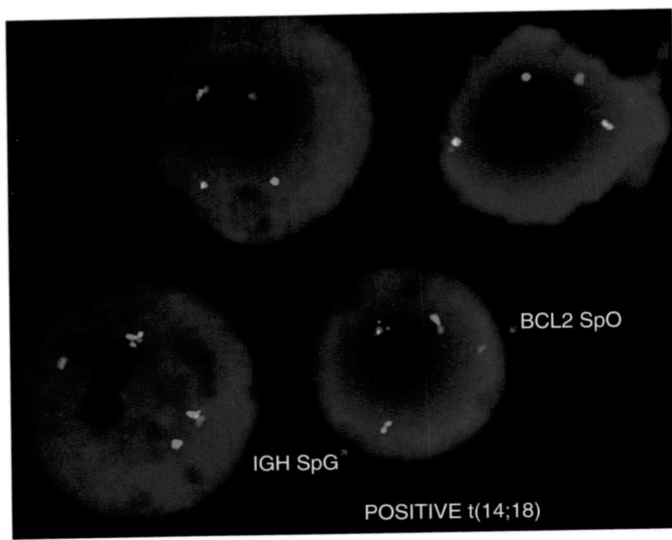

Figure 14.6 FISH analysis for t(14;18) using a colocalization assay. The red probe localizes to the *BCL2* gene on chromosome 18 with the green probe localizing to the *IGH* gene on chromosome 14. The presence of the translocation brings these probes together, resulting in a fusion (yellow) signal. A normal cell would have two red and two green signals.

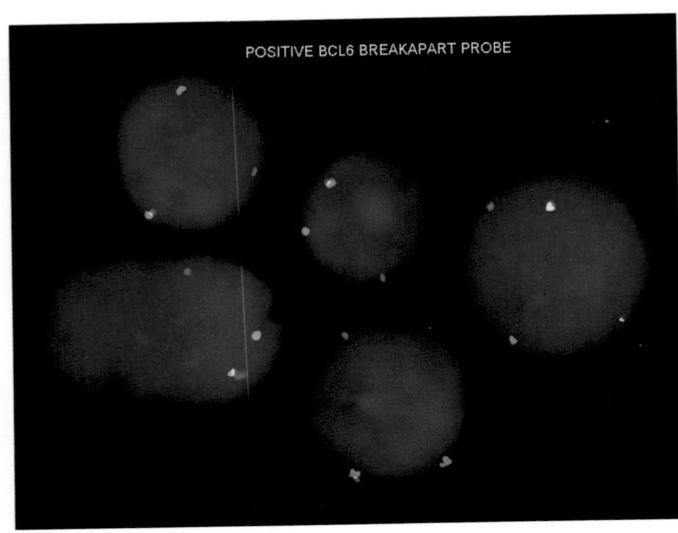

Figure 14.7 FISH analysis of the *BCL6* gene at chromosome 3q27, using a breakapart assay. Two probes, red and green, span the region of interest creating a yellow signal. A disruption of the genetic locus by a translocation is demonstrated by a separation of the probes resulting in distinct green and red signals.

germinal center B lymphocytes. BCL-2 is a potent antiapoptotic factor, giving the malignant cells a survival but not a proliferative advantage. Rare variant translocations can occur involving the immunoglobulin light chain genes and can be considered as biologic equivalents. These include t(2;18) bringing *BCL2* under the control of *IGK* and t(18;22) involving *IGL*. In approximately 10% of FL cases, BCL2 protein cannot be demonstrated by immunohistochemistry, raising the possibility of alternative antiapoptotic mechanisms.[66] Other B-cell lymphomas also demonstrate overexpression of BCL2.[67] However, this is a result of various other mechanisms for upregulation, rather than the classic t(14;18).

The breakpoints on chromosome 14 occur within the J-region of the *IGH* locus. Most breakpoints on chromosome 18 are clustered within a 150-bp segment at the 3′ untranslated end of exon 3 of *BCL2*, which is known as the major breakpoint region (MBR).[58] Additional breakpoints have also been identified approximately 20 Kb 3′ of the MBR in a region termed the minor cluster region (MCR).[68] Recently, several new breakpoints have been identified in an intermediate cluster region (ICR) in a large segment of DNA between the MBR and the MCR.[69] The ICR is now recognized to be more common than MCR breakpoints.[70]

PCR approaches can be used to detect t(14;18) using a primer 5′ to the MBR and a consensus J-region *IGH* primer. This approach is able to detect approximately 60–70% of rearrangements.[71–73] Primer sets that target the additional breakpoints can increase the detection rate.[70] FISH has proven to be more sensitive than PCR as it is capable of detecting breakpoints that lie outside the regions covered by the PCR strategy and because absolute sequence complementarity is not required.[74,75] (See Figure 14.6.) Conventional cytogenetics still provides the most complete documentation of karyotypic abnormalities found in FL. However, due to disadvantages including the requirement for fresh tissue and the low metaphase yield due to the indolent nature of low-grade NHLs, this technique is not always employed.

BCL6

The *BCL6* gene acts as a regulator and is involved in important cellular functions including cell cycle control, lymphocyte differentiation, and immune response through B-cell activation and inflammation. Its initial identification came about because of its involvement in chromosomal translocations affecting 3q27, present in a group of FL and DLBCL.[76,77] (See Figure 14.7.) *BCL6* expression is not exclusive to lymphocytes as its mRNA can be detected in different cell types,[78,79] but its protein product seems to be expressed at higher levels in lymphocytes. As a result, *BCL6* and its oncogenic properties have been studied primarily in the lymphoid system.

BCL6 is expressed by both B and T cells in the germinal center and is required for germinal center formation and T-cell-dependent antigen responses.[80] It is also found in scattered lymphocytes in the interfollicular area, and is also found in cortical thymocytes.[81–83] Due to the fact that BCL6 is expressed by germinal center B cells, it is useful as a marker for lymphomas that are derived from the germinal center. BCL6 is expressed in lymphomas that are thought to arise from follicle center cells, such as FL (almost 100%), Burkitt lymphoma (BL) (100%), a majority of DLBCLs (80%), and nodular lymphocyte predominant Hodgkin lymphoma (NLPHL) (80%).[81–83]

BCL6 is usually expressed in cells with a high proliferation index. Therefore, for the most part, it is not expressed by low-growth fraction lymphomas. The exception is FL where BCL6 is present in the proliferating cells of the germinal center and is downregulated in the interfollicular compartment, where the proliferation rate is also lower. In the case of NLPHL, the lymphocyt predominant (LP) or "popcorn" cells have a high proliferation rate and also demonstrate BCL6 expression.

BCL6 rearrangements (chromosomal translocations involving the *BCL6* 5′-noncoding region in 3q27) occur at a frequency of 20–40% in DLBCL and 6–14% in FL.[84] In contrast, rearrangements of *BCL6* (as well as those affecting *BCL2* or *MYC*) are very rare in primary mediastinal B-cell lymphoma, which suggests that this tumor is a separate type of DLBCL arising by different pathogenetic mechanisms.[85] These translocations contribute to *BCL6* deregulation. However, the level of BCL6 expression seems to depend on the partner involved in the translocation, as tumors in which *BCL6* is translocated to an *IG* locus express higher levels of BCL6 mRNA than those with non-*IG/BCL6* translocation, and also overexpression of BCL6 is often independent of chromosomal translocations.[86]

The *BCL6* gene is also altered by somatic hypermutation, analogous to *IGH* genes.[87,88] As these *BCL6* mutations occur in normal germinal center B cells, the same mutations are then present in tumors that are derived from germinal center or post-germinal center B cells.[89,90] Most of the mutations are present in the 5′ region in intron 1 although a second region in exon 1 is described.[89,91,92] Some of these mutations can lead to deregulated *BCL6* expression. These *BCL6* mutations are detected in 50–60% of all DLBCL cases.[88,90,93] The germinal center B-cell-like (GCB) subgroup and the primary mediastinal (PMBCL) subgroup of DLBCL have a higher frequency of mutated cases than the activated B-cell-like (ABC) subgroup.[93]

CCND1/cyclin D1

The t(11;14)(q13;q32) translocation that characterizes mantle cell lymphoma (MCL) juxtaposes the proto-oncogene *CCND1*, which encodes cyclin D1, at chromosome 11q13, to the *IG* heavy chain J-region at chromosome 14q32. This translocation results in over-expression of cyclin D1, which is not normally expressed in B lymphocytes. Cyclin D1 plays a key role in cell cycle regulation during the G1/S transition. Overexpression of cyclin D1 drives cellular proliferation.[94,95] This genetic alteration is thought to be the primary event in the pathogenesis of MCL. However, deregulation of cyclin D1 may also have oncogenic potential independently of its cell cycle regulatory function as it is known to participate in the regulation of several transcription factors and transcriptional coregulators.[96,97]

It was previously thought that t(11;14) was found occasionally in chronic lymphocytic leukemia (CLL), B-cell prolymphocytic leukemia (B-PLL), and in splenic B-cell marginal zone lymphoma (SMZL). However, with further studies, most of these cases represent morphologic variants of MCL, many being the blastoid variant.[98–100]

Two common methods for detecting t(11;14) are routinely employed in the laboratory. The simplest method is the use of an immunohistochemical stain for cyclin D1 in paraffin tissue sections. As was mentioned previously, normal B and T lymphocytes lack expression of cyclin D1. Therefore, positive nuclear staining of B cells with the correct histologic appearance confirms overexpression of the protein. The second method is FISH analysis for the translocation. (See Figure 14.8.) This is routinely performed on peripheral blood specimens but can also be performed on fresh or fixed tissue specimens. PCR has a limited role due to the very high false-positive rate.

t(11;18)/*API2-MALT1*

In most cases of extranodal marginal zone lymphoma of mucosa-associated lymphoid tissue (MALT lymphoma) with a detectable translocation, t(11;18) is the sole aberration.[101–103] As well, t(11;18) appears to be specifically associated with MALT lymphoma and has not been detected in nodal or splenic marginal zone B-cell lymphoma nor in other NHLs.[104–106] It has been reported very rarely in DLBCL, although they all appear to be a high-grade transformation from MALT lymphoma.[107,108] The translocation occurs at variable frequencies depending on the site where the MALT lymphoma arises. The highest frequencies appear in the lung (25–40%) and stomach (20–30%) with lower frequency in the conjunctiva and orbit.[109,110] It is also rarely found in transformed MALT lymphomas, as the presence of the translocation seems to denote cytogenetically stable disease not at risk to transform.[102,111] t(11;18) is not found in uncomplicated *Helicobactes pylori*-associated gastritis and is significantly associated with more advanced-stage gastric MALT lymphoma.[106] Of clinical importance, gastric MALT lymphomas with an associated t(11;18) do not respond to *H. pylori* eradication.[112–114]

This translocation causes a fusion of the *API2* gene on chromosome 11 with the *MALT1* gene on chromosome 18. API2 is believed to be an inhibitor of apoptosis whereas MALT1 is involved in the activation of the nuclear factor-kappa B(NF-κB) pathway. By themselves, neither wild-type API2 nor MALT1 are able to activate NF-κB but the fusion product can dimerize and activate this transcription factor.[115]

t(11;18) can be detected by RT-PCR but the breakpoints are extremely heterogeneous in both genes requiring a comprehensive primer strategy, limiting the clinical utility of this detection method. FISH analysis is currently the best clinical method for detection of this translocation.

t(8;14)/*C-MYC-IGH*

The defining feature of BL is a chromosomal translocation that involves a recombination between the *IG* heavy-chain locus and the *MYC* oncogene.[116–118] This translocation has been found in both Epstein–Barr virus (EBV)-positive and EBV-negative BL and in all variants of the disease. The classic t(8;14), combining the *MYC* gene on chromosome 8 with the *IGH* gene on chromosome 14, has been observed in nearly 85% of BL. Two variant chromosome translocations, t(2;8) and t(8;22) combining the *MYC* locus with the kappa light chain gene on chromosome 2 or the lambda light chain gene on chromosome 22, have been observed in approximately 10% of cases.[119,120] *MYC* translocations are not exclusive to BL as DLBCLs may also harbor this abnormality.[121–123]

(a)

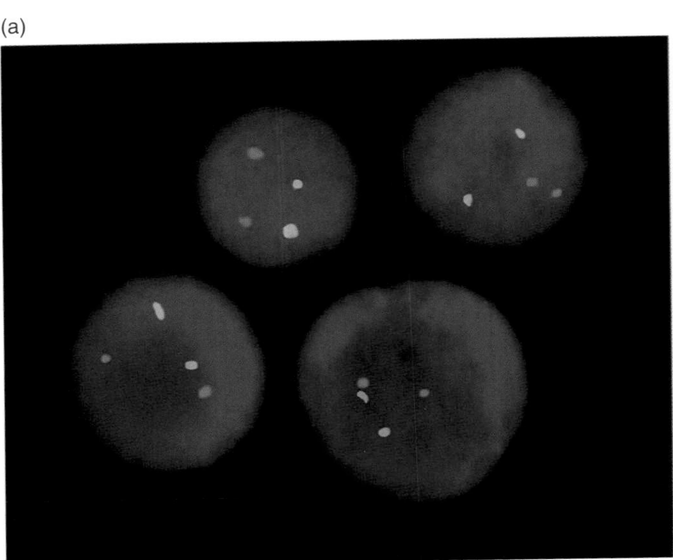

(b)

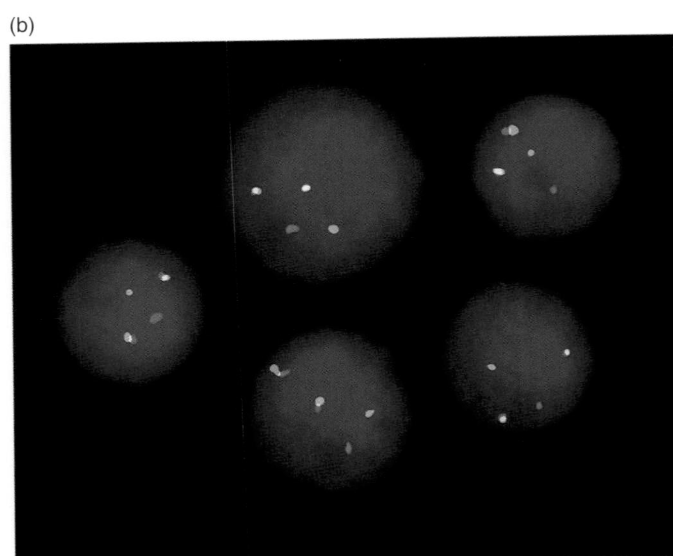

Figure 14.8 FISH analysis for t(11;14) using a colocalization assay. (a) A normal signal constellation with two red probes localizing to the two alleles of the *CCND1* gene on chromosome 11 and two green probes localizing to the *IGH* gene on chromosome 14. (b) A case with a t(11;14) translocation, resulting in a fused signal (yellow).

The chromosomal breakpoints in *MYC* differ and can assist in distinguishing endemic from sporadic variants.[124,125] Endemic variants have *MYC* breakpoints far upstream from the gene with the corresponding *IGH* break occurring in the J-region. This variant is also highly associated with EBV. In sporadic variants, the *MYC* break occurs immediately 5′ of the gene with the *IGH* break occurring in the heavy chain switch region, in keeping with a later stage in B-cell differentiation. No matter what breakpoints occur, the result is an overexpression of MYC, a transcription factor that regulates cell growth, cell proliferation, cell cycle, and apoptosis.[126] Normal expression of *MYC* is tightly regulated but translocations render the rearranged gene unable to respond normally to regulatory factors. The overexpression of Myc protein drives cells into S phase of the cell cycle leading to increased growth and proliferation of cells, hence the high proliferation rate in BL.

Standard DNA PCR methods are not practical for the detection of *MYC* translocations due to the large intervening DNA regions and lack of significant breakpoint clustering. Therefore, FISH analysis is the method of choice. FISH probes for t(8;14) span large segments of the *MYC* gene and the *IGH* region. Therefore, detection of the many different breakpoints in *MYC* is possible. As well, breakapart probes spanning the *MYC* gene are able to identify rearrangements arising from variant translocations. Often, probes for both t(8;14) and *MYC* breakapart are done so that a *MYC* rearrangement is not missed. There is some evidence in the literature that translocations of *MYC* that involve non-*IG* partners may result in slightly less aggressive disease.

Dual translocation lymphoma

A subgroup of NHL cases contain concurrent t(14;18) and *C-MYC* rearrangements and are termed dual translocation or "double hit" lymphomas.[127,128] One of the original descriptions of this dual translocation occurred in a patient with precursor B-cell acute lymphoblastic lymphoma.[129] In aggregate, these double-hit lymphomas/leukemias arise by one of two pathways; (1) following a diagnosis of antecedent FL or (2) *de novo* where all metaphases show both translocations.[130–132] The histologic features of these lymphomas are heterogeneous, with described cases mimicking DLBCL, atypical BL, so-called Burkitt-like lymphomas with features intermediate between BL and DLBCL (gray-zone), TdT+ lymphoblastic lymphoma, surface immunoglobulin-positive acute lymphoblastic leukemia, and rarely blastic or blastoid FL. The presence of a t(14;18) precludes a diagnosis of classic BL. Moreover, virtually all of the double-hit lymphomas strongly express BCL2 protein. This form of lymphoma should be considered whenever there is discordance between the morphology and the immunophenotype, particularly in patients with preexisting FL, or in *de novo* presentations of aggressive lymphomas when classification is difficult. Gene expression profiling data show that dual translocation lymphomas have a molecular signature different to that of BL and constitute a heterogeneous subgroup of high-grade lymphomas.[122,123] Many studies have concluded that patients with dual translocation lymphomas have an aggressive clinical presentation and a very poor prognosis.[127,128,130] This would be expected based on the molecular consequences of these two translocations.

Gene expression subgroups within DLBCL

DLBCL is a heterogeneous category of lymphoma with respect to morphology, phenotype, and molecular and clinical outcome. Gene expression profiling studies have been able to identify distinct molecular subgroups of DLBCL.[133–136] These three subgroups have been termed GCB, ABC, and PMBCL. These DLBCL

Table 14.2. Features of DLBCL subgroups

	GCB DLBCL	ABC DLBCL	PMBCL
Cell of origin	Germinal center B cell	Post-germinal center B cell	Asteroid B cell (thymic)
Clinical features	Typically older patients	Typically older patients > 60	Typically affects younger women
	Increased likelihood of bone marrow and extranodal involvement	Increased likelihood of bone marrow and extranodal involvement	Commonly bulky mass (> 10 cm) with local spread
	Favorable outcome 60% 5-yr OS in CHOP era, significantly improved with R-CHOP	Poorer performance status ECOG > 2	Distant spread and bone marrow involvement infrequent Favorable outcome, late relapses not seen
		Poor outcome – 35% 5-yr OS in CHOP era, improved with R-CHOP	
Chromosomal alterations	t(14;18)	t(3;14) and variants	Gains of 2p and 9p
	Gains of 12q13	Trisomy 3	Losses of 1p13.2 and 17p12
	MYC translocations	Gains of 3q	
		Gains of 18q21-q22	
		Deletion of 6q21-q22	
Oncogenic mechanisms	*BCL2* translocation	Constitutive NF-κB activation	Constitutive NF-κB activation
	Amplification of *c-rel* locus on chromosome 2p	*BLIMP1* inactivation	
		CARD11 activating mutations *SPIB* amplification	

Note: GCB DLBCL: germinal center B-cell-like diffuse large B-cell lymphoma; ABC DLBCL: activated B-cell-like diffuse large B-cell lymphoma; PMBCL: primary mediastinal B-cell lymphoma; OS: overall survival; CHOP: cyclophosphamide, doxorubicin, vincristine, and prednisone; R-CHOP: CHOP plus rituximab.

subgroups can be considered distinct entities as they originate from B cells at different stages of differentiation, have different oncogenic mechanisms, and differ in their survival rates and patterns of relapse following chemotherapy (see Table 14.2).

GCB DLBCLs demonstrate a gene expression profile that clusters with normal germinal center B cells, whereas ABC DLBCLs have downregulated these genes.[133,137] These genes not only encode for germinal center B-cell surface markers such as CD10 but also include various transcription factors and signaling molecules. ABC DLBCLs appear to be derived from a B cell that is in the process of differentiating from a germinal center B cell to a plasma cell as a number of genes that are characteristically expressed in plasma cells show higher expression in ABC DLBCL than GCB DLBCL.[137] However, these cells appear to be blocked from undergoing terminal plasma cell differentiation, as reflected by the oncogenic alterations that characterize a subset of ABC-type DLBCL. Previously, PMBCL was defined mainly by clinical criteria but gene expression profiling has shown a distinct molecular signature, allowing it to be differentiated from ABC and GCB DLBCL.[136,138] Of interest, over one-third of genes more highly expressed in PMBCL than other DLBCL subgroups are also found to be expressed in Hodgkin lymphoma cell lines.

These three subgroups have shown distinct differences in the frequency of certain recurrent translocations, chromosomal aberrations, and oncogenic signaling pathways, supporting the idea that these are distinct entities with differing pathogenic mechanisms. The t(14;18) translocation involving *BCL2* and amplification of the *c-rel* locus at 2p16 are present in a percentage of GCB DLBCL, but are not seen in ABC DLBCL.[134] Amplification of *c-rel* is also a feature of PMBCL. However, many ABC DLBCLs have high *BCL2* expression in the absence of t(14;18). A key difference between the subgroups is the activation of the NF-κB pathway, a pro-survival pathway. It is found to be constitutively activated in ABC DLBCL and PMBCL but not typically in GCB DLBCL.[136,138,139] The *BCL2* gene is an important target of NF-κB and thus the dominant mechanism leading to overexpression of BCL2 protein in ABC DLBCLs. An increase of *BCL2* copy number also underlies some of the increase in BCL2 expression and is mutually exclusive of the t(14;18).

Somatic hypermutation in B-cell lymphoma

As was mentioned previously, somatic hypermutation of the *IGHV* region occurs in the germinal center to increase the affinity of the antibody to its cognate antigen. The presence of these mutations suggests that the cell has been through the germinal center. This information has shed light on the cellular origin of many B-cell malignancies.[140] As well, the mutational status has been found to have prognostic implications in certain B-cell lymphomas. In CLL, those patients with CLL cells containing mutated *IGHV* genes have better prognosis than those with unmutated *IGHV* genes.[141,142] More recent studies have shown that MCL consists of two subsets, the majority of which have unmutated *IGHV* genes with a smaller subset (20–30% of cases) having mutated *IGHV* genes.[143–145] The presence of mutations suggests either exposure to a germinal center environment or alternatively, that somatic hypermutations have been acquired in a non-germinal context, possibly in the marginal zone. However, the data so far have been inconclusive as to the effect of mutational status on prognosis.

Molecular genetics of T-cell non-Hodgkin lymphomas

t(2;5)/*NPM/ALK*

The t(2;5)(p23;q35) genetic abnormality is a characteristic feature present in a subset of T-cell anaplastic large cell lymphoma (T-ALCL).[146,147] This translocation couples the nucleophosmin gene (*NPM*) on chromosome 5 with a tyrosine kinase gene designated anaplastic lymphoma kinase (*ALK*) on chromosome 2.[148,149] ALK is a signal transduction protein that is not expressed in normal lymphocytes. The gene fusion results in a chimeric protein leading to the constitutive expression of the ALK protein. ALK expression is detected in approximately 40–60% of ALCL tumors of T-cell or null-cell immunophenotype, or significantly more frequently if strict diagnostic criteria are applied.[150] In 80% of these cases, ALK expression results from t(2;5)(p23;q35) and results in a characteristic nuclear and cytoplasmic staining pattern. A large number of variant translocations occur where ALK is fused to other partners, typically resulting in unique staining patterns that differ from the t(2;5). Recent CGH analysis shows that ALK-positive ALCL cases have frequent secondary chromosomal imbalances, including losses of chromosome 4, 11q, and 13q, and gains of 7, 17p, and 17q.[151] ALK-negative ALCL cases have different secondary genetic alterations, suggesting that they are a different biologic entity.

Again, many methods are available for detecting *ALK* abnormalities. Likely the most information is provided by conventional cytogenetic analysis as it allows detection of the t(2;5) or any other translocation or inversion involving *ALK*.[152] As well, additional abnormalities can be detected if present. FISH analysis, using a dual-color/breakapart probe spanning the *ALK* breakpoint region at 2p23, can detect t(2;5) as well as other *ALK* translocation variants. However, the partner gene cannot be identified. Reverse-transcriptase or long-range PCR can be used but neither method will detect the variant translocations.[153] The most convenient method for detection of ALK overexpression is by immunohistochemical staining on paraffin sections.[154] A positive result by staining has similar meaning to a positive FISH result and is less laborious with faster turnaround time.

Other rarer T-cell chromosomal aberrations

The majority of T-cell lymphomas lack a recurrent defining translocation. However, some novel chromosomal translocations have been demonstrated in certain subtypes of T-cell lymphoma. t(5;9)(q33;q22) has been described in a small number of cases of peripheral T-cell lymphoma, not otherwise specified (PTCL, NOS). This results in the fusion of the *ITK* gene on chromosome 5 with the *SYK* gene on chromosome 9. SYK is a non-receptor protein kinase that serves as a key regulator of multiple biochemical signal transduction events.[155] This translocation leads to constitutive activation of the *SYK* gene. Cases of PTCL, NOS with t(5;9) have shown a characteristic follicular or perifollicular growth pattern.[156–158]

In enteropathy-associated T-cell lymphoma (EATL), numerous recurrent chromosomal gains and losses have been identified. However, the most common chromosomal alteration has been gain of 9q33-q34. The terminal part of 9q harbors many genes potentially involved in lymphomagenesis, which may be key in the pathogenesis of EATL. In one series, this alteration has been detected in 64% of 72 EATL cases studied.[159] Chromosomal gains on 9q33-q34 appear to characterize EATL and are only rarely detectable in other types of peripheral T-cell lymphomas.[160]

Molecular genetics common to B-cell and T-cell non-Hodgkin lymphoma

TP53

p53 is a transcription factor that regulates the cell cycle and functions as a tumor suppressor. *TP53* is located on chromosome 17 (17p13.1). p53 has many important functions including activation of DNA repair proteins, inhibition of the cell cycle at the G1/S regulation point until DNA damage can be repaired, and initiation of apoptosis if the DNA damage is irreparable. It also plays a role in the inhibition of angiogenesis. Mutations or deletions of the *TP53* gene lead to loss of the tumor suppressor function and loss of its regulatory effects. It is mutated in at least half of all human tumors and is frequently mutated in B-and T-cell lymphomas.

Mutations of the *TP53* gene and loss of heterozygosity in 17p are found in approximately 10–15% of CLL/SLL cases.[161,162] A higher frequency of p53 alterations is observed after transformation of CLL/SLL to Richter's syndrome,[161] suggesting that p53 may be involved in the genetic mechanisms underlying CLL/SLL progression. A subset of MCL has been shown to accumulate alterations in *TP53*, leading to the generation of blastoid variants characterized by higher proliferative activity and more aggressive clinical behavior.[163–165] Mutations of *TP53* are detected in 17–25% of cases of DLBCL[166–169] and 30–40% of BL cases.[161,170] This frequency is relatively low compared with other types of cancer but is still significantly higher than indolent lymphomas, supporting the hypothesis that p53 inactivation is one of the events leading to high-grade progression.

p53 overexpression is commonly present in some forms of T- or NK-cell lymphomas including anaplastic large cell lymphomas and, to a lesser extent, nodal peripheral T-cell lymphomas and nasal NK/T lymphomas.[171–173] However, mutations in *TP53* are rare and often a late event associated with tumor progression.

p16$^{\mathrm{INK4a}}$

p16^{INK4a} is a tumor suppressor gene located on 9p21 and is the most frequently altered locus in human cancer after *TP53*. The p16$^{\mathrm{INK4a}}$ protein associates with and inhibits cyclin/cyclin-dependent kinase (CDK) complexes, which promote the progression of the cell cycle.[174] p16$^{\mathrm{INK4a}}$ protein is present in reactive lymphoid tissue, with a slight increase in the germinal centers and interfollicular areas and a decrease in the mantle zone, which mainly consists of resting lymphocytes.[175] Indolent B-cell lymphomas display normal p16$^{\mathrm{INK4a}}$ expression whereas in more aggressive B-cell lymphomas, more than 50% show partial or total loss of expression of p16$^{\mathrm{INK4a}}$ protein.[166,176,177] This finding is often associated with alterations in the *p16^{INK4a}* gene, predominantly by 9p21 deletion/loss of heterozygosity or promoter hypermethylation. Point mutations of *p16^{INK4a}* are infrequent.

p16^{INK4a} inactivation appears to play a role in the transformation of lymphoma. The progression of FL to an aggressive large cell lymphoma is frequently accompanied by 9p21 deletions, often resulting in reduction or loss of p16$^{\mathrm{INK4a}}$ expression.[178] In MCL, *p16^{INK4a}* deletions are associated with aggressive variants.[179] In composite tumors comprised of an indolent and higher-grade component, the indolent component tends to express p16$^{\mathrm{INK4a}}$, but the larger transformed cells usually demonstrate loss of p16$^{\mathrm{INK4a}}$ expression.[175] Cutanteous T-cell lymphomas including mycosis fungoides (MF) and Sézary syndrome have relatively high frequencies of loss of p16$^{\mathrm{INK4a}}$ expression, again showing more frequent loss with progression from plaque to tumor stage in MF.[180–182]

Inactivation of *p16^{INK4a}* may also play a role in the development of Hodgkin lymphoma HL, as many Hodgkin lymphoma cases show selective loss of p16$^{\mathrm{INK4a}}$ expression by Reed–Sternberg (RS) cells.[183]

Practical application of molecular genetics

Differentiating between CLL and MCL

One of the common problems in lymphoma pathology is the differentiation between CLL and MCL in peripheral blood smears. The morphologic appearance can point towards a diagnosis but is not foolproof, partly due to the heterogeneity of CLL cells but also as a result of the blood smear preparation and the age of the blood specimen arriving at referral hospital laboratories. Typical CLL cells will reveal small mature lymphocytes with round nuclei, clumped chromatin, and scant amounts of cytoplasm. Occasional cases can show plasmacytoid features with more abundant cytoplasm. Most cases reveal at least some prolymphocytes, and thus are best described as dimorphic. MCL cells in the peripheral blood will typically show more heterogeneity than CLL. There may be some small lymphocytes resembling CLL cells but often there is a spectrum including larger cells with more irregular nuclei, slightly open chromatin, and occasional small nucleoli. Virtually all cases show some blast cells, a key distinguishing feature from CLL. Flow cytometric analysis can often aid in distinguishing between these two entities. Both will show coexpression of CD5 on the B cells but other antigens and intensity of expression for several antigens is unique. CLL will typically show dim expression of CD20 and surface light chains. These cells typically express CD23 and will be negative for FMC-7. CD11c expression is variable. MCL cells will typically show brighter expression of CD20 and surface light chains, and be positive for FMC-7 but negative for CD23. MCL is typically negative for CD11c. However, not all cases are straightforward and considerable overlap may be observed. The most definitive method for differentiating between these entities is FISH analysis for t(11;14), present in MCL but absent in CLL. One caveat is the potential for cyclin D1-negative MCL cases. The existence of such cases has been controversial in the past. However, gene expression profiling data has proven that this entity does exist and shows the typical gene expression signature of MCL.[184,185] Importantly, a confident diagnosis of cyclin D1-negative MCL would require gene expression profiling. Expression of either cyclin D2 or D3 would not suffice.

Nodal marginal zone lymphoma versus follicular lymphoma

There can often be difficulty in distinguishing cases of nodal marginal zone B-cell lymphomas (NMZL) from FL. Histologically, some NMZL can show a nodular pattern, similar to FL with enlarged, densely packed, malignant appearing follicles. However, the nodular pattern is a result of malignant marginal zone B cells moving into and colonizing the follicle as opposed to growth of malignant germinal center B cells in FL. The large cells that appear as centroblasts are in fact residual benign germinal center B cells, infiltrated by the marginal zone cells. These marginal zone B cells will lack CD10 and BCL6 expression by immunohistochemistry, helping to distinguish between these two entities in the majority of cases, but CD10/BCL6-negative FL cases do exist. As well, many NMZL will demonstrate overexpression of the BCL2 protein, again mimicking FL by immunohistochemistry as the follicles will be positive. FISH analysis for the presence of t(14;18) is therefore invaluable in these cases as 80% to 90% of FL cases will be positive for this translocation.

MALT lymphoma with t(14;18) versus FL

In rare cases of MALT lymphoma, mainly involving liver, lung, or ocular adnexa, a t(14;18) translocation is found.[186,187] The translocation occurs at band 18q21 as in FL, but it is the *MALT1* gene rather than *BCL2* that is subsequently juxtaposed to the *IGH* gene on 14q32. By conventional cytogenetic analysis, the t(14;18) in FL and in MALT cannot be distinguished. As the translocation in FL is much more frequent, an incorrect diagnosis could be made on a case of MALT with t(14;18). This problem can be overcome by FISH analysis. As the *MALT1* gene is 500 kb centromeric of *BCL2*, specific probes for the *BCL2* locus and the *MALT1* locus can be used to distinguish which gene is involved in the translocation.

Limitations of molecular diagnostics in lymphoma

As with any diagnostic test, the clinician and pathologist must realize the limitations of the test and its interpretation. PCR is a very sensitive test able to detect DNA abnormalities present at very low levels. However, these results must never be interpreted in isolation. Due to the enhanced sensitivity of PCR, there is a high risk of false positives, as a tiny amount of carryover from a positive sample can render a negative sample positive. However, good laboratory practice should have procedures in place to minimize the risk of contamination. Other types of false positives are difficult to control for. Otherwise normal individuals may have a small number of cells that carry translocations such as t(14;18).[188] Most individuals carrying these *BCL2* gene rearrangements do not have FL and even fewer go on to develop it. These assays can be set up so as to be used preferentially for diagnosis by avoiding the pitfalls of nested PCR strategies that utilize many rounds of amplification. It is these latter approaches that run the risk of false-positive results.

When looking at *IGH* or *TCR* rearrangements by PCR, a monoclonal population is not always synonymous with malignancy. Clones of lymphoid cells have been detected by PCR analysis in individuals without evidence of malignancy, including congenital immune deficiency disorders, autoimmune diseases, in the setting of iatrogenic immunosuppression following organ transplantation, and in acquired immunodeficiency syndrome (AIDS).[189] The distinction between a reactive versus a malignant condition is often difficult in these cases as many of these conditions predispose to development of lymphoma. Another frequent problem encountered, especially with small biopsies and biopsies with limited amounts of lymphoid tissue, is false-positive results due to limiting DNA template. The high sensitivity of PCR can cause the amplification of the few *IG* or *TCR* gene rearrangements derived from the limited number of B or T cells in the tissue sample analyzed, leading to an apparent monoclonal population. Therefore the results of molecular analysis must always be correlated in the laboratory with the histologic appearance of the tissue or the morphology of the blood smear and clinically with the patient's symptoms and clinical findings.

References

1. Davis MM, Bjorkman PJ. T-cell antigen receptor genes and T-cell recognition. *Nature* 1988;**334**(6181):395–402.
2. Borst J, Brouns GS, de Vries E, *et al.* Antigen receptors on T and B lymphocytes: parallels in organization and function. *Immunol Rev* 1993;**132**:49–84.
3. Lefranc MP. IMGT databases, web resources and tools for immunoglobulin and T cell receptor sequence analysis, http://imgt.cines.fr. *Leukemia* 2003;**17**(1):260–6.
4. Desiderio SV, Yancopoulos GD, Paskind M, *et al.* Insertion of N regions into heavy-chain genes is correlated with expression of terminal deoxytransferase in B cells. *Nature* 1984;**311**(5988):752–5.
5. Berek C, Milstein C. Mutation drift and repertoire shift in the maturation of the immune response. *Immunol Rev* 1987;**96**:23–41.
6. Rajewsky K, Forster I, Cumano A. Evolutionary and somatic selection of the antibody repertoire in the mouse. *Science* 1987;**238**(4830):1088–94.
7. Greaves MF. Differentiation-linked leukemogenesis in lymphocytes. *Science* 1986;**234**(4777):697–704.
8. van Dongen JJ, Wolvers-Tettero IL. Analysis of immunoglobulin and T cell receptor genes. Part II: Possibilities and limitations in the diagnosis and management of lymphoproliferative diseases and related disorders. *Clin Chim Acta* 1991;**198**(1–2):93–174.
9. Campbell LJ. Cytogenetics of lymphomas. *Pathology* 2005;**37**(6):493–507.
10. Juneja S, Lukeis R, Tan L, *et al.* Cytogenetic analysis of 147 cases of non-Hodgkin's lymphoma: non-random chromosomal abnormalities and histological correlations. *Br J Haematol* 1990;**76**(2):231–7.
11. Cleary ML, Chao J, Warnke R, *et al.* Immunoglobulin gene rearrangement as a diagnostic criterion of B-cell lymphoma. *Proc Natl Acad Sci U S A* 1984;**81**(2):593–7.
12. Korsmeyer SJ, Waldmann TA. Immunoglobulin genes: rearrangement and translocation in human lymphoid malignancy. *J Clin Immunol* 1984;**4**(1):1–11.
13. Toyonaga B, Mak TW. Genes of the T-cell antigen receptor in normal and malignant T cells. *Annu Rev Immunol* 1987;**5**:585–620.
14. Spagnolo DV, Ellis DW, Juneja S, *et al.* The role of molecular studies in lymphoma diagnosis: a review. *Pathology* 2004;**36**(1):19–44.
15. Rockman SP. Determination of clonality in patients who present with diagnostic dilemmas: a laboratory experience and review of the literature. *Leukemia* 1997;**11**(6):852–62.
16. Kamat D, Laszewski MJ, Kemp JD, *et al.* The diagnostic utility of immunophenotyping and immunogenotyping in the pathologic evaluation of lymphoid proliferations. *Mod Pathol* 1990;**3**(2):105–12.
17. Kearney L. The impact of the new FISH technologies on the cytogenetics of

haematological malignancies. *Br J Haematol* 1999;**104**(4):648–58.

18. Vaandrager JW, Schuuring E, Raap T, *et al.* Interphase FISH detection of BCL2 rearrangement in follicular lymphoma using breakpoint-flanking probes. *Genes Chromosomes Cancer* 2000;**27**(1):85–94.
19. Frater JL, Tsiftsakis EK, Hsi ED, *et al.* Use of novel t(11;14) and t(14;18) dual-fusion fluorescence in situ hybridization probes in the differential diagnosis of lymphomas of small lymphocytes. *Diagn Mol Pathol* 2001;**10** (4):214–22.
20. Haralambieva E, Kleiverda K, Mason DY, *et al.* Detection of three common translocation breakpoints in non-Hodgkin's lymphomas by fluorescence in situ hybridization on routine paraffin-embedded tissue sections. *J Pathol* 2002;**198**(2):163–70.
21. Paternoster SF, Brockman SR, McClure RF, *et al.* A new method to extract nuclei from paraffin-embedded tissue to study lymphomas using interphase fluorescence in situ hybridization. *Am J Pathol* 2002;**160**(6):1967–72.
22. Martin-Subero JI, Harder L, Gesk S, *et al.* Interphase FISH assays for the detection of translocations with breakpoints in immunoglobulin light chain loci. *Int J Cancer* 2002; **98**(3):470–4.
23. Sanchez-Izquierdo D, Siebert R, Harder L, *et al.* Detection of translocations affecting the BCL6 locus in B cell non-Hodgkin's lymphoma by interphase fluorescence in situ hybridization. *Leukemia* 2001;**15** (9):1475–84.
24. Arber DA. Molecular diagnostic approach to non-Hodgkin's lymphoma. *J Mol Diagn* 2000;**2**(4):178–90.
25. Pan LX, Diss TC, Isaacson PG. The polymerase chain reaction in histopathology. *Histopathology* 1995;**26** (3):201–17.
26. Segal GH, Hussey CE, Wittwer CT. PCR for T-cell rearrangements. *Diagn Mol Pathol* 1996;**5**(4):297–8.
27. Cairns SM, Taylor JM, Gould PR, *et al.* Comparative evaluation of PCR-based methods for the assessment of T cell clonality in the diagnosis of T cell lymphoma. *Pathology* 2002; **34**(4):320–5.
28. van Dongen JJ, Langerak AW, Bruggemann M, *et al.* Design and standardization of PCR primers and protocols for detection of clonal immunoglobulin and T-cell receptor gene recombinations in suspect lymphoproliferations: report of the BIOMED-2 Concerted Action BMH4-CT98–3936. *Leukemia* 2003; **17**(12):2257–317.
29. Theriault C, Galoin S, Valmary S, *et al.* PCR analysis of immunoglobulin heavy chain (IgH) and TcR-gamma chain gene rearrangements in the diagnosis of lymphoproliferative disorders: results of a study of 525 cases. *Mod Pathol* 2000;**13**(12):1269–79.
30. Krafft AE, Taubenberger JK, Sheng ZM, *et al.* Enhanced sensitivity with a novel TCRgamma PCR assay for clonality studies in 569 formalin-fixed, paraffin-embedded (FFPE) cases. *Mol Diagn* 1999;**4**(2):119–33.
31. Hoeve MA, Krol AD, Philippo K, *et al.* Limitations of clonality analysis of B cell proliferations using CDR3 polymerase chain reaction. *Mol Pathol* 2000;**53**(4):194–200.
32. Inagaki H, Nonaka M, Nagaya S, *et al.* Monoclonality in gastric lymphoma detected in formalin-fixed, paraffin-embedded endoscopic biopsy specimens using immunohistochemistry, in situ hybridization, and polymerase chain reaction. *Diagn Mol Pathol* 1995;**4** (1):32–8.
33. Wan JH, Sykes PJ, Orell SR, *et al.* Rapid method for detecting monoclonality in B cell lymphoma in lymph node aspirates using the polymerase chain reaction. *J Clin Pathol* 1992; **45**(5):420–3.
34. Chen YT, Mercer GO, Chen Y. Polymerase chain reaction-based detection of B-cell monoclonality in cytologic specimens. *Arch Pathol Lab Med* 1993;**117**(11):1099–103.
35. Sukpanichnant S, Vnencak-Jones CL, McCurley TL. Detection of clonal immunoglobulin heavy chain gene rearrangements by polymerase chain reaction in scrapings from archival hematoxylin and eosin-stained histologic sections: implications for molecular genetic studies of focal pathologic lesions. *Diagn Mol Pathol* 1993;**2**(3):168–76.
36. Alkan S, Lehman C, Sarago C, *et al.* Polymerase chain reaction detection of immunoglobulin gene rearrangement and bcl-2 translocation in archival glass slides of cytologic material. *Diagn Mol Pathol* 1995;**4**(1):25–31.
37. Pan LX, Diss TC, Peng HZ, *et al.* Clonality analysis of defined B-cell populations in archival tissue sections using microdissection and the polymerase chain reaction. *Histopathology* 1994;**24**(4):323–7.
38. Wan JH, Trainor KJ, Brisco MJ, *et al.* Monoclonality in B cell lymphoma detected in paraffin wax embedded sections using the polymerase chain reaction. *J Clin Pathol* 1990; **43**(11):888–90.
39. Reed TJ, Reid A, Wallberg K, *et al.* Determination of B-cell clonality in paraffin-embedded lymph nodes using the polymerase chain reaction. *Diagn Mol Pathol* 1993;**2**(1):42–9.
40. Chen YT, Whitney KD, Chen Y. Clonality analysis of B-cell lymphoma in fresh-frozen and paraffin-embedded tissues: the effects of variable polymerase chain reaction parameters. *Mod Pathol* 1994;**7**(4):429–34.
41. Greer CE, Lund JK, Manos MM. PCR amplification from paraffin-embedded tissues: recommendations on fixatives for long-term storage and prospective studies. *PCR Methods Appl* 1991;**1**(1):46–50.
42. Greer CE, Peterson SL, Kiviat NB, *et al.* PCR amplification from paraffin-embedded tissues. Effects of fixative and fixation time. *Am J Clin Pathol* 1991;**95** (2):117–24.
43. Speicher MR, Gwyn Ballard S, Ward DC. Karyotyping human chromosomes by combinatorial multi-fluor FISH. *Nat Genet* 1996;**12**(4):368–75.
44. Schrock E, du Manoir S, Veldman T, *et al.* Multicolor spectral karyotyping of human chromosomes. *Science* 1996;**273** (5274):494–7.
45. Bayani JM, Squire JA. Applications of SKY in cancer cytogenetics. *Cancer Invest* 2002;**20**(3):373–86.
46. Nordgren A, Sorensen AG, Tinggaard-Pedersen N, *et al.* New chromosomal breakpoints in non-Hodgkin's lymphomas revealed by spectral karyotyping and G-banding. *Int J Mol Med* 2000;**5**(5):485–92.
47. Houldsworth J, Chaganti RS. Comparative genomic hybridization: an overview. *Am J Pathol* 1994;**145** (6):1253–60.
48. Pinkel D, Segraves R, Sudar D, *et al.* High resolution analysis of DNA copy

number variation using comparative genomic hybridization to microarrays. *Nat Genet* 1998;**20**(2):207–11.

49. Wessendorf S, Schwaenen C, Kohlhammer H, *et al.* Hidden gene amplifications in aggressive B-cell non-Hodgkin lymphomas detected by microarray-based comparative genomic hybridization. *Oncogene* 2003;**22** (9):1425–9.

50. Wessendorf S, Fritz B, Wrobel G, *et al.* Automated screening for genomic imbalances using matrix-based comparative genomic hybridization. *Lab Invest* 2002;**82**(1):47–60.

51. de Leeuw RJ, Davies JJ, Rosenwald A, *et al.* Comprehensive whole genome array CGH profiling of mantle cell lymphoma model genomes. *Hum Mol Genet* 2004;**13**(17):1827–37.

52. Deleeuw RJ, Zettl A, Klinker E, *et al.* Whole-genome analysis and HLA genotyping of enteropathy-type T-cell lymphoma reveals 2 distinct lymphoma subtypes. *Gastroenterology* 2007;**132** (5):1902–11.

53. Golub TR, Slonim DK, Tamayo P, *et al.* Molecular classification of cancer: class discovery and class prediction by gene expression monitoring. *Science* 1999;**286**(5439):531–7.

54. Staudt LM. Molecular diagnosis of the hematologic cancers. *N Engl J Med* 2003;**348**(18):1777–85.

55. Wiestner A, Staudt LM. Towards molecular diagnosis and targeted therapy of lymphoid malignancies. *Semin Hematol* 2003;**40**(4):296–307.

56. Tsujimoto Y, Finger LR, Yunis J, *et al.* Cloning of the chromosome breakpoint of neoplastic B cells with the t(14;18) chromosome translocation. *Science* 1984;**226**(4678):1097–9.

57. Bakhshi A, Jensen JP, Goldman P, *et al.* Cloning the chromosomal breakpoint of t(14;18) human lymphomas: clustering around JH on chromosome 14 and near a transcriptional unit on 18. *Cell* 1985;**41**(3):899–906.

58. Cleary ML, Sklar J. Nucleotide sequence of a t(14;18) chromosomal breakpoint in follicular lymphoma and demonstration of a breakpoint-cluster region near a transcriptionally active locus on chromosome 18. *Proc Natl Acad Sci U S A* 1985;**82**(21):7439–43.

59. Tsujimoto Y, Cossman J, Jaffe E, *et al.* Involvement of the bcl-2 gene in human follicular lymphoma. *Science* 1985;**228** (4706):1440–3.

60. Bende RJ, Smit LA, van Noesel CJ. Molecular pathways in follicular lymphoma. *Leukemia* 2007;**21**(1):18–29.

61. Weiss LM, Warnke RA, Sklar J, *et al.* Molecular analysis of the t(14;18) chromosomal translocation in malignant lymphomas. *N Engl J Med* 1987;**317**(19):1185–9.

62. Aisenberg AC, Wilkes BM, Jacobson JO. The bcl-2 gene is rearranged in many diffuse B-cell lymphomas. *Blood* 1988;**71**(4):969–72.

63. Offit K, Koduru PR, Hollis R, *et al.* 18q21 rearrangement in diffuse large cell lymphoma: incidence and clinical significance. *Br J Haematol* 1989;**72** (2):178–83.

64. Gascoyne RD, Adomat SA, Krajewski S, *et al.* Prognostic significance of BCL2 protein expression and BCL2 gene rearrangement in diffuse aggressive non-Hodgkin's lymphoma. *Blood* 1997;**90**(1):244–51.

65. Iqbal J, Neppalli VT, Wright G, *et al.* BCL2 expression is a prognostic marker for the activated B-cell-like type of diffuse large B-cell lymphoma. *J Clin Oncol* 2006;**24**(6):961–8.

66. de Jong D. Molecular pathogenesis of follicular lymphoma: a cross talk of genetic and immunologic factors. *J Clin Oncol* 2005;**23**(26):6358–63.

67. Zutter M, Hockenbery D, Silverman G, *et al.* Immunolocalization of the BCL2 protein within hematopoietic neoplasms. *Blood* 1991;**78**(4):1062–8.

68. Cleary ML, Galili N, Sklar J. Detection of a second t(14;18) breakpoint cluster region in human follicular lymphomas. *J Exp Med* 1986;**164**(1):315–20.

69. Albinger-Hegyi A, Hochreutener B, Abdou MT, *et al.* High frequency of t(14;18)-translocation breakpoints outside of major breakpoint and minor cluster regions in follicular lymphomas: improved polymerase chain reaction protocols for their detection. *Am J Pathol* 2002;**160**(3):823–32.

70. Weinberg OK, Ai WZ, Mariappan MR, *et al.* 'Minor' BCL2 breakpoints in follicular lymphoma: frequency and correlation with grade and disease presentation in 236 cases. *J Mol Diagn* 2007;**9**(4):530–7.

71. Liu J, Johnson RM, Traweek ST. Rearrangement of the BCL-2 gene in follicular lymphoma. Detection by PCR in both fresh and fixed tissue samples. *Diagn Mol Pathol* 1993;**2**(4):241–7.

72. Horsman DE, Gascoyne RD, Coupland RW, *et al.* Comparison of cytogenetic analysis, southern analysis, and polymerase chain reaction for the detection of t(14;18) in follicular lymphoma. *Am J Clin Pathol* 1995;**103** (4):472–8.

73. Barrans SL, Evans PA, O'Connor SJ, *et al.* The detection of t(14;18) in archival lymph nodes: development of a fluorescence in situ hybridization (FISH)-based method and evaluation by comparison with polymerase chain reaction. *J Mol Diagn* 2003;**5**(3):168–75.

74. Jiang F, Lin F, Price R, *et al.* Rapid detection of IgH/BCL2 rearrangement in follicular lymphoma by interphase fluorescence in situ hybridization with bacterial artificial chromosome probes. *J Mol Diagn* 2002;**4**(3):144–9.

75. Matsumoto Y, Nomura K, Matsumoto S, *et al.* Detection of t(14;18) in follicular lymphoma by dual-color fluorescence in situ hybridization on paraffin-embedded tissue sections. *Cancer Genet Cytogenet* 2004;**150** (1):22–6.

76. Baron BW, Nucifora G, McCabe N, *et al.* Identification of the gene associated with the recurring chromosomal translocations t(3;14) (q27;q32) and t(3;22)(q27;q11) in B-cell lymphomas. *Proc Natl Acad Sci U S A* 1993;**90**(11):5262–6.

77. Kerckaert JP, Deweindt C, Tilly H, *et al.* LAZ3, a novel zinc-finger encoding gene, is disrupted by recurring chromosome 3q27 translocations in human lymphomas. *Nat Genet* 1993; **5**(1):66–70.

78. Bajalica-Lagercrantz S, Piehl F, Lagercrantz J, *et al.* Expression of LAZ3/BCL6 in follicular center (FC) B cells of reactive lymph nodes and FC-derived non-Hodgkin lymphomas. *Leukemia* 1997;**11**(4):594–8.

79. Fukuda T, Miki T, Yoshida T, *et al.* The murine BCL6 gene is induced in activated lymphocytes as an immediate early gene. *Oncogene* 1995;**11**(8):1657–63.

80. Ye BH, Cattoretti G, Shen Q, *et al.* The BCL-6 proto-oncogene controls germinal-center formation and Th2-type inflammation. *Nat Genet* 1997;**16** (2):161–70.

81. Onizuka T, Moriyama M, Yamochi T, *et al.* BCL-6 gene product, a 92- to 98-kD nuclear phosphoprotein, is highly expressed in germinal center B cells and their neoplastic counterparts. *Blood* 1995;**86**(1):28–37.

82. Flenghi L, Bigerna B, Fizzotti M, *et al.* Monoclonal antibodies PG-B6a and PG-B6p recognize, respectively, a highly conserved and a formol-resistant epitope on the human BCL-6 protein amino-terminal region. *Am J Pathol* 1996;**148**(5):1543–55.

83. Dogan A, Bagdi E, Munson P, *et al.* CD10 and BCL-6 expression in paraffin sections of normal lymphoid tissue and B-cell lymphomas. *Am J Surg Pathol* 2000;**24**(6):846–52.

84. Diaz-Alderete A, Doval A, Camacho F, *et al.* Frequency of BCL2 and BCL6 translocations in follicular lymphoma: relation with histological and clinical features. *Leuk Lymphoma* 2008; **49**(1):95–101.

85. Tsang P, Cesarman E, Chadburn A, *et al.* Molecular characterization of primary mediastinal B cell lymphoma. *Am J Pathol* 1996;**148**(6):2017–25.

86. Ueda C, Uchiyama T, Ohno H. Immunoglobulin (Ig)/BCL6 versus non-Ig/BCL6 gene fusion in diffuse large B-cell lymphoma corresponds to a high- versus low-level expression of BCL6 mRNA. *Blood* 2002;**99**(7):2624–5.

87. Migliazza A, Martinotti S, Chen W, *et al.* Frequent somatic hypermutation of the 5' noncoding region of the BCL6 gene in B-cell lymphoma. *Proc Natl Acad Sci U S A* 1995;**92**(26):12 520–4.

88. Vitolo U, Botto B, Capello D, *et al.* Point mutations of the BCL-6 gene: clinical and prognostic correlation in B-diffuse large cell lymphoma. *Leukemia* 2002;**16**(2):268–75.

89. Pasqualucci L, Migliazza A, Fracchiolla N, *et al.* BCL-6 mutations in normal germinal center B cells: evidence of somatic hypermutation acting outside Ig loci. *Proc Natl Acad Sci U S A* 1998;**95**(20):11 816–21.

90. Capello D, Vitolo U, Pasqualucci L, *et al.* Distribution and pattern of BCL-6 mutations throughout the spectrum of B-cell neoplasia. *Blood* 2000;**95**(2):651–9.

91. Artiga MJ, Saez AI, Romero C, *et al.* A short mutational hot spot in the first intron of BCL-6 is associated with increased BCL-6 expression and with longer overall survival in large B-cell lymphomas. *Am J Pathol* 2002;**160**(4):1371–80.

92. Pasqualucci L, Migliazza A, Basso K, *et al.* Mutations of the BCL6 proto-oncogene disrupt its negative autoregulation in diffuse large B-cell lymphoma. *Blood* 2003;**101**(8):2914–23.

93. Iqbal J, Greiner TC, Patel K, *et al.* Distinctive patterns of BCL6 molecular alterations and their functional consequences in different subgroups of diffuse large B-cell lymphoma. *Leukemia* 2007;**21**(11):2332–43.

94. Hunter T, Pines J. Cyclins and cancer. II: Cyclin D and CDK inhibitors come of age. *Cell* 1994;**79**(4):573–82.

95. Jares P, Colomer D, Campo E. Genetic and molecular pathogenesis of mantle cell lymphoma: perspectives for new targeted therapeutics. *Nat Rev Cancer* 2007;**7**(10):750–62.

96. Fu M, Wang C, Li Z, *et al.* Minireview: Cyclin D1: normal and abnormal functions. *Endocrinology* 2004;**145**(12):5439–47.

97. Coqueret O. Linking cyclins to transcriptional control. *Gene* 2002;**299**(1–2):35–55.

98. Wong KF, So CC, Chan JK. Nucleolated variant of mantle cell lymphoma with leukemic manifestations mimicking prolymphocytic leukemia. *Am J Clin Pathol* 2002;**117**(2):246–51.

99. Schlette E, Bueso-Ramos C, Giles F, *et al.* Mature B-cell leukemias with more than 55% prolymphocytes. A heterogeneous group that includes an unusual variant of mantle cell lymphoma. *Am J Clin Pathol* 2001;**115**(4):571–81.

100. Ruchlemer R, Parry-Jones N, Brito-Babapulle V, *et al.* B-prolymphocytic leukaemia with t(11;14) revisited: a splenomegalic form of mantle cell lymphoma evolving with leukaemia. *Br J Haematol* 2004;**125**(3):330–6.

101. Horsman D, Gascoyne R, Klasa R, *et al.* t(11;18)(q21;q21.1): a recurring translocation in lymphomas of mucosa-associated lymphoid tissue (MALT)? *Genes Chromosomes Cancer* 1992; **4**(2):183–7.

102. Ott G, Katzenberger T, Greiner A, *et al.* The t(11;18)(q21;q21) chromosome translocation is a frequent and specific aberration in low-grade but not high-grade malignant non-Hodgkin's lymphomas of the mucosa-associated lymphoid tissue (MALT-) type. *Cancer Res* 1997;**57**(18):3944–8.

103. Auer IA, Gascoyne RD, Connors JM, *et al.* t(11;18)(q21;q21) is the most common translocation in MALT lymphomas. *Ann Oncol* 1997;**8**(10):979–85.

104. Rosenwald A, Ott G, Stilgenbauer S, *et al.* Exclusive detection of the t(11;18)(q21;q21) in extranodal marginal zone B cell lymphomas (MZBL) of MALT type in contrast to other MZBL and extranodal large B cell lymphomas. *Am J Pathol* 1999;**155**(6):1817–21.

105. Remstein ED, James CD, Kurtin PJ. Incidence and subtype specificity of API2-MALT1 fusion translocations in extranodal, nodal, and splenic marginal zone lymphomas. *Am J Pathol* 2000;**156**(4):1183–8.

106. Liu H, Ye H, Dogan A, *et al.* T(11;18)(q21;q21) is associated with advanced mucosa-associated lymphoid tissue lymphoma that expresses nuclear BCL10. *Blood* 2001;**98**(4):1182–7.

107. Chuang SS, Lee C, Hamoudi RA, *et al.* High frequency of t(11;18) in gastric mucosa-associated lymphoid tissue lymphomas in Taiwan, including one patient with high-grade transformation. *Br J Haematol* 2003;**120**(1):97–100.

108. Tan SY, Ye H, Liu H, *et al.* t(11;18)(q21;q21)-positive transformed MALT lymphoma. *Histopathology* 2008; **52**(6):777–80.

109. Ye H, Liu H, Attygalle A, *et al.* Variable frequencies of t(11;18)(q21;q21) in MALT lymphomas of different sites: significant association with CagA strains of *H. pylori* in gastric MALT lymphoma. *Blood* 2003;**102**(3):1012–18.

110. Streubel B, Simonitsch-Klupp I, Mullauer L, *et al.* Variable frequencies of MALT lymphoma-associated genetic aberrations in MALT lymphomas of different sites. *Leukemia* 2004;**18**(10):1722–6.

111. Baens M, Maes B, Steyls A, *et al.* The product of the t(11;18), an API2-MLT fusion, marks nearly half of gastric MALT type lymphomas without large cell proliferation. *Am J Pathol* 2000;**156**(4):1433–9.

112. Liu H, Ruskon-Fourmestraux A, Lavergne-Slove A, *et al.* Resistance of t(11;18) positive gastric mucosa-associated lymphoid tissue lymphoma

to *Helicobacter pylori* eradication therapy. *Lancet* 2001;**357**(9249):39–40.

113. Sugiyama T, Asaka M, Nakamura T, *et al.* API2-MALT1 chimeric transcript is a predictive marker for the responsiveness of *H. pylori* eradication treatment in low-grade gastric MALT lymphoma. *Gastroenterology* 2001;**120**(7):1884–5.
114. Liu H, Ye H, Ruskone-Fourmestraux A, *et al.* T(11;18) is a marker for all stage gastric MALT lymphomas that will not respond to *H. pylori* eradication. *Gastroenterology* 2002;**122**(5):1286–94.
115. Lucas PC, Yonezumi M, Inohara N, *et al.* Bcl10 and MALT1, independent targets of chromosomal translocation in malt lymphoma, cooperate in a novel NF-κB signaling pathway. *J Biol Chem* 2001;**276**(22):19 012–19.
116. Taub R, Kirsch I, Morton C, *et al.* Translocation of the c-myc gene into the immunoglobulin heavy chain locus in human Burkitt lymphoma and murine plasmacytoma cells. *Proc Natl Acad Sci U S A* 1982;**79**(24):7837–41.
117. Hamlyn PH, Rabbitts TH. Translocation joins c-myc and immunoglobulin gamma 1 genes in a Burkitt lymphoma revealing a third exon in the c-myc oncogene. *Nature* 1983;**304**(5922):135–9.
118. Battey J, Moulding C, Taub R, *et al.* The human c-myc oncogene: structural consequences of translocation into the IgH locus in Burkitt lymphoma. *Cell* 1983;**34**(3):779–87.
119. Emanuel BS, Selden JR, Chaganti RS, *et al.* The 2p breakpoint of a 2;8 translocation in Burkitt lymphoma interrupts the V kappa locus. *Proc Natl Acad Sci U S A* 1984;**81**(8):2444–6.
120. Hollis GF, Mitchell KF, Battey J, *et al.* A variant translocation places the lambda immunoglobulin genes 3' to the c-myc oncogene in Burkitt's lymphoma. *Nature* 1984;**307**(5953):752–5.
121. Ladanyi M, Offit K, Jhanwar SC, *et al.* C-MYC rearrangement and translocations involving band 8q24 in diffuse large cell lymphomas. *Blood* 1991;**77**(5):1057–63.
122. Hummel M, Bentink S, Berger H, *et al.* A biologic definition of Burkitt's lymphoma from transcriptional and genomic profiling. *N Engl J Med* 2006;**354**(23):2419–30.
123. Dave SS, Fu K, Wright GW, *et al.* Molecular diagnosis of Burkitt's lymphoma. *N Engl J Med* 2006;**354**(23):2431–42.
124. Pelicci PG, Knowles DM 2nd, Magrath I, *et al.* Chromosomal breakpoints and structural alterations of the c-myc locus differ in endemic and sporadic forms of Burkitt lymphoma. *Proc Natl Acad Sci U S A* 1986;**83**(9):2984–8.
125. Shiramizu B, Barriga F, Neequaye J, *et al.* Patterns of chromosomal breakpoint locations in Burkitt's lymphoma: relevance to geography and Epstein-Barr virus association. *Blood* 1991;**77**(7):1516–26.
126. Adhikary S, Eilers M. Transcriptional regulation and transformation by Myc proteins. *Nat Rev Mol Cell Biol* 2005;**6**(8):635–45.
127. Macpherson N, Lesack D, Klasa R, *et al.* Small noncleaved, non-Burkitt's (Burkitt-like) lymphoma: cytogenetics predict outcome and reflect clinical presentation. *J Clin Oncol* 1999;**17**(5):1558–67.
128. Le Gouill S, Talmant P, Touzeau C, *et al.* The clinical presentation and prognosis of diffuse large B-cell lymphoma with t(14;18) and 8q24/c-C-MYC rearrangement. *Haematologica* 2007;**92**(10):1335–42.
129. Mufti GJ, Hamblin TJ, Oscier DG, *et al.* Common ALL with pre-B-cell features showing (8;14) and (14;18) chromosome translocations. *Blood* 1983;**62**(5):1142–6.
130. Kanungo A, Medeiros LJ, Abruzzo LV, *et al.* Lymphoid neoplasms associated with concurrent t(14;18) and 8q24/c-C-MYC translocation generally have a poor prognosis. *Mod Pathol* 2006;**19**(1):25–33.
131. McDonnell TJ, Korsmeyer SJ. Progression from lymphoid hyperplasia to high-grade malignant lymphoma in mice transgenic for the t(14;18). *Nature* 1991;**349**(6306):254–6.
132. Yano T, Jaffe ES, Longo DL, *et al.* C-MYC rearrangements in histologically progressed follicular lymphomas. *Blood* 1992;**80**(3):758–67.
133. Alizadeh AA, Eisen MB, Davis RE, *et al.* Distinct types of diffuse large B-cell lymphoma identified by gene expression profiling. *Nature* 2000;**403**(6769):503–11.
134. Rosenwald A, Wright G, Chan WC, *et al.* The use of molecular profiling to predict survival after chemotherapy for diffuse large-B-cell lymphoma. *N Engl J Med* 2002;**346**(25):1937–47.
135. Shipp MA, Ross KN, Tamayo P, *et al.* Diffuse large B-cell lymphoma outcome prediction by gene-expression profiling and supervised machine learning. *Nat Med* 2002;**8**(1):68–74.
136. Savage KJ, Monti S, Kutok JL, *et al.* The molecular signature of mediastinal large B-cell lymphoma differs from that of other diffuse large B-cell lymphomas and shares features with classical Hodgkin lymphoma. *Blood* 2003;**102**(12):3871–9.
137. Wright G, Tan B, Rosenwald A, *et al.* A gene expression-based method to diagnose clinically distinct subgroups of diffuse large B cell lymphoma. *Proc Natl Acad Sci U S A* 2003;**100**(17):9991–6.
138. Rosenwald A, Wright G, Leroy K, *et al.* Molecular diagnosis of primary mediastinal B cell lymphoma identifies a clinically favorable subgroup of diffuse large B cell lymphoma related to Hodgkin lymphoma. *J Exp Med* 2003;**198**(6):851–62.
139. Davis RE, Brown KD, Siebenlist U, *et al.* Constitutive nuclear factor kappaB activity is required for survival of activated B cell-like diffuse large B cell lymphoma cells. *J Exp Med* 2001;**194**(12):1861–74.
140. Kuppers R, Klein U, Hansmann ML, *et al.* Cellular origin of human B-cell lymphomas. *N Engl J Med* 1999;**341**(20):1520–9.
141. Damle RN, Wasil T, Fais F, *et al.* Ig V gene mutation status and CD38 expression as novel prognostic indicators in chronic lymphocytic leukemia. *Blood* 1999;**94**(6):1840–7.
142. Hamblin TJ, Davis Z, Gardiner A, *et al.* Unmutated Ig V(H) genes are associated with a more aggressive form of chronic lymphocytic leukemia. *Blood* 1999;**94**(6):1848–54.
143. Camacho FI, Algara P, Rodriguez A, *et al.* Molecular heterogeneity in MCL defined by the use of specific VH genes and the frequency of somatic mutations. *Blood* 2003;**101**(10):4042–6.
144. Kienle D, Krober A, Katzenberger T, *et al.* VH mutation status and VDJ rearrangement structure in mantle cell lymphoma: correlation with genomic aberrations, clinical characteristics, and outcome. *Blood* 2003;**102**(8):3003–9.

145. Lai R, Lefresne SV, Franko B, *et al.* Immunoglobulin VH somatic hypermutation in mantle cell lymphoma: mutated genotype correlates with better clinical outcome. *Mod Pathol* 2006;**19**(11):1498–505.

146. Rimokh R, Magaud JP, Berger F, *et al.* A translocation involving a specific breakpoint (q35) on chromosome 5 is characteristic of anaplastic large cell lymphoma ('Ki-1 lymphoma'). *Br J Haematol* 1989;**71** (1):31–6.

147. Le Beau MM, Bitter MA, Larson RA, *et al.* The t(2;5)(p23;q35): a recurring chromosomal abnormality in Ki-1-positive anaplastic large cell lymphoma. *Leukemia* 1989;**3**(12):866–70.

148. Morris SW, Kirstein MN, Valentine MB, *et al.* Fusion of a kinase gene, ALK, to a nucleolar protein gene, NPM, in non-Hodgkin's lymphoma. *Science* 1994;**263**(5151):1281–4.

149. Shiota M, Fujimoto J, Semba T, *et al.* Hyperphosphorylation of a novel 80 kDa protein-tyrosine kinase similar to Ltk in a human Ki-1 lymphoma cell line, AMS3. *Oncogene* 1994;**9** (6):1567–74.

150. Falini B, Bigerna B, Fizzotti M, *et al.* ALK expression defines a distinct group of T/null lymphomas ("ALK lymphomas") with a wide morphological spectrum. *Am J Pathol* 1998;**153**(3):875–86.

151. Salaverria I, Bea S, Lopez-Guillermo A, *et al.* Genomic profiling reveals different genetic aberrations in systemic ALK-positive and ALK-negative anaplastic large cell lymphomas. *Br J Haematol* 2008;**140**(5):516–26.

152. Medeiros LJ, Elenitoba-Johnson KS. Anaplastic large cell lymphoma. *Am J Clin Pathol* 2007;**127**(5):707–22.

153. Sarris AH, Luthra R, Cabanillas F, *et al.* Genomic DNA amplification and the detection of t(2;5)(p23;q35) in lymphoid neoplasms. *Leuk Lymphoma* 1998;**29**(5–6):507–14.

154. Shiota M, Fujimoto J, Takenaga M, *et al.* Diagnosis of t(2;5)(p23;q35)-associated Ki-1 lymphoma with immunohistochemistry. *Blood* 1994;**84** (11):3648–52.

155. Bolen JB, Brugge JS. Leukocyte protein tyrosine kinases: potential targets for drug discovery. *Annu Rev Immunol* 1997;**15**:371–404.

156. Streubel B, Vinatzer U, Willheim M, *et al.* Novel t(5;9)(q33;q22) fuses ITK to SYK in unspecified peripheral T-cell lymphoma. *Leukemia* 2006;**20** (2):313–18.

157. Rudiger T, Ichinohasama R, Ott MM, *et al.* Peripheral T-cell lymphoma with distinct perifollicular growth pattern: a distinct subtype of T-cell lymphoma? *Am J Surg Pathol* 2000;**24** (1):117–22.

158. de Leval L, Savilo E, Longtine J, *et al.* Peripheral T-cell lymphoma with follicular involvement and a CD4+/bcl-6+ phenotype. *Am J Surg Pathol* 2001;**25**(3):395–400.

159. Zettl A, Ott G, Makulik A, *et al.* Chromosomal gains at 9q characterize enteropathy-type T-cell lymphoma. *Am J Pathol* 2002;**161**(5):1635–45.

160. Zettl A, Rudiger T, Konrad MA, *et al.* Genomic profiling of peripheral T-cell lymphoma, unspecified, and anaplastic large T-cell lymphoma delineates novel recurrent chromosomal alterations. *Am J Pathol* 2004;**164**(5):1837–48.

161. Gaidano G, Ballerini P, Gong JZ, *et al.* p53 mutations in human lymphoid malignancies: association with Burkitt lymphoma and chronic lymphocytic leukemia. *Proc Natl Acad Sci U S A* 1991;**88**(12):5413–17.

162. Gaidano G, Newcomb EW, Gong JZ, *et al.* Analysis of alterations of oncogenes and tumor suppressor genes in chronic lymphocytic leukemia. *Am J Pathol* 1994;**144**(6):1312–19.

163. Louie DC, Offit K, Jaslow R, *et al.* P53 overexpression as a marker of poor prognosis in mantle cell lymphomas with t(11;14)(q13;q32). *Blood* 1995;**86** (8):2892–9.

164. Hernandez L, Fest T, Cazorla M, *et al.* P53 gene mutations and protein overexpression are associated with aggressive variants of mantle cell lymphomas. *Blood* 1996;**87**(8):3351–9.

165. Wlodarska I, Pittaluga S, Hagemeijer A, *et al.* Secondary chromosome changes in mantle cell lymphoma. *Haematologica* 1999;**84**(7):594–9.

166. Sanchez-Beato M, Saez AI, Navas IC, *et al.* Overall survival in aggressive B-cell lymphomas is dependent on the accumulation of alterations in p53, p16, and p27. *Am J Pathol* 2001;**159** (1):205–13.

167. Moller MB, Ino Y, Gerdes AM, *et al.* Aberrations of the p53 pathway components p53, MDM2 and CDKN2A appear independent in diffuse large B cell lymphoma. *Leukemia* 1999; **13**(3):453–9.

168. Ichikawa A, Kinoshita T, Watanabe T, *et al.* Mutations of the p53 gene as a prognostic factor in aggressive B-cell lymphoma. *N Engl J Med* 1997;**337** (8):529–34.

169. Koduru PR, Raju K, Vadmal V, *et al.* Correlation between mutation in P53, p53 expression, cytogenetics, histologic type, and survival in patients with B-cell non-Hodgkin's lymphoma. *Blood* 1997;**90**(10):4078–91.

170. Bhatia KG, Gutierrez MI, Huppi K, *et al.* The pattern of p53 mutations in Burkitt's lymphoma differs from that of solid tumors. *Cancer Res* 1992;**52** (15):4273–6.

171. Matsushima AY, Cesarman E, Chadburn A, *et al.* Post-thymic T cell lymphomas frequently overexpress p53 protein but infrequently exhibit p53 gene mutations. *Am J Pathol* 1994; **144**(3):573–84.

172. Pescarmona E, Pignoloni P, Santangelo C, *et al.* Expression of p53 and retinoblastoma gene in high-grade nodal peripheral T-cell lymphomas: immunohistochemical and molecular findings suggesting different pathogenetic pathways and possible clinical implications. *J Pathol* 1999;**188** (4):400–6.

173. Petit B, Leroy K, Kanavaros P, *et al.* Expression of p53 protein in T- and natural killer-cell lymphomas is associated with some clinicopathologic entities but rarely related to p53 mutations. *Hum Pathol* 2001;**32** (2):196–204.

174. Serrano M, Hannon GJ, Beach D. A new regulatory motif in cell-cycle control causing specific inhibition of cyclin D/CDK4. *Nature* 1993;**366** (6456):704–7.

175. Villuendas R, Sanchez-Beato M, Martinez JC, *et al.* Loss of p16/INK4A protein expression in non-Hodgkin's lymphomas is a frequent finding associated with tumor progression. *Am J Pathol* 1998;**153** (3):887–97.

176. Koduru PR, Zariwala M, Soni M, *et al.* Deletion of cyclin-dependent kinase 4 inhibitor genes P15 and P16 in non-Hodgkin's lymphoma. *Blood* 1995;**86** (8):2900–5.

177. Klangby U, Okan I, Magnusson KP, *et al.* p16/INK4a and p15/INK4b gene methylation and absence of p16/INK4a mRNA and protein expression in Burkitt's lymphoma. *Blood* 1998;**91**(5):1680–7.

178. Elenitoba-Johnson KS, Gascoyne RD, Lim MS, *et al.* Homozygous deletions at chromosome 9p21 involving p16 and p15 are associated with histologic progression in follicle center lymphoma. *Blood* 1998;**91**(12):4677–85.

179. Pinyol M, Hernandez L, Cazorla M, *et al.* Deletions and loss of expression of p16INK4a and p21Waf1 genes are associated with aggressive variants of mantle cell lymphomas. *Blood* 1997;**89**(1):272–80.

180. Navas IC, Ortiz-Romero PL, Villuendas R, *et al.* p16(INK4a) gene alterations are frequent in lesions of mycosis fungoides. *Am J Pathol* 2000;**156**(5):1565–72.

181. Scarisbrick JJ, Woolford AJ, Calonje E, *et al.* Frequent abnormalities of the p15 and p16 genes in mycosis fungoides and sezary syndrome. *J Invest Dermatol* 2002;**118**(3):493–9.

182. Zhang C, Toulev A, Kamarashev J, *et al.* Consequences of p16 tumor suppressor gene inactivation in mycosis fungoides and Sezary syndrome and role of the bmi-1 and ras oncogenes in disease progression. *Hum Pathol* 2007;**38**(7):995–1002.

183. Garcia JF, Villuendas R, Algara P, *et al.* Loss of p16 protein expression associated with methylation of the p16INK4A gene is a frequent finding in Hodgkin's disease. *Lab Invest* 1999;**79**(12):1453–9.

184. Rosenwald A, Wright G, Wiestner A, *et al.* The proliferation gene expression signature is a quantitative integrator of oncogenic events that predicts survival in mantle cell lymphoma. *Cancer Cell* 2003;**3**(2):185–97.

185. Fu K, Weisenburger DD, Greiner TC, *et al.* Cyclin D1-negative mantle cell lymphoma: a clinicopathologic study based on gene expression profiling. *Blood* 2005;**106**(13):4315–21.

186. Streubel B, Lamprecht A, Dierlamm J, *et al.* T(14;18)(q32;q21) involving IGH and MALT1 is a frequent chromosomal aberration in MALT lymphoma. *Blood* 2003;**101**(6):2335–9.

187. Sanchez-Izquierdo D, Buchonnet G, Siebert R, *et al.* MALT1 is deregulated by both chromosomal translocation and amplification in B-cell non-Hodgkin lymphoma. *Blood* 2003;**101**(11):4539–46.

188. Limpens J, de Jong D, van Krieken JH, *et al.* BCL2/JH rearrangements in benign lymphoid tissues with follicular hyperplasia. *Oncogene* 1991;**6**(12):2271–6.

189. Knowles DM. Immunodeficiency-associated lymphoproliferative disorders. *Mod Pathol* 1999;**12**(2):200–17.

Chapter 15

International staging and response criteria for lymphomas

Bruce D. Cheson

Introduction

The goal of lymphoma therapy is to improve the outcome of patients by reducing the size of or completely eradicating the disease, and/or by causing a decrease in disease-related symptoms. Although major progress has been made in the treatment of patients with lymphoma, many still fail to achieve a response or subsequently relapse. Thus, new therapies are needed to improve patient outcome. In order to identify promising regimens and reliably compare the results with existing therapies, it is critical to have uniform definitions of the extent of disease prior to therapy and measurements of efficacy following treatment. In the absence of active agents, response criteria are irrelevant. However, because of the increasing number of effective treatment options for lymphoma, standardized response criteria are necessary to assess and compare the activity of various therapies within and among studies, and facilitate the evaluation of new treatments by regulatory agencies.

In 1999, an international working group (IWG) of clinicians, radiologists, and pathologists with expertise in the evaluation and management of patients with lymphoma developed guidelines that standardized a number of important components of patient assessment.[1] Since response is most often measured by the change in size of lymph nodes, the first goal was to define the size of a "normal" node, which previously had varied widely among studies. Even minor variations in what is considered "normal" lymph node size can result in major differences in the complete response rate following therapy. Grillo-López *et al.* analyzed a database of 166 patients treated with rituximab for relapsed or refractory follicular and low-grade non-Hodgkin lymphoma (NHL) defining "normal" as either 1 by 1 cm, 1.5 by 1.5 cm, or 2 by 2 cm.[2] Whereas the overall response rate remained the same at 48%, the complete remission rate increased from 6% to 18% to 28%, respectively. Using computed tomography (CT) scanning or autopsy, the size of a normal node ranges from an upper limit of normal of about 8–12 mm in the short axis, with greater variation in the long axis. Nevertheless, normal mediastinal nodes may be as large as 12 mm, 11 mm in the abdomen, and up to 15 mm in the pelvis.[3–7] The IWG recommendation was to consider a pretreatment node greater than 1 cm in its longest diameter as likely to be involved with lymphoma.[1,8]

Additional recommendations included when and how responses should be assessed following therapy, and definitions of complete remission (CR), complete remission unconfirmed (CRu), partial remission (PR), stable disease (SD), relapsed disease (RD), and progressive disease (PD).[1] These recommendations were rapidly and widely accepted by clinicians and used by regulatory agencies for approval of new agents.

As the IWG criteria were used in clinical trials over the next few years, it became apparent that revisions were necessary. For example, the IWG criteria relied on relatively insensitive methods of assessment including physical examination, CT scans, and single photon emission computed tomography (SPECT) gallium scans, the latter no longer widely used.

While CT scans provide relatively high sensitivity and specificity in pretreatment staging,[9,10] specificity in response assessment following therapy is relatively low.[11–14] One problem reflects the inability of the CT to distinguish scar tissue or fibrosis from viable tumor. As lymphomatous nodes shrink in size following treatment, fibrosis, necrosis, or inflammation may result in a persistent enlargement of a node that does not necessarily indicate the presence of residual disease.[11–13,15]

Another problem with the original IWG criteria was that certain terms were misinterpreted. For example, CRu was intended to designate two specific types of responses to treatment: first were those patients with potentially curable lymphomas, primarily Hodgkin lymphoma (HL) and diffuse large B-cell lymphoma, with a large mass prior to treatment, and for whom treatment resulted in disappearance of all detectable tumor except that the mass persisted but had decreased by at least 75% on CT scan. Prior studies had demonstrated that in as many as 90% of cases, these patients remained free of disease for prolonged periods, and biopsies demonstrated that the masses represented scar tissue or fibrosis.[13,16] Instead, the

Management of Hematologic Malignancies, ed. Susan M. O'Brien, Julie M. Vose, and Hagop M. Kantarjian. Published by Cambridge University Press.

designation CRu was often inappropriately applied to a decrease in the sum of the product of the diameters (SPD) of multiple nodes by at least 75%, even in patients with incurable histologies, which should be considered a PR. The result was that PRs were included as CRu and the CR rate was artificially inflated. The second type of CRu included patients with bone marrow involvement prior to treatment who fulfilled all of the conditions for a CR following therapy except that rebiopsy of the bone marrow was considered by the pathologist to be morphologically indeterminate. Instead, the term was also assigned to patients who did not undergo a confirmatory posttreatment bone marrow biopsy.

One of the most compelling arguments for revising the IWG criteria was the increased availability of newer and more sensitive technologies which enhanced the distinction between lymphoma and normal tissue, including 18-fluoro deoxyglucose positron emission tomography (FDG-PET) scanning, and bone marrow immunohistochemistry and flow cytometry. CT scans provide information on size, shape, and location of lesions, while FDG-PET scans add the dimension of a study that identifies metabolically active tissues by their FDG-avidity. A role for FDG-PET has been suggested in staging, restaging posttreatment, midtreatment, and for posttreatment surveillance. However, the amount of available information is far greater than its demonstrated usefulness.

FDG-PET for staging of lymphoma

Pretreatment staging determines the extent of disease, helps direct therapy, and provides a baseline against which results following therapy can be compared. The four-stage Ann Arbor classification most commonly used was initially designed to distinguish patients with Hodgkin lymphoma who might be candidates for radiation therapy from those who were more suitable for systemic treatment.[17] It was originally based on physical examination and bone marrow assessment, but CT scans were subsequently incorporated. The value of this system to direct therapy has diminished with the increased use of systemic treatments and a reduction in the number of patients who receive radiation.

FDG-PET is clearly more sensitive and specific than CT scan; nevertheless, whether PET should be incorporated into the Ann Arbor staging system is controversial. In favor of this change in practice is that FDG-PET is more sensitive than CT scan in detecting nodal and extranodal involvement by most histologic subtypes of lymphoma.[9,10,18–32]

FDG-PET and CT are concordant 80–90% of the time in staging of patients with diffuse large B-cell lymphoma, follicular lymphoma, and mantle cell lymphoma.[21,23] In patients with discordant results, FDG-PET typically results in upstaging due to the identification of additional sites of disease. In contrast, concordance of FDG-PET and CT in determining clinical stage occurs in only about 60–80% of patients with HL. Discordant findings occur with a comparable frequency in both directions.[22,25–30] However, while FDG-PET identifies more lesions than CT, FDG-PET alone cannot replace CT for pretreatment staging.[22,25,27,29]

In a meta-analysis of FDG-PET in staging of patients with lymphoma,[32] the pooled sensitivity for 14 studies with patient-based data was 90.9% (95% confidence intervals [CI] = 88.0–93.4) with a false-positive rate of 10.3% (95% CI = 7.4–13.8). The maximum joint sensitivity and specificity was 87.8% (95% CI = 85.0–90.7) with an apparently higher sensitivity and false-positive rate in patients with HL compared with NHL. The pooled sensitivity for seven studies with lesion-based data was 95.6% (95% CI = 93.9–97.0) with a false-positive rate of only 1.0% (95% CI = 0.6–1.3). The maximum sensitivity and specificity was 95.6% (95% CI = 93.1–98.1).

FDG-PET can detect bone or bone marrow involvement even when the iliac crest trephine bone marrow biopsy is negative.[33–35] However, whereas FDG-PET is typically positive in patients with extensive bone/bone marrow involvement by lymphoma, FDG-PET is unreliable in detecting limited bone marrow involvement.[35] Moreover, diffusely increased bone marrow uptake on PET may also be due to reactive hyperplasia, such as with the use of myeloid growth factors.[34] FDG-PET-positive bone marrow findings must be confirmed by biopsy if a change in treatment will be based on these findings. Thus, FDG-PET cannot substitute for bone marrow biopsy in lymphoma staging.

Although FDG-PET is more sensitive for staging than CT scans, the additional sites identified modify clinical stage in only a small percentage of patients (~15–30%), and this modification influences treatment in only ~10–15% of patients, with no data that patient outcome is improved.[18,21,36–38]

FDG-PET/CT provides more sensitive and specific imaging than either modality alone.[31,39–43] PET/CT combines a full-ring detector PET scanner with a multidetector helical CT such that the PET scan is acquired immediately after the CT scan. The images are fused to provide precise localization of abnormal lesions. PET/CT is considerably faster than the combination of emission and transmission PET scans required to obtain attenuation-corrected PET images. FDG-PET/CT performed even without intravenous contrast (unenhanced FDG-PET/CT) with the CT portion typically acquired as low-dose CT is more sensitive and specific than contrast-enhanced full-dose CT for evaluation of nodal and extranodal lymphomatous involvement.[31,39] Tatsumi *et al.* evaluated 1537 anatomic sites in 20 patients with HL and 33 patients with NHL on an unenhanced low-dose FDG-PET/CT scanner.[39] There were 1489 sites concordant between FDG-PET and CT, and among the 48 discordant sites, FDG-PET correctly identified 40 sites as true positives or true negatives by biopsy or clinical follow-up.

Kwee *et al.* conducted a systematic review of 19 studies of CT and FDG-PET in staging of lymphomas.[44] Nine of 17 studies that incorporated FDG-PET included patients with HL, but in only one of these was it part of initial staging, with sensitivity and specificity of 87.5% and 100%, respectively. In the single study including patients with NHL, the sensitivity was 83.3% with 100% lesion-based specificity. Four studies evaluated PET/CT fusion scans, but only one for initial staging.[45] The authors concluded that CT remains the standard for staging, with FDG-PET being superior for restaging. While PET/CT was found to be superior to either modality alone, they felt that further study was needed to determine the most accurate and cost-effective method for lymphoma staging.

FDG-PET for restaging

Restaging of lymphoma is defined as an assessment that is performed following completion of treatment in order to detect residual tumor or suspected recurrence, or to determine the extent of known recurrence.[46] This term differs from monitoring of therapy, which occurs during the course of treatment. However, as risk-adapted treatment strategies evolve, and response evaluation occurs earlier in the course of treatment, the distinction between monitoring and restaging will begin to blur.

FDG-PET is most useful in the restaging of the curable lymphomas.[47–53] PET is more accurate than CT in this setting because it distinguishes between viable tumor and necrosis or fibrosis in residual mass(es). Thus, the outcome of patients who are FDG-PET-negative after therapy is superior to those who are still positive regardless of the presence of a residual mass.[47–52]

In general, FDG-PET has a consistently high negative predictive value (NPV) averaging about 85% across studies including patients with HL and/or diffuse large B-cell NHL (DLBCL).[47–53] The approximately 15% false-negative rate with PET is mostly related to its inability to detect microscopic disease resulting in future relapse. The positive predictive value (PPV) of PET is generally lower and considerably more variable averaging about 70–80%, with generally lower average values in patients with HL (~65%) compared with NHL (~85%).[47–52] The PPV of FDG-PET is substantially higher than CT, which has a reported PPV in patients with aggressive NHL of about 40–50% and in HL of only about 20%. The NPV of FDG-PET is similar to that of CT resulting in a considerably higher accuracy of FDG-PET for response assessment compared with CT (approximately 80% vs. 50%).

Recent studies may be more accurate because they utilized currently standard attenuation-corrected FDG-PET to evaluate the predictive value of PET.

Thus, while a positive test following therapy is generally considered a strong predictor of failure, such results should be interpreted in conjunction with the history, physical examination, and CT scans. False-positive results have been reported in more than 20% of patients serially studied following therapy as a consequence of infection, inflammation, tumor necrosis, or other causes.[54,55] Thus, in general, major treatment decisions should not be based on a single imaging study. Either a biopsy should be performed of the FDG-avid lesion, or the study should be repeated in 2–3 months to confirm residual disease.

FDG-PET during treatment

Numerous studies have demonstrated that PET scans performed after one or more cycles of chemotherapy predict progression-free and overall survival.[50,56–60] Unfortunately, no available data demonstrate that altering treatment on the basis of PET results improves patient outcome. Moskowitz *et al.* reported on 87 patients with DLBCL who underwent four cycles of a dose-intense R-CHOP (cyclophosphamide, doxorubicin, vincrinstine, and prednisone, plus rituximab) every 14 days followed by a PET scan.[61] Those with a negative scan received three cycles of ifosfamide, carboplatin, and etoposide (ICE) and observation. Patients with a positive interim PET scan underwent a biopsy. Those with a negative biopsy received three cycles of ICE. Patients with a positive biopsy were to receive ICE for two cycles, rituximab plus ICE for one cycle, and autologous stem cell transplantation. The NPV of the PET scan was 89%. However, the PPV was only 26%. There were 4 positive biopsies, but 27 were negative, giving an 87% false-positive rate. There was no difference in event-free survival between patients with a positive or negative PET scan.

Recently Terasawa *et al.* published a systematic review of the published literature to characterize the prognostic accuracy of FDG-PET for interim response assessment.[62] They identified 13 studies including 360 patients with advanced-stage HL and 311 patients with DLBCL. They found that FDG-PET had an overall sensitivity of 0.81 (95% CI = 0.72–0.89) and a specificity of 0.97 (95% CI = 0.94–0.99) in HL and a sensitivity of 0.78 (95% CI = 0.64–0.87) and specificity of 0.87 (95% CI = 0.75–0.93) in DLBCL. They were unable to identify factors that influenced the prognostic accuracy of the procedure. They concluded that interim PET was not currently of demonstrated usefulness and it should be limited to further study in clinical trials.

The International Harmonization Project and revised response criteria

Juweid *et al.* were the first to evaluate the impact of integrating FDG-PET into the IWG response criteria of 1999.[52] They reported a retrospective analysis of 54 patients with aggressive NHL treated with CHOP-based chemotherapy, who were evaluated by CT and FDG-PET, and followed for at least 18 months posttreatment. FDG-PET increased the number of CRs by converting not only PRs into CRs, but also by more accurately characterizing the subset of patients who would have been considered CRu. The 18-month progression-free survival was similar whether patients were considered to be in a CR by CT or FDG-PET and CT. However, the major difference was in patients considered PR for whom the median progression-free survival was 70% with IWG recommendation and 22% when FDG-PET was included.

In 2005, the German Competence Network Malignant Lymphoma sponsored a workshop at the International Conference on Malignant Lymphomas (ICML, Lugano,

Switzerland) to determine compliance with the IWG response criteria. Numerous discrepancies were identified in compliance with the IWG criteria amongst nine international lymphoma study groups.[63] As a consequence, the International Harmonization Project (IHP) was convened to bring together an international committee of lymphoma investigators, pathologists, and nuclear medicine physicians. The IWG criteria and other available response schemes were reassessed. Assouline *et al.*[64] had proposed a modified Response Evaluation Criteria in Solid Tumors (RECIST) criteria for lymphoma using unidimensional measurements of lymph nodes and masses and reported a high concordance with the IWG criteria; however, the concordance was high only in those studies with low response rates.[65]

Following extensive deliberations, the International Harmonization Workshop developed two consensus reports: one that standardized the performance and interpretation of PET in lymphoma clinical trials[66] and the other that revised the IWG response criteria by integrating FDG-PET and bone marrow immunohistochemistry.[8]

The IHP defined a positive scan using visual assessment as focal or diffuse FDG uptake above background in a location incompatible with normal anatomy or physiology. Exceptions include mild and diffusely increased FDG uptake at the site of moderate or large-sized masses with an intensity that is lower than or equal to the mediastinal blood pool, hepatic or splenic nodules 1.5 cm with FDG uptake lower than the surrounding liver/spleen uptake, and diffusely increased bone marrow uptake within weeks following treatment.[66] Areas of necrosis may be FDG-avid within an otherwise negative residual mass and a follow-up scan in a few months is often indicated to confirm this clinical impression. The proportion of a reduction in maximum standard uptake value (SUV_{max}) that best correlates with response is currently being evaluated.

FDG-PET and response assessment

The new IHP response criteria recommendations took into account differences in clinical behavior and FDG-avidity among the various lymphoma histologic subtypes, and the relevant endpoints of clinical trials (Table 15.1). For example, PET was strongly encouraged prior to treatment of patients with routinely FDG-avid, potentially curable lymphomas (e.g., DLBCL, HL) to better delineate the extent of disease and provide a baseline for posttreatment comparisons. For the incurable but FDG-avid histologies (e.g., follicular and low-grade lymphoma, and mantle cell lymphoma) PET was not recommended prior to treatment unless response rate, particularly CR, was a primary endpoint of the trial since time-dependent endpoints (e.g., progression-free survival) are generally more relevant for these diseases. FDG-PET was also recommended for patients with clinical stage I disease for whom local radiation therapy was being considered to rule out the possibility of other sites of disease. In addition, FDG-PET may be useful to identify the preferred node to biopsy in a patient with an indolent lymphoma suspected of having transformed to a more aggressive histology.

Table 15.1. Recommended indications for FDG-PET

Histology	Pre-treatment	Mid-treatment	Restaging	Surveillance
Hodgkin	Yes	No[a]	Yes	No
DLBCL	Yes	No[a]	Yes	No
Follicular	No[b]	No	No[b,c]	No
Mantle cell	No[b]	No	No[b,c]	No
CLL/SLL	No[d]	No	No	No
Other indolent	No[b]	No	No[b,c]	No
T-NHL	No[b]	No	No[b,c]	No

Note: CLL/SLL: chronic lymphocytic leukemia/small lymphocytic lymphoma.
[a]Except in studies looking at risk-directed strategies.
[b]Unless complete response is a study endpoint.
[c]Unless complete response is a study endpoint and the PET scan was positive prior to treatment.
[d]Unless Richter's transformation is suspected.

The timing of PET scans following the completion of treatment is an important consideration. In general, PET scans should not be performed until 6–8 weeks following completion of therapy to reduce the likelihood of a false-positive result.[66]

Revised response criteria

Given these considerations, the new response criteria were developed to incorporate PET (Table 15.2.)[8]

Complete remission (CR) requires:

1. Complete disappearance of all clinical evidence of disease and disease-related symptoms.
2. a. Typically FDG-avid lymphoma. In patients with no pretreatment PET scan or when the FDG-PET scan was positive prior to therapy: a posttreatment residual mass of any size is permitted as long as it is PET-negative.
   b. Variably FDG-avid lymphomas/FDG-avidity unknown. In patients without a pretreatment PET scan, or if a pretreatment PET scan was negative: all lymph nodes and nodal masses must have regressed on CT to normal size (≤ 1.5 cm in their greatest transverse diameter for nodes > 1.5 cm prior to therapy). Previously involved nodes that were 1.1–1.5 cm in their long axis and > 1.0 cm in their short axis prior to treatment must have decreased to ≤ 1.0 cm in their short axis after treatment.
3. The spleen and/or liver, if considered enlarged prior to therapy on the basis of a physical examination or CT scan,

Table 15.2. Response definitions for clinical trials

Response	Definition	Nodal masses	Spleen/liver	Bone marrow
Complete remission	Disappearance of all evidence of disease	a. FDG-avid or PET+ prior to therapy: FDG-negative mass of any size	Not palpable, no nodules	No involvement
		b. Variably FDG-avid, PET-neg, or no PET: normal CT scan		
Partial remission	Regression of measurable disease, no new sites	≥ 50% decrease in SPD of up to 6 largest masses. No increase in other nodes a. FDG-avid or PET+ prior to therapy: ≥ 1 PET+ previously involved sites	No increase in liver/spleen ≥ 50% decrease in SPD of nodules or transverse diameter if single nodule	Irrelevant if positive prior to therapy
		b. Variably FDG-avid or PET-neg: regression on CT		
Stable disease	Failure to attain CR, PR, or progression	a. FDG-avid or PET+ prior to therapy: PET+ at prior sites of disease, no new sites		
		b. Variably avid or PET-neg: no change on CT		
Relapsed or progressive disease	Any new lesion or increase by ≥ 50% from nadir in previously involved sites	New lesion > 1.5 cm in any axis	≥ 50% increase from nadir in SPD of previous lesions or longest diameter if only a single lesion	New or recurrent involvement
		≥ 50% increase in longest diameter of previous node > 1 cm in short axis or in SPD of > 1 node		
		PET+ if FDG-avid or + prior to therapy		

Note: SPD: sum of the product of the diameters.
Source: Adapted from Cheson *et al.*[8]

should not be palpable on physical examination and should be considered normal size by imaging studies, and nodules related to lymphoma should disappear. However, determination of splenic involvement is not always reliable as a spleen considered normal in size may still contain lymphoma, whereas an enlarged spleen may reflect variations in anatomy, blood volume, the use of hematopoietic growth factors, or other causes rather than lymphoma.

4. If the bone marrow was involved by lymphoma prior to treatment, the infiltrate must have cleared on repeat bone marrow biopsy. The biopsy sample on which this determination is made must be adequate (with a goal of ≥ 20 mm unilateral core). If the sample is indeterminate by morphology, it should be negative by immunohistochemistry. A sample that is negative by immunohistochemistry but demonstrating a small population of clonal lymphocytes by flow cytometry will be considered a CR until data become available demonstrating a clear difference in patient outcome.

Complete remission/unconfirmed (CRu): Using the above definition for CR and that below for PR eliminates the category of CRu.

Partial remission (PR) requires all of the following:

1. ≥ 50% decrease in sum of the product of the diameters (SPD) of up to six of the largest dominant nodes or nodal masses. These nodes or masses should be selected according to all of the following: (a) they should be clearly measurable in at least two perpendicular dimensions; (b) if possible, they should be from disparate regions of the body; (c) they should include mediastinal and retroperitoneal areas of disease whenever these sites are involved.
2. No increase in the size of other nodes, liver, or spleen.

3. Splenic and hepatic nodules must regress by $\geq 50\%$ in their SPD or, for single nodules, in the greatest transverse diameter.
4. With the exception of splenic and hepatic nodules, involvement of other organs is usually evaluable and not measurable disease.
5. Bone marrow assessment is irrelevant for determination of a PR if the sample was positive prior to treatment. However, if positive, the cell type should be specified, e.g., large cell lymphoma or small neoplastic B cells. Patients who achieve a CR by the above criteria but who have persistent morphologic bone marrow involvement will be considered partial responders.
   In cases where the bone marrow was involved prior to therapy that resulted in a clinical CR, but with no bone marrow assessment following treatment, patients should be considered partial responders.
6. No new sites of disease.
7. Typically FDG-avid lymphoma: For patients with no pretreatment PET scan or if the PET scan was positive prior to therapy, the posttreatment PET should be positive in at least one previously involved site.
8. Variably FDG-avid lymphomas/FDG-avidity unknown: For patients without a pretreatment PET scan, or if a pretreatment PET scan was negative, CT criteria should be used.

Stable disease:

1. Failing to attain the criteria needed for a CR or PR, but not fulfilling those for progressive disease (see below).
2. Typically FGD-avid lymphomas: The FDG-PET should be positive at prior sites of disease with no new areas of involvement on the posttreatment CT or PET.
3. Variably FDG-avid lymphomas/FDG-avidity unknown: For patients without a pretreatment PET scan or if the pretreatment PET was negative, there must be no change in the size of the previous lesions on the posttreatment CT scan.

Relapsed disease (after CR)/progressive disease (after PR, SD):

Lymph nodes should be considered abnormal if the long axis is > 1.5 cm regardless of the short axis. If a lymph node has a long axis of 1.1–1.5 cm it should only be considered abnormal if its short axis is > 1.0 cm. Lymph nodes ≤ 1.0 cm by ≤ 1.0 cm will not be considered as abnormal for relapse or progressive disease.

1. Appearance of any new lesion > 1.5 cm in any axis during or at the end of therapy, even if others are decreasing in size. Increased FDG uptake in a previously unaffected site should only be considered relapsed or progressive disease after confirmation with other modalities. In patients with no prior history of pulmonary lymphoma, new lung nodules identified by CT are mostly benign. Thus, a therapeutic decision should not be made solely on the basis of the PET without histologic confirmation.
2. $\geq 50\%$ increase from nadir in the SPD of any previously involved nodes, or in a single involved node, or the size of other lesions (e.g., splenic or hepatic nodules). To be considered progressive disease, a lymph node with a diameter of the short axis of < 1.0 cm must increase by $\geq 50\%$ and to a size of 1.5×1.5 cm or > 1.5 cm in the long axis.
3. $\geq 50\%$ increase in the longest diameter of any single previously identified node > 1 cm in its short axis.
4. Lesions should be PET-positive if a typical FDG-avid lymphoma or one that was PET-positive prior to therapy unless the lesion is too small to be detected with current PET systems (< 1.5 cm in its long axis by CT).

In clinical trials where PET is not available to the vast majority of participants, or where PET is deemed neither necessary nor appropriate, response should be assessed as above, but only using CT scans. In this setting, residual masses should not be considered a CRu, but should be designated as PR.

These response criteria have now been adopted internationally by study groups and regulatory agencies. Brepoels *et al.* validated the new response criteria in 69 patients with aggressive or indolent NHL and confirmed that the new response criteria were superior to the IWG criteria alone, although PET was of less value in the indolent NHL.[67]

Follow-up

After completion of therapy, the manner in which patients are followed may differ considerably between a clinical trial and clinical practice, by histologic subtype, and whether treatment was initiated with curative or palliative intent. The National Comprehensive Cancer Network published recommendations for follow-up of patients with NHL:[68] for patients with a history of follicular or other indolent histology in a complete remission, the recommendation for follow-up was every 3 months for a year then every 3–6 months. For DLBCL, the guidelines proposed assessment every 3 months for 24 months then every 6 months for 36 months with imaging studies performed when clinically indicated. For patients with HL in an initial CR, an interim history and physical examination every 2–4 months for 1–2 years, then every 3–6 months for the next 3–5 years, with annual monitoring for late effects after 5 years. Imaging studies should be performed when clinically indicated.[69]

Although widely used in clinical practice, there is no evidence to support regular surveillance CT or PET scans and this practice is discouraged. A number of studies in the pre-PET era demonstrated that the patient or physician identifies the relapse more than 80% of the time.[70–73] There is no apparent role for surveillance PET scans in the follow-up of patients with NHL. Jerusalem *et al.* reported on 36 patients who underwent PET following therapy and every 4–6 months thereafter.[74] There were five events detected by PET, one in a patient with known residual disease. Two of the four patients whose relapse 5–24 months following treatment was identified by PET already had developed disease-related symptoms. In addition, there were six false-positive studies.

Zinzani *et al.* conducted a prospective evaluation of 160 patients with HL, 183 with aggressive NHL, and 78 with indolent lymphoma who underwent regular follow-up evaluation as well as FDG-PET at 6, 12, 18, and 24 months post-therapy, then annually.[55] For patients with HL, the likelihood of relapse was negligible after 12 months and after 18 months for the aggressive NHLs. Scans were interpreted as positive for relapse, negative for relapse, or inconclusive when they were considered equivocal. All patients with an inconclusive study underwent biopsy; in only 33% was there suspected relapse on CT scan as well. Among the patients who were PET+/CT−, there was a 42% false-positive rate. There was a continuous risk of relapse for the indolent NHLs. Patients with suspected relapse underwent biopsy with a 33% false-positive rate of PET scans. There was no benefit from continued surveillance studies after 12 months for HL and 18 months for DLBCL. Importantly, the likelihood of a true positive was greatest in patients considered to be at highest risk for recurrence. However, the cost-effectiveness of such monitoring has not yet been demonstrated.

Conclusions

FDG-PET is the most sensitive and specific imaging modality currently available for patients with lymphoma. However, despite the increasing use of FDG-PET, its role in clinical management remains to be defined. Risk-directed studies are needed to validate preliminary observations that suggest that a negative PET may permit a decrease in the amount of chemotherapy or radiation therapy required, especially in patients with limited-stage disease that is responding to therapy, or increase efficacy by leading to an alteration of therapy in patients with less responsive disease.[75,76] There are currently no data to support routine surveillance with CT or PET scans. Clearly, PET scans provide additional information regarding the status of activity of lymphoma; however, the impact of this technology on patient management is still being clarified in clinical research trials. Integration of PET into the revised response criteria for clinical trials will hopefully improve the ability to accurately define efficacy of therapy, facilitate drug approval by regulatory agencies, and improve the outcome for patients with lymphoma.

References

1. Cheson BD, Horning SJ, Coiffier B, *et al.* Report of an international workshop to standardize response criteria for non-Hodgkin's lymphomas. *J Clin Oncol* 1999;**17**:1244–53.
2. Grillo-López AJ, Cheson BD, Horning SJ, *et al.* Response criteria for NHL: importance of "normal" lymph node size and correlations with response rates. *Ann Oncol* 2000;**11**: 399–408.
3. Dorfman RE, Alpern MB, Gross BH, *et al.* Upper abdominal lymph nodes: criteria for normal size determined with CT. *Radiology* 1991;**180**:319–22.
4. Einstein DM, Singer AA, Chilcote WA, *et al.* Abdominal lymphadenopathy: spectrum of CT findings. *RadioGraphics* 1991;**11**:457–72.
5. Glazer GM, Gross BH, Quint LE, *et al.* Normal mediastinal lymph nodes: number and size according to American Thoracic Society mapping. *AJR Am J Roentgenol* 1985;**144**:261–5.
6. Kiyono K, Sone S, Sakai F, *et al.* The number and size of normal mediastinal lymph nodes: a postmortem study. *AJR Am J Roentgenol* 1988; **150**:771–6.
7. Steinkamp HJ, Hosten N, Richter C, *et al.* Enlarged cervical lymph nodes at helical CT. *Radiology* 1994;**191**:795–8.
8. Cheson BD, Pfistner B, Juweid ME, *et al.* Revised response criteria for malignant lymphoma. *J Clin Oncol* 2007;**25**:579–86.
9. Newman JS, Francis JR, Kaminski MS, *et al.* Imaging of lymphoma with PET with 2-[F-18]-fluoro-2-deoxy-D-glucose: correlation with CT. *Radiology* 1994;**190**:111–16.
10. Thill R, Neuerburg J, Fabry U, *et al.* Comparison of findings with 18-FDG PET and CT in pretherapeutic staging of malignant lymphoma. *Nuklearmedizin* 1997;**36**:234–9.
11. Fuks JZ, Aisner J, Wiernik PH. Restaging laparotomy in the management of the non-Hodgkin lymphomas. *Med Pediatr Oncol* 1982;**10**:429–38.
12. Stewart FM, Williamson BR, Innes DJ, *et al.* Residual tumor masses following treatment for advanced histiocytic lymphoma. *Cancer* 1985;**55**:620–3.
13. Surbone A, Longo DL, DeVita VT Jr, *et al.* Residual abdominal masses in aggressive non-Hodgkin's lymphoma after combination chemotherapy: significance and management. *J Clin Oncol* 1988;**6**:1832–7.
14. Stumpe KD, Urbinelli M, Steinert HC, *et al.* Whole-body positron emission tomography using fluorodeoxyglucose for staging of lymphoma: effectiveness and comparison with computed tomography. *Eur J Nucl Med* 1998;**25**:721–8.
15. Longo DL, DeVita VT Jr, Duffey PL, *et al.* Superiority of ProMACE-CytaBOM over ProMACE-MOPP in the treatment of advanced diffuse aggressive lymphoma: results of a prospective randomized trial. *J Clin Oncol* 1991;**9**:25–38.
16. Radford JA, Cowan RA, Flanagan M, *et al.* The significance of residual mediastinal abnormality on the chest radiograph following treatment for Hodgkin's disease. *J Clin Oncol* 1988;**6**:940–6.
17. Carbone PP, Kaplan HS, Musshoff K, *et al.* Report of the Committee on Hodgkin's Disease Staging Classification. *Cancer Res* 1971;**31**:1860–1.
18. Jerusalem G, Warland V, Najjar F, *et al.* Whole-body 18F-FDG PET for the evaluation of patients with Hodgkin's disease and non-Hodgkin's lymphoma. *Nucl Med Commun* 1999;**20**:13–20.
19. Moog F, Bangerter M, Diederichs CG, *et al.* Lymphoma: role of whole-body 2-deoxy-2-[F-18]-D-glucose (FDG) PET in nodal staging. *Radiology* 1997;**203**:795–800.
20. Moog F, Bangerter M, Diederichs CG, *et al.* Extranodal malignant lymphoma:

detection with FDG PET versus CT. *Radiology* 1998;**206**:475–81.

21. Buchmann I, Reinhardt M, Elsner K, *et al.* 2-(fluorine-18)fluoro-2-deoxy-D-glucose positron emission tomography in the detection and staging of malignant lymphoma. A bicenter trial. *Cancer* 2001;**91**:889–99.
22. Bangerter M, Moog F, Buchmann I, *et al.* Whole-body 2-[18F]-fluoro-2-deoxy-D-glucose positron emission tomography (FDG-PET) for accurate staging of Hodgkin's disease. *Ann Oncol* 1998;**9**:1117–22.
23. Jerusalem G, Beguin Y, Najjar F, *et al.* Positron emission tomography (PET) with 18F-fluorodeoxyglucose (18F-FDG) for the staging of low-grade non-Hodgkin's lymphoma (NHL). *Ann Oncol* 2001;**12**:825–30.
24. Blum RH, Seymour JF, Wirth A, *et al.* Frequent impact of [18F] fluorodeoxyglucose positron emission tomography on the staging and management of patients with indolent non-Hodgkin's lymphoma. *Clin Lymphoma* 2004;**4**:43–9.
25. Jerusalem G, Beguin Y, Fassotte MF, *et al.* Whole-body positron emission tomography using 18F-fluorodeoxyglucose compared to standard procedures for staging patients with Hodgkin's disease. *Haematologica* 2001;**86**:266–73.
26. Partridge S, Timothy A, O'Doherty MJ, *et al.* 2-Fluorine-18-fluoro-2-deoxy-D glucose positron emission tomography in the pretreatment staging of Hodgkin's disease: influence on patient management in a single institution. *Ann Oncol* 2000;**11**:1273–9.
27. Weihrauch MR, Re D, Bischoff S, *et al.* Whole-body positron emission tomography using 18F-fluorodeoxyglucose for initial staging of patients with Hodgkin's disease. *Ann Hematol* 2002;**81**:20–5.
28. Menzel C, Dobert N, Mitrou P, *et al.* Positron emission tomography for the staging of Hodgkin's lymphoma – increasing the body of evidence in favor of the method. *Ann Oncol* 2002; **41**:430–6.
29. Naumann R, Beuthien-Baumann B, Reiss A, *et al.* Substantial impact of FDG PET imaging on the therapy decision in patients with early-stage Hodgkin's lymphoma. *Br J Cancer* 2004;**90**:620–5.
30. Hutchings M, Loft A, Hansen M, *et al.* Positron emission tomography with or without computed tomography in the primary staging of Hodgkin's lymphoma. *Haematologica* 2006;**91**:482–9.
31. Schaefer NG, Hany TF, Taverna C, *et al.* Non-Hodgkin lymphoma and Hodgkin disease: coregistered FDG PET and CT at staging and restaging – do we need contrast-enhanced CT? *Radiology* 2004;**232**:823–9.
32. Isasi CR, Lu P, Blaufox MD. A metaanalysis of ^{18}F-2-deoxy-2-fluoro-D-glucose positron emission tomography in the staging and restaging of patients with lymphoma. *Cancer* 2005;**104**:1066–74.
33. Moog F, Bangerter M, Kotzerke J, *et al.* 18-F-fluorodeoxyglucose-positron emission tomography as a new approach to detect lymphomatous bone marrow. *Blood* 1998;**16**:603–9.
34. Carr R, Barrington SF, Madan B, *et al.* Detection of lymphoma in bone marrow by whole-body positron emission tomography. *Blood* 1998;**91**:3340–6.
35. Pakos EE, Fotopoulos AD, Ioannidis JP. 18F-FDG PET for evaluation of bone marrow infiltration in staging of lymphoma: a meta-analysis. *J Nucl Med* 2005;**46**:958–63.
36. Munker R, Glass J, Griffeth LK, *et al.* Contribution of PET imaging to the initial staging and prognosis of patients with Hodgkin's disease. *Ann Oncol* 2004;**15**:1699–704.
37. Karam M, Novak L, Cyriac J, *et al.* Role of fluorine-18 fluoro-deoxyglucose positron emission tomography scan in the evaluation and follow-up of patients with low-grade lymphoma. *Cancer* 2006;**107**:175–183.
38. Rigacci L, Vitolo U, Nassi L, *et al.* Positron emission tomography in the staging of patients with Hodgkin's lymphoma. A prospective multicentric study by the Intergruppo Italiano Linfomi. *Ann Hematol* 2007;**86**: 897–903.
39. Tatsumi M, Cohade C, Nakamoto Y, *et al.* Direct comparison of FDG PET and CT findings in patients with lymphoma: initial experience. *Radiology* 2005;**237**:1038–45.
40. Raanani P, Shasha Y, Perry C, *et al.* Is CT scan still necessary for staging in Hodgkin and nonHodgkin lymphoma patients in the PET/CT era? *Ann Oncol* 2006;**17**:117–22.
41. la Fougère C, Hundt W, Bröckel N, *et al.* Value of PET/CT versus PET and CT performed as separate investigations in patients with Hodgkin's disease and non-Hodgkin's lymphoma. *Eur J Nucl Med Mol Imaging* 2006.
42. Querellou S, Valette F, Bodet-Milin C, *et al.* FDG-PET/CT predicts outcome in patients with aggressive non-Hodgkin's lymphoma and Hodgkin's disease. *Ann Hematol* 2006;**85**:759–67.
43. Allen-Auerbach M, Quon A, Weber WA, *et al.* Comparison between 2-deoxy-2-[18F]fluoro-D-glucose positron emission tomography and positron emission tomography/computed tomography hardware fusion for staging of patients with lymphoma. *Mol Imaging Biol* 2004;**6**:411–16.
44. Kwee TC, Kwee RM, Nievelstein RA. Imaging in staging of malignant lymphoma: a systematic review. *Blood* 2008;**111**:504–16.
45. la Fougere C, Hundt W, Brockel N, *et al.* Value of PET/CT versus PET and CT performed as separate investigations in patients with Hodgkin's disease and non-Hodgkin's lymphoma. *Eur J Nucl Med Mol Imaging* 2006;**33**:1417–25.
46. Juweid M, Cheson BD. Positron emission tomography (PET) in post-therapy assessment of cancer. *New Engl J Med* 2006;**354**:496–507.
47. Jerusalem G, Beguin Y, Fassotte MF, *et al.* Whole-body positron emission tomography using 18F-fluorodeoxyglucose for posttreatment evaluation in Hodgkin's disease and non-Hodgkin's lymphoma has higher diagnostic and prognostic value than classical computed tomography scan imaging. *Blood* 1999;**94**:429–33.
48. Zinzani PL, Magagnoli M, Chierichetti F, *et al.* The role of positron emission tomography (PET) in the management of lymphoma patients. *Ann Oncol* 1999;**10**:1141–3.
49. Weihrauch MR, Re D, Scheidhauer K, *et al.* Thoracic positron emission tomography using ^{18}F-fluorodeoxyglucose for the evaluation of residual mediastinal Hodgkin disease. *Blood* 2001;**98**:2930–4.
50. Spaepen K, Stroobants S, Dupont P, *et al.* Prognostic value of positron emission tomography (PET) with fluorine-18 fluorodeoxyglucose ([^{18}F]

FDG) after first-line chemotherapy in non-Hodgkin's lymphoma: Is [^{18}F] FDG-PET a valid alternative to conventional diagnostic methods? *J Clin Oncol* 2001;**19**:414–19.

51. Spaepen K, Stroobants S, Dupont P, *et al.* Can positron emission tomography with [18F]-fluorodeoxyglucose after first-line treatment distinguish Hodgkin's disease patients who need additional therapy from others in whom additional therapy would mean avoidable toxicity? *Br J Haematol* 2001;**115**:272–8.

52. Juweid M, Wiseman GA, Vose JM, *et al.* Response assessment of aggressive non-Hodgkin's lymphoma by integrated International Workshop Criteria (IWC) and 18F-fluorodeoxyglucose positron emission tomography (PET). *J Clin Oncol* 2005;**23**:4652–61.

53. Zijlstra JM, Lindauer-van der Werf G, Hoekstra OS, *et al.* ^{18}F-fluoro-deoxyglucose positron emission tomography for post-treatment evaluation of malignant lymphoma: a systematic review. *Haematologica* 2006;**91**:522–9.

54. Castellucci P, Nanni C, Farsad M, *et al.* Potential pitfalls of ^{18}F-FDG PET in a large series of patients treated for malignant lymphoma: prevalence and scan interpretation. *Nucl Med Commun* 2005;**26**:689–94.

55. Zinzani PL, Stefoni V, Tani M, *et al.* Role of [18F] Fluorodeoxy glucose positron emission tomography scan in the follow-up of lymphoma. *J Clin Oncol* 2009;**27**:1781–7.

56. Spaepen K, Stroobants S, Dupont P, *et al.* Prognostic value of pretransplantation positron emission tomography using fluorine 18-fluorodeoxyglucose in patients with aggressive lymphoma treated with high-dose chemotherapy and stem cell transplantation. *Blood* 2003;**102**:53–9.

57. Spaepen K, Stroobants S, Dupont P, *et al.* Early restaging positron emission tomography with 18F-fluorodeoxyglucose predicts outcome in patients with aggressive non-Hodgkin's lymphoma. *Ann Oncol* 2002;**13**:1356–63.

58. Haioun C, Itti E, Rahmouni A, *et al.* [^{18}F]fluoro-2-deoxy-D-glucose positron emission tomography (FDG-PET) in aggressive lymphoma: an early prognostic tool for predicting patient outcome. *Blood* 2005;**106**:1376–81.

59. Zinzani PL, Tani M, Fanti S, *et al.* Early positron emission tomography (PET) restaging: a predictive final response in Hodgkin's disease patients. *Ann Oncol* 2006;**17**:1296–300.

60. Kostakoglu L, Goldsmith SJ, Leonard JP, *et al.* FDG-PET after 1 cycle of therapy predicts outcome in diffuse large cell lymphoma and classic Hodgkin disease. *Cancer* 2006;**107**:2678–87.

61. Moskowitz C, Hamlin PA, Horwitz SM, *et al.* Phase II trial of dose-dense R-CHOP followed by risk-adapted consolidation with either ICE or ICE and ASCT, based upon the results of biopsy confirmed abnormal interim restaging PET scan, improves outcome in patients with advanced stage DLBCL. *Blood* 2006;**108**(part 1):161a (Abstract 532).

62. Terasawa T, Lau J, Bardet S, *et al.* Fluorine-18-fluorodeoxyglucose positron emission tomography for interim response assessment of advanced-stage Hodgkin's lymphoma and diffuse large B-cell lymphoma: a systematic review. *J Clin Oncol* 2009;**27**:1906–14.

63. Pfistner B, Diehl V, Cheson B. International harmonization of trial parameters in malignant lymphoma. *Eur J Haematol Suppl* 2005;**66**: 53–4.

64. Assouline S, Meyer RM, Infante-Rivard C, *et al.* Development of adapted RECIST criteria to assess response in lymphoma and their comparison to the International Workshop Criteria. *Leuk Lymphoma* 2007;**48**:513–20.

65. Cheson BD. Overcoming mechanisms of RECISTance in lymphoma. *Leuk Lymphoma* 2007;**48**:447–8.

66. Juweid ME, Stroobants S, Hoekstra OS, *et al.* Use of positron emission tomography for response assessment of lymphoma: consensus recommendations of the Imaging Subcommittee of the International Harmonization Project in Lymphoma. *J Clin Oncol* 2007;**25**:571–8.

67. Brepoels L, Stroobants S, De Wever W, *et al.* Aggressive and indolent non-Hodgkin's lymphoma: response assessment by integrated international workshop criteria. *Leuk Lymphoma* 2007;**48**:1522–30.

68. Zelenetz AD, Advani RH, Buadi F, *et al.* Non-Hodgkin's lymphoma: clinical practice guidelines in oncology. *J Natl Compr Canc Netw* 2006;**4**(3): 258–310.

69. Hoppe RT, Advani RH, Bierman PJ, *et al.* Hodgkin disease/lymphoma. Clinical practice guidelines in oncology. *J Natl Comp Canc Netw* 2006;**4**(3): 210–30.

70. Weeks JC, Yeap BY, Canellos GP, *et al.* Value of follow-up procedures in patients with large-cell lymphoma who achieve a complete remission. *J Clin Oncol* 1991;**9**:1196–203.

71. Oh YK, Ha CS, Samuels BI, *et al.* Stages I-III follicular lymphoma: role of CT of the abdomen and pelvis in follow-up studies. *Radiology* 1999;**210**:483–6.

72. Foltz LM, Song KW, Connors JM. Who actually detects relapse in Hodgkin lymphoma: patient or physician? *Blood* 2004;**104**(part 1):853–4a (Abstract 3124).

73. Liedtke M, Hamlin PA, Moskowitz CH, *et al.* Surveillance imaging during remission identifies a group of patients with more favorable aggressive NHL at time of relapse: a retrospective analysis of a uniformly-treated patient population. *Ann Oncol* 2006;**17**: 909–13.

74. Jerusalem G, Beguin Y, Fassotte MF, *et al.* Early detection of relapse by whole-body positron emission tomography in the follow-up of patients with Hodgkin's disease. *Ann Oncol* 2003;**14**:123–30.

75. Sehn LH, Savage K, Hoskins P, *et al.* Limited-stage DLBCL patients with a negative PET scan following three cycles of R-CHOP have an excellent outcome following abbreviated immuno-chemotherapy. *Ann Oncol* 2008;**19** Suppl 4: Abstract 052.

76. Sehn LH, Hoskins P, Klasa R, *et al.* FDG-PET scan guided consolidative radiation therapy may improve outcome in patients with advanced-stage aggressive NHL with residual abnormalities on CT scan following chemotherapy. *Ann Oncol* 2008;**19** Suppl 4:Abstract 126.

Chapter 16

Treatment approach to diffuse large B-cell lymphomas

Sonali M. Smith and Julie M. Vose

Introduction

Non-Hodgkin lymphoma (NHL) is a heterogeneous cancer encompassing several dozen distinct clinicopathologic diseases. The incidence of NHL appears to be rising independent of the aging of the population, and NHL currently ranks as the fifth most common cancer in both men and women with 71 380 new cases in 2007 and nearly 20 000 estimated deaths.[1] Diffuse large B-cell lymphoma (DLBCL), accounting for approximately one-third of all new cases, is both the most common histologic subtype of NHL and the prototype of aggressive lymphomas.

There are several histologic variants and clinical subtypes of DLBCL that are recognized (Figure 16.1). Histologic variants include immunoblastic, centroblastic, and anaplastic morphologies, whereas distinct clinical subtypes have included primary mediastinal large B-cell lymphoma (PMBL), intravascular large B-cell lymphoma, and primary effusion lymphoma, among others.[3] The latter two entities occur primarily in immunocompromised hosts and are associated with human herpesvirus 8. The histologic heterogeneity of DLBCL is complicated by the recent identification of molecular heterogeneity discovered by gene expression profiling, and is discussed in more detail below with an emphasis on its prognostic potential.

In general, DLBCL is a chemosensitive disease with a substantial portion of patients achieving cure with frontline chemoimmunotherapy. Unfortunately, many patients continue to relapse and are in need of further treatment. Patients with chemosensitive disease at relapse can achieve long-term disease control with autologous stem cell transplant, but others will succumb to DLBCL. Patients with refractory disease, those who relapse following transplant, and those who are not candidates for transplantation have no true curative options and most will ultimately die of lymphoma. The development of new agents and new treatment strategies, including improvement of existing transplant regimens and exploring allogeneic approaches, is an important area of ongoing research and is discussed below.

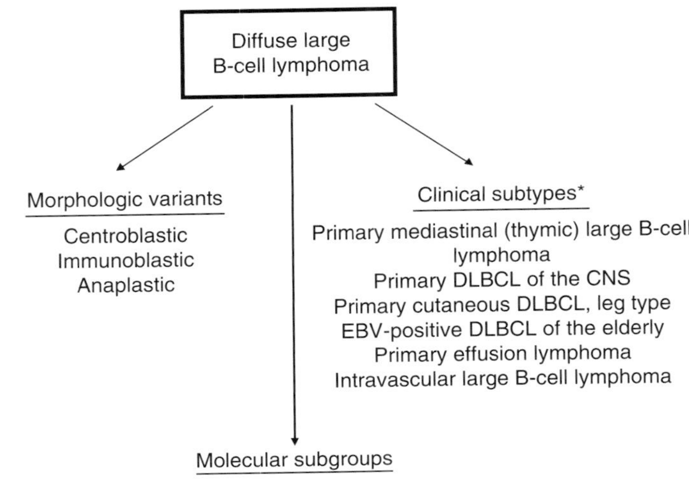

Figure 16.1 Morphologic, molecular, and selected clinical subtypes of DLBCL. (*See WHO 2008[2] for complete list.)

Clinical presentation, diagnosis, and staging

DLBCL occurs in all age groups, including children; however, the incidence of DLBCL increases with age, and the median age at presentation is the sixth decade of life. Men are affected slightly more often than women.[4] There are no known racial differences in incidence. The etiology of DLBCL, as with many cancers, is unknown for most patients. However, there are several well-established risk factors, including acquired and iatrogenic states of immunosuppression. NHL commonly occurs in patients with human immunodeficiency virus (HIV), and has been an AIDS-defining illness since 1985. Although most HIV-infected patients will develop aggressive subtypes, including DLBCL, there are new trends in both histology and behavior of these lymphomas due to increased availability of HAART (highly active antiretroviral therapy), and the increased incidence of HIV in heterosexual, minority, and female populations.[5] Among non-immunocompromised

Management of Hematologic Malignancies, ed. Susan M. O'Brien, Julie M. Vose, and Hagop M. Kantarjian. Published by Cambridge University Press.

(a)

(b)

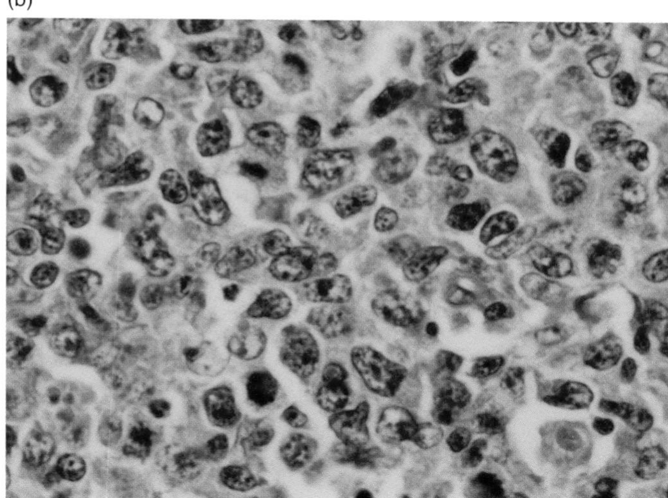

Figure 16.2 Low-power (a) and high-power (b) view of DLBCL. Lymph node architecture has been completely effaced by large lymphoid cells that are classically CD20+, CD19+, CD22+, and CD79a+. Photo courtesy of John Anastasi.

populations, a genetic component has been proposed, with some intriguing observations, but these remain active areas of investigation for the present time.[6] Viruses, autoimmune disorders, and other environmental factors may also increase the risk of DLBCL.[6,7]

In contrast to indolent lymphomas which are often incidentally diagnosed, most patients with DLBCL come to medical attention due to lymphoma-related symptoms. The symptoms can be systemic, such as classical B symptoms, but also include pain or organ dysfunction due to local consequences of rapidly enlarging adenopathy or infiltration. B symptoms include fevers, night sweats, or unintentional weight loss of greater than 10%. Although nodal involvement is most common, nearly every body part can be involved, and approximately 30–50% of newly diagnosed DLBCL includes at least one extranodal site.

The diagnosis of DLBCL requires adequate histologic examination. The increasing use of minimally invasive techniques or interventional radiology procedures unfortunately provides scant material for both morphologic assessment and immunohistochemical analysis. A fine needle aspirate (FNA) does not allow the ability to determine prognosis or biologic subtypes within DLBCL (see discussion below). The optimal biopsy specimen is an excisional or incisional lymph node biopsy, but large-bore core-needle biopsies are occasionally sufficient if the architecture is preserved. The usual morphologic appearance is sheets of intermediate- to large-sized cells obliterating the normal follicular architecture (Figure 16.2).[3] The malignant cells express mature B-cell markers including CD20, CD19, CD79a, and CD22, which can be detected by both flow cytometry and immunohistochemical analysis. Rarely, DLBCL will coexpress CD5, ALK protein, or the Myc oncoprotein, all of which portend an unfavorable prognosis. Cytogenetic analysis shows translocation of t(14;18), leading to BCL2 overexpression, or 3q27 abnormalities, leading to BCL6 abnormalities, in approximately one-third of cases. Cytogenetics currently are diagnostic in intent, and do not generally carry prognostic significance. However, a recently identified subtype carrying both the t(14;18) translocation and 8q24/*c-MYC* rearrangement has an extremely aggressive behavior with a poor prognosis.[8,9]

Table 16.1. Ann Arbor staging classification of lymphomas (Cotswold revision)

Stage I	Involvement of a single lymph node region or a lymph node structure or a single extralymphatic site
Stage II	Involvement of two or more lymph node regions on the same side of the diaphragm or localized contiguous involvement of an extralymphatic site and lymph node organ
Stage III	Involvement of lymph node regions on both sides of the diaphragm
Stage IV	Diffuse or disseminated involvement of one or more extranodal organs or tissues, with or without associated lymph node involvement
A	Absence of B symptoms
B	Presence of B symptoms (fevers, drenching night sweats, weight loss > 10% of body weight)
E	Extranodal disease or extension from known nodal site of disease
X	Bulky disease: > 1/3 widening of the mediastinum at T5–T6, or maximum of nodal mass > 10 cm

Once the diagnosis of DLBCL is established, a staging evaluation is performed to determine the extent of disease and extranodal involvement. The Ann Arbor classification remains the standard staging system (Table 16.1). The staging evaluation consists of ^{18}F-fluorodeoxyglucose positron emission tomography (FDG-PET) or FDG-PET/CT scans of the chest, abdomen, and pelvis, along with a bone marrow aspirate and core biopsy. In many centers, bilateral bone marrow biopsies are preferred, but a single biopsy of at least 2 cm may be acceptable.[10] A lumbar puncture is suggested for patients with a higher risk of central nervous system (CNS) relapse including those with marrow involvement by large cell lymphoma, elevated lactate dehydrogenase (LDH), DLBCL of the sinuses or head and neck, testicular lymphoma, breast lymphoma, and high-risk disease by the International Prognostic Index (IPI) (see discussion below). An assessment of cardiac function in anticipation of anthracycline-based chemotherapy is also routinely performed. Laboratory testing should include an LDH, complete blood count (CBC) with differential, hepatic function tests, renal function tests, and uric acid. FDG-PET scans have dramatically improved the sensitivity of radiologic imaging, and are currently recommended at baseline and following treatment to evaluate response in DLBCL.[11] DLBCL is a strongly FDG-PET-avid disease, and many investigators have proposed that a mid-treatment negative FDG-PET connotes a favorable prognostic significance.[12–15] A prospective multicenter French study found that a negative FDG-PET scan following two cycles of therapy carried a 2-year event-free survival (EFS) of 82% versus only 43% for FDG-PET-positive patients ($p < 0.001$); similarly, overall survival (OS) was improved (91% vs. 60%, $p = 0.006$).[12] However, the results of an interim PET do not currently change treatment approaches and should not be done outside of a clinical trial. Details on the use of FDG-PET imaging in lymphomas are discussed in Chapter 15.

Prognosis in DLBCL

Despite being a potentially curable disease, there is vast heterogeneity in patient outcomes, much of which can be attributed to pretreatment variables. The landmark evaluation of prognostic factors in DLBCL is the IPI, published by an international task force in 1993.[16] Over 2000 patients receiving anthracycline-based treatment were retrospectively analyzed for clinical features potentially predictive of outcome including sex, age, Ann Arbor stage, performance status, presence or absence of B symptoms, sites of lymphoma involvement, number of extranodal disease sites, tumor size, LDH, albumin, and β_2-microglobulin. The only five factors retaining independent prognostic significance in multivariate analysis include age ≥ 60 years, tumor stage (I or II versus III or IV), performance status ≥ 2, serum LDH level, and the presence of greater than one extranodal site of involvement. The IPI is essentially a scoring system in which these five clinical features are tallied to categorize patients into one of four prognostic groups that correlate with both relapse-free and overall survival. In addition to providing prognostic guidance at an individual patient level, the IPI provides a common language for clinical trials to allow homogeneity when comparing patient groups. Some groups have proposed to revise the prognostic potential of the IPI since the standard of care for frontline treatment has now evolved to include both rituximab and anthracycline-based chemotherapy.[17] The Vancouver group evaluated 345 unselected patients reported to a regional registry. The standard IPI could only identify two prognostic groups instead of four groups; by regrouping the same five risk factors, however, patients could be once again separated into four groups with different outcomes. The authors propose this revised IPI (R-IPI) for use in patients treated with R-CHOP (rituximab plus cyclophosphamide, doxorubicin, vincristine, and prednisone) type regimens. It is worthwhile to note the excellent prognosis of patients with 0 risk factors, with 94% survival at 4 years. In contrast, patients with 3–5 risk factors, comprising 45% of the sampled population, had a 4-year OS of only 55%. For now, the IPI and R-IPI remain the most clinically useful tools to predict prognosis.

In addition to clinical heterogeneity captured by the IPI and R-IPI, there is recent awareness of molecular heterogeneity within DLBCL that influences prognosis.[18–20] The National Cancer Institute (NCI) first published their findings of distinct mRNA gene expression profiles with disparate clinical outcomes: germinal center B-cell-like DLBCL (GCB) and activated B-cell-like DLBCL (ABC).[18] Patients with the GCB phenotype had a 5-year OS of 76% versus only 16% for patients with the ABC phenotype. Not only did the gene expression profile (GEP) correlate with the IPI (i.e., low- versus high-risk patients) but it could also distinguish differential outcomes within risk groups (Figure 16.3). This powerful analysis proposes that DLBCL is actually two distinct diseases with differing prognoses. The Lymphoma/Leukemia Molecular Profiling Project (LLMPP) and others have reported similar findings using a variety of microarray techniques such as hierarchical clustering and supervised learning algorithms applied to mRNA platforms.[19,20] Of the thousands of genes within each signature, six genes were most predictive of survival in DLBCL patients treated with CHOP-like chemotherapy: *LMO2, BCL6, FN1, CCND2, SCYA3,* and *BCL2*.[21] *LMO2, BCL6,* and *FN1* were associated with a longer survival whereas *CCND2, SCYA3,* and *BCL2* were associated with a shorter survival.

A major limitation of gene expression profiling is that, for now, it is a costly and still experimental technique that is not widely available. Furthermore, mRNA gene expression profiling via microarrays requires frozen material and cannot be performed on paraffin-embedded tumor specimens. As an alternative, immunohistochemical algorithms have been proposed as a surrogate, which may correctly identify GCB versus non-GCB at least two-thirds of the time.[22,23] Using a tissue microarray of paraffin-embedded tissue and staining for a variety of markers, Hans and colleagues found that three immunohistochemical markers correlated with either GCB or non-GCB subtypes identified by gene expression profiling on frozen counterparts in 152 patients: CD10, BCL6, and MUM-1 (Figure 16.4).[23] Patients with GCB using this

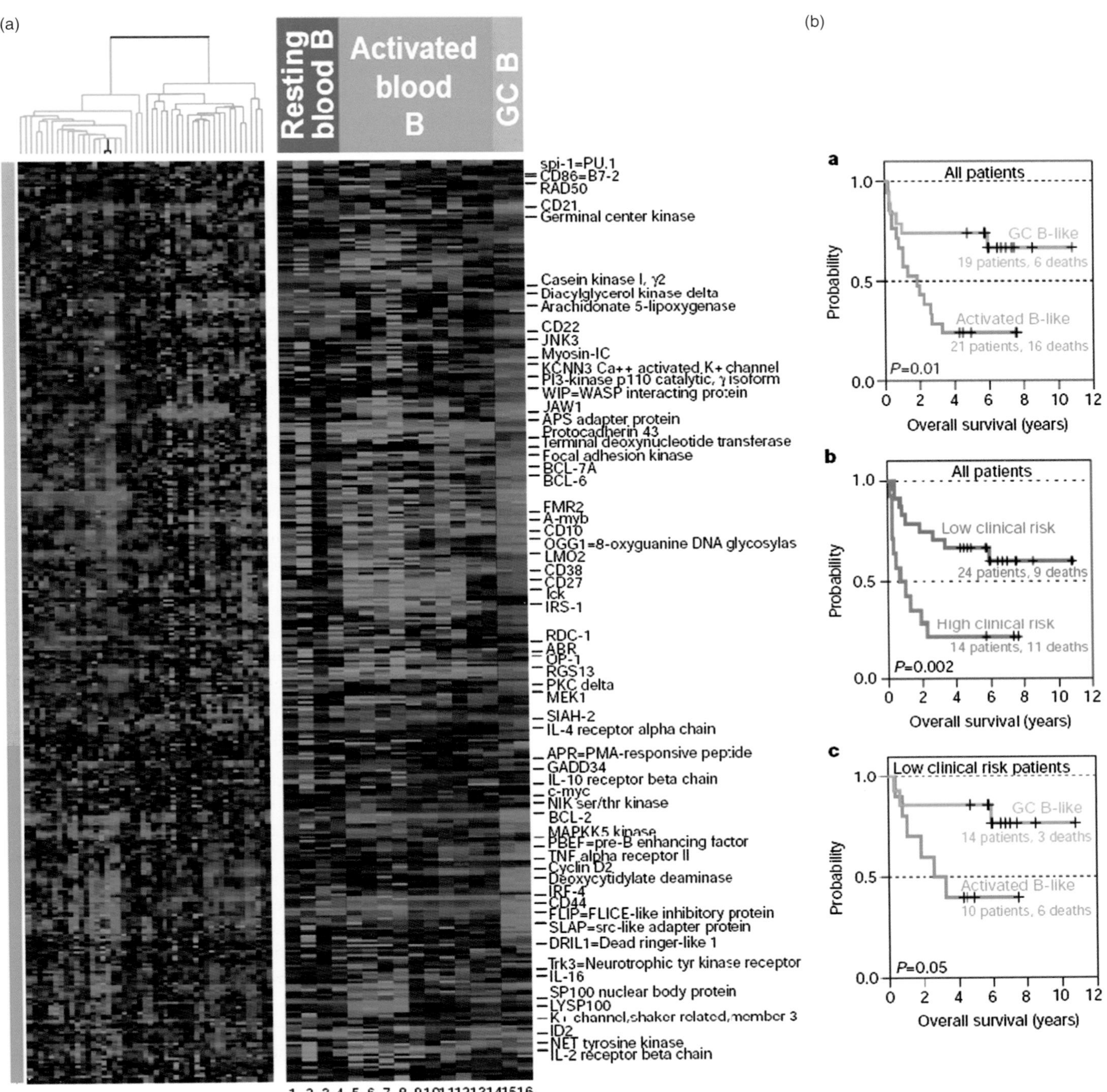

Figure 16.3 (a) Relationship between DLBCL subgroups and normal B-cell stages of differentiation using gene expression profiling. At least two molecular subtypes of DLBCL are identified. With permission from Alizadeh *et al.*, *Nature* 2000; **403**:503–11.[18] (b) Clinical outcome for a test group of patients with GCB-like versus activated B-like gene expression for all patients (panel a), by IPI (panel b), and for low clinical risk groups (panel c).

immunohistochemical algorithm had a 5-year OS of 76% versus 34% for the non-GCB group ($p < 0.001$). Another group found that many patients express both germinal center markers such as CD10 and/or BCL6 along with activation markers such as MUM-1 or CD138.[22] They developed an alternative immunohistochemical algorithm, and categorized patients into either GCB, *activated* GCB, and activated non-GCB. In this analysis, the presence of any activation marker irrespective of germinal center markers resulted in a less favorable outcome.

A second challenge to the interpretation of microarray data in DLBCL is the applicability of findings to patients being treated with chemoimmunotherapy (i.e., anthracycline-based

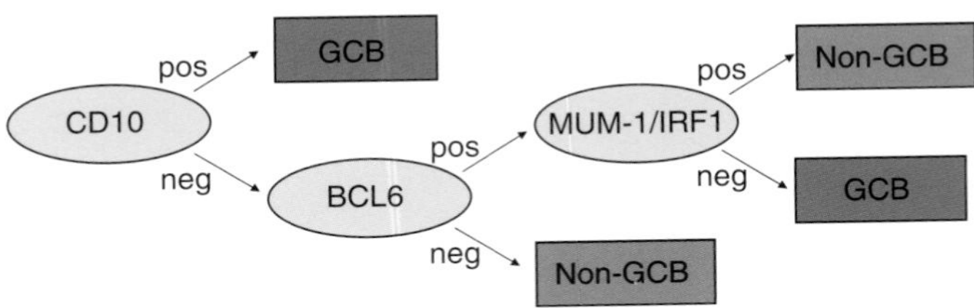

Figure 16.4 Immunohistochemical algorithm to identify germinal center B-cell-like DLBCL (GCB) from non-germinal center B-cell-like DLBCL. IRF1: interferon regulating factor 1. With permission from Hans *et al.*, *Blood* 2004;**103**(1):275–82.[23] © The American Society of Hematology.

chemotherapy plus rituximab as opposed to anthracycline-based chemotherapy alone). It is possible that changes in therapy will cause a re-assessment of previously accepted prognostic factors. In order to test this assumption, there are several international collaborative efforts to test the prognostic significance of GCB versus non-GCB phenotype in patients treated with R-CHOP or similar regimens. One recently published report suggests that the same six-gene model found in CHOP-treated patients retains its prognostic significance in R-CHOP treated patients.[24]

Outside of GEP, other biologic features also carry prognostic significance. Perhaps one of the most powerful is BCL2, where overexpression of this antiapoptotic protein leads to shortened EFS and OS in patients with DLBCL.[25,26] The prognostic significance of BCL2 in DLBCL has been called into question with the introduction of rituximab. A subanalysis of GELA98–5 shows that rituximab overcomes the negative prognostic significance of BCL2 protein overexpression.[27] In this study, 193 elderly patients with BCL2 overexpression were compared to 99 patients without BCL2 overexpression. Of the BCL2-positive patients, R-CHOP improved the EFS from 32% to 58% ($p < 0.001$) and the OS from 48% to 67% ($p = 0.004$). In contrast, there was no statistically significant improvement by the addition of rituximab for the BCL2-negative group. It should be noted that the mechanism of BCL2 activation is different in GCB and non-GCB subtypes of DLBCL, which may explain some differences in prognostic significance.[26] In the GCB subtype, BCL2 overexpression is due to t(14;18) and does not appear to have a major prognostic role. In activated/non-GCB subtypes, BCL2 overexpression is due to 18q21 amplification or activation from the nuclear factor-kappa B (NF-κB) pathway, and reduces OS.

BCL6 normally portends a positive effect on EFS and OS, but its prognostic potential has also been challenged by the use of rituximab. In ECOG 4494, the use of R-CHOP overcame the negative prognostic significance of BCL6 negativity. Of 199 elderly DLBCL patients, R-CHOP improved the failure-free survival (FFS) from 9% to 76% ($p < 0.001$) and OS from 17% to 79% ($p < 0.001$) in BCL6-negative patients.[28] Expression of a third protein, LMO2, appears to influence outcome in a positive manner in patients treated with both CHOP and R-CHOP, and may actually be one of the most powerful predictors of survival of markers studied to date.[29,30] In summary, it is clear that reevaluation of traditional prognostic markers is needed as the standard of care for frontline DLBCL evolves. The use of GCB versus non-GCB nomenclature is being actively incorporated into ongoing trials which will prospectively test their validity in patients being treated with rituximab plus anthracycline-based chemotherapy.

Initial therapy of localized DLBCL

Approximately 30% of patients with DLBCL present with initially localized disease that can be either nodal or primary extranodal in origin.[16] Primary extranodal DLBCL accounts for approximately half of all patients with stage I and II disease, with head and neck organs most commonly involved.[31,32] The management of primary extranodal DLBCL typically follows treatment paradigms of nodal stage I and II disease, although several exceptions include primary testicular DLBCL, which requires radiation, and primary mediastinal lymphoma, which is discussed in detail below. Although many patients with localized DLBCL have an excellent prognosis, subgroups with higher-risk disease can be identified using modifications of the IPI. Miller and colleagues found that a stage-modified IPI was highly predictive of outcome, with age greater than 60 years, stage II disease, elevated LDH, and decreased performance status all correlating with inferior progression-free survival (PFS) and OS.[33] In this study, patients with 0–1 risk factors had a 5-year PFS of 77% compared to 60% for patients with 2 risk factors, and 34% with 3 risk factors. A British Columbia population-based analysis confirmed the utility of the stage-modified IPI in identifying three groups with 5-year OS ranging from 90% (0 risk factors), 77% (1 or 2 risk factors), to 58% (3 or 4 risk factors). Thus, these studies suggest that there is substantial heterogeneity even amongst patients with limited disease at presentation.

The mainstay of therapy is anthracycline-based chemotherapy with or without consolidative radiotherapy. Historically, radiation alone was used but has an unacceptably high failure rate approaching 70%, and should not be used alone unless there is a significant contraindication to systemic treatment.[31] The success of combination chemotherapy for advanced-stage DLBCL in the 1980s and 1990s initially led investigators to use chemotherapy alone in the management of early-stage DLBCL with hopes of improving systemic control. However, many questioned the need for protracted chemotherapy in early-stage patients, especially given the more favorable prognosis and concern regarding cardiotoxicity. The Southwest Oncology Group (SWOG) conducted an influential randomized controlled trial comparing CHOP $\times 8$ ($n = 201$) versus CHOP $\times 3$ ($n = 200$) followed by 40–55 Gy radiation in patients with localized intermediate- and high-grade lymphomas and at least one adverse risk factor.[33] Their initial report favored the combined modality arm, with better PFS (77% vs. 64%, $p = 0.03$) and OS (82% vs. 72%, $p = 0.02$) at 4.4 years median follow-up time. Furthermore, more patients on the chemotherapy-only arm were unable to complete the full course of treatment due to toxicity.

The authors concluded that the addition of consolidative radiation therapy safely allowed a reduction in chemotherapy cycles, leading to fewer toxic effects ($p = 0.06$) and avoiding cardiotoxicity ($p = 0.02$). Other studies at the time confirmed the promising efficacy of combined modality therapy with limited chemotherapy followed by RT. A Surveillance, Epidemiology, and End Results (SEER) database analysis of over 13 000 patients also found that the use of radiation in early-stage DLBCL improved the disease-specific survival and OS in all age groups in both univariate and multivariate analysis; unfortunately, this study is limited by the lack of any information regarding chemotherapy used and number of cycles.[34]

However, longer follow-up of SWOG 8736 shows that the failure-free survival (FFS) and OS curves cross at 7 years, and that patients on the combined modality arm continue to relapse between 5 and 10 years following therapy with no obvious plateau on the survival curve.[35] Subgroup analysis shows that most of the relapses occur in patients with at least one risk factor on the stage-modified IPI (non-bulky stage II disease, age greater than 60 years, elevated LDH, PS > 1). The continuous risk of relapse is surprising, and suggests that these patients require better systemic therapies. The role of consolidative irradiation has also been questioned by other groups. The GELA performed two large-scale randomized controlled trials, one in younger patients and one in patients greater than 60 years of age without adverse risk factors.[36,37] For younger patients, the intensive regimen ACVBP (doxorubicin, cyclophosphamide, vindesine, bleomycin, predrisone $\times 4$ cycles with 4 intrathecal injections of methotrexate followed by sequential consolidation with high-dose methotrexate, ifosfamide, etoposide, and cytarabine) ($n = 318$) without radiation proved superior to CHOP $\times 3$ followed by 40 Gy radiation therapy (RT) ($n = 329$) with respect to EFS (82% vs. 74%, $p < 0.001$) and OS (90% vs. 81%, $p = 0.001$) at 7.7 years median follow-up time. The median time to relapse was only 15 months in the combined modality therapy (CMT) arm compared to 21 months for the chemotherapy-only arm, with nearly one-third of relapses occurring in the radiation field. A multivariate analysis of all patients showed that bulky disease, assignment to the CMT arm, and stage II disease predicted an inferior outcome. For older patients without adverse risk factors, CHOP $\times 4$ ($n = 271$) proved equivalent to CHOP $\times 4$ followed by RT ($n = 299$), again with 7 years median follow-up time. The local failure rate was higher in the non-radiation arm (47% vs. 21%), but this did not impact either EFS or OS which were approximately 60% and 70%, respectively, in both groups. ECOG 1484 evaluated the role of consolidative low-dose RT (30 Gy) in patients achieving complete remission to CHOP $\times 8$, as well as the ability of RT (40 Gy) to convert partial responders to complete responders.[38] Although the addition of radiotherapy altered the pattern of relapse by improving local control, OS was not impacted.

The advent of chemoimmunotherapy with rituximab has reinvigorated the question of number of chemotherapy cycles and the role of radiation in patients with early-stage DLBCL. Although there are no prospectively conducted randomized trials specifically evaluating the impact of rituximab with anthracycline-based therapy in localized DLBCL, the MabThera International Trial (MInT) had nearly 70% of its population comprised of patients with either stage I or II disease.[39] This trial compared CHOP-like chemotherapy $\times 6$ cycles with or without rituximab, and found an improved 2-year EFS (79% vs. 59%, $p < 0.0001$) and OS (93% vs. 84%, $p = 0.0001$). All patients with bulky disease received consolidative radiation per the treating physician's discretion. Patients with non-bulky early-stage disease and no risk factors had a 98% OS with rituximab plus chemotherapy for six cycles, prompting the next set of studies to evaluate a reduction in the number of chemoimmunotherapy cycles. The question of consolidative RT was not directly asked, but the addition of rituximab removed the adverse prognostic significance of bulky disease even in patients with maximum tumor masses up to 9 cm;[40] future prospective trials will be needed to clarify the need for RT following rituximab plus chemotherapy. Outside of the MInT trial, SWOG 0014 is a phase II study of rituximab plus CHOP $\times 3$ followed by 40–46 Gy involved-field radiation therapy (IFRT).[41] This single-arm study found a promising 4-year PFS and OS of 88% and 92%, respectively, in 60 patients with early-stage disease. However, five of eight patients relapsed outside the radiation field, again hinting that better systemic control is needed. PET scans may help influence decisions regarding radiation, as shown by a population-based analysis in British Columbia, Canada. Practice patterns in British Columbia were set in 2005 as R-CHOP $\times 3$ for all patients with stage I or II DLBCL without B symptoms and without bulky disease (mass < 10 cm); a PET scan following the third cycle determined if patients would receive one further cycle of R-CHOP (if PET negative) or IFRT (if PET positive). Patients with a negative PET had an excellent outcome, with 97% PFS and OS at 2 years, suggesting that a favorable subgroup can be identified in order to avoid radiation.[42] However, this study has thus far been presented in preliminary form and only a prospective trial would help confirm the ability of PET to determine treatment options.

In summary, the prognosis of patients with localized DLBCL is generally favorable, but careful risk stratification will identify patients for whom abbreviated chemotherapy is insufficient. Accordingly, a subgroup of patients with an excellent outcome can also be identified using a stage-modified IPI. The current standard treatment ranges from four to six cycles of R-CHOP with or without IFRT. Patients with at least one risk factor probably require more than four cycles of chemotherapy.

Initial therapy of advanced DLBCL

DLBCL is a potentially curable disease, with major improvements achieved in the past decade. The backbone of treatment is the CHOP regimen, initially proposed for aggressive lymphomas in the 1970s.[43,44] In the era prior to routine radiographic imaging, CHOP produced a response rate of 40% in all patients, and an unprecedented 90% response rate in patients with nodal disease only.[43] For much of the 1980s and 1990s, a variety of intensified combination chemotherapy regimens were proposed in phase II trials as being superior to CHOP, including m-BACOD (methotrexate with leucovorin, bleomycin, doxorubicin, cyclophosphamide, vincristine, and dexamethasone), Pro-MACE-CytaBOM (cyclophosphamide, doxorubicin, etoposide, cytarabine, bleomycin, vincristine, methotrexate, and prednisone), and MACOP-B (methotrexate followed by leucovorin, doxorubicin, cyclophosphamide, vincristine, prednisone, and bleomycin). A pivotal intergroup study eventually found that clinical outcomes were actually similar in all groups, but that toxicity of the CHOP regimen was less, thus establishing CHOP given on a 21-day schedule as the standard of care for frontline management of advanced DLBCL for the next decade.[45] In this trial, Fisher and colleagues found a 3-year disease-free survival (DFS) and OS of 41% and 54%, respectively, setting the benchmarks for future studies.

A major shift in the frontline management of DLBCL has been the addition of the monoclonal chimeric antibody against CD20, rituximab, to anthracycline-based chemotherapy. Rituximab has several putative mechanisms of action, including direct induction of apoptosis and both complement-mediated lysis and antibody-dependent cellular cytotoxicity.[46] As a single agent in relapsed or refractory DLBCL, rituximab has a response rate of approximately 30%, with few complete remissions and a short median response duration.[47] However, when combined with chemotherapy, there is marked synergy with substantial gains in both PFS and OS, and there are now several large-scale randomized trials demonstrating superiority of rituximab-containing regimens for both older and younger patients.[39,48–50] The LNH98-5 trial of the GELA randomized elderly patients between 60 and 80 years old with previously untreated DLBCL to receive either CHOP $\times$ 8 (n = 197) or CHOP plus rituximab $\times$ 8 (n = 202). There was no planned consolidative radiation. This was a high-risk population with more than half of patients on either arm having an IPI score greater than 2, and a median age of 69 years. With a median follow-up of 24 months, patients on the rituximab-containing arm had a superior 2-year EFS (57% vs. 38%, $p < 0.001$) and OS (70% vs. 57%, $p = 0.007$). These benefits persist with longer follow-up as well,[48,51] with 7-year data continuing to show a better EFS (42% vs. 25%, $p < 0.0001$) and fewer deaths in the rituximab-containing arm. An intergroup study (ECOG 4494) from the United States questioned the role of rituximab in both induction and maintenance of remission in frontline DLBCL in elderly patients by randomizing patients first to CHOP or CHOP plus rituximab, followed by a second randomization to either observation or rituximab maintenance.[50] This was again a study focusing on elderly patients with a median age 69 years in the R-CHOP group and 70 years in the CHOP group. In contrast to the GELA 98–5 study, there was no difference in response rate (77% vs. 76%) by induction. The addition of maintenance rituximab improved FFS, but only in patients who had initially received CHOP, and not in patients treated with R-CHOP. When comparing all four groups, patients receiving CHOP induction without maintenance rituximab had the worst outcome (2-year FFS 45%) compared to all other groups (2-year FFS 74–79%). It should be noted that both of these large multi-institutional trials focused on elderly patients with adverse risk factors.

The MInT evaluated CHOP-like chemotherapy $\times$ 6 cycles with or without rituximab in younger patients, ages 18–60 years, and with no more than one risk factor. This large-scale international trial enrolled over 800 patients, and allowed treating physicians to select an anthracycline-based regimen of their choice prior to randomization. With a median follow-up time of 34 months, the 3-year EFS (79% vs. 59%, $p < 0.0001$) and OS (93% vs. 84%, $p = 0.0001$) were superior in the chemoimmunotherapy arm. The incremental benefit of rituximab was seen in all subgroups (IPI 0 vs. IPI 1, bulky vs. non-bulky) but was most pronounced in the highest-risk patients who had both an IPI 1 and bulky disease with an improvement in 3-year EFS from 44% to 74% ($p < 0.0001$). Patients with an IPI 0 and no bulky disease had a remarkable outcome with 97% EFS and 100% OS at 3 years.[39] Finally, a population-based analysis in British Colombia evaluated the role of rituximab within a provincial region where regulatory bodies did not approve rituximab with chemotherapy for DLBCL until 2000. In this study, Sehn and colleagues evaluated the PFS and OS of patients treated in the 18 months immediately prior to this change, and in the 18 months following the change.[17] Although all age groups were included in the analysis, the median age was 63 years, reflecting the expected population. Patients treated prior to the introduction of rituximab had an inferior 2-year PFS (51% vs. 69%, $p = 0.002$) and OS (52% vs. 78%, $p < 0.0001$). The benefit was most pronounced in patients greater than 60 years. Thus, the bulk of data supports a substantial gain in both EFS and OS for patients receiving rituximab plus CHOP or CHOP-like chemotherapy for previously untreated DLBCL of all ages, and R-CHOP is currently considered the standard frontline treatment regimen.

However, it is important to recognize that subgroups with varying outcomes following R-CHOP can be identified using both biologic and clinical factors. A secondary analysis of the GELA98–5 trial found that addition of rituximab provided most benefit to patients with BCL2 protein overexpression, a known adverse prognostic factor correlated with shorter EFS and OS in DLBCL.[27] In contrast, patients without BCL2 overexpression had a much smaller margin of benefit, a finding confirmed by others.[52] A secondary analysis of ECOG 4494 showed that rituximab could overcome the negative prognostic significance of BCL6 negativity, whereas BCL6-positive patients fared well irrespective of rituximab.[28] Future studies will hopefully incorporate biologic features into treatment paradigms that will help individualize therapies, using rituximab when it is most beneficial and allowing newer agents to be developed for other groups of patients.

Can we improve upon R-CHOP?

Despite the improvements seen with R-CHOP, it is clear that subgroups with a worse prognosis remain, and attempts at improving upon R-CHOP continue. Several approaches are being evaluated, including shortening the cycle length from 21 to 14 days to increase dose intensity, using infusional regimens with dose escalation, adding more cytotoxic agents, and adding maintenance or "adjuvant" treatments following R-CHOP.

The standard delivery of R-CHOP is every 21 days, initially based on the time required for marrow recovery following cytotoxic therapies. The introduction of hematopoietic growth factors, as well as general improvements in supportive care, allow a reduction in cycle length which escalates relative dose intensity. Many studies evaluating intensification of CHOP regimens were performed prior to the addition of rituximab, which complicates their interpretation for modern treatment paradigms.[53–55] The largest phase III investigation of shortened treatment cycles was done by the German High-Grade non-Hodgkin Lymphoma Study Group (DSHNHL), which applied a 2×2 trial design in both younger (NHL-B1) and older (NHL-B2) patients with randomization to either CHOP versus CHOEP (addition of etoposide 100 mg/m^2 on days 1–3 of each cycle) given every 14 versus 21 days; all patients on the 14-day treatment arms received hematopoietic growth factor support.[56,57] The NHL-B1 trial randomized over 700 patients younger than 60 years old and with favorable prognosis to either CHOP-21, CHOP-14, CHOEP-21, or CHOEP-14. Both the addition of etoposide and reduction of cycle length benefited patients. The addition of etoposide improved the complete remission rate (from 79.4% to 87.6%, $p = 0.003$) and EFS (from 57.6% to 69.2%, $p = 0.004$) whereas shortening the interval between treatments improved the OS ($p = 0.05$). Their NHL-B2 trial randomized 689 patients between the ages of 61 and 75 years to receive either CHOP-21, CHOP-14, CHOEP-21, or CHOEP-14. The addition of etoposide was highly toxic in this group, especially when delivered on the accelerated schedule. However, CHOP-14 had an acceptable toxicity profile, and conferred 34% risk reduction in EFS and 42% risk reduction in OS compared to all three of the other groups. As treatment paradigms have evolved, however, the relevance of NHL-B1 and NHL-B2 (which did not include rituximab) and other attempts at dose intensification have had to be re-evaluated. The RICOVER-60 trial addresses this issue, and had two major objectives: to compare the additional effect of rituximab over CHOP-14, and to compare eight versus six cycles of treatment, all in elderly patients. Over 1200 patients were randomized at 203 European centers.[58] Compared to CHOP-14 $\times$ 6, all three of the other arms (CHOP-14 $\times$ 8, R-CHOP-14 $\times$ 6, R-CHOP-14 $\times$ 8) were superior with no further improvement by delivering eight cycles of chemotherapy. With a median follow-up of 34.5 months, the 3-year EFS and OS were highest for the R-CHOP-14 $\times$ 6 arm at 66.5% and 78.1%, respectively. Comparing across trials to the NHL-B2 study, the authors observe that the incremental benefit by the addition of rituximab to CHOP-14 is less than that observed when rituximab is added to CHOP-21. Furthermore, in contrast to the GELA98–5 study, the margin of benefit by adding rituximab was similar in both low-risk and high-risk groups. The authors propose that both intensification of chemotherapy and rapid escalation of serum rituximab levels contributed to the improved outcomes. The DSHNHL has extended these observations to their next generation of trials in which rituximab is given more frequently on a CHOP-14 backbone based on pharmacokinetic modeling ("DENSER" trial).[59] It should be noted that these data do not answer the question of whether R-CHOP-14 is superior to R-CHOP-21; this is being evaluated by GELA (NHL-03–6B).

A second approach is to increase exposure to cytotoxic agents by altering from bolus to infusional administration. The NCI developed the EPOCH (doxorubicin, etoposide, vincristine, cyclophosphamide, and prednisone) regimen in the 1990s based on the premise that prolonged exposure of antineoplastic agents breeds less drug resistance as compared to brief, but higher, doses of chemotherapy. Initial trials in patients failing CHOP-like regimens showed an overall response rate in excess of 70%.[60] The finding of variable drug concentrations formed the basis for dose-adjusted EPOCH (DA-EPOCH) in which chemotherapy doses are adjusted to achieve a neutrophil nadir below 0.5×10^9/L. This type of individualized manipulation proved highly effective in phase II trials of previously untreated DLBCL with complete responses observed in over 90% of patients, and PFS and OS rates greater than 70% at a median follow-up time of 62 months.[61] The addition of rituximab to DA-EPOCH is feasible,[62,63] and consistent with a subanalysis of GELA98–5 discussed above, overcomes the negative prognostic significance of BCL2 overexpression. An ongoing intergroup study is comparing R-CHOP to DA-EPOCH-R with an important tissue collection component in which biologic DLBCL subtypes (activated B-cell type versus germinal center phenotype) will be evaluated as predictors of outcome on both arms.

A third approach has been the application of strategies to reduce minimal residual disease following initial therapy with CHOP or CHOP-like regimens, with hopes of prolonging remission and increasing the cure rate. Careful evaluation of frontline studies shows that, although many patients can achieve long-term disease control, patients with high-risk disease have an unacceptably high failure rate. In the GELA98–5 study, over 50% of patients had a high IPI/age-adjusted IPI, corresponding to a 5-year EFS of only 41% even in the rituximab-containing arm.[49,51] Similarly, the British Colombia Cancer Agency (BCCA) analysis of patients with DLBCL showed that 45% of their population had an IPI 3–5 and a 4-year EFS and OS of only 50% even when treated with R-CHOP.[17] Even more concerning is the apparent inability to salvage high-risk elderly patients relapsing after R-CHOP; these patients respond poorly to salvage measures and have a median survival of approximately one year. These results are in stark contrast to long-term disease control in over 80% of patients with lower-risk disease, and justify efforts to reduce persistent disease following standard induction chemotherapy with R-CHOP or similar regimens.

Several groups have proposed the application of biologic agents, including rituximab, following induction chemotherapy. ECOG 4494, as discussed above, was an intergroup study of elderly patients with previously untreated DLBCL randomized to either CHOP or R-CHOP, and a second randomization to either observation or maintenance rituximab.[50] The use of maintenance rituximab improved FFS, but only in patients receiving CHOP induction; there was no additional benefit to maintenance rituximab in patients receiving R-CHOP. Others have hypothesized that radioimmunotherapy, using anti-CD20-directed therapies, will be more beneficial. There are currently two US Food and Drug Administration (FDA)-approved radioimmunoconjugates in lymphomas, both of which are directed against CD20: ^{90}Y-labeled ibritumomab tiuxetan (Zevalin) and ^{131}I-tositumomab (Bexxar). A phase II pilot study showed the feasibility and promising efficacy of adding ^{90}Y-labeled ibritumomab tiuxetan to CHOP induction in elderly patients, with a 95% complete response rate.[64] Follow-up is short, but the 2-year PFS is 75%, and we await mature data. A variety of other biologic agents, including protein kinase C (PKC)-beta inhibitors and mTOR inhibitors, are also being actively tested in this setting.

An alternative approach that was extensively studied in the past decade is to perform an autologous stem cell support as part of frontline management in order to eradicate residual disease and extend disease-free and overall survival. This is discussed in detail below.

High-dose chemotherapy followed by autologous stem cell support: is there a role in frontline management of DLBCL?

Autologous stem cell transplant (ASCT) as consolidation treatment in newly diagnosed DLBCL patients has been tested in several randomized studies, with the results highly dependent on patient selection and the timing of transplantation. The two major settings investigated include ASCT following an abbreviated course of induction chemotherapy,[65–69] or ASCT following a full course of induction chemotherapy.[70–72] Still others compare treatment arms that are quite dissimilar.[73–76] Interpretation and application of the current body of literature is difficult given the vast heterogeneity in patient selection (high risk versus low risk, inclusion of histologies other than DLBCL), induction regimens, and transplant regimens. The LNH87–2 by the GELA randomized 236 patients in a complete remission following either ACVB (doxorubicin, cyclophosphamide, vinblastine, bleomycin) or NCVB (mitoxantrone, cyclophosphamide, vinblastine, bleomycin) to either intensive consolidation (methotrexate, ifosfamide, etoposide, L-asparaginase, cytarabine) or methotrexate and CBV (cyclophosphamide, carmustine [BCNU], etoposide) high-dose chemotherapy and autologous bone marrow transplant (ABMT).[70] The transplant arm was superior to sequential chemotherapy, primarily for the high-risk patients where 8-year EFS increased from 39% to 55% ($p = 0.02$) and 8-year OS improved from 49% to 64% ($p = 0.04$). Similarly, a multicenter randomized Italian study of VACOP-B (etoposide, doxorubicin, cyclophosphamide, vincristine, prednisone, and bleomycin) versus VACOP-B plus ABMT found significant gains only for high-intermediate and high-IPI groups undergoing ABMT.[72] The European Organization for Research and Treatment of Cancer (EORTC) as well found no advantage for ABMT consolidation of response to a full course of induction chemotherapy in low or low-intermediate groups, and only borderline benefit for higher-risk groups.[71] In each of these three studies, patients received a uniform and full (i.e., at least six cycles) course of induction chemotherapy, and most patients had chemosensitive disease.

Can transplant benefit patients without a complete response or supplant standard chemotherapy in patients with slowly responsive disease? Most studies have found minimal benefit to this approach.[65–69] Verdonck and colleagues treated 286 patients with CHOP × 3 cycles; patients with either a complete remission (CR) or a partial remission (PR) but with bone marrow involvement were randomized to five more cycles of CHOP whereas patients with a PR and no bone marrow involvement were randomized to one more cycle of CHOP followed by ABMT using a cyclophosphamide and TBI (total body irradiation) conditioning regimen.[69] With 4-year follow-up time, the DFS, EFS, and OS were similar in both groups with no advantage for ABMT. Similarly, a German multicenter study reported by Kaiser *et al.* showed no advantage for BEAM (carmustine, etoposide, cytarabine, melphalan) transplant following CHOEP (CHOP plus etoposide) × 2 cycles over CHOEP × 5 cycles without transplant.[66] In contrast, GOELAMS 072 compared CHOP times eight cycles versus CEEP (cyclophosphamide 1200 mg/m^2, epirubicin 100 mg/m^2, vindesine 3 mg/m^2, prednisone 80 mg/m^2) plus intravenous methotrexate and cytarabine and ASCT (BEAM preparative regimen), and did find a benefit in terms of EFS. In this study, all patients had chemosensitive disease after either CHOP × 4 or after CEEP × 2, and were stratified by age-adjusted IPI. With a median follow-up of 4 years, patients in the transplant arm had a higher 5-year EFS (37% vs. 55%, $p = 0.037$) but OS was not significantly different (56% vs. 71%, $p = 0.076$) on an intent-to-treat basis. Subgroup analysis, however, shows that patients with an age-adjusted IPI 2–3 had important gains in both EFS (56% vs. 28%, $p = 0.003$) and OS (74% vs. 44%, $p = 0.001$) without improvements observed for patients with low or low-intermediate risk.

Unfortunately, these disparate results are difficult to reconcile. It seems clear that transplant as part of frontline therapy does not provide benefit for low-risk patients, but the results in high-risk patients are more problematic. Additional limitations in the applicability of these trials include that these were all performed prior to chemoimmunotherapy (i.e., R-CHOP), and that the definition of response has been greatly improved by modern imaging modalities. Thus we do not know how many "resistant" patients or "partial responders" actually might have been in a PET-negative remission, and in turn, how many patients with small residual masses may have had residual PET-avid lymph nodes. The challenge in interpreting these randomized trials is underscored in a meta-analysis that evaluated over 2200 patients to determine whether or not a benefit for ASCT in first remission exists.[77] The authors of the meta-analysis conclude that there are insufficient data to support ASCT in first remission at this time, specifically due to the heterogeneity in trials reported to date. For now, ASCT is not routinely used in frontline management of DLBCL and new randomized studies comparing the efficacy and toxicity of R-CHOP versus R-CHOP plus ASCT will need to be performed. A recently completed intergroup study (SWOG 9704) of CHOP versus R-CHOP versus R-CHOP followed by ASCT may help address the issue once mature results are available.

Management of primary refractory DLBCL

Patients with refractory disease or an incomplete response to frontline therapy generally have a poor outcome with only 10–15% long-term survivors. However, if chemosensitivity can be demonstrated to salvage measures, these patients can substantially benefit from ASCT. The ability to demonstrate some chemosensitivity is critical. An Autologous Blood and Marrow Transplant Registry (ABMTR) analysis showed that patients with primary refractory disease, defined as achieving less than a CR to initial therapy, derive benefit from subsequent ASCT if the high-dose chemotherapy successfully converts their incomplete responses to CRs.[78] Patients converting to CR following ASCT had a 3-year OS of 68% compared to only 11% for those achieving a PR or less to ASCT ($p < 0.0001$). Partial chemosensitivity remained the most important predictor of outcome following ASCT. The group at Memorial Sloan Kettering Cancer Center (MSKCC) treated 85 patients with partial response to induction chemotherapy or refractory disease with ICE (ifosfamide, carboplastin, etoposide) salvage chemotherapy.[79] Among 42 responding patients who were eventually transplanted, EFS and OS were 44% and 53%, respectively, at 3 years, suggesting that initially refractory patients demonstrating chemosensitivity to salvage chemotherapy may still benefit from ASCT. A Spanish registry analysis on 114 patients similarly shows 5-year survival of 43% for patients failing to achieve a CR to frontline therapies, but subsequently responding to salvage measures.[80] Thus, if immediate salvage chemotherapy identifies a chemosensitive subset, such patients may benefit from ASCT as consolidation therapy, even if they had failed their initial chemotherapy. Unfortunately, in each of these studies, patients with chemoresistance to salvage measures continued to have a poor outcome, with rare long-term survivors. These patients should be considered for alternative treatments and participation in clinical trials.

CNS recurrence of DLBCL

Secondary CNS involvement by DLBCL is an uncommon event, but portends a grave prognosis with a median survival of the order of months. The overall incidence is estimated to be approximately 2–5%, but high-risk subgroups may have up to a 25% incidence.[81–85] Several groups have performed either retrospective analyses or re-analyses of prospectively conducted clinical trials in order to identify risk factors predictive of CNS relapse. The MD Anderson Cancer Center (MDACC) found 24 (4.5%) DLBCL patients with CNS recurrence out of 605 patients enrolled on prospective trials that did *not* include any CNS prophylaxis.[85] Multivariate analysis found an elevated LDH and greater than one extranodal site to be the most important predictors of CNS relapse; patients with both of these risk factors had a 17.4% CNS recurrence rate. A GELA study of 974 patients in which *all* patients received both intrathecal and systemic methotrexate showed that the overall incidence was 1.6%, but that patients with an elevated IPI (H-HI), increased LDH, or greater than one extranodal site had a 4.1% risk (compared to only 0.6% for L-LI risk groups).[84] Re-analysis of the DSHNHL studies shows 37 of 1693 (2.2%) of patients developing CNS recurrence.[81] Again, multivariate analysis found increased LDH and greater than one extranodal site to be the most important risk factors. Elderly patients with both of these risk factors had up to a 20% incidence of CNS recurrence. Neither CNS prophylaxis nor shortening the cycle length (i.e., from 21 to 14 days) reduced the CNS relapse rate, but use of etoposide in the CHOEP regimen appeared to provide benefit (relative risk [RR] 0.4, $p = 0.017$). In addition to these clinical risk factors, unique biologic subtypes of DLBCL, such as primary testicular lymphoma and primary breast lymphoma, also are associated with a high risk of CNS relapse.[86]

The median time to CNS relapse is generally short, at approximately 4–8 months following frontline therapy. The only study showing later relapses is an international collaborative effort of the International Primary CNS Lymphoma group which retrospectively gathered 113 cases of CNS recurrence, and found a median time to brain relapse of 1.8 years.[87] However, most studies show an extremely quick time to CNS relapse, often during primary therapy, suggesting that these patients may have had occult involvement at the time of diagnosis.[81–83,85,88] The prognosis of CNS relapse is grim, with median survival across series of 2–6 months despite aggressive chemotherapy or radiotherapy.

It's unclear if the addition of rituximab to frontline regimens has reduced the risk of CNS relapse. Rituximab does not cross the blood–brain barrier, and it would seem unlikely that it should have an impact. However, analysis of the RICOVER-60 trial in which elderly patients were randomized to CHOP-14 with or without rituximab for six versus eight cycles found that rituximab decreased the risk (RR 0.5).[58] The overall incidence of CNS recurrences was 4.8% in this study, with most patients relapsing at a median 8 months following treatment. In multivariate analysis, an elevated LDH, greater than one extranodal site, and the presence of B symptoms retained their adverse prognostic value. Patients with all three risk factors had a 24% CNS recurrence rate, irrespective of rituximab. The median survival following CNS relapse was only 3 months. In contrast, GELA98-5 performed a similar analysis on 399 elderly patients randomized to CHOP with or without rituximab, and found a 5% CNS relapse rate but no influence of rituximab.

If a patient with high-risk disease (i.e., high IPI, elevated LDH, greater than one extranodal site) is identified, does prophylaxis help? Both the RICOVER-60 and DSHNHL studies showed that etoposide reduced the risk (RR 0.4, $p = 0.017$). Furthermore, the risk of CNS relapse was significantly reduced in patients receiving planned intrathecal prophylaxis with 15 mg methotrexate (twice within first two cycles of treatment), with a RR of 0.3 ($p = 0.023$).[82] The GELA, which has long used the intensive ACVBP regimen, has shown in a prospective trial that CNS recurrences were more common in the CHOP arm, and occurred primarily during therapy.[88] In this trial, Tilly and colleagues showed that intrathecal and systemic methotrexate substantially reduced the risk of CNS recurrence particularly in high-risk patients; they conclude that patients with low-risk disease do not need intrathecal prophylaxis. In general, options for CNS prophylaxis range from intrathecal methotrexate and/or cytarabine given on day 1 of each cycle of systemic therapy to intravenous methotrexate either following induction chemotherapy or as part of the ACVBP regimen. There are no firm guidelines on either the route of prophylaxis or the number of doses required, both of which are badly needed.

Management of relapsed DLBCL

Despite substantial gains in initial management described above, approximately 50% of patients with DLBCL either relapse following R-CHOP-type regimens or never respond to frontline measures. The major decision point in the management of relapsed DLBCL is to determine whether or not the patient is a candidate for high-dose chemotherapy and ASCT. As outlined below, ASCT is able to salvage approximately 30–50% of relapsed patients. Patients who are unable to undergo ASCT, however, have a poor prognosis with a median survival typically less than one year.

The rationale for ASCT in DLBCL is a well-established steep dose–response curve to intensive chemotherapy. The Parma trial, now published more than a decade ago, remains one of the few prospective randomized trials comparing ABMT versus salvage chemotherapy alone. In this trial, 215 patients with relapsed DLBCL received DHAP (dexamethasone, cytarabine, cisplatin) salvage for two cycles; 109 patients with chemosensitive disease (i.e., either a CR or PR) were subsequently randomized to either two additional cycles of DHAP or ABMT. Patients in the transplant arm had a superior EFS (46% vs. 12%, $p = 0.001$) and OS (53% vs. 32%, $p = 0.038$).

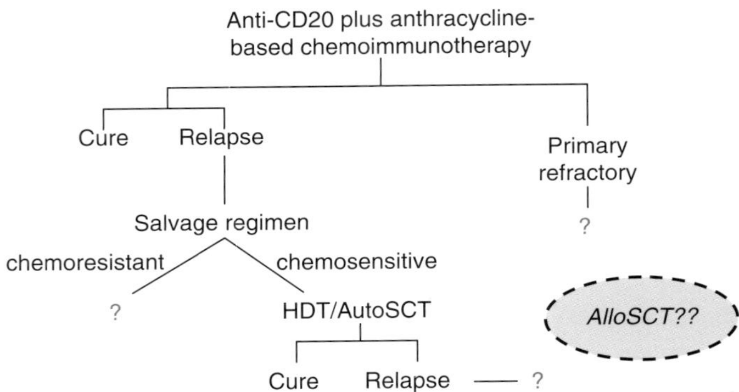

Figure 16.5 Conceptual treatment approach to patients with DLBCL.

The applicability of the Parma trial has been critiqued, however, for excluding patients with refractory disease or marrow involvement, and for excluding patients with less than a PR to DHAP salvage. Furthermore, response in the Parma study was based on CT criteria of the time, and we do not know how many patients on either arm had residual disease based on modern response criteria that incorporate PET.[11] In addition, CHOP has been supplanted by R-CHOP, and patients relapsing after R-CHOP may be an entirely different population compared to those included in the Parma trial (see discussion below).

Despite these caveats and limitations, however, the Parma trial provides a basic framework with which to approach patients with relapsed DLBCL (Figure 16.5). The ABMTR reported on 429 patients with diffuse aggressive lymphomas in first relapse or second CR transplanted between 1989 and 1996, and showed 3-year PFS and OS of 31% and 44%, respectively.[89] A multi-institutional German study found 2-year freedom from second failure and OS of 35% and 58%, respectively, for chemosensitive patients with relapsed aggressive lymphomas.[90]

Based on these reports and others, an international consensus panel currently recommends ASCT for patients with relapsed aggressive lymphomas demonstrating chemosensitivity to salvage regimens.[91] However, long-term disease control in only one-third of patients is clearly suboptimal, justifying efforts to improve upon the status quo by either optimizing patient selection, identifying more effective salvage regimens, improving preparative regimens, and/or applying post-transplant therapies to eliminate minimal residual disease following ASCT.

ASCT for relapsed DLBCL: patient and disease characteristics

Although high-dose chemotherapy and autologous stem cell rescue has evolved into a standard treatment approach in relapsed DLBCL, it is clear that not all patients derive equal benefit. A reanalysis of the original Parma study, for example, showed that autologous transplantation did not provide a survival advantage over conventional salvage chemotherapy for patients with an IPI of 0 (5-year OS, 51% vs. 48%, $p = 0.59$).[92] In contrast, patients with an IPI > 0 had a significantly superior survival if treated with autologous transplantation ($p < 0.05$). This IPI at relapse, also termed the second-line IPI (sIPI), has shown strong prognostic significance in other studies as well. A review of 150 relapsed and refractory DLBCL patients enrolled on three sequential autologous transplant studies at MSKCC and treated with a uniform salvage regimen (ICE), showed that, for patients with chemosensitive disease, a sAA-IPI score of 0, 1, or ≥ 2 correlated with a 4-year PFS of 69%, 46%, and 26% ($p < 0.001$), respectively, and 4-year OS of 83%, 55%, and 26% ($p < 0.001$), respectively.[93] Patients not responding to ICE had a dismal outcome with a median survival of only 4 months. A multivariate analysis of prognostic features performed at the MDACC of 97 relapsed patients found decreasing 3-year OS with higher AA-IPI (3-year OS, 16% vs. 44% vs. 71% for AA-IPI of 2, 1, and 0, respectively; $p = 0.00003$).[94] The Mayo Clinic found that the sIPI predicts outcome in older patients undergoing ASCT as well. Of 80 patients with a median age of 62 years, the sIPI was highly predictive of OS.[95] Patients with an sIPI ≥ 3 had a median survival of 23.3 months versus not reached for patients with a more favorable sIPI ($p = 0.01$). Thus, the IPI at relapse provides important prognostic information regarding ASCT outcomes.

Perhaps the most critical determinant of patient outcome following ASCT is the ability to demonstrate chemosensitivity to salvage regimens. In addition, many have shown that the *degree* of chemosensitivity (i.e., CR versus PR) influences outcome. For example, a large registry analysis of 429 patients by the ABMTR showed that a CR versus PR versus resistant disease after salvage chemotherapy affected 3-year OS and PFS following ASCT, with OS decreasing from 55% to 40% to 28%, and PFS decreasing from 38% to 25% to 23%, respectively ($p < 0.001$ for all comparisons).[89] An MSKCC analysis of 163 patients (118 with DLBCL) similarly showed that CR versus PR versus failure to ICE salvage chemotherapy was highly correlated with both EFS and OS.[96] Specifically, EFS in patients who achieved CR versus PR versus no response was 54%, 29%, and 0%, respectively; OS was 65%, 30%, and 15%, respectively. These observations suggest that improved salvage regimens may induce deeper responses and in more patients, thus potentially allowing ASCT to benefit a greater number of patients. Means of improving salvage regimens are discussed below.

The availability of FDG-PET imaging has greatly improved our ability to detect residual disease in DLBCL, and thus more accurately identify chemosensitive disease. A pre-transplant FDG-PET is highly predictive for both FFS and OS, although most series are retrospective in nature and include several lymphoma subtypes.[97–100] Spaepen and colleagues reviewed pre-ASCT FDG-PET images in 60 patients with relapsed lymphomas.[101] Of 30 patients with a negative FDG-PET, 25 remain in an ongoing remission as compared to only 4 of 30 patients with residual FDG-PET-positive disease. This translated into an improved 2-year PFS (96% vs. 23%, $p < 0.000001$) and OS (100% vs. 55%, $p < 0.00002$) for patients with a negative versus positive pre-ASCT FDG-PET. Furthermore, the median time to relapse was only 432 days in the FDG-PET-positive group, as compared to 1466 days in the FDG-PET-negative group. Similarly, a retrospective analysis of 50 patients at the University of Pennsylvania and University of Michigan reported 1-year PFS of 54% versus 7% in patients with negative versus positive pre-ASCT FDG-PET, respectively;[99] they also found that patients with a positive pre-transplant FDG-PET had a median survival of only 19 months, identifying an extremely poor-prognostic group of patients. A major challenge in interpreting FDG-PET data, however, is the high number of patients with residual uptake that is either low-level or indeterminate in nature. To address this intermediate group, one analysis of 101 patients (60 with DLBCL) categorized FDG-PET responses as either complete, partial, or non-response and had two blinded and independent reviewers reinterpret the scans without knowledge of clinical outcomes. Patients with NHL showed differential 2-year PFS of 72%, 38%, and 10% for complete, partial, and non-responders, respectively.[97]

Does metabolic imaging supplement or replace information already obtained by clinical parameters such as the sAA-IPI?[97] In 117 patients with relapsed lymphomas, Schot and colleagues report that univariate analysis found LDH ($p = 0.003$), primary refractory disease ($p < 0.001$), clinical risk score ($p < 0.001$), and FDG-PET response ($p < 0.001$) as highly predictive of outcome.[97] A multivariate analysis, however, identified only sAA-IPI and FDG-PET as independent prognostic risk factors for progression. When combined into a new model, patients with a risk score of 0 to 1 had a 2-year FFS in excess of 80%, as compared to less than 10% for patients with a score of 4 or 5.

In summary, a variety of pre-transplant patient and disease characteristics can predict outcome and be used to guide patient selection. It is interesting to note that there are no validated prognostic biologic markers correlating with outcome following ASCT for relapsed DLBCL. In contrast to the strong prognostic significance of gene expression profiles in patients with previously untreated DLBCL,[18] a similar evaluation of 150 transplant eligible relapsed and primary refractory DLBCL patients showed no significant difference in EFS or OS.[102] Most investigators have shown that a shorter time to relapse after initial remission, increased number of chemotherapy regimens prior to transplant, heavy tumor burden, decreased performance status, poor response to salvage chemotherapy, and elevated LDH all contribute to an inferior outcome. In the best-risk patients, as identified by a negative PET and low sIPI, autologous transplant produces long-term disease control in excess of 70% of patients. Unfortunately, a significant portion of patients do not fall into one of these favorable categories, justifying ongoing efforts to improve upon the status quo.

ASCT for relapsed DLBCL: salvage regimens

Despite evidence that better and deeper remissions lead to improved outcomes following transplant, there are almost no prospective randomized trials showing superiority of any one salvage regimen, and most salvage measures are selected based on toxicity profiles and physician/patient preference. There are a variety of available salvage regimens that are either platinum-based, ifosfamide-based, or gemcitabine-based, and all appear to have high overall response rates and comparable mobilization kinetics.[94,96,103] A major advance in eliciting more responses has been the addition of rituximab to salvage regimens, which should translate to better disease control post-ASCT. The prospectively conducted HOVON-44 randomized relapsed and refractory B-cell lymphomas to DHAP-VIM (etoposide, ifosfamide, methotrexate)-DHAP salvage with or without rituximab, with ASCT planned for all patients.[104] Only 4% of 225 eligible patients had received prior rituximab. The addition of rituximab led to a statistically significant improvement in response to salvage, FFS, and PFS, but not OS. The authors hypothesize that the total rituximab dose may have been too low to affect survival, since only three pre-ASCT doses were delivered; nevertheless, the improvements in FFS and PFS were substantial. When compared to historical control groups, the addition of rituximab to salvage regimens also shows improved outcomes.[105,106] The group at MSKCC compared the outcome of 37 rituximab-naïve patients with relapsed DLBCL receiving rituximab plus ICE (R-ICE) salvage to 107 historical control patients receiving ICE alone.[105] The overall response rate was similar in the two groups, but the percentage of patients achieving a CR increased from 27% to 53% ($p = 0.01$) in all patients, and from 19% to 53% ($p = 0.01$) in high-risk patients. A German study similarly added rituximab to DHAP in 22 largely rituximab-naïve patients and compared their outcome to 45 historical controls treated with DHAP alone. They found an improvement in freedom from second treatment failure and OS at 2 years (74% vs. 33%, $p = 0.0424$) in a matched-pair analysis. Finally, Fenske and colleagues from the Center for International Blood and Marrow Transplant Research (CIBMTR) recently presented a registry analysis on 1006 patients (818 no rituximab, 188 receiving rituximab) undergoing ASCT between 1996 and 2003 to determine the impact of pre-ASCT rituximab on outcome.[107] The addition of rituximab did not increase transplant-related mortality or engraftment. Both 3-year PFS (49% vs. 38%, $p = 0.01$) and OS (57% vs. 45%, $p = 0.003$) were significantly improved in the group receiving rituximab prior to ASCT. Thus, there are now prospective, registry, and retrospective data suggesting that a more effective salvage regimen incorporating rituximab improves response rates, PFS, and perhaps, overall survival.

However, whether or not the apparent superior efficacy of rituximab-containing frontline regimens persists in patients already failing rituximab-containing frontline treatments remains unknown. The ongoing prospective Cardiovascular Outcomes in Renal Atherosclerotic Lesions (CORAL) study may answer some of these issues.[108] The CORAL study is an international multicenter phase III trial randomizing patients with relapsed DLBCL after one prior regimen to either R-ICE or R-DHAP. Patients are stratified by prior exposure to rituximab, relapsed versus refractory disease, and relapse less than or greater than 12 months from frontline therapy. Responding patients proceed to ASCT with BEAM preparative regimen. Following transplant, there is a second randomization comparing rituximab maintenance (375 mg/m^2 every 8 weeks) versus observation. An interim analysis on 194 patients shows that factors negatively influencing EFS include the following: less than 12 months since first-line treatment (36% vs. 68%, $p < 0.001$), sIPI 2–3 versus 0–1 (39% vs. 56%, $p = 0.03$), and prior rituximab (34% vs. 66%, $p = 0.001$). This final finding is worrisome, suggesting that patients relapsing after frontline rituximab-containing regimens may be more difficult to salvage with rituximab-containing second-line combinations. However, these are results of an interim analysis, and we await mature results of the CORAL study on the entire cohort of 400 patients.

ASCT for relapsed DLBCL: conditioning regimens

Analogous to the dilemma with salvage regimens, the optimal preparative or conditioning regimen for DLBCL is not known, and there are no prospective comparative studies. The ideal conditioning or preparative regimen used during ASCT should be capable of eliminating all residual malignant cells and minimize toxicity to non-hematopoietic organs. Most regimens can be divided into TBI-based (Cy [cyclophosphamide]/TBI), BCNU-based (BEAC [carmustine, cytarabine, etoposide, cyclophosphamide], CBV, BEAM), platinum-based, or other. Although TBI-containing regimens are highly effective, there are concerns about an increased risk of veno-occlusive disease, cardiopulmonary toxicity, and secondary leukemias.[109,110] To circumvent bystander toxicity to normal organs, radiolabeled monoclonal antibodies are being actively investigated as part of transplant preparative regimens. Radiolabeled monoclonal antibodies have the potential of delivering radiation directly to the tumor and minimizing non-hematopoietic toxicities. The major toxicity of radiolabeled antibodies is myelosuppression, and these are thus ideal agents to test in an autologous transplant setting where hematopoietic stem cell rescue is planned. There are currently two available radiolabeled monoclonal antibodies, ^{90}Y-labeled ibritumomab tiuxetan and ^{131}I-labeled tositumomab, with nearly a dozen preliminary or ongoing trials evaluating them in combination with standard preparative regimens. The studies can generally be divided into those that escalate the dose of radioimmunotherapy and those that deliver standard (non-myeloablative) doses of radioimmunotherapy, either with or without a standard conditioning regimen.

Both ^{131}I-tositumomab and ^{90}Y-labeled ibritumomab tiuxetan have been evaluated. The University of Nebraska group performed a phase I study with escalating doses of ^{131}I-tositumomab (up to 0.75 Gy total body dose) combined with BEAM chemotherapy.[111] Half of the patients had refractory disease.

The 3-year EFS and OS were 39% and 55%, respectively, which is quite promising for this poor-risk population. Importantly, there was no significant added toxicity, and a subsequent phase II study in a relapsed and largely chemosensitive population shows remarkable results with 3-year PFS of 70% and OS of 81%.[112] These encouraging results are now being tested in an ongoing prospective randomized Blood and Marrow Transplant (BMT) Clinical Trial Network (CTN) trial comparing rituximab plus BEAM versus ^{131}I-tositumomab plus BEAM.

^{90}Y-labeled ibritumomab tiuxetan has similarly been studied in conjunction with high-dose chemotherapy.[113–115] A phase I/II trial showed that up to 71.6 mCi of ^{90}Y-labeled ibritumomab tiuxetan (compared to the standard dose of 32 mCi without stem cell rescue) could be safely delivered with high-dose cyclophosphamide and etoposide using dosimetric techniques.[114] At a median follow-up of 22 months, the 2-year estimated relapse-free survival and OS rates are 78% and 92%, respectively, with no increase in transplant-related mortality or delayed engraftment. Another dosimetric approach (using the liver as the critical organ of exposure) by Winter and colleagues also showed successful escalation of ^{90}Y-labeled ibritumomab tiuxetan to deliver 1500 cGy without a significant increase in toxicity.[116] In order to facilitate outpatient transplants, the City of Hope group conducted a phase II trial of ^{90}Y-labeled ibritumomab tiuxetan in combination with BEAM chemotherapy. This exploratory study showed encouraging 2-year outcomes (PFS 69% and OS 89%) without added toxicity. Similar promising results were shown by an Israeli study delivering standard-dose ^{90}Y-labeled ibritumomab tiuxetan with BEAM chemotherapy to a chemorefractory group of patients with estimated 2-year PFS and OS at 52% and 67%, respectively. Finally, the MDACC group added ^{90}Y-labeled ibritumomab tiuxetan to high-dose rituximab delivered peri-transplant (RZ-BEAM versus R-BEAM) in a preliminary report, with encouraging activity compared to historical control patients.[117]

"Adjuvant" strategies to reduce minimal residual disease after ASCT

Although ASCT is effective for many patients with relapsed disease, those who are destined to relapse typically do so within the first 1–2 years following transplant.[118–120] The MSKCC group found that the median time to progression, even in patients with favorable and chemosensitive disease prior to transplant, was only 5.1 months. These data suggest the presence of residual disease following high-dose chemotherapy that is below the current level of detection. There is no current standard "adjuvant" strategy to eliminate minimal residual disease following transplant, and most patients are expectantly followed with serial CT scans.

In general, two strategies have been investigated: post-ASCT anti-CD20 directed therapies (i.e., rituximab) and post-ASCT immune modulatory agents. The use of post-ASCT immune modulating drugs such as ciclosporin, interferons, and interleukins (see comprehensive review by Kline *et al.*[121]) has been limited mainly to small reports and case series. Most recently, the SWOG published long-term data on a phase III randomized trial of ASCT for relapsed lymphoma patients with or without adjuvant interleukin-2 (IL-2).[122] They did not find improvements in PFS or OS, and concluded that the dose and schedule of IL-2 administered did not benefit patients. The use of immune modulating agents and vaccines remains exploratory and investigational at this time.

Increasingly, rituximab following ASCT is being evaluated. MDACC treated 67 consecutive patients with relapsed aggressive lymphomas with high-dose rituximab (1000 mg/m^2) both prior to and immediately following (day+1 and day+8) autologous stem cell reinfusion.[123] Compared to a group of 30 historical control patients not receiving any rituximab, they found significant improvements in both actuarial DFS (67% vs. 43%, $p = 0.004$) and OS (80% vs. 53%, $p = 0.002$) favoring the group receiving high-dose rituximab in the peri-transplant period. However, there was a statistically significant delay in time to both neutrophil and platelet recovery, although this did not translate into clinical complications. The Stanford group delivered extended "maintenance" rituximab with four weekly doses at day+42 and again at 6 months following ASCT in a pilot study of 35 patients (25 with DLBCL).[124] Although most patients were rituximab-naïve, the 2-year EFS and OS of 21 patients with DLBCL was 81% and 85%, respectively, which is superior to other published reports on this population.

As with any adjuvant strategy, it is important to minimize toxicities of prolonged administrations of drugs. Unfortunately, the data thus far show that rituximab following ASCT is associated with delayed and prolonged neutropenia and hypogammaglobulinemia, as well as varicella and cytomegalovirus (CMV) reactivation.[125–127] In addition, we do not know which doses, schedules, and agents will be most helpful in eliminating minimal residual disease and preventing relapse without increasing toxicity. The ongoing CORAL study (see above) includes a post-transplant randomization between either observation or rituximab 375 mg/m^2 given once every 8 weeks for 1 year, and should help clarify the efficacy and toxicity of adjuvant rituximab, especially in patients with prior rituximab exposure.

Relapsed DLBCL: allogeneic stem cell transplantation

Although the concept of "graft-versus-lymphoma" is well-established, the role of allogeneic stem cell transplant remains least well-defined for aggressive lymphomas, including DLBCL. This can be attributed to several issues. First, the success of autologous transplant approaches for relapsed DLBCL implies that most patients considered for allogeneic transplant have either already failed an ASCT (and thus are heavily pretreated) or are poor candidates for an ASCT (and thus are also poor candidates for an allogeneic approach). Second, the magnitude of graft-versus-lymphoma appears partially dependent on histology, with aggressive lymphomas generally faring worse than indolent subtypes.[128–130] Third, allogeneic transplant approaches generally have higher transplant-related morbidity and mortality even with reduced intensity approaches in this population.[131–134]

Reduced intensity transplants (RIT) and non-myeloablative stem cell transplants (NMSCT) rely on sufficient immunosuppression and moderate myelosuppression to allow donor stem cells to coexist with the patient's own stem cell population (i.e., mixed chimerism). By reducing the intensity of the preparative regimen, early transplant-related mortality can be lowered, but may come at the cost of increased relapse. For example, a small retrospective comparison of 16 patients with aggressive NHL undergoing conventional myeloablative transplant to 12 patients undergoing reduced intensity regimens showed a higher 2-year relapse rate with RIT (44% vs. 12%, $p = 0.02$).[135] The poorer outcome of aggressive histologies has also been noted. Of 62 patients with aggressive lymphomas undergoing RIT, the European Group for Blood and Marrow Transplantation (EBMT) found that patients with aggressive subtypes had only a 32% 1-year PFS, which was inferior to patients with indolent histologies.[130] A multicenter report from the United Kingdom showed similar results in a smaller group of patients; aggressive lymphomas had a higher relapse risk compared to low-grade lymphomas (67.9% vs 10%, $p = 0.014$), leading to a dismal 16% 2-year EFS.[128] Finally, Morris and colleagues showed that patients with high-grade lymphomas fared much worse than indolent subtypes in terms of PFS (34% vs. 65%, $p = 0.002$), OS (34% vs. 73%, $p < 0.001$), and treatment-related mortality (RR, 2.3; $p = 0.02$).[129] The increase in toxicity for aggressive subtypes was unexplained, but may have been due to intensive prior treatments.

The relative success of ASCT in relapsed DLBCL as discussed above implies that patients considered for allogeneic approaches are more likely to have either failed a prior ASCT or are not optimal candidates for any transplant approach. The outcome of patients undergoing allogeneic stem cell transplant after failing a prior autologous transplant has mixed reports. The CIBMTR found no plateau in terms of PFS for lymphoma patients relapsing after an autologous transplant and subsequently receiving a fully myeloablative transplant.[136] Branson and colleagues used fludarabine, melphalan, and alemtuzumab conditioning in a heterogeneous group of NHL patients (10 with high-grade NHL) and demonstrated PFS and OS of 50% and 53%, respectively, with a median follow-up of 14 months.[137] The Fred Hutchinson Cancer Research Center (FHCRC) reported a 3-year PFS and OS of 28% and 31%, respectively, with no plateau in terms of relapse in a group of 147 patients (including 24 with aggressive NHL) treated with fludarabine and low-dose TBI. The presence of acute graft-versus-host disease (GVHD) increased toxicity but did not confer benefit, whereas chronic GVHD correlated with improved PFS. In contrast, Escalon and colleagues from the MDACC presented pilot data on 20 patients with NHL relapsing after a prior ASCT, including 10 with DLBCL.[138] Most patients had minimal disease burden and a good performance status. Using fludarabine, cyclophosphamide, and rituximab, the authors showed an encouraging 95% 3-year PFS with a median follow-up of 25 months. The CIBMTR is currently conducting a large registry analysis of NMSCT after ASCT, with results not yet available.

There are many remaining questions about the use of allogeneic stem cell transplant in DLBCL. We do not know which patient subsets are most likely to benefit, whether or not allogeneic approaches are superior to autologous transplant, and whether or not RIT provides sufficient disease control. It appears that some patients with aggressive lymphoma benefit from RIT with approximately 30% long-term disease control, expecially if chemosensitivity is demonstrated. However, allogeneic stem cell transplant remains investigational at this time for DLBCL.

Relapsed DLBCL: non-transplant eligible patients

It is clear that ASCT can effectively salvage some patients with relapsed DLBCL, especially if chemosensitivity can be demonstrated. Unfortunately, patients who are ineligible for transplant either due to advanced age or chemoresistant disease have a suboptimal outcome and the vast majority will die of progressive lymphoma. The median survival following relapse is partly dependent upon the initial IPI, with high-risk patients surviving less than one year.[139] A variety of salvage regimens have been used, but none is curative. Compared to the transplant arm, patients randomized to DHAP in the original Parma trial had a dismal 5-year survival of less than 15%. Whether or not modern salvage regimens that include rituximab can prolong survival is under active investigation. A clinical trial is the best option for these patients, with several new agents on the horizon including proteosome inhibitors, immunomodulatory agents, mTOR inhibitors, BCL2 inhibitors, and many other potentially active drugs.

Primary mediastinal B-cell lymphoma

Primary mediastinal B-cell lymphoma (PMBL) is a unique clinicopathologic subset of DLBCL, first recognized over 25 years ago, and accounts for approximately 5% of all lymphomas.[140,141] The median age of presentation is in the third decade of life, sharply contrasting with most DLBCL which present in the sixth or even seventh decade of life. Most patients present with signs and symptoms related to local invasion of mediastinal and thoracic structures by a prominent anterior mediastinal mass. This may include shortness of breath, chest pain, superior vena cava syndrome, or pericardial/pleural effusions with or without classic B symptoms. The staging evaluation shows a strongly PET-avid large anterior mediastinal mass, and bone marrow involvement is distinctly uncommon occurring in less than 5% of patients.[142–144] The pattern of dissemination is unusual for NHL, with frequent distant organ and CNS involvement reminiscent of hematogenous spread. A challenge to optimal staging is that some physicians consider invasion of mediastinal structures as stage IVE disease, whereas others consider localized PMBL as either stage I or II disease; this has particular relevance when interpreting clinical trial results or applying the IPI.

Histologically, PMBL arises from thymic B cells and is characterized by intermediate-sized lymphocytes interspersed with dense bands of fibrosis.[3] The significant fibrosis can make a pathologic diagnosis difficult, and a core biopsy or larger tissue sample may be required; a fine needle aspirate is usually insufficient. The frequent infiltration of inflammatory cells, including eosinophils and benign lymphocytes, can be confused with nodular sclerosis Hodgkin lymphoma. Immunophenotyping shows a population of CD20+, CD19+, CD45+, CD5−, CD10− B cells, and helps to distinguish PMBL from Hodgkin lymphoma which lacks CD45 and other mature B-cell surface markers. PMBL is genomically unique compared to other DLBCL subtypes, and in fact shares a gene expression profile more closely aligned with Hodgkin lymphoma.[145] Despite the biologic similarity to Hodgkin lymphoma, however, the treatment of PMBL follows that of other DLBCL. Several recurring genetic and biologic alterations have been observed, including gains of chromosome 9p occurring in 70% of cases, BCL6 translocations and mutations, c-rel amplification (with nuclear accumulation of rel protein), nuclear factor-kappa B pathway activation, and Jak/Stat abnormalities.[146,147]

In general, the prognosis for PMBL appears favorable compared to other DLBCL subtypes.[148–150] Savage and colleagues compared the outcome of 153 PMBL patients to that of 1273 DLBCL patients. As expected, the median age of the PMBL group was much younger at 37 years compared to 64 years for DLBCL. The 10-year PFS and OS were better in the PMBL group (69% vs. 43%, $p = 0.0001$; and 66% vs. 43%, $p = 0.00001$) following a variety of anthracycline-containing regimens. Of interest, the authors found that the vast majority of relapses occurred within the first year after treatment with no relapses beyond 2.5 years. In contrast, there was no clear plateau in terms of EFS or OS for other DLBCL subtypes. Others have also observed that relapse in PMBL is generally a quick phenomenon, with a median time to relapse of 6–18 months.[142,151,152]

The treatment of PMBL generally follows guidelines established for other DLBCL subtypes as described above. However, PMBL appears quite sensitive to dose intensification, as reported by several groups, and may benefit from augmented regimens. A single-center retrospective review of 141 patients at MSKCC by Hamlin *et al.* found that patients receiving either an intensified chemotherapy regimen (NHL-15) or front line ASCT had a superior EFS and OS compared to patients treated with CHOP alone.[142] This is echoed in several other reports showing that intensified regimens (i.e., MACOP-B, VACOP-B) or autologous transplantation is superior to CHOP.[143,144,150] However, each of these reports was prior to rituximab being available, and the high response rates with R-CHOP in this disease may imply that intensive frontline approaches are no longer needed for most patients.

A major therapeutic question is whether or not consolidative radiation is needed in PMBL. As with many bulky lymphomas, there is frequently a residual mass at the end of treatment. Many groups have advocated radiation, showing that local recurrence can be reduced without substantial additive toxicity.[143–144,151–153] In contrast, others have found similar rates of in-field and distant relapses irrespective of radiation. Lazzarino and colleagues retrospectively reported on 99 evaluable patients and found that the relapse rate did not significantly differ between patients receiving RT and those who did not.[151] Furthermore, 11 of 12 relapses in the RT group were intrathoracic. A French group reported that patients achieving only a PR to frontline chemotherapy did not further respond to RT.[154] The Vancouver group also found no added benefit to routine use of radiation to 5-year PFS or OS.[150] Similar to debates in other DLBCL and in Hodgkin lymphoma, the increasing use of PET-scanning further complicates the decision regarding radiation, remembering that consolidative radiation to bulky masses was based on eliminating residual disease not detected by CT scans alone. PET provides increased sensitivity in disease detection not previously available, and it remains to be seen if radiation can further improve outcomes in patients with PET-negative residual masses.

Conclusions

DLBCL is a potentially curable disease, with curability highly dependent on clinical and biologic features. Increased understanding of heterogeneity within DLBCL will hopefully lead to the study and future implementation of risk-based therapies. For now, the standard frontline regimen is rituximab plus an anthracycline as in the R-CHOP regimen, which achieves cure in more than half of newly diagnosed patients. Up to 90% of patients with low-risk disease can be considered cured. Relapsed DLBCL can be effectively treated by ASCT in approximately 40–50% of patients, particularly if chemosensitivity to salvage regimens is observed. Despite substantial gains in overall outcomes, however, intensive investigation in improving both the frontline and salvage approaches is ongoing with many promising agents and approaches on the horizon.

References

1. American Cancer Society Atlanta. *Cancer Facts and Figures: 2007.* www.cancer.org/docroot.
2. Swerdlow S, Campo E, Harris N, *et al.* (eds.) *WHO Classification of Tumours of Haematopoietic and Lymphoid Tissues*, 4th edn. Lyon, France, IARC Press, 2008.
3. Jaffe ES, Harris NL, Stein H, *et al.* (eds.) *World Health Organization Classification of Tumours: Pathology and Genetics of Tumours of Haematopoietic and Lymphoid Tissues.* Lyon, France, IARC Press, 2001.
4. Jemal A, Siegel R, Ward E, *et al.* Cancer statistics, 2008. *CA Cancer J Clin* 2008;**58**:71–96.
5. Levine AM, Seneviratne L, Espina BM, *et al.* Evolving characteristics of AIDS-related lymphoma. *Blood* 2000;**96**:4084–90.
6. Altieri A, Bermejo JL, Hemminki K. Familial risk for non-Hodgkin lymphoma and other lymphoproliferative malignancies by histopathologic subtype: the Swedish Family-Cancer Database. *Blood* 2005;**106**:668–72.

7. Morton LM, Wang SS, Cozen W, *et al.* Etiologic heterogeneity among non-Hodgkin lymphoma subtypes. *Blood* 2008;**112**:5150–60.

8. Kanungo A, Medeiros LJ, Abruzzo LV, *et al.* Lymphoid neoplasms associated with concurrent t(14;18) and 8q24/c-MYC translocation generally have a poor prognosis. *Mod Pathol* 2006;**19**:25–33.

9. Le Gouill S, Talmant P, Touzeau C, *et al.* The clinical presentation and prognosis of diffuse large B-cell lymphoma with t(14;18) and 8q24/c-MYC rearrangement. *Haematologica* 2007;**92**:1335–42.

10. Cheson BD, Horning SJ, Coiffier B, *et al.* Report of an international workshop to standardize response criteria for non-Hodgkin's lymphomas. NCI Sponsored International Working Group. *J Clin Oncol* 1999;**17**:1244.

11. Cheson BD, Pfistner B, Juweid ME, *et al.* Revised response criteria for malignant lymphoma. *J Clin Oncol* 2007;**25**:579–86.

12. Haioun C, Itti E, Rahmouni A, *et al.* [18F]fluoro-2-deoxy-D-glucose positron emission tomography (FDG-PET) in aggressive lymphoma: an early prognostic tool for predicting patient outcome. *Blood* 2005;**106**:1376–81.

13. Kostakoglu L, Goldsmith SJ, Leonard JP, *et al.* FDG-PET after 1 cycle of therapy predicts outcome in diffuse large cell lymphoma and classic Hodgkin disease. *Cancer* 2006;**107**:2678–87.

14. Ng AP, Wirth A, Seymour JF, *et al.* Early therapeutic response assessment by (18)FDG-positron emission tomography during chemotherapy in patients with diffuse large B-cell lymphoma: isolated residual positivity involving bone is not usually a predictor of subsequent treatment failure. *Leuk Lymphoma* 2007;**48**:596–600.

15. Seam P, Juweid ME, Cheson BD. The role of FDG-PET scans in patients with lymphoma. *Blood* 2007;**110**:3507–16.

16. The International Non-Hodgkin's Lymphoma Prognostic Factors Project. A predictive model for aggressive non-Hodgkin's lymphoma. *N Engl J Med* 1993;**329**:987–94.

17. Sehn LH, Berry B, Chhanabhai M, *et al.* The revised International Prognostic Index (R-IPI) is a better predictor of outcome than the standard IPI for patients with diffuse large B-cell lymphoma treated with R-CHOP. *Blood* 2007;**109**:1857–61.

18. Alizadeh AA, Eisen MB, Davis RE, *et al.* Distinct types of diffuse large B-cell lymphoma identified by gene expression profiling. *Nature* 2000;**403**:503–11.

19. Rosenwald A, Wright G, Chan WC, *et al.* The use of molecular profiling to predict survival after chemotherapy for diffuse large-B-cell lymphoma. *N Engl J Med* 2002;**346**:1937–47.

20. Shipp MA, Ross KN, Tamayo P, *et al.* Diffuse large B-cell lymphoma outcome prediction by gene-expression profiling and supervised machine learning. *Nat Med* 2002;**8**:68–74.

21. Lossos IS, Czerwinski DK, Alizadeh AA, *et al.* Prediction of survival in diffuse large-B-cell lymphoma based on the expression of six genes. *N Engl J Med* 2004;**350**:1828–37.

22. Chang CC, McClintock S, Cleveland RP, *et al.* Immunohistochemical expression patterns of germinal center and activation B-cell markers correlate with prognosis in diffuse large B-cell lymphoma. *Am J Surg Pathol* 2004;**28**:464–70.

23. Hans CP, Weisenburger DD, Greiner TC, *et al.* Confirmation of the molecular classification of diffuse large B-cell lymphoma by immunohistochemistry using a tissue microarray. *Blood* 2004;**103**(1):275–82.

24. Malumbres R, Chen J, Tibshirani R, *et al.* Paraffin-based 6-gene model predicts outcome in diffuse large B-cell lymphoma patients treated with R-CHOP. *Blood* 2008;**111**:5509–14.

25. Gascoyne RD, Adomat SA, Krajewski S, *et al.* Prognostic significance of Bcl-2 protein expression and Bcl-2 gene rearrangement in diffuse aggressive non-Hodgkin's lymphoma. *Blood* 1997;**90**:244–51.

26. Iqbal J, Neppalli VT, Wright G, *et al.* BCL2 expression is a prognostic marker for the activated B-cell-like type of diffuse large B-cell lymphoma. *J Clin Oncol* 2006;**24**:961–8.

27. Mounier N, Briere J, Gisselbrecht C, *et al.* Rituximab plus CHOP (R-CHOP) overcomes bcl2-associated resistance to chemotherapy in elderly patients with diffuse large B-cell lymphoma (DLBCL). *Blood* 2003;**101**:4279–84.

28. Winter JN, Weller EA, Horning SJ, *et al.* Prognostic significance of Bcl-6 protein expression in DLBCL treated with CHOP or R-CHOP: a prospective correlative study. *Blood* 2006;**107**:4207–13.

29. Natkunam Y, Farinha P, Hsi ED, *et al.* LMO2 protein expression predicts survival in patients with diffuse large B-cell lymphoma treated with anthracycline-based chemotherapy with and without rituximab. *J Clin Oncol* 2008;**26**:447–54.

30. Natkunam Y, Zhao S, Mason DY, *et al.* The oncoprotein LMO2 is expressed in normal germinal-center B cells and in human B-cell lymphomas. *Blood* 2007;**109**:1636–42.

31. Spicer J, Smith P, Maclennan K, *et al.* Long-term follow-up of patients treated with radiotherapy alone for early-stage histologically aggressive non-Hodgkin's lymphoma. *Br J Cancer* 2004;**90**:1151–5.

32. Shenkier TN, Voss N, Fairey R, *et al.* Brief chemotherapy and involved-region irradiation for limited-stage diffuse large-cell lymphoma: an 18-year experience from the British Columbia Cancer Agency. *J Clin Oncol* 2002;**20**:197–204.

33. Miller TP, Dahlberg S, Cassady JR, *et al.* Chemotherapy alone compared with chemotherapy plus radiotherapy for localized intermediate- and high-grade non-Hodgkin's lymphoma. *N Engl J Med* 1998;**339**:21–6.

34. Ballonoff A, Rusthoven KE, Schwer A, *et al.* Outcomes and effect of radiotherapy in patients with stage I or II diffuse large B-cell lymphoma: a surveillance, epidemiology, and end results analysis. *Int J Radiat Oncol Biol Phys* 2008;**72**:1465–71.

35. Miller TP, LeBlanc M, Spier CM, *et al.* CHOP alone compared to CHOP plus radiotherapy for early stage aggressive non-Hodgkin's lymphomas: update of the Southwest Oncology Group (SWOG) randomized trial. *Blood* 2001;**98**:724a.

36. Bonnet C, Fillet G, Mounier N, *et al.* CHOP alone compared with CHOP plus radiotherapy for localized aggressive lymphoma in elderly patients: a study by the Groupe d'Etude des Lymphomes de l'Adulte. *J Clin Oncol* 2007;**25**:787–92.

37. Reyes F, Lepage E, Ganem G, *et al.* ACVBP versus CHOP plus radiotherapy for localized aggressive lymphoma. *N Engl J Med* 2005;**352**:1197–205.

38. Horning SJ, Weller E, Kim K, *et al.* Chemotherapy with or without radiotherapy in limited-stage diffuse aggressive non-Hodgkin's lymphoma: Eastern Cooperative Oncology Group study 1484. *J Clin Oncol* 2004;**22**:3032–8.

39. Pfreundschuh M, Trumper L, Osterborg A, *et al.* CHOP-like chemotherapy plus rituximab versus CHOP-like chemotherapy alone in young patients with good-prognosis diffuse large-B-cell lymphoma: a randomised controlled trial by the MabThera International Trial (MInT) Group. *Lancet Oncol* 2006;**7**:379–91.

40. Pfreundschuh M, Ho AD, Cavallin-Stahl E, *et al.* Prognostic significance of maximum tumour (bulk) diameter in young patients with good-prognosis diffuse large-B-cell lymphoma treated with CHOP-like chemotherapy with or without rituximab: an exploratory analysis of the MabThera International Trial Group (MInT) study. *Lancet Oncol* 2008;**9**:435–44.

41. Persky DO, Unger JM, Spier CM, *et al.* Phase II study of rituximab plus three cycles of CHOP and involved-field radiotherapy for patients with limited-stage aggressive B-cell lymphoma: Southwest Oncology Group study 0014. *J Clin Oncol* 2008;**26**:2258–63.

42. Sehn HL, Savage KJ, Hoskins P, *et al.* Limited-stage diffuse large B-cell lymphoma (DLBCL) patients with a negative PET scan following three cycles of R-CHOP can be effectively treated with abbreviated chemoimmunotherapy alone. *Blood* 2007;**110**:787a.

43. Elias L, Portlock CS, Rosenberg SA. Combination chemotherapy of diffuse histiocytic lymphoma with cyclophosphamide, adriamycin, vincristine and prednisone (CHOP). *Cancer* 1978;**42**:1705–10.

44. McKelvey EM, Gottlieb JA, Wilson HE, *et al.* Hydroxyldaunomycin (Adriamycin) combination chemotherapy in malignant lymphoma. *Cancer* 1976;**38**:1484–93.

45. Fisher RI, Gaynor ER, Dahlberg S, *et al.* Comparison of a standard regimen (CHOP) with three intensive chemotherapy regimens for advanced non-Hodgkin's lymphoma. *N Engl J Med* 1993;**328**:1002–6.

46. Cartron G, Watier H, Golay J, Solal-Celigny P. From the bench to the bedside: ways to improve rituximab efficacy. *Blood* 2004;**104**:2635–42.

47. Coiffier B, Haioun C, Ketterer N, *et al.* Rituximab (anti-CD20 monoclonal antibody) for the treatment of patients with relapsing or refractory aggressive lymphoma: a multicenter phase II study. *Blood* 1998;**92**:1927–32.

48. Coiffier B, Feugier P, Mounier N, *et al.* Long-term results of the GELA study comparing R-CHOP and CHOP chemotherapy in older patients with diffuse large B-cell lymphoma show good survival in poor-risk patients. *J Clin Oncol* 2007;**25**:Abstract 8009.

49. Coiffier B, Lepage E, Briere J, *et al.* CHOP chemotherapy plus rituximab compared with CHOP alone in elderly patients with diffuse large-B-cell lymphoma. *N Engl J Med* 2002;**346**:235–42.

50. Habermann TM, Weller EA, Morrison VA, *et al.* Rituximab-CHOP versus CHOP alone or with maintenance rituximab in older patients with diffuse large B-cell lymphoma. *J Clin Oncol* 2006;**24**:3121–7.

51. Feugier P, Van Hoof A, Sebban C, *et al.* Long-term results of the R-CHOP study in the treatment of elderly patients with diffuse large B-cell lymphoma: a study by the Groupe d'Etude des Lymphomes de l'Adulte. *J Clin Oncol* 2005;**23**:4117–26.

52. Wilson KS, Sehn LH, Berry B, *et al.* CHOP-R therapy overcomes the adverse prognostic influence of BCL-2 expression in diffuse large B-cell lymphoma. *Leuk Lymphoma* 2007;**48**:1102–9.

53. Blayney DW, LeBlanc ML, Grogan T, *et al.* Dose-intense chemotherapy every 2 weeks with dose-intense cyclophosphamide, doxorubicin, vincristine, and prednisone may improve survival in intermediate- and high-grade lymphoma: a phase II study of the Southwest Oncology Group (SWOG 9349). *J Clin Oncol* 2003;**21**:2466–73.

54. Portlock CS, Qin J, Schaindlin P, *et al.* The NHL-15 protocol for aggressive non-Hodgkin's lymphomas: a sequential dose-dense, dose-intense regimen of doxorubicin, vincristine and high-dose cyclophosphamide. *Ann Oncol* 2004;**15**:1495–503.

55. Wunderlich A, Kloess M, Reiser M, *et al.* Practicability and acute haematological toxicity of 2- and 3-weekly CHOP and CHOEP chemotherapy for aggressive non-Hodgkin's lymphoma: results from the NHL-B trial of the German High-Grade Non-Hodgkin's Lymphoma Study Group (DSHNHL). *Ann Oncol* 2003; **14**:881–93.

56. Pfreundschuh M, Trumper L, Kloess M, *et al.* Two-weekly or 3-weekly CHOP chemotherapy with or without etoposide for the treatment of elderly patients with aggressive lymphomas: results of the NHL-B2 trial of the DSHNHL. *Blood* 2004;**104**:634–41.

57. Pfreundschuh M, Trumper L, Kloess M, *et al.* Two-weekly or 3-weekly CHOP chemotherapy with or without etoposide for the treatment of young patients with good-prognosis (normal LDH) aggressive lymphomas: results of the NHL-B1 trial of the DSHNHL. *Blood* 2004;**104**:626–33.

58. Pfreundschuh M, Schubert J, Ziepert M, *et al.* Six versus eight cycles of bi-weekly CHOP-14 with or without intuximab in elderly patients with aggressive CD20+ B-cell lymphomas: a randomised controlled trial (RICOVER-60). *Lancet Oncol* 2008;**9**:105–16.

59. Pfreundschuh M, Zeynalova S, Poeschel V, *et al.* Improved outcome of elderly patients with poor-prognosis diffuse large B-cell lymphoma (DLBCL) after dose-dense rituximab: results of the DENSE-R-CHOP-14 trial of the German High-Grade Non-Hodgkin Lymphoma Study Group (DSHNHL). *J Clin Oncol* 2008;**20** Suppl: Abstract 8508.

60. Gutierrez M, Chabner BA, Pearson D, *et al.* Role of a doxorubicin-containing regimen in relapsed and resistant lymphomas: an 8-year follow-up study of EPOCH. *J Clin Oncol* 2000; **18**:3633–42.

61. Wilson WH, Grossbard ML, Pittaluga S, *et al.* Dose-adjusted EPOCH chemotherapy for untreated large B-cell lymphomas: a pharmacodynamic approach with high efficacy. *Blood* 2002;**99**:2685–93.

62. Garcia-Suarez J, Banas H, Arribas I, *et al.* Dose-adjusted EPOCH plus rituximab is an effective regimen in patients with poor-prognostic untreated diffuse large B-cell lymphoma: results from a prospective observational study. *Br J Haematol* 2007;**136**:276–85.

63. Wilson WH, Dunleavy K, Pittaluga S, *et al.* Phase II study of dose-adjusted EPOCH and rituximab in untreated diffuse large B-cell lymphoma with analysis of germinal center and post-germinal center biomarkers. *J Clin Oncol* 2008;**26**:2717–24.

64. Zinzani PL, Tani M, Fanti S, *et al.* A phase II trial of CHOP chemotherapy followed by yttrium 90 ibritumomab tiuxetan (Zevalin) for previously untreated elderly diffuse large B-cell lymphoma patients. *Ann Oncol* 2008;**19**:769–73.

65. Baldissera RC, Nucci M, Vigorito AC, *et al.* Frontline therapy with early intensification and autologous stem cell transplantation versus conventional chemotherapy in unselected high-risk, aggressive non-Hodgkin's lymphoma patients: a prospective randomized GEMOH report. *Acta Haematol* 2006;**115**:15–21.

66. Kaiser U, Uebelacker I, Abel U, *et al.* Randomized study to evaluate the use of high-dose therapy as part of primary treatment for "aggressive" lymphoma. *J Clin Oncol* 2002;**20**:4413–19.

67. Martelli M, Gherlinzoni F, De Renzo A, *et al.* Early autologous stem-cell transplantation versus conventional chemotherapy as front-line therapy in high-risk, aggressive non-Hodgkin's lymphoma: an Italian multicenter randomized trial. *J Clin Oncol* 2003;**21**:1255–62.

68. Martelli M, Vignetti M, Zinzani PL, *et al.* High-dose chemotherapy followed by autologous bone marrow transplantation versus dexamethasone, cisplatin, and cytarabine in aggressive non-Hodgkin's lymphoma with partial response to front-line chemotherapy: a prospective randomized Italian multicenter study. *J Clin Oncol* 1996;**14**:534–42.

69. Verdonck LF, van Putten WL, Hagenbeek A, *et al.* Comparison of CHOP chemotherapy with autologous bone marrow transplantation for slowly responding patients with aggressive non-Hodgkin's lymphoma. *N Engl J Med* 1995;**332**:1045–51.

70. Haioun C, Lepage E, Gisselbrecht C, *et al.* Survival benefit of high-dose therapy in poor-risk aggressive non-Hodgkin's lymphoma: final analysis of the prospective LNH87–2 protocol–a groupe d'Etude des lymphomes de l'Adulte study. *J Clin Oncol* 2000;**18**:3025–30.

71. Kluin-Nelemans HC, Zagonel V, Anastasopoulou A, *et al.* Standard chemotherapy with or without high-dose chemotherapy for aggressive non-Hodgkin's lymphoma: randomized phase III EORTC study. *J Natl Cancer Inst* 2001;**93**:22–30.

72. Santini G, Salvagno L, Leoni P, *et al.* VACOP-B versus VACOP-B plus autologous bone marrow transplantation for advanced diffuse non-Hodgkin's lymphoma: results of a prospective randomized trial by the non-Hodgkin's Lymphoma Cooperative Study Group. *J Clin Oncol* 1998;**16**:2796–802.

73. Gianni AM, Bregni M, Siena S, *et al.* High-dose chemotherapy and autologous bone marrow transplantation compared with MACOP-B in aggressive B-cell lymphoma. *N Engl J Med* 1997;**336**:1290–7.

74. Gisselbrecht C, Lepage E, Molina T, *et al.* Shortened first-line high-dose chemotherapy for patients with poor-prognosis aggressive lymphoma. *J Clin Oncol* 2002;**20**:2472–9.

75. Milpied N, Deconinck E, Gaillard F, *et al.* Initial treatment of aggressive lymphoma with high-dose chemotherapy and autologous stem-cell support. *N Engl J Med* 2004;**350**:1287–95.

76. Vitolo U, Liberati AM, Cabras MG, *et al.* High dose sequential chemotherapy with autologous transplantation versus dose-dense chemotherapy MegaCEOP as first line treatment in poor-prognosis diffuse large cell lymphoma: an "Intergruppo Italiano Linfomi" randomized trial. *Haematologica* 2005;**90**:793–801.

77. Strehl J, Mey U, Glasmacher A, *et al.* High-dose chemotherapy followed by autologous stem cell transplantation as first-line therapy in aggressive non-Hodgkin's lymphoma: a meta-analysis. *Haematologica* 2003;**88**:1304–15.

78. Vose JM, Zhang MJ, Rowlings PA, *et al.* Autologous transplantation for diffuse aggressive non-Hodgkin's lymphoma in patients never achieving remission: a report from the Autologous Blood and Marrow Transplant Registry. *J Clin Oncol* 2001;**19**:406–13.

79. Kewalramani T, Zelenetz AD, Hedrick EE, *et al.* High-dose chemoradiotherapy and autologous stem cell transplantation for patients with primary refractory aggressive non-Hodgkin lymphoma: an intention-to-treat analysis. *Blood* 2000;**96**:2399–404.

80. Rodriguez J, Caballero MD, Gutierrez A, *et al.* Autologous stem-cell transplantation in diffuse large B-cell non-Hodgkin's lymphoma not achieving complete response after induction chemotherapy: the GEL/TAMO experience. *Ann Oncol* 2004;**15**:1504–9.

81. Boehme V, Zeynalova S, Kloess M, *et al.* Incidence and risk factors of central nervous system recurrence in aggressive lymphoma–a survey of 1693 patients treated in protocols of the German High-Grade Non-Hodgkin's Lymphoma Study Group (DSHNHL). *Ann Oncol* 2007;**18**:149–57.

82. Boehme V, Zeynalova S, Lengfelder E, *et al.* CNS-disease in elderly patients treated with modern chemotherapy (CHOP-14) with or without rituximab: an analysis of CNS events in the RICOVER-60 trial of the German High-Grade Non-Hodgkin's Lymphoma Study Group (DSHNHL). *Blood* 2007;**110**:Abstract 519.

83. Feugier P, Virion JM, Tilly H, *et al.* Incidence and risk factors for central nervous system occurrence in elderly patients with diffuse large-B-cell lymphoma: influence of rituximab. *Ann Oncol* 2004;**15**:129–33.

84. Haioun C, Besson C, Lepage E, *et al.* Incidence and risk factors of central nervous system relapse in histologically aggressive non-Hodgkin's lymphoma uniformly treated and receiving intrathecal central nervous system prophylaxis: a GELA study on 974 patients. Groupe d'Etudes des Lymphomes de l'Adulte. *Ann Oncol* 2000;**11**:685–90.

85. van Besien K, Ha CS, Murphy S, *et al.* Risk factors, treatment, and outcome of central nervous system recurrence in adults with intermediate-grade and immunoblastic lymphoma. *Blood* 1998;**91**:1178–84.

86. Hill QA, Owen RG. CNS prophylaxis in lymphoma: who to target and what therapy to use. *Blood Rev* 2006;**20**:319–32.

87. Doolittle ND, Abrey LE, Shenkier TN, *et al.* Brain parenchyma involvement as isolated central nervous system relapse of systemic non-Hodgkin lymphoma: an International Primary CNS Lymphoma Collaborative Group report. *Blood* 2008;**111**:1085–93.

88. Tilly H, Lepage E, Coiffier B, *et al.* Intensive conventional chemotherapy (ACVBP regimen) compared with standard CHOP for poor-prognosis aggressive non-Hodgkin lymphoma. *Blood* 2003;**102**:4284–9.

89. Vose JM, Rizzo DJ, Tao-Wu J, *et al.* Autologous transplantation for diffuse aggressive non-Hodgkin lymphoma

in first relapse or second remission. *Biol Blood Marrow Transplant* 2004;**10**:116–27.

90. Josting A, Sieniawski M, Glossmann JP, *et al.* High-dose sequential chemotherapy followed by autologous stem cell transplantation in relapsed and refractory aggressive non-Hodgkin's lymphoma: results of a multicenter phase II study. *Ann Oncol* 2005;**16**:1359–65.

91. Shipp MA, Abeloff MD, Antman KH, *et al.* International Consensus Conference on High-Dose Therapy with Hematopoietic Stem Cell Transplantation in Aggressive Non-Hodgkin's Lymphomas: report of the jury. *J Clin Oncol* 1999;**17**:423–9.

92. Blay J, Gomez F, Sebban C, *et al.* The International Prognostic Index correlates to survival in patients with aggressive lymphoma in relapse: analysis of the PARMA trial. Parma Group. *Blood* 1998;**92**:3562–8.

93. Hamlin PA, Zelenetz AD, Kewalramani T, *et al.* Age-adjusted International Prognostic Index predicts autologous stem cell transplantation outcome for patients with relapsed or primary refractory diffuse large B-cell lymphoma. *Blood* 2003;**102**:1989–96.

94. van Besien K, Rodriguez A, Tomany S, *et al.* Phase II study of a high-dose ifosfamide-based chemotherapy regimen with growth factor rescue in recurrent aggressive NHL. High response rates and limited toxicity, but limited impact on long-term survival. *Bone Marrow Transplant* 2001;**27**:397–404.

95. Costa LJ, Micallef IN, Inwards DJ, *et al.* Time of relapse after initial therapy significantly adds to the prognostic value of the IPI-R in patients with relapsed DLBCL undergoing autologous stem cell transplantation. *Bone Marrow Transplant* 2008;**41**:715–20.

96. Moskowitz CH, Bertino JR, Glassman JR, *et al.* Ifosfamide, carboplatin, and etoposide: a highly effective cytoreduction and peripheral-blood progenitor-cell mobilization regimen for transplant-eligible patients with non-Hodgkin's lymphoma. *J Clin Oncol* 1999;**17**:3776–85.

97. Schot BW, Zijlstra JM, Sluiter WJ, *et al.* Early FDG-PET assessment in combination with clinical risk scores determines prognosis in recurring lymphoma. *Blood* 2007;**109**:486–91.

98. Spaepen K, Stroobants S, Dupont P, *et al.* Early restaging positron emission tomography with (18)F-fluorodeoxyglucose predicts outcome in patients with aggressive non-Hodgkin's lymphoma. *Ann Oncol* 2002;**13**:1356–63.

99. Svoboda J, Andreadis C, Elstrom R, *et al.* Prognostic value of FDG-PET scan imaging in lymphoma patients undergoing autologous stem cell transplantation. *Bone Marrow Transplant* 2006;**38**:211–16.

100. Crocchiolo R, Canevari C, Assanelli A, *et al.* Pre-transplant 18FDG-PET predicts outcome in lymphoma patients treated with high-dose sequential chemotherapy followed by autologous stem cell transplantation. *Leuk Lymphoma* 2008;**49**:727–33.

101. Spaepen K, Stroobants S, Dupont P, *et al.* Prognostic value of pretransplantation positron emission tomography using fluorine 18-fluorodeoxyglucose in patients with aggressive lymphoma treated with high-dose chemotherapy and stem cell transplantation. *Blood* 2003; **102**:53–9.

102. Moskowitz CH, Zelenetz AD, Kewalramani T, *et al.* Cell of origin, germinal center versus nongerminal center, determined by immunohistochemistry on tissue microarray, does not correlate with outcome in patients with relapsed and refractory DLBCL. *Blood* 2005;**106**:3383–85.

103. Corazzelli G, Russo F, Capobianco G, *et al.* Gemcitabine, ifosfamide, oxaliplatin and rituximab (R-GIFOX), a new effective cytoreductive/mobilizing salvage regimen for relapsed and refractory aggressive non-Hodgkin's lymphoma: results of a pilot study. *Ann Oncol* 2006; **17** Suppl 4:iv18–24.

104. Vellenga E, van Putten WL, van't Veer MB, *et al.* Rituximab improves the treatment results of DHAP-VIM-DHAP and ASCT in relapsed/progressive aggressive CD20+ NHL: a prospective randomized HOVON trial. *Blood* 2008;**111**:537–43.

105. Kewalramani T, Zelenetz AD, Nimer SD, *et al.* Rituximab and ICE as second-line therapy before autologous stem cell transplantation for relapsed or primary refractory diffuse large B-cell lymphoma. *Blood* 2004;**103**:3684–8.

106. Sieniawski M, Staak O, Glossmann JP, *et al.* Rituximab added to an intensified salvage chemotherapy program followed by autologous stem cell transplantation improved the outcome in relapsed and refractory aggressive non-Hodgkin lymphoma. *Ann Hematol* 2007;**86**:107–15.

107. Fenske TS, Hari PN, Carreras J, *et al.* Impact of pre-transplant rituximab on survival after autologous hematopoietic stem cell transplantation for diffuse large B cell lymphoma. *Biol Blood Marrow Transplant* 2009;**15**:1455–64.

108. Gisselbrecht C, Schmitz N, Mounier N, *et al.* R-ICE versus R-DHAP in relapsed patients with CD20 diffuse large B-cell lymphoma (DLBCL) followed by stem cell transplantation and maintenance treatment with rituximab or not: first interim analysis on 200 patients. CORAL Study. *Blood* 2007;**110**:517a.

109. Friedberg JW, Neuberg D, Stone RM, *et al.* Outcome in patients with myelodysplastic syndrome after autologous bone marrow transplantation for non-Hodgkin's lymphoma. *J Clin Oncol* 1999;**17**:3128–35.

110. Milligan DW, Ruiz De Elvira MC, Kolb HJ, *et al.* Secondary leukaemia and myelodysplasia after autografting for lymphoma: results from the EBMT. EBMT Lymphoma and Late Effects Working Parties. European Group for Blood and Marrow Transplantation. *Br J Haematol* 1999;**106**:1020–6.

111. Vose JM, Bierman PJ, Enke C, *et al.* Phase I trial of iodine-131 tositumomab with high-dose chemotherapy and autologous stem-cell transplantation for relapsed non-Hodgkin's lymphoma. *J Clin Oncol* 2005;**23**:461–7.

112. Vose J, Bierman PJ, Bociek G, *et al.* Radioimmunotherapy with 131-I tositumomab enhanced survival in good prognosis relapsed and high-risk diffuse large B-cell lymphoma (DLBCL) patients receiving high-dose chemotherapy and autologous stem cell transplantation. *J Clin Oncol (2007 ASCO Annual Meeting Proceedings Part 1)* 2007;**25**(185): Abstract 8013.

113. Krishnan A, Nademanee A, Fung HC, *et al.* Phase II trial of a transplantation regimen of yttrium-90 ibritumomab tiuxetan and high-dose chemotherapy in patients with non-Hodgkin's lymphoma. *J Clin Oncol* 2008; **26**:90–5.

114. Nademanee A, Forman S, Molina A, *et al.* A phase 1/2 trial of high-dose yttrium-90-ibritumomab tiuxetan in combination with high-dose etoposide and cyclophosphamide followed by autologous stem cell transplantation in patients with poor-risk or relapsed non-Hodgkin lymphoma. *Blood* 2005;**106**:2896–902.

115. Shimoni A, Zwas ST, Oksman Y, *et al.* Yttrium-90-ibritumomab tiuxetan (Zevalin) combined with high-dose BEAM chemotherapy and autologous stem cell transplantation for chemo-refractory aggressive non-Hodgkin's lymphoma. *Exp Hematol* 2007;**35**:534–40.

116. Winter JN, Inwards DJ, Spies S, *et al.* 90Y Ibritumomab tiuxetan (Zevalin®; 90YZ) doses calculated to deliver up to 1500 cGy to critical organs may be safely combined with high-dose BEAM and autotransplant in NHL. *Blood* 2006;**108**:330a.

117. Alousi AM, Hosing C, Saliba R, *et al.* Zevalin®/BEAM/rituximab vs BEAM/ rituximab and autologous stem cell transplantation (ASCT) for relapsed chemosensitive diffuse large B-cell lymphoma (DLBCL): impact of the IPI and PET status. *Blood* 2007;**110**:620a.

118. Kewalramani T, Nimer SD, Zelenetz AD, *et al.* Progressive disease following autologous transplantation in patients with chemosensitive relapsed or primary refractory Hodgkin's disease or aggressive non-Hodgkin's lymphoma. *Bone Marrow Transplant* 2003;**32**:673–9.

119. Philip T, Guglielmi C, Hagenbeek A, *et al.* Autologous bone marrow transplantation as compared with salvage chemotherapy in relapses of chemotherapy-sensitive non-Hodgkin's lymphoma. *N Engl J Med* 1995;**333**:1540–5.

120. Vose JM, Bierman PJ, Anderson JR, *et al.* Progressive disease after high-dose therapy and autologous transplantation for lymphoid malignancy: clinical course and patient follow-up. *Blood* 1992;**80**:2142–8.

121. Kline J, Subbiah S, Lazarus HM, *et al.* Autologous graft-versus-host disease: harnessing anti-tumor immunity through impaired self-tolerance. *Bone Marrow Transplant* 2008;**41**:505–13.

122. Thompson JA, Fisher RI, Leblanc M, *et al.* Total body irradiation, etoposide, cyclophosphamide, and autologous peripheral blood stem-cell transplantation followed by randomization to therapy with interleukin-2 versus observation for patients with non-Hodgkin lymphoma: results of a phase 3 randomized trial by the Southwest Oncology Group (SWOG 9438). *Blood* 2008;**111**: 4048–54.

123. Khouri IF, Saliba RM, Hosing C, *et al.* Concurrent administration of high-dose rituximab before and after autologous stem-cell transplantation for relapsed aggressive B-cell non-Hodgkin's lymphomas. *J Clin Oncol* 2005;**23**:2240–7.

124. Horwitz SM, Negrin RS, Blume KG, *et al.* Rituximab as adjuvant to high-dose therapy and autologous hematopoietic cell transplantation for aggressive non-Hodgkin lymphoma. *Blood* 2004;**103**:777–83.

125. Lee MY, Chiou TJ, Hsiao LT, *et al.* Rituximab therapy increased post-transplant cytomegalovirus complications in non-Hodgkin's lymphoma patients receiving autologous hematopoietic stem cell transplantation. *Ann Hematol* 2008;**87**:285–9.

126. Lemieux B, Tartas S, Traulle C, *et al.* Rituximab-related late-onset neutropenia after autologous stem cell transplantation for aggressive non-Hodgkin's lymphoma. *Bone Marrow Transplant* 2004;**33**:921–3.

127. Shortt J, Spencer A. Adjuvant rituximab causes prolonged hypogamma-globulinaemia following autologous stem cell transplant for non-Hodgkin's lymphoma. *Bone Marrow Transplant* 2006;**38**:433–6.

128. Faulkner RD, Craddock C, Byrne JL, *et al.* BEAM-alemtuzumab reduced-intensity allogeneic stem cell transplantation for lymphoproliferative diseases: GVHD, toxicity, and survival in 65 patients. *Blood* 2004;**103**:428–34.

129. Morris E, Thomson K, Craddock C, *et al.* Outcomes after alemtuzumab-containing reduced-intensity allogeneic transplantation regimen for relapsed and refractory non-Hodgkin lymphoma. *Blood* 2004;**104**:3865–71.

130. Robinson SP, Goldstone AH, Mackinnon S, *et al.* Chemoresistant or aggressive lymphoma predicts for a poor outcome following reduced-intensity allogeneic progenitor cell transplantation: an analysis from the Lymphoma Working Party of the European Group for Blood and Bone Marrow Transplantation. *Blood* 2002;**100**:4310–16.

131. Peniket AJ, Ruiz de Elvira MC, Taghipour G, *et al.* An EBMT registry matched study of allogeneic stem cell transplants for lymphoma: allogeneic transplantation is associated with a lower relapse rate but a higher procedure-related mortality rate than autologous transplantation. *Bone Marrow Transplant* 2003;**31**:667–78.

132. van Besien KW, de Lima M, Giralt SA, *et al.* Management of lymphoma recurrence after allogeneic transplantation: the relevance of graft-versus-lymphoma effect. *Bone Marrow Transplant* 1997;**19**:977–82.

133. Dhedin N, Giraudier S, Gaulard P, *et al.* Allogeneic bone marrow transplantation in aggressive non-Hodgkin's lymphoma (excluding Burkitt and lymphoblastic lymphoma): a series of 73 patients from the SFGM database. Societ Francaise de Greffe de Moelle. *Br J Haematol* 1999;**107**:154–61.

134. Doocey RT, Toze CL, Connors JM, *et al.* Allogeneic haematopoietic stem-cell transplantation for relapsed and refractory aggressive histology non-Hodgkin lymphoma. *Br J Haematol* 2005;**131**:223–30.

135. Rodriguez R, Nademanee A, Ruel N, *et al.* Comparison of reduced-intensity and conventional myeloablative regimens for allogeneic transplantation in non-Hodgkin's lymphoma. *Biol Blood Marrow Transplant* 2006; **12**:1326–34.

136. Freytes CO, Loberiza FR, Rizzo JD, *et al.* Myeloablative allogeneic hematopoietic stem cell transplantation in patients who experience relapse after autologous stem cell transplantation for lymphoma: a report of the International Bone Marrow Transplant Registry. *Blood* 2004;**104**:3797–803.

137. Branson K, Chopra R, Kottaridis PD, *et al.* Role of nonmyeloablative allogeneic stem-cell transplantation after failure of autologous transplantation in patients with lymphoproliferative malignancies. *J Clin Oncol* 2002;**20**:4022–31.

138. Escalon MP, Champlin RE, Saliba RM, *et al.* Nonmyeloablative allogeneic hematopoietic transplantation: a promising salvage therapy for patients

with non-Hodgkin's lymphoma whose disease has failed a prior autologous transplantation. *J Clin Oncol* 2004;**22**:2419–23.

139. Coiffier B, Feugier P, Mounier N, *et al.* Long-term results of the GELA study comparing R-CHOP and CHOP chemotherapy in older patients with diffuse large B-cell lymphoma show good survival in poor-risk patients. *J Clin Oncol (2007 ASCO Annual Meeting Proceedings)* 2007;**25**(18S): Abstract 8009.

140. Lichtenstein AK, Levine A, Taylor CR, *et al.* Primary mediastinal lymphoma in adults. *Am J Med* 1980;**68**:509–14.

141. Miller JB, Variakojis D, Bitran JD, *et al.* Diffuse histiocytic lymphoma with sclerosis: a clinicopathologic entity frequently causing superior venacaval obstruction. *Cancer* 1981;**47**:748–56.

142. Hamlin PA, Portlock CS, Straus DJ, *et al.* Primary mediastinal large B-cell lymphoma: optimal therapy and prognostic factor analysis in 141 consecutive patients treated at Memorial Sloan Kettering from 1980 to 1999. *Br J Haematol* 2005;**130**:691–9.

143. Todeschini G, Secchi S, Morra E, *et al.* Primary mediastinal large B-cell lymphoma (PMLBCL): long-term results from a retrospective multicentre Italian experience in 138 patients treated with CHOP or MACOP-B/VACOP-B. *Br J Cancer* 2004;**90**:372–6.

144. Zinzani PL, Martelli M, Bertini M, *et al.* Induction chemotherapy strategies for primary mediastinal large B-cell lymphoma with sclerosis: a retrospective multinational study on 426 previously untreated patients. *Haematologica* 2002;**87**:1258–64.

145. Rosenwald A, Wright G, Leroy K, *et al.* Molecular diagnosis of primary mediastinal B cell lymphoma identifies a clinically favorable subgroup of diffuse large B cell lymphoma related to Hodgkin lymphoma. *J Exp Med* 2003;**198**:851–62.

146. Iqbal J, Greiner TC, Patel K, *et al.* Distinctive patterns of BCL6 molecular alterations and their functional consequences in different subgroups of diffuse large B-cell lymphoma. *Leukemia* 2007;**21**:2332–43.

147. Weniger MA, Gesk S, Ehrlich S, *et al.* Gains of REL in primary mediastinal B-cell lymphoma coincide with nuclear accumulation of REL protein. *Genes Chromosomes Cancer* 2007;**46**:406–15.

148. Abou-Elella AA, Weisenburger DD, Vose JM, *et al.* Primary mediastinal large B-cell lymphoma: a clinicopathologic study of 43 patients from the Nebraska Lymphoma Study Group. *J Clin Oncol* 1999;**17**:784–90.

149. Cazals-Hatem D, Lepage E, Brice P, *et al.* Primary mediastinal large B-cell lymphoma. A clinicopathologic study of 141 cases compared with 916 nonmediastinal large B-cell lymphomas, a GELA ("Groupe d'Etude des Lymphomes de l'Adulte") study. *Am J Surg Pathol* 1996;**20**:877–88.

150. Savage KJ, Al-Rajhi N, Voss N, *et al.* Favorable outcome of primary mediastinal large B-cell lymphoma in a single institution: the British Columbia experience. *Ann Oncol* 2006;**17**:123–30.

151. Lazzarino M, Orlandi E, Paulli M, *et al.* Treatment outcome and prognostic factors for primary mediastinal (thymic) B-cell lymphoma: a multicenter study of 106 patients. *J Clin Oncol* 1997;**15**:1646–53.

152. Nguyen LN, Ha CS, Hess M, *et al.* The outcome of combined-modality treatments for stage I and II primary large B-cell lymphoma of the mediastinum. *Int J Radiat Oncol Biol Phys* 2000;**47**:1281–5.

153. Zinzani PL, Martelli M, Magagnoli M, *et al.* Treatment and clinical management of primary mediastinal large B-cell lymphoma with sclerosis: MACOP-B regimen and mediastinal radiotherapy monitored by (67)Gallium scan in 50 patients. *Blood* 1999; **94**:3289–93.

154. Haioun C, Gaulard P, Roudot-Thoraval F, *et al.* Mediastinal diffuse large-cell lymphoma with sclerosis: a condition with a poor prognosis. *Am J Clin Oncol* 1989;**12**:425–9.

Chapter

17 Mantle cell lymphoma

Andre Goy

Introduction

Since its addition to the Revised European–American Lymphoma classification, in 1994, mantle cell lymphoma (MCL) has been recognized as carrying both features of indolent lymphoma (incurable) and a more aggressive course with short response to standard chemotherapy and common chemoresistance over time leading to very poor long-term prognosis. The disease presents typically in the elderly male population, with advanced-stage and constant extranodal involvement. There is still no consensus in the treatment of MCL; dose-intensification approaches with or without stem cell transplantation are commonly used in younger patients (<65 years), though unfortunately patients still relapse over time. In the relapsed setting, the field is marked by the development of a large number of novel agents, especially biologicals or targeted therapies. The integration of these new agents to frontline conventional therapies will hopefully improve patients' outcome. On the other hand, evidence is mounting on the complexity and heterogeneity of MCL, which might be best described as a spectrum of diseases (based essentially on the degree of proliferation). The landmark t(11;14)(q13;q32) translocation, responsible for cyclin D1 overexpression, is in virtually all cases accompanied by additional secondary genomic alterations (genomic instability), which vary among patients and strongly impact clinical course and prognosis. Though the overall survival seems to have improved (doubled) in the last three decades, a better stratification of patients is needed as well as an effort for participation in clinical trials. Given its relative rarity and impressive heterogeneity, MCL might represent an opportunity to design smaller "molecularly relevant" clinical trials in the future, a step towards more rational therapeutics.

Epidemiology

MCL represents 4–6% of all non-Hodgkin lymphoma (NHL) overall with an incidence of about 2500–3800 new cases a year in the USA and a similar number in Europe.[1,2] The apparent increasing incidence of MCL over the last two decades[3] likely reflects a higher awareness and improved diagnosis methods since its recognition in the early 1990s.[4,5] A recent Surveillance, Epidemiology, and End Results (SEER) database survey confirms that MCL is more common in men and in the white population than in African Americans;[3] however, geographic differences suggested in some reports are difficult to interpret given the difficulties in MCL diagnosis and often small series.[6,7]

An aging population does not seem to be the only factor to explain the increasing incidence of NHL (about 80%) over the last 30 years.[8,9] Chronic antigenic stimulation has been implicated in several subtypes of NHL,[10] though most MCL appear to derive from an antigen-naïve pregerminal center cell. Rare cases have been reported associated with hepatitis C including a case report with response to antiviral therapy[11] or more recently association with borrelia infection[12] of yet unclear significance. Familial clustering has been reported in patients with several subtypes of lymphoid malignancies, including rare cases with MCL, but the genetic basis for this familial clustering remains unknown.[13,14] MCL carries typically DNA repair defects with mutation/deletion of ATM gene (ataxia telangiectasia mutated), which was not found in those rare "familial" observations. On the other hand, some studies suggest an increased rate of additional malignancies in patients with MCL, especially urologic malignancies.[15]

Pathology/diagnosis

MCL is a distinct clinicopathologic subtype of B-cell lymphoma with the following classical immunophenotype of a mature B-cell expressing CD19, CD20, and CD22 with coexpression of CD5, CD43, and FMC7 as well as surface immunoglobulin (sIg) but negative for CD10, CD23, and BCL6. A subset of MCL lacking or with discordant (among different tissues) expression of CD23 or CD5 was recently reported,[16,17] though these cases carried the same morphological features and expression of cyclin-D1. Unique among all non-Hodgkin lymphomas, MCL expresses more commonly λ than κ light chain. A subset of MCL cases coexpress sIgG and IgM

Management of Hematologic Malignancies, ed. Susan M. O'Brien, Julie M. Vose, and Hagop M. Kantarjian. Published by Cambridge University Press.

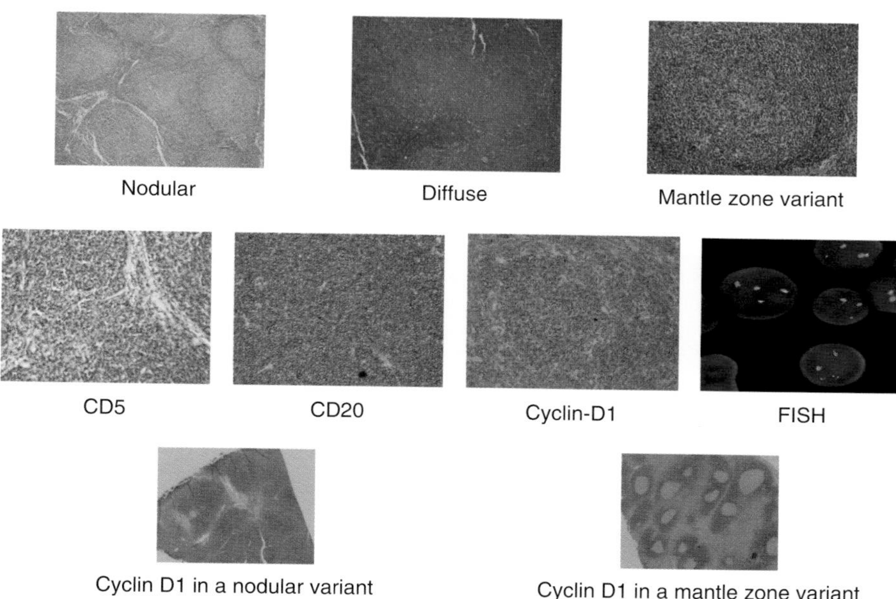

Figure 17.1 MCL diagnosis criteria. FISH: fluorescence *in situ* hybridization.

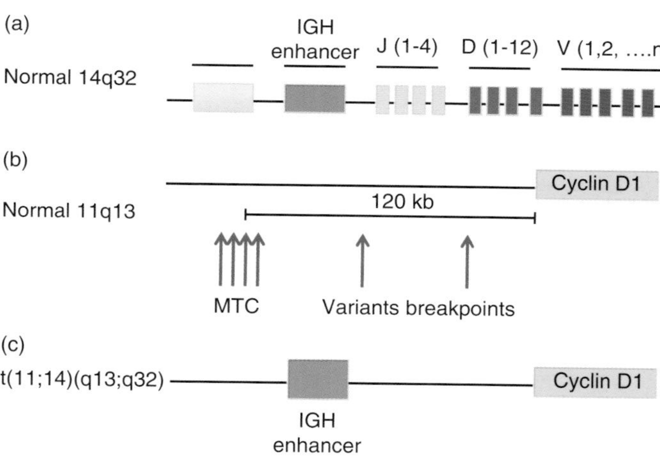

Figure 17.2 Translocation t(11;14)(q13;q32) in MCL.

suggesting they can still undergo isotype switching.[18] The morphology and IHC (immunohistochemistry) typical pattern of MCL is shown in Figure 17.1 while morphological variants will be discussed below.

Cyclin D1 is overexpressed in MCL as a result of the landmark t(11;14)(q13;q32) translocation (Figure 17.2).[19] The t(11;14) translocation breakpoint can occur over a wide DNA region[20] beyond the most common breakpoint called MTC (major translocation cluster).[21,22] Multiple alternative additional breakpoints have been reported[23,24] (with more distinct breakpoints than initially expected [E. Campo personal communication, Lymphoma Research Foundation (LRF) MCL consortium Dallas 2008]). Consequently, the breakpoint can be found more easily in the clinic by cytogenetics (70%)[25] or fluorescence *in situ* hybridization (FISH) (95%)[26,27] rather than by polymerase chain reaction (PCR) (40%);[28–31] as a result also minimal residual disease (MRD) studies will require the use of CDR3 clonotypic primers[32] when the t(11;14) is not amplifiable.

MCL, initially described as centrocytic lymphoma,[33] is recognized histologically with two main subtypes, nodular or diffuse pattern;[34] the mantle zone variant is much less common and considered more indolent. Cytological variants have also been reported: typical and blastoid (Figure 17.3). Typical cases show a proliferation of small to intermediately sized lymphoid cells with irregular nuclei and scarce cytoplasm. Blastic variants include a spectrum of intermediate to large cells with round or irregular nuclei and finely dispersed chromatin. These cases have a higher proliferative activity, are often associated with a mutation/deletion of p53, and show a more aggressive clinical course.[35,36] A pleiomorphic variant also reported (mix of small cells and blastoid-like cells) illustrates well the heterogeneity encompassed within the MCL entity, and the spectrum of diseases[37] now recognized through a better understanding of the molecular features of MCL.[38]

Pathogenesis

The pathogenesis of MCL can be summarized as a combination or resultant of three key features illustrated in Figure 17.4: cell cycle dysregulation (proliferation index), DNA damage response defect (more than 80–90% of MCL cases develop additional secondary genomic alterations over time) and dysregulation of survival pathways (chemoresistance).

Cell of origin

MCL cells are mature B lymphocytes which express markers of naïve B cells/sIgD and T-cell-associated antigen CD5. They seem derived from a small population of cells producing low-affinity polyreactive antibodies, which colonize the normal

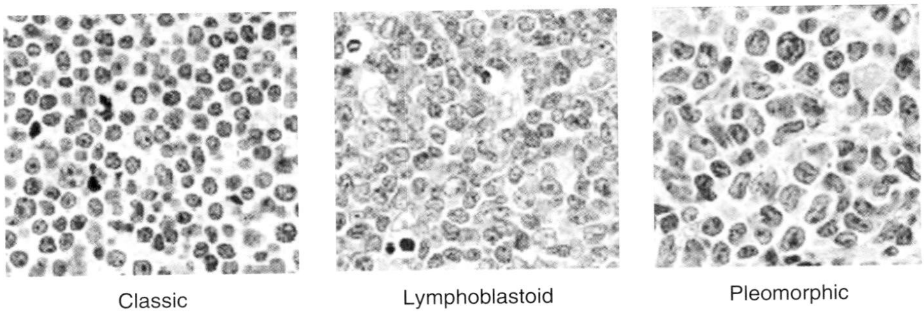

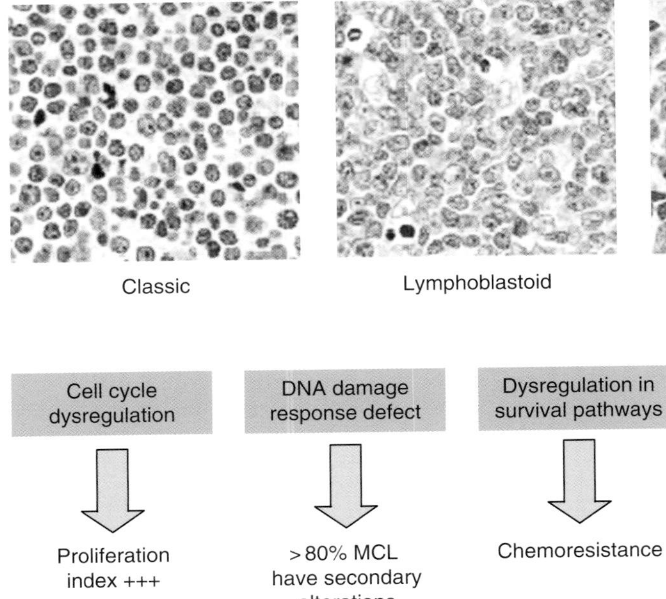

Figure 17.3 MCL: cytological variants.

Cell cycle dysregulation → Proliferation index +++
DNA damage response defect → >80% MCL have secondary alterations
Dysregulation in survival pathways → Chemoresistance

Figure 17.4 Summary of MCL pathogenesis.

mantle zone of follicles (rationale for term mantle cell lymphoma) and tend to recirculate. The initial oncogenic event, that is the t(11;14)(q13;q32) translocation, occurs in early B cells and fully develops into a selective oncogenic advantage when the cells attain the differentiation stage of a mature naïve pregerminal center B cell.[39]

Concordant with their pregerminal center B cells, most cases of MCL carry no or few somatic mutations in the V-gene sequences of Ig (VH) genes. About one-quarter of MCLs carry some degree of mutations but compared to chronic lymphocytic leukemia (CLL)[40,41] the incidence of somatic mutations overall is lower (15–40% depending on the series) and when mutated, the load or percentage of mutations is less than in CLL and does not correlate with Zap-70 expression. In addition, the presence of mutations does not seem to be predictive of outcome as in CLL[42–44] and in particular does not correlate with less intraclonal evolution over time contrary to CLL.

There is no correlation between the presence of somatic mutations and the histological or cytological subtype.[45,46] The ongoing mutations identified in a subset of MCL indicate that some tumors originate in cells that have undergone the influence of the mutational machinery of the follicular germinal center.[47,48] Similarly a restricted usage of individual V(H) genes has been reported in some MCL series with preferential usage of VH3–21, VH3–23, VH3–34, VH3–07, V(H)4–34, VH4–59, and V(H)5–51.[37,44,46,49,50] This occasional somatic mutations pattern[41] and non-random usage of IgV(H) segments suggest a possible involvement of antigen stimulation in the clonal expansion of a proportion of MCLs.[49–52] Though still debated the prognostic value of somatic mutations in MCL does not seem to be as prognostic as in CLL,[44,53] and likely again reflects more the heterogeneity of the disease itself.

Initial oncogenic event

MCL is genetically characterized by the t(11;14)(q13;q32) translocation that juxtaposes the proto-oncogene *CCND1* initially called *PRAD-1* to the Ig heavy chain gene at chromosome 14q32. The role of the *PRAD-1* (parathyroid adenomatosis 1) gene in human tumorigenesis was demonstrated by its initial cloning from the breakpoint region on chromosome band 11q13 of the inv(11)(p15q13) in a subset of parathyroid adenomas (hence its name) and also by the demonstration of its likely role as the elusive and long-sought BCL1 oncogene in t(11;14)-bearing B-cell lymphoma. The gene product of *PRAD-1*, identified to be cyclin D1, is then brought to the proximity of the IGH enhancer region (see Figure 17.2), and becomes constitutively overexpressed while it is usually *not* expressed in normal lymphocytes.[21,54] Very rare cases of variants of alternative rearrangement of *CCND1* locus with light chain Ig locus have been reported which also overexpress cyclin D1[55] while cases have also been reported with an amplification of the *CCND1/IGH* fusion gene in addition to the translocated allele.[56]

The t(11;14)(q13;q32) translocation is thought to be the primary event in the pathogenesis of the tumor, probably facilitating the deregulation of the cell cycle at the G1–S phase transition.[57,58] Analysis of the breakpoint regions in the two chromosomes has suggested that this translocation occurs in the bone marrow in an early B cell at the pre-B stage of differentiation[29,59] when the cell is initiating the Ig gene rearrangement with the recombination of the V(D)J segments.[60,61] Though the intrinsic mechanisms involved in the DNA double-strand breaks (DSBs) and repair involved during the recombination of the V(D)J segments of the Ig are not well known,[62,63] the topologic location of the Ig and *CCND1* loci in the nucleus has revealed a physical proximity of these two chromosomal regions in immature lymphoid B cells,[52,64,65] which may facilitate the occurrence of recurrent translocations and erroneous rearrangements.

Cyclin D1 overexpression

The t(11;14)(q13;q32) translocation deregulating cyclin D1 is present in virtually all cases of MCL.[66,67] Cyclin D1 is encoded by two major mRNA transcripts of approximately 4.5 and 1.5 kb, which differ in the length of the 3′ untranslated region

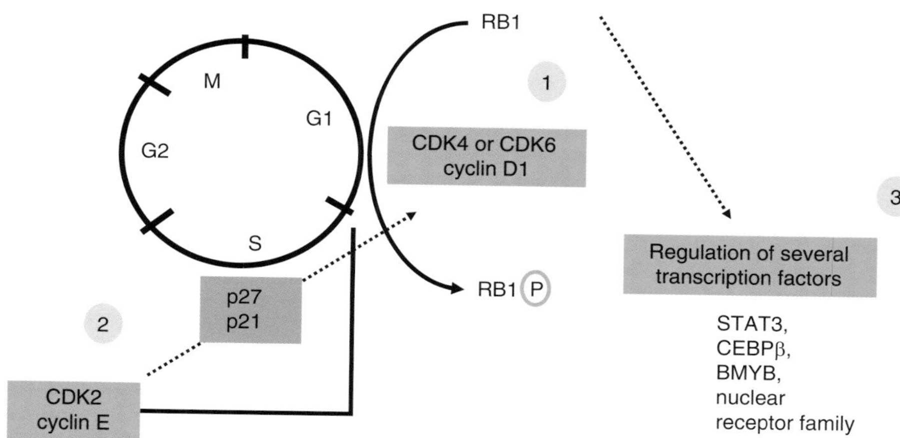

Figure 17.5 Threefold consequences of cyclin D1 overexpression.

(UTR) but contain the whole coding region that generates a polypeptide of 36 kDa (isoform a). About 4–10% of MCLs lack the 4.5-kb transcript and instead express aberrant mRNAs with shorter 3′ UTRs that lack destabilizing AUUUA sequences. The loss of these regulatory sequences is caused by additional rearrangements in the 3′ region of the gene with microdeletions[68] or point mutations.[69] These aberrant transcripts have an increased half-life and the tumors have very high levels of cyclin D1 expression, high proliferation, and a more aggressive clinical behavior.[70] Of note the deleted 3′ UTR contains important micro-RNA (miR) binding sites especially miR-16-1 (regulator of cyclin D1).[71] A less abundant noncanonical isoform (isoform b) that lacks the C-terminal region is generated by an alternative splicing that skips the whole exon 5. This exon contains important regulatory motifs including a residue that promotes the nuclear export of the cyclin when phosphorylated.[70] Although the cyclin D1b isoform seems to have a higher transforming capacity in cultured cells, its oncogenic mechanisms are not well understood and it is not clear how relevant this is *in vivo*.[72]

The consequences of cyclin D1 expression are threefold, as shown in Figure 17.5. Cyclin D1 binds to two cyclin-dependent kinases (CDK4 and CDK6),[73] the complexes lead to phosphorylation of retinoblastoma 1 (RB1), hence inactivation of the natural Rb1 suppressor effect on cell cycle progression.[74] The hyperphosphorylation of RB1 by cyclin D1-CDK4 and cyclin D1-CDK6 will lead to the release of E2F transcription factors and the subsequent progression of the cell into S phase. RB1 is hyperphosphorylated in MCL, particularly in highly proliferative variants; however, recently reported intragenic deletions[75] of RB1 leading to a total lack of protein expression in some cases of MCL would suggest that cyclin D1 may also have an additional role independently of RB1 in these tumors. The excess of CDK4-cyclin D1 complexes seem to trap/titer p27 away from cyclin E-CDK2[76] leading also to progression into G1–S transition. This is reinforced by a frequent overdegradation of p27 by the proteasome reported in MCL, which correlates with outcome.[77] In addition, at least in experimental models, cyclin D1 can participate in the regulation of several transcription factors and transcriptional coregulators including STAT3 (signal transducer and activator of transcription 3), CEBPβ (CCAAT/enhancer binding protein β), BMYB (MYB-related gene B), and members of the nuclear receptor superfamily, which can also participate in lymphomagenesis, though its relevance in vivo remains unclear.[78]

Cyclin D1-negative MCL

A subset of MCL does not express cyclin D1 and represents less than 5% of cases overall. These cases have now been confirmed to have similar morphology, presentation, gene profiling by microarray studies,[38] and outcome, suggesting they correspond to *the same disease*.[79] Of notice these cases have high expression of cyclin D2 or cyclin D3.[38,80] Although the mechanism deregulating these cyclins is not well understood, some cases carry a t(2;12)(p11;p13)/IGK-CCND2 translocation fusing cyclin D2 to the light Ig chain gene locus[81] or a t(6;14)(p21;q32)/IGH-CCND3.[82] These cyclin D1-negative MCL cases are uncommon but they highlight the relevance of the oncogenic dysregulation of the G1 phase of the cell cycle in the pathogenesis of MCL.

Secondary genomic alterations

Notwithstanding the key role of the t(11;14) translocation and cyclin D1 overexpression in the development of MCL, several observations suggest that these mechanisms may not be sufficient for transformation or maintenance of the MCL phenotype. The t(11;14)(q13;q32) translocation has been reported in a small (∼ 1%) number of normal individuals[83,84] consistent with the fact this is not a sufficient event in itself as confirmed by murine models.[85] The forced overexpression of cyclin D1 in transgenic mice through Eμ enhancer suggests that additional events are required from cyclin D1/MYC double transgenic mice[86] to secondary genomic alterations involving p53 or BCL2 as oncogeneic cooperative events or combination models with BCL2, nuclear factor-kappa B (NF-κB), MCL-1, MYC, or Blys.[87] More recent studies established the role of additional signaling pathways disrupted in MCL including

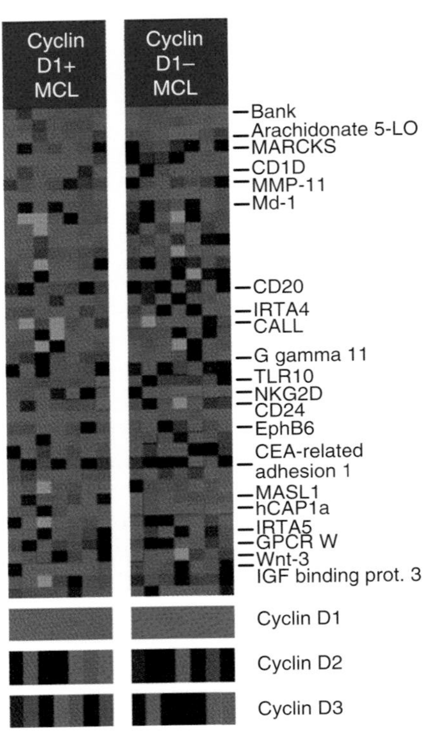

Figure 17.6 Cyclin D1-negative MCL have similar molecular profiles to cyclin D1-positive MCL.

phosphatidyl inositol 3-kinase (PI3K)/AKT,[88] transforming growth factor beta (TGFβ),[89] and WNT.[90] The WNT signaling pathway is a highly conserved system that has a key role in embryonic development and in the growth and maintenance of normal tissues. Recent data show that the WNT canonical pathway (especially WNT3 and WNT10) is constitutively activated in a subset of MCL where it appears to promote tumorigenesis.[90] An interesting murine model using interleukin 14 (IL-14) (often expressed in high grade NHL) and MYC double-transgenic model showed the development of 100% "blastoid variant looking" MCL.[91] In addition specific lentiviral shRNA-mediated knockdown of cyclin D1 in MCL cell lines has minimal effects on proliferation and survival of MCL cells and reveals a compensatory regulatory circuit with cyclin D2 overexpression.[92]

The collaboration of these multiple defects in MCL lymphomagenesis is well illustrated in the clinic with frequent accumulation of multiple secondary genetic defects in MCL in up to 80% of MCL cases[93,94] and often complex karyotypes (tetraploidies).[95–97] Among the most common genes/loci involved are *ATM* deletion/mutations (*ATM* encodes a phosphoprotein kinase that belongs to the PI3K-related superfamily and has a central role in the cellular response to DNA damage, such as DNA double-strand break [DSB] formation).[98] ATM mutations have been detected in 40–75% of MCLs and are usually associated with the loss of the other allele.[99,100] The high frequency of inactivating *ATM* mutations in MCL is intriguing because they are uncommon in other B-cell lymphomas. The fact that they occur throughout the spectrum of MCL cytological variants, including tumors with low and high proliferation rates, suggests this is an important and early event. Cases with ATM mutations tend to accumulate even more secondary genomic defects over time. Other commonly observed genomic defects seen in MCL are deletion of INK4/ARF at locus 9q21, mutations/deletions of p53, rare mutations of CHK-1 or CHK-2 (two kinases that act downstream of ATM and prevent cell cycle progression in response to ATM and ATR activation following DNA damage), and loss of p16 or p27.[101] As shown in Figure 17.7, these deletions/mutations will synergize with the underlying cell cycle dysregulation hallmark of MCL to promote further cell proliferation and chemoresistance.

The list of gains or losses seen in MCL is growing impressively[93,102,103] including a large number of loci affecting in many cases unknown genes as yet. These genomic imbalances in some reports correlate with clinical features, for example leukemic phase vs. nodal presentation[104,105] or outcome with a subset of emerging prognostic probes including 1p21, 9q21-q22, 9p21.3, and 17p13.1.

Dysregulation of survival pathways

The accumulation and correlation of genomic data including CHG-BAC profiling[24,104,106–108] and expression profiles[38,93,109] confirm the significance of genes related to DNA repair, chromosome stability, cell cycle, energy metabolism, and survival pathways, which might influence response to chemotherapy. Ongoing proteomic work confirms again the importance of cell cycle regulators, HSP, BCL-X, and MDM2[110] as well as MCL-1[111] or NF-κB and PI3K-mTOR, MAPK1, CK2, CK1, PKCζ, and PKCε as important players in the disrupted pathways of MCL.[112] Some of these pathways are summarized in Table 17.1.

In summary MCL lymphomagenesis is a complex integration of cell cycle dysruption, secondary genomic imbalances (more than in other NHL), and dysregulation of survival pathways. The actual sequence of events remains elusive but could be summarized as follows.

The early event of t(11;14) leads to overexpression of cyclin D1 in B cells in the mantle zone followed by mutations/inactivation/deletion of ATM/CHK-2, which leads to actual MCL cells with evolving more complex karyotypes. Further gains or losses (more losses in MCL) lead to worsening of the proliferation signature and towards blastoid variants. This occurs as a *spectrum of disease* as confirmed by molecular profiling of clinical samples.[38] This also is consistent with the challenges encountered in the management of MCL patients who often develop chemoresistance over time and carry a poor outcome.

MCL clinical presentation

Patients with MCL are typically older adults (median age early to mid 60s) with a male predominance (ratio 3/1) and usually advanced stage (more than 75%), though B symptoms are seen in only one-third to one-half of patients.[119,120] Patients present with lymphadenopathy, splenomegaly, and a variable degree of

Table 17.1. Some of the genes involved in dysregulation of survival pathways in MCL

Pathway	Pattern in MCL	Comment
Apoptosis	Amplification of BCL2[113]	Chemoresistance
	BIM-1 deletion[114]	Proapoptotic BH3 family member Homozygous deletion in MCL cell lines Relevance in vivo unclear
NF-κB	Constitutive activation both in cell lines and primary samples with overexpression of downstream targets such as FADD-like apoptosis regulator[115]	Chemoresistance
PI3K/AKT	Akt was phosphorylated in aggressive blastoid MCL due to loss of PTEN (not mutation of PI3K)[88]	Especially in blastoid variants 12/12 patients and 4/4 MCL cell lines 5/16 typical MCL
INK4-RB1 and ARF-MDM2-p53	Control of cell senescence[105,116,117]	Correlates with highly proliferative MCL
HSP (HSP90)	Stress response[110,118]	Chemoresistance, proteasome resistance
Mitochondrial signaling	Energy metabolism[109,112]	Apoptosis

Note: FADD: Fas-associated protein with death domain; PTEN: phosphatase and tensin homolog.

leukemic phase (virtually all patients have detectable circulating MCL cells by flow cytometry);[25,121,122] but almost constant extranodal involvement, which includes bone marrow (BM), liver, and characteristically gastrointestinal (GI) involvement. The GI tract involvement can vary from extensive and symptomatic polyposis coli[123,124] to just random biopsies positive in more than 90% of patients at baseline.[125,126] Consequently baseline endoscopies are not necessary but would be recommended as part of restaging studies to confirm response although they are not part of the official restaging guidelines. Rare cases with orbits,[127] testis,[128] or skin involvement[129,130] in MCL have also been reported. On rare occasions patients will present with localized disease, but typically after extensive workup other sites of disease will be identified including peripheral blood (flow cytometry) or GI tract; consistent with the fact that this is a systemic disease and should be approached and treated likewise.

Though patients have extensive extranodal disease and virtually all have some degree of leukemic phase, current clinical evaluations do not routinely include assessment of the cerebrospinal fluid (CSF) for lymphomatous infiltration at presentation.[131] More recent reports suggest that CSF involvement might be underestimated[132,133] and might become more common as patients' survival has clearly improved over the last two decades. In a retrospective analysis of 82 patients by Ferrer *et al.*,[133] 11 patients were found with central nervous system (CNS) involvement by MCL (one at baseline asymptomatic as routine staging maneuver, the other 10 with neurological signs prompting evaluation). The authors report an actuarial 5-year risk of CNS involvement of 26% while another series of 108 patients reviewed suggested around 9%.[132]

Prognostic factors in MCL

Conventional prognostic factors used in NHL do not apply as easily in MCL, since most patients present with advanced stage and frequent multiple extranodal involvement.[134] The FLIPI

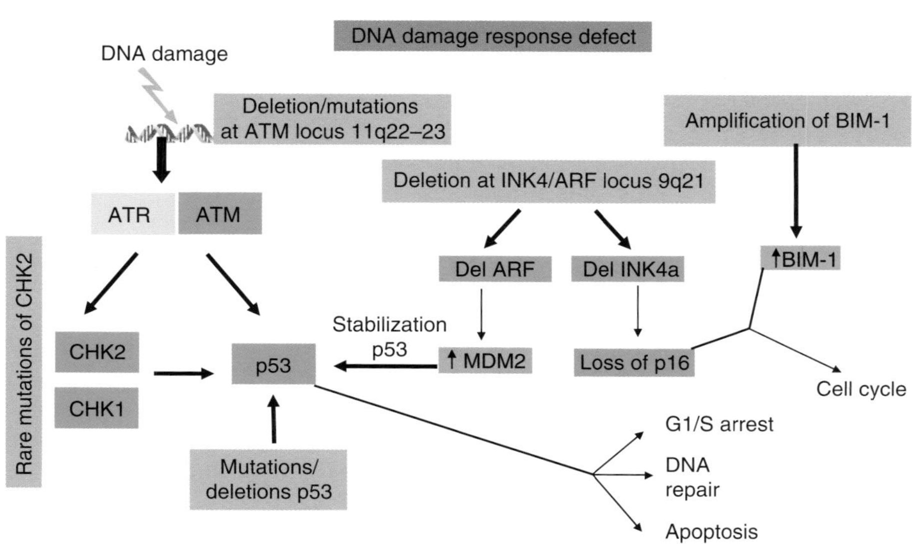

Figure 17.7 Accumulation of (secondary) genomic defects in MCL.

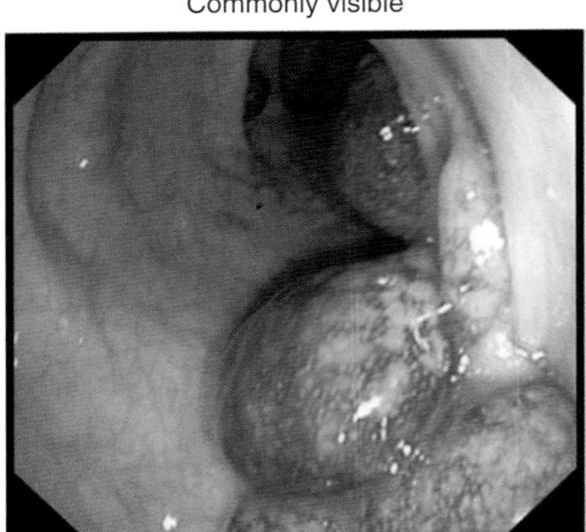
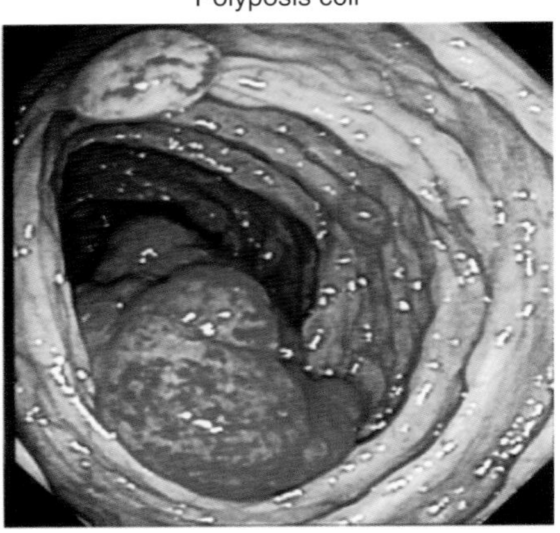
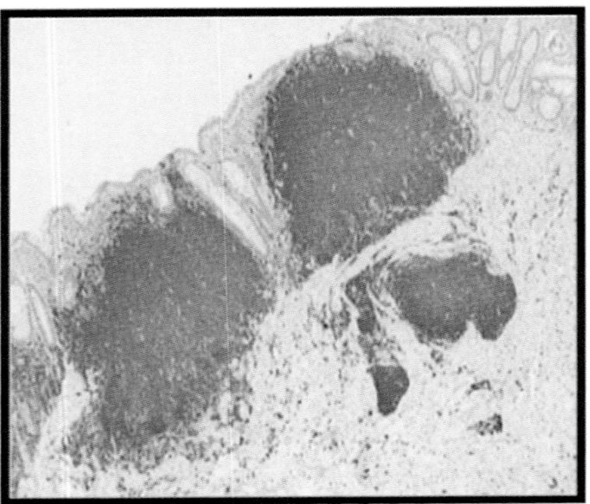

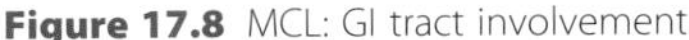
Figure 17.8 MCL: GI tract involvement.

(Follicular Lymphoma International Prognostic Index) might be more useful than the IPI,[135] which separates only the low risk patients from the rest as shown in Figure 17.9. A modified prognostic index called MIPI (white blood cell [WBC] count, age, lactate dehydrogenase [LDH], Eastern Cooperative Oncology Group performance status [ECOGPS]) was recently reported,[136] which includes leukemic phase [122,137] besides other clinical parameters used in the IPI.

Other prognostic factors include the proliferation index (Ki-67),[138] blastoid variant,[35,139] cytogenetic abnormalities as detailed above, and beta-2 microglobulin.[140] Molecular studies with microarrays profiling showed that the proliferation gene expression signature in MCL is a quantitative integrator of oncogenic events that predicts survival in MCL (see Figure 17.10). This signature allowed the separation of patients into four groups with a median overall survival (OS) of 0.7 years to more than 7.0 years in 90 patients treated essentially with an anthracycline-based chemotherapy regimen (before rituximab).[38] This proliferation signature can be reproduced to a certain degree by the proliferation index defined by Ki-67 (MIB-1) by immunohistochemistry (Figure 17.11). The prognostic relevance of Ki-67 was confirmed in the era of R-CHOP (rituximab plus cyclophosphamide, doxorubicin, vincristine, prednisone)-based chemotherapy.[141] Additional markers relevant to cell proliferation or mitotic index evaluable by IHC have been reported also in the post-rituximab era and with the use of high-dose therapy including PIM-1[142] and survivin.[143] The limitations for quantification and reproducibility inherent to IHC apply to Ki-67. Besides the difficulty for quantification, Ki-67 is a *continuous* variable with different cutoff depending on the series. In a series of 134 cases Katzenberger *et al.* divided patients into proliferation groups with Ki-67 indices of 20% or less (n = 62), 21–40% (n = 32), 41–60% (n = 25), and more than 60% (n = 15), showing that 70% of patients had less than 40% and the rest were spread with a small number of cases with high proliferation index.[138] In addition Ki-67 can also vary depending on the area of the slide quite significantly (slide scanning),[144] which obviously can be of concern when using tissue microarrays.

MCL shows a clear distinct profile from the other subtypes of NHL: small lymphocytic lymphoma (SLL), GC (germinal center)- and ABC-DLBCL (activated B-cell-like diffuse large B-cell lymphoma). Also, within the MCL group contrary to DLBCL there are no distinct profiles but a spectrum of diseases based on the proliferation signature, which predicts outcome with four groups from 0.7 year median OS to more than 7 years median OS.[38]

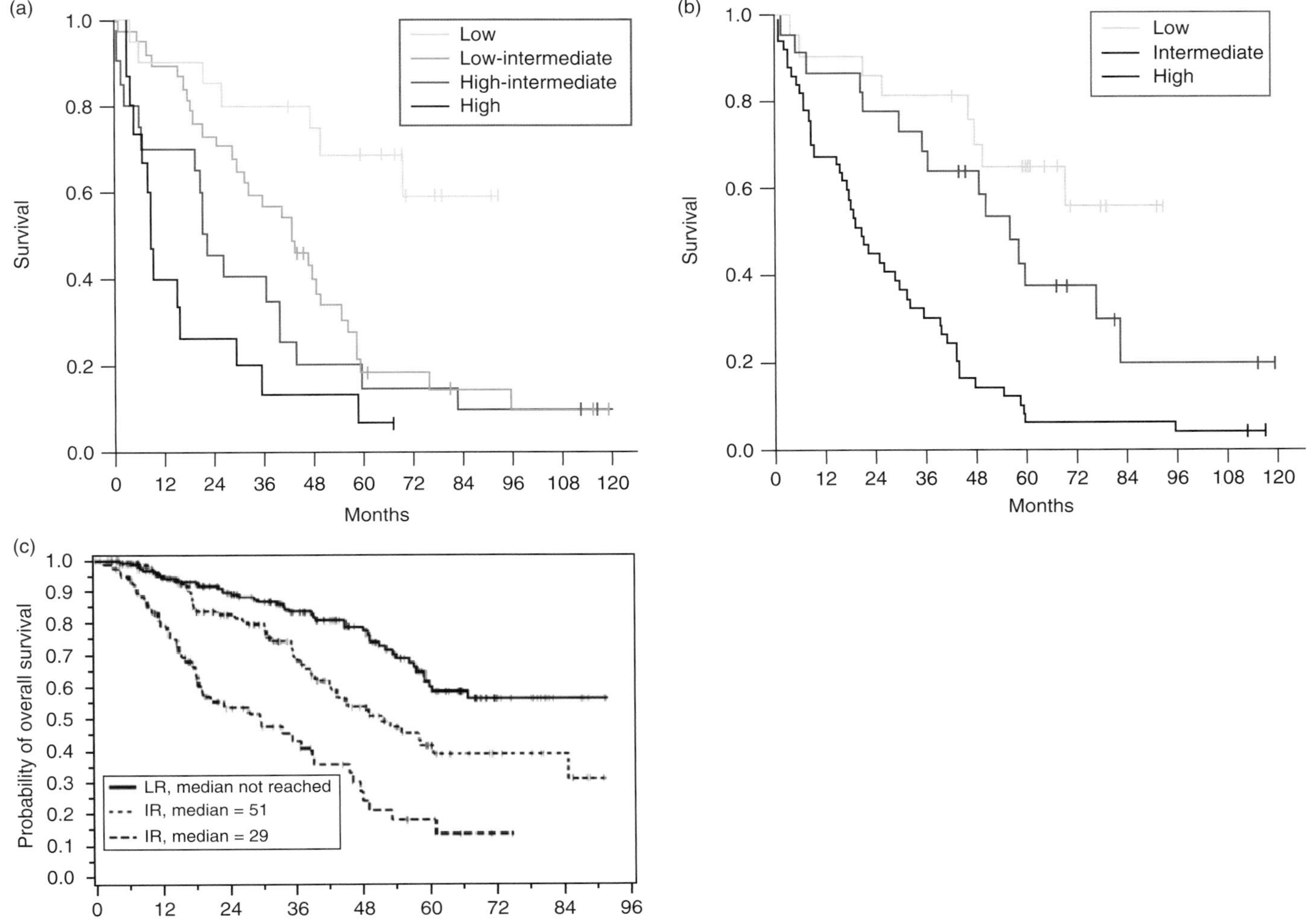

Figure 17.9 Lymphoma prognostic index applied to MCL: (A) IPI, (B) FLIPI, and (C) new index MIPI.

In the MIPI index described above, the addition of Ki-67 remained independently significant from the MIPI clinical score (regression coefficient 0.02142, $p < 0.001$) and inclusion of Ki-67 did not substantially change the regression coefficient of the MIPI score (0.9554, $p < 0.001$).

An elegant model using real-time PCR was recently reported looking at the expression of 33 genes with potential prognostic and pathogenetic impact in MCL. This gene set was analyzed using quantitative reverse-transcription PCR (qRT-PCR) in a low-density array format in frozen tumor samples from 73 patients with MCL.[145] Based on the results, a prognostic model was defined as an optimized survival predictor composed of five genes: RAN, MYC, TNFRSF10B, POLE2, and SLC29A2. Furthermore, this model was validated for application in formalin-fixed paraffin-embedded tissue samples and appeared superior to the immunohistochemical marker Ki-67 itself by IHC.

Other prognostic factors include single-nucleotide polymorphisms (SNPs) (which affect chemotherapy drugs metabolism as well as detoxification and will be discussed later) and miR. As mentioned briefly above, miR are a new class of abundant small RNAs that play important regulatory roles at the posttranscriptional level by binding to the 3′ UTR of mRNAs blocking either their translation or initiating their degradation; for example recent data showed that miR-16-1 regulates CCND1 expression.[71] Contrary to CLL, the presence of somatic mutations in MCL, as mentioned above, is not as common and does not correlate with ZAP-70 expression either, which is found only in a minority of MCL (10–15%).[146,147] The prognostic value of somatic mutations, well established (mutated vs. unmutated) in CLL, is still debated in MCL. It appears that the mutation status involves only a subset of MCL, illustrating again the heterogeneity of the disease, and has no correlation with clinical presentation or outcome.[53] Regarding the VH usage bias also there are no firm conclusions though there was no VH3–23 rearrangement in long-term survivors with MCL in the largest series.[49] The role of MRD in MCL has also been associated with outcome in some reports whereas other studies suggested that molecular complete remission (CR) in MCL after high-dose therapy

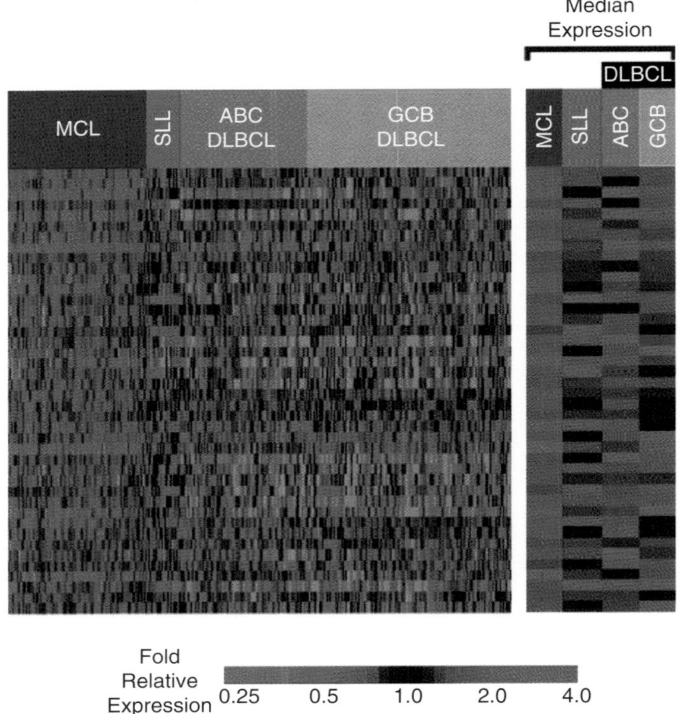

Figure 17.10 The proliferation gene expression signature is a quantitative integrator of oncogenic events that predicts survival in mantle cell lymphoma.

(HDT) and autologous stem cell transplantation (ASCT) did not hold as well as in follicular lymphoma.[148] In a recent report[149] MRD and MIPI appeared as the most significant predictive factors in large ongoing European randomized trials with HDT-ASCT in patients < 65 years (using two different induction regimens to look at the impact of high-dose cytarabine) and R-CHOP vs. FCR (fludarabine, cyclophosphamide, rituximab) in > 65-year-old patients. Table 17.2 summarizes classical clinical and new prognostic markers in MCL.

MCL treatment

There is no consensus therapy in MCL and, despite response rates to many regimens in the 50–70% range, patients still progress after chemotherapy with a median survival time of approximately 3–5 years. However, the treatment paradigm of MCL is evolving, from dose intensification of conventional chemotherapy to a growing number of novel biologic agents, which by targeting specific pathways may represent a step towards more rational therapeutics. Since there is no clear standard approach for treating MCL patients, it is critical that they be enrolled in clinical trials to help build guidelines that will likely include novel therapies early on in the treatment of the disease.

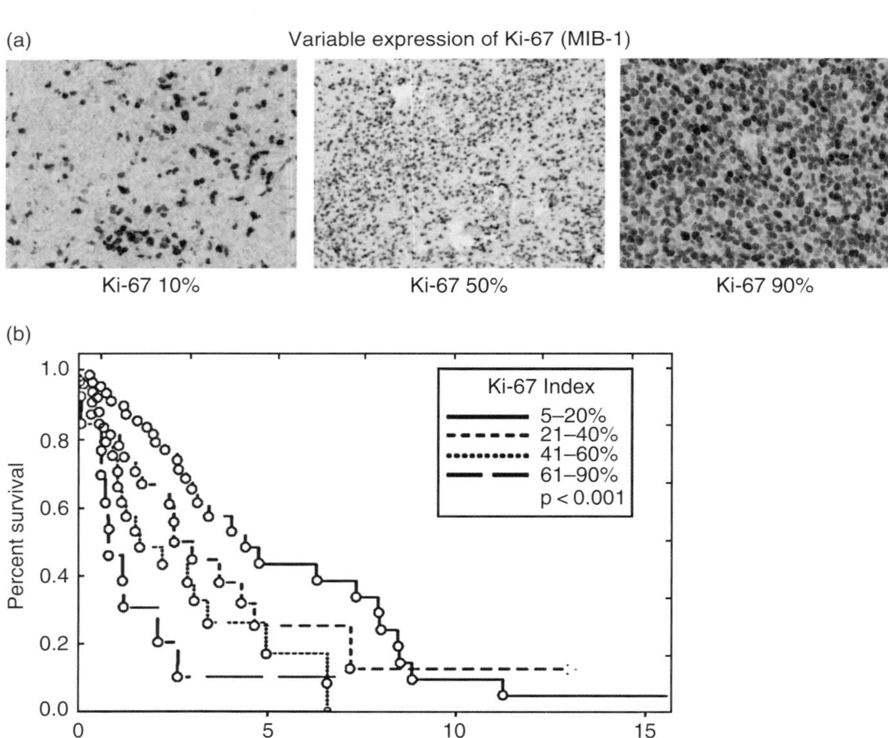

Figure 17.11 (a) Variable expression of Ki-67 (MIB-1) in MCL patients; (b) Impact of Ki-67 (MIB-1) expression on outcome.

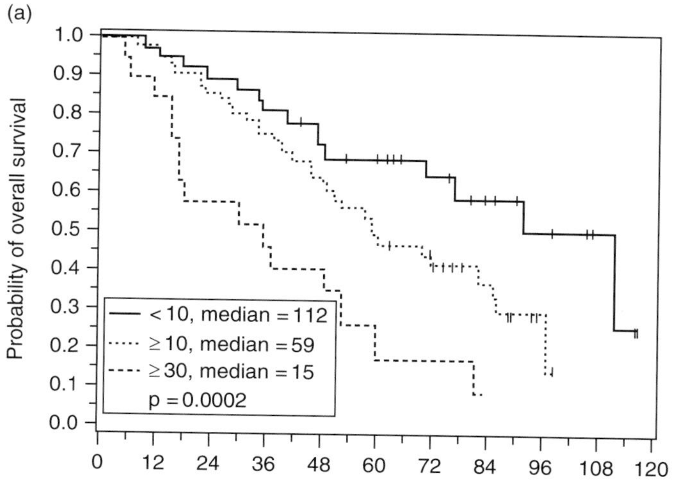

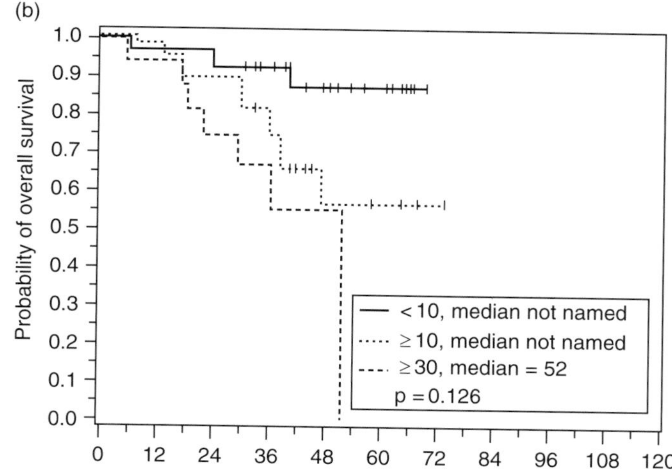

Figure 17.12 Impact of Ki-67 (MIB-1) on overall survival: (a) pre-rituximab and (b) post-rituximab era. Kaplan–Meier plot for OS of patients treated with CHOP (a) and R-CHOP (b) stratified in three groups according to the Ki-67 index of less than 10% (< 10), 10% to less than 30% (≥ 10), and 30% or more (≥ 30) Ki-67-positive cells.

Table 17.2. Prognostic factors in MCL (classical and "new" evolving parameters)

Parameter	Comment
Leukemic phase	Detectable by flow in most patients, value as prognostic cutoff unclear
New mantle IPI (MIPI)[a] (variant of IPI/FLIPI)	WBC High, Age, LDH, ECOG PS
β_2-microglobulin	Might be superior to LDH in MCL
p53 status	More common in blastoid variants
MIB-1/Ki-67 overexpression	Proliferation signature (10%, 10% to 30%, and > 30%) remains valid after R-CHOP ++
Cyclin D1 transcripts	3′ UTR deletions/mutations have > half-life and higher level of cyclin D1
MRD	Issue with breakpoint/FISH
Additional cytogenetic abnormalities	Comparative genomic hybridization showed value of gains: 3q, 2q; loss: 9q, 13q, 17p
New model qRT-PCR (5 genes)	Might be > Ki-67
Other	Somatic mutations SNPs
PET scan	Still under evaluation

Note: [a]Calculation of MIPI is as per formula: MIPI score = [0.03535 × age (years)] × age (years)] + 0.6978 (if ECOG PS > 1) + [1.367 × log10 (LDH/ULN)] + [0.9393 × log10 (WBC count)]

Conventional chemotherapy

Standard CHOP

CHOP-based chemotherapy remains by default often the standard of care in MCL. Given that rituximab itself had shown some activity in relapsed MCL,[150] it was added to CHOP where it showed a higher CR rate but the median progression-free survival (PFS) remained in the same range of 16–18 months.[151] In addition, in a series of 40 newly diagnosed MCL treated with R-CHOP × 6, patients who achieved a molecular remission (MRD measured in peripheral blood and/or BM) had similar PFS to patients without molecular CR (16.5 vs. 18.8 months, p = 0.51).[151] A German randomized study with 122 previously untreated patients with advanced-stage MCL compared six cycles of CHOP (n = 60) vs. R-CHOP (n = 62). Patients up to 65 years of age achieving a partial remission (PR) or CR underwent a second randomization to either myeloablative radiochemotherapy (cyclophosphamide/total body radiation [Cy/TBI]) followed by ASCT or interferon alpha (IFN-α) maintenance (6×10^6 U subcutaneously three times weekly continued until progression or until the occurrence of intolerable side effects). As expected, there was no difference between the two arms in terms of toxicity during induction therapy and R-CHOP was significantly superior to CHOP in terms of overall response rate (ORR) (94% vs. 75%; p = 0.0054), CR rate (34% vs. 7%; p = 0.00024), and time to treatment failure (TTF; median, 21 vs. 14 months; p = 0.0131) but there was no difference in PFS[152] as shown below.

EPOCH regimen

The National Cancer Institute (NCI) group has piloted the principle of dose-adjusted chemotherapy using the EPOCH regimen (doxorubicin 15 mg/m^2 as a continuous IV infusion on days 2–4, etoposide 65 mg/m^2 as a continuous IV infusion on days 2–4, vincristine 0.5 mg as a continuous IV infusion on days 2–4, cyclophosphamide 750 mg/m^2 IV on day 5, and prednisone 60 mg/m^2 orally on days 1–14). Pharmacokinetic analyses (etoposide and doxorubicin) showed significant interpatient variations in steady-state plasma concentrations and suggested the need for individual-patient dose adjustment.[153] This was translated into dose-adjustments based on nadir post

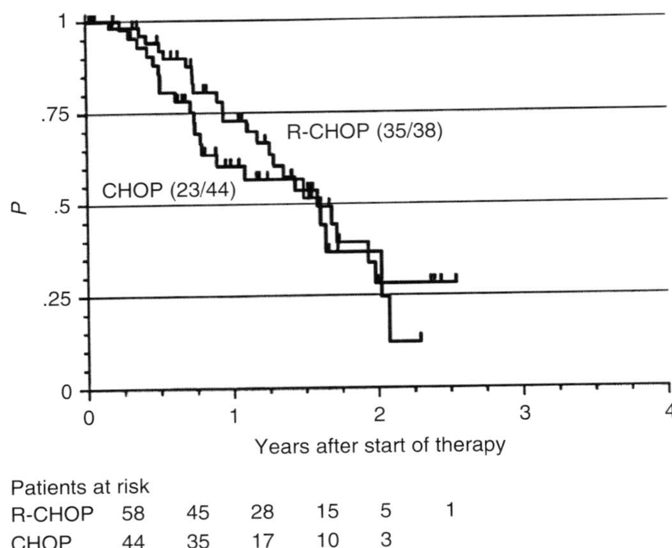

Figure 17.13 PFS with CHOP vs. R-CHOP induction in MCL.

chemotherapy (reach an absolute neutrophil count [ANC] ≤ 0.5) as surrogate marker or drug exposure in vivo. This regimen combined with rituximab was tested as induction therapy in MCL followed by an anti-idiotype vaccine in a series of 26 MCL patients with unfortunately a reported median PFS still less than 2 years. Though both B- and T-cell tumor-specific immune responses could be detected (delayed for humoral response until B-cell recovery post rituximab), a detectable immune response had no impact on the outcome.[154] In addition, in that study the proliferation signature was not found prognostic, contrary to the experience previously seen using the same infusional therapy in DLBCL.[153]

HyperCVAD

Initially developed at the MD Anderson Cancer Center (MDACC) for acute lymphocytic leukemia,[155] this regimen was used in MCL as an induction therapy (four cycles) prior to consolidation with HDT followed by ASCT.[156] A subset of patients who refused or could not proceed to HDT and ASCT were continued from four to eight cycles and did reasonably well, providing a rationale for using the regimen in MCL by itself. HyperCVAD (hyperfractionated cyclophosphamide, vincristine, doxorubicin, and dexamethasone alternating with high-dose methotrexate [MTX] and cytarabine [cytosine arabinoside; Ara-C]) was later on combined with rituximab as induction therapy in a series of 99 patients, median age 60 (range: 41–80), all stage IV disease, 89% diffuse histology, 11% nodular and 14% blastoid variants; a quarter of patients had high LDH, and 55% high β2-microglobulin.[140] Patients received the classical rituximab-HyperCVAD (R-HyperCVAD) with rituximab on day 1 of each cycle (rituximab was delayed in patients with high WBC count at diagnosis); cycles were repeated every 21 days up to six or eight cycles. For patients > 60 years of age, the cytarabine dose was reduced

Table 17.3. Hematologic toxicity of R-HyperCVAD

Grade 3–4 toxicity	Number (%)
Neutropenic fever*	80 (13%)
R-HyperCVAD	20 (7%)
R-MTX/Ara-C	60 (20%)
Infection*	35 (6%)

Table 17.4. Age-related responses to HyperCVAD

Age group	No.	CR (%)	PR (%)
All ages	97	87	11
≤ 65 years	66	88	9
> 65 years	31	84	16

from 3 g/m^2 to 1 g/m^2 due to concerns of CNS toxicity. Patients were restaged every two cycles (i.e., after cycle 1A and 1B) as previously described, with restaging including both upper and lower endoscopies in all patients.[125] If patients had a CR after two cycles, they completed six cycles, if not eight cycles. Patients did not receive HDT-ASCT unless they had not achieved a CR after six cycles. Toxicity with R-HyperCVAD was as expected mainly hematologic and is summarized in Table 17.3.

The toxicity was significantly higher after R-methotrexate-cytarabine ($p = 0.00001$) compared to the part A of R-HyperCVAD but there was no difference in numbers of infections or fever neutropenia for patients ≤ 65 years and patients > 65 years. Five patients in that series died: sepsis (three), hemorrhage (one), unknown (one), and five patients developed secondary myelodysplastic syndrome (MDS) (in CR).

The ORR was 97% including 87% CR/complete remission unconfirmed (CRu) and the 3-year failure-free survival (FFS) was 64% and OS 82% with a median follow-up time of 40 months. These results were superior in patients ≤ 65 years old, where the 3-year FFS was 73%. Patients more than 65 years seemed to benefit from R-HyperCVAD only if they had a normal β2-microglobulin at baseline, otherwise their median PFS was just around 2 years. A recent update confirmed that with a 9.8-year follow-up after R-HyperCVAD regimen, the FFS was still 52% for patients < 65 years.[157]

Several prognostic factors emerged for FFS after R-HyperCVAD including age (> 65), LDH (> normal), beta-2 (≥ 3 mg/L), and IPI (but not MIPI),[158] while all of these factors were prognostic for OS. Patients > 65 years with low beta-2 still did significantly better than high beta-2 (> 3 mg) for both FFS and OS ($p = 0.001$). Cytological (blastoid, nodular, diffuse) subtypes had no impact, and in the blastoid variant group (small number of patients though) there was no relapse after 2 years.[159] A subset of patients with available material for Ki-67 staining showed no impact of proliferation index measured by IHC of MIB-1.[157]

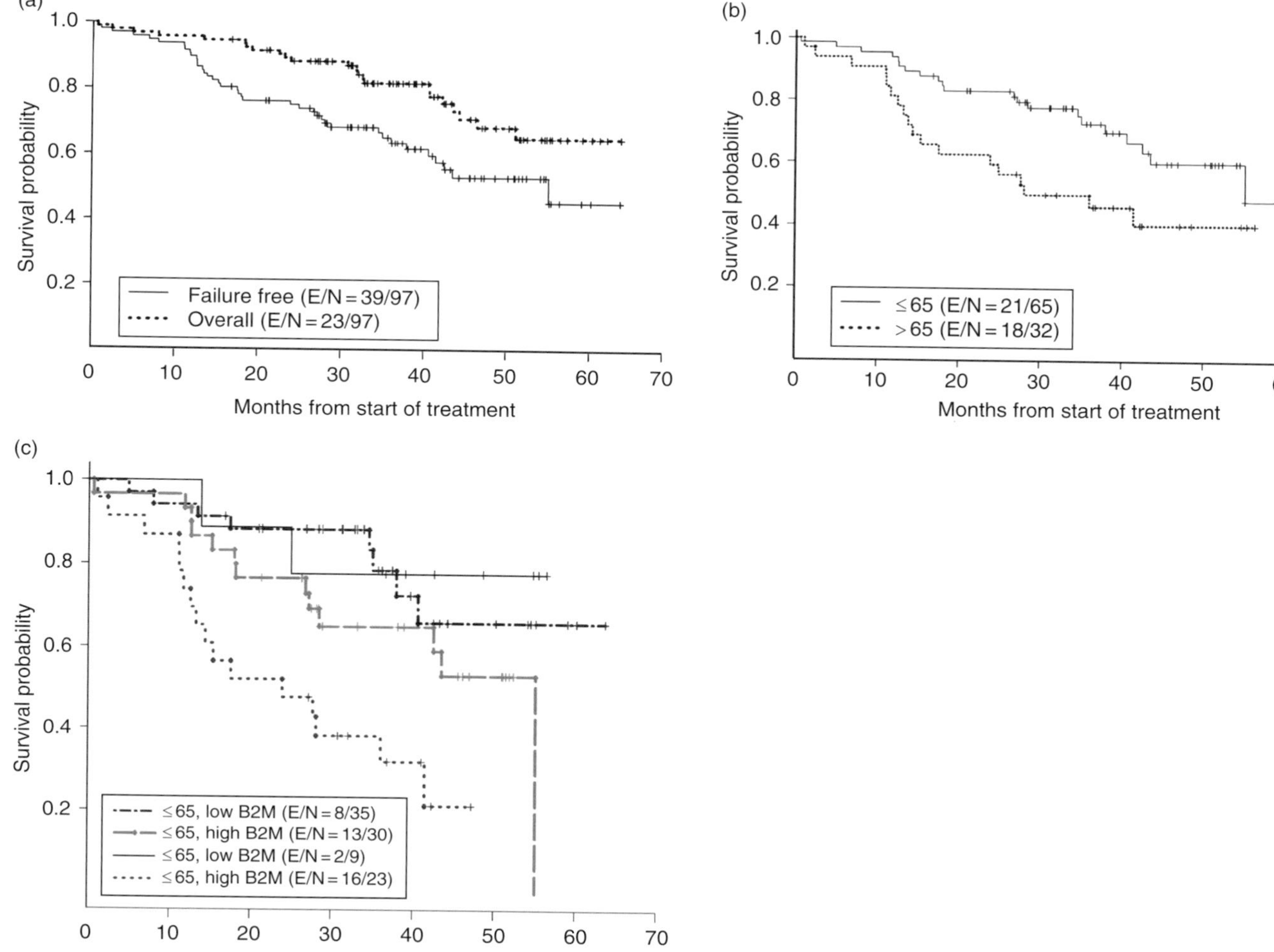

Figure 17.14 Outcome with R-HyperCVAD in MCL frontline (MDACC) in 97 patients with newly diagnosed aggressive mantle cell lymphoma treated with rituximab plus fractionated cyclophosphamide, vincristine, doxorubicin, and dexamethasone (HyperCVAD) alternating with rituximab plus methotrexate-cytarabine. (a) FFS and OS with a median follow-up of 40 months; the 3-year FFS and OS were 64% and 82%, respectively. E: events; N: total patients. (b) FFS by age subgroup with a median follow-up of 40 months; the 3-year FFS rate for patients more than 65 years old is 50% compared with 73% for patients 65 years or younger ($p = 0.02$). E: events; N: total patients. (c) FFS by age subgroup according to pretreatment serum ß2-microglobulin levels. The levels were of prognostic importance only for patients more than 65 years old ($p = 0.02$). E: events; N: total patients; B2M: ß2-microglobulin.

An attempt to expand on the concept of R-HyperCVAD was reported by the Southwest Oncology Group (SWOG)[160] in a series of 49 patients, median age 57, with an unusual proportion of mantle zone variant subtypes (more than half the patients). The study showed a 2-year PFS of 63% and 42% of patients stopped because of toxicity. The overall toxicity of R-HyperCVAD certainly is a challenge depending on the setting, especially in the elderly. In the > 65 years group in the MDACC experience, the median PFS was only 26 months, illustrating the need for new strategies in that patient population. This was the rationale for a modified R-HyperCVAD (no methotrexate or Ara-C, no vincristine on day 11), with cycles given every 28 days for four to six cycles total. The regimen included scheduled rituximab maintenance[161] in responding patients (PR and CR) with four weekly doses every 6 months for 2 years. Of 22 patients, the ORR was 77% and the CR rate 64%. With a median follow-up time of 37 months in surviving patients, the median PFS was 37 months. The achievement of a molecular remission did not correlate with improved outcome as seen with R-CHOP above. The major toxicity was as expected myelosuppression. When compared to historical controls, both the original and modified R-HyperCVAD regimens provided a much higher CR rate than R-CHOP (87%, 64%, 34–48%, respectively) and considerably longer median PFS (> 60 months, 37 months, 16–20 months).[162]

Nucleoside analogs

Fludarabine single-agent activity in MCL showed an ORR of 30–40%[163] compared with 63% when in combination with cyclophosphamide.[164,165] Multiple other combination studies including a regimen with fludarabine, cyclophosphamide, and mitoxantrone with or without rituximab showed a clear benefit for the rituximab-arm combination.[166] A randomized study comparing R-CHOP and FCR is ongoing in Europe in patients >65 years. Other purine analogs include cladribine (2-chlorodeoxyadenosine [2-CDA]) which also showed activity as a single agent[167] or combined with mitoxantrone[168] or with rituximab (RC),[169] whereas clofarabine showed some activity in preliminary studies and is currently being evaluated in larger trials[170] in combination trials, as well as an oral form of clofarabine in relapsed MCL.

Novel cytotoxics

Multiple new or "revisited" cytotoxics are being developed in NHL including in MCL with bendamustin, previously known as SDX-105 (developed in the German Democratic Republic as Cytostasan since the 1970s). This "old-new" drug has generated great interest as it contains both a nitrogen mustard group and a benzimidazole ring, which may act as a purine analog. Bendamustin has been shown to have single-agent activity in MCL and is now being integrated in other regimens including in combination with rituximab (B-R) (16 patients: ORR $= 75\%$, CR $= 50\%$)[171] or with mitoxantrone[172] or fludarabine, all ongoing. A study comparing as frontline therapy B-R vs. R-CHOP in indolent NHL and MCL showed similar response rates and no difference in outcome, including in a subset of MCL cases with an ORR of 88%/96% and CR 42%/41%.[173] Pixantrone (BBR2778) is a novel anthracenedione analog (derivative of mitoxantrone) with preclinical evidence of reduced cardiotoxicity and activity as single agent in NHL in phase II studies including in MCL. It is currently being tested as part of FPR or R-CPOP vs. R-CHOP (RAPID trial) as well as single agent against investigators' choice among predefined options in relapse/refractory NHL. Among other agents being tested are the new microtubule inhibitors with the epothilone derivatives from ixabepilone with preliminary evidence of activity in MCL[174] to CY-2121 (SB-743921) in earlier development. On the other hand some of the revisited approaches looked at low-dose oral agents administered (PEPC [prednisone, etoposide, procarbazine, and cyclophosphamide] regimen) in combination for continuous, prolonged periods with minimal drug-free intervals (so called metronomic therapy) as a potential option in the relapsed setting in elderly patients.[175]

High-dose therapy (HDT) and stem cell transplantation (SCT)

Given the poor results seen with conventional standard chemotherapy regimens, HDT has been studied extensively in MCL initially in the relapse setting but also in frontline as consolidation.[176,177] A large randomized trial from the European mantle cell lymphoma network compared in the frontline setting CHOP-IFN-α vs. CHOP-HDT-ASCT. Responding patients to CHOP-like chemotherapy (four to six cycles) were randomized to IFN-α maintenance vs. HDT-ACST consolidation using Cy/TBI as conditioning regimen. The HDT arm showed a significantly longer PFS of 39 months compared with 17 months for patients in the IFN-α arm ($p = 0.0108$) (see Figure 17.15).[178] A recent update with more mature data confirmed a longer PFS and TTTF but no difference in OS (5.4 years vs. 7.5 years; $p = 0.075$).[179] Out of 232 patients enrolled, 144 were evaluable as per the protocol (75 ASCT arm; 69 IFN-α arm) illustrating the potential patient selection bias in such trials as well. Similar results were reported from the GITMO multicenter prospective trial with a high-dose sequential therapy (R-HDS) in follicular and mantle cell lymphoma. HDS ensured superior disease control and molecular outcome to R-CHOP, but no OS improvement. Other series have shown similar results with prolonged PFS[180] but still questions around durable long-term remissions.[181]

Overall the results of studies using consolidation with HDT and ACST have been mixed and though most studies show a benefit over standard-dose therapy in terms of CR rate and PFS, there is no confirmed indication that the procedure is curative. In addition it is difficult to design and conduct prospective randomized trials in this "non-consensus disease" and relatively rare disease. Some of the issues to be addressed in future studies are listed below.[180,182]

What is the optimal induction regimen in MCL?

Preliminary results suggest that the role of high-dose Ara-C is important as part of the induction/consolidation therapy in MCL[183] serving as a basis for an ongoing large randomized study in Europe, which is more than halfway completed.

The timing for stem cell transplantation:

Several reports suggest that the best results are obtained when the HDT-ASCT is performed in first CR (CR1),[184,185] particularly after an induction using R-HyperCVAD prior to ASCT,[186] which appears very promising when compared to R-CHOP as shown in Table 17.5.[187,188]

What is the role of TBI in the conditioning regimen?

MCL is a very radiation-sensitive disease and TBI is more commonly used in Europe than the USA (which might explain some differences in results among studies). This would be consistent with the promising results seen with high-dose radioimmunotherapy detailed below[189] though in small studies so far but heavily pretreated patients.

How to optimize the use of rituximab peri-transplantation to improve MRD and risk of recurrence post-ASCT[190,191]

The experience reported by the NORDIC group was very impressive using the MCL-2 regimen: an R-CHOP-based therapy alternating with cytarabine (Ara-C 3 g/m^2 bid d1–2) for six cycles followed by carmustine, etoposide, cytarabine, and melphalan/carmustine, etoposide, cytarabine, and cyclophosphamide (BEAM/BEAC)-ASCT and maintenance rituximab in "presumptive relapse." In this large multicenter trial of 160 patients in the MCL-2 arm, patients were monitored by RQ-PCR for MRD and given rituximab accordingly. The results were compared to the previous regimen from the same

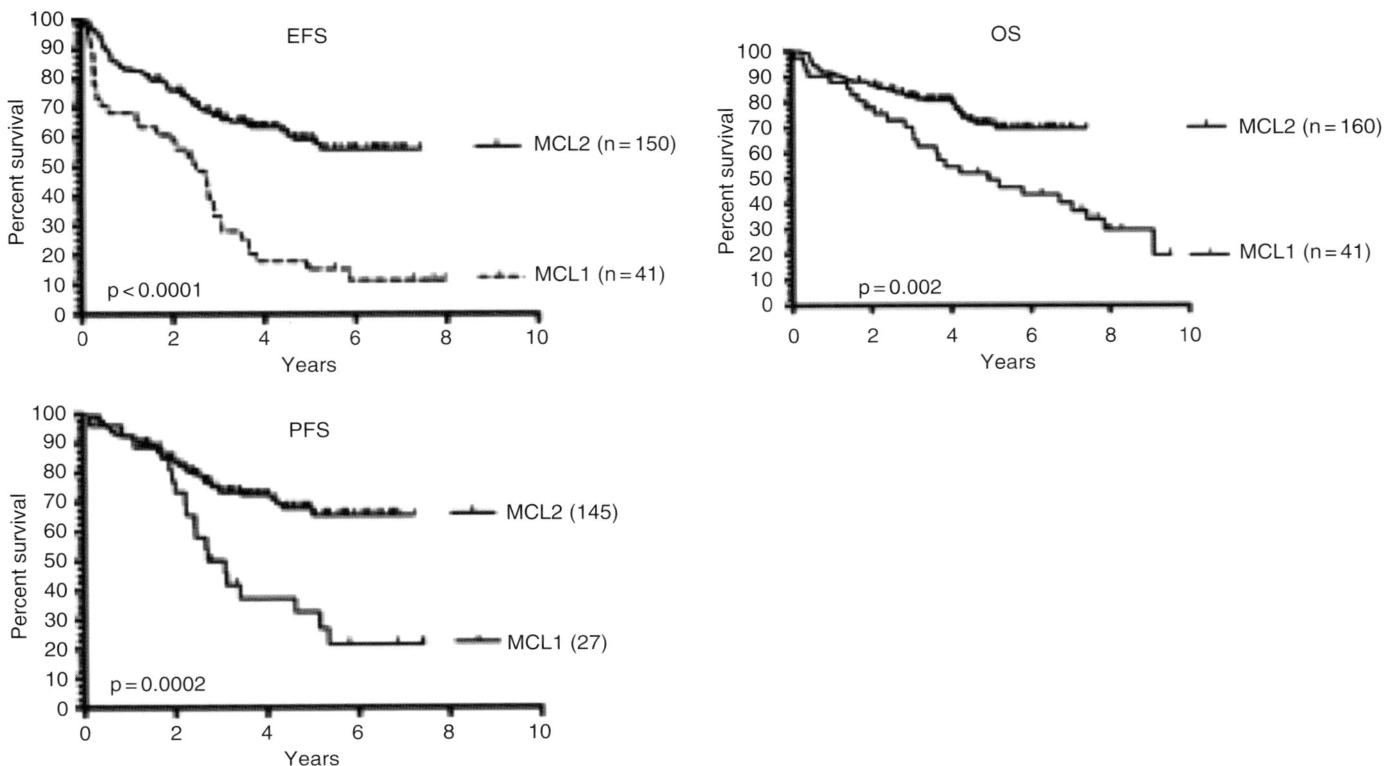

Figure 17.15 Frontline consolidation with high-dose therapy and stem cell transplant in MCL. CHOP-IFN-α vs. CHOP→ HDT-ASCT (German Lymphoma Study Group [GSLG]): improvement of PFS but no difference in OS.

Table 17.5. Outcome by induction therapy

Outcome	AutoPSC with CHOP-like regimen (n = 48)	AutoPSC with HyperCVAD (n = 32)	
PFS 1 yr	76%	97%	
PFS 3 yr	55%	78%	p = 0.05
OS 1 yr	94%	97%	
OS 3 yr	68%	97%	p = 0.01

group (MCL-1: a CHOP-like chemotherapy for four cycles followed by BEAM/BEAC + peripheral blood stem cell [PBSC]). As shown in Figure 17.16 the MCL-2 regimen was dramatically better for EFS, PFS, and OS, though the median follow-up for the MCL-2 group was only 3.5 years. In addition patients who relapsed molecularly were not taken as events in the outcome analysis while they were converted to molecular CR with additional rituximab, some of them more than one year post-transplantation.[192]

Another European approach using a tandem HDT (high-dose sequential therapy) and in vivo purging as well with rituximab also reported impressive results though the series was smaller (28 patients).[193] With a long follow-up, the survival is impressive, the EFS curves did not show a plateau, and there was no significant difference between high-risk and good-risk patients. The 10-year OS estimate of the patients treated with the R-HDS regimen at 120 months was 76.2% for the low-risk group, and 68% for the intermediate-high-risk group. The 10-year EFS rate was 57% for the low-risk group, 34% for the intermediate-high-risk group.

Table 17.6 summarizes the results of three large studies reported using either HDT-ASCT or dose intense therapy (R-HyperCVAD). The pooled data represent a total of more than 350 MCL patients treated with Ara-C-containing induction regimens. The 5-year EFS or FFS and OS are remarkably in the same range when comparing the "younger" patient groups underlying again the benefit of high-dose or dose intense therapy as induction in MCL.[194]

The relative rarity of MCL and lack of consensus for its management makes it difficult to develop large prospective randomized trials to confirm these promising results, though such trials are feasible, based on the very impressive experience in Europe. The difficulty in the interpretation of the data in MCL also relates often to small studies or single-institution experience and potential patient selection issues. On the other hand, recent reports from a single-institution retrospective analysis suggest that less aggressive approaches can still lead to prolonged survival[195] adding to the controversy. Though dose-intensified approaches, type R-HyperCVAD, or induction chemotherapy with HDT upfront remain the current standard approach in younger patients up to 65 years,[194] this represents only about half of the patient pool with MCL

Table 17.6. Ara-C-containing inductions in MCL

Study	Therapy	n	Age limit (years)	5-yr EFS	5-yr OS	Follow-up (mo)
Nordic ASH 07	MCL-2 (R+ Ara-C cont)	160	< 66	63%	74%	60
GITL ASH 07	(R) HDS-ASCT	77	< 61	61%	74%	50
MDACC	R-HyperCVAD	97	Up to 80 (1/3 > 65)	48%/FFS	65%	50
			< 65	60%/FFS	76%	50

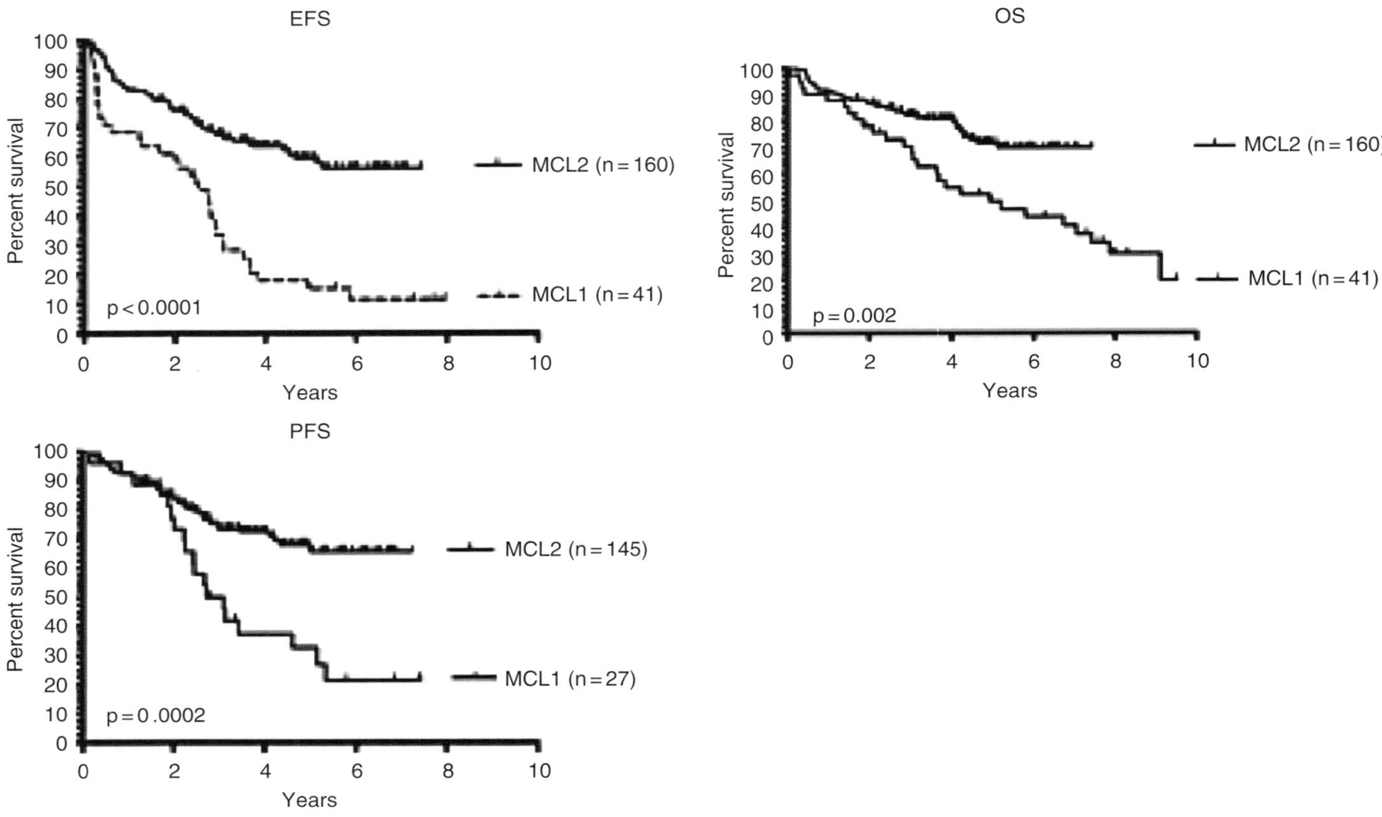

Figure 17.16 PFS and OS in the NORDIC MCL-1 and MCL-2 regimens.

at diagnosis. Novel strategies are needed for the more than 65 years group; hopefully the integration of novel therapies discussed below with conventional therapies into multimodal approaches will help overcome the still disappointing long-term prognosis of MCL.[196]

Immune-based therapy in the management of MCL

Monoclonal antibodies (mAbs)

Rituximab

Though rituximab does not have the same single-agent activity in MCL compared to follicular lymphoma (FL), its combination with conventional chemotherapy is now well accepted as beneficial from large studies with fludarabine, cyclophosphamide, and mitoxantrone (FCM) alone or combined with rituximab (R-FCM)[166] among others. This large study (with a double randomization) showed that R-FCM was superior to FCM and that rituximab maintenance appears effective after salvage with rituximab chemotherapy as it significantly prolongs response duration in patients with relapsed or refractory FL or MCL.[197] This observation was not true when rituximab was given as maintenance after rituximab induction as single agent consistent with the modest activity of rituximab by itself in MCL.[198] The question remains of how long rituximab maintenance should be carried out and will require additional (some ongoing) trials.

New monoclonal antibodies

A variety of novel second-and third-generation anti-CD20 mAbs are currently being evaluated with the rationale of humanized anti-CD20 antibodies (to improve infusion reaction and potentially antibody-dependent cell-mediated cytotoxicity), stronger

Table 17.7. Summary of new anti-CD20 mAbs

New anti-CD20 mAb	Antibody	Results/comments
Modification of Fc portion	AME-133v	Ongoing
	PRO-131921	Phase I completed
	GA-101 (glycoengineered + modified elbow hinge)	Type II Ab/reduced CDC and > direct induction of apoptosis, > 50% activity in phase I at all dose levels
Modification of Fab	Ofatumumab (HuMAxCD20)	Most advanced in development/ impressive activity in refractory/relapsed CLL/ORR 47–58%; median DOR 5.6–7 months
	Veltuzumab (IMMU-106/hA20)	Phase I completed
	Ocrelizumab (PRO70769)	36% RR in relapsed FL previously treated with rituximab

Note: DOR: duration of response.

binding (modification of Fab portion), altered complement-dependent cytotoxicity activity, or improved direct induction of apoptosis. Though these antibodies are still being tested, early data suggest they might be superior to rituximab especially in CLL.[199] These new anti-CD20 mAbs will certainly be evaluated as well in MCL[200] where rituximab had only a modest impact. The early results of ongoing studies with these new anti-CD20 mAbs are summarized in Table 17.7.

Other mAbs still under investigation include anti-CD52 (alentuzumab), which is mostly used as part of conditioning regimen in allotransplant[201] and anti-CD22 (epratuzumab), which has not been as effective as a single agent.[202] However, given its rapid internalization after binding to CD22, epratuzumab might be more useful as "drug shuttle," or as immunotoxin, providing a rationale for ongoing studies with calicheamycin (CMC-544) in B-cell NHL including in MCL.[203] Other mAbs include anti-HLA-DR or anti-CD40, which can induce ADCC and inhibit proliferation in preclinical models in a variety of B-cell lymphoma cell lines.[204] Multiple other mAbs are in development including antibodies against cell surface death receptors targeting the Fas/TRAIL pathway as detailed below.[205]

Idiotype vaccine

In order to prevent recurrence of disease in MCL after chemotherapy (at the stage of MRD), active immunization studies using anti-idiotype vaccines have been attempted in MCL. The main study was done using an induction with R-EPOCH chemotherapy followed by a conventional anti-idiotype vaccine.[154] Results showed the induction of T-cell CD4+ and CD8+ antitumor type-I cytokines responses in most patients but tumor-specific humoral responses occurred only in a subset of these patients and after peripheral blood B-cell recovery (post-rituximab). However, the immune responses that were observed did not translate into clear clinical benefit or reduction of risk of MCL recurrence. MCL is still overall a rather aggressive disease, making it a challenging subtype for vaccine approaches, which remain also time consuming and where likely the humoral response will be critical as seen in other NHL. Additional schedules and other vaccine models (autologous tumor cells and GM.CD40L intradermally plus low-dose IL-2) are being evaluated and might benefit subsets of patients. In this setting the recent data on the BiTE antibody (a new single-chain bispecific mAb: BiTE Ab [BiTE = Bispecific T-cell engager molecules]) binds CD19 and CD3 and then bypasses the regular T-cell activation requirement. The first one being tested is MT103, which showed very promising activity including in some MCL patients in the phase I study.[206] Finally trying to break the immune tolerance to tumors is the rationale for testing CTLA-4-Ig (ipilimumab) (anti-CD152), which has been done as single agent but also in the relapse setting after allogeneic transplantation including in MCL cases.[207]

Allotransplantation

The presence of a graft-versus-tumor (GVT) effect has now been well established in a variety of hematologic malignancies including indolent lymphomas and MCL. Given the median age of MCL is in the mid-60s, the risks of conventional allotransplantation make it a very rarely valid option. The development of non-myeloablative regimens has changed the outcome of such patients and though results certainly vary depending on the studies,[208,209] some patients showed prolonged disease-free survival (DFS) suggesting that "minitransplant" might be the only potentially curative option in MCL.[210,211] Consequently a donor search should be initiated in all patients with MCL especially in the younger population with poor prognostic features at baseline or certainly in the first or second relapse. Unfortunately, the incidence of chronic graft-versus-host (cGVH) disease in more than 50% of patients in this setting remains a serious concern. Alternative approaches with donor Th-2 lymphocyte enrichment prior to transplantation appear promising reducing GVH incidence and preserving graft-versus-leukemia (GVL) effect.[212]

Radioimmunotherapy (RIT)

Promising activity has been shown as single agent and in combination for both available RIT agents: ibritumomab tiuxetan (Zevalin®) and tositumomab (Bexxar®). In a small series, 5/15 relapsed MCL responded to ibritumomab (33%)

including 3 CR and 2 CRu, though the median response duration of CR/CRu patients was only 5.7 months.[213,214] Combination of RIT with standard chemotherapy as frontline therapy has been explored either as sequential tositumomab followed by CHOP[215] or R-CHOP followed by ibritumomab tiuxetan (ECOG 1499), just recently completed. In the ECOG study, 50 evaluable patients with newly diagnosed MCL received four cycles of R-CHOP followed by consolidation with ibritumomab tiuxetan.[216] Results showed that consolidation with ibritumomab tiuxetan after R-CHOP chemotherapy increased (tripled) the CR rate, though more follow-up is needed to see how these responses are sustained (in an otherwise relatively short chemotherapy induction).

The most impressive results of RIT in MCL have been as part of the conditioning regimen prior to ASCT in MCL[189,217] using high-dose ^{131}I-tositumomab, etoposide, cyclophosphamide with stem cell support in 16 patients with relapsed MCL. The ORR was 100% with 91% CR; 93% survival at 3 years and 61% DFS at 3 years. This approach to replace TBI has also been explored in other settings as part of the conditioning regimen[218,219] or at reduced dose as part of non-myeloablative allogenic SCT regimens.[220]

New biologic agents

Proteasome inhibitors

The proteasome is a large multiunit protease complex, which processes the vast majority of intracellular proteins including abnormal proteins (more common in cancer cells) and short-lived proteins (33% of nascent proteins have a half-life of less than 10 minutes) which are typically involved in critical functions such as cell cycle, cell growth, differentiation, and/or apoptosis.[221] Proteasome inhibition results in the disruption of a variety of pathways and checkpoints leading to apoptosis. Bortezomib, the first in the class of proteasome inhibitors, is a small molecule with potent selective and reversible inhibition of the chymotrypsine-like enzyme (one of the three enzymes located within the core of the proteasome).[222]

Bortezomib initial activity seen in MCL in the phase I (at the highest dose tested one PR in refractory MCL) was rapidly confirmed in four phase II studies: two in the USA,[223,224] one in Canada,[225] and one in the UK[226] with a remarkable consistency showing an ORR in the 40% range altogether. The multicenter pivotal trial (PINNACLE study with 155 patients enrolled) confirmed the activity of bortezomib in patients with relapsed or refractory MCL in the multicenter setting with a final ORR of 33% (including 8% CR/CRu) and a median DOR of 9.2 months.[227] In the subset of patients who achieved a CR/CRu, a recent update showed a median DOR not reached at 27 months.[228] The activity of bortezomib was confirmed in primary refractory patients and patients who had failed prior HDT; in addition responses were seen and maintained regardless of the number of prior therapies as shown in our previous experience at MD Anderson.[223,229] Moreover, similar response rate was found in untreated versus treated MCL in the Canadian experience.[230] All phase II studies showed similar toxicity profiles with fatigue, GI toxicity, neuropathy, and thrombocytopenia. The similar ORR range (35–45%) to bortezomib across all studies underlines the need to define biomarkers predictive of response to bortezomib in MCL. Preliminary results suggest that NF-κB expression (p65) and p27 level are potential biomarkers for patients receiving bortezomib as single agent in B-cell NHL including MCL, while Ki-67 did not correlate with response but with time to progression.[231,232] Elegant work looking at differences of response to bortezomib among B-cell NHL in preclinical models suggests that bortezomib induces distinct changes in MCL compared to other types of lymphoma including the overexpression of MCL-1 (an antiapoptotic protein described as myeloid cell leukemia 1) and induction of apoptosis through NOXA (a protein called Noxa for 'damage') and ROS (reactive oxygen species).[233,234]

Ongoing studies are also exploring the use of bortezomib in combination with a variety of other chemotherapy regimens including R-CHOP[235,236] and classic R-HyperCVAD[237] as well as with the modified R-HyperCVAD.[238] In the latter study, 30 newly diagosed MCL received bortezomib on days 1 and 4 of R-HyperCVAD A only ×6 cycles followed by maintenance rituximab as described previously.[161] After the addition of bortezomib, the ORR was 90% with 77% CR/CRu (60% in the prior modified HyperCVAD no bortezomib). The toxicities were as expected hematologic primarily, though the neuropathy incidence led to dose reduction at 1.3 mg/m^2 for bortezomib and 1 mg for vincristine. This study was expanded through ECOG in the multicenter setting (ECOG-1405), which enrolled 70 patients and was just completed. Numerous other regimens are combining bortezomib with induction regimens including R-CBoRP (replacement of vincristine by bortezomib in the R-CVP [rituximab plus cyclophosphamide, vincristine, and prednisone] regimen) ongoing,[239] a large randomized trial in >60 years old with R-CHOP vs. R-CHBzP (replacing vincristine by bortezomib in the R-CHOP), and as part of HDT and ASCT (Cancer and Leukemia Group B [CALGB]) all ongoing. The NCI study with R-EPOCH-Bz combination explores a window of opportunity as single agent (with biomarkers analysis on circulating leukemic cells) as well as maintenance with bortezomib post-completion of therapy. Other combinations in the relapsed setting in MCL include fludarabine-based therapy, high-dose cytarabine, and lenalidomide as well as other biologicals and small molecules as detailed below. The mechanisms of resistance to proteasome inhibition appear to involve heat-shock proteins (HSP; especially HSP90)[240] providing a rationale for combination with HSP inhibitors, some of which have also shown preliminary evidence of activity in lymphoma on their own as well (e.g. 17-allylamino-17-demethoxy geldanamycin [17AAG] or geldanamycin). Interestingly many of these combinations using bortezomib and other agents appear to be schedule dependent,[241] which might impact the design of our clinical trials.

Second-generation proteasome inhibitors include: NPI-0052, which can inhibit all three enzymes of the 20S unit of the proteasome and is just entering the clinic, and PR171 or carfilzomib, a novel, irreversible proteasome inhibitor under investigation in phase I–II studies. In spite of being irreversible, preclinical data showed that the half-life of recovery from proteasome inhibition by carfilzomib in tissues was approximately 24 hours. PR-171 was found to be more potent than bortezomib in preclinical models and is currently being tested with so far only anecdotal responses in MCL.[242] The next-generation drugs targeting the proteasome include ligase-specific inhibitors as well as immunoproteasome inhibitors that might increase the therapeutic index by targeting preferentially lymphoid cells.[243]

mTOR inhibitors

The mammalian target of rapamycin (mTOR) is a downstream effector of the PI3K/AKT (protein kinase B) signaling pathway, which mediates cell survival and proliferation. mTOR regulates essential signal-transduction pathways, in particular the coupling of growth stimuli and nutrient status with cell cycle progression and initiation of mRNA translation (sometimes hence called an "integrator of cell environment conditions"). The mTOR kinase regulates protein translation by phosphorylation of two critical substrates: the eukaryotic initiation factor 4E and the p70S6 kinase, which will control the final step in protein translation including that of cyclin D1, an important potential target in MCL. The activity of mTOR can be inhibited by rapamycin analogs, several of which are currently being evaluated in lymphomas especially in MCL.

Temsirolimus (CCI-779) has been shown to be active in relapsed or refractory MCL using 250 mg intravenously weekly as a single agent, with an ORR of 38% with one CR (3%) and 12 PR (35%) and a median DOR of 6.9 months.[244] Hematological toxicities were the most common, with 81% grade 3–4 especially thrombocytopenia. Though this was reversible, lower doses (25 mg weekly) were subsequently tested and showed a maintained activity and less myelosuppression with thrombocytopenia in a quarter of patients.[245] A large international three-arms randomized trial was recently presented comparing temsirolimus (two dosings) against treatment of choice (among a defined set of options) in relapsed/refractory MCL. The end point of the trial was reached in favor of temsirolimus, though the response rate in the control arm was surprisingly low (2%).[246] Temsirolimus is now being tested in combination with rituximab or cladribine among others. As in other biologicals, it will become important to define which subsets of patients might benefit most from mTOR inhibitors. Recent data confirm that the PI3K/AKt signaling pathway is a relevant target in MCL especially in blastoid variant[88] though based on small numbers this has not translated into the clinic, illustrating the difficulty of extrapolation from the preclinical setting to patients.

Other mTOR inhibitors include AP23573, a non-prodrug rapamycin analog tested in early trials (12.5 mg IV daily × 5 days, every 2 weeks) and well tolerated with no thrombocytopenia. Efficacy was seen in leukemia and it is currently being evaluated in lymphoma including MCL.[247] Everolimus (RAD001) is an oral derivative of rapamycin, which appeared to be well tolerated from phase I study[248,249] and has shown activity in about one-third of patients;[250] it is currently being evaluated in a large international trial in patients who failed bortezomib.

Inhibitors of angiogenesis

Based on its activity on the microenvironment and activity in other B-cell malignancies including multiple myeloma (MM), thalidomide was tested in MCL. The preliminary activity of thalidomide seen in MCL cases led to testing its combination with rituximab standard dose at 375 mg/m^2 weekly for four doses concomitantly with thalidomide (200 mg daily, with a dose increment up to 400 mg on day 15), which was continued as maintenance therapy until progression or toxicity.[251] The ORR was 81% with 31% CR and a median PFS $>$ 20 months making it a potential good option in elderly patients (though a large number of patients in that study were rituximab naïve). Additional studies are looking at thalidomide in the frontline setting with R-CHOP or other regimens (R-PEPC) as well as the role of maintenance with thalidomide in MCL after chemotherapy induction. Similarly CC-5013, a derivative immunomodulatory drug (IMiD) (lenalidomide), showed activity as single agent[252] in NHL including in MCL with an ORR of 41% in the multicenter setting and a median DOR $>$ 1 year.[253] Lenalidomide is currently also being tested in combination with rituximab[254] and/or other agents in relapsed MCL including planned trials for maintenance post-R-CHOP chemotherapy induction in the elderly.

Alternative approaches to target angiogenesis have been through mAbs including bevacizumab and VGEF-trap currently being tested also in B-cell NHL including MCL, again with rituximab or in combination with chemotherapy with R-CHOP in the frontline setting.[255]

Small molecules targeting apoptosis

Targeting apoptosis is an obvious appealing goal in anticancer therapy resulting in a plethora of small molecules currently in development.

Antisense approach

One of the first approaches used was through antisense oligonucleotides (ASO) against BCL2, which is commonly overexpressed in a variety of lymphomas including MCL and classically associated with chemoresistance. Though there was preclinical evidence of activity of the first one tested, G3139 or oblimersen sodium (Genasense),[256] this compound did not show convincing activity in the clinic with only so far modest activity in CLL from a phase I–II study.[257] Preclinical data are supporting additive or even synergistic effect with a variety of other agents including rituximab, cytotoxics, and bortezomib[258,259] providing a rationale for additional studies, although future research with this compound remains unclear given negative recommendation by the advisory US Food and Drug Administration (FDA) committee. Other antisenses such as against BCX-L or bispecific antisense against BCL2 and BCL-XL are in early development.[260]

Pan family inhibitors

These represent another way to induce apoptosis by interacting with several BCL2 family members. The antiapoptotic BCL2 family includes BCL2, BCL-XL, A1, BCL-W, and MCL-1. These are multidomain proteins with sequence similarity across BH-1 through BH-4 domains. The proapoptotic BCL2 family members differ based on structural and functional differences. They include multidomain Bax-like proteins (which include Bax, Bak, and Bok), which share BH-1, BH-2, and BH-3 domains in common with the antiapoptotic proteins. Other proapoptotic proteins include BH-3 only members such as Bid and Bim, which can induce apoptosis directly, and Bad and NOXA, which act more as sensitizers to apoptosis.[261] A hydrophobic groove is present at the surface of the antiapoptotic proteins BCL2, BCL-XL, and MCL-1; this groove forms the binding site of the BH-3-region of proapoptotic proteins. This provides a good target for BH-3-only small molecules mimicking the proapoptotic activities of BH-3-only proteins. Among them AT-101, an orally bioavailable derivative of gossypol, and ABT-737, a small molecule also a pan-BCL2 inhibitor, both showed preclinical activity in B-cell malignancies alone or in combination with other agents. ABT-263 – an oral pan-BCL2 inhibitor – has recently shown promising activity as single agent in the phase I setting especially in small lymphocytic leukemia (SLL)/CLL; the main toxicity being thrombocytopenia.[262] Of notice the pan-BCL2 inhibitors differ by the subset of BCL2 family members they can inhibit.[263] GX15–070 is another pan-BCL2 inhibitor, which has the ability to also inhibit MCL-1 (which is not affected by ABT-263). Evidence of synergy was found between these new BCL2 inhibitors and a variety of other agents including specifically GX15–070 and bortezomib in MCL cells,[264] providing a rationale for combining obatoclax and Bz in relapsed/refractory MCL in an ongoing study with preliminary promising results including in patients who failed prior bortezomib.[265]

Agents targeting the extrinsic pathway

Additional compounds can target apoptosis including its extrinsic pathway through stimulation of cell surface death receptors, which include tumor necrosis factor receptors (TNFR1), FAS (also known as CD95), and death receptors DR4 and DR5. The corresponding ligands for these receptors are TNF, FAS ligand (also known as CD95 ligand), or TNF-related apoptosis-inducing ligands (TRAILS) (also known as APO2 ligands). TRAIL R1, which targets DR4, and TRAIL R2, which targets DR5, are both agonist antibodies, which can induce apoptosis in cancer cells but not in normal cells.[266] They are also both currently in early development in the clinic including AMG 655 tested in combination with Bz and HDAC inhibitors.

Other ways to target apoptosis

IAPs are important regulators of apoptosis that function by binding and inhibiting caspases; the family includes XIAP (which inhibits caspases 3, 7, and 9); survivin (only expressed in tumor cells and has also a role in cell cycle); and SMACs peptides, which can inhibit IAPs (hence SMAC peptidomimetics can enhance apoptosis). MDM2 is a protein that binds to p53 and negatively regulates its activity and stability. Therefore the MDM2-mediated loss of p53 will impair the cell's ability to block cell cycle progression and induce apoptosis in response to DNA damage. This provides a rationale to design small peptides that are antagonists of MDM2, several of which are currently in preclinical phase including the nutlins groups which showed activity in xenografts models.

Histone deacetylase (HDAC) inhibitors

The chromatin structure (open versus closed chromatin) affects gene transcription. This occurs as a result of the opposing activities of two types of enzymes: the HDACs (that remove acetylation residues) and the histone acetyl-transferases (HATs) (that add more acetylation residues). The regulation or balance of acetylation of histones will then impact gene transcription and it is estimated that HDACs will alter the transcription of about 2–10% of expressed genes (increased or decreased). Inhibitors of HDAC represent a new class of targeted anticancer agents with now several structural classes of HDAC inhibitors developed, including the short-chain fatty acids (the benzamides [MS-275]), the cyclic peptide depsipeptide (FK-228), and suberoylanilide hydroxamic acid (SAHA). HDAC inhibitors have been shown to cause cultured, transformed cells to undergo growth arrest, terminal differentiation, and apoptosis. So far the activity of HDAC inhibitors has been mostly in cutaneous T-cell leukemia (CTCL) and there is preliminary evidence of activity in other B-cell NHL as well.[267] However, HDAC inhibitors have also been found to be additive and in some instances synergistic with a number of anticancer agents including radiation, anthracyclines, flavopiridol, and proteasome inhibitors[258,268] providing a rationale for additional ongoing studies which include MCL[268] where preclinical models show a downregulation of cyclin D1. The aggresome, which can also be inhibited by HDAC (especially HDAC6), is an important target in this setting. Proteins are sequestered and stabilized within the aggresome, in response to stress, including endoplasmic reticulum stress in response to proteasome inhibition. Aggresome disruption (through targeting of HDAC6 especially) as shown in recent models provides also new rationale for future combinations.[269]

Other agents

Flavopiridol (alvocidib)

The overexpression of cyclin D1 in MCL makes it an attractive target for potential therapeutic agents. Flavopiridol, a synthetic *N*-methylpiperidinyl, chlorophenyl flavone compound, has been found to block several cyclin-dependent kinases (CDKs) including complex CDK4-cyclin D1. Extensive preclinical work including in MCL cell lines showed activity of flavopiridol supporting its use in the clinic. The initial clinical experience was disappointing in terms of efficacy (11% ORR only PR).[270,271] Pharmacokinetic elegant work led to new schedules (bolus + 3 hours infusion)[272] with impressive preliminary results as single agent in CLL and MCL alone or in combination with rituximab and/or fludarabine.[273,274] Several second-generation CDK inhibitors are in development including PD0–332991, which selectively inhibits CDK4/6, and is being tested in MCL as well.

Protein kinase C (PKC) inhibitors

Bryostatin, which seems to have both cytotoxic and immunomodulatory properties, has been in early clinic development for several years and has not yet proven of substantial benefit as single agent. Other PKC inhibitors including enzastaurin[275] are being evaluated and preclinical studies suggest that these compounds might be more potent in the combination setting with other cytotoxics as seen for other biologicals.

IKB kinase (IKK)/NF-κB stabilizers

Nuclear factor-kappa B (NF-κB) is a collective term that refers to a small class of dimeric transcription factors that control a number of genes, including growth factors, angiogenesis modulators, cell-adhesion molecules, and antiapoptotic factors. The most common p50-RelA (p65) dimer known specifically as NF-κB is relatively abundant, controls the expression of numerous genes and seems involved in chemoresistance. The NF-κB complex exists as an inactive cytoplasmic dimer bound to inhibitory proteins of the IKB family. The inactive NF-κB-IKB complex is activated by a variety of stimuli, including proinflammatory cytokines, mitogens, growth factors, and stress-inducing agents (including chemotherapy and radiation). The phosphorylation of IKB induces the release of NF-κB, which can then translocate to the nucleus, where it promotes cell survival by initiating the transcription of genes encoding stress-response enzymes, cell-adhesion molecules, proinflammatory cytokines, and antiapoptotic proteins. Constitutive activation of NF-κB in the nucleus is observed in several types of lymphoma including MCL where it appears to be a great target for novel therapies,[115] though contrary to the initial thinking, NF-κB does not appear to be a significant player in proteasome inhibition efficacy in MCL as suggested by biomarkers results. Several small molecule inhibitors of the IKB kinase (PS115; BAY 11–7082 and AS602868) (which would trap NF-κB) are currently in development with a strong rationale for trials in several subtypes of NHL including MCL.[276,277]

Conclusions

1. The biology of MCL results from the combination of three factors: cell cycle disruption (proliferation index +++), DNA damage response defect (> 80% MCL have secondary genomic alterations), and dysregulation in survival pathways (chemoresistance).
2. There is NO standard and effective or curative therapy yet defined in MCL, which typically presents as advanced disease.
3. The overall prognostic of MCL remains poor especially in the relapse setting, though the median OS has doubled in the last two decades.
4. Dose-intense approaches such as R-HyperCVAD or R-chemo induction followed by HDT-ASCT are routinely used in patients < 65 years. They clearly prolong PFS but are still debated (patient selection and questionable impact on OS).
5. New strategies are needed in the elderly given the median age at diagnosis (mid 60s); this represents half of MCL patients.
6. Rituximab appears beneficial in combination with chemotherapy, and as part of consolidation with ASCT; its role in OR maintenance is still being evaluated. New anti-CD20 mAbs are currently being tested and might improve on the modest contribution of rituximab in MCL.
7. Allotransplantation especially "miniallo" might be curative in a subset of patients though cGVH occurs in > 50% of patients.
8. A multitude of novel agents are currently being tested in MCL, including proteasome inhibitors (bortezomib), mTOR inhibitors (temsirolimus, RAD-001), and IMiDs (lenalidomide), which all have clear single-agent activity.
9. The integration of these novel or biologic/targeted therapies with other regimens remains to be defined, underlining again a much-needed effort to enroll MCL patients on clinical trials.
10. A better understanding of the heterogeneity of MCL might allow a better stratification of patients and help develop novel therapies targeting relevant biologic mechanisms. This overall will hopefully in the future guide our treatment algorithm and improve patients' outcomes.

Acknowledgements

Thanks to Dr Pritish Bhattacharyya and Dr Xiao Yang from the Hematopathology Division at Hackensuck University Medical Center, for providing all pathology slides for this chapter.

References

1. Velders GA, Kluin-Nelemans JC, De Boer CJ, *et al.* Mantle-cell lymphoma: a population-based clinical study. *J Clin Oncol* 1996;**14**:1269–74.
2. Andersen NS, Jensen MK, de Nully Brown P, *et al.* A Danish population-based analysis of 105 mantle cell lymphoma patients: incidences, clinical features, response, survival and prognostic factors. *Eur J Cancer* 2002;**38**:401–8.
3. Zhou Y, Wang H, Fang W, *et al.* Incidence trends of mantle cell lymphoma in the United States between 1992 and 2004. *Cancer* 2008;**113**:791–8.
4. Banks PM, Chan J, Cleary ML, *et al.* Mantle cell lymphoma. A proposal for unification of morphologic, immunologic, and molecular data. *Am J Surg Pathol* 1992;**16**:637–40.
5. Weisenburger DD, Armitage JO. Mantle cell lymphoma– an entity comes of age. *Blood* 1996;**87**:4483–94.
6. Chim CS, Chan AC, Choo CK, *et al.* Mantle cell lymphoma in the Chinese: clinicopathological features and treatment outcome. *Am J Hematol* 1998;**59**:295–301.
7. Chuang SS, Huang WT, Hsieh PP, *et al.* Mantle cell lymphoma in Taiwan: clinicopathological and molecular study of 21 cases including one cyclin D1-negative tumor expressing cyclin D2. *Pathol Int* 2006;**56**:440–8.
8. Anderson JR, Armitage JO, Weisenburger DD. Epidemiology of the non-Hodgkin's lymphomas: distributions of the major subtypes differ by geographic locations. Non-Hodgkin's Lymphoma Classification Project. *Ann Oncol* 1998;**9**:717–20.
9. Mitterlechner T, Fiegl M, Muhlbock H, *et al.* Epidemiology of non-Hodgkin lymphomas in Tyrol/Austria from 1991 to 2000. *J Clin Pathol* 2006;**59**:48–55.
10. Fisher SG, Fisher RI. The epidemiology of non-Hodgkin's lymphoma. *Oncogene* 2004;**23**:6524–34.
11. Levine AM, Shimodaira S, Lai MM. Treatment of HCV-related mantle-cell lymphoma with ribavirin and pegylated interferon alfa. *N Engl J Med* 2003;**349**:2078–9.
12. Schollkopf C, Melbye M, Munksgaard L, *et al.* Borrelia infection and risk of non-Hodgkin lymphoma. *Blood* 2008;**111**:5524–9.
13. Tort F, Camacho E, Bosch F, *et al.* Familial lymphoid neoplasms in patients with mantle cell lymphoma. *Haematologica* 2004;**89**:314–19.
14. Marti GE. Familial lymphoid neoplasms in patients with mantle cell lymphoma. *Haematologica* 2004;**89**:262–3.
15. Barista I, Cabanillas F, Romaguera JE, *et al.* Is there an increased rate of additional malignancies in patients with mantle cell lymphoma? *Ann Oncol* 2002;**13**:318–22.
16. Kelemen K, Peterson LC, Helenowski I, *et al.* CD23+ mantle cell lymphoma: a clinical pathologic entity associated with superior outcome compared with CD23- disease. *Am J Clin Pathol* 2008;**130**:166–77.
17. Liu Z, Dong HY, Gorczyca W, *et al.* CD5- mantle cell lymphoma. *Am J Clin Pathol* 2002;**118**:216–24.
18. Babbage G, Garand R, Robillard N, *et al.* Mantle cell lymphoma with t(11;14) and unmutated or mutated VH genes expresses AID and undergoes isotype switch events. *Blood* 2004;**103**:2795–8.
19. de Boer CJ, van Krieken JH, Kluin-Nelemans HC, *et al.* Cyclin D1 messenger RNA overexpression as a marker for mantle cell lymphoma. *Oncogene* 1995;**10**:1833–40.
20. Vaandrager JW, Kluin P, Schuuring E. The t(11;14) (q13;q32) in multiple myeloma cell line KMS12 has its 11q13 breakpoint 330 kb centromeric from the cyclin D1 gene. *Blood* 1997;**89**:349–50.
21. Bosch F, Jares P, Campo E, *et al.* PRAD-1/cyclin D1 gene overexpression in chronic lymphoproliferative disorders: a highly specific marker of mantle cell lymphoma. *Blood* 1994;**84**:2726–32.
22. de Boer CJ, Loyson S, Kluin PM, *et al.* Multiple breakpoints within the BCL-1 locus in B-cell lymphoma: rearrangements of the cyclin D1 gene. *Cancer Res* 1993;**53**:4148–52.
23. Degan M, Doliana R, Gloghini A, *et al.* A novel bcl-1/JH breakpoint from a patient affected by mantle cell lymphoma extends the major translocation cluster. *J Pathol* 2002;**197**:256–63.
24. Salaverria I, Espinet B, Carrio A, *et al.* Multiple recurrent chromosomal breakpoints in mantle cell lymphoma revealed by a combination of molecular cytogenetic techniques. *Genes Chromosomes Cancer* 2008;**47**:1086–97.
25. Argatoff LH, Connors JM, Klasa RJ, *et al.* Mantle cell lymphoma: a clinicopathologic study of 80 cases. *Blood* 1997;**89**:2067–78.
26. Li JY, Gaillard F, Moreau A, *et al.* Detection of translocation t(11;14)(q13;q32) in mantle cell lymphoma by fluorescence in situ hybridization. *Am J Pathol* 1999;**154**:1449–52.
27. Siebert R, Matthiesen P, Harder S, *et al.* Application of interphase cytogenetics for the detection of t(11;14)(q13;q32) in mantle cell lymphomas. *Ann Oncol* 1998;**9**:519–26.
28. Chibbar R, Leung K, McCormick S, *et al.* bcl-1 gene rearrangements in mantle cell lymphoma: a comprehensive analysis of 118 cases, including B-5-fixed tissue, by polymerase chain reaction and Southern transfer analysis. *Mod Pathol* 1998;**11**:1089–97.
29. Vaandrager JW, Schuuring E, Zwikstra E, *et al.* Direct visualization of dispersed 11q13 chromosomal translocations in mantle cell lymphoma by multicolor DNA fiber fluorescence in situ hybridization. *Blood* 1996;**88**:1177–82.
30. Fan H, Gulley ML, Gascoyne RD, *et al.* Molecular methods for detecting t(11;14) translocations in mantle-cell lymphomas. *Diagn Mol Pathol* 1998;**7**:209–14.
31. Rimokh R, Berger F, Delsol G, *et al.* Detection of the chromosomal translocation t(11;14) by polymerase chain reaction in mantle cell lymphomas. *Blood* 1994;**83**:1871–5.
32. Kurokawa T, Kinoshita T, Murate T, *et al.* Complementarity determining region-III is a useful molecular marker for the evaluation of minimal residual disease in mantle cell lymphoma. *Br J Haematol* 1997;**98**:408–12.
33. Swerdlow SH, Williams ME. From centrocytic to mantle cell lymphoma: a clinicopathologic and molecular review of 3 decades. *Hum Pathol* 2002;**33**:7–20.
34. Campo E, Raffeld M, Jaffe ES. Mantle-cell lymphoma. *Semin Hematol* 1999;**36**:115–27.
35. Ott G, Kalla J, Hanke A, *et al.* The cytomorphological spectrum of mantle cell lymphoma is reflected by distinct

biological features. *Leuk Lymphoma* 1998;**32**:55–63.

36. Hernandez L, Fest T, Cazorla M, *et al.* p53 gene mutations and protein overexpression are associated with aggressive variants of mantle cell lymphomas. *Blood* 1996;**87**:3351–9.
37. Yin CC, Medeiros LJ, Cromwell CC, *et al.* Sequence analysis proves clonal identity in five patients with typical and blastoid mantle cell lymphoma. *Mod Pathol* 2007;**20**:1–7.
38. Rosenwald A, Wright G, Wiestner A, *et al.* The proliferation gene expression signature is a quantitative integrator of oncogenic events that predicts survival in mantle cell lymphoma. *Cancer Cell* 2003;**3**:185–97.
39. Jares P, Colomer D, Campo E. Genetic and molecular pathogenesis of mantle cell lymphoma: perspectives for new targeted therapeutics. *Nat Rev Cancer* 2007;**7**:750–62.
40. Hummel M, Tamaru J, Kalvelage B, *et al.* Mantle cell (previously centrocytic) lymphomas express VH genes with no or very little somatic mutations like the physiologic cells of the follicle mantle. *Blood* 1994;**84**:403–7.
41. Du MQ, Diss TC, Xu CF, *et al.* Ongoing immunoglobulin gene mutations in mantle cell lymphomas. *Br J Haematol* 1997;**96**:124–31.
42. Cogliatti SB, Bertoni F, Zimmermann DR, *et al.* IgV H mutations in blastoid mantle cell lymphoma characterize a subgroup with a tendency to more favourable clinical outcome. *J Pathol* 2005;**206**:320–7.
43. Walsh SH, Thorselius M, Johnson A, *et al.* Mutated VH genes and preferential VH3–21 use define new subsets of mantle cell lymphoma. *Blood* 2003;**101**:4047–54.
44. Lai R, Lefresne SV, Franko B, *et al.* Immunoglobulin VH somatic hypermutation in mantle cell lymphoma: mutated genotype correlates with better clinical outcome. *Mod Pathol* 2006;**19**:1498–505.
45. Pittaluga S, Tierens A, Pinyol M, *et al.* Blastic variant of mantle cell lymphoma shows a heterogenous pattern of somatic mutations of the rearranged immunoglobulin heavy chain variable genes. *Br J Haematol* 1998;**102**:1301–6.
46. Laszlo T, Nagy M, Kelenyi G, *et al.* Immunoglobulin V(H) gene mutational analysis suggests that blastic variant of mantle cell lymphoma derives from different stages of B-cell maturation. *Leuk Res* 2000;**24**:27–31.
47. Thorselius M, Walsh S, Eriksson I, *et al.* Somatic hypermutation and V(H) gene usage in mantle cell lymphoma. *Eur J Haematol* 2002;**68**:217–24.
48. Varade W, Marin E, Milano M, *et al.* VH gene repertoire of mantle cell lymphomas. *Ann N Y Acad Sci* 1995;**764**:504–6.
49. Camacho FI, Algara P, Rodriguez A, *et al.* Molecular heterogeneity in MCL defined by the use of specific VH genes and the frequency of somatic mutations. *Blood* 2003;**101**:4042–6.
50. Kienle D, Krober A, Katzenberger T, *et al.* VH mutation status and VDJ rearrangement structure in mantle cell lymphoma: correlation with genomic aberrations, clinical characteristics, and outcome. *Blood* 2003;**102**:3003–9.
51. Orchard J, Garand R, Davis Z, *et al.* A subset of t(11;14) lymphoma with mantle cell features displays mutated IgVH genes and includes patients with good prognosis, nonnodal disease. *Blood* 2003;**101**:4975–81.
52. Welzel N, Le T, Marculescu R, *et al.* Templated nucleotide addition and immunoglobulin JH-gene utilization in t(11;14) junctions: implications for the mechanism of translocation and the origin of mantle cell lymphoma. *Cancer Res* 2001;**61**:1629–36.
53. Schraders M, Oeschger S, Kluin PM, *et al.* Hypermutation in mantle cell lymphoma does not indicate a clinical or biological subentity. *Mod Pathol* 2009;**22**:416–25.
54. Ott MM, Helbing A, Ott G, *et al.* bcl-1 rearrangement and cyclin D1 protein expression in mantle cell lymphoma. *J Pathol* 1996;**179**:238–42.
55. Wlodarska I, Meeus P, Stul M, *et al.* Variant t(2;11)(p11;q13) associated with the IgK-CCND1 rearrangement is a recurrent translocation in leukemic small-cell B-non-Hodgkin lymphoma. *Leukemia* 2004;**18**:1705–10.
56. Gruszka-Westwood AM, Atkinson S, Summersgill BM, *et al.* Unusual case of leukemic mantle cell lymphoma with amplified CCND1/IGH fusion gene. *Genes Chromosomes Cancer* 2002;**33**:206–12.
57. Callanan M, Leroux D, Magaud JP, *et al.* Implication of cyclin D1 in malignant lymphoma. *Crit Rev Oncog* 1996;**7**:191–203.
58. Donnellan R, Chetty R. Cyclin D1 and human neoplasia. *Mol Pathol* 1998;**51**:1–7.
59. Williams ME, Meeker TC, Swerdlow SH. Rearrangement of the chromosome 11 bcl-1 locus in centrocytic lymphoma: analysis with multiple breakpoint probes. *Blood* 1991;**78**:493–8.
60. Stamatopoulos K, Kosmas C, Belessi C, *et al.* Molecular analysis of bcl-1/IgH junctional sequences in mantle cell lymphoma: potential mechanism of the t(11;14) chromosomal translocation. *Br J Haematol* 1999;**105**:190–7.
61. Chesi M, Bergsagel PL, Brents LA, *et al.* Dysregulation of cyclin D1 by translocation into an IgH gamma switch region in two multiple myeloma cell lines. *Blood* 1996;**88**:674–81.
62. Seto M. Molecular mechanisms of lymphomagenesis through transcriptional disregulation by chromosome translocation. *Int J Hematol* 2002;**76** Suppl 1:323–6.
63. Difilippantonio MJ, Petersen S, Chen HT, *et al.* Evidence for replicative repair of DNA double-strand breaks leading to oncogenic translocation and gene amplification. *J Exp Med* 2002;**196**:469–80.
64. Roix JJ, McQueen PG, Munson PJ, *et al.* Spatial proximity of translocation-prone gene loci in human lymphomas. *Nat Genet* 2003;**34**:287–91.
65. Pederson T. Gene territories and cancer. *Nat Genet* 2003;**34**:242–3.
66. Williams ME, Swerdlow SH. Cyclin D1 overexpression in non-Hodgkin's lymphoma with chromosome 11 bcl-1 rearrangement. *Ann Oncol* 1994;**5** Suppl 1:71–3.
67. Yatabe Y, Suzuki R, Tobinai K, *et al.* Significance of cyclin D1 overexpression for the diagnosis of mantle cell lymphoma: a clinicopathologic comparison of cyclin D1-positive MCL and cyclin D1-negative MCL-like B-cell lymphoma. *Blood* 2000;**95**:2253–61.
68. Rimokh R, Berger F, Bastard C, *et al.* Rearrangement of CCND1 (BCL1/PRAD1) 3' untranslated region in mantle-cell lymphomas and t(11q13)-associated leukemias. *Blood* 1994;**83**:3689–96.
69. Wiestner A, Tehrani M, Chiorazzi M, *et al.* Point mutations and genomic

deletions in CCND1 create stable truncated cyclin D1 mRNAs that are associated with increased proliferation rate and shorter survival. *Blood* 2007;**109**:4599–606.

70. Sander B, Flygare J, Porwit-Macdonald A, *et al.* Mantle cell lymphomas with low levels of cyclin D1 long mRNA transcripts are highly proliferative and can be discriminated by elevated cyclin A2 and cyclin B1. *Int J Cancer* 2005;**117**:418–30.

71. Chen RW, Bemis LT, Amato CM, *et al.* Truncation in CCND1 mRNA alters miR-16–1 regulation in mantle cell lymphoma. *Blood* 2008;**112**:822–9.

72. Solomon DA, Wang Y, Fox SR, *et al.* Cyclin D1 splice variants. Differential effects on localization, RB phosphorylation, and cellular transformation. *J Biol Chem* 2003;**278**:30 339–47.

73. Hunter T, Pines J. Cyclins and cancer. II: Cyclin D and CDK inhibitors come of age. *Cell* 1994;**79**:573–82.

74. Ewen ME, Sluss HK, Sherr CJ, *et al.* Functional interactions of the retinoblastoma protein with mammalian D-type cyclins. *Cell* 1993;**73**:487–97.

75. Pinyol M, Bea S, Pla L, *et al.* Inactivation of RB1 in mantle-cell lymphoma detected by nonsense-mediated mRNA decay pathway inhibition and microarray analysis. *Blood* 2007;**109**:5422–9.

76. Quintanilla-Martinez L, Davies-Hill T, Fend F, *et al.* Sequestration of p27Kip1 protein by cyclin D1 in typical and blastic variants of mantle cell lymphoma (MCL): implications for pathogenesis. *Blood* 2003; **101**:3181–7.

77. Chiarle R, Budel LM, Skolnik J, *et al.* Increased proteasome degradation of cyclin-dependent kinase inhibitor p27 is associated with a decreased overall survival in mantle cell lymphoma. *Blood* 2000;**95**:619–26.

78. Fu M, Wang C, Li Z, *et al.* Minireview: Cyclin D1: normal and abnormal functions. *Endocrinology* 2004;**145**:5439–47.

79. Fu K, Weisenburger DD, Greiner TC, *et al.* Cyclin D1-negative mantle cell lymphoma: a clinicopathologic study based on gene expression profiling. *Blood* 2005;**106**:4315–21.

80. Wlodarska I, Dierickx D, Vanhentenrijk V, *et al.* Translocations targeting CCND2, CCND3, and MYCN do occur in t(11;14)-negative mantle cell lymphomas. *Blood* 2008;**111**:5683–90.

81. Gesk S, Klapper W, Martin-Subero JI, *et al.* A chromosomal translocation in cyclin D1-negative/cyclin D2-positive mantle cell lymphoma fuses the CCND2 gene to the IGK locus. *Blood* 2006;**108**:1109–10.

82. Sonoki T, Harder L, Horsman DE, *et al.* Cyclin D3 is a target gene of t(6;14)(p21.1;q32.3) of mature B-cell malignancies. *Blood* 2001;**98**:2837–44.

83. Jiang Y, Thomaides A, Rassidakis G, *et al.* Detection of the t(11;14) translocation in peripheral blood (PB) of healthy individuals. *Blood* 2002;**11**:4266.

84. Hirt C, Schuler F, Dolken L, *et al.* Low prevalence of circulating t(11;14)(q13;q32)-positive cells in the peripheral blood of healthy individuals as detected by real-time quantitative PCR. *Blood* 2004;**104**:904–5.

85. Gladden AB, Woolery R, Aggarwal P, *et al.* Expression of constitutively nuclear cyclin D1 in murine lymphocytes induces B-cell lymphoma. *Oncogene* 2006;**25**:998–1007.

86. Lovec H, Grzeschiczek A, Kowalski MB, *et al.* Cyclin D1/bcl-1 cooperates with myc genes in the generation of B-cell lymphoma in transgenic mice. *EMBO J* 1994;**13**:3487–95.

87. Smith MR, Joshi I, Jin F, *et al.* Murine model for mantle cell lymphoma. *Leukemia* 2006;**20**:891–3.

88. Rudelius M, Pittaluga S, Nishizuka S, *et al.* Constitutive activation of Akt contributes to the pathogenesis and survival of mantle cell lymphoma. *Blood* 2006;**108**:1668–76.

89. Rizzatti EG, Falcao RP, Panepucci RA, *et al.* Gene expression profiling of mantle cell lymphoma cells reveals aberrant expression of genes from the PI3K-AKT, WNT and TGFbeta signalling pathways. *Br J Haematol* 2005;**130**:516–26.

90. Gelebart P, Anand M, Armanious H, *et al.* Constitutive activation of the Wnt canonical pathway in mantle cell lymphoma. *Blood* 2008;**112**:5171–9.

91. Ford RJ, Shen L, Lin-Lee YC, *et al.* Development of a murine model for blastoid variant mantle-cell lymphoma. *Blood* 2007;**109**:4899–906.

92. Klier M, Anastasov N, Hermann A, *et al.* Specific lentiviral shRNA-mediated knockdown of cyclin D1 in mantle cell lymphoma has minimal effects on cell survival and reveals a regulatory circuit with cyclin D2. *Leukemia* 2008;**22**: 2097–105.

93. Salaverria I, Zettl A, Bea S, *et al.* Specific secondary genetic alterations in mantle cell lymphoma provide prognostic information independent of the gene expression-based proliferation signature. *J Clin Oncol* 2007;**25**:1216–22.

94. Bea S, Ribas M, Hernandez JM, *et al.* Increased number of chromosomal imbalances and high-level DNA amplifications in mantle cell lymphoma are associated with blastoid variants. *Blood* 1999;**93**:4365–74.

95. Neben K, Ott G, Schweizer S, *et al.* Expression of centrosome-associated gene products is linked to tetraploidization in mantle cell lymphoma. *Int J Cancer* 2007;**120**:1669–77.

96. Ott G, Kalla J, Ott MM, *et al.* Blastoid variants of mantle cell lymphoma: frequent bcl-1 rearrangements at the major translocation cluster region and tetraploid chromosome clones. *Blood* 1997;**89**:1421–9.

97. Daniel MT, Tigaud I, Flexor MA, *et al.* Leukaemic non-Hodgkin's lymphomas with hyperdiploid cells and t(11;14)(q13;q32): a subtype of mantle cell lymphoma? *Br J Haematol* 1995;**90**:77–84.

98. Shiloh Y. ATM and related protein kinases: safeguarding genome integrity. *Nat Rev Cancer* 2003;**3**:155–68.

99. Fang NY, Greiner TC, Weisenburger DD, *et al.* Oligonucleotide microarrays demonstrate the highest frequency of ATM mutations in the mantle cell subtype of lymphoma. *Proc Natl Acad Sci U S A* 2003;**100**:5372–7.

100. Camacho E, Hernandez L, Hernandez S, *et al.* ATM gene inactivation in mantle cell lymphoma mainly occurs by truncating mutations and missense mutations involving the phosphatidylinositol-3 kinase domain and is associated with increasing numbers of chromosomal imbalances. *Blood* 2002;**99**:238–44.

101. Fernandez V, Hartmann E, Ott G, *et al.* Pathogenesis of mantle-cell lymphoma: all oncogenic roads lead to dysregulation of cell cycle and DNA damage response pathways. *J Clin Oncol* 2005;**23**:6364–9.

102. Bea S, Salaverria I, Armengol L, *et al.* Uniparental disomies, homozygous deletions, amplifications and target genes in mantle cell lymphoma revealed by integrative high-resolution whole genome profiling. *Blood* 2009;**113**:3059–69.

103. Jares P, Campo E. Advances in the understanding of mantle cell lymphoma. *Br J Haematol* 2008;**142**:149–65.

104. Rubio-Moscardo F, Climent J, Siebert R, *et al.* Mantle-cell lymphoma genotypes identified with CGH to BAC microarrays define a leukemic subgroup of disease and predict patient outcome. *Blood* 2005;**105**:4445–54.

105. Solenthaler M, Matutes E, Brito-Babapulle V, *et al.* p53 and mdm2 in mantle cell lymphoma in leukemic phase. *Haematologica* 2002;**87**:1141–50.

106. Kohlhammer H, Schwaenen C, Wessendorf S, *et al.* Genomic DNA-chip hybridization in t(11;14)-positive mantle cell lymphomas shows a high frequency of aberrations and allows a refined characterization of consensus regions. *Blood* 2004;**104**:795–801.

107. Jarosova M, Papajik T, Holzerova M, *et al.* High incidence of unbalanced chromosomal changes in mantle cell lymphoma detected by comparative genomic hybridization. *Leuk Lymphoma* 2004;**45**:1835–46.

108. Allen JE, Hough RE, Goepel JR, *et al.* Identification of novel regions of amplification and deletion within mantle cell lymphoma DNA by comparative genomic hybridization. *Br J Haematol* 2002;**116**:291–8.

109. Schraders M, Jares P, Bea S, *et al.* Integrated genomic and expression profiling in mantle cell lymphoma: identification of gene-dosage regulated candidate genes. *Br J Haematol* 2008;**143**:210–21.

110. Ghobrial IM, McCormick DJ, Kaufmann SH, *et al.* Proteomic analysis of mantle-cell lymphoma by protein microarray. *Blood* 2005;**105**:3722–30.

111. Khoury JD, Medeiros LJ, Rassidakis GZ, *et al.* Expression of Mcl-1 in mantle cell lymphoma is associated with high-grade morphology, a high proliferative state, and p53 overexpression. *J Pathol* 2003;**199**:90–7.

112. Cecconi D, Zamo A, Bianchi E, *et al.* Signal transduction pathways of mantle cell lymphoma: a phosphoproteome-based study. *Proteomics* 2008; **8**:4495–506.

113. Tucker CA, Kapanen AI, Chikh G, *et al.* Silencing Bcl-2 in models of mantle cell lymphoma is associated with decreases in cyclin D1, nuclear factor-kappaB, p53, bax, and p27 levels. *Mol Cancer Ther* 2008;**7**:749–58.

114. Tagawa H, Karnan S, Suzuki R, *et al.* Genome-wide array-based CGH for mantle cell lymphoma: identification of homozygous deletions of the proapoptotic gene BIM. *Oncogene* 2005;**24**:1348–58.

115. Pham LV, Tamayo AT, Yoshimura LC, *et al.* Inhibition of constitutive NF-kappa B activation in mantle cell lymphoma B cells leads to induction of cell cycle arrest and apoptosis. *J Immunol* 2003;**171**:88–95.

116. Haidar JH, Neiman RS, Orazi A, *et al.* mdm-2 oncoprotein expression associated with deletion of the long arm of chromosome 12 in a case of mantle cell lymphoma with blastoid transformation [corrected]. *Mod Pathol* 1996;**9**:355–9.

117. Louie DC, Offit K, Jaslow R, *et al.* p53 overexpression as a marker of poor prognosis in mantle cell lymphomas with t(11;14)(q13;q32). *Blood* 1995;**86**:2892–9.

118. Georgakis GV, Li Y, Younes A. The heat shock protein 90 inhibitor 17-AAG induces cell cycle arrest and apoptosis in mantle cell lymphoma cell lines by depleting cyclin D1, Akt, Bid and activating caspase 9. *Br J Haematol* 2006;**135**:68–71.

119. Fisher RI. Mantle-cell lymphoma: classification and therapeutic implications. *Ann Oncol* 1996;**7** Suppl 6: S35–9.

120. Armitage JO. Management of mantle cell lymphoma. *Oncology (Williston Park)* 1998;**12**:49–55.

121. Wong KF, Chan JK, So JC, *et al.* Mantle cell lymphoma in leukemic phase: characterization of its broad cytologic spectrum with emphasis on the importance of distinction from other chronic lymphoproliferative disorders. *Cancer* 1999;**86**:850–7.

122. Schlette E, Lai R, Onciu M, *et al.* Leukemic mantle cell lymphoma: clinical and pathologic spectrum of twenty-three cases. *Mod Pathol* 2001;**14**:1133–40.

123. Michopoulos S, Petraki K, Matsouka C, *et al.* Mantle-cell lymphoma (multiple lymphomatous polyposis) of the entire GI tract. *J Clin Oncol* 2008;**26**:1555–7.

124. Mar N, Khaled S, Kencana F, *et al.* Multiple lymphomatous polyposis as a sole presentation of mantle cell lymphoma. *J Clin Gastroenterol* 2006;**40**:653–4.

125. Romaguera JE, Medeiros LJ, Hagemeister FB, *et al.* Frequency of gastrointestinal involvement and its clinical significance in mantle cell lymphoma. *Cancer* 2003;**97**:586–91.

126. Tamura S, Ohkawauchi K, Yokoyama Y, *et al.* Non-multiple lymphomatous polyposis form of mantle cell lymphoma in the gastrointestinal tract. *J Gastroenterol* 2004;**39**:995–1000.

127. Looi A, Gascoyne RD, Chhanabhai M, *et al.* Mantle cell lymphoma in the ocular adnexal region. *Ophthalmology* 2005;**112**:114–9.

128. Iwuanyanwu E, Medeiros LJ, Romaguera JE, *et al.* Mantle cell lymphoma with a rare involvement of the testicle. *Leuk Lymphoma* 2007;**48**:1242–3.

129. Motegi S, Okada E, Nagai Y, *et al.* Skin manifestation of mantle cell lymphoma. *Eur J Dermatol* 2006;**16**:435–8.

130. Sen F, Medeiros LJ, Lu D, *et al.* Mantle cell lymphoma involving skin: cutaneous lesions may be the first manifestation of disease and tumors often have blastoid cytologic features. *Am J Surg Pathol* 2002;**26**:1312–18.

131. Montserrat E, Bosch F, Lopez-Guillermo A, *et al.* CNS involvement in mantle-cell lymphoma. *J Clin Oncol* 1996;**14**:941–4.

132. Valdez R, Kroft SH, Ross CW, *et al.* Cerebrospinal fluid involvement in mantle cell lymphoma. *Mod Pathol* 2002;**15**:1073–9.

133. Ferrer A, Bosch F, Villamor N, *et al.* Central nervous system involvement in mantle cell lymphoma. *Ann Oncol* 2008;**19**:135–41.

134. Raty R, Franssila K, Joensuu H, *et al.* Ki-67 expression level, histological subtype, and the International Prognostic Index as outcome predictors

in mantle cell lymphoma. *Eur J Haematol* 2002;**69**:11–20.

135. Moller MB, Pedersen NT, Christensen BE. Mantle cell lymphoma: prognostic capacity of the Follicular Lymphoma International Prognostic Index. *Br J Haematol* 2006;**133**:43–9.

136. Hoster E, Dreyling M, Klapper W, *et al.* A new prognostic index (MIPI) for patients with advanced-stage mantle cell lymphoma. *Blood* 2008;**111**:558–65.

137. Tiemann M, Schrader C, Klapper W, *et al.* Histopathology, cell proliferation indices and clinical outcome in 304 patients with mantle cell lymphoma (MCL): a clinicopathological study from the European MCL Network. *Br J Haematol* 2005;**131**:29–38.

138. Katzenberger T, Petzoldt C, Holler S, *et al.* The Ki67 proliferation index is a quantitative indicator of clinical risk in mantle cell lymphoma. *Blood* 2006;**107**:3407.

139. Parrens M, Belaud-Rotureau MA, Fitoussi O, *et al.* Blastoid and common variants of mantle cell lymphoma exhibit distinct immunophenotypic and interphase FISH features. *Histopathology* 2006;**48**:353–62.

140. Romaguera JE, Fayad L, Rodriguez MA, *et al.* High rate of durable remissions after treatment of newly diagnosed aggressive mantle-cell lymphoma with rituximab plus hyper-CVAD alternating with rituximab plus high-dose methotrexate and cytarabine. *J Clin Oncol* 2005; **23**:7013–23.

141. Determann O, Hoster E, Ott G, *et al.* Ki-67 predicts outcome in advanced-stage mantle cell lymphoma patients treated with anti-CD20 immunochemotherapy: results from randomized trials of the European MCL Network and the German Low Grade Lymphoma Study Group. *Blood* 2008;**111**:2385–7.

142. Hsi ED, Jung SH, Lai R, *et al.* Ki67 and PIM1 expression predict outcome in mantle cell lymphoma treated with high dose therapy, stem cell transplantation and rituximab: a Cancer and Leukemia Group B 59909 correlative science study. *Leuk Lymphoma* 2008; **49**:2081–90.

143. Martinez A, Bellosillo B, Bosch F, *et al.* Nuclear survivin expression in mantle cell lymphoma is associated with cell proliferation and survival. *Am J Pathol* 2004;**164**:501–10.

144. Weigert O, Dreyling M. Prognosis of mantle cell lymphoma: is it all about proliferation? *Leuk Lymphoma* 2008;**49**:2029–30.

145. Hartmann E, Fernandez V, Moreno V, *et al.* Five-gene model to predict survival in mantle-cell lymphoma using frozen or formalin-fixed, paraffin-embedded tissue. *J Clin Oncol* 2008;**26**:4966–72.

146. Sup SJ, Domiati-Saad R, Kelley TW, *et al.* ZAP-70 expression in B-cell hematologic malignancy is not limited to CLL/SLL. *Am J Clin Pathol* 2004;**122**:582–7.

147. Admirand JH, Rassidakis GZ, Abruzzo LV, *et al.* Immunohistochemical detection of ZAP-70 in 341 cases of non-Hodgkin and Hodgkin lymphoma. *Mod Pathol* 2004;**17**:954–61.

148. Corradini P, Ladetto M, Zallio F, *et al.* Long-term follow-up of indolent lymphoma patients treated with high-dose sequential chemotherapy and autografting: evidence that durable molecular and clinical remission frequently can be attained only in follicular subtypes. *J Clin Oncol* 2004;**22**:1460–8.

149. Pott C, Hoster E, Böttcher S, *et al.* Molecular remission after combined immunochemotherapy is of prognostic relevance in patients with MCL: results of the Randomized Intergroup Trials of the European MCL Network. *Blood* 2008;**112**:

150. Ghielmini M, Schmitz SF, Burki K, *et al.* The effect of Rituximab on patients with follicular and mantle-cell lymphoma. Swiss Group for Clinical Cancer Research (SAKK). *Ann Oncol* 2000;**11** Suppl 1:123–6.

151. Howard OM, Gribben JG, Neuberg DS, *et al.* Rituximab and CHOP induction therapy for newly diagnosed mantle-cell lymphoma: molecular complete responses are not predictive of progression-free survival. *J Clin Oncol* 2002;**20**:1288–94.

152. Lenz G, Dreyling M, Hoster E, *et al.* Immunochemotherapy with rituximab and cyclophosphamide, doxorubicin, vincristine, and prednisone significantly improves response and time to treatment failure, but not long-term outcome in patients with previously untreated mantle cell lymphoma: results of a prospective randomized trial of the German Low Grade Lymphoma Study Group (GLSG). *J Clin Oncol* 2005;**23**:1984–92.

153. Wilson WH, Grossbard ML, Pittaluga S, *et al.* Dose-adjusted EPOCH chemotherapy for untreated large B-cell lymphomas: a pharmacodynamic approach with high efficacy. *Blood* 2002;**99**:2685–93.

154. Neelapu SS, Kwak LW, Kobrin CB, *et al.* Vaccine-induced tumor-specific immunity despite severe B-cell depletion in mantle cell lymphoma. *Nat Med* 2005;**11**:986–91.

155. Cortes J, O'Brien SM, Pierce S, *et al.* The value of high-dose systemic chemotherapy and intrathecal therapy for central nervous system prophylaxis in different risk groups of adult acute lymphoblastic leukemia. *Blood* 1995;**86**:2091–7.

156. Khouri IF, Romaguera J, Kantarjian H, *et al.* Hyper-CVAD and high-dose methotrexate/cytarabine followed by stem-cell transplantation: an active regimen for aggressive mantle-cell lymphoma. *J Clin Oncol* 1998; **16**:3803–9.

157. Romaguera J, Fayad L, Rodriguez A, *et al.* Rituximab (R) + hypercvad alternating with R-methotrexate/ cytarabine after 9 years: continued high rate of failure-free survival in untreated mantle cell lymphoma (MCL). *Blood* 2008;**112**:833.

158. Shah JJ, Fayad L, Romaguera J. Mantle Cell International Prognostic Index (MIPI) not prognostic after R-hyper-CVAD. *Blood* 2008;**112**:2583; author reply 2583–4.

159. Fayad L, Thomas D, Romaguera J. Update of the M. D. Anderson Cancer Center experience with hyper-CVAD and rituximab for the treatment of mantle cell and Burkitt-type lymphomas. *Clin Lymphoma Myeloma* 2007;**8** Suppl 2:S57–62.

160. Epner E, Unger J, Miller T, *et al.* A multi center trial of hyperCVAD+rituxan in patients with newly diagnosed mantle cell lymphoma. *Blood* 2007;**110**:

161. Kahl BS, Longo WL, Eickhoff JC, *et al.* Maintenance rituximab following induction chemoimmunotherapy may prolong progression-free survival in mantle cell lymphoma: a pilot study from the Wisconsin Oncology Network. *Ann Oncol* 2006;**17**:1418–23.

162. Dreyling M. Hyper-CVAD in mantle-cell lymphoma: really "hyper" or just hype? *Leuk Lymphoma* 2008; **49**:1017–18.

163. Decaudin D, Bosq J, Tertian G, *et al.* Phase II trial of fludarabine monophosphate in patients with mantle-cell lymphomas. *J Clin Oncol* 1998;**16**:579–83.

164. Foran JM, Rohatiner AZ, Coiffier B, *et al.* Multicenter phase II study of fludarabine phosphate for patients with newly diagnosed lymphoplasmacytoid lymphoma, Waldenstrom's macroglobulinemia, and mantle-cell lymphoma. *J Clin Oncol* 1999; **17**:546–53.

165. Cohen BJ, Moskowitz C, Straus D, *et al.* Cyclophosphamide/fludarabine (CF) is active in the treatment of mantle cell lymphoma. *Leuk Lymphoma* 2001;**42**:1015–22.

166. Forstpointner R, Dreyling M, Repp R, *et al.* The addition of rituximab to a combination of fludarabine, cyclophosphamide, mitoxantrone (FCM) significantly increases the response rate and prolongs survival as compared with FCM alone in patients with relapsed and refractory follicular and mantle cell lymphomas: results of a prospective randomized study of the German Low-Grade Lymphoma Study Group. *Blood* 2004;**104**:3064–71.

167. Rummel MJ, Chow KU, Jager E, *et al.* Treatment of mantle-cell lymphomas with intermittent two-hour infusion of cladribine as first-line therapy or in first relapse. *Ann Oncol* 1999;**10**:115–17.

168. Rummel MJ, Chow KU, Karakas T, *et al.* Reduced-dose cladribine (2-CdA) plus mitoxantrone is effective in the treatment of mantle-cell and low-grade non-Hodgkin's lymphoma. *Eur J Cancer* 2002;**38**:1739–46.

169. Robak T, Smolewski P, Cebula B, *et al.* Rituximab combined with cladribine or with cladribine and cyclophosphamide in heavily pretreated patients with indolent lymphoproliferative disorders and mantle cell lymphoma. *Cancer* 2006;**107**:1542–50.

170. Goy A. New directions in the treatment of mantle cell lymphoma: an overview. *Clin Lymphoma Myeloma* 2006;**7** Suppl 1:S24–32.

171. Rummel MJ, Al-Batran SE, Kim SZ, *et al.* Bendamustine plus rituximab is effective and has a favorable toxicity profile in the treatment of mantle cell and low-grade non-Hodgkin's lymphoma. *J Clin Oncol* 2005; **23**:3383–9.

172. Weide R, Hess G, Koppler H, *et al.* High anti-lymphoma activity of bendamustine/mitoxantrone/rituximab in rituximab pretreated relapsed or refractory indolent lymphomas and mantle cell lymphomas. A multicenter phase II study of the German Low Grade Lymphoma Study Group (GLSG). *Leuk Lymphoma* 2007;**48**:1299–306.

173. Rummel M, von Gruenhagen U, Niederle N, *et al.* Bendamustine plus rituximab versus CHOP plus rituximab in the first-line treatment of patients with indolent and mantle cell lymphomas – first interim results of a randomized phase III study of the StiL (Study Group Indolent Lymphomas, Germany). *Blood* 2007;**110**:

174. O'Connor OA, Portlock C, Moskowitz C, *et al.* A multicentre phase II clinical experience with the novel aza-epothilone Ixabepilone (BMS247550) in patients with relapsed or refractory indolent non-Hodgkin lymphoma and mantle cell lymphoma. *Br J Haematol* 2008;**143**:201–9.

175. Coleman M, Martin P, Ruan J, *et al.* Low-dose metronomic, multidrug therapy with the PEP-C oral combination chemotherapy regimen for mantle cell lymphoma. *Leuk Lymphoma* 2008;**49**:447–50.

176. Jacobsen E, Freedman A. An update on the role of high-dose therapy with autologous or allogeneic stem cell transplantation in mantle cell lymphoma. *Curr Opin Oncol* 2004;**16**:106–13.

177. Sweetenham JW. Stem cell transplantation for mantle cell lymphoma: should it ever be used outside clinical trials? *Bone Marrow Transplant* 2001;**28**:813–20.

178. Dreyling M, Lenz G, Hoster E, *et al.* Early consolidation by myeloablative radiochemotherapy followed by autologous stem cell transplantation in first remission significantly prolongs progression-free survival in mantle-cell lymphoma: results of a prospective randomized trial of the European MCL Network. *Blood* 2005;**105**:2677–84.

179. Dreyling M, Hoster E, Van Hoof A, *et al.* Early consolidation with myeloablative radiochemotherapy followed by autologous stem cell transplantation in first remission in mantle cell lymphoma: long term follow up of a randomized trial of GSLG. *Blood* 2008;**112**:769.

180. Vose JM, Bierman PJ, Weisenburger DD, *et al.* Autologous hematopoietic stem cell transplantation for mantle cell lymphoma. *Biol Blood Marrow Transplant* 2000;**6**:640–5.

181. van't Veer MB, de Jong D, Mackenzie M, *et al.* High-dose Ara-C and beam with autograft rescue in R-CHOP responsive mantle cell lymphoma patients. *Br J Haematol* 2009; **144**:524–30.

182. Ganti AK, Bierman PJ, Lynch JC, *et al.* Hematopoietic stem cell transplantation in mantle cell lymphoma. *Ann Oncol* 2005;**16**:618–24.

183. Lefrere F, Delmer A, Levy V, *et al.* Sequential chemotherapy regimens followed by high-dose therapy with stem cell transplantation in mantle cell lymphoma: an update of a prospective study. *Haematologica* 2004;**89**:1275–6.

184. Vandenberghe E, Ruiz de Elvira C, Loberiza FR, *et al.* Outcome of autologous transplantation for mantle cell lymphoma: a study by the European Blood and Bone Marrow Transplant and Autologous Blood and Marrow Transplant Registries. *Br J Haematol* 2003;**120**:793–800.

185. Till BG, Gooley TA, Crawford N, *et al.* Effect of remission status and induction chemotherapy regimen on outcome of autologous stem cell transplantation for mantle cell lymphoma. *Leuk Lymphoma* 2008;**49**:1062–73.

186. Vose J, Loberiza F, Bierman P, *et al.* Mantle cell lymphoma (MCL): induction therapy with hyperCVAD/high-dose methotrexate and cytarabine (M-C) (±rituximab) improves results of autologous stem cell transplant in first remission. *J Clin Oncol* 2006;**24**:7511.

187. Villanueva ML, Vose JM. The role of hematopoietic stem cell transplantation in non-Hodgkin lymphoma. *Clin Adv Hematol Oncol* 2006;**4**:521–30.

188. Evens AM, Winter JN, Hou N, *et al.* A phase II clinical trial of intensive chemotherapy followed by consolidative stem cell transplant: long-term follow-up in newly diagnosed

mantle cell lymphoma. *Br J Haematol* 2008;**140**:385–93.

189. Gopal AK, Rajendran JG, Petersdorf SH, *et al.* High-dose chemo-radioimmunotherapy with autologous stem cell support for relapsed mantle cell lymphoma. *Blood* 2002;**99**:3158–62.

190. Gianni AM, Cortelazzo S, Magni M, *et al.* Rituximab: enhancing stem cell transplantation in mantle cell lymphoma. *Bone Marrow Transplant* 2002;**29** Suppl 1:S10–13.

191. Brugger W, Hirsch J, Grunebach F, *et al.* Rituximab consolidation after high-dose chemotherapy and autologous blood stem cell transplantation in follicular and mantle cell lymphoma: a prospective, multicenter phase II study. *Ann Oncol* 2004;**15**:1691–8.

192. Geisler CH, Kolstad A, Laurell A, *et al.* Long-term progression-free survival of mantle cell lymphoma after intensive front-line immunochemotherapy with in vivo-purged stem cell rescue: a nonrandomized phase 2 multicenter study by the Nordic Lymphoma Group. *Blood* 2008;**112**:2687–93.

193. Magni M, Di Nicola M, Carlo-Stella C, *et al.* High-dose sequential chemotherapy and in vivo rituximab-purged stem cell autografting in mantle cell lymphoma: a 10-year update of the R-HDS regimen. *Bone Marrow Transplant* 2009;**43**:509–11.

194. Dreyling M, Hiddemann W. Dose-intense treatment of mantle cell lymphoma: can durable remission be achieved? *Curr Opin Oncol* 2008;**20**:487–94.

195. Martin P, Chadburn A, Christos P, *et al.* Intensive treatment strategies may not provide superior outcomes in mantle cell lymphoma: overall survival exceeding 7 years with standard therapies. *Ann Oncol* 2008;**19**:1327–30.

196. Martin P, Coleman M, Leonard JP. Progress in mantle-cell lymphoma. *J Clin Oncol* 2009;**27**:481–3.

197. Forstpointner R, Unterhalt M, Dreyling M, *et al.* Maintenance therapy with rituximab leads to a significant prolongation of response duration after salvage therapy with a combination of rituximab, fludarabine, cyclophosphamide, and mitoxantrone (R-FCM) in patients with recurring and refractory follicular and mantle cell lymphomas: results of a prospective randomized study of the German Low Grade Lymphoma Study Group (GLSG). *Blood* 2006;**108**:4003–8.

198. Ghielmini M, Rufibach K, Salles G, *et al.* Single agent rituximab in patients with follicular or mantle cell lymphoma: clinical and biological factors that are predictive of response and event-free survival as well as the effect of rituximab on the immune system: a study of the Swiss Group for Clinical Cancer Research (SAKK). *Ann Oncol* 2005;**16**:1675–82.

199. Osterborg A, Kipps T, Mayer J, *et al.* Ofatumumab (HuMax-CD20), a novel CD20 monoclonal antibody, is an active treatment for patients with CLL refractory to both fludarabine and alemtuzumab or bulky fludarabine-refractory disease: results from the planned interim analysis of an international pivotal trial. 2008.

200. Salles G, Morschhauser F, Cartron G, *et al.* A phase I/II study of RO5072759 (GA101) in patients with relapsed/refractory CD20+ malignant disease. *Blood* 2008;**112**:234.

201. Morris E, Thomson K, Craddock C, *et al.* Outcomes after alemtuzumab-containing reduced-intensity allogeneic transplantation regimen for relapsed and refractory non-Hodgkin lymphoma. *Blood* 2004;**104**:3865–71.

202. Leonard JP, Coleman M, Ketas JC, *et al.* Epratuzumab, a humanized anti-CD22 antibody, in aggressive non-Hodgkin's lymphoma: phase I/II clinical trial results. *Clin Cancer Res* 2004; **10**:5327–34.

203. DiJoseph JF, Dougher MM, Kalyandrug LB, *et al.* Antitumor efficacy of a combination of CMC-544 (inotuzumab ozogamicin), a CD22-targeted cytotoxic immunoconjugate of calicheamicin, and rituximab against non-Hodgkin's B-cell lymphoma. *Clin Cancer Res* 2006;**12**:242–9.

204. Advani R, Furman R, Rosenblatt J, *et al.* A phase I study of humanized anti-CD40 immunotherapy with SGN-40 in non-Hodgkin's lymphoma. *Blood* 2005;**106**: Abstract 1504.

205. Younes Y, Vose J, Zelenetz A, *et al.* Results of a phase 2 trial of HGS-ETR1 (agonistic human monoclonal antibody to TRAIL receptor 1) in subjects with relapsed/refractory non-Hodgkin's lymphoma (NHL). *Blood* 2005;**106**: Abstract 489.

206. Bargou R, Kufer P, Goebeler M, *et al.* Sustained response duration seen after treatment with single agent blinatumomab (MT103/MEDI-538) in the ongoing phase I study MT103-104 in patients with relapsed NHL. *Blood* 2008;**112**:

207. Bashey A, Medina B, Corringham S, *et al.* CTLA4 blockade with ipilimumab to treat relapse of malignancy after allogeneic hematopoietic cell transplantation. *Blood* 2009; **113**:1581–8.

208. Khouri IF, Lee MS, Saliba RM, *et al.* Nonablative allogeneic stem-cell transplantation for advanced/recurrent mantle-cell lymphoma. *J Clin Oncol* 2003;**21**:4407–12.

209. Maris MB, Sandmaier BM, Storer BE, *et al.* Allogeneic hematopoietic cell transplantation after fludarabine and 2 Gy total body irradiation for relapsed and refractory mantle cell lymphoma. *Blood* 2004;**104**:3535–42.

210. Tam CS, Bassett R, Ledesma C, *et al.* Mature results of the MD Anderson Cancer Center risk-adapted transplantation strategy in mantle cell lymphoma. *Blood* 2009;

211. Maloney D. Allogeneic transplantation following nonmyeloablative conditioning for aggressive lymphoma. *Bone Marrow Transplant* 2008;**42** Suppl 1:S35–6.

212. Fowler DH, Odom J, Steinberg SM, *et al.* Phase I clinical trial of costimulated, IL-4 polarized donor CD4+ T cells as augmentation of allogeneic hematopoietic cell transplantation. *Biol Blood Marrow Transplant* 2006;**12**:1150–60.

213. Adams J, Kauffman M. Development of the proteasome inhibitor Velcade (Bortezomib). *Cancer Invest* 2004;**22**:304–11.

214. Weigert O, Jurczak CW, Von Schilling V, *et al.* Efficacy of radioimmunotherapy with (90Y) ibritumomab tiuxetan is superior as consolidation in relapsed or refractory mantle cell lymphoma: results of two phase II trials of the European MCL Network and the PLRG. *J Clin Oncol* 2006;**24**:7533.

215. Zelenetz A. Tositumomab followed by CHOP in sequential therapy for mantle cell lymphoma. *Blood* 2003; Abstract 1477.

216. Smith M, Chen H, Gordon L, *et al.* Phase II study of rituximab + CHOP followed by 90Y-ibritumomab tiuxetan in patients with previously untreated mantle cell lymphoma: an Eastern Cooperative Oncology Group Study (E1499). *J Clin Oncol* 2006; Abstract 7503.

217. Behr TM, Griesinger F, Riggert J, *et al.* High-dose myeloablative radioimmunotherapy of mantle cell non-Hodgkin lymphoma with the iodine-131-labeled chimeric anti-CD20 antibody C2B8 and autologous stem cell support. Results of a pilot study. *Cancer* 2002;**94**:1363–72.

218. Nademanee A, Forman S, Molina A, *et al.* A phase 1/2 trial of high-dose yttrium-90-ibritumomab tiuxetan in combination with high-dose etoposide and cyclophosphamide followed by autologous stem cell transplantation in patients with poor-risk or relapsed non-Hodgkin lymphoma. *Blood* 2005;**106**:2896–902.

219. Krishnan A, Nademanee A, Fung HC, *et al.* Phase II trial of a transplantation regimen of yttrium-90 ibritumomab tiuxetan and high-dose chemotherapy in patients with non-Hodgkin's lymphoma. *J Clin Oncol* 2008;**26**:90–5.

220. Fietz T, Uharek L, Gentilini C, *et al.* Allogeneic hematopoietic cell transplantation following conditioning with 90Y-ibritumomab-tiuxetan. *Leuk Lymphoma* 2006;**47**:59–63.

221. Adams J. The proteasome: a suitable antineoplastic target. *Nat Rev Cancer* 2004;**4**:349–60.

222. Adams J, Palombella VJ, Sausville EA, *et al.* Proteasome inhibitors: a novel class of potent and effective antitumor agents. *Cancer Res* 1999;**59**:2615–22.

223. Goy A, Younes A, McLaughlin P, *et al.* Phase II study of proteasome inhibitor bortezomib in relapsed or refractory B-cell non-Hodgkin's lymphoma. *J Clin Oncol* 2005;**23**:667–75.

224. O'Connor OA, Wright J, Moskowitz C, *et al.* Phase II clinical experience with the novel proteasome inhibitor bortezomib in patients with indolent non-Hodgkin's lymphoma and mantle cell lymphoma. *J Clin Oncol* 2005;**23**:676–84.

225. Belch A, Kouroukis CT, Crump M, *et al.* A phase II study of bortezomib in mantle cell lymphoma: the National Cancer Institute of Canada Clinical Trials Group trial IND.150. *Ann Oncol* 2007;**18**:116–21.

226. Strauss SJ, Maharaj L, Hoare S, *et al.* Bortezomib therapy in patients with relapsed or refractory lymphoma: potential correlation of in vitro sensitivity and tumor necrosis factor alpha response with clinical activity. *J Clin Oncol* 2006;**24**:2105–12.

227. Fisher RI, Bernstein SH, Kahl BS, *et al.* Multicenter phase II study of bortezomib in patients with relapsed or refractory mantle cell lymphoma. *J Clin Oncol* 2006;**24**:4867–74.

228. Goy A, Bernstein SH, Kahl BS, *et al.* Bortezomib in patients with relapsed or refractory mantle cell lymphoma: updated time-to-event analyses of the multicenter phase 2 PINNACLE study. *Ann Oncol* 2009;**20**:520–5.

229. Goy A, Bernstein S, Kahl BS, *et al.* Bortezomib in relapsed or refractory mantle cell lymphoma (MCL): results of the PINNACLE study. *J Clin Oncol (2006 ASCO Annual Meeting Proceedings Part I)* 2006;**24**(185): Abstract 7512.

230. Belch A, Kouroukis C, Crump M, *et al.* Phase II trial of bortezomib in mantle cell lymphoma. *Blood* 2004;**104**: Abstract 608.

231. Goy A, Bernstein S, McDonald A, *et al.* Immunohistochemical analyses for potential biomarkers of bortezomib activity in mantle cell lymphoma from the PINNACLE phase 2 trial. *Blood* 2004;**110**:2573.

232. Gerecitano J, Gounder S, Feldstein J, *et al.* Pre-treatment p27 and Bcl-6 staining levels correlate with response to bortezomib in non-Hodgkin lymphoma: results from a tissue microarray analysis. *Blood* 2008;**210**:1294.

233. Perez-Galan P, Roue G, Villamor N, *et al.* The BH3-mimetic GX15-070 synergizes with bortezomib in mantle cell lymphoma by enhancing Noxa-mediated activation of Bak. *Blood* 2007;**109**:4441–9.

234. Perez-Galan P, Roue G, Villamor N, *et al.* The proteasome inhibitor bortezomib induces apoptosis in mantle-cell lymphoma through generation of ROS and Noxa activation independent of p53 status. *Blood* 2006;**107**:257–64.

235. Mounier N, Ribrag V, Haioun C, *et al.* Efficacy and toxicity of two schedules of R-CHOP plus bortezomib in front-line B lymphoma patients: a randomized phase II trial from the Groupe d'Etude des Lymphomes de l'Adulte (GELA). *J Clin Oncol* 2007;**25**:8010.

236. Leonard J, Furman R, Feldman E, *et al.* Phase I/II trial of bortezomib + CHOP-rituximab in diffuse large B cell (DLBCL) and mantle cell lymphoma (MCL): phase I results. *Blood* 2005;**104**: Abstract 491.

237. Romaguera J, Fayad L, McLaughlin P, *et al.* Phase I trial of bortezomib in combination with rituximab-hyperCVAD/methotrexate and cytarabine for untreated mantle cell lymphoma. *Blood* 2008;**112**:3051.

238. Kahl B, Chang J, Eickhoff J, *et al.* VcR-CVAD produces a high complete response rate in untreated mantle cell lymphoma: a phase II study from the Wisconsin Oncology Network. 2008.

239. Gerecitano J, Portlock C, Hamlin P, *et al.* A phase I study evaluating two dosing schedules of bortezomib (Bor) with rituximab (R), cyclophosphamide (C) and prednisone (P) in patients with relapsed/refractory indolent and mantle cell lymphomas. *J Clin Oncol* 2008;**26**:8512.

240. Mitsiades N, Mitsiades CS, Richardson PG, *et al.* The proteasome inhibitor PS-341 potentiates sensitivity of multiple myeloma cells to conventional chemotherapeutic agents: therapeutic applications. *Blood* 2003;**101**:2377–80.

241. Goy A, Remache Y, Barkoh, *et al.* Sensitivity, schedule-dependence and molecular effects of the proteasome inhibitor bortezomib in non-Hodgkin's lymphoma cells. *Blood* 2004;**104**:389a.

242. Stewart K, O'Connor O, Alsina M, *et al.* Phase I evaluation of carfilzomib (PR-171) in hematological malignancies: responses in multiple myeloma and Waldenstrom's macroglobulinemia at well-tolerated doses. *J Clin Oncol* 2007;**25**:8003.

243. Yewdell JW. Immunoproteasomes: regulating the regulator. *Proc Natl Acad Sci U S A* 2005;**102**:9089–90.

244. Witzig TE, Geyer SM, Ghobrial I, *et al.* Phase II trial of single-agent temsirolimus (CCI-779) for relapsed mantle cell lymphoma. *J Clin Oncol* 2005;**23**:5347–56.

245. Ansell SM, Inwards DJ, Rowland KM Jr, *et al.* Low-dose, single-agent temsirolimus for relapsed mantle cell

lymphoma: a phase 2 trial in the North Central Cancer Treatment Group. *Cancer* 2008;**113**:508–14.

246. Hess G, Romaguera J, Verhoef G, *et al.* Phase III study of patients with relapsed, refractory mantle cell lymphoma treated with temsirolimus compared with investigator's choice therapy. *J Clin Oncol* 2008;**26**:8513.
247. Feldman E, Giles F, Roboz G, *et al.* A phase 2 clinical trial of AP23573, an mTOR inhibitor, in patients with relapsed or refractory hematologic malignancies. *J Clin Oncol* 2005;**23**:6631.
248. Yee KW, Zeng Z, Konopleva M, *et al.* Phase I/II study of the mammalian target of rapamycin inhibitor everolimus (RAD001) in patients with relapsed or refractory hematologic malignancies. *Clin Cancer Res* 2006;**12**:5165–73.
249. Haritunians T, Mori A, O'Kelly J, *et al.* Antiproliferative activity of RAD001 (everolimus) as a single agent and combined with other agents in mantle cell lymphoma. *Leukemia* 2007;**21**:333–9.
250. Reeder C, Gornet M, Habermann T, *et al.* A phase II trial of the oral mTOR inhibitor everolimus (RAD001) in relapsed aggressive non-Hodgkin lymphoma (NHL). *Blood* 2007;**110**:121.
251. Kaufmann H, Raderer M, Wohrer S, *et al.* Antitumor activity of rituximab plus thalidomide in patients with relapsed/refractory mantle cell lymphoma. *Blood* 2004;**104**:2269–71.
252. Wiernik PH, Lossos IS, Tuscano JM, *et al.* Lenalidomide monotherapy in relapsed or refractory aggressive non-Hodgkin's lymphoma. *J Clin Oncol* 2008;**26**:4952–7.
253. Zinzani P, Witzig T, Vose J, *et al.* Confirmation of the efficacy and safety of lenalidomide oral monotherapy in patients with relapsed or refractory mantle-cell lymphoma: results of an international study (NHL-003). *Blood* 2008;**112**:262.
254. Wang M, Fayad L, Hagemeister F, *et al.* A phase I/II study of lenalidomide (Len) in combination with rituximab (R) in relapsed/refractory mantle cell lymphoma (MCL) with early evidence of efficacy. *J Clin Oncol* 2007;**25**:8030.
255. Kahl B. Chemotherapy combinations with monoclonal antibodies in non-Hodgkin's lymphoma. *Semin Hematol* 2008;**45**:90–4.
256. Ramanarayanan J, Hernandez-Ilizaliturri FJ, Chanan-Khan A, *et al.* Pro-apoptotic therapy with the oligonucleotide Genasense (oblimersen sodium) targeting Bcl-2 protein expression enhances the biological anti-tumor activity of rituximab. *Br J Haematol* 2004;**127**:519–30.
257. O'Brien SM, Cunningham CC, Golenkov AK, *et al.* Phase I to II multicenter study of oblimersen sodium, a Bcl-2 antisense oligonucleotide, in patients with advanced chronic lymphocytic leukemia. *J Clin Oncol* 2005;**23**:7697–702.
258. O'Connor OA, Smith EA, Toner LE, *et al.* The combination of the proteasome inhibitor bortezomib and the Bcl-2 antisense molecule oblimersen sensitizes human B-cell lymphomas to cyclophosphamide. *Clin Cancer Res* 2006;**12**:2902–11.
259. Chanan-Khan A. BCL2 antisense therapy in B-cell malignancies. *Blood Rev* 2005;**19**:213–21.
260. Masui T, Hosotani R, Ito D, *et al.* Bcl-XL antisense oligonucleotides coupled with antennapedia enhances radiation-induced apoptosis in pancreatic cancer. *Surgery* 2006;**140**:149–60.
261. Rizzatti EG, Mora-Jensen H, Weniger MA, *et al.* Noxa mediates bortezomib induced apoptosis in both sensitive and intrinsically resistant mantle cell lymphoma cells and this effect is independent of constitutive activity of the AKT and NF-kappaB pathways. *Leuk Lymphoma* 2008;**49**:798–808.
262. Wilson W, O'Connor O, Czuczman M, *et al.* Phase 1 study of ABT-263, a Bcl-2 family inhibitor, in relapsed or refractory lymphoid malignancies. *Blood* 2008;**112**:2108.
263. Deng J, Carlson N, Takeyama K, *et al.* BH3 profiling identifies three distinct classes of apoptotic blocks to predict response to ABT-737 and conventional chemotherapeutic agents. *Cancer Cell* 2007;**12**:171–85.
264. Patricia Perez Galan GR, Neus Villamor, Elias Campo, Dolors Colomer. The small molecule Pan-Bcl-2 inhibitor GX15–070 induces apoptosis in vitro in mantle cell lymphoma (MCL) cells and exhibits a synergistic effect in combination with the proteasome inhibitor bortezomib. *Blood* 2005;**106**:Abstract 1490.
265. Goy A, Ford P, Feldman T, *et al.* A phase 1 trial of the Pan Bcl-2 family inhibitor obatoclax mesylate (GX15–070) in combination with bortezomib in patients with relapsed/refractory mantle cell lymphoma. *Blood* 2007;**110**:2569.
266. Ichikawa K, Liu W, Zhao L, *et al.* Tumoricidal activity of a novel anti-human DR5 monoclonal antibody without hepatocyte cytotoxicity. *Nat Med* 2001;**7**:954–60.
267. O'Connor OA, Heaney ML, Schwartz L, *et al.* Clinical experience with intravenous and oral formulations of the novel histone deacetylase inhibitor suberoylanilide hydroxamic acid in patients with advanced hematologic malignancies. *J Clin Oncol* 2006; **24**:166–73.
268. Eucker J, Sterz J, Krebbel H, *et al.* Peroxisome proliferator-activated receptor-gamma ligands inhibit proliferation and induce apoptosis in mantle cell lymphoma. *Anticancer Drugs* 2006;**17**:763–9.
269. Nawrocki ST, Carew JS, Pino MS, *et al.* Aggresome disruption: a novel strategy to enhance bortezomib-induced apoptosis in pancreatic cancer cells. *Cancer Res* 2006;**66**:3773–81.
270. Kouroukis CT, Belch A, Crump M, *et al.* Flavopiridol in untreated or relapsed mantle-cell lymphoma: results of a phase II study of the National Cancer Institute of Canada Clinical Trials Group. *J Clin Oncol* 2003;**21**:1740–5.
271. Lin TS, Howard OM, Neuberg DS, *et al.* Seventy-two hour continuous infusion flavopiridol in relapsed and refractory mantle cell lymphoma. *Leuk Lymphoma* 2002;**43**:793–7.
272. Brown JR. Chronic lymphocytic leukemia: a niche for flavopiridol? *Clin Cancer Res* 2005;**11**:3971–3.
273. Byrd JC, Lin TS, Dalton JT, *et al.* Flavopiridol administered using a pharmacologically derived schedule is associated with marked clinical efficacy in refractory, genetically high-risk chronic lymphocytic leukemia. *Blood* 2007;**109**:399–404.

274. Lin T, Fischer B, Moran M, *et al.* Flavopiridol, fludarabine and rituximab is a highly active regimen in indolent B-cell lymphoproliferative disorders including mantle cell lymphoma. *Blood* 2005;**106**:944.

275. Graff JR, McNulty AM, Hanna KR, *et al.* The protein kinase Cbeta-selective inhibitor, Enzastaurin (LY317615.HCl), suppresses signaling through the AKT pathway, induces apoptosis, and suppresses growth of human colon cancer and glioblastoma xenografts. *Cancer Res* 2005; **65**:7462–9.

276. Lam LT, Davis RE, Pierce J, *et al.* Small molecule inhibitors of IkappaB kinase are selectively toxic for subgroups of diffuse large B-cell lymphoma defined by gene expression profiling. *Clin Cancer Res* 2005;**11**: 28–40.

277. Rabson AB, Weissmann D. From microarray to bedside: targeting NF-kappaB for therapy of lymphomas. *Clin Cancer Res* 2005; **11**:2–6.

Chapter

18 Follicular lymphomas

Francisco J. Hernandez-Ilizaliturri and Myron S. Czuczman

Introduction

Follicular lymphoma (FL) is the most common type of indolent B-cell lymphoma diagnosed in the United States. A better understanding of the biology of disease and the development of novel targeted agents are challenging prior dogmatic concepts regarding the standard therapeutic approach to FL.

In recent years, the lymphoma field has seen significant progress with respect to the identification of clinical, tumor-associated, and host-associated prognostic factors, as well as the development of novel functional imaging (e.g., positron emission tomography [PET] scans). Improvements in molecular diagnostics allow a clearer distinction between various lymphoma subtypes. Perhaps the single most important advance has been the development and integration of monoclonal antibodies (mAbs) into the treatment of B-cell lymphoma which has resulted in a steady improvement in progression-free survival (PFS) and overall survival (OS) of patients. This chapter summarizes the advances achieved in the last two decades that have led to the current approach and management of patients with FL.

Pathogenesis of FL

As technology and its applications have improved over the last two decades, there has been a parallel improvement in our understanding of the molecular mechanisms responsible not only for the development of FL, but also to explain its clinical heterogeneity. Ontologically, FL arises from germinal B cells usually as a result of deregulation in the apoptotic machinery. FL was one of the first lymphomas in which a molecular defect was defined.[1] The characteristic t(14;18) translocation that deregulates the *BCL2* gene, a key regulator of the cell death process, was recognized in FL patients in the early 1980s and the translocation partners were cloned and identified by several investigators.[2–4]

In contrast to normal germinal B cells, FL harboring the t(14;18) or similar genetic aberrations evade programmed cell death upon antigenic selection and become immortalized. The t(14;18) translocates the *BCL2* gene to the immunoglobulin heavy chain (IGH) gene locus, placing the *BCL2* gene under the influence of the IGH enhancer, resulting in the overexpression of BCL2 protein. While the majority of the FL will express higher levels of BCL2 (90%) this can also be the result of other less common observed genetic translocations such as t(2;18) and t(18;22).[5–7] Approximately 10% of the FL do not express BCL2, suggesting the existence of alternative mechanisms for preventing apoptosis (e.g., survivin, Mcl-1, BCL-XL, etc.).[7,8] It has been demonstrated that BCL2-negative FL may produce BCL2 protein in a mutated but functional form that does not react with commonly used anti-BCL2 antibodies for immunohistochemistry (IHC) or Western blotting.[9]

The t(14;18) or similar genetic aberrations are necessary but not sufficient alone for the transformation of a germinal B cell into a malignant state. BCL2 transgenic mice develop polyclonal B-cell hyperplasia of long-living resting B cells.[10] Transformation into a monoclonal B-cell lymphoma occurs only after a long period of latency where the acquisition of secondary genetic "hits" takes place.[11]

Similar to what was observed in the transgenic mice models, the majority of patients with FL show at least one additional karyotypic abnormality in addition to the t(14;18) with an average of six alterations.[12] These findings support a natural selection model of accumulation of genetic abnormalities and clonal selection in the development and progression of FL. The complexity of the genetic alterations increases parallel to the histologic grade and degree of transformation.[12–14] Studies from the British Columbia Cancer Agency have identified cytogenetic abnormalities present early in the course of the disease such as −6q, dup der(18)t(14;18), and +7/+8 as compared to del17, +12, +1q, and −1p which are observed as late events.[15]

High-output technologies such as gene microarrays are providing insightful information in the biology and prognosis of B-cell lymphomas, including FL.[16–21] The tumor microenvironment appears to play an important role in the development, maintenance, and progression of FL.[19–21] Recently available

Management of Hematologic Malignancies, ed. Susan M. O'Brien, Julie M. Vose, and Hagop M. Kantarjian. Published by Cambridge University Press.

gene expression data demonstrated the existence of two gene signature profiles that reflect two subtypes of non-malignant tumor-infiltrating immune cells. The first gene-signature profile was named immune response 1 and is characterized by high expression of T-cell marker genes. The second gene signature was named immune response 2 and is characterized by genes preferentially expressed by dendritic cells (DC) and/or macrophages.[19]

The delicate balance between the type and activation state of DC, T-cells, and macrophages that results in the genetic signatures detected by microarray technology (e.g., immune response 1 vs. immune response 2) can be potentially driven by the genetic alterations observed in the FL cells and potentially impact clinical behavior, "sensitivity" to rituximab therapy, and transformation risk. In her seminal paper, Dr. de Jong postulated a model for the development of FL that incorporates the information obtained from cytogenetic studies and microarray gene profiling.[22] She proposes the existence of a dual model for FL. The initial event is the resistance to apoptosis upon antigen selection secondary to BCL2 overexpression driven by the t(14;18) or equivalent genetic aberrations. Subsequently, early secondary alterations will affect the tumor microenvironment resulting in the progression of FL into two separate subtypes of FL. The first one is a poor-prognosis pathway characterized by the induction of activated DC and activated T cells and manifested by rapid clinical progression and early transformation into diffuse large B-cell lymphoma. The second one is a good-prognosis pathway that results in a resting DC and T-cell network manifested by genetic stability and slow clinical progression. Therefore, FL is likely a disease of functional B cells in which the clinical behavior is determined by the intrinsic characteristics of the malignant cells and their interactions with surrounding immunologic cells.[19,21] Current research will likely further elucidate the important relationship between FL and the tumor microenvironment and concomitantly lead to the development of therapeutic strategies with novel mechanisms of action and improved therapeutic indices compared to standard chemotherapeutic agents.

Risk stratification and prognostic factors in FL

The clinical course of FL while manifested by multiple relapses varies from patient to patient. It is unclear to physicians and scientists why some FL patients have a long and indolent disease course while others have a more aggressive course or even early transformation and death. In addition, as the spectrum of therapeutic approaches for FL patients is becoming as diverse and varied as the course of the disease (e.g., from "watchful waiting" to high-dose chemotherapy and autologous or allogeneic stem cell transplantation [SCT]), it has become a major challenge to determine the optimal type of therapy (e.g., immunotherapy, chemoimmunotherapy, radioimmunotherapy, SCT, etc.) and its optimal sequencing for an individual patient.

Development of clinical predictors of outcome in FL patients

The development and validation of an accurate and easily available prognostic index for FL has facilitated the development of treatment algorithm plans, enabled crosstalk between investigators, and improved the understanding of the results of clinical studies.[23–25] At the beginning the International Prognostic Index (IPI) criteria, originally developed for patients with diffuse large B-cell lymphoma, was applied to FL. Early enthusiasm for the use of IPI in FL was followed by the realization that it was lacking in its ability to distribute patients between all risk groups.[23,24] Subsequently, a multinational effort resulted in the development and validation of the Follicular Lymphoma International Prognostic Index (FLIPI). The FLIPI score has evolved into a valuable tool for assessing FL risk and in helping to assess the comparability of patient populations between different clinical trials.[25] Briefly, the FLIPI score was designed by studying clinical characteristics of 1795 newly diagnosed FL between 1985 and 1992 across 27 different cancer centers that were treated with various chemotherapeutic approaches. Several clinical parameters known to affect the outcome of FL patients were tested in the patient population using a univariate and multivariate analysis. The statistical analysis identified five variables that strongly and independently were associated with a poor clinical outcome: age $>$ 60 years, Ann Arbor stage III–IV, hemoglobin level $<$ 12 g/dL, LDH $>$ upper limit of normal (ULN), and $>$ 4 nodal sites of disease (Figure 18.1). Based on this clinical characteristic FL patients could be categorized in three risk groups with different 5- and 10-year survival rates: "low-risk" (0–1 adverse factor present) with 5- and 10-year survival rates of 90.6% and 70.7%, respectively; "intermediate risk" (2 factors present) with 5- and 10-year survival rates of 77.6% and 50.9%, respectively; and "high-risk" ($\geq$ 3 risk factors present) with 5- and 10-year survival rates of 52.5% and 35.2%, respectively (Figure 18.1). The clinical outcome estimated by the FLIPI score was subsequently validated in 919 consecutive FL patients by the same group of investigators, proved superior to IPI, and sustained its predictive value even in patients receiving front-line chemoimmunotherapy (i.e., R-CHOP [rituximab plus cyclophosphamide, doxorubicin, vincristine, and prednisone]).[25,26]

While the development of the FLIPI score has aided in improving the categorization of FL patients in clinical studies, there exists an important goal to further risk-stratify FL patients by incorporating biologic information into risk calculations. An initial effort was the use of morphological parameters in the biopsy specimen (e.g., histologic grade or the presence of diffuse areas). However, because of lack of reproducibility these factors were not widely accepted. One notable exception to this is the "poor-risk" distinction of grade 3B FL from the rest of FL since this subset has a clinical behavior similar to patients with diffuse large B-cell lymphoma (DLBCL).[27–29]

Recent and ongoing studies looking at gene expression profiles and proteomic arrays are potentially more powerful and innovative strategies for risk stratification, but require validation and standardization before they are implemented in clinical practice.

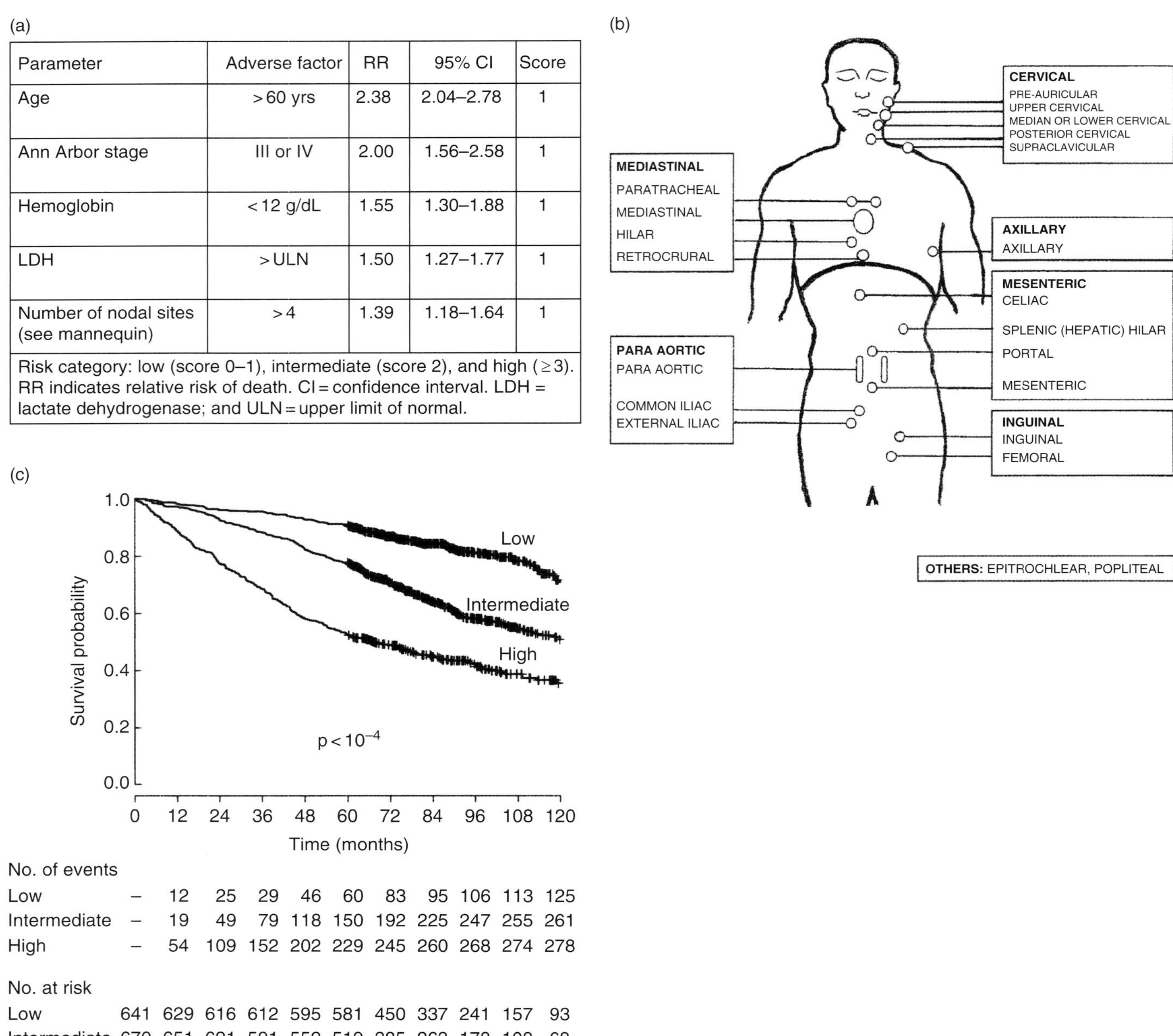

(a)

Parameter	Adverse factor	RR	95% CI	Score
Age	> 60 yrs	2.38	2.04–2.78	1
Ann Arbor stage	III or IV	2.00	1.56–2.58	1
Hemoglobin	< 12 g/dL	1.55	1.30–1.88	1
LDH	> ULN	1.50	1.27–1.77	1
Number of nodal sites (see mannequin)	> 4	1.39	1.18–1.64	1

Risk category: low (score 0–1), intermediate (score 2), and high (≥3). RR indicates relative risk of death. CI = confidence interval. LDH = lactate dehydrogenase; and ULN = upper limit of normal.

No. of events	0	12	24	36	48	60	72	84	96	108	120
Low	–	12	25	29	46	60	83	95	106	113	125
Intermediate	–	19	49	79	118	150	192	225	247	255	261
High	–	54	109	152	202	229	245	260	268	274	278

No. at risk	0	12	24	36	48	60	72	84	96	108	120
Low	641	629	616	612	595	581	450	337	241	157	93
Intermediate	670	651	621	591	552	519	385	263	178	108	68
High	484	430	375	332	282	255	193	139	98	56	33

Figure 18.1 The Follicular Lymphoma International Prognostic Index (FLIPI) score. The score was developed from analyzing clinical and demographic characteristics of 1795 patients with follicular lymphoma. Five parameters were associated with an adverse clinical outcome and used to develop a risk category score (a and b). The FLIPI score was able to identify three groups of patients with different clinical outcome as determined by overall survival after systemic chemotherapy (c). Adapted with permission from Solal-Celigny *et al. Blood* 2004;**104**:1258–65[25] and Buske *et al. Blood* 2006;**108**:1504–8.[26]

Prediction of survival in FL based on gene expression signatures and validation studies

Dave *et al.* on behalf of the Leukemia Lymphoma Molecular Profiling Project (LLMPP) consortium reported the identification of two main gene signature profiles that were independently associated with FL survival.[19] The investigators of the LLMPP consortium conducted a whole-genome microarray analysis of nucleic acids in 286 FL specimens using affymetrix microarrays. Of the two main gene signature profiles, immune response 1 included genes encoding for T-cell markers and the immune response 2 included genes associated with DC and macrophage markers. The investigators built and validated a molecular predictor score based on these two gene signatures and were able to classify patients in four risk-categories with different survival (Figure 18.2).[19] Of interest, the genetic alterations observed in the microarray analysis by the LLMPP consortium were restricted to the non-malignant

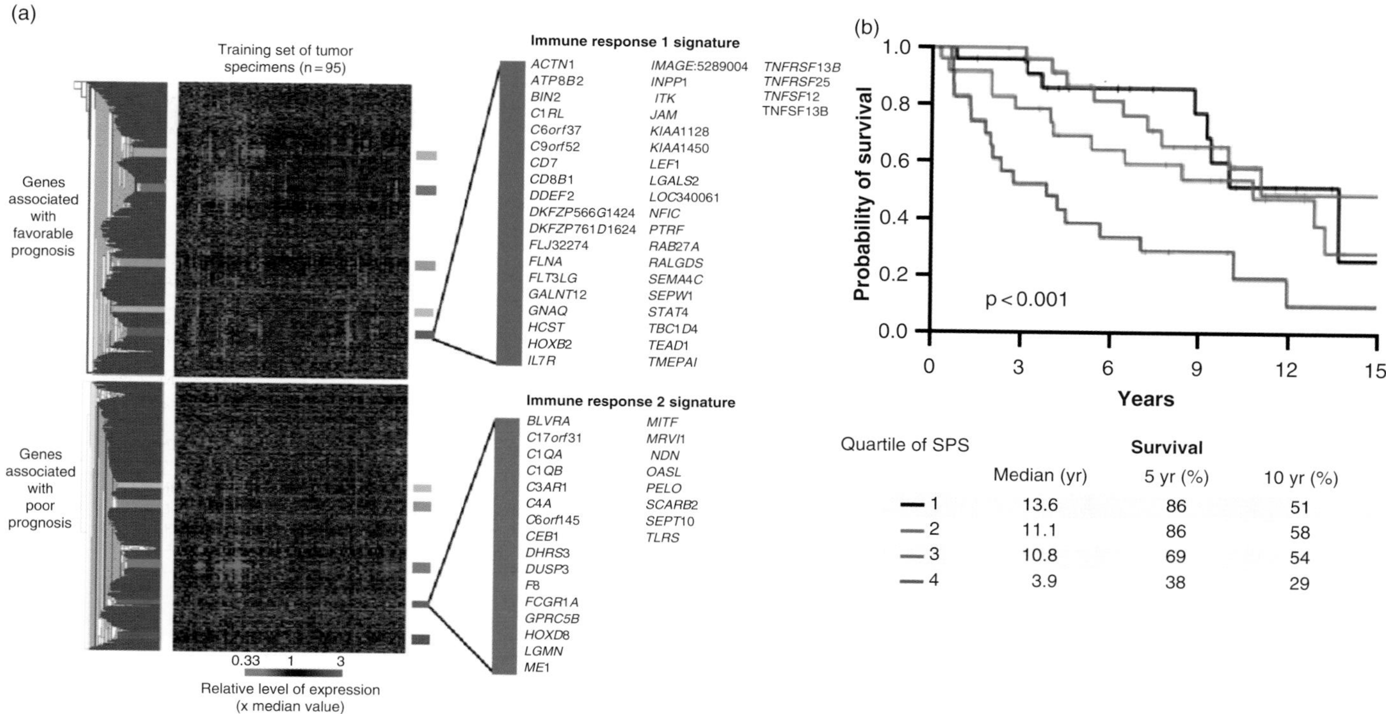

Figure 18.2 Gene-profiling microarrays to predict the clinical outcome of patients with follicular lymphoma (FL). Gene profiling was performed in the training set of 95 FL biopsy specimens (a). The data are represented in a grid format in which each column represents a single case of FL, and each row a single gene. The relative level of gene expression is depicted according to the color scale shown. To the right, the genes making up the immune response 1 and immune response 2 signatures that formed the survivor predictor model are listed (a). The two signatures were used to create a model in the training set in which a survival-predictor score (SPS) was assigned to each patient. Patients' SPS were separated into quartiles. There was a direct relationship between the SPS and the 5- and 10-year survival in patients with FL (b). Adapted with permission from Dave *et al. N Engl J Med* 2004;**351**:2159–69.[19]

tumor-infiltrating cells, stressing the likely importance of the tumor microenvironment in the development, maintenance, and progression of FL. It is important to note that the specimens obtained in this study consisted of lymphoma specimens treated in the pre-rituximab era when extrapolating data in today's immunotherapy-based therapies and need further prospective validation in the context of well-designed clinical trials.

Recently, Harjunpää *et al.* attempted to differentiate the clinical outcomes of 64 FL patients treated with R-CHOP using oligonucleotide microarrays.[30] In this innovative study, the investigators were able to identify and validate via quantitative polymerase chain reaction (qPCR) and IHC three genes associated with differences in duration of response following R-CHOP therapy. High levels of EPHA1 (a tyrosine kinase involved in trans-epithelial migration) and low levels of SMAD1 (a transcription factor) and MARCO (a scavenger receptor on macrophages) were associated with better PFS. Although the patient population study was small and validation studies were not consistent, their data demonstrated that non-tumor immune cells appear to play a major role in sensitivity to R-CHOP chemoimmunotherapy.[30]

Additional studies using whole-genome microarrays have focused on evaluating the risk of transformation and/or responsiveness to rituximab immunotherapy. The results obtained from these studies further support the importance of immune cells surrounding the malignant B cell in the clinical behavior of FL patients.[20,31]

Finally, an elegant study recently addressed the influence of the cytokine environment in the clinical outcome of patients with FL. The investigators postulated that germline single nucleotide polymorphisms (SNPs) present in immune genes can be responsible for differences in the survival of patients with FL. Using an extremely complicated statistical analysis, the investigators were able to identify four SNPs in the interleukin (IL)-8, IL-2, IL-12B, and IL-1RN (IL-1 receptor antagonist) genes associated with survival. Using these four SNPs the investigators were able to create a risk score and classify patients in three groups, low, intermediate, and high risk associated with different 5-year survival (i.e., 96%, 72%, and 58%, respectively).[32] The potential value of this study lies with the wide availability of the technique used for SNPs detection. However, further studies to confirm this finding in independent cohorts are underway before it is recommended for clinical practice.

Attempts to extrapolate data from gene profiling studies to immunohistochemical biomarker studies to predict prognosis in FL

The results obtained from gene microarray studies prompted several investigators to attempt to validate the prognostic factors at the protein level using less expensive, readily available laboratory techniques (e.g., IHC).[33–37] One group of investigators reported that a high number of tumor-infiltrating macrophages (TAM), as determined by CD68 staining, was associated with a poor clinical outcome in FL patients treated with systemic chemotherapy.[33] Subsequently, this observation was also noted by other researchers in patients receiving rituximab in combination with systemic chemotherapy +/− interferon.[34] Of interest, Taskinen *et al.* reported that a high number of TAM was associated with a better clinical outcome, whereas a higher number of tumor-infiltrating mast cells (MC) was associated with a worse prognosis in FL patients receiving R-CHOP chemoimmunotherapy.[35,37] The conflictive result observed in IHC studies stresses not only the limitation of currently available laboratory techniques, but also how rituximab therapy may change the predictive value of previously validated prognostic factors which utilized different therapy. The ongoing challenge is to identify and prospectively validate predictor factors that can be implemented to different therapeutic interventions, so that they can be used in tailoring treatments for FL patients. The establishment of tissue banks at academic centers to preserve lymphatic tissue at time of diagnosis and relapse (e.g., especially "paired" specimens) is critical in order to provide researchers with ample material that can be used in the future development and validation of biomarkers in FL.

Management of FL: changing the natural course of the disease

In contrast to aggressive forms of B-cell lymphomas, FL has long been considered an incurable disease. The historical course of the FL is classically characterized by initial response to a given therapy, followed by subsequent relapses with shorter periods of remission and subsequent development of refractory disease. Outcomes were not significantly altered by the use of standard chemotherapy +/− radiotherapy approaches.

The use of single-agent chemotherapy agents (e.g., alkylating compounds, nucleoside analogs), or combination chemotherapy regimens (e.g., CHOP or cyclophosphamide, vincristine, and prednisone [CVP]) were felt to be promising initially, but did not result in a prolonged duration of response or improvement in OS in FL. In fact, a standard systemic chemotherapy approach did not extend OS beyond what could be obtained by initial "watchful waiting" followed by palliative therapy upon development of symptomatic disease.

As a result of the data generated from these early clinical trials, a dogma regarding the incurability of FL dominated the medical field for several decades. The development and integration of promising targeted therapies (e.g., initially rituximab and radioconjugated anti-CD20 mAbs) appear to be changing the historic treatment paradigm in FL patients today.

There are several challenges encountered by the oncologist managing patients with FL. Controversies exist regarding the best time to start therapy, how to choose between varied treatment options, how to balance the efficacy versus toxicity when making treatment decisions, and which end points (e.g., palliation of symptoms versus long-term disease-free survival [DFS]) are to be achieved.

Table 18.1. Criteria for starting a cytotoxic treatment in patients with follicular lymphoma (FL)

The Groupe pour l'Etude de Lymphome Folliculaire (GELF)	The British National Lymphoma Investigation (BNLI)
High tumor bulk defined by either: A tumor > 7 cm 3 nodes in 3 distinct areas each > 3 cm	Rapid generalized disease progression in the preceding 3 months
Symptomatic spleen enlargement	
Organ compression	
Ascites or pleura effusion	
Presence of systemic symptoms	Life-threatening organ involvement
ECOG performance status > 1	Renal infiltration
Serum LDH or β_2-microglobulin above normal values	Bone lesions
	Presence of systemic symptoms: Hemoglobin < 10 g/dL or WBC count < 1.5 × 10^9/L, or platelet counts < 100 × 10^9/L; related to bone marrow involvement

Notes: LDH: lactate dehydrogenase; WBC: white blood cell; ECOG: Eastern Cooperative Oncology Group.

Challenges in determining the best time to initiate local or systemic therapy in patients with FL

Some clinical scenarios are associated with relatively straightforward treatment decisions: (1) Stage I or II FL (refers to World Health Organization [WHO] follicular lymphoma, grade 1 or 2 throughout this text, unless otherwise specified) treated with involved-field radiation therapy (IFRT); or (2) advanced-stage FL patients with progressive/symptomatic disease treated with systemic therapy. The Groupe pour l'Etude de Lymphome Folliculaire (GELF) and The British National Lymphoma Investigation (BNLI) had proposed and used defined criteria for patients for whom immediate therapy is necessary (Table 18.1).[38,39] For the relatively lucky 15–30% of FL patients to be diagnosed with stage I or II disease, upfront IFRT has been shown to give long-term local control and possible cure in a significant subset of patients.[40,41] More commonly, FL patients are found to have asymptomatic, advanced-stage disease at presentation. As mentioned above, few physicians would question the necessity of initiating therapy in those FL patients with symptomatic and/or rapidly progressive disease at time of diagnosis. However, the accepted and long-honored practice of "watchful waiting" of asymptomatic advanced-stage FL patients needs to be reanalyzed and revalidated in today's era of targeted therapies. In the pre-rituximab era, standard chemotherapy-based treatments, whether single-versus multiagent (e.g., oral cyclophosphamide; CVP; CHOP; fludarabine $\pm$ mitoxantrone $\pm$ dexamethasone [FMD], etc.), did not appear to change the natural relapsing history or OS for FL patients. Historically, patients with advanced-stage FL were found to have a median OS of 8–10 years.[42] The delay of "toxic" therapy until "needed" allowed patients to maintain a better quality of life by avoiding acute chemotherapy-associated side effects and perhaps even long-term toxicities by limiting cumulative doses of drugs +/− IFRT associated with the development of secondary myelodysplastic syndromes (MDS) or acute myelogenic leukemia (AML).

In view of the ability to achieve prolonged (i.e., $\geq$ 5 years) remission duration from recent trials evaluating upfront immunotherapy/radioimmunotherapy alone or in combination with standard chemotherapeutic regimens brings the age-old practice of watchful waiting for the majority of asymptomatic FL patients into question yet again. Several important clinical trials addressing the issues of watchful waiting versus immediate treatment with "conventional" therapy need to be briefly reviewed. The US National Cancer Institute (NCI) studied 104 advanced indolent lymphoma patients in a randomized clinical trial as follows: 44 were randomly assigned to "watch-and-wait"; 45 assigned to aggressive, upfront combination chemotherapy with prednisone, methotrexate, doxorubicin, cyclophosphamide, plus etoposide plus mechlorethamine, vincristine, procarbazine, prednisone (ProMACE-MOPP), followed by total nodal irradiation (TNI); and 15 "symptomatic" patients requiring therapy received the aggressive combination chemotherapy without randomization.[43] Of note, patients in the "watch-and-wait" arm could receive palliative RT to control localized disease and remain in the "watch-and-wait" group, but would be treated with ProMACE-MOPP for non-localized progressive disease. Initial results demonstrated OS at 5 years of greater than 75% in both arms, but of interest was a 4-year DFS of 51% vs. 12% and "continuous" DFS of 51% vs. 0% noted in favor of the initial aggressive therapy arm vs. watchful-waiting arm, respectively. As part of a commentary on a FL review article, principal investigator Dr. Dan Longo briefly updated this NCI trial: he noted that in 1997, with a median follow-up of 13 years, no difference in OS was seen between arms; however, 75% of patients assigned to aggressive treatment who were alive were "continuously" cancer-free, in contrast to 75% of the patients in the watch-and-wait arm who were alive with lymphoma.[44] Brice *et al.* from the GELF randomized low-tumor-burden FL patients between initial watch-and-wait, predimustine (200 mg/m^2 per day for 5 days per month $\times$ 18 months), or interferon alpha (IFN-α) (5 MU/day for 3 months, then 5 MU thrice weekly $\times$ 15 months).[38] Deferred therapy was found to not adversely affect 5-year OS, which was 78%, 70%, and 84% in arms 1, 2, and 3, respectively. However, neither single-agent predimustine, nor IFN-α would be considered as standard therapies for treatment of FL by oncologists today. A multicenter trial done by the BNLI randomized more than 300 asymptomatic, advanced-stage indolent (204 FL) lymphoma patients to immediate chlorambucil (up to 10 mg po qd until complete response [CR]) versus delayed chlorambucil (i.e., started at time of clinical progression).[39] Following a median follow-up of 16 years, OS was similar in both groups (i.e., 5.9 years with immediate chlorambucil and 6.7 years with observation). Of interest was the observation that immediate-therapy patients had higher CR rates (i.e., 63% CR) compared with delayed-therapy patients (i.e., CR rate of 27%). These data suggest that asymptomatic FL may be more sensitive to oral alkylator therapy earlier on as compared to later on during its natural history. It is unknown whether a lower CR rate in prior watch-and-wait patients is associated with a reduced efficacy of subsequent therapies. Lastly, Peterson *et al.* published a Cancer and Leukemia Group B (CALGB) study in which 228 newly diagnosed stage III/IV follicular small cleaved cell (FSCC) and follicular mixed lymphoma (FML) patients were randomized between one of two immediate-treatment arms: oral cyclophosphamide versus CHOP-bleomycin combination chemotherapy.[45] No treatment advantage was seen in either group: at 10 years overall time to failure was found to be 25% versus 33% ($p = 0.107$) and OS of 44% versus 46% ($p = 0.79$) between the two arms, respectively. Approximately 50% of the patients in both arms were asymptomatic. In an unplanned subgroup analysis, it was found that FML patients who received combination CHOP-bleomycin had improvement in disease control and survival compared to patients treated with oral alkylator therapy. At the current time it would be extremely tedious, if not nearly impossible, to attempt to go back and re-examine individual patients and data from the aforementioned trials with respect to: reassigning pathology using current WHO classification criteria; utilizing and documenting the FLIPI score of each study patient to ensure that we are comparing "similar" populations between treatment arms and different studies; applying the same response criteria in all studies; and comparing the restaging methods and schedule between all studies to determine their potential impact on outcomes. A plausible explanation as to why OS was not impacted between treatment arms in the aforementioned studies is that pure chemotherapy-based non-myeloablative therapies lack "curative" potential. Comparing today's novel target-specific therapeutic approach and optimistic results from recent chemoimmunotherapy and radioimmunotherapy trials, the results from earlier studies could be summarized as: "*Suboptimal therapy in = suboptimal results out!*" In order to help answer the original question: "When is the best time to start therapy for patients with FL?" a large national/international watchful-waiting versus immediate "chemoimmunotherapy-based" clinical trial in advanced-stage asymptomatic FL patients with monitoring of well-described clinical, laboratory, and pathological features is warranted. Possibly, newly diagnosed FL patients with "good-risk" disease may prove to be the optimal subgroup to benefit from today's novel biological-based treatments.

Navigating the treatment options for patients with FL

Once the decision to start therapy has been made, the practicing oncologist is faced with the challenge of which therapy to use first and how to balance the benefit:risk ratio for each FL patient. Before definitive guidelines can be developed, additional information with respect to a better understanding of the optimal antitumor activity of agents for a given subset of FL patients, as well as their optimal "sequencing" in order to not diminish the number of future therapeutic options, is needed. At the current time, the "aggressiveness" of either initial or subsequent treatment is largely dependent on several factors: (1) tumor characteristics (rate of tumor growth, tumor bulk, etc.); (2) clinical/laboratory characteristics (e.g., FLIPI score; elevated LDH, etc.); and (3) patient characteristics (e.g., comorbid medical problems, "goal of therapy," patient's wishes). Recent publications that evaluate prognostic factors associated with response to a specific therapy (e.g., rituximab monotherapy or combined chemoimmunotherapy)[46–48] will hopefully help guide future treatment decisions. Furthermore, a review of the literature on radioimmunotherapy (RIT) strongly suggests that patients achieving CRs (e.g., more prevalent in low tumor burden and/or non-bulky disease) are the subgroup that achieve the longest DFS from this treatment modality.[49,50] In general, it is our opinion that the ideal upfront treatment strategy to use is an induction regimen that (based on the patient's clinical and biologic characteristics) will hopefully achieve the highest rate of complete molecular response (Figure 18.3).

Biologic agents

Historically, cytokines were one of the first targeted agents utilized against non-Hodgkin lymphoma (NHL). IFN-α is a cytokine with various effects in both immunoeffector and cancer cells. In effector cells, IFN-α increases the expression of MHC class I antigens, stimulates the secretion of other cytokines, and/or augments the cytotoxic activity of natural killer (NK) cells.[51] On the other hand, IFN-α lowers the sensitivity threshold to the action of other cytokines in tumor cells.[51] In vitro studies revealed that IFN-α enhances the antitumor activity of anti-idiotype antibodies or immunotoxins; the synergistic effects observed are via upregulation of antigen expression and/or enhanced cellular cytotoxicity.[52–55] IFN-α has been used, with modest antitumor activity, in patients with low-grade NHL as a single agent or in combination with anthracycline-containing regimens.[56,57] A major obstacle to the practical use of IFN-α is its toxicity profile and limited antitumor activity.

IL-2 is a cytokine produced by T cells that affects the function of normal B lymphocytes, NK cells, and monocytes. In vitro studies had demonstrated NK cell expansion and activation occurs following IL-2 exposure.[58,59] In addition, multiple preclinical models have demonstrated that IL-2 enhances the antitumor activity of various monoclonal antibodies including rituximab.[60–62] Clinical trials are exploring alternate IL-2 formulations, dosing, and/or schedules of administration in rituximab-refractory lymphoma patients.[63,64]

The development of monoclonal antibodies (mAbs) for the treatment of FL

The concept of using mAbs to treat lymphoma was initially tested in the early 1980s when two independent groups of investigators reported the first cases of lymphoma patients responding to a mouse anti-idiotype antibody.[65,66] However, other early clinical studies proved disappointing. Several factors contributed to poor outcomes: (1) suboptimal antigen selection (i.e., modulation of the antibody–antigen complex or antigen shedding); (2) rapid clearance of antibody; and/or (3) development of host immune response to the murine mAb (i.e., production of human anti-mouse antibodies by the host).[67,68] Advances in molecular biotechnology and tumor immunology have led to the development of chimeric or humanized/human mAbs with increased biologic activity, longer half-lives, and less immunogenicity. Results from recent clinical trials have confirmed the improved antitumor activity of these newer mAbs, particularly rituximab.[69–71]

Rituximab is an IgGκ chimeric mAb directed against the CD20 antigen expressed on normal B cells and the majority of B-cell NHLs.[15] Four weekly doses of rituximab are well tolerated and result in clinically meaningful responses in up to 50% of previously treated indolent NHL patients.[70,71] As a result of the initial clinical studies, rituximab became the first mAb to be approved by the US Food and Drug Administration (FDA) to treat patients with B-cell lymphoma.[69] However, in ~50% of previously chemotherapy-treated indolent NHL patients treated with rituximab, little to no clinical benefit can be demonstrated. Scientific efforts to improve its antitumor activity are based on improving the understanding of the biology of the CD20 target and the mechanisms of action of rituximab.

Several biologic effects have been postulated as rituximab's primary mechanism of antitumor activity, including: antibody-dependent cellular cytotoxicity (ADCC), complement-mediated cytotoxicity (CMC), and induction of apoptosis/anti-proliferation. A major area of research is the study of intracellular signals that result in apoptosis of lymphoma cells following binding of rituximab to the CD20 antigen and factors associated with activation of the innate immune system.[72–83] Currently, the function(s) of CD20 has not been identified. Previous CD20 knockout mice studies failed to show an abnormal murine phenotype.[84] Exposure of lymphoma cells to rituximab results in the activation of the Src-family of protein tyrosine kinases, leading to phosphorylation of PLCγ2 and increased cytoplasmic Ca^{++}.[73–79] These early signal transduction events activate caspase 3 to promote apoptotic cell death of NHL B cells.[77] In addition, in vitro exposure

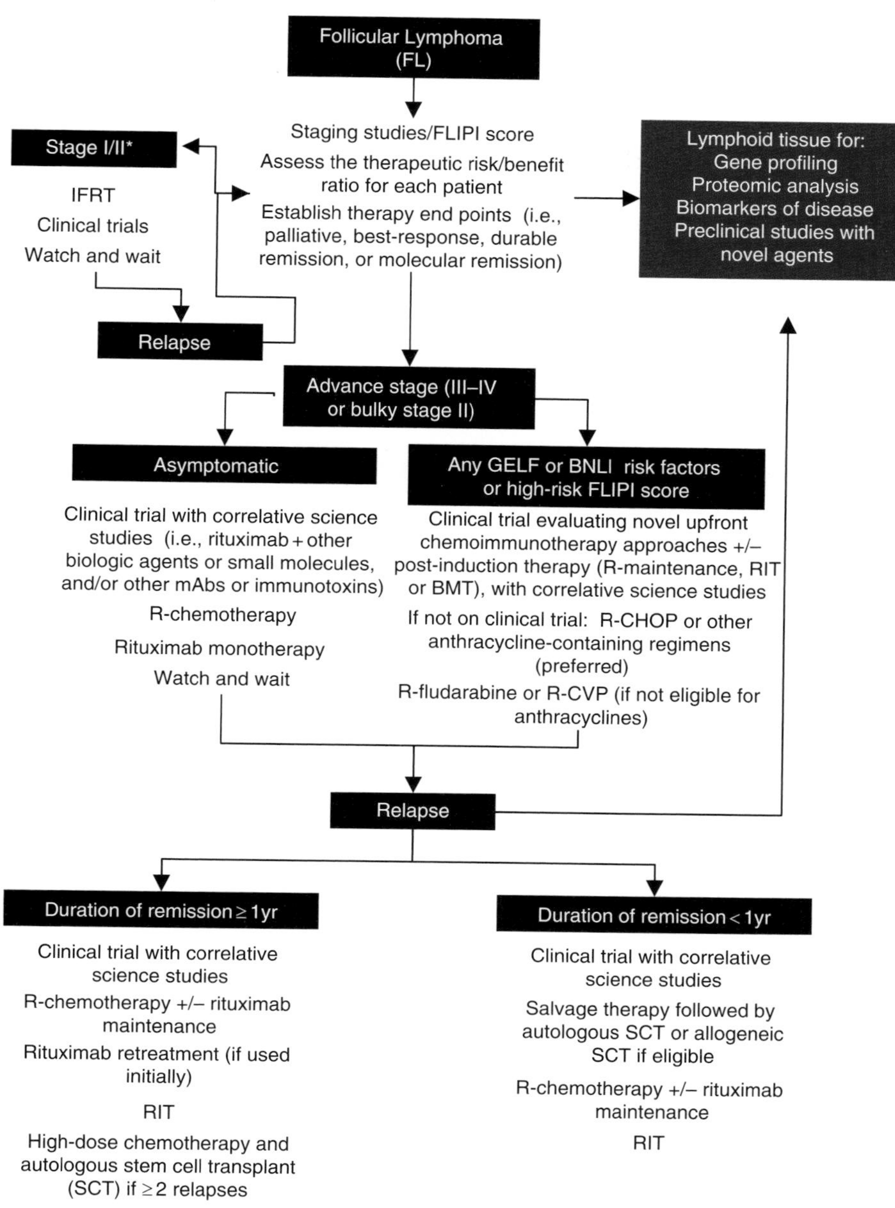

Figure 18.3 Algorithm that simplifies the approach to patients with follicular lymphoma (FL). FLIPI: Follicular Lymphoma International Prognostic Index; IFRT: involved-field radiation therapy; GELF: Groupe pour l'Etude de Lymphome Folliculaire; BNLI: British National Lymphoma Investigation; BMT: bone marrow transplant; RIT: radio immunotherapy; SCT: stem cell transplantation.

of lymphoma cell lines to rituximab is associated with a sustained phosphorylation of p38-MAP, JNK, and ERK kinases.[78] Signaling had been demonstrated in lymphoma cells primarily following cross-linking of rituximab with a secondary antibody (usually a goat anti-mouse or mouse anti-human) or by Fc-receptor-bearing accessory cells[79] (Figure 18.4). We have recently demonstrated that neutrophils may be necessary for optimal antitumor activity of rituximab, corroborating findings reported by other investigators.[82,83] Reorganization of the CD20 receptor into lipid raft domains occurs following rituximab binding and precedes the aforementioned signaling events.[85,86] Structural changes in CD20 antigen may affect cellular responses to rituximab. Specific mutations and deletions in the intracellular domain of CD20 were transfected into Molt-4 lymphoblastic T cells and resulted in a significant decrease in CD20 reorganization into lipid raft domains and reduction in signaling events, without affecting the extracellular binding of rituximab.[86]

Preclinical studies demonstrate augmented antitumor activity between rituximab and chemotherapy agents.[87,88] Inhibition of IL-10 by rituximab results in downregulation of BCL2 and sensitization of NHL cells to chemotherapy-induced apoptosis.[87] Moreover, pretreatment of "resistant" B-cell lymphoma cell lines with fludarabine results in down regulation of CD59, a complement inhibitory protein, and increased sensitivity to rituximab-induced CMC.[88]

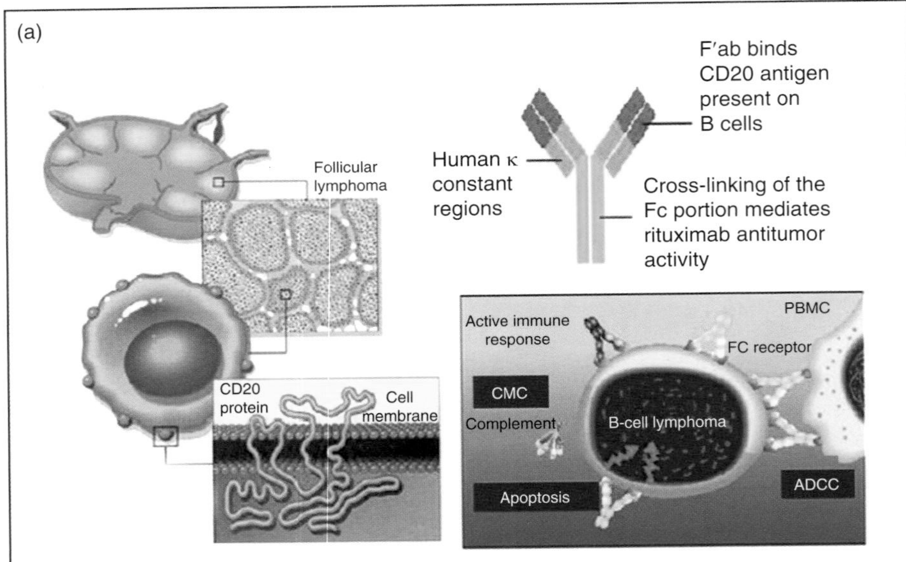

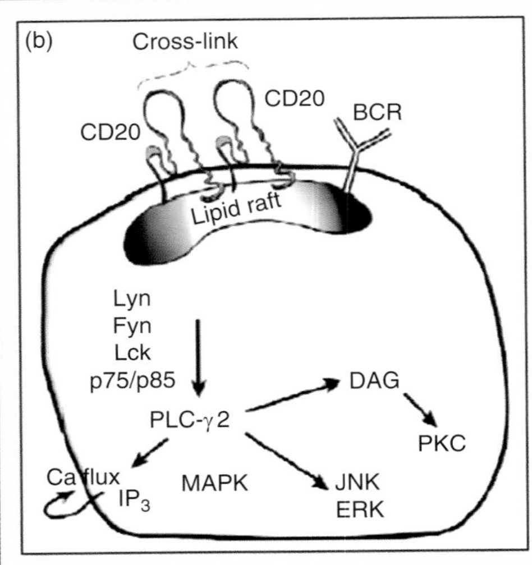

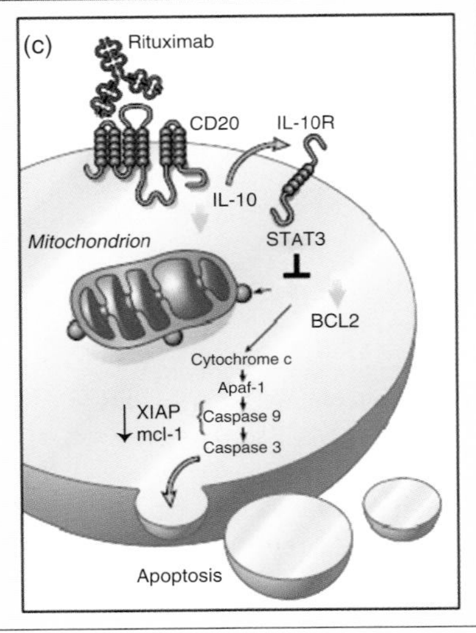

Figure 18.4 Proposed mechanisms of action of rituximab (a). Signaling events following rituximab binding to CD20 (b and c). Recruitment of CD20 into lipid raft domains followed by activation of the Src family of protein tyrosine kinases, leading to phosphorylation of phospholipase C-γ2 and increased cytoplasmic Ca^{++}. Cleavage of caspase 3 promotes apoptosis of NHL B cells. Phosphorylation of p38-MAP and ERK kinases occurs (b). Inhibition of interleukin-10 with subsequent downregulation of BCL2 has been demonstrated (c). ADCC: antibody-dependent cellular cytotoxicity; CMC: complement-mediated cytotoxicity; PBMC: peripheral blood mononuclear cell; IL: interleukin; NHL: non-Hodgkin lymphoma; BCR: B-cell receptor; PKC: protein kinase C; PLC: phospholipase C; DAG: diacylglycerol; IP_3: inositol triphosphate.

Rituximab monotherapy in B-cell lymphomas

Rituximab monotherapy was initially tested in relapsed and refractory B-cell lymphoma then subsequently in the frontline setting. The initial pivotal trial included refractory/relapsed indolent lymphomas, including FL, and demonstrated that four doses of rituximab administered at weekly intervals produced a response rate of 50% with a median duration of response of 12 months.[71] A subsequent study determined that a subset of FL patients (40%) could be successfully retreated with a second course of rituximab at the time of disease progression. Moreover, the duration of the second response in this group of patients exceeded the duration of the first response (18 months versus 12 months).[89] Several clinical observations noted from the initial rituximab clinical trials were used to design subsequent clinical studies such as: (1) response rate was higher among patients receiving rituximab "earlier than later" (e.g., as second-line therapy compared to third-line or greater); and (2) response rate inversely correlated with the bulk of the disease.

Two groups of investigators studied the use of rituximab as frontline in FL patients. Approximately two-thirds of the patients (72–73%) achieved a clinical response and 26–35% of the patients achieved a CR or unconfirmed CR (CRu).[90,91] In contrast to previously treated patients, the duration of response lasted an average of 26 months; some patients with low-bulk disease without evidence of PCR-detectable minimal residual disease (MRD) remained in CR for more than 7 years.[92] It is important to note that patients enrolled into these two clinical trials consisted of patients with FL grade 1 or 2, normal LDH, and low FLIPI or IPI scores.

Ongoing research is aimed to further characterize the subset of FL patients most likely to benefit from rituximab monotherapy in an attempt to reduce unnecessary therapy-related toxicity from concurrent chemotherapy. Recently published in vivo studies demonstrate that FcγR receptor expression is necessary to eradicate NHL in a murine animal model, suggesting that ADCC plays a significant role in rituximab's activity.[82] Furthermore, certain polymorphisms in the FcγRIIIa gene have been associated with a clinical and molecular response to anti-CD20 mAb therapy in patients with indolent NHL.[83,93]

Rituximab extended schedules: maximizing clinical benefit against the potential risk for development of rituximab resistance

Rituximab maintenance following rituximab monotherapy

Pharmacokinetic analysis of data from the pivotal trial indicated that steady state serum concentrations are not achieved after four doses of rituximab at 375 mg/m^2.[94] Steady state serum concentrations could potentially be reached by increasing the rituximab dose or duration of treatment. Although there is significant heterogeneity between patients with regard to rituximab clearance, patients ultimately classified as responders to rituximab tend to have significantly higher serum rituximab levels than non-responders at 1 week, 1 month, and 3 months post-treatment with rituximab. Unlike regimens using chemotherapy agents, the treatment-related toxicity is usually mild and limited with some exceptions to infusion-related symptoms. Pharmacokinetic data obtained during the pivotal trial and analyzed by Berinstein *et al.* demonstrated a significant correlation between the serum concentration of rituximab and antitumor response and was the rationale for investigating prolonged rituximab-dose/schedule regimens.[94]

Gordan *et al.* conducted a phase II trial to determine the feasibility of individualized pharmacokinetic dosing of rituximab and compare the response rate (RR) and PFS to that achieved in historical trials. Thirty-one patients were treated with 4 weekly infusions of rituximab at 375 mg/m^2. Rituximab's serum levels were obtained immediately prior to the first and after the fourth doses, and then monthly for 1 year. A single dose of rituximab (375 mg/m^2) was administered when rituximab serum levels dropped below 25 μg/mL during the follow-up period. The overall response rate (ORR) and CR rate in patients with low-grade NHL were 59% and 27%, respectively. Only 4/22 (18%) evaluable patients with low-grade NHL had disease progression after a median follow-up period of 14 months. The median number of rituximab maintenance doses in 15 evaluable patients was 2 (range, 0–5).[95] While the clinical results are interesting, the data are difficult to compare to other maintenance regimens since long-term response and PFS data are not yet available. However, this study paved the road for the subsequent development of rituximab maintenance trials.

Rituximab maintenance programs had been tested clinically in the following clinical scenarios: (1) following rituximab single-agent therapy upfront/relapsed low-grade lymphomas; (2) following systemic chemotherapy or chemoimmunotherapy in patients with relapsed/refractory B-cell indolent lymphomas; (3) in previously untreated FL patients upon completion of CVP therapy; (4) in previously untreated diffuse large B-cell lymphoma; and (5) in relapsed/refractory mantle cell lymphomas.[96–100] While the efficacy of rituximab maintenance varied within each clinical trial, the general consensus is that while extended use of rituximab may produce some degree of clinical benefit (improvement in time to progression), its use has not been associated with an improved OS in patients with B-cell lymphoma treated with upfront rituximab-based chemoimmunotherapy and raises the potential risk for the development of rituximab resistance.[101,102] In this section we will focus on the current data available for rituximab maintenance in FL (Table 18.2).

The first reported randomized trial of rituximab maintenance therapy was conducted at The Sarah Cannon Cancer Center (SCCC), in Nashville TN. The initial goal of the study was to compare the benefit of rituximab maintenance versus rituximab retreatment. In this phase II study, previously treated FL or small lymphocytic lymphoma (SLL) responding to standard rituximab therapy were randomized to retreatment upon progression versus a rituximab maintenance regimen. The experimental arm was designed on the observation that rituximab serum concentrations are maintained for approximately 6 months and that disease progression tends to occur after that time period in most patients who initially respond to rituximab. Therefore, the rituximab maintenance arm consisted of four additional full courses of rituximab (375 mg/m^2 weekly × 4) at 6-month intervals for 2 years. This trial showed that the response of an initial four-dose course of rituximab (ORR 47%, with 7% CR rate) was improved with maintenance courses of rituximab given at 6-month intervals in responding patients (ORR to 73%, with 37% CR rate). The median PFS was 37 months (range, 23 months to not reached [NR]) for patients in the maintenance program versus 7.4 months in the observation arm. However, the "duration of rituximab benefit" (defined as the date of the first treatment until the date that the patient developed progressive lymphoma and required other treatment) was similar in both arms: 31.3 months versus 27.4 months, respectively. The 3-year survival for the maintenance group was 72% versus 68% for the retreatment group (p = NS).[96] Whereas patients in the maintenance group received a total of 114 additional courses of rituximab after the induction regimen, with most patients receiving three maintenance courses, the patients in the retreatment group received only 83 additional courses with most patients requiring only a single course of rituximab retreatment. In summary, while maintenance therapy produces superior results in terms of ORR, CR, and PFS, retreatment of patients with rituximab at the time of disease progression results in the same duration of "benefit" and appears to utilize less rituximab.[96]

In an attempt to minimize the amount of rituximab utilized, but at the same time explore the concept of rituximab maintenance, the Swiss Group for Clinical Cancer Research (SAKK) conducted a randomized clinical trial to determine if

Table 18.2. Summary of clinical studies evaluating the efficacy of rituximab maintenance in different schedules of administration in patients with FL

Investigator	Phase	Induction regimen	Population	Response	Cumulative rituximab dose	Progression-free survival (median)	Overall survival
Gordan *et al.*[95]	II	Rituximab weekly × 4 follow by rituximab monthly as needed if rituximab levels < 25 µg/mL	Previously treated NHL	ORR in low-grade NHL 69% CR in low-grade NHL 27%	2250 mg/m^2	NR	NR
Hainsworth *et al.*[96] (Lym-5)	II	Rituximab weekly × 4 follow by retreatment upon progression vs. rituximab weekly × 4 every 6 months for 2 years	Untreated and relapsed indolent NHL (n = 114 patients) (75% FL)	ORR 67% vs. 61% CR 27% vs. 4%	6000 mg/m^2	7.4 months (before retreatment) vs. 31.3 months 27.4 months (after retreatment) vs. 31.3 months	3-yr survival 68% vs. 72% (p = NS)
Ghielmini *et al.*[97] (SAKK)	III	Rituximab weekly × 4 vs. rituximab weekly × 4 followed by rituximab q, 2months for 4 doses	Previously untreated and treated FL or MCL	At 12 weeks: ORR = 67% vs. 62% CR = 8% vs. 12% At 12 months: ORR = 44% vs. 60%	3000 mg/m^2	Event-free survival 11.8 vs. 23.2 months	NS
Hochster *et al.*[98] (ECOG 1496)	III	CVP × 6–8, if no progression rituximab weekly × 4 every 6 months vs. observation	Untreated FL		6000 mg/m^2	15 months vs. 52 months ($p < 0.001$)	3-yr survival 83% vs. 93% ($p = 0.03$)
Forstpointner *et al.*[100]	III	FCM × 4 (arm closed after 147 pts) vs. R-FCM × 4 follow by second randomization to observation vs. rituximab weekly × 4 after 3 and 6 months post-induction	Relapsed/ refractory FL and MCL	Reponses observed in FL: ORR for R-FCM = 94% vs. FCM = 70% ($P = 0.011$). CR for R-FCM = 40% vs. FCM = 23%	4500 mg/m^2	Limited to FL: R-FCM not reached vs. FCM = 21 months ($p = 0.0139$)	Not reached at 2 yrs in both groups
van Oers *et al.*[99] (EORTC 20981)	III	CHOP vs. R-CHOP × 6 and if no progression observation vs. rituximab weekly × 4 every 6 months	Rituximab naïve, previously treated FL	ORR CHOP vs. R-CHOP: 72.3% vs. 85.1% CR CHOP vs. R-CHOP: 15.6% vs. 29.5%	6000 mg/m^2	Observation vs. RM 51.5 vs. 14.9 months CHOP + Obs. = 11.6 months CHOP → RM = 42.2 months R-CHOP → Obs. = 23 months R-CHOP → RM = 51.8 months	% at 3 yrs 77.1% (Obs.) vs. 85.1% (RM) ($p = 0.011$)

Notes: NHL: non-Hodgkin lymphoma; FL: follicular lymphoma; MCL: mantle cell lymphoma;
R: rituximab; CHOP: cyclophosphamide, doxorubucin, vincristine, and prednisone; FCM: fludarabine, cyclophosphamide, and mitoxantrone; CVP: cyclophosphamide, vincristine, and prednisone; RM: rituximab maintenance; ORR: overall response rate; CR: complete response; NR: not reached.

extending induction treatment with rituximab delivered at a different dosing regimen could improve outcome compared to the standard 4-week course alone.[97] The study enrolled a total of 185 eligible and evaluable patients with untreated or previously chemotherapy-treated B-cell indolent lymphoma including FL and mantle cell lymphomas (MCL). All patients were given induction therapy with rituximab 375 mg/m^2 per week for 4 weeks and evaluated for response after 12 weeks following initial treatment. Responders and patients with stable disease (SD) were subsequently randomized to either observation (78 patients) or four additional doses of rituximab at 375 mg/m^2 given 2 months apart each (73 patients). The end point of the study was event-free survival (EFS) defined as the time from first induction infusion to progression, relapse, second tumor, or death from any cause.

At 3 months after the randomization, the ORR and CR rate among the patients allocated to observation or maintenance rituximab were similar at 67% and 8% versus 62% and 12%, respectively. However, only 53% of the patients in the observation group maintained a response at 7 months, and by 12 months, the ORR had dropped to 44%. By contrast, in the maintenance rituximab group, the ORR had increased to 67% (18% CR rate) at month 7; by month 12, the ORR was 60% (26% CR rate). The median EFS was prolonged from 11.8 months in the observation group to 23.2 months in the maintenance rituximab group ($p = 0.024$). The difference was particularly more noticeable in chemotherapy-naïve patients (19 vs. 36 months; $p = 0.009$) and in patients responding to induction treatment (16 months vs. 36 months; $p = 0.004$).[97]

Rituximab maintenance therapy following chemotherapy

At the 2005 annual meeting of the American Society of Hematology (ASH), the Eastern Cooperative Oncology Group (ECOG) presented results of the first randomized trial that shows a clear and definitive benefit for rituximab maintenance therapy versus observation following induction chemotherapy. The ECOG 1496 was launched with the initial goal of comparing first-line induction chemotherapy with fludarabine and cyclophosphamide (FC) or CVP, which was then to be followed by a second randomization to either observation or rituximab maintenance. Because of an increased toxic death rate, accrual to the FC arm was discontinued, and the primary objective became evaluating the effect of rituximab maintenance therapy post-CVP induction chemotherapy for patients with indolent NHL.[98]

Patients were initially treated with six to eight cycles of CVP consisting of cyclophosphamide at 1000 mg/m^2 and vincristine at 1.4 mg/m^2 on day 1 with prednisone at 100 mg/m^2 administered on days 1–5. Patients who achieved a response (PR or CR) or SD after induction therapy were then randomized to observation or maintenance therapy with rituximab 375 mg/m^2 per week for 4 weeks administered every 6 months for 2 years. The study was terminated early when the PFS difference for CVP followed by maintenance rituximab versus CVP alone crossed statistical significance. Patients who received maintenance rituximab after CVP had significantly higher PFS at 2.5 and 4.5 years (74% and 58%, respectively) compared to those who received only induction CVP (42% and 34%, respectively).[98]

Although a statistically significant difference in OS was not detectable at the early analysis (median follow-up 1.2 years), the results of the trial provided the first definitive evidence that providing scheduled rituximab therapy to patients who achieve a response or SD to frontline chemotherapy can extend the period of clinical benefit. Ultimately, since most of the patients with B-cell lymphoma, including FL, are currently being treated with upfront combined chemoimmunotherapy, the findings of this study have become much less relevant to current clinical practice.

Rituximab maintenance therapy following chemoimmunotherapy

Several studies have demonstrated superior clinical end points by combining rituximab and systemic chemotherapy when compared to chemotherapy alone in FL patients treated in the frontline or relapsed setting (Table 18.3). The use of rituximab-chemotherapy has been adopted by the majority of practicing oncologists worldwide as the new standard of care of FL patients. Despite the impressive CR rates (including molecular CRs) and length of response duration a significant number of FL patients relapse after systemic chemoimmunotherapy (especially those patients with high FLIPI scores). In an attempt to prolong the duration of remission, rituximab maintenance has been studied in FL patients treated with rituximab-chemotherapy-based regimens, originally in relapsed patients and currently in untreated FL.

The first of two studies addressing the role of rituximab maintenance following chemoimmunotherapy was conducted by the European Organization for Research and Treatment of Cancer (EORTC). In 1998, the EORTC opened a phase III randomized study (EORTC 20981) to evaluate the response rates between CHOP versus R-CHOP in patients with relapsed/refractory rituximab-naïve FL patients and to explore the effect of rituximab maintenance on PFS in responding patients to CHOP or R-CHOP.[99] Eligible patients were randomized to receive six cycles of CHOP or R-CHOP. Responding patients were subsequently randomized again to observation or rituximab maintenance in a schedule similar to the one proposed by the SCCC.[96]

As expected, R-CHOP induction resulted in an increased ORR when compared with CHOP chemotherapy (85.1% vs. 72.3%, $p < 0.001$). The median PFS from the first randomization was 20.2 months after CHOP chemotherapy and 33.1 months after R-CHOP ($p < 0.001$). Rituximab maintenance yielded a longer PFS from second randomization when compared to observation alone; 51.5 months vs. 14.9 months ($p < 0.001$). Of interest, the improvement in PFS by rituximab maintenance was observed regardless of the type of induction received (i.e., R-CHOP or CHOP). The 3-year OS from the pooled patients demonstrated that rituximab maintenance increased the 3-year OS rates from 77.1% in the observation arm to 85.1% in the maintenance group ($p = 0.011$, log-rank test). It appeared that a benefit was derived not only for patients treated with induction CHOP followed by rituximab maintenance, but also in patients receiving R-CHOP that were randomized to rituximab maintenance.[99]

The second study was reported by Forstpointner *et al.* on behalf of the German Low Grade Lymphoma Study.[100] In this particular study 319 patients with recurrent/relapsed indolent B-cell lymphomas (including 29% MCL patients) were randomized to fludarabine, cyclophosphamide, mitoxantrone

Table 18.3. Selected clinical studies with rituximab in combination with systemic chemotherapy in indolent lymphomas

Investigator	Phase	Induction regimen	Consolidation regimen	Disease	Response rate	Time to progression (median)	Overall survival (median)
Czuczman *et al.*[103]	II	R-CHOP	None	Untreated and relapsed indolent NHL (40 pts)	ORR = 100% CR/CRu = 87%	82.3 months	NR after 8 yrs of follow-up
Czuczman *et al.*[104]	II	R-F	None	Untreated and relapsed indolent NHL (40 pts)	ORR = 90%	NR at 44 months	NR at 44 months
Zinzani *et al.*[105]	III	CHOP vs. FM	Observation (MCR) Rituximab × 4 (< MCR or ≥ PR)	Previously untreated FL (151 pts)	CR = 68% (FM) vs. 42% (CHOP) p = 0.003	Estimated 3-yr RFS rate FM = 71% vs. CHOP = 54% (p = 0.20)	94% at 3 yrs for the entire group
Forstpointner *et al.*[106] on behalf of the GLSG	III	FCM vs. R-FCM	None	Relapsed FL or MCL (147 pts)	ORR R-FCM = 79% vs. FCM = 58% (p = 0.01)	R-FCM = 16 months vs. FCM = 10 months (p = 0.003)	R-FCM = NR vs. FCM = 24 months (p = 0.003)
Marcus *et al.*[107]	III	CVP vs. R-CVP	None	Untreated FL (321 pts)	CRR R-CVP = 81% vs. CVP 41% (p < 0.001)	R-CVP = 27 months vs. CVP = 15 months (p < 0.001)	No difference observed at 3 yrs
Hiddemann *et al.*[108] on behalf of the GLSG	III	CHOP vs. R-CHOP	< 60 yrs ASCT vs. IFN > 60 yrs high-dose IFN vs. low-dose IFN	Untreated FL or MCL (789 pts)	ORR FL R-CHOP (97%) vs. CHOP (91%) (p = 0.005) ORR MCL R-CHOP = 93% vs. CHOP = 76% (p = 0.015)	FL R-CHOP not reached vs. CHOP = 2 yrs (p = 0.001) MCL R-CHOP = 2 yrs vs. CHOP = 1 yr (p = 0.0131)	No differences observed at 4 yrs of follow-up
Herold *et al.*[109]	III	MCP vs. R-MCP	IFN-α until PD	Previously untreated indolent lymphomas and MCL	ORR MCP = 75% vs. R-MCP = 92% (p = 0.009) CR MCP = 25% vs. R-MCP = 50% (p = 0.004)	MCP = 28.8 months vs. R-MCP = NR after 47 months (p < 0.001)	MCP = 74% vs. R-MCP = 87% (p = 0.0096)
Salles *et al.*[110]	III	CHVP + I vs. R-CHVP + I	None	Untreated high tumor burden indolent lymphomas	ORR CHVP + I = 85% with 49% CR/CRu vs. R-CHVP + I = 94% with 76% CR/CRu (p < 0.001)	35 months vs. NR at 60 months (p = 0.004)	5 yr OS CHVP + I = 79% vs. R-CHVP + I = 84% (p = NS) Survival benefit from R-CHVP + I was statistically significant in FL with FLIPI score ≥ 3

Notes: NHL: non-Hodgkin lymphoma; FL: follicular lymphoma; MCL: mantle cell lymphoma;
R: rituximab; CHOP: cyclophosphamide, doxorubicin, vincristine, and prednisone; FCM: fludarabine, cyclophosphamide, and mitoxantrone; F: fludarabine; FM: fludarabine and mitoxantrone; CVP: cyclophosphamide, vincristine, and prednisone; ASCT: autologous stem cell transplantation; IFN: interferon; CHVP + I: cyclophosphamide, doxorubicin, tenoposide, and prednisone plus interferon. MCP: mitoxantrone, chlorambucil, and prednisolone; GLSG: German Low Grade Lymphoma Study Group; ORR: overall response rate; CRR: complete response rate; CR: complete response; CRu: unconfirmed complete response; PR: partial response; MCR: molecular complete response; NR: not reached; pts: patients.

(FCM) alone or with concurrent rituximab for four cycles. Patients who achieved a CR or PR were randomized to observation (control arm) or rituximab maintenance regimen (rituximab 375 mg/m^2 per week $\times 4$, administered 3 and 9 months post-chemotherapy). Again, as noted by other chemoimmunotherapy trials, the addition of rituximab to FCM resulted in higher response rates (79%) when compared to FCM alone (58%) and resulted in the termination of the randomization to FCM arm alone in 2001. All subsequent patients received R-FCM followed by either observation or rituximab maintenance. After a median observation time of 26 months, a significantly longer duration of response was noted in the patients in the maintenance arm (not reported at the time of publication) versus 17 months for patients in the observation arm. This analysis, however, includes 38 patients treated with FCM alone as initial therapy and includes patients with both FL and MCL. Subset analysis of FL patients treated with R-FCM as induction therapy demonstrated that rituximab maintenance translated to a longer duration of remission (not reached) when compared to observation (26 months). At the time of this report, no published differences in OS were noted between rituximab maintenance or observation groups following FCM or R-FCM for either FL or MCL.[100]

These results were consistent with the data reported by the EORTC and supported the use of rituximab maintenance following salvage rituximab-chemotherapy in indolent lymphomas. However, the benefit of extending rituximab must be weighed against its potential long-term risk. While maintenance therapy produces superior results in terms of RR, CR, and PFS, re-treating patients with rituximab at the time of disease progression results in the same duration of benefit and may require less resource utilization. Moreover, an objective survival benefit in favor of rituximab maintenance following rituximab or rituximab-chemotherapy treatment has not yet been demonstrated. It is possible that as the observation period of enrolled subjects increases over time, differences in survival between treatment arms may emerge. In the meantime, clinicians should be wary that the prolonged use of rituximab may potentially increase the risk for development of rituximab resistance and of the potential deleterious effects of prolonged B-cell depletion (e.g., possible increased risk of infections, etc.).[101,102]

It is postulated that chronic exposure to rituximab may lead to the development of rituximab resistance. The impact of rituximab resistance in responses to subsequent biologic or chemotherapy treatment in lymphoma patients is unknown. Indeed, the emergence of rituximab resistance is a current clinical concern and scientific efforts focused on defining cellular pathways associated with it, as well as novel therapeutic strategies to overcome it, are ongoing.

In our previous work, we developed and characterized several rituximab-resistant cell lines and found that the acquirement of rituximab resistance was also associated with resistance to multiple chemotherapeutic agents commonly used to treat B-cell lymphoma.[101,102] These data suggest the possible existence of shared pathways of resistance to both biologic and chemotherapeutic agents that can negatively impact on the sensitivity to salvage therapies in these patients in the future.

Ongoing clinical trials seek to define the role of rituximab maintenance following chemoimmunotherapy and the impact of rituximab resistance in subsequent therapies. The MAXIMA study is a phase II clinical trial that has completed enrollment, and included patients with untreated or relapsed/refractory indolent lymphomas responding to chemoimmunotherapy. Patients in this study received maintenance rituximab every 8 weeks for 1 or 2 years. The results of this study are expected to be released in the near future.

In the primary rituximab and maintenance study (PRIMA), patients with FL are being treated with upfront chemoimmunotherapy (R-CHOP, R-CVP, or R-FCM) followed by a randomization to observation or rituximab maintenance. The maintenance regimen consists of a single dose of rituximab at 375 mg/m^2 every 2 months for 2 years. Finally the SAKK 35/03 is enrolling patients with untreated or chemotherapy relapsed/refractory FL. All patients will receive an induction treatment consisting of four standard doses of rituximab given weekly. Responding patients will be randomized to two maintenance schedules, a single dose of rituximab (375 mg/m^2) every 2 months for four doses or a single dose of rituximab every 2 months for 5 years or until disease progression or unacceptable toxicity.

Novel monoclonal antibodies in FL

An important lesson learned from the clinical development of rituximab is that the rational design of therapies for lymphomas based on targeting specific targets on neoplastic cells can be achieved. In addition to rituximab, other mAbs targeting cell surface antigens present in various subtypes of B-cell neoplasms are being actively studied in ongoing clinical trials (e.g., alemtuzumab, epratuzumab, mapatumumab [HGS-ETR1], and galiximab [IDEC114]).

Alemtuzumab (anti-CD52 mAbs, Campath-1H)

CD52 is a 21- to 28-kDa cell surface glycophosphatidyl inositol linked glycoprotein with only 12 amino acids. It is expressed on most normal and malignant lymphocytes, monocytes, and macrophages but not on hematopoietic stem cells, platelets, or granulocytes.[111] It is also expressed on a large proportion of lymphoid malignancies.[112] The function of CD52 is not known; however, T-cell activation and downstream signaling have been demonstrated in T cells from blocking antibody studies.[113–116] Initially, there were two main categories of Campath-1 (Cambridge Pathology) antibodies: Campath-1M (IgM) and Campath-1G (includes IgG1a and IgG2b mAbs). Campath-1M and -1G were produced from the rat using hybridoma techniques. Early in vitro and in vivo studies demonstrated that Campath-1H IgG2b induced more prolonged lymphopenia than other antibody formulations.[117] Based on initial studies, a humanized form of Campath-1G was formulated, alemtuzumab (Campath-1H), by grafting the hypervariable regions from heavy and light chain variable domains of the rat monoclonal antibody Campath-1G on to human IgG1k, as the IgG1 isotype had greater complement lysing capacity and cell-mediated killing.[118,119]

Currently, alemtuzumab is approved by the FDA for the treatment of fludarabine-refractory CLL. In contrast to its significant antitumor activity in CLL, alemtuzumab possesses a more limited therapeutic effect against B-cell lymphomas.

Response rates from alemtuzumab in NHL have been disappointing since the majority of the responses seen were limited primarily to the peripheral blood, bone marrow, and/or spleen, and were often transient.[120] The lymph nodes appeared to be less responsive even though they expressed the CD52 antigen to a similar extent to the other lymphoid tissues, implying the variable biodistribution of the antibody into the different tissues.[120] Interestingly, Campath-1H has been shown to result in significant and durable responses in small subsets of patients with indolent lymphoma with non-bulky or minimal residual disease.[121] In a phase II multicenter trial by Khorana *et al.* 16 patients with relapsed non-bulky B-cell NHL and 2 patients with minimal disease were treated with alemtuzumab for 6 weeks; 2 of the 16 patients with non-bulky NHL achieved CR and one patient achieved a PR. One of the two patients with minimal residual NHL achieved a molecular CR. The duration of response was variable: two patients continue to be in clinical remission for greater than 4.5–5+ years.[121]

A second multicenter alemtuzumab trial was reported by Lundin *et al.* in 50 previously treated low-grade NHL patients: 6 (12%) patients with B-cell lymphoma achieved a PR.[122] The response was demonstrated in the bone marrow and peripheral blood as previously described by others.[84] Seven of ten patients with cutaneous involvement by various subtypes of lymphomas responded to alemtuzumab (four CR and three PR). Again, patients with nodal disease were less responsive to Campath-1 (i.e., only 15% achieving a clinical objective response). The duration of response was short in most patients.[122]

In addition to the limited antitumor activity observed in alemtuzumab clinical trials, significant adverse events have significantly hampered the further development of anti-CD52 antibodies. The administration of alemtuzumab results in significant depletion of T- and B-cell lymphocytes leading to pronounced immunosuppression which predisposes patients to the development of opportunistic infections (i.e., cytomegalovirus [CMV], viremia, etc.).[123] Similar to other monoclonal antibodies, infusion-related side effects such as rigors, fever, rash, urticaria, and hypotension have been observed with the intravenous infusion of alemtuzumab, likely related to the sudden release of cytokines such as interferonγ, tumor necrosis factor beta (TNFβ), and IL-6.[124]

Innovative dosing schemas such as a subcutaneous (sq) route of administration or combining alemtuzumab with other biologic antibodies such as rituximab have been explored in clinical trials.[125]

Faderl *et al.* in a phase I/II trial combined alemtuzumab and rituximab to treat the patients with relapsed or refractory lymphoid malignancies. The rationale for this combination was the fact that these tumors coexpress CD20 and CD52 and the suboptimal efficacy of each single-agent antibody in patients with bulky organomegaly (alemtuzumab) or bone marrow (rituximab), respectively. Forty-eight patients with relapsed or refractory chronic lymphoid malignancies were treated; ORR was 52%, with median survival of 11 months. The combination had an acceptable safety profile and established clinical activity in a poor prognostic patient population.[126]

Anti-CD22 mAbs

Similar to CD20, CD22 is also expressed in the majority of B-cell malignancies. CD22 is a 135-kDa B-cell-specific membrane-bound sialoglycoprotein from the immunoglobulin superfamily. It is expressed on the cell surface in all IgM-positive and IgD-positive B cells, whereas in pre-B cells it is expressed only in the cytoplasm and is lost during maturation into plasma cells. Nodal expression of CD22 is strong in the follicular, mantle, and marginal zone of B cells. Although the germinal center has the maximum concentration of CD22 mRNA, the protein expression is weak on the cell surface.[127]

CD22 is associated with the B-cell receptor. In vitro studies have demonstrated that monoclonal antibodies to CD22 can induce apoptosis in multiple Burkitt lymphoma cell lines.[128] CD22 is not normally shed from the cell surface; however, upon antibody binding, it rapidly internalizes within hours and reappears slowly in days following modulation.[129] This feature of CD22 enables it to potentially serve as an ideal target to deliver radioisotopes or toxins by using anti-CD22 monoclonal antibody conjugates against neoplastic B cells.[130–132]

Clinical trials using epratuzumab as single agent or in combination with other biologic agents have been explored. The initial phase I/II clinical study conducted in patients with relapsed and refractory B-cell malignancies demonstrated that epratuzumab was well tolerated with minimal infusion-related toxicities.[133] Clinical responses were observed at doses ranging from 360 to 480 mg/m^2 among patients with indolent (three CRs and six PRs) or aggressive (five objective responses, including three CRs) B-cell lymphomas. The median duration of response in the indolent group was 47+ weeks and median time to progression was 103+ weeks; for aggressive lymphoma, the median duration of response was 38+ weeks and median time to progression was 35+ weeks. Durable antitumor activity was seen even in a subset of patients with extensive prior chemotherapy and autologous stem cell transplantation.[133]

A second phase I/II dose escalation was conducted in patients with indolent lymphomas.[134] Fifty-five previously treated lymphoma patients received the epratuzumab (half of the patients received prior rituximab) at doses ranging from 360 to 1000 mg/m^2 per week × 4 doses. Nine of the 51 patients had an objective response and 20 patients had SD. The mean duration of response was 79.3 weeks and median time to progression was 86.6 weeks.[134]

The use of epratuzumab in combination with another biologically active mAb such as rituximab or chemotherapy drugs is being currently investigated. Results from a single-institution pilot study conducted in 19 patients with NHL demonstrated that the combination of epratuzumab (360 mg/m^2 per week) with rituximab (375 mg/m^2 per week) was well tolerated.[135] Response rates were similar to historical control patients treated with rituximab monotherapy. However, a higher number of patients achieved a CR suggesting a possible augmented interaction between rituximab and epratuzumab.[135] Similar results were reported by Emmanouilides in a multicenter phase II clinical study evaluating the combination of rituximab and epratuzumab.[136] Several phase I/II clinical trials with epratuzumab are underway to better define its role in the treatment paradigm of B-cell malignancies.

Clinical development of radio-immunoconjugates and immunotoxins using anti-CD22 mAbs

Initial clinical studies conducted with a murine iodine-131 (^{131}I)-labeled anti-LL2 (i.e., anti-CD22) mAb by Goldenberg *et al.* in patients with refractory B-cell NHL demonstrated significant antitumor activity.[137] The ^{131}I was subsequently substituted by yttrium-90 (^{90}Y) due to its "better" pharmacokinetic profile (i.e., the longer retention time of the heavy metal ^{90}Y within cells).[138] A humanized form of LL2 (hLL2) with reduced immunogenicity was assessed in a pilot study comparing ^{131}I- and ^{90}Y-labeled hLL2 mAbs with regards to their pharmacokinetics, dosimetry, and immunogenicity in relapsed or refractory NHL. ^{90}Y-hLL2 revealed favorable tumor dosimetry compared to ^{131}I-hLL2.[139] In addition, hLL2 mAb was found to be superior to murine LL2 mAb with respect to immunogenicity. Objective tumor responses were seen in 2 of 13 and 2 of 7 patients given ^{131}I-hLL2 or ^{90}Y-hLL2, respectively.[139–141]

Of note was the observation that the CD22 target internalizes following antibody binding. Use of anti-CD22 to deliver toxins inside lymphoma cells has been explored in preclinical models and clinical trials. In a phase I dose escalation clinical trial an anti-CD22 antibody coupled to chemically deglycosylated ricin A chain was administered to 15 patients with refractory B-cell lymphoma.[131] The toxicities included vascular leak syndrome, fever, and anorexia. The patients with peripheral but not retroperitoneal adenopathy showed antitumor responses.[131] Conjugating several *Pseudomonas aeruginosa* exotoxins (BL22 or PE38) to hLL2 mAb has demonstrated significant antitumor activity against lymphoma preclinical in vitro or mouse models.[142] Other investigators have noted that the immunotoxin containing anti-CD22 conjugated to BL22 truncated pseudomonas exotoxin induced CR in patients with hairy cell leukemia resistant to purine analogs.[143]

CMC-544 is an IgG4 CD22-humanized targeted immunoconjugate of calicheamicin. Upon CD22 binding, CMC-544 internalizes inducing cell apoptosis in vitro/in vivo against NHL with minimal modulation of the immune system. We previously demonstrated that CMC-544 is an active agent against rituximab-chemotherapy resistant cell lines and is capable of enhancing rituximab activity in preclinical models. Ongoing clinical studies are evaluating its antitumor activity as a single agent or in combination with rituximab in patients with indolent and aggressive B-cell lymphomas.[144,145]

RNAse A was found to be cytotoxic against cancer cell lines in vitro and has been evaluated in several clinical trials for solid tumors. The activity of anti-CD22 RNAse was evaluated in lymphoma preclinical models with promising activity.[146]

Targeting CD80: galiximab

An initial phase I/II study with galiximab as a single agent in patients with relapsed FL, published by Czuczman *et al.*, demonstrated its safety and antitumor activity and provided a framework for future studies.[147] Leonard *et al.* conducted the first phase I/II study with galiximab in combination with rituximab in patients with relapsed/refractory FL. The primary end point of the study was safety and secondary end points consisted of pharmacokinetics studies, efficacy, and biomarkers of response (e.g., CD80 expression in tumor cells) and positive antitumor activity[148] led to a current international randomized phase III trial comparing rituximab plus galiximab to rituximab plus placebo.

Of interest, and in contrast with what had been observed with other biologic agents, the time to best response for responding patients was significantly delayed in a subset of patients, suggesting an alternative mechanism of action (i.e., possible changes in cellular immunity and/or tumor microenvironment) other than the traditional ADCC, apoptosis, and/or CMC. Ongoing and future studies plan to further evaluate galiximab in vivo mechanism(s) of action, as well as further study its therapeutic role in the treatment of FL, Hodgkin lymphoma, and other subtypes of NHL (both as a single agent and in combination with other agents).

Targeting the death receptor pathway

As has been demonstrated by other investigators, the death receptor pathway is intact and functional in various types of cancers, including B-cell lymphomas.[149,150] Moreover, binding and subsequent activation of the TNF death family receptors, by either ligands or antibodies, results in significant apoptosis and antitumor activity in a variety of solid tumor malignancies.[151–156] Targeting the extrinsic apoptotic pathway using agonist antibodies is another attractive strategy by which to treat FL patients. Mapatumumab and lexatumumab are fully human, high-affinity IgG1λ mAbs that target/activate the TNF-related apoptosis-inducing ligand (TRAIL) receptor-1 (TRAIL-R1) and receptor-2 (TRAIL-R2), respectively.

A phase II clinical study with mapatumumab was previously reported in patients with relapsed/refractory B-cell lymphomas. Patients included on the study had relapsed/refractory NHL of any histologic subtype, and were heavily pretreated. Mapatumumab was administered at two dose levels: 3 mg/kg (8 subjects) or 10 mg/kg (32 subjects) every 21 days in the absence of disease progression or prohibitive toxicity for up to six cycles. Preliminary reports in efficacy and toxicity demonstrated that mapatumumab was well tolerated with patients experiencing primarily grade 1 or 2 toxicities. In addition, objective antitumor responses were demonstrated in a subset of patients, all with follicular histologies. Moreover, 30% of all patients had disease stabilization following mapatumumab therapy.[157] Our lab has studied the interactions between mapatumumab and rituximab in preclinical models. Our positive findings support the ongoing evaluation of this unique combination (i.e., mapatumumab and rituximab) in clinical trials of patients with CD20-positive B-cell lymphomas.[158]

Humanized CD20 mAbs

A new generation of humanized/human mAbs targeting CD20 with significant antitumor activity is undergoing clinical testing. Currently, the most extensively studied human anti-CD20 mAb is ofatumumab, known to bind to a unique epitope present in the CD20 antigen as compared to rituximab. Preclinical studies with ofatumumab suggest differences in its biologic antitumor activity when compared to rituximab: (1) higher affinity for the CD20 antigen, (2) longer duration of antigen binding, and (3) greater degree of antitumor activity as measured by CMC assays (even in rituximab-resistant cell lines) and primary neoplastic B cells.[159–163] Initial clinical studies in patients with indolent lymphomas and chronic lymphocytic leukemia (CLL) demonstrated significant antitumor activity and tolerability.[162,163] Ongoing studies are evaluating the single-agent efficacy and toxicity of ofatumumab in rituximab-resistant B-cell neoplasms, as well as its activity in combination with CHOP or fludarabine/cyclophosphamide chemotherapy in patients with FL or CLL, respectively.

Other second- and third-generation humanized/human anti-CD20 mAbs are undergoing evaluation in preclinical models and early clinical trials and include: veltuzumab (Immunomedics, Inc.), GA101 (Roche), AME-133v (Eli Lilly and Co.), PRO131921 (Genentech), and ocrelizumab (Genentech).

Rituximab in combination with chemotherapy for follicular lymphomas

Historically, we reported on the first multicenter study evaluating rituximab in combination with standard doses of CHOP.[103,164] The study was a multi-institutional phase II clinical trial that evaluated the safety and efficacy of rituximab in combination with CHOP and enrolled 40 patients with either newly diagnosed or previously treated low-grade or follicular B-cell NHL expressing CD20. Patients with bulky disease (defined as any single mass >10 cm in its greater diameter) or with prior anthracycline therapy were excluded.[164] The results of our study were impressive as initially reported and then updated after a 9-year follow-up period.[103,164] The ORR was 95% and 22 patients (55%) achieved a CR and 16 patients (40%) a PR. In the subsequent and final analysis of the study, responses were updated using the International Workshop Response Criteria (IWRC) developed for lymphomas as described.[165] According to IWRC, the overall response rate was 100%, with 87% of the patients achieving a CR or CRu and 13% a PR. The median time to progression in all patients was 82.3 months (range 4.5 to 105.6+ months) and the median duration of response was 83.5 months (range 3.1 to 105.1+ months). At the time of the final analysis 42% of the patients continue to be on long-term remission. The toxicity profile of the combination was comparable to that observed for CHOP alone. Moreover, the addition of rituximab to CHOP did not compromise the CHOP dose intensity or density.[103,164]

Subsequent clinical studies were aimed to evaluate rituximab in combination with other chemotherapy regimens with better toxicity profile than CHOP, such as fludarabine-based regimens (Table 18.3). An Italian multicenter clinical trial evaluated the biologic effect of rituximab administered in patients failing to achieve molecular remission after induction chemotherapy with either CHOP or fludarabine/mitoxantrone (FM) combination.[105] The study reported by Zinzani *et al.* enrolled only previously untreated patients with stage II–IV FL, grade 1 and 2 according to the Revised European–American Lymphoma (REAL) classification expressing CD20, with detectable BCL2/Ig gene rearrangement by PCR analysis in peripheral blood or bone marrow. Patients were randomized to receive standard doses of CHOP or fludarabine at 25 mg/m^2 on days 1 to 3 and mitoxantrone 10 mg/m^2 on day 1. Both regimens were administered at 21-day intervals. On completion of the clinical and molecular re-staging (6 weeks after the last cycle of chemotherapy) only responding patients that did not achieve a molecular CR subsequently received four weekly doses of rituximab at 375 mg/m^2. Patients with molecular CR were observed and those with no response or progressive disease were removed from the study.[105] The study enrolled 151 patients of whom 140 were randomized to CHOP (68 patients) or FM (72 patients). The overall clinical response was similar between the two arms. However, the CR rate was higher in patients receiving FM (68%) than CHOP (42%) ($p = 0.003$). The rate of molecular responses was also higher in the FM arm (39%) than in the CHOP arm (19%) ($p = 0.001$). In accordance with the protocol, 95 patients (41 from the FM arm and 54 from the CHOP arm) received rituximab. In the overall study population, rituximab led to a significant improvement in terms of both CR rate (from 57% to 86%) and combined clinical and molecular response rate (from 29% to 61%) ($p < 0.001$). At a median follow-up of 19 months at the time of the publication, the OS for the cohort was 94% and the PFS was 63%. No differences in survival or PFS were noted between the treatment arms.[105]

Our group conducted the first phase II study evaluating the safety and efficacy of rituximab in combination with fludarabine in patients with untreated or previously treated low-grade/follicular lymphoma.[104] Eligible patients received six cycles of fludarabine at 25 mg/m^2 for five days repeated every 28 days, along with seven infusions of rituximab administered at 375 mg/m^2. After the initial analysis of the first ten enrolled patients demonstrated an unexpectedly high hematologic toxicity, the protocol was amended to reduce the dose of fludarabine by 40% in cases of prolonged cytopenia, as well as to discontinue the use of prophylactic trimethoprim-sulfamethoxazole, and limit the use of growth factor support.[104] The study accrued a total of 40 patients; 38 were evaluable for response. All patients had advanced-stage (III, IV) disease and the majority were previously untreated (68%). The majority of patients (65%) were IWFB (International Working Formulation B, i.e. follicular small cleave low-grade lymphoma). The median patient age was 53 years (range: 40–77 years). The most frequent extranodal site of disease was bone marrow (65%). Half the patients had IPI scores of 0 or 1, and the others had IPI scores of ≥ 2. Efficacy data were analyzed on two subsets of patients: subgroup #1 (included the first 10 patients) and subgroup #2 (included the next 30 patients following changes in the study design).[104] The ORR (CR and PR) was equal to 90% (95% confidence intervals [CI] = 76–97%); no significant differences were noted between the two subgroups of patients. Two patients in the entire sample had progressive disease secondary to transformed lymphoma before completion of therapy. For the whole group, the median duration of response, time to progression, and OS had not been reached after a median follow-up time of 44 months (range: 15–66 months). At last follow-up, 22 of 36 (61%) patients had ongoing responses. At the time of the first publication of this report six patients had died due to NHL.[104]

The toxicity profile of the combination was acceptable especially after the protocol was amended. The majority of the toxicity was hematologic with most of the patients experiencing grade 1 or 2 anemia or thrombocytopenia. However, 76% of the entire cohort developed grade 3/4 neutropenia which in general was transient and reversible. Overall, infectious complications (especially no occurrence of *Pneumocystis carinii* pneumonia or other serious opportunistic infection) seen in the intent-to-treat group appeared to be similar to that expected in a similar population treated with fludarabine alone. However, aciclovir prophylaxis was subsequently prescribed to all treated patients for 6–12 months post-completion of therapy because of the relatively high incidence of herpes infections (6 of 40 patients = 15%) believed secondary to T-cell depletion from fludarabine. No patient on aciclovir prophylaxis developed herpes infection.[104]

Mature data from randomized clinical studies have demonstrated the superiority of rituximab in combination with chemotherapy against chemotherapy alone in terms of response rates, time to progression, and OS[106–108] in patients with indolent lymphomas. The German Lymphoma Study Group (GLSG) conducted a prospective, randomized trial comparing FCM versus rituximab in combination with FCM in patients with relapsed follicular or mantle cell lymphoma. The FCM regimen consisted of fludarabine at 25 mg/m^2 per day on days 1 to 3, cyclophosphamide 200 mg/m^2 per day on days 1 to 3, and mitoxantrone 8 mg/m^2 on day 1. Chemotherapy was repeated every 4 weeks for a total of four cycles. Patients randomized to the R-FCM arm received in addition rituximab at 375 mg/m^2 72 hours prior to each cycle of chemotherapy.[106] A total of 147 patients were randomized of which 128 were evaluable for study end points; 62 were randomized for FCM and 66 for R-FCM. R-FCM-treated patients had an ORR higher (78%, 33% CR, 45% PR) than for patients treated with FCM alone (58%, 13% CR, 45% PR; $p = 0.01$), with similar results in a subgroup analysis of FL (94% vs. 70%) and MCL (58% vs. 46%). In the total group, the R-FCM arm was significantly superior concerning PFS ($p = 0.0381$) and OS ($p = 0.0030$). In FL, PFS was significantly longer in the R-FCM arm ($p = 0.0139$) whereas in MCL a significantly longer OS was observed ($p = 0.0042$). There were no differences in clinically relevant side effects in both study arms. This study is considered one of the first randomized clinical studies where the addition of rituximab to systemic and adequate chemotherapy was shown to significantly improve the outcome of relapsed or refractory FL and MCL.[106]

A second randomized study evaluated the effect of rituximab in combination with CVP versus CVP alone. The study as reported by Marcus *et al.* enrolled previously untreated CD20 expressing stage III/IV FL.[107] Eligible patients were randomized to R-CVP or CVP alone. Systemic chemotherapy consisted of a combination of cyclophosphamide at 750 mg/m^2 on day 1, vincristine at 1.4 mg/m^2 up to a maximal dose of 2 mg on day 1, and prednisone at 40 mg/m^2 daily for days 1–5. Patients randomized to R-CVP also received rituximab at 375 mg/m^2 on day 1 of each cycle. The treatments were administered every 21 days in both groups for a maximum of eight cycles. No crossover between the two arms was planned. A total of 321 eligible patients were randomized to R-CVP (162 patients) or CVP (159 patients). The ORR and CR rates were 81% and 41% in the R-CVP arm, versus 57% and 10% in the CVP arm, respectively ($p < 0.001$). After a median follow-up of 30 months, the time to progression was statistically longer in patients receiving R-CVP (27 months) than patients treated with CVP (15 months) ($p < 0.001$). No differences in toxicity profiles were observed between treatment arms. The OS was not different between treatment arms at 3 years. Despite the encouraging results, a concern raised by investigators was a "lower" dose of cyclophosphamide used in this study compared to other CVP regimens used by other groups.[106]

Hiddemann *et al.* have reported results from a randomized study comparing rituximab plus CHOP versus CHOP alone in patients with untreated FL. Despite the difficult interpretation of the data due to a second randomization to interferon or autologous stem cell transplantation, the median PFS observed in patients receiving induction R-CHOP was superior to that seen by CHOP alone.[108]

Two additional studies demonstrated that adding rituximab to systemic chemotherapy followed by biologic therapy with IFN-α resulted in improved clinical outcomes when compared to chemotherapy and IFN-α alone.[109,165] The East German Study Group (EGSG) compared the efficacy of rituximab added to first-line mitoxantrone, chlorambucil, and prednisolone (MCP) followed by IFN-α maintenance versus MCP + IFN-α, and included previously untreated patients with FL grade 1 and 2, lymphoplasmacytic lymphoma, and MCL. Patients were

Table 18.4. Clinical trials using radio-immunoconjugates in relapsed/refractory follicular lymphomas: non-myeloablative clinical trials

Author	Agent	Phase	n	Patient population	Response rate	Duration of response (DR)
Kaminski *et al.*[169]	^{131}I-labeled tositumomab	I/II	42	Relapsed or refractory CD20+ B-cell low- and intermediate-grade NHL	ORR = 71% CR = 32%	Median PFS = 12 months
Vose *et al.*[170]	^{131}I-labeled tositumomab	II	47	Relapsed or refractory CD20+ B-cell low-grade and transformed NHL	ORR = 57% CR = 32%	Median DR = 9.9 months
Kaminski *et al.*[50]	^{131}I-labeled tositumomab	II	60	Relapsed or refractory CD20+ B-cell low-grade and transformed NHL	ORR = 65% CR = 20%	Median DR = 6.5 months
Witzig *et al.*[172]	^{90}Y-labeled ibritumomab tiuxetan	I/II	51	Relapsed or refractory CD20+ B-cell low- and intermediate-grade NHL or MCL	ORR = 67% CR = 26%	Estimated DR = 11.7 months
Witzig *et al.*[173]	^{90}Y-labeled ibritumomab tiuxetan	III	143	Relapsed or refractory low-grade FL or transformed NHL	ORR = 80% CR = 30% CRu = 4%	Estimated DR = 14.2 months
Wiseman *et al.*[171]	^{90}Y-labeled ibritumomab tiuxetan	II	30	Relapsed or refractory low-grade FL or transformed NHL and mild thrombocytopenia	ORR = 83% CR = 37% CRu = 6%	Estimated TTP = 9.4 months
Witzig *et al.*[174]	^{90}Y-labeled ibritumomab tiuxetan	II	54	Rituximab-refractory FL	ORR = 74% CR = 15%	Estimated TTP = 6.8 months

Notes: PFS: progression-free survival; ORR: overall response rate; CR: complete response; CRu: unconfirmed complete response; FL: follicular lymphoma; MCL: mantle cell lymphoma; NHL: non-Hodgkin lymphoma; TTP: time to progression.

randomized to eight cycles of R-MCP or MCP followed by IFN-α maintenance until progression. The addition of rituximab to MCP resulted in higher ORR, CR, and PR when compared to MCP alone. Moreover, after a median follow-up period of 47 months, the PFS and the OS was significantly prolonged in patients receiving R-MCP, for both FL and MCL (Table 18.3).[1] The GELA-GOELAMS compared the efficacy of 12 cycles of the chemotherapy regimen CHVP + I (cyclophosphamide, adriamycin, etoposide, and prednisolone plus IFN-α) versus six cycles of R-CHVP + I in patients with untreated high tumor burden FL. All the therapy was delivered over 18 months in both arms. Once again, the results of the study favored the addition of rituximab in terms of ORR, CR/CRu, and PR rates, EFS, and PFS that has been maintained after 5 years of follow-up. Of interest, a benefit in OS favoring the addition of rituximab to this regimen was only observed in FL with FLIPI scores ≥ 3 (Table 18.3).[165]

Radiolabeled monoclonal antibodies: the challenge to find the optimal positioning of radioimmunotherapy in the treatment algorithm of FL patients

Because of the inherent and high sensitivity to radiation therapy observed in FL, along with the high number of potential target antigens on the cell surface, RIT represents an attractive therapeutic concept.[50,166–174] Currently, two available radio-immunoconjugates targeting the CD20 are approved by the FDA for clinical use in B-cell lymphomas: ^{90}Y-labeled ibritumomab tiuxetan and the ^{131}I-labeled tositumomab. In addition, several radio-immunoconjugates targeting other B-cell surface antigens or novel delivery of the radioisotope in two steps known as pre-targeted therapy are being studied in preclinical and clinical studies.[137–139,175]

^{90}Y-labeled ibritumomab tiuxetan and ^{131}I-labeled tositumomab combine the specific tumor targeting of mature B-cell neoplasms by anti-CD20-mAbs with the therapeutic effects of radiation therapy from conjugated radioisotopes. There are however some differences between the two agents: ^{90}Y-labeled ibritumomab tiuxetan is a pure β-emitter of high energy, with a short half-life (64 hours), and is suitable for outpatient use without the need for dosimetry. In contrast, ^{131}I-labeled tositumomab has both β- and γ-emissions, with longer half-life (193 hours), that requires precautions for radio-protection and dosimetric individualized dosing.

Both RIT agents have been tested in the non-myeloablative and myeloablative (e.g., stem cell transplant) settings with comparable efficacy and toxicity. In this chapter we will focus on the non-myeloablative use of RIT in FL. RIT had been studied as a single treatment modality in various clinical trials in patients with "relapsed/refractory" FL (Table 18.4).

Response rates range from 60% to 80%, with CR rates of about 20–30%. When compared to rituximab therapy, RIT has been shown to potentially induce higher response rates, including CR rates, but no significant differences in the duration of response or PFS.[169–174]

RIT has also been studied as frontline therapy. Kaminski *et al.* reported their experience with upfront ^{131}I-labeled tositumomab in patients with untreated FL. The study included FL patients with favorable prognostic profiles that likely contributed to the impressively high and durable remission rate observed after a single treatment of ^{131}I-labeled tositumomab (ORR of 95%, CR of 75%).[175] Notably, after 4 years of follow-up, 59% of the patients continue to be free of disease. Similarly, Sweetenham *et al.* reported an ORR of 100% and CR rate of 62% in FL patients treated with ^{90}Y-labeled ibritumomab tiuxetan in the frontline setting.[177]

Recent studies had investigated the role of RIT as consolidation strategy following chemotherapy (either CHOP or fludarabine ± rituximab). Most of these studies had shown that the addition of RIT is associated with an improvement in the response rate and the quality of the response. Of interest, the Southwest Oncology Group (SWOG) conducted a phase II study with patients with advanced FL treated with six cycles of CHOP chemotherapy followed by ^{131}I-labeled tositumomab. The response rate of the entire regimen was 90%, including 67% CR/CRu. The estimated 5-year OS was 87% and the PFS was 67%.[178] While the results are impressive and similar to that observed with rituximab-chemotherapy regimens, the use of RIT is limited by the side effects observed. Of interest, both RIT regimens induce considerable myelosuppression with delayed nadirs occurring 6–10 weeks post-treatment. Their administration is limited currently to patients with less than 25% bone marrow involvement.

Two important prospective studies are comparing RIT with other therapeutic strategies. The US Intergroup trial is prospectively randomizing FL patients between six upfront cycles of R-CHOP versus six cycles of CHOP followed by ^{131}I-labeled tositumomab whereas the RIT international study is comparing the administration of ^{90}Y-labeled ibritumomab tiuxetan versus observation as adjuvant therapy in FL patients responding to upfront induction chemotherapy. The results of these studies will provide clinicians/researchers with more insights regarding the true value of RIT in the treatment of FL patients.

High-dose chemotherapy and autologous or allogeneic hematopoetic stem cell transplantation (SCT) in FL

Unlike patients with DLBCL, the role of high-dose chemotherapy followed by autologous SCT (ASCT) is less defined, as the clear benefit is often masked by the historic observation of an increased risk of secondary malignancies. Usually, ASCT is reserved for physically fit patients with relapsed/refractory FL. The use of ASCT in patients with high-risk disease measured by the FLIPI score remains controversial.[178] Previous work reported by investigators at the Dana Farber Cancer Institute suggested that FL patients undergoing ASCT with BCL2 PCR-negative grafts had higher PFS rates at 8 years (83%) than patients that received BCL2-positive grafts (19%) and suggested the importance of achieving a molecular CR in FL undergoing ASCT.[180] The important of "ex vivo" purging of autologous bone marrow harvests in the past appears to have lost its potential value in the current era of being able to achieve "in vivo" purging via the use of rituximab-based chemoimmunotherapy regimens. As therapeutic options for patients with FL are increasing with better antitumor activity and improved toxicity profiles, two schools of thought are forming: one is a group of physicians willing to reinvestigate the role of ASCT in patients with high-risk disease (as measured by gene-profiling or FLIPI score), and the other "group" is abandoning its use in favor of sequential administration of less toxic non-myeloablative regimens.

For patients with relapsed/refractory FL considering ASCT, there are several phase II studies that consistently demonstrated improved DFS and sustained remission in patients that received salvage chemotherapy followed by ASCT.[179] However, no definitive benefit in terms of OS was observed until recently. A European group of investigators conducted a randomized study where 140 relapsed FL patients were randomized to chemotherapy alone, or ASCT with an unpurged or ASCT with a purged autograft. The 2-year PFS was 46%, 71%, and 77%, respectively. Of interest, the OS at 4 years was significantly prolonged in patients receiving purged (58%) or unpurged (55%) ASCT when compared to patients treated with chemotherapy alone (26%).[181] This is the first study to demonstrate an OS benefit of ASCT in patients with relapsed but chemosensitive FL. Rituximab was not part of the treatment utilized in this cohort of patients, and therefore this has dampened the enthusiasm for the observed results.[181]

The role of ASCT in the first-line setting of FL continues to be a subject of controversy and is not recommended outside clinical trials. There is limited information available in the current era of rituximab chemoimmunotherapy. Recently, investigators from the Gruppo Italiano Trapianto di Midollo Osseo (GITMO) and the Intergruppo Italiano Linfomi (IIL) published results comparing six courses of CHOP followed by four doses of rituximab to rituximab supplemented with high-dose sequential chemotherapy and autografting (R-HSD) in previously untreated patients with high-risk FL.[182] In this study the standard arm consisted of six cycles of CHOP followed by 4 weekly infusions of rituximab (CHOP-R). In the R-HSD arm, the regimen consisted of three phases: (1) induction with two full-dose doxorubicin, vincristine, and prednisone (APO) followed (if less than CR) by two additional courses of high-dose cytarabine, cisplatin, and dexamethasone (DHAP); (2) high-dose chemotherapy consisting of etoposide followed by two doses of rituximab, high-dose cyclophosphamide, and two additional doses of rituximab. Subsequently, peripheral blood stem cell (PBSC) mobilization and graft were purged with rituximab; (3) autograft conditioning regimen consisted of mitoxantrone and melphalan as previously described.[182]

The R-HSD arm resulted in higher CRs (85%) when compared to CHOP-R (62%, $p < 0.001$). Differences in molecular RRs were noted in R-HSD-treated patients (80%) when compared to the control arm (44%, $p < 0.001$). While the 4-year EFS was 61% in the R-HSD versus 26% for those patients treated with CHOP-R, it did not translate into an improvement in OS. It is important to note that 71% of the patients initially treated with the CHOP-R subsequently crossed over to R-HSD upon progression with excellent CR rates (85%) and 3-year EFS (68%).[182]

Allogeneic SCT represents what could be considered as a more radical form of immunotherapy for patients with FL, but also is the only treatment modality with proven curative potential. Allogeneic SCT has been evaluated in patients with refractory/relapsed FL in several clinical studies with variable degrees of success. However, the benefits are counterweighed by the high transplant-related mortality (TRM). The International Bone Marrow Transplant Registry (IBMTR) reported a descriptive analysis of the results observed with SCT in 904 patients with FL who received allogeneic SCT, purged-HCT, or unpurged-HCT. The risk of relapse was 54% lower in the allogeneic recipients and 26% lower in recipients of purged-HCT when compared to unpurged-HCT ($p < 0.001$ and $p = 0.04$, respectively).[183] However, in a multivariate analysis, the risk of TRM was 4.4 times higher after allogeneic HCT than in ASCT. This resulted in compatible 5-year probabilities of OS: 52% after allogeneic HCT, 62% after purged-HCT, and 55% after unpurged-HCT.[183]

The development of reduced-intensity chemotherapy (RIC) regimens in preparation for allogeneic SCT had been tested in patients with FL with some degree of success (increase of 3-year PFS to about 65%), particularly due to a reduction in TRM. Non-myeloablative or reduced-intensity allogeneic transplant relies upon graft-versus-lymphoma effect and uses fludarabine or alemtuzumab in the preparative regimens.[179] The results observed with reduced-intensity allogeneic SCT are encouraging with less upfront toxicity, but with a significant risk for chronic graft-versus-host disease. Longer follow-up is necessary to fully evaluate its long-term effect on the natural history of FL.

Novel chemotherapy agents and/or small molecules in FL

While a significant number of patients benefit from rituximab-based therapies, a high percentage of patients fail to respond or relapse after initial remission as a result of intrinsic or acquired resistance. Scientific efforts must now be focused not only on defining these pathways in lymphoma cells, but also ways by which to best prevent or decrease their incidence. Concurrently ongoing preclinical and clinical studies also seek to evaluate novel strategies to improve the antitumor activity of rituximab-based regimens (e.g., extending rituximab administration after induction chemoimmunotherapy, or incorporating novel target-specific therapies such as immunotoxins, BCL2 inhibitors, hypomethylating agents, and/or proteasome inhibitors).

The discovery and functional characterization of the ubiquitin–proteasome pathway as the major system for extra-lysosomal protein degradation has delineated its importance for regulating the selective and temporal proteolysis of key regulatory proteins.[184] Over the past couple of years, a significant number of proteins that regulate cell cycle, apoptosis, and cell proliferation and differentiation have been found to undergo processing and functional limitation by entering the ubiquitin–proteasome pathway.[185–186] Several groups of investigators have reported data suggesting that deregulation of the ubiquitin–proteasome system contributes to the pathogenesis of several malignancies (e.g., lymphoma, gliomas, colon, and lung carcinomas).[189–192]

Abnormal proteolysis of tumor suppressor oncoproteins, proapoptotic proteins, and cell cycle regulators had been associated with the development and progression of certain malignancies.[193,194] In addition, several transmembrane receptors undergo ubiquitinization and proteasome degradation such as FcγRI and HLA-class II molecules. Given the varied spectrum of proteasome substrates, it is not surprising that inhibition of the proteasome affects many cellular pathways (i.e., NF-κB, p44/42 mitogen-activated protein kinase [MAPK], or p53 pathways)[194,195] and has led to the scientific development of various proteasome inhibitors (i.e., MG132, lactacystin, and bortezomib). To date, the first and only proteasome inhibitor entered into clinical trials is bortezomib (PS-341, Velcade), a peptide boronic acid derivative that reversibly inhibits the chymotrypsin-like activity of the proteasome.[197]

Preclinical studies have demonstrated that bortezomib possesses significant antitumor activity against various subtypes of lymphomas including MCL, and is capable of enhancing the biologic activity of other target-specific therapies such as rituximab or antisense oligonucleotides targeting BCL2.[198–200] Moreover, proteasome inhibition could potentially overcome chemotherapy resistance as demonstrated in several preclinical cancer models.[201,202]

Reports from two single-institution phase II clinical trials evaluating the efficacy of bortezomib in patients with NHL have been published.[203,204] O'Connor *et al.* evaluated the antitumor activity of bortezomib in patients with refractory/relapsed indolent lymphomas. Twenty-four patients with relapsed indolent lymphomas received bortezomib at 1.5 mg/m^2 twice a week for 2 weeks every 21 days. Responses were observed in patients with FL (1 CR and 5 PRs), MCL (5 PRs), and marginal zone lymphomas (2 PRs). Toxicities were manageable and dose reduction occurred in 7/20 patients.[204]

Similarly, early antitumor activity has been observed with BCL2 inhibitors, a new class of agents entering into clinical trials. BCL2 inhibitors are BH3-mimic compounds that are capable of binding and inactivating several members of the BCL2 family proteins such as Mcl-1, BCL-XL, and BCL-W and increasing the cancer cells' proapoptotic potential.[205,206] Early results from phase I/II studies in B-cell lymphomas are encouraging and further support these exciting agents' clinical development.

Development of targeted therapy has broadened the treatment options for patients with B-cell lymphomas. Targeting apoptosis, signaling pathways, and the proteasome-ubiquitin system using small molecules such as BCL2 inhibitors or bortezomib has demonstrated antitumor activity with manageable toxicities. While early results are encouraging, more clinical studies addressing dosing, route of administration, or combination strategies are necessary to better optimize the efficacy of these exciting new agents.

Establishing goals of treatment: are we moving from palliation only or possible cure?

With improvement in treatment outcomes (i.e., more durable time to progression and better "quality" CRs) being seen with current novel immunologic-based therapies, we need to rethink our goals associated with treatment of FL: (1) Palliation only? or (2) Potential "cure" in a subset of patients? Ultimately, "cure" may not be achievable in this disease, but "optimal" palliation by which patients receive therapies which induce long periods of durable remissions while limiting the development of long-term toxicity (e.g., MDS, therapy-related [t]-AML, secondary solid tumors) and/or "cross-resistance" to future therapies, which may be a very close "second." Another important advantage associated with prolonged remissions between treatments, which should not be overlooked, is improvement in quality-of-life for patients for the prolonged periods during which they are not receiving "active" therapy. However, for the optimists amongst ourselves, "cure" in at least "good-risk" subsets of FL treated early with chemoimmunotherapy-based treatments is very likely an achievable goal in our lifetime.

Conclusions

Prior to the development of rituximab, the general approach to the treatment of FL was watchful-waiting until development of symptomatic/progressive disease at which time there was recurrent use of a limited number of "standard" chemotherapeutic agents utilized at different levels of intensity +/− radiotherapy to achieve primarily palliative effects. Over the past decade there has been a significant amount of information obtained from basic/translational research and clinical trials that supports the addition of rituximab to frontline chemotherapy for patients with indolent lymphomas. The effect of rituximab in combination with chemotherapy as measured by time to progression, median duration of response, time to treatment failure, response rates, time to next treatment, and OS have been improved and translate into an overall better quality of life in patients and may even result in "cures" in a subset of patients. Two recently published retrospective analyses suggest that the use of mAbs targeting CD20 (rituximab) in combination with systemic polychemotherapy improves the overall survival in patients with FL when compared to chemotherapy alone.[166,167]

As described in this current chapter, an existing large number of active novel chemotherapeutic and target-specific small molecules, second- and third-generation anti-CD20 and numerous other non-CD20 mAbs with potentially unique mechanisms of action, are under study. The largest "obstacle" facing clinicians and researchers today is how best to streamline the evaluation of a large number of effective therapies in order to determine their "optimal" use and sequencing in order to continue to improve both the quantity- and quality-of-life of FL patients not only today, but also for future generations of lymphoma patients.

References

1. Bende RJ, Smit LA, van Noesel CJ. Molecular pathways in follicular lymphoma. *Leukemia* 2007;**21**: 18–29.
2. Tsujimoto Y, Finger LR, Yunis J, *et al.* Cloning of the chromosome breakpoint of neoplastic B cells with the t(14;18) chromosome translocation. *Science* 1994;**226**:1097–9.
3. Cleary ML, Sklar J. Nucleotide sequence of a t(14;18) chromosomal breakpoint in follicular lymphoma and demonstration of a breakpoint-cluster region near a transcriptionally active locus on chromosome 18. *Proc Natl Acad Sci U S A* 1985;**82**:7439–43.
4. Bakhshi A, Jensen JP, Goldman P, *et al.* Cloning the chromosomal breakpoint of t(14;18) human lymphomas: clustering around JH on chromosome 14 and near a transcriptional unit on 18. *Cell* 1985;**41**:899–906.
5. Meijerink JPP. t(14:18): a journey to eternity. *Leukemia* 1997;**11**:2175–87.
6. Ross CW, Ouillette PD, *et al.* Comprehensive analysis of copy number and allele status identifies multiple chromosome defects underlying follicular lymphoma pathogenesis. *Clin Cancer Res* 2007;**13**:4777–85.
7. Danial NN. BCL-2 family proteins: critical checkpoints of apoptotic cell death. *Clin Cancer Res* 2007; **13**:7254–63.
8. Zha H, Raffeld M, Charboneau L, *et al.* Similarities of prosurvival signals in Bcl-2-positive and Bcl-2-negative follicular lymphomas identified by reverse phase protein microarray. *Lab Invest* 2004;**84**:235–44.
9. Schraders M, de Jong D, Kluin P, *et al.* Lack of Bcl-2 expression in follicular lymphoma may be caused by mutations in the BCL2 gene or by absence of the t(14;18) translocation. *J Pathol* 2005; **205**:329–35.
10. McDonnell TJ, Deane N, Platt FM, *et al.* BCL2-immunoglobulin transgenic mice demonstrate extended B cell survival and follicular lymphoproliferation. *Cell* 1989;**57**:79–88.
11. Strasser A, Harris AW, Bath ML, *et al.* Novel primitive lymphoid tumours induced in transgenic mice by cooperation between myc and BCL2. *Nature* 1990;**348**:331–3.
12. Horsman DE, Connors JM, Pantzar T, *et al.* Analysis of secondary chromosomal alterations in 165 cases of follicular lymphoma with t(14;18). *Genes Chromosomes Cancer* 2001;**30**:375–82.
13. Yunis JJ, Frizzera G, Oken MM, *et al.* Multiple recurrent genomic defects in follicular lymphoma. A possible model for cancer. *N Engl J Med* 1987;**316**:79–84.
14. Speaks SL, Sanger WG, Linder J, *et al.* Chromosomal abnormalities in

indolent lymphoma. *Cancer Genet Cytogenet* 1987;**27**:335–44.

15. Höglund M, Sehn L, Connors JM, *et al.* Identification of cytogenetic subgroups and karyotypic pathways of clonal evolution in follicular lymphomas. *Genes Chromosomes Cancer* 2004; **39**:195–204.

16. Alizadeh AA, Eisen MB, Davis RE, *et al.* Distinct types of diffuse large B-cell lymphoma identified by gene expression profiling. *Nature* 2000; **403**:503–11.

17. Davis RE, Brown KD, Siebenlist U, *et al.* Constitutive nuclear factor kappaB activity is required for survival of activated B cell-like diffuse large B cell lymphoma cells. *Exp Med* 2001; **194**:1861–74.

18. de Jong D, Rosenwald A, Chhanabhai M, *et al.* Immunohistochemical prognostic markers in diffuse large B-cell lymphoma: validation of tissue microarray as a prerequisite for broad clinical applications–a study from the Lunenburg Lymphoma Biomarker Consortium. *J Clin Oncol* 2007;**25**:805–12.

19. Dave SS, Wright G, Tan B, *et al.* Prediction of survival in follicular lymphoma based on molecular features of tumor-infiltrating immune cells. *N Engl J Med* 2004;**351**:2159–69.

20. Bohen SP, Troyanskaya OG, Alter O, *et al.* Variation in gene expression patterns in follicular lymphoma and the response to rituximab. *Proc Natl Acad Sci U S A* 2003;**100**:1926–30.

21. Glas AM, Kersten MJ, Delahaye LJ, *et al.* Gene expression profiling in follicular lymphoma to assess clinical aggressiveness and to guide the choice of treatment. *Blood* 2005;**105**:301–7.

22. de Jong D. Molecular pathogenesis of follicular lymphoma: a cross talk of genetic and immunologic factors. *J Clin Oncol* 2005;**23**:6358–63.

23. Hermans J, Krol AD, van Groningen K, *et al.* International Prognostic Index for aggressive non-Hodgkin's lymphoma is valid for all malignancy grades. *Blood* 1995;**86**:1460–3.

24. López-Guillermo A, Montserrat E, Bosch F, *et al.* Applicability of the International Index for aggressive lymphomas to patients with low-grade lymphoma. *J Clin Oncol* 1994;**12**:1343–8.

25. Solal-Céligny P, Roy P, Colombat P, *et al.* Follicular lymphoma international prognostic index. *Blood* 2004;**104**: 1258–65.

26. Buske C, Hoster E, Dreyling M, *et al.* The Follicular Lymphoma International Prognostic Index (FLIPI) separates high-risk from intermediate- or low-risk patients with advanced-stage follicular lymphoma treated front-line with rituximab and the combination of cyclophosphamide, doxorubicin, vincristine, and prednisone (R-CHOP) with respect to treatment outcome. *Blood* 2006;**108**:1504–8.

27. Winter JN, Gascoyne RD, Van Besien K. Low-grade lymphoma. *Hematology Am Soc Hematol Educ Program* 2004;203–20.

28. Hans CP, Weisenburger DD, Vose JM, *et al.* A significant diffuse component predicts for inferior survival in grade 3 follicular lymphoma, but cytologic subtypes do not predict survival. *Blood* 2003;**101**:2363–7.

29. Ganti AK, Weisenburger DD, Smith LM, *et al.* Patients with grade 3 follicular lymphoma have prolonged relapse-free survival following anthracycline-based chemotherapy: the Nebraska Lymphoma Study Group Experience. *Ann Oncol* 2006;**17**:920–7.

30. Harjunpää A, Taskinen M, Nykter M, *et al.* Differential gene expression in non-malignant tumour microenvironment is associated with outcome in follicular lymphoma patients treated with rituximab and CHOP. *Br J Haematol* 2006;**135**:33–42.

31. Glas AM, Knoops L, Delahaye L, *et al.* Gene-expression and immunohistochemical study of specific T-cell subsets and accessory cell types in the transformation and prognosis of follicular lymphoma. *J Clin Oncol* 2007;**25**:390–8.

32. Cerhan JR, Wang S, Maurer MJ, *et al.* Prognostic significance of host immune gene polymorphisms in follicular lymphoma survival. *Blood* 2007;**109**:5439–46.

33. Farinha P, Masoudi H, Skinnider BF, *et al.* Analysis of multiple biomarkers shows that lymphoma-associated macrophage (LAM) content is an independent predictor of survival in follicular lymphoma (FL). *Blood* 2005;**106**:2169–74.

34. Canioni D, Salles G, Mounier N, *et al.* High numbers of tumor-associated macrophages have an adverse prognostic value that can be circumvented by rituximab in patients with follicular lymphoma enrolled onto the GELA-GOELAMS FL-2000 trial. *J Clin Oncol* 2008;**26**:440–6.

35. Taskinen M, Karjalainen-Lindsberg ML, Nyman H, *et al.* A high tumor-associated macrophage content predicts favorable outcome in follicular lymphoma patients treated with rituximab and cyclophosphamide-doxorubicin-vincristine-prednisone. *Clin Cancer Res* 2007;**13**:5784–9.

36. Kelley T, Beck R, Absi A, *et al.* Biologic predictors in follicular lymphoma: importance of markers of immune response. *Leuk Lymphoma* 2007; **48**:2403–11.

37. Taskinen M, Karjalainen-Lindsberg ML, Leppä S. Prognostic influence of tumor-infiltrating mast cells in patients with follicular lymphoma treated with rituximab and CHOP. *Blood* 2008;**111**:4664–7.

38. Brice P, Bastion Y, Lepage E, *et al.* Comparison in low-tumor-burden follicular lymphomas between an initial no-treatment policy, prednimustine, or interferon alfa: a randomized study from the Groupe d'Etude des Lymphomes Folliculaires. Groupe d'Etude des Lymphomes de l'Adulte. *J Clin Oncol* 1997;**15**:1110–17.

39. Ardeshna KM, Smith P, Norton A, *et al.* British National Lymphoma Investigation. Long-term effect of a watch and wait policy versus immediate systemic treatment for asymptomatic advanced-stage non-Hodgkin lymphoma: a randomised controlled trial. *Lancet* 2003;**362**:516–22.

40. Wilder RB, Jones D, Tucker SL, *et al.* Long-term results with radiotherapy for stage I–II follicular lymphomas. *Int J Radiat Oncol Biol Phys* 2001;**51**:1219–27.

41. Tsang RW, Gospodarowicz MK. Radiation therapy for localized low-grade non-Hodgkin's lymphomas. *Hematol Oncol* 2005;**23**:10–17.

42. Horning SJ. Natural history of and therapy for the indolent non-Hodgkin's lymphomas. *Semin Oncol* 1993;**20**:75–88.

43. Young RC, Longo DL, Glatstein E, *et al.* The treatment of indolent lymphomas: watchful waiting v aggressive combined modality treatment. *Semin Hematol* 1988;**25**:11–16.

44. Ganti AK, Bociek RG, Bierman PJ, *et al.* Follicular lymphoma: expanding

therapeutic options. *Oncology (Williston Park)* 2005;**19**:213–28; discussion 228, 233–6, 239.

45. Peterson BA, Petroni GR, Frizzera G, *et al.* Prolonged single-agent versus combination chemotherapy in indolent follicular lymphomas: a study of the cancer and leukemia group B. *J Clin Oncol* 2003;**21**:5–15.

46. Ghielmini M, Rufibach K, Salles G, *et al.* Factors prognostic for response and event free survival and treatment related toxicity in 306 patients with follicular or mantle cell lymphoma randomized to single agent rituximab given at the standard or at a prolonged schedule. *Ann Oncol* 2005;**16**:1675–82.

47. Czuczman M, Grillo-Lopez A, Alkuzweny B, *et al.* Prognostic factors for non-Hodgkin's lymphoma patients treated with chemotherapy may not predict outcome in patients treated with rituximab. *Leuk Lymphoma* 2006; **47**:1830–40.

48. Solal-Celigny P, Salles GA, Brousse N, *et al.* Single 4-dose rituximab treatment for low-tumor burden follicular lymphoma (FL): survival analyses with a follow-up (F/Up) of at least 5 years. *Blood* 2004;**104**:169a.

49. Gokhale AS, Mayadev J, Pohlman B, *et al.* Gamma camera scans and pretreatment tumor volumes as predictors of response and progression after Y-90 anti-CD20 radioimmunotherapy. *Int J Radiat Oncol Biol Phys* 2005;**63**:194–201.

50. Kaminski MS, Zelenetz AD, Press OW, *et al.* Pivotal study of iodine I 131 tositumomab for chemotherapy-refractory low-grade or transformed low-grade B-cell non-Hodgkin's lymphomas. *J Clin Oncol* 2001; **19**:3918–28.

51. Herberman RR, Ortaldo JR, Bonnard GD. Augmentation by interferon of human natural and antibody-dependent cell-mediated cytotoxicity. *Nature* 1979;**277**:221–3.

52. Basham TY, Kaminski MS, Kitamura K, *et al.* Synergistic anti-tumor activity with IFN and anti idiotype monoclonal antibody in murine lymphoma. *J Immunol* 1986;**137**:3019–24.

53. Nakamura K, Kubo A, Hosokawa S, *et al.* Effect of α-interferon on anti-α-fetoprotein-monoclonal antibody targeting of hepatoma. *Oncology* 1993;**50**:35–40.

54. Murray JL, Zukiwski AA, Mujoo K, *et al.* Recombinant α-interferon enhances tumor targeting of an anti-melanoma monoclonal antibody in vivo. *J Biol Response Mod* 1990;**9**:556–63.

55. Yokota S, Hara H, Luo Y, *et al.* Synergistic potentiation of in vivo anti-tumor activity of anti-human T-leukemia immunotoxins by recombinant α-interferon. *Cancer Res* 1990;**50**:32–7.

56. Hagenbeek A, Carde P, Meerwaldt JH, *et al.* Maintenance of remission with human recombinant interferon-α 2a in patients with stages III and IV low-grade malignant non-Hodgkin's lymphoma. European Organization for Research and Treatment of Cancer Lymphoma Cooperative Group. *J Clin Oncol* 1990;**16**:41–7.

57. Solal-Celigny P, Lepage E, Brousse N, *et al.* Doxorubicin-containing regimen with or without interferon-α 2b for advanced follicular lymphomas: final analysis of survival and toxicity in the Groupe d'Etude des Lymphomes Folliculaires 86 Trial. *J Clin Oncol* 1998;**16**:2332–8.

58. Albertsson PA, Basse PH, Hokland M, *et al.* NK cells and the tumor microenvironment: implications for NK-cell function and anti-tumour activity. *Trends Immunol* 2003;**24**:603–9.

59. Cooper MA, Fehniger TA, Fuchs A, *et al.* NK cell and DC interactions. *Trends Immunol* 2004;**25**:47–52.

60. Berinstein N, Levy R. Treatment of a murine B cell lymphoma with monoclonal antibodies and IL 2. *J Immunol* 1987;**139**:971–6.

61. Berinstein N, Starnes CO, Levy R. Specific enhancement of the therapeutic effect of anti-idiotype antibodies on a murine B cell lymphoma by IL-2. *J Immunol* 1988;**140**:2839–45.

62. Golay J, Manganini M, Facchinetti V, *et al.* Rituximab-mediated antibody-dependent cellular cytotoxicity against neoplastic B cells is stimulated strongly by interleukin-2. *Haematologica* 2003;**88**:1002–12.

63. Friedberg JW, Neuberg D, Gribben JG, *et al.* Combination immunotherapy with rituximab and interleukin2 in patients with relapsed or refractory follicular non-Hodgkin's lymphoma. *Br J Haematol* 2002;**117**:828–34.

64. Berdeja JG, Hess A, Ambinder RF, *et al.* Lymphokine activated killer cells augment rituximab antibody dependent cellular cytotoxicity in patients with rituximab refractory lymphoma. *Blood* 2002;**100**:2264a.

65. Nadler LM, Stashenko P, Hardy R, *et al.* Serotherapy of a patient with a monoclonal antibody directed against a human lymphoma-associated antigen. *Cancer Res* 1980;**40**:3147–54.

66. Miller RA, Maloney DG, Warnke R, *et al.* Treatment of B-cell lymphoma with monoclonal anti-idiotype antibody. *N Engl J Med* 1982;**306**:517–22.

67. Kohler G, Milstein C. Continuous cultures of fused cells secreting antibody of predefined specificity. *Nature* 1975;**256**:495–7.

68. Barinaga M. From bench top to bedside. *Science* 1997;**278**:1036–9.

69. Leget GA, Czuczman MS. Use of rituximab, the new FDA-approved antibody. *Curr Opin Oncol* 1998;**10**:548–51.

70. Piro LD, White CA, Grillo-Lopez AJ, *et al.* Extended rituximab (anti-CD20 monoclonal antibody) therapy for relapsed or refractory low-grade or follicular non-Hodgkin's lymphoma. *Ann Oncol* 1999;**10**:655–61.

71. McLaughlin P, Grillo-Lopez AJ, Link BK, *et al.* Chimeric anti-CD20 monoclonal antibody therapy for relapsed indolent lymphoma: half of patients respond to a 4-dose, 22-day treatment program. *J Clin Oncol* 1998;**16**:2825–33.

72. Deans JP, Schieven GL, Shu GL, *et al.* Association of tyrosine and serine kinases with B cell surface antigen CD20. *J Immunol* 1993;**151**:4494–504.

73. Shan D, Ledbetter JA, Press OW. Apoptosis of malignant human B cell by ligation of CD20 with monoclonal antibodies. *Blood* 1998;**91**:1644–52.

74. Shan D, Ledbetter JA, Press OW. Signaling events involved in anti-CD20-induced apoptosis of malignant human B-cells. *Cancer Immunol Immunother* 2000;**48**:673–83.

75. Popoff IJ, Savage JA, Blake J, *et al.* The association between CD20 and Src-family tyrosine kinases requires an additional factor. *Mol Immunol* 1998; **35**:207–14.

76. Taji H, Kagami Y, Okada Y, *et al.* Growth inhibition of CD20-positive B lymphoma cell lines by IDEC-C2B8 anti-CD20 monoclonal antibody. *Jpn J Cancer Res* 1998;**89**:748–56.

77. Holder M, Grafton G, MacDonald I, *et al.* Engagement of CD20 suppress apoptosis in germinal center B cells. *Eur J Immunol* **25**:3160–4.

78. Mathas S, Rickers A, Bommert K, *et al.* Anti-CD20 and B-cell receptor-mediated apoptosis: evidence for shared intracellular signaling pathways. *Cancer Res* 2000;**60**:7170–6.

79. Hofmeister JK, Cooney D, Coggeshall KM. Clustered CD20 induced apoptosis: Src-family kinase, the proximal regulator of tyrosine phosphorylation, calcium influx, and caspase 3-dependent apoptosis. *Blood Cells, Mol Dis* 2000;**26**:133–43.

80. Harjunpaa A, Junnikkala S, Meri S. Rituximab (anti-CD20) therapy of B-cell lymphomas: direct complement killing is superior to cellular effector mechanisms. *Scand J Immunol* 2000;**51**:634–41.

81. Cragg MS, French RR, Glennie MJ. Signaling antibodies in cancer therapy. *Curr Opin Immunol* 1999;**11**:541–7.

82. Hernandez-Ilizaliturri FJ, Jupudy V, Oflazoglu E, *et al.* Neutrophils contribute to the biological anti-tumor activity of rituximab in a non-Hodgkin's lymphoma severe combined immunodeficiency (SCID) mouse model. *Clin Cancer Res* 2003;**9**: 5866–73.

83. Clynes RA, Towers TL, Presta LG, *et al.* Inhibitory Fc receptors modulate in vivo cytotoxicity against tumor targets. *Nat Med* 2000;**4**:443–6.

84. O'Keefe TL, Williams GT, Davies SL, *et al.* Mice carrying a CD20 gene disruption. *Immunogenetics* 1998;**48**:125–32.

85. Semac I, Palomba C, Kulangara K, *et al.* Anti-CD20 therapeutic antibody rituximab modifies the functional organization of rafts/microdomains of B lymphoma cells. *Cancer Res* 2003;**63**:534–40.

86. Polyak M, Tailor SH, Deans JP. Identification of a cytoplasmic region of CD20 required for its distribution to a detergent-insoluble membrane compartment. *J Immunol* 1998;**161**: 3242–8.

87. Alas S, Emmanouilides C, Bonavida B. Inhibition of interleukin 10 by rituximab results in down-regulation of Bcl-2 and sensitization of B-cell non-Hodgkin's lymphoma to apoptosis. *Clin Cancer Res* 2001;**7**:709–23.

88. Di Gaetano N, Xiao Y, Erba E, *et al.* Synergism between fludarabine and rituximab revealed in a follicular lymphoma cell line resistant to the cytotoxic activity of either drug alone. *Br J Haematol* 2001;**114**:800–9.

89. Davis TA, Grillo-López AJ, White CA, *et al.* Rituximab anti-CD20 monoclonal antibody therapy in non-Hodgkin's lymphoma: safety and efficacy of re-treatment. *J Clin Oncol* 2000; **18**(17):3135–43.

90. Colombat P, Salles G, Brousse N, *et al.* Rituximab (anti-CD20 monoclonal antibody) as single first-line therapy for patients with follicular lymphoma with a low tumor burden: clinical and molecular evaluation. *Blood* 2001;**97**:101–6.

91. Hainsworth JD, Litchy S, Burris HA 3rd, *et al.* Rituximab as first-line and maintenance therapy for patients with indolent non-hodgkin's lymphoma. *J Clin Oncol* 2002;**20**:4261–7.

92. Colombat P, Brousse N, Morschhauser F, *et al.* Single treatment with rituximab monotherapy for low-tumor burden follicular lymphoma (FL): survival analyses with extended follow-up (F/Up) of 7 years. *ASH Annual Meeting Abstracts* 2006;**108**:486.

93. Ghielmini M, Rufibach K, Salles G, *et al.* Single agent rituximab in patients with follicular or mantle cell lymphoma: clinical and biological factors that are predictive of response and event-free survival as well as the effect of rituximab on the immune system: a study of the Swiss Group for Clinical Cancer Research (SAKK). *Ann Oncol* 2005;**16**:1675–82.

94. Berinstein NL, Grillo-López AJ, White CA, *et al.* Association of serum rituximab (IDEC-C2B8) concentration and anti-tumor response in the treatment of recurrent low-grade or follicular non-Hodgkin's lymphoma. *Ann Oncol* 1998;**9**:995–1001.

95. Gordan LN, Grow WB, Pusateri A, *et al.* Phase II trial of individualized rituximab dosing for patients with CD20-positive lymphoproliferative disorders. *J Clin Oncol* 2005;**23**:1096–102.

96. Hainsworth JD, Litchy S, Shaffer DW, *et al.* Maximizing therapeutic benefit of rituximab: maintenance therapy versus re-treatment at progression in patients with indolent non-Hodgkin's lymphoma–a randomized phase II trial of the Minnie Pearl Cancer Research Network. *J Clin Oncol* 2005;**23**:1088–95.

97. Ghielmini M, Schmitz SF, Cogliatti SB, *et al.* Prolonged treatment with rituximab in patients with follicular lymphoma significantly increases event-free survival and response duration compared with the standard weekly x 4 schedule. *Blood* 2004;**103**:4416–23.

98. Hochster HS, Weller E, Gascoyne RD, *et al.* Maintenance rituximab after CVP results in superior clinical outcome in advanced follicular lymphoma (FL): results of the E1496 Phase III Trial from the Eastern Cooperative Oncology Group and the Cancer and Leukemia Group B. *ASH Annual Meeting Abstracts* 2005;**106**:349.

99. van Oers MH, Klasa R, Marcus RE, *et al.* Rituximab maintenance improves clinical outcome of relapsed/resistant follicular non-Hodgkin lymphoma in patients both with and without rituximab during induction: results of a prospective randomized phase 3 intergroup trial. *Blood* 2006;**108**:3295–301.

100. Forstpointner R, Unterhalt M, Dreyling M, *et al.* German Low Grade Lymphoma Study Group (GLSG). Maintenance therapy with rituximab leads to a significant prolongation of response duration after salvage therapy with a combination of rituximab, fludarabine, cyclophosphamide, and mitoxantrone (R-FCM) in patients with recurring and refractory follicular and mantle cell lymphomas: results of a prospective randomized study of the German Low Grade Lymphoma Study Group (GLSG). *Blood* 2006;**108**(13):4003–8.

101. Czuczman MS, Olejniczak S, Gowda A, *et al.* Acquirement of rituximab resistance in lymphoma cell lines is associated with both a global CD20 gene and protein down-regulation regulated at the pre- and post-transcriptional level. *Clin Cancer Res* 2008;**14**:1561–70.

102. Olejniczak S, Hernandez-Ilizaliturri FJ, Clements JL, *et al.* Acquired resistance to rituximab is associated with chemotherapy resistance resulting from down-regulation of Bax and Bak. *Clin Cancer Res* 2008;**14**:1550–60.

103. Czuczman MS, Weaver R, Alkuzweny B, *et al.* Prolonged clinical and molecular remission in patients with low-grade or follicular non-Hodgkin's lymphoma treated with rituximab plus CHOP chemotherapy: 9-year follow-up. *J Clin Oncol* 2004;**22**:4711–16.

104. Czuczman MS, Koryzna A, Mohr A, *et al.* Rituximab in combination with fludarabine chemotherapy in low-grade or follicular lymphoma. *J Clin Oncol* 2005;**23**:694–704.

105. Zinzani PL, Pulsoni A, Perrotti A, *et al.* Fludarabine plus mitoxantrone with and without rituximab versus CHOP with and without rituximab as front-line treatment for patients with follicular lymphoma. *J Clin Oncol* 2004;**22**:2654–61.

106. Forstpointner R, Dreyling M, Repp R, *et al.* The addition of rituximab to a combination of fludarabine, cyclophosphamide, mitoxantrone (FCM) significantly increases the response rate and prolongs survival as compared with FCM alone in patients with relapsed and refractory follicular and mantle cell lymphomas: results of a prospective randomized study of the German Low-Grade Lymphoma Study Group. *Blood* 2004;**104**: 3064–71.

107. Marcus R, Imrie K, Belch A, *et al.* CVP chemotherapy plus rituximab compared with CVP as first-line treatment for advanced follicular lymphoma. *Blood* 2005;**105**:1417–23.

108. Hiddemann W, Kneba M, Dreyling M, *et al.* Frontline therapy with rituximab added to the combination of cyclophosphamide, doxorubicin, vincristine, and prednisone (CHOP) significantly improves the outcome for patients with advanced-stage follicular lymphoma compared with therapy with CHOP alone: results of a prospective randomized study of the German Low-Grade Lymphoma Study Group. *Blood* 2005;**106**:3725–32.

109. Herold M, Haas A, Srock S, *et al.* East German Study Group Hematology and Oncology Study. Rituximab added to first-line mitoxantrone, chlorambucil, and prednisolone chemotherapy followed by interferon maintenance prolongs survival in patients with advanced follicular lymphoma: an East German Study Group Hematology and Oncology Study. *J Clin Oncol* 2007;**25**:1986–92.

111. Hale G, Gia MQ, Tighe HP, *et al.* The CAMPATH-1 antigen (CDw52). *Tissue Antigens* 1990;**35**:118–27.

112. Ginaldi L, De Martinis M, Matutes E, *et al.* Levels of expression of CD52 in normal and leukemic B and T cell. *Leuk Res* 1998;**22**:185–91.

113. Hale C, Bartholomew M, Taylor V, *et al.* Recognition of CD52 allelic gene products by Campath-1H antibodies. *Immunology* 1996;**88**:183–90.

114. Rowan WC, Hale G, Tite JP, *et al.* Cross-linking of the Campath-1 antigen (CD52) triggers activation of normal human T lymphocytes. *Int Immunol* 1995;**7**:69–77.

115. Rowan W, Tite J, Topley P, *et al.* Cross-linking of the Campath-1 antigen (CD52) mediates growth inhibition in human B- and T-lymphoma cell lines, and subsequent emergence of CD52-deficient cells. *Immunology* 1998; **95**:427–36.

116. Flynn J, Byrd JC. Campath-1H monoclonal antibody therapy. *Curr Opin Oncol* 2000;**12**:574–81.

117. Gilleece MH, Dexter TM. Effect of Campath 1-H antibody on human hematopoietic progenitors in vitro. *Blood* 1993;**82**:807–12.

118. Riechmann L, Clark MR, Waldmann H, *et al.* Reshaping human antibodies for therapy. *Nature* 1998;**332**:323–7.

119. Bindon CI, Hale G, Bruggemann M, *et al.* Human monoclonal IgG antibodies differ in complement activation function at the level of C4 as well as C1q. *J Exp Med* 1988;**268**;127–52.

120. Lim S, Davey G, Marcus R. Differential response in a patient treated with Campath-1H monoclonal antibody for refractory NHL. *Lancet* 1993;**341**:432–3.

121. Khorana A, Bunn P, Mclaughlin P, *et al.* A phase II multicenter study of Campath-1H antibody in previously treated patients with nonbulky non-Hodgkin's lymphoma. *Leuk Lymphoma* 2001;**41**:77–87.

122. Lundin J, Osterborg A, Brittinger G, *et al.* Campath-1H monoclonal antibody in therapy for previously treated low-grade non-Hodgkin's lymphomas: a phase II multicenter study. European Study Group of Campath-1H Treatment in Low-Grade Non-Hodgkin's Lymphoma. *J Clin Oncol* 1998;**16**:3257–63.

123. Tang SC, Hewitt K, Reis MD, *et al.* Immunosuppressive toxicity of CAMPATH1H monoclonal antibody in the treatment of patients with recurrent low grade lymphoma. *Leuk Lymphoma* 1996;**24**:93–101.

124. Moreau T, Coles A, Wing M, *et al.* Transient increase in symptoms associated with multiple sclerosis. *Brain* 1996;**119**:225–37.

125. Lundin J, Kimby E, Bjorkholm M, *et al.* Phase II trial of subcutaneous anti-CD52 monoclonal antibody alemtuzumab (Campath-1H) as first-line treatment for patients with B-cell chronic lymphocytic leukemia (B-CLL). *Blood* 2002;**100**:768–73.

126. Faderl S, Thomas DA, O'Brien S, *et al.* Experience with alemtuzumab plus rituximab in patients with relapsed and refractory lymphoid malignancies. *Blood* 2003;**101**:3413–15.

127. Dorken B, Moldenhauer G, Pezzutto A, *et al.* HD39 (B3), a B lineage-restricted antigen whose cell surface expression is limited to resting and activated human B lymphocytes. *J Immunol* 1986;**136**:4470–9.

128. Tuscano JM, Riva A, Toscano SN, *et al.* CD22 cross-linking generates B-cell antigen receptor-independent signals that activate the JNK/SAPK signaling cascade. *Blood* 1999;**94**:1382–92.

129. Shih LB, Lu HH, Xuan H, *et al.* Internalization and intracellular processing of an anti-B cell lymphoma monoclonal antibody, LL2. *Int J Cancer* 1994;**56**:538–45.

130. Kreitman RJ, Hansen HJ, Jones AL, *et al.* Pseudomonas exotoxin-based immunotoxins containing the antibody LL2 or LL2-Fab' induce regression of subcutaneous human B-cell lymphoma in mice. *Cancer Res* 1993;**53**:819–25.

131. Vitetta ES, Stone M, Amlot P, *et al.* Phase I immunotoxin trial in patients with B-cell lymphoma. *Cancer Res* 1991;**51**:4052–8.

132. Goldenberg DM, Horowitz JA, Sharkey RM, *et al.* Targeting, dosimetry, and radioimmunotherapy of B-cell lymphoma with iodine-131-labeled LL2 monoclonal antibody. *J Clin Oncol* 1991;**9**:548–64.

133. Leonard JP, Coleman M, Matthews JC, *et al.* Phase I/II trial of epratuzumab in non-Hodgkin's lymphoma. *Blood* 2002;**100**:1388a.

134. Leonard JP, Coleman M, Ketas JC, *et al.* Phase I/II trial of epratuzumab (humanized anti-CD22 antibody) in indolent non-Hodgkin's lymphoma. *J Clin Oncol* 2003;**21**:3051–9.

135. Leonard JP, Coleman M, Matthews JC, *et al.* Combination monoclonal antibody therapy for lymphoma: treatment with epratuzumab (anti-CD22) and

rituximab (anti-CD20) is well tolerated. *Blood* 2001;**98**:3506a.

136. Emmanouilides C, Leonard JP, Schuster SJ, *et al.* A multicenter, phase 2 study of combination antibody therapy with epratuzumab plus rituximab in recurring low-grade NHL. *Blood* 2003;**102**:233a.
137. Goldenberg DM, Horowitz JA, Sharkey RM, *et al.* Targeting, dosimetry, and radioimmunotherapy of B-cell lymphomas with iodine-131-labeled LL2 monoclonal antibody. *J Clin Oncol* 1991;**9**:548–64.
138. Mattes MJ, Griffiths GL, Difil H, *et al.* Processing of antibody–radioisotope conjugates after binding to the surface of tumor cells. *Cancer* 1994;**73**:787–93.
139. Vose JM, Colcher D, Gobar L, *et al.* Phase I/II trial of multiple dose 131 iodine-Mab LL2 (CD22) in patients with recurrent non-Hodgkin's lymphoma. *Leuk Lymphoma* 2000;**38**:91–101.
140. Juweid M, Sharkey RM, Behr T, *et al.* Treatment of non Hodgkin's lymphoma with radiolabeled murine, chimeric or humanized LL2 monoclonal antibody. *Cancer Res* 1995;**55**:5899–907.
141. Juweid ME, Stadtmauer E, Hajjar G, *et al.* Pharmacokinetics, dosimetry and initial therapeutic results with (I131) and In111-/Y90 labeled humanized LL2 anti CD22 monoclonal antibody in patients with relapsed, refractory NHL. *Clin Cancer Res* 1999;**5**:3292–303.
142. Salvatore G, Beers R, Margulies I, *et al.* Improved cytotoxic activity toward cell lines and fresh leukemia cells of a mutant anti-CD22 immunotoxin obtained by antibody phage display. *Clin Cancer Res* 2002;**8**:996–1002.
143. Kreitman RJ, Wilson WH, Bergeron K, *et al.* Efficacy of the anti-CD22 recombinant immunotoxin BL22 in chemotherapy resistant hairy cell leukemia. *N Engl J Med* 2001;**345**:241–7.
144. DiJoseph JF, Dougher MM, Kalyandrug LB, *et al.* Antitumor efficacy of a combination of CMC-544 (inotuzumab ozogamicin), a CD22-targeted cytotoxic immunoconjugate of calicheamicin, and rituximab against non-Hodgkin's B-cell lymphoma. *Clin Cancer Res* 2006;**12**:242–9.
145. Hernandez-Ilizaliturri FJ, Devineni S, Arora S, *et al.* Targeting CD20 and CD22 with rituximab in combination with CMC-544 results in improved anti-tumor activity against non-Hodgkin's lymphoma (NHL) pre-clinical models. *ASH Annual Meeting Abstracts* 2005;**106**:1473.
146. Hursey M, Newton DL, Hansen HJ, *et al.* Specifically targeting the CD22 receptor of human B-cell lymphomas with RNA damaging agents; a new generation of therapeutics. *Leuk Lymphoma* 2002;**43**:953–9.
147. Czuczman MS, Thall A, Witzig TE, *et al.* A phase I/II study of galiximab, an anti-CD80 antibody, for relapsed or refractory, follicular lymphoma. *J Clin Oncol* 2005;**23**(19):4390–8.
148. Leonard JP, Friedberg JW, Younes A, *et al.* A phase I/II study of galiximab (an anti-CD80 monoclonal antibody) in combination with rituximab for relapsed or refractory, follicular lymphoma. *Ann Oncol* 2007;**18**:216–23.
149. Georgakis GV, Li Y, Humphreys R, *et al.* Activity of selective fully human agonistic antibodies to the TRAIL death receptors TRAIL-R1 and TRAIL-R2 in primary and cultured lymphoma cells: induction of apoptosis and enhancement of doxorubicin- and bortezomib-induced cell death. *Br J Haematol* 2005;**130**:501–10.
150. Snell V, Clodi K, Zhao S, *et al.* Activity of TNF-related apoptosis-inducing ligand (TRAIL) in haematological malignancies. *Br J Haematol* 1997;**99**:618–24.
151. Walczak H, Miller RE, Ariail K, *et al.* Tumoricidal activity of tumor necrosis factor-related apoptosis-inducing ligand in vivo. *Nat Med* 1999;**5**:157–63.
152. Pitti RM, Marsters SA, Ruppert S, *et al.* Induction of apoptosis by Apo-2 ligand, a new member of the tumor necrosis factor cytokine family. *J Biol Chem* 1996;**271**:12 687–90.
153. Pukac L, Kanakaraj P, Humphreys R, *et al.* Mapatumumab, a fully human TRAIL-receptor 1 monoclonal antibody, induces cell death in multiple tumour types in vitro and in vivo. *Br J Cancer* 2005;**92**:1430–41.
154. Cretney E, Shanker A, Yagita H, *et al.* TNF-related apoptosis-inducing ligand as a therapeutic agent in autoimmunity and cancer. *Immunol Cell Biol* 2006;**84**:87–98.
155. Keane MM, Ettenberg SA, Nau MM, *et al.* Chemotherapy augments TRAIL-induced apoptosis in breast cell lines. *Cancer Res* 1999;**59**:734–41.
156. Griffith TS, Lynch DH. TRAIL: a molecule with multiple receptors and control mechanisms. *Curr Opin Immunol* 1998;**10**:559–63.
157. Younes A, Vose JM, Zelenetz AD, *et al.* Results of a phase 2 trial of HGSETR1 (agonistic human monoclonal antibody to TRAIL receptor 1) in subjects with relapsed/refractory non-Hodgkin's lymphoma (NHL). *Blood* 2005;**106**:146a.
158. Maddipatla S, Hernandez-Ilizaliturri FJ, Knight J, *et al.* Augmented anti-tumor activity against B-cell lymphoma by a combination of monoclonal antibodies (mAbs) targeting TRAIL-R1 and CD20. *Clin Cancer Res* 2007;**13**:4556–64.
159. Teeling JL, French RR, Cragg MS, *et al.* Characterization of new human CD20 monoclonal antibodies with potent cytolytic activity against non-Hodgkin lymphomas. *Blood* 2004;**104**:1793–800.
160. Beum PV, Lindorfer MA, Beurskens F, *et al.* Complement activation on B lymphocytes opsonized with rituximab or ofatumumab produces substantial changes in membrane structure preceding cell lysis. *J Immunol* 2008;**181**:822–32.
161. Glennie MJ, French RR, Cragg MS, *et al.* Mechanisms of killing by anti-CD20 monoclonal antibodies. *Mol Immunol* 2007;**44**:3823–37.
162. Hagenbeek A, Gadeberg O, Johnson P, *et al.* First clinical use of ofatumumab, a novel fully human anti-CD20 monoclonal antibody in relapsed or refractory follicular lymphoma: results of a phase 1/2 trial. *Blood* 2008; **111**:5486–95.
163. Coiffier B, Lepretre S, Pedersen LM, *et al.* Safety and efficacy of ofatumumab, a fully human monoclonal anti-CD20 antibody, in patients with relapsed or refractory B-cell chronic lymphocytic leukemia: a phase 1–2 study. *Blood* 2008;**111**:1094–100.
164. Czuczman MS, Grillo-Lopez AJ, White CA, *et al.* The treatment of patients with low-grade B-cell lymphoma with the combination of chimeric anti-CD20 monoclonal antibody (rituxan, rituximab) and CHOP chemotherapy. *J Clin Oncol* 1999;**17**:268–76.
165. Cheson BD, Horning SJ, Coiffier B, *et al.* Report of an international workshop to standardize response criteria for non-Hodgkin's lymphoma. *J Clin Oncol* 1999;**17**:1244–53.

166. Salles GA, Mounier N, de Guibert S, *et al.* Rituximab combined with chemotherapy and interferon in follicular lymphoma patients: results of the GELA-GOELAMS FL2000 study. *Blood* 2008;**112**:4824–31.

167. Fisher RI, LeBlanc M, Press OW, *et al.* New treatment options have changed the survival of patients with follicular lymphoma. *J Clin Oncol* 2005;**23**:8447–52.

168. Liu Q, Fayad L, Cabanillas F, *et al.* Improvement of overall and failure-free survival in stage IV follicular lymphoma: 25 years of treatment experience at The University of Texas M.D. Anderson Cancer Center. *J Clin Oncol* 2006;**24**:1582–9.

169. Kaminski MS, Estes J, Zasadny KR, *et al.* Radioimmunotherapy with iodine ^{131}I tositumomab for relapsed or refractory B-cell non-Hodgkin lymphoma: updated results and long-term follow-up of the University of Michigan experience. *Blood* 2000;**96**:1259–66.

170. Vose JM, Wahl RL, Saleh M, *et al.* Multicenter phase II study of iodine-131 tositumomab for chemotherapy-relapsed/refractory low-grade and transformed low grade B-cell non-Hodgkin's lymphomas. *J Clin Oncol* 2000;**18**:1316–23.

171. Wiseman GA, Gordon LI, Multani PS, *et al.* Ibritumomab tiuxetan radioimmunotherapy for patients with relapsed or refractory non-Hodgkin lymphoma and mild thrombocytopenia: a phase II multicenter trial. *Blood* 2002;**99**:4336–42.

172. Witzig TE, White CA, Wiseman GA, *et al.* Phase I/II trial of IDEC-Y2B8 radioimmunotherapy for treatment of relapsed or refractory CD20(+) B-cell non-Hodgkin's lymphoma. *J Clin Oncol* 1999;**17**:3793–803.

173. Witzig TE, Gordon LI, Cabanillas F, *et al.* Randomized controlled trial of yttrium-90-labeled ibritumomab tiuxetan radioimmunotherapy versus rituximab immunotherapy for patients with relapsed or refractory low-grade, follicular, or transformed B-cell non-Hodgkin's lymphoma. *J Clin Oncol* 2002;**20**:2453–63.

174. Witzig TE, Flinn IW, Gordon LI, *et al.* Treatment with ibritumomab tiuxetan radioimmunotherapy in patients with rituximab-refractory follicular non-Hodgkin's lymphoma. *J Clin Oncol* 2002;**20**:3262–9.

175. Kaminski MS, Tuck M, Estes J, *et al.* 131I-tositumomab therapy as initial treatment for follicular lymphoma. *N Engl J Med* 2005;**352**:441–9.

176. Green DJ, Pagel JM, Pantelias A, *et al.* Pretargeted radioimmunotherapy for B-cell lymphomas. *Clin Cancer Res* 2007;**13**(18 Pt 2):5598s–603s.

177. Sweetenham JW, Dicke K, Arcaroli J, *et al.* Efficacy and safety of yttrium 90 (90Y) ibritumomab tiuxetan (Zevalin (R)) therapy with rituximab maintenance in patients with untreated low-grade follicular lymphoma. *ASH Annual Meeting Abstracts* 2004;**104**:2633.

178. Press OW, Unger JM, Braziel RM, *et al.* Southwest Oncology Group. Phase II trial of CHOP chemotherapy followed by tositumomab/iodine I-131 tositumomab for previously untreated follicular non-Hodgkin's lymphoma: five-year follow-up of Southwest Oncology Group Protocol S9911. *J Clin Oncol* 2006;**24**:4143–9.

179. Laport GG. The role of hematopoietic cell transplantation for follicular non-Hodgkin's lymphoma. *Biol Blood Marrow Transplant* 2006;**12**(1 Suppl 1): 59–65.

180. Freedman AS, Neuberg D, Mauch P, *et al.* Long-term follow-up of autologous bone marrow transplantation in patients with relapsed follicular lymphoma. *Blood* 1999;**94**:3325–33.

181. Montoto S, Canals C, Rohatiner AZ, *et al.* EBMT Lymphoma Working Party. Long-term follow-up of high-dose treatment with autologous haematopoietic progenitor cell support in 693 patients with follicular lymphoma: an EBMT registry study. *Leukemia* 2007;**21**:2324–31.

182. Ladetto M, De Marco F, Benedetti F, *et al.* Gruppo Italiano Trapianto di Midollo Osseo (GITMO); Intergruppo Italiano Linfomi (IIL). Prospective, multicenter randomized GITMO/IIL trial comparing intensive (R-HDS) versus conventional (CHOP-R) chemoimmunotherapy in high-risk follicular lymphoma at diagnosis: the superior disease control of R-HDS does not translate into an overall survival advantage. *Blood* 2008;**111**:4004–13.

183. van Besien K, Loberiza FR Jr, Bajorunaite R, *et al.* Comparison of autologous and allogeneic hematopoietic stem cell transplantation for follicular lymphoma. *Blood* 2003;**102**(10):3521–9.

184. Ciechanover A, Schwarz AL. The ubiquitin-proteasome pathway: the complexity and myriad function of proteins death. *Proc Natl Acad Sci U S A* 1998;**95**:2727–30.

185. Hauser HP, Bardroff M, Pyrowolakis G, *et al.* A giant ubiquitin-conjugating enzyme related to IAP apoptosis inhibitors. *J Cell Biol* 1998;**141**:1415–22.

186. Palombella VJ, Rando OJ, Goldberg AL, *et al.* The ubiquitin-proteasome pathway is required for processing the NF-kappa B1 precursor protein and the activation of NF-kappa B. *Cell* 1994;**78**:773–85.

187. Peters JM. Proteasomes: protein degradation machines of the cell. *Trends Biochem Sci* 1994;**19**:377–82.

188. Coux O, Tanaka K, Goldberg AL. Structure and functions of the 20S and 26S proteasomes. *Annu Rev Biochem* 1996;**65**:801–47.

189. Gray DA, Inazawa J, Gupta K, *et al.* Elevated expression of Unph, a proto-oncogene at 3p21.3 in human lung tumors. *Oncogene* 1995;**10**:2179–83.

190. Keyomarsi K, Conte D, Toyofuku W, *et al.* Deregulation of cyclin *E* in breast cancer. *Oncogene* 1995;**11**:941–50.

191. Masdehors P, Merle-Beral H, Maloum K, *et al.* Deregulation of the ubiquitin system and p53 proteolysis modify the apoptotic response in B-cell lymphocytes. *Blood* 2000;**96**:269–74.

192. Jeremias I, Kupatt C, Bauman B. Inhibition of nuclear factor κB activation attenuates apoptosis resistance in lymphoid cells. *Blood* 1998;**91**:4624–31.

193. Blagosklonny MV, Wu GS, Omura S, *et al.* Proteasome-dependent regulation of p21WAF1/CIP1 expression. *Biochem Biophys Res Commun* 1996;**227**:564–9.

194. Pagano M, Tam SW, Theodoras AM, *et al.* Role of the ubiquitin-proteasome pathway in regulating abundance of the cyclin-dependent kinase inhibitor p27. *Science* 1995;**269**:682–5.

195. Drexler HC. Activation of the cell death program by inhibition of proteasome function. *Proc Natl Acad Sci U S A* 2002;**99**:16 220–5.

196. Lops UG, Erhardt P, Yao R, *et al.* p53-dependent induction of apoptosis by proteasome inhibitors. *J Biol Chem* 1997;**272**:12 893–6.

197. Voorhees PM, Dees CE, O'Neil B, *et al.* The proteasome as a target for

cancer therapy. *Clin Cancer Res* 2003; **9**:6316–25.

198. Pham LV, Tamayo AT, Yoshimura LC, *et al.* Inhibition of constitutive NF-kappa B activation in mantle cell lymphoma B cells leads to induction of cell cycle arrest and apoptosis. *J Immunol* 2003;**171**:88–95.
199. Hernandez-Ilizaliturri FJ, Kotowski A, Czuczman MS. PS341 inhibits cell proliferation, induces apoptosis of and enhances the biological effects of rituximab on non-Hodgkin's lymphoma (NHL) cell lines and lymphoma xenografts. *Blood* 2003; **102**:3359a.
200. O' Connor O, Srinivasan S, Hernandez F, *et al.* Oblimersen (Bcl-2 antisense) enhances the antitumor activity of bortezomib (Bor) in multiple myeloma (MM) and non-Hodgkin's lymphoma (NHL) preclinical models. *Blood* 2003;**102**:628a.
201. Ma MH, Yang HH, Parker K, *et al.* The proteasome inhibitor PS-341 markedly enhances sensitivity of multiple myeloma tumor cells to chemotherapeutic agents. *Clin Cancer Res* 2003;**9**:1136–44.
202. Cusack JC, Liu R, Houston M, *et al.* Enhanced chemosensitivity to CPT-11 with proteasome inhibitor PS-341: implications for systemic nuclear factor-B inhibition. *Cancer Res* 2001;**61**:3535–40.
203. Goy A, Younes A, McLaughlin P, *et al.* Phase II study of proteasome inhibitor bortezomib in relapsed or refractory B-cell non-Hodgkin's lymphoma. *J Clin Oncol* 2005;**23**:667–75.
204. O'Connor O, Wright J, Moskowitz C, *et al.* Phase II clinical experience with the novel proteasome inhibitor bortezomib in patients with indolent non-Hodgkin's lymphoma and mantle cell lymphoma. *J Clin Oncol* 2005;**23**:676–84.
205. Tse C, Shoemaker AR, Adickes J, *et al.* ABT-263: a potent and orally bioavailable Bcl-2 family inhibitor. *Cancer Res* 2008;**68**:3421–8.
206. Konopleva M, Watt J, Contractor R, *et al.* Mechanisms of antileukemic activity of the novel Bcl-2 homology domain-3 mimetic GX15–070 (obatoclax). *Cancer Res* 2008;**68**: 3413–20.

Chapter 19

Hodgkin lymphoma: epidemiology, diagnosis, and treatment

Andrew M. Evens and Sandra J. Horning

Introduction

Hodgkin disease/lymphoma is a malignancy with deep-rooted history. Thomas Hodgkin described the clinical history and post-mortem findings of lymphadenopathy and splenomegaly in six patients in 1832.[1] In 1865, Sir Samuel Wilks published a second paper entitled "Cases of the enlargement of the lymphatic glands and spleen (or Hodgkin's disease) with remarks."[2] In that report, Wilks described a disease that may remain in the lymph nodes for years and is associated with anemia, fevers, and weight loss. Over the next 30 years, several physicians (W. S. Greenfield 1878, Carl Sternberg 1879, and Dorothy Reed 1902) provided the first pathologic descriptions of the characteristic malignant cells.[3–5] Physicians initially believed that Hodgkin disease was caused by an infection, such as tuberculosis. Despite studies in the early twentieth century confirming the malignant nature of this disease, it has only been in the last 10–15 years that the malignant cells were shown to be derived from clonal B cells,[6–8] hence the current World Health Organization (WHO) designation as "Hodgkin lymphoma."[9]

Prior to the 1960s, patients with advanced-stage Hodgkin lymphoma were typically treated with single-agent chemotherapy, resulting in a median survival of approximately 1 year and 5-year overall survival (OS) of $< 5\%$.[10] Major success in Hodgkin lymphoma has been achieved by radiation treatment and moreover by the development of multi-agent poly-chemotherapy. In 1950, Peters reported 70–80% 10-year OS rates for patients with stage I disease treated with high-dose, fractionated radiation therapy (RT).[11] In 1964, investigators at the National Cancer Institute (NCI) pioneered a four-drug combination chemotherapy program, MOPP (nitrogen mustard, vincristine [Oncovin], procarbazine, and prednisone). They reported a 5-year OS rate of approximately 50% using MOPP for the treatment of advanced-stage Hodgkin lymphoma.[12] Over the past several decades, newer chemotherapy regimens have been developed leading to a multitude of large randomized clinical trials that have helped refine the treatment options for patients with newly diagnosed Hodgkin lymphoma. In addition, increased insight has been gained into the acute and long-term toxicities, in particular secondary cancers and cardiopulmonary disease, caused by Hodgkin lymphoma therapy. More recently, significant progress has been made into the understanding of the epidemiology, etiology, biology, and translational science of Hodgkin lymphoma.

Epidemiology

Descriptive epidemiology

United States

In 2008, it was estimated that 8220 new cases of Hodgkin lymphoma were diagnosed in the United States, while approximately 1350 persons died from the disease.[13] The male-to-female ratio of Hodgkin lymphoma is 1.5:1.0. Hodgkin lymphoma is more common in whites (age-adjusted incidence rate 3.38/100 000) compared with blacks (2.86/100 000) or Hispanics (2.45/100 000).[a] Hodgkin lymphoma has been associated with a bimodal age-incidence of disease, historically with the highest peak in the third decade of life and a second, smaller peak after the age of 50 years. Data from a recent Surveillance, Epidemiology, and End Results (SEER) analysis (SEER 17) show a continued bimodal peak with the first peak occurring at age 20–24 years (4.25/100 000) with a second prominent peak at 75–79 years of age (4.46/100 000) as shown in Figure 19.1. Further, these age-specific incidence

[a]Incidence source: SEER 17 areas (San Francisco, Connecticut, Detroit, Hawaii, Iowa, New Mexico, Seattle, Utah, Atlanta, San Jose-Monterey, Los Angeles, Alaska Native Registry, Rural Georgia, California excluding SF/SJM/LA, Kentucky, Louisiana, and New Jersey). Rates are per 100 000 and are age-adjusted to the 2000 US Std Population (19 age groups – Census P25–1130). The modeled rates are the point estimates for the regression lines calculated by the Joinpoint Regression Program (Version 3.3, April 2008, National Cancer Institute). Incidence data for Hispanics and non-Hispanics are based on NHIA and exclude cases from the Alaska Native Registry and Kentucky.

Management of Hematologic Malignancies, ed. Susan M. O'Brien, Julie M. Vose, and Hagop M. Kantarjian. Published by Cambridge University Press.

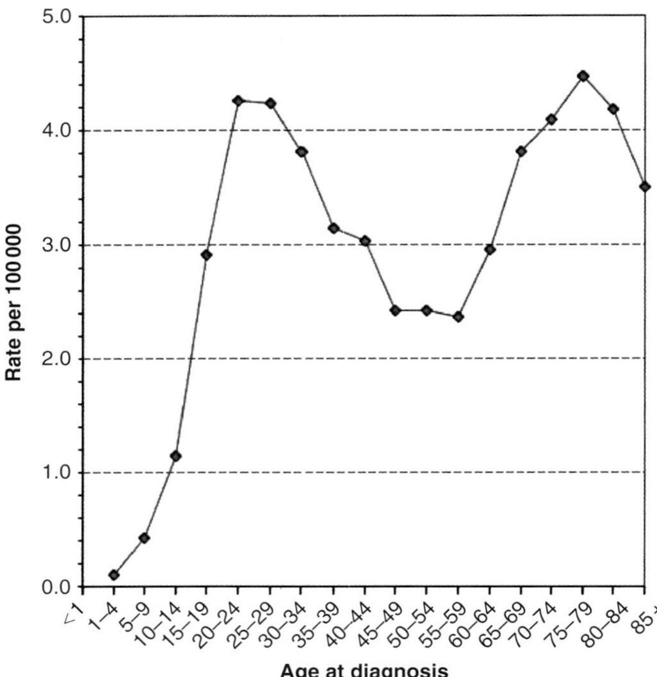

Figure 19.1 SEER incidence rate of Hodgkin lymphoma in the United States based on age (2000–5). Incidence source: SEER 17 areas (San Francisco [SF], Connecticut, Detroit, Hawaii, Iowa, New Mexico, Seattle, Utah, Atlanta, San Jose-Monterey [SJM], Los Angeles [LA], Alaska Native Registry, Rural Georgia, California excluding SF/SJM/LA, Kentucky, Louisiana, and New Jersey). Rates are per 100 000.

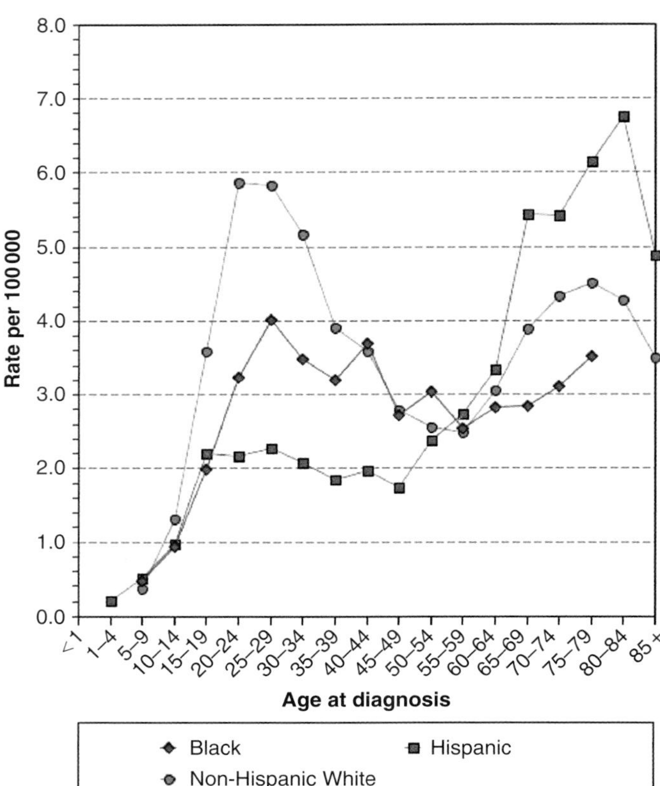

Figure 19.2 SEER incidence rate of Hodgkin lymphoma in the United States based on race/ethnicity (2000–5). Incidence source: SEER 17 areas (San Francisco [SF], Connecticut, Detroit, Hawaii, Iowa, New Mexico, Seattle, Utah, Atlanta, San Jose-Monterey [SJM], Los Angeles [LA], Alaska Native Registry, Rural Georgia, California excluding SF/SJM/LA, Kentucky, Louisiana, and New Jersey). Rates are per 100 000. Incidence data for Hispanics and non-Hispanics are based on NHIA (NAACCR [North American Association of Central Cancer Registries] Hispanic Identification Algorithm) and exclude cases from the Alaska Native Registry and Kentucky.

rates vary widely according to race/ethnicity as shown in Figure 19.2. In non-Hispanic whites, the second peak is smaller (age 20–24 years: 5.86/100 000 and age 75–79 years: 4.52/100 000), while in Hispanics the second peak is much more prominent compared with the first (age 25–29 years: 2.28/100 000 and age 80–84 years: 6.72/100 000).

Worldwide differences

The incidence of Hodgkin lymphoma varies greatly throughout the world. The highest rates of Hodgkin lymphoma are seen in the United States, Canada, and Eastern and Northern Europe, with markedly lower rates in China, Korea, and Japan (Figures 19.3 and 19.4).[14] The age-standardized incidence rate of Asian immigrants to the USA is slightly higher than their homeland, but still less frequent than non-immigrants (whites or blacks). Au *et al.* found that the incidence of Hodgkin lymphoma among immigrants of Chinese descent in British Columbia, Canada was significantly lower than expected from the British Columbia background population (24 observed vs. 71 expected cases; standardized incidence ratio [SIR] = 0.34; 90% confidence interval [CI] = 0.24–0.48; $p < 0.0001$), although the incidence was higher compared with the Hong Kong Chinese population (24 observed vs. 8.5 expected cases; SIR = 2.81; 90% CI = 1.94–3.95; $p < 0.0001$).[15] These data suggest that genetic and environmental factors play a role in the pathogenesis of Hodgkin lymphoma. In the 1970s, it was suggested that the international variation was due to economic development with increased incidence in developed countries compared with developing countries.[16] Later reports from the 1990s showed that the incidence rates for young adults had increased in less developed countries while they remained static in Western countries.[17] The incidence rate of Hodgkin lymphoma in the USA over the last 30 years has been overall stable with an age-adjusted incidence rate (per 100 000) of 3.08 in 1975 and 2.96 in 2005.[b]

[b]Incidence source: SEER 9 areas (San Francisco, Connecticut, Detroit, Hawaii, Iowa, New Mexico, Seattle, Utah, and Atlanta). Rates are per 100 000 and are age-adjusted to the 2000 US Std Population (19 age groups – Census P25–1130). Regression lines are calculated using the Joinpoint Regression Program Version 3.3, April 2008, National Cancer Institute.

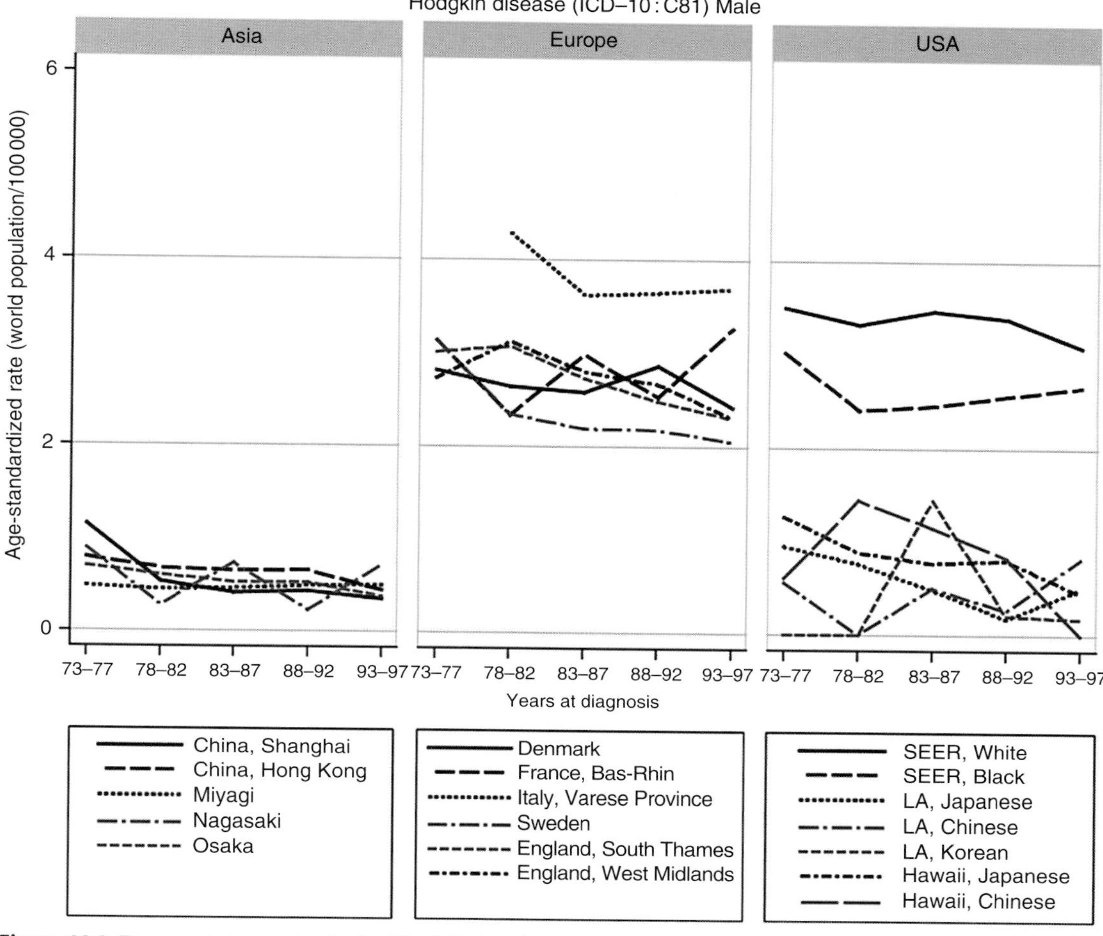

Figure 19.3 Time trends in age-standardized Hodgkin lymphoma incidence rate in 18 cancer registries in East Asia, Europe, and USA, males.

Etiologic epidemiology

Familial factors

The cause of Hodgkin lymphoma remains largely unknown. Genetic factors have been shown to be a likely component of Hodgkin lymphoma pathogenesis. Siblings of young adults with Hodgkin lymphoma have an approximate five- to tenfold excess risk of developing the disease,[18–21] the risk being higher for same-sex siblings.[18] Further, the monozygotic twin of a patient with Hodgkin lymphoma has an almost 100-fold risk of developing Hodgkin lymphoma, whereas the risk of a dizygotic twin is minimal.[22] The latter may be related in part to inherited interleukin-6 polymorphism genotypes.[23] Family history of hematopoietic malignancy in a first-degree relative has been shown to be associated with an approximate two- to threefold increased risk of Hodgkin lymphoma.[21,24–27] Anderson *et al.* studied the prognosis of familial Hodgkin lymphoma and found that survival appeared to be similar to sporadic patients.[26] The increased incidence of Hodgkin lymphoma in young adults in Westernized more affluent countries with smaller family size and growing up in a single-family house have suggested a role for an infectious and/or environmental agent in the etiology of this disease.[20,28] The hypothesis of delayed exposure to infection as an etiologic factor for Hodgkin lymphoma in young adults is strongest in Epstein–Barr virus (EBV)-positive Hodgkin lymphoma.[29,30] Accordingly, early exposure to other children at nursery school or day care was shown to be associated with decreased risk of Hodgkin lymphoma, possibly by facilitating exposure to common infections with associated promotion of cellular immunity.[27]

Infection

Despite the implications of EBV as an etiologic factor,[29–32] its role as a causative agent in Hodgkin lymphoma is not clear. The EBV genome is detected in 30–50% of tumor biopsies of Hodgkin lymphoma patients (as identified by latent membrane protein 1 [LMP-1] or EBV-encoded RNA [EBER] immunostaining of Hodgkin and Reed–Sternberg [H-RS] cells),[33–35] while a history of infectious mononucleosis is associated with an approximate three- to fourfold increased likelihood of developing Hodgkin lymphoma.[29,30,32] The risk of Hodgkin lymphoma appears to occur at a median of 3–4 years after EBV infection,[29,30] while some data support the idea that

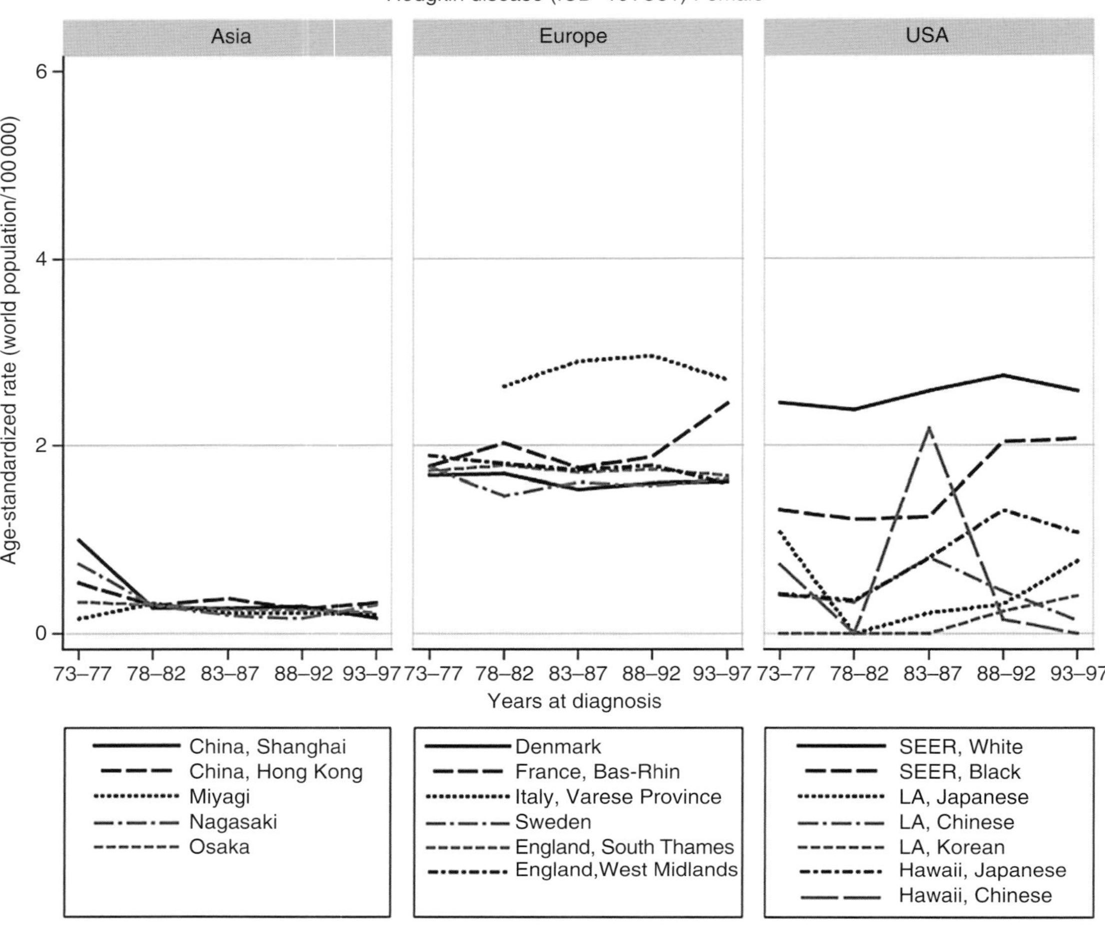

Figure 19.4 Time trends in age-standardized Hodgkin lymphoma incidence rate in 18 cancer registries in East Asia, Europe, and USA, females.

the risk may remain elevated for two decades after infection.[32] In young adults, Hodgkin lymphoma in underdeveloped countries and low socioeconomic groups is more likely to be EBV positive compared with developed countries and higher socioeconomic status.[33,34,36] Further, mixed-cellularity subtype, Hispanic ethnicity (vs. whites), male gender (vs. women), HIV-related, and older Hodgkin lymphoma patients (> age 60 years) are more likely to be EBV-associated.[36–38]

The risk of Hodgkin lymphoma in patients with human immunodeficiency virus (HIV) infection is approximately 10- to 20-fold increased compared with the general population.[39–42] The increased risk associated with HIV/AIDS is more pronounced than with iatrogenic immunosuppression (e.g., solid organ transplant recipients). A recent meta-analysis compared the risk of Hodgkin lymphoma, which was increased in both, slightly higher in HIV/AIDS (SIR 11.03) than post-transplant (SIR 3.89).[43] The effect of highly active antiretroviral therapy (HAART) on the incidence of HIV-related Hodgkin lymphoma has been investigated. Unlike non-Hodgkin lymphoma (NHL), Hodgkin lymphoma occurs more often at moderate levels of immunosuppression,[44] and there are emerging data suggesting that the corresponding relative risk of developing Hodgkin lymphoma increases following immune reconstitution when on HAART.[45] A Swiss report found no evidence of changed incidence patterns among HIV-positive patients using HAART,[46] while a recent British analysis found a significantly increased risk of Hodgkin lymphoma temporally associated with HAART therapy (SIR from 1983 to 1995 [pre-HAART era]: 4.5; from 1996 to 2001 [early HAART era]: 11.1; and from 2002 to 2007 [HAART widely available]: 32.4).[47]

Autoimmune and other factors

Autoimmune diseases have been linked with an increased risk of Hodgkin lymphoma. In a Scandinavian population-based analysis Landgren *et al.* show that personal history of the autoimmune conditions rheumatoid arthritis (odds ratio [OR] = 2.7; 95% CI = 1.9–4.0), systemic lupus erythematosus (OR = 5.8; 95% CI = 2.2–15.1), sarcoidosis (OR = 14.1; 95% CI = 5.4–36.8), and immune thrombocytopenic purpura (OR = infinity; p = 0.002) increased the risk of developing Hodgkin lymphoma.[48] Family history of sarcoidosis (OR = 1.8; 95% CI = 1.01–3.1) or ulcerative colitis (OR = 1.6; 95% CI = 1.02–2.6) was also associated with increased risk of Hodgkin lymphoma.

Several studies have shown that cigarette smoking is associated with Hodgkin lymphoma;[27,49–51] the mechanisms of susceptibility are not clear but may be related to non-specific immunologic abnormalities such as impaired humoral and cellular responses and/or direct carcinogenic effect. Other associations with increased risk of Hodgkin lymphoma that have been investigated but without a consistent causal association include Jewish ethnicity,[27] occupational exposures such as wood dust and chemicals such as phenoxy herbicides and chlorophenols,[52] and personal history of multiple sclerosis. Familial clustering of multiple sclerosis has been reported with young adult-onset Hodgkin lymphoma with the hypothesis of shared environmental and constitutional etiologies among the two conditions (e.g., EBV),[53] although not all studies have supported this association.[54]

Fewer data are available compared with non-Hodgkin lymphoma, but genetic features have been recently examined regarding risk of Hodgkin lymphoma. El-Zein *et al.* showed that germline polymorphisms in several DNA repair genes contributed to the susceptibility of developing Hodgkin lymphoma.[55] HLA class I region polymorphisms predicted risk of Hodgkin lymphoma.[56] Niens *et al.* found that the HLA-A*02 allele was associated with a reduced risk of developing EBV+ Hodgkin lymphoma, while individuals carrying the HLA-A*01 allele had an increased risk.[56] Lastly, deletions in glutathione *S*-transferase (GST) have been associated with increased risk of Hodgkin lymphoma, particularly among women less than 45 years of age.[57]

Biology

Clonal B cells

Significant knowledge of the genetic characteristics and transcriptional alterations of H-RS cells of classical Hodgkin lymphoma and "lymphocytic and histiocytic" (L&H) cells of nodular lymphocyte predominant Hodgkin lymphoma (NLPHL) has been acquired over the last decade, including recent information regarding transforming mechanisms and signaling pathways that contribute to the anti-apoptotic phenotype of H-RS and L&H cells.[58,59] H-RS cells show coexpression of markers normally expressed by different cell types, such as dendritic cells, granulocytes and monocytes (CD15), B cells (Pax-5), plasma cells (multiple myeloma oncogene-1-protein, CD138), and activated lymphocytes (CD30). H-RS cells generally do not express CD20 nor do they exhibit light chain restriction. The origin of the H-RS cells was finally established when single H-RS cells, microdissected from immunostained tissue sections, were analyzed for immunoglobulin (Ig) variable region (VAR) gene rearrangements. Monoclonal VAR gene rearrangements were found in nearly all cases of classical Hodgkin lymphoma, demonstrating that these malignant cells are derived from B cells.[6–8]

Transcription

Gene expression profiling studies of Hodgkin lymphoma cell lines extended the finding that H-RS cells lack expression of markers characteristic for B-lineage cells by a global downregulation of the B-cell phenotype.[60] The downregulation of several B-cell-specific transcription factors (i.e., Oct-2, Bob-1, and Pu.1) has been described,[61,62] and this likely contributes to the lost B-cell phenotype of H-RS cells as well as the downregulation of Ig expression. The suspected tumor cells of NLPHL, L&H cells, show an immunophenotype indicating B-cell origin including CD20 and CD79a, while the B-cell-specific transcription factors Pax-5, Oct-2, and Bob-1, and Ig are also expressed.[62,63] The germinal center B-cell origin had also been confirmed through single cell microdissection of L&H cells finding clonal and somatically mutated VAR Ig rearrangements.[7,64,65] Increasing knowledge has been gained regarding the transforming mechanisms involved in the pathogenesis of classical Hodgkin lymphoma. A hallmark of classical Hodgkin lymphoma H-RS cells is the constitutive activity of nuclear factor-kappa B (NF-κB) transcription factor that functions as an important survival signal. This activity may in part be due to signaling through members of the tumor necrosis factor (TNF) receptor family (CD30, CD40), and there is also evidence that EBV can mimic CD40 signaling. One of the main functions of virally encoded oncogene *LMP1* is activation of NF-K(κ)B, such that *LMP1* expression by EBV-infected H-RS cells represents a mechanism for constitutive NF-K(κ)B activity. The latent membrane protein 2A (*LMP-2A*), which is also expressed by EBV-infected H-RS cells, mimics a B-cell receptor, and it has been speculated that *LMP-2A* plays an important role in the rescue of EBV-positive H-RS cells from apoptosis.[66]

Apoptotic pathways

Several transcriptional signaling pathways are involved in the anti-apoptotic phenotype of H-RS and L&H cells. The major inhibitory molecules that prevent proper downstream caspase 3 activation in H-RS cells are c-FLICE inhibitory protein (*c-FLIP*)[67–70] and X-linked inhibitor of apoptosis proteins (*XIAP*),[71] blocking the extrinsic and intrinsic apoptotic pathways, respectively. The relevance of the CD95 pathway for the pathogenesis of HL came from the observation that H-RS cells are resistant to apoptosis and harbor clonal somatic CD95 mutations in some instances.[72] Additional evidence for the role of the extrinsic pathway in Hodgkin lymphoma pathogenesis is that c-FLIP expression has been shown to inhibit CD95,[67,70] and TNF receptor apoptosis-inducing ligand (*TRAIL*)-induced apoptosis in H-RS cells.[68,69] Many other factors, including multiple cytokine and chemokine interactions, as well as the Hodgkin lymphoma tumor microenvironment,[73] are also involved in the pathogenesis of Hodgkin lymphoma and have been reviewed elsewhere in detail.[58,59]

Staging

History

Following confirmation of pathologic diagnosis of Hodgkin lymphoma, complete staging is warranted to determine the extent of disease prior to the initiation of cytotoxic chemotherapy. Recommended clinical, laboratory, radiologic, and other testing prior to the start of treatment is depicted in Table 19.1. In 1939, Gilbert noted the propensity of Hodgkin lymphoma to spread by contiguity from one lymph nodal chain to adjacent nodal sites,[74] a concept later confirmed by Peters[11,75] and Austin-Seymour *et al.*[76] In part, staging laparotomy was used extensively to document the involvement and extent of abdominal disease in order to define fields of radiotherapy, the primary treatment modality at that time.[77] Clinical factors that predict for disease below the diaphragm include constitutional (B) symptoms of weight loss, fever, and night sweats, mixed cellularity or lymphocytic depletion (LD) histology, number of supradiaphragmatic sites greater than or equal to two, male sex, and age ≥ 40 years.[78] An analysis by the German Hodgkin Lymphoma Study Group (GHSG) found that among 391 patients diagnosed from 1988 to 1993, 21% had subdiaphragmatic disease.[79] On multivariate analysis, left cervical involvement, mediastinal disease, histology (mixed cellularity/lymphocyte depleted), and low performance status predicted for subdiaphragmatic disease whereas mediastinal disease reduced the risk. With the evolution of chemotherapy over the past 20–30 years, staging laparotomy is no longer warranted.

Table 19.1. Staging studies for Hodgkin lymphoma

Clinical	Detailed history with evaluation of B symptoms and pruritis; physical examination with complete lymph node exam, inspection of Waldeyer's ring, and evaluation of liver and spleen size
Laboratory	CBC with differential, ESR, metabolic panel including albumin and liver function tests
Radiologic	CT of chest, abdomen, and pelvis (neck included if not able to be detailed on physical examination)[a] Nuclear scan (PET scan)[b] CXR (PA and lateral) for patients with large mediastinal mass
Other	Pulmonary function tests (PFTs) with diffusion lung capacity of oxygen (DLCO) MUGA (to determine ejection fraction) Bone marrow aspirate and biopsy (bilateral)
Additional tests for patients at risk	HIV testing, TB test with anergy panel, and hepatitis B testing (surface antigen and core antibody)

Note: [a]Number of lymph node sites should be documented, especially for stage II disease.
[b]If combined FDG-PET/CTs performed, dedicated CTs should be obtained unless oral and intravenous contrast were given with FDG-PET/CT.
CBC: complete blood count; ESR: erythrocyte sedimentation rate; PET: positron emission tomography; CXR: chest X-ray; PA: posterior-anterior; PFT: pulmonary function tests; DLCO: carbon monoxide diffusing capacity; MUGA: multi-gated acquisition scan; TB: tuberculosis; HIV: human immunodeficiency virus.

FDG-PET

Prior to the 1990s, lymphangiography and ^{64}gallium scanning were commonly used for staging, especially to evaluate disease below the diaphragm.[77] These studies have been largely replaced by high-resolution CT scanning and ^{18}F-fluorodeoxyglucose positron emission tomography (FDG-PET).[80–82] FDG-PET scanning is helpful to evaluate for less commonly involved extranodal sites (e.g., bone, liver), but also to assist in the evaluation of response to therapy since residual radiographic abnormality on CT images is common after the completion of therapy. Combined FDG-PET/CT scanning has become popular recently. It is important to note that it is still recommended that dedicated CT scans be obtained in addition to FDG-PET/CT as CT scans with contrast are the most precise determinant of tumor size and location. Revised response guidelines were published through the International Harmonization Project incorporating FDG-PET into definitions of response.[83] Hodgkin lymphoma clinical trials now incorporate these FDG-PET guidelines, which better differentiate complete remission (CR) and partial remission (PR) and have eliminated the category of CR unconfirmed (CRu). There are several issues, however, that need to be considered with FDG-PET, such as technical variability and false positivity (e.g., infection, thymic hyperplasia, brown fat, diffuse marrow uptake with hematopoietic growth factors, etc.).

Bone marrow

The incidence of bone marrow involvement at diagnosis ranges from 5% to 13%.[84–88] Of note, trephine biopsy is indicated for some presentations,[86] whereas flow cytometric analysis is not useful. Several studies have examined the utility and predictability of bone marrow involvement.[85,89] A Greek group reported on independent prognostic factors associated with bone marrow involvement: presence of B symptoms, stage III/IV prior to marrow biopsy, anemia, blood leukocyte count $< 6000/\mu L$, iliac/inguinal node involvement, and age ≥ 35 years.[88] Stage I/IIA without any of these risk factors had a $< 0.5\%$ risk of bone marrow involvement and most authorities no longer support bone marrow biopsy in this group.

Other testing

Other warranted tests prior to initiating chemotherapy include pulmonary function testing with carbon monoxide diffusing capacity (DLCO) and assessment of ejection fraction (e.g., multi-gated acquisition scan [MUGA]) in anticipation of use of bleomycin- and anthracycline-based chemotherapy (Table 19.1). Patients with pulmonary or cardiac impairment may need decreased dosing or alteration of the planned chemotherapy regimen and/or may need these tests to be repeated intermittently during chemotherapy.

Classification

The same four-stage system applies to Hodgkin and the non-Hodgkin lymphomas. The Ann Arbor system and the later Cotswolds modification are used for Hodgkin disease staging/classification.[83,90] (Table 19.2). Stage IIIA/B and IVA/B are considered advanced stage, while some groups also consider/include stage IIB (with or without bulk disease) in advanced-stage clinical trials. Staging reflects extent and location of disease; presence or absence of B symptoms; occurrence of extranodal disease; and tumor bulk.

Clinical presentation

The median age of patients presenting with Hodgkin lymphoma is approximately 35 years; however, within population-based studies, the proportion of Hodgkin lymphoma patients over age 60 years has ranged between 15% and 30%.[91–96] The majority of Hodgkin lymphoma patients present with enlarged lymph nodes most commonly in the cervical region/supraclavicular (60–70%), axillary (15–20%), and/or mediastinal areas. Uncommon nodal sites of involvement are Waldeyer's ring, occipital, and epitrochlear. Lymph nodes are typically painless, although they may uncommonly become painful shortly after alcohol ingestion.

The majority of patients present with supradiaphragmatic disease. Approximately 15–20% of patients present with disease below the diaphragm. As discussed before, Hodgkin lymphoma classically starts as a localized process and spreads to "contiguous" lymphoid structures. Constitutional symptoms such as: B symptoms defined above, pruritus (typically in absence of rash, may be severe, and may precede diagnosis by months), fatigue, malaise, and weakness are seen in approximately one-third of all patients on presentation. When including only patients with stage III and IV disease, approximately 50–60% present with presence of B symptoms.[97–102] Uncommonly, patients will present with symptoms due to compressive lymph node disease such as shortness of breath, cough, and chest pain (due to very large mediastinal mass) or rarely superior vena cava or spinal cord syndrome.

Note: Stage extranodal disease sites. Besides palpable lymphadenopathy, signs on physical examination and laboratory abnormalities include splenomegaly, hepatomegaly, anemia (normochromic, normocytic), leukocytosis, thrombocytosis, eosinophilia, lymphopenia, elevated alkaline phosphatase, and elevated erythrocyte sedimentation rate (ESR). Laboratory abnormalities resolve once therapy is initiated. Extranodal disease may represent extension in a limited area (e.g., chest wall, lung) or be disseminated in nature. Among advanced-stage patients, approximately 10–20% will have two or more extranodal sites present at diagnosis.[100,102,103] Involvement of the liver is rare, and when present, almost always occurs with concomitant splenic involvement. When extranodal pulmonary disease is present, it typically occurs together with hilar nodal disease. Other uncommon clinical presentations of this disease include autoimmune hemolytic anemia and immune thrombocytopenic purpura,[104] Hodgkin lymphoma-related vanishing bile duct syndrome and idiopathic cholestasis,[105] hypothermia,[106] nephrotic syndrome,[107] and paraneoplastic neurologic syndromes.[108]

Table 19.2. Cotswolds classification staging system

Stage	Description
I	Involvement of a single lymph node region or lymphoid structure (e.g., spleen, thymus, Waldeyer's ring) or involvement of a single extralymphatic site
II	Involvement of two or more lymph node regions on the same side of the diaphragm (hilar nodes, when involved on both sides, constitute stage II disease); localized contiguous involvement of only one extranodal organ or site and lymph node region(s) on the same side of the diaphragm (IIE). The number of anatomic regions involved should be indicated by a subscript (e.g., II_3)
III	Involvement of lymph node regions on both sides of the diaphragm (III), which may also be accompanied by involvement of the spleen (III_S) or by localized contiguous involvement of only one extranodal organ site (III_E) or both (III_{SE}) III_1 With or without involvement of splenic, hilar, celiac, or portal nodes III_2 With involvement of para-aortic, iliac, and mesenteric nodes
IV	Diffuse or disseminated involvement of one or more extranodal organs or tissues, with or without associated lymph node involvement
Additional designations (applicable to any stage)	A = absence of B symptoms; B = + presence of B symptoms (fever/temperature > 38 °C, drenching night sweats, unexplained loss of > 10% body weight within preceding 6 months) E = involvement of a single extranodal site that is contiguous or proximal to the known nodal site X = bulky disease: ratio > one-third largest transverse diameter of thorax on standing posterior-anterior chest radiograph or > 10 cm maximal dimension of nodal mass

Prognosis

Early-stage Hodgkin lymphoma: definition and prognosis

Early-stage Hodgkin lymphoma is frequently subdivided into "favorable" early-stage and "unfavorable" (or intermediate) early-stage disease based on presence or absence of adverse prognostic factors (Table 19.3). This has been especially important for design of homogenous patient populations for prospective clinical trials. In Europe, the GHSG defines clinical stage I–II (supradiaphragmatic only) patients as unfavorable (intermediate) if any of the following four factors are present: (1) large mediastinal mass (LMM), (2) extranodal disease, (3) elevated ESR (≥ 50 without or ≥ 30 with B symptoms), and/or (4) ≥ 3 involved nodal regions.[109,110] The European Organisation for Research and Treatment of Cancer (EORTC) differs substituting age ≥ 50 years (in place of extranodal) and ≥ 4 involved regions (vs. ≥ 3).[111]

The National Cancer Institute of Canada (NCI-C) and the Eastern Cooperative Oncology Group (ECOG) in their early-stage trial subdivided early-stage Hodgkin lymphoma into risk categories with "low risk" being: NLPHL and nodular sclerosis histology, age < 40 years, ESR < 50, and ≤ 3 disease regions; "high risk": all others in stages I–II, excluding bulky disease > 10 cm, which is assigned advanced-stage disease.[112] In the GHSG, all stage III and IV patients plus stage I–IIB with LMM or E-lesions (extralymphatic extension of the disease) are included in the "advanced" group (Table 19.3).

Table 19.3. Definition of treatment groups according to risk factors

GHSG risk factors	EORTC/GELA risk factors
Large mediastinal mass	Large mediastinal mass
Elevated ESR[a]	Elevated ESR[a]
3 or more involved nodal regions	4 or more involved nodal regions
Extranodal disease	Age ≥ 50 years
Early-stage favorable: I–II with no risk factors	*Early-stage favorable*: I–II (supradiaphragmatic only) with no risk factors
Early-stage intermediate: I–IIA with 1 or more risk factors or I/IIB with elevated ESR and/or 3 or more involved nodal regions	*Early-stage intermediate*: I–II (supradiaphragmatic only) with 1 or more risk factors
Advanced stage: III/IV or I/IIB with large mediastinal mass and/or extranodal disease	*Advanced stage*: III/IV

Note: [a]ESR: ≥ 50 without or ≥ 30 with B symptoms.
ESR: erythrocyte sedimentation rate; GHSG: German Hodgkin Lymphoma Study Group; EORTC: European Organization for Research and Treatment of Cancer; GELA: Groupe d'Etude des Lymphomes de l'Adulte.

Advanced-stage Hodgkin lymphoma

An international effort involving more than 5000 patients, led by Hasenclever and Diehl, identified prognostic factors in advanced-stage classical Hodgkin lymphoma.[113] Seven factors were recognized on multivariate analysis, each of which contributed about a 7% reduction in freedom from progression (FFP) at 5 years: stage IV, male sex, age, hemoglobin, white blood count, lymphocyte count, and albumin (Table 19.4). One of the seven adverse prognostic factors included age over 45 years. It should also be noted, however, that only 9% of patients were > 55 years of age and no patients $>$ age 65 years were included (Volker Diehl, personal communication, 2010).

In a subsequent analysis of 462 patients, the GHSG reported that severe leukopenia during chemotherapy was associated with improved freedom from treatment failure (FFTF) by multivariate analysis ($p < 0.001$).[114] Interestingly, women had more frequent severe leukopenia and an improved survival compared with men. It is not clear if actual delivered dose intensity would have the same prognostic impact.

Table 19.4. International prognostic score (IPS): advanced-stage disease

Number of risk factors[a]	Percent of population	Freedom from disease progression at 5 years (%)
0	7	84
1	22	77
2	29	67
3	23	60
4	12	51
5+	7	42

Note: [a]Risk factors: stage IV disease; male gender; age > 45 years; hemoglobin < 10.5 g/dL; WBC $> 15\,000/\mu L$; lymphocytes $< 8\%$ or absolute lymphocyte count $600/\mu L$; albumin < 4 g/dL.

FDG-PET to predict outcome in Hodgkin lymphoma

As discussed before, FDG-PET has become a standard imaging modality complementing CT scans in the diagnosis and management of Hodgkin lymphoma.[115–118] In advanced-stage Hodgkin lymphoma, treatment intensification could theoretically benefit the proportion of patients who respond insignificantly to therapy as determined by interim FDG-PET scanning. Several early studies of both non-Hodgkin lymphoma and Hodgkin lymphoma showed that early FDG-PET was a strong indicator of survival.[81,115,118–121] Hutchings and colleagues reported that FDG-PET after two cycles standard ABVD chemotherapy (see below) (PET-2) was significantly predictive of survival; the 2-year progression-free survival (PFS) for FDG-PET-2-negative patients was 96% compared with 0% for FDG-PET-2-positive patients.[122] In this prospective study, there was no appreciable difference between the prognostic value of FDG-PET after two vs. four cycles or compared to FDG-PET at the end of therapy. Gallamini and colleagues reported on the prognostic importance of "early FDG-PET" after two of six planned chemotherapy cycles (doxorubicin, bleomycin, inblastine, and dacarbazine [ABVD] in 96%) for 108 patients with advanced-stage HL.[123] The 2-year PFS rate for patients with a negative FDG-PET-2 compared with a positive FDG-PET-2 were 96% and 6%, respectively ($p < 0.01$). A compilation of the Italian and Danish data further showed that FDG-PET-2 has prognostic value independent of IPS risk stratification.[124] Early FDG-PET assessment has been less well studied with more aggressive chemotherapy regimens routinely incorporating growth factors. Dann and colleagues studied early FDG-PET in two different Hodgkin lymphoma risk groups following two cycles of BEACOPP (bleomycin, etoposide, doxorubicin [Adriamycin], cyclophosphamide, vincristine, procarbazine, and prednisone) chemotherapy (see below).[125] Early positive FDG-PET was used to decrease or intensify therapy based on FDG-PET-2 outcome. These data support the concept of early risk assessment using FDG-PET imaging in the study of newly diagnosed Hodgkin lymphoma. Several issues regarding FDG-PET response-adapted therapy need to be considered, however, including consistent definitions of FDG-PET-negativity vs. positivity and strategy of trial design with appropriate control arms. It is also important to note that the vast majority of early FDG-PET data has been studied in patients with advanced-stage disease.

Emerging factors

EBV

There are emerging pathologic and genetic factors in Hodgkin lymphoma with potential etiologic and prognostic importance.[36,37,94] Two population-based studies showed that the survival of older patients with EBV-positive tumors was significantly inferior compared with EBV-negative tumors.[94,96] Among 922 classical Hodgkin lymphoma patients, Keegan *et al.* showed that the presence of EBV independently predicted inferior survival for older adults (age 45–96 years) with significantly increased Hodgkin lymphoma-specific mortality (hazard ratio for death 2.5).[126] Interestingly, presence of EBV predicted for superior survival for patients < 15 years of age. In a prospective population-based elderly Hodgkin lymphoma study, Stark *et al.* reported that 34% of cases were EBV positive by LMP staining and that EBV status correlated with stage at presentation (EBV positive: 9% early stage vs. 50% advanced stage, $p = 0.0006$).[96] Moreover, EBV-positive Hodgkin lymphoma was associated with inferior OS compared with EBV-negative cases (median OS 20 months vs. not reached, respectively; $p = 0.007$). Others have confirmed the correlation of inferior survival for older patients with EBV-positive Hodgkin lymphoma.[127,128] Although the basis for this association is unknown, it may reflect reduced EBV-specific cellular immunity of older patients. The weaker immunocompetence in older patients may allow increased proliferation of an EBV-related tumor and/or EBV antigens might induce a less robust immune response.[129,130]

Other factors

Kelley and colleagues reported that Hodgkin lymphoma patients with more intra-tumor T-cell regulatory cells (Tregs), and fewer activated cytotoxic T/natural killer (NK) lymphocytes, had superior survival.[131] Older age (> 45 years) in that analysis was associated with decreased forkhead box P3 (FOXP3) Tregs and increased granzyme-B-positive cells compared with younger patients. Maggio *et al.* reported that the lack of HLA class II cell surface expression on H-RS cells was associated with inferior failure-free survival (FFS) and OS.[67] This factor was significant on multivariate analysis with a relative risk of death of 2.55. The only other factor in that study associated with increased risk of death was older age (> age 65: relative risk of death 6.47). A recent pharmacogenetic study related various enzyme gene polymorphisms with outcome. Ribrag *et al.* showed that patients who carried one or two UGT1A1*28 alleles had a significantly better FFP, time to treatment failure (TTF), and OS compared with patients homozygous for the UGT1A1 allele.[132] In addition to influencing risk of Hodgkin lymphoma, at least one glutathione S-transferase (GST) deletion (*GSTM1* or *GSTT1*) associated with improved disease-free survival (DFS) in the study of Hohaus *et al.*[57]

Treatment

Major success was achieved initially by refinement in radiation techniques, and more recently, by the development of multiagent polychemotherapy. DeVita and Carbone pioneered the combination of nitrogen mustard, vincristine (Oncovin), procarbazine, and prednisone (MOPP) for the treatment of advanced-stage Hodgkin lymphoma in the late 1960s which was followed by the ABVD (doxorubicin, bleomycin, vinblastine, dacarbazine) combination developed by Bonadonna *et al.* in the 1970s, both landmark events in oncology.[133] Over the last 10–15 years, other chemotherapy regimens have been developed leading to a number of prospective clinical trials that have shaped the treatment for current patients with newly diagnosed Hodgkin lymphoma (Table 19.5).

Favorable early-stage disease

Overview

High cure rates are achieved in favorable stage I–II patients treated with combined modality strategies using chemotherapy followed by RT. Many of the completed and ongoing early-stage studies[109–112,134–146] were developed in an attempt to reduce the long-term morbidity and potentially fatal side effects of treatment, in particular secondary tumors[147–153] and cardiovascular toxicity,[147,154–159] without compromising the high cure rate. These studies include evaluation of the optimal chemotherapy regimen,[111,135,139,141,143] the optimal number of chemotherapy cycles,[112,137–141] and determination of the optimal RT volume and dose in combination with chemotherapy.[111,112,134,136–138,140–144,146]

Table 19.5. Multiagent chemotherapy regimens used in Hodgkin lymphoma

Drug	Dose (mg/m^2)	Route	Cycle schedule (days)	Cycle length
ABVD				
Adriamycin (doxorubicin)	25	IV	1, 15	28 days
Bleomycin	10	IV	1, 15	
Vinblastine	6	IV	1, 15	
Dacarbazine	375	IV	1, 15	
BCVPP				
Carmustine (BCNU)	100	IV	1	28 days
Cyclophosphamide	600	IV	1	
Vinblastine	5	IV	1	
Procarbazine	50	PO	1	
	100	PO	2–10	
Prednisone	60	PO	1–10	
BEACOPP (baseline)				
Bleomycin	10	IV	8	21 days
Etoposide	100	IV	1–3	
Adriamycin (doxorubicin)	25	IV	1	
Cyclophosphamide	650	IV	1	
Oncovin (vincristine)	1.4[a]	IV	8	
Procarbazine	100	PO	1–7	
Prednisone	40	PO	1–14	
BEACOPP (escalated)				
Bleomycin	10	IV	8	21 days
Etoposide	200	IV	1–3	
Adriamycin (doxorubicin)	35	IV	1	
Cyclophosphamide	1250	IV	1	
Oncovin (vincristine)	1.4[a]	IV	8	
Procarbazine	100	PO	1–7	
Prednisone	40	PO	1–14	
G-CSF	+	SQ	8+	
BEACOPP-14				
Bleomycin	10	IV	8	14 days
Etoposide	100	IV	1–3	
Adriamycin (doxorubicin)	25	IV	1	
Cyclophosphamide	650	IV	1	
Oncovin (vincristine)	1.4[a]	IV	8	
Procarbazine	100	PO	1–7	
Prednisone	40	PO	1–7	
G-CSF	+	SQ	8–13	

Table 19.5. *(cont.)*

Drug	Dose (mg/m^2)	Route	Cycle schedule (days)	Cycle length
ChlVPP				
Chlorambucil	6	PO	1–14	28 days
Vinblastine	6	IV	1, 8	
Procarbazine	100	PO	1–14	
Prednisone	40 total	PO	1–14	
Stanford V				
Mechlorethamine	6	IV	Wk 1, 5, 9	12 weeks
Adriamycin (doxorubicin)	25	IV	Wk 1, 3, 5, 9, 11	
Vinblastine	6	IV	Wk 1, 3, 5, 9, 11	
Vincristine	1.4[a]	IV	Wk 2, 4, 6, 8, 10, 12	
Bleomycin	5	IV	Wk 2, 4, 6, 8, 10, 12	
Etoposide	60	IV	Wk 3, 7, 11	
Prednisone	40	IV	Wk 1–9 qod, then taper	
G-CSF	+	SQ	If dose reduction or delay	

Note: [a]Vincristine dose capped at 2 mg.
IV: intravenous; PO: oral; SQ: subcutaneous; G-CSF: granulocyte colony-stimulating factor; wk: week.

Clinical trials

ABVD is the standard chemotherapeutic regimen for clinical stage I–II patients. Based on pivotal studies in Milan, Italy and Stanford, California, combined modality studies in early-stage, favorable Hodgkin lymphoma have focused on brief chemotherapy (typically two to four cycles) followed by involved-field radiation therapy (IFRT) at a reduced dosage of 20–30 Gy (Table 19.6).[109,111,112,135–138,140,143,144,160] Recently, the GHSG HD10 trial completed a phase III 2 × 2 factorial design trial (four arms) for early-stage favorable disease that randomized 1370 patients to 2 or 4 cycles of ABVD and then 20 Gy vs. 30 Gy IFRT.[137] At 53-month median follow-up, there was no significant difference in outcome according to the number of ABVD cycles or RT dose with FFTF of 91–92% and OS of 96–97%. Continued follow-up is important to confirm these preliminary findings as several of the aforementioned early-stage clinical trials have been reported only in abstract form.[24,25,27,28,29,31]

Radiation considerations

The volume, field, and technical aspects of RT have evolved together with the combined application of chemotherapy. IFRT, which encompasses the initially involved "nodal region," is the current standard radiation technique employed for most patients. The rationale for IFRT goes back to the original MOPP series in which relapses occurred in involved, particularly bulky disease sites. Several groups have supported the concept of further reduction of the volume of RT to involved-nodal radiation therapy (INRT),[161–163] to include only the initially involved lymph nodes. Of note, differences in IFRT and INRT are closely related to disease distribution and require expert planning and definition by function imaging (see FDG-PET).

Intermediate (unfavorable) early-stage disease

Combined modality therapy is the accepted standard for intermediate, unfavorable (I and II with risk factors) Hodgkin lymphoma based on historical observations that relapse rate was unacceptably high in patients treated with either modality alone.[110,111,112,139,141,164] The prognostic impact of a single risk factor, the number of chemotherapy cycles, the dosage of radiation, and whether chemotherapy may be used alone (i.e., no radiation) are subjects of ongoing studies and continuing debates (Table 19.7). ABVD has been the standard chemotherapy regimen used in combination with IFRT for intermediate early-stage Hodgkin lymphoma. Attempts to modify ABVD chemotherapy, to date, have fallen short. The EORTC H7U randomized patients to six cycles of epirubicin, bleomycin, vinblastine, and prednisone (EBVP) vs. six cycles MOPP/ABV, both with IFRT. EBVP was an inferior regimen with significantly lower 10-year event-free survival (EFS) and OS.[111] Similarly, EVE (epirubicin, vinblastine, and etoposide) + RT was inferior to ABVD + RT in a smaller randomized trial with 5-year FFS rates of 90% for ABVD and 73% for EVE ($p < 0.05$).[166]

The EORTC H8U study established that four cycles of MOPP/ABV plus IFRT were as effective as a longer course of chemotherapy and more extensive RT. The subsequent H9U trial demonstrated that four cycles of ABVD was associated

Table 19.6. Favorable early-stage I–II Hodgkin lymphoma: recent randomized studies[a]

Trial	No. patients	Treatment regimens	Outcome	
			7-yr FFTF	*7-yr OS*
GHSG HD7[136]	650	EFRT (30 Gy) + IFRT (10 Gy)	67%	94%
		2 ABVD + same RT	88%	92%
			$p < 0.0001$	$p = 0.43$
			5-yr EFS	*10-yr OS*
EORTC H8F[138]	542	3 MOPP/ABV + IFRT (36 Gy)	98%	97%
		STLI	74%	92%
			$p < 0.001$	$p = 0.001$
			4-yr EFS	*4-yr OS*
EORTC/GELA H9F[143]	783	6 EBVP + IFRT (36 Gy)	88%	98%
		6 EBVP + IFRT (20 Gy)	85%	100%
		6 EBVP (no RT)	69%	98%
			$p < 0.001$	$p = 0.241$
			'No RT' arm closed due to elevated relapse rate	
GHSG HD10[137]	1370	2 ABVD + IFRT (30 Gy) 2 ABVD + IFRT (20 Gy) 4 ABVD + IFRT (30 Gy) 4 ABVD + IFRT (20 Gy)	Median follow-up 53 months, no survival differences between number of ABVD cycles or radiation dose (FFTF 91–92%, *OS* 96–97%)	
			5-yr EFS	*5-yr OS*
NCI-C/ECOG[112]	123	ABVD 4–6 cycles	87%	97%
		STLI	88%	100%
			p = NS	p = NS
GHSG HD13	Ongoing	2 ABVD + 30 Gy IFRT 2 ABV + 30 Gy IFRT 2 AVD + 30 Gy IFRT 2 AV + 30 Gy IFRT	AV and ABV arms closed September 2006 due to elevated relapse rate	

Note: [a]See text for definitions of favorable early-stage category. Minimum Hodgkin lymphoma favorable early-stage study size 120 patients.
No: number; yr: year; EORTC: European Organisation for Research and Treatment of Cancer; Gy: gray; EBVP: epirubicin, bleomycin, vinblastine, prednisone; IFRT: involved-field radiation therapy; EFS: event-free survival; OS: overall survival; GHSG: German Hodgkin Study Group; FFTF: freedom from treatment failure; ABVD: doxorubicin, vinblastine, bleomycin, dacarbazine; STLI: subtotal nodal irradiation; NS: not significant; RT: radiation therapy; EFRT: external-field radiation therapy.

with outcomes no different than those with six cycles or four cycles of standard BEACOPP regimen, all in combination with IFRT.[139] The chemotherapy question was also addressed in the GHSG HD11 trial, together with RT dose, in a 2×2 factorial design. After a median observation time of 30 months, there was no FFS difference between the chemotherapy arms or IFRT doses with 97% OS for all patients.[141] From 1/03 to 1/07, the GHSG HD14 study randomized 1216 patients to either four ABVD with 30 Gy IFRT vs. two BEACOPP-escalated followed by two ABVD and 30 Gy IFRT. In preliminary results, the 3-year FFTF is improved for the BEACOPP-containing arm as shown in Table 19.7.[165] Continued follow-up of this and other preliminary early-stage Hodgkin lymphoma clinical trial reports is critical in order to confirm if efficacy differences persist, and to examine potential toxicity differences, especially fertility and secondary malignancies.

Chemotherapy alone for early-stage Hodgkin lymphoma

Chemotherapy alone for early-stage Hodgkin lymphoma represents a less well-studied treatment option that is attractive for those for whom the risk(s) of acute and/or long-term RT toxicity is deemed unacceptable.[112,142,143,146,164,167–169] A study from India randomized 179 patients in CR following six cycles of ABVD to IFRT or no RT.[168] The trial included a heterogeneous patient population (stages I–IV; 53% of report with stage I/II); >80% had mixed cellularity or NLPHL

Table 19.7. Intermediate early-stage I–II Hodgkin lymphoma: randomized chemotherapy studies[a]

Trial	No. patients	Treatment regimens	Outcome	
			10-yr FFS	*10-yr OS*
EORTC H6U[135]	316	3 MOPP + Mantle + 3 MOPP	77%	87%
		3 ABVD + Mantle + 3 ABVD	88%	87%
			p < 0.0001	p = 0.52
EORTC H7U[111]	316		*6-yr EFS*	*6-yr OS*
		6 EBVP + IFRT (36 Gy)	68%	79%
		6 MOPP/ABV + IFRT	88%	87%
			p < 0.001	p = 0.0175
GHSG HD11[141]	1422	4 ABVD + IFRT (30 Gy) 4 ABVD + IFRT (20 Gy) 4 BEACOPP-base + IFRT (30 Gy) 4 BEACOPP-base + IFRT (20 Gy)	Median follow-up 30 months: no differences between ABVD and BEACOPP (FFS 89% and 91%, respectively), or between 20 Gy and 30 Gy IFRT (FFS 91% and 93%, respectively)	
EORTC H8U[138]	996		*5-yr EFS*	*5-yr OS*
		6 MOPP/ABV + IFRT (36 Gy)	84%	88%
		4 MOPP/ABV + IFRT (36 Gy)	88%	85%
		4 MOPP/ABV + STLI	87%	84%
			p = NS	p = NS
NCI-C/ECOG[112]	276		*5-yr EFS*	*5-yr OS*
		ABVD 4–6 cycles	88%	95%
		ABVD 2 cycles + STLI	92%	92%
			p = 0.09	p = NS
EORTC H9U[139]	808		*4-yr EFS*	*4-yr OS*
		6 ABVD + IFRT (30 Gy)	91%	95%
		4 ABVD + IFRT (30 Gy)	87%	94%
		4 BEACOPP-base + IFRT (30 Gy)	90%	93%
			p = NS	p = NS
GHSG HD14[165]	1216	4 ABVD + IFRT (30 Gy) 2 BEACOPP-esc + 2 ABVD + IFRT (30 Gy)	Preliminary report: 3-year FFTF for ABVD alone 90% vs. 96% for BEACOPP/ABVD	

Note: [a]See text for definitions of intermediate early-stage category. Minimum study size 250 patients.
No: number; yr: year; EORTC: European Organisation for Research and Treatment of Cancer; GHSG: German Hodgkin Study Group; NCI-C: National Cancer Institute of Canada; ECOG: Eastern Cooperative Oncology Group; MOPP: mechlorethamine, vincristine, procarbazine, prednisone; ABVD: doxorubicin, vinblastine, bleomycin, dacarbazine; BEACOPP: bleomycin, etoposide, doxorubicin (Adriamycin), cyclophosphamide, vincristine, procarbazine, and prednisone; esc: escalated; base: baseline; FFS: failure-free survival; OS: overall survival; Gy: gray; IFRT: involved-field radiation therapy; STLI: subtotal nodal irradiation; EFS: event-free survival; FFTF: freedom from treatment failure; NS: not significant.

histology, and half of the patients were aged over 15 years. No EFS or OS differences were detected for stage I–II patients (8-year EFS and OS of chemotherapy alone 94% and 98%, respectively, vs. 97% and 100% for chemotherapy and IFRT, p values 0.29 for EFS and 0.26 for OS). A multivariate subgroup analysis of all patients showed EFS superiority for IFRT with B symptoms, bulky disease, age < 15, and advanced stages. Surprisingly, RT provided more EFS benefit for patients without mediastinal involvement. For OS, the IFRT arm was superior in the patient subgroups with B symptoms, stage III–IV disease, and patients < 15 years, but not for patients with bulky disease.

The NCI-C/ECOG HD6 trial evaluated 399 Hodgkin lymphoma patients with early stage I–II disease, excluding patients with LMM or bulky disease (> 10 cm).[112] Favorable patients were randomized to STLI vs. four to six cycles of ABVD (two cycles beyond CR) without RT, while unfavorable patients were randomized to two cycles ABVD with STLI vs. four to six total cycles of ABVD alone. With both prognostic groups combined, FFP and EFS were superior in patients who received radiation (5-year FFP 93% vs. 87% and EFS 88% vs. 86%, $p = 0.006$ and $p = 0.06$, respectively), while OS was similar (94% and 96%, $p = 0.40$). Differences were less apparent when examining the prognostic subgroups separately (Tables 19.6 and 19.7).

The EORTC–GELA H9F trial randomized 783 patients to six cycles EBVP with 20 Gy IFRT, six cycles EBVP with 36 Gy IFRT, or six cycles EBVP without radiation.[143] The arm without radiation was stopped early due to high relapse rate. As discussed before with the EORTC H7U data, it is apparent that EBVP is an inferior regimen compared with ABVD. At median follow-up of 33 months, there are no differences between radiation dosing and OS is $\geq 98\%$ in all arms (Table 19.6). Straus and colleagues reported a single-institution trial of 152 patients comparing six cycles of ABVD alone vs. six cycles ABVD with 36 Gy IFRT for Hodgkin lymphoma patients with stages I–II and IIIA disease.[146] There were no differences in FFS or OS, although the sample size of the trial might have limited the ability to detect a small difference.

Ongoing early-stage data

The GHSG HD13 was initiated as a four-arm phase III trial for favorable, early-stage disease randomizing patients to two cycles each of ABVD, AVD, ABV, or AV with all arms followed by 30 Gy IFRT. In preliminary analysis, the two non-dacarbazine-containing arms, ABV and AV, were closed prematurely because of increased relapse rates. Accrual continues to the ABVD and AVD arms. It seems that dacarbazine is an important therapeutic agent in the treatment of early-stage Hodgkin lymphoma. For early-stage intermediate Hodgkin lymphoma, the GHSG HD14 trial is comparing two courses of intensified BEACOPP followed by two cycles ABVD vs. four cycles ABVD, with both arms followed by 30 Gy IFRT.

The United Kingdom and EORTC have incorporated FDG-PET response-adapted therapy into early-stage Hodgkin lymphoma trial designs. The ongoing United Kingdom trial treats all early-stage patients with three ABVD cycles, which is followed by PET restaging. PET-negative patients are randomized to 30 Gy IFRT vs. no RT, while PET-positive patients receive a fourth ABVD cycle followed by IFRT. The recently initiated EORTC–GELA H10 Intergroup trial compares "standard therapy" to PET-based response-adapted therapy (PET after two cycles ABVD). Favorable early-stage patients are randomized to standard therapy (three cycles ABVD and 30 Gy IFRT) vs. PET-based therapy: four cycles ABVD alone (no RT) for PET-negative patients or two cycles ABVD and two cycles BEACOPP-escalated followed by 30 Gy IFRT for PET-positive disease. Intermediate group early-stage patients are randomized to standard therapy (four cycles ABVD and 30 Gy IFRT) vs. PET-based treatment with six cycles ABVD (no RT) for PET-negative disease or two cycles ABVD and two cycles BEACOPP-escalated followed by 30 Gy IFRT for PET-positive disease.

Advanced-stage disease

Initial chemotherapy studies

In a landmark report, DeVita and Carbone showed for patients with advanced Hodgkin lymphoma disease that more than 80% achieved remission and approximately 50% were alive at 5 years with MOPP combination chemotherapy.[12] Other trials studying MOPP showed long-term FFP rates of 36–52% and OS of 50–64%.[12,170,171] Several groups subsequently examined alternative treatment regimens in an attempt to further improve long-term survival and/or to reduce toxicity (sterility, neurologic toxicity, and secondary acute leukemia). Several MOPP variants were studied including the substitution of vinblastine for vincristine (MVPP), which was comparable to MOPP in remission and OS.[172,173] In a randomized trial, the British National Lymphoma Investigation (BNLI) substituted nitrogen mustard with chlorambucil (leukeran; LOPP) and compared it to MOPP.[174] The LOPP regimen was less toxic, and no significant survival differences were seen. The United Kingdom also substituted chlorambucil for mustard developing the chlorambucil, vinblastine, procarbazine, and prednisolone regimen (ChlVPP);[175] this regimen appeared comparable to MOPP, although a randomized trial was not performed.

In a randomized study, the ECOG compared a regimen containing carmustine (BCNU), cyclophosphamide, vinblastine, procarbazine, and prednisone (BCVPP) with MOPP.[176] At 5 years, BCVPP had a significantly higher FFP (50% vs. 33%, respectively) and OS (83% vs. 75%, respectively). Hematologic toxicity was similar, although BCVPP caused less non-hematologic toxicity (gastrointestinal and neurologic). Bonadonna and colleagues introduced the ABVD regimen[133] in 1975 in order to develop a non-cross resistant regimen for patients who had relapsed following MOPP. The Milan group subsequently compared three cycles of MOPP and three cycles ABVD preceding and following extended-field RT in 232 previously untreated Hodgkin lymphoma patients.[177] A significant improvement in outcome for ABVD was noted over MOPP with superior 7-year FFP and OS rates (Table 19.8).

Hybrid regimens

The theoretic basis for multidrug regimens is based on the model by Goldie and Coldman[183] of the advantage to early introduction of all active agents to avoid resistant tumor cell clones. The Milan group randomized 88 patients to MOPP vs. MOPP alternating monthly with ABVD and found significantly superior 8-year FFP rates of 65% for MOPP/ABVD vs. 36% for MOPP and OS of 84% vs. 64%, respectively ($p = 0.06$).[170] Investigators in Vancouver[182] and Milan[183] designed two hybrids of MOPP and ABVD. The NCI-C compared the MOPP-ABV hybrid with alternating MOPP/ABVD in patients with stage IIIB or IV Hodgkin lymphoma.[184] At 5 years, there was no significant difference in OS; however, the hybrid regimen was associated with higher hematologic and non-hematologic toxicities.

Table 19.8. Advanced-stage Hodgkin lymphoma: ABVD and BEACOPP randomized trials

Trial	No. patients	Treatment regimens	Outcome	
Milan[177]	232		*7-yr EFS*	*7-yr OS*
		ABVD 6 cycles + STLI	81%	77%
		MOPP 6 cycles + STLI	63%	68%
			p < 0.002	p < 0.03
CALGB[178]	361		*5-yr FFS*	*5-yr OS*
		ABVD 6–8 cycles	61%	73%
		MOPP 6–8 cycles	50%	66%
		MOPP/ABVD 12 cycles	65%	75%
			p = 0.03	p = NS
CALGB[99]	856		*5-yr FFS*	*5-yr OS*
		ABVD 8–10 cycles	63%	82%
		MOPP-ABV 8–10 cycles	66%	81%
			p = NS	p = NS
GHSG HD9[101]	1201		*5-yr FFTF*	*5-yr OS*
		COPP/ABVD × 8 cycles + IFRT[a]	69%	83%
		BEACOPP-baseline × 8 cycles + IFRT[a]	76%	88%
		BEACOPP-escalated × 8 cycles + IFRT[a]	87%	91%
			p < 0.002	p < 0.002
United Kingdom[102]	807		*3-yr EFS*	*3-yr OS*
		ABVD 6 cycles + 30–35 Gy[a]	75%	90%
		MDR regimen (ChlVPP/PABIOE or ChlVPP/EVA) 6 cycles + 30–35 Gy[a]	75%	88%
			p = NS	p = NS
GHSG HD12[179,180]	1661		*4-yr FFTF*	*4-yr OS*
		BEACOPP-escalated × 8 cycles	86%	88%
		BEACOPP × 4 esc and 4 base cycles	91%	91%
		BEACOPP + 30 Gy IFRT	91%	95%
		BEACOPP without RT	88%	95%
			p = NS	p = NS
Italy[100]	355		*5-yr PFS*	*5-yr OS*
		ABVD × 6 cycles + IFRT (RT 62% of pts)[a]	85%	90%
		MOPPEBVCAD × 6 cycles + IFRT (RT 66%)[a]	94%	89%
		Stanford V × 3 cycles + IFRT (RT 47%)[a]	73%	82%
			p < 0.01	p < 0.04
Italy[97]	307[b]		*5-yr PFS*	*5-yr OS*
		ABVD × 6 cycles (RT 46%)	68%	84%
		COPPEBVCAD × 6 cycles (RT 43%)	78%	91%
		EscBEACOPP × 4, baseBEACOPP × 2 (RT 44%)	81%	92%
			p < 0.038	p = NS

Table 19.8. *(cont.)*

Trial	No. patients	Treatment regimens	Outcome	
United Kindgom[181]	520		*5-yr PFS*	*5-yr OS*
		Stanford V × 12 weeks	74%	92%
		ABVD 6–8 cycles	76%	90%
			p = NS	p = NS
GHSG HD15[182]	1500	BEACOPP-esc × 8 cycles +/− 30 Gy IFRT[a]	All pts: FFTF 86% and OS 95% at median follow-up 21 months	
		BEACOPP-esc × 6 cycles +/− 30 Gy IFRT[a]		
		BEACOPP-14 × 8 cycles +/− 30 Gy IFRT[a]		
EORTC 20012	Ongoing	*For patients IPS 4–7 only:* ABVD × 8 cycles	Open – target sample size 550	
		BEACOPP × 4 esc and 4 base cycles		

Notes: Minimum study size 230 patients.
[a]Radiation delivered to sites of initial bulk disease or partial remission after chemotherapy. For GHSG HD15, radiation was given only to patients with disease > 2.5 cm following chemotherapy that was PET positive.
[b]Patients with less than partial response (PR) after the first three cycles of chemotherapy were taken off study (considered as progressing).
No: number; IFRT: involved-field radiation therapy; STLI: subtotal nodal irradiation; EFS: event-free survival; OS: overall survival; FFS: failure-free survival; FFTF: freedom from treatment failure; MOPP: mechlorethamine, vincristine, procarbazine, prednisone; ABVD; doxorubicin, bleomycin, vinblastine, dacarbazine; MDR: multidrug resistant; ChlVPP/PABIOE: chlorambucil, vinblastine, procarbazine, prednisone/prednisolone, doxorubicin, bleomycin, vincristine, etoposide; EVA: etoposide, vincristine, and doxorubicin; GHSG: German Hodgkin Study Group; BEACOPP: bleomycin, etoposide, doxorubicin (Adriamycin), cyclophosphamide, vincristine, procarbazine, prednisone; esc: escalated; base: baseline; MOPPEBVCAD: mechlorethamine, vincristine, procarbazine, prednisone, epidoxirubicin, bleomycin, vinblastine, lomustine, doxorubicin, and vindesine; COPPEBVCAD: same as MOPPEBVCAD but cyclophosphamide instead of mechlorethamine; IPS: international prognostic score; NS: not significant; RT: radiation therapy; pts: patients.

The Milan group randomized 427 patients with pathologic stage IB, IIA bulky, IIB, and III/IV disease to MOPP/ABVD alternating monthly and alternating one-half cycles of MOPP and ABVD.[185] No survival differences were detected among these two regimens with 67–69% without progression and 72–74% alive at 10 years. Large multicenter trials in the United States and Europe studied other comparisons.[186,187] The CALGB investigated sequential MOPP/ABV vs. MOPP-ABV hybrid in newly diagnosed and first relapsed advanced-stage Hodgkin lymphoma.[186] FFS and OS were significantly better with the hybrid regimen. The EORTC compared two courses of MOPP alternating with two courses of ABVD to total of eight vs. MOPP.[187] MOPP/ABVD was associated with significantly higher FFP (60% vs. 43%, respectively).

As a conclusion to these comparative trials, as reported by Canellos *et al.*[167] and then later by Duggan *et al.*,[99] randomized phase III trials showed that ABVD alone was equally effective as MOPP/ABVD and MOPP-ABV hybrid, but less toxic, and all regimens were more effective than MOPP alone (Table 19.8). In addition, ABVD had less acute toxicity, especially no sterility and few or no secondary acute myeloid leukemia/myelodysplastic syndrome (AML/MDS). At present, it is internationally accepted that ABVD should be the standard regimen against which all experimental combinations should be tested.

Other chemotherapy regimens

Stanford V, a seven-drug regimen, was developed as a short-duration, reduced-toxicity program including doxorubicin, vinblastine, mechlorethamine, bleomycin, vincristine, etoposide, and prednisone. Stanford V is given weekly over 12 weeks and consolidative RT is applied to tumors ≥ 5 cm.[98] In an Italian multicenter phase III trial, 334 patients were randomized to ABVD, Stanford V, or MOPPEBVCAD (mechlorethamine, vincristine, procarbazine, prednisone, epidoxirubicin, bleomycin, vinblastine, lomustine, doxorubicin, and vindesine).[100] The dose intensities varied slightly between the regimens with ABVD 83%, Stanford V 81%, and MOPPEBVCAD 73%. An important consideration in interpreting the results of this trial is that RT was administered on a more limited basis for Stanford V patients (66%) compared with > 90% in the original Stanford program.[98] The 5-year FFS and PFS rates were inferior for Stanford V compared to ABVD and MOPPEBVCAD, while ABVD had improved OS vs. Stanford V ($p < 0.04$). A preliminary report from the United Kingdom found no difference between Stanford V and ABVD in a 520-patient randomized trial (Table 19.8).[181] RT was given to 72% of Stanford V patients and to 53% of the ABVD cohort (RT was not required for ABVD patients who achieved CR). The North American Intergroup phase III trial randomizing Stanford V vs. ABVD has completed accrual and follow-up of patient events continues.

In a UK randomized trial, the abbreviated 11-week chemotherapy program, VAPEC-B (vincristine, doxorubicin, prednisone, etoposide, cyclophosphamide, bleomycin), was compared with the hybrid ChlVPP-EVA (etoposide, vincristine, and doxorubicin) regimen with radiation applied to initial bulk or residual disease.[188] The study was stopped after 26 months due to a threefold increase in the rate of progression after

VAPEC-B. The UK trial subsequently randomized 807 patients over 42 months to ABVD vs. two multidrug regimens (MDR), ChlVPP alternating with PABIOE (prednisolone, doxorubicin, bleomycin, vincristine, and etoposide) or ChlVPP/EVA.[102] The 3-year EFS and OS rates at a median follow-up of 52 months were similar for ABVD compared with the MDRs (Table 19.8). Of note, EFS and OS for patients aged greater than 45 years were significantly better with ABVD vs. the MDRs.

Chemotherapy strategies/regimens increasing dose intensity

High dose intensity of MOPP-based therapy (i.e., full chemotherapy doses and no treatment delays) was associated with significant improvement in DFS and OS.[189,190] As discussed before, the GHSG showed that the overall degree of hematologic toxicity was an independent predictor of survival in Hodgkin lymphoma as severe leukopenia during treatment was associated with superior OS.[114] It is not clear if that association was a patient-specific or a treatment-specific phenomenon. Consolidative autologous hematopoietic stem cell transplantation (ASCT) as a part of initial therapy for Hodgkin lymphoma has been studied.[191–193] Updated results of an Italian randomized study of conventional chemotherapy vs. chemotherapy and ASCT for newly diagnosed unfavorable Hodgkin lymphoma found no difference in 10-year relapse-free survival (89% and 88%, respectively) or FFS (75% and 79%, respectively).[191]

In 1992, the GHSG designed the BEACOPP regimen with similar drugs as in the COPP/ABVD regimen, but included etoposide instead of vinblastine and dacarbazine. The GHSG designed the HD9 trial, which compared COPP/ABVD, BEACOPP-baseline, and BEACOPP-escalated in 1201 patients with advanced-stage Hodgkin lymphoma.[101] RT was prescribed for bulky disease at diagnosis (30 Gy) or for residual disease (40 Gy) after eight cycles of chemotherapy; about two-thirds of patients received IFRT. FFTF was significantly higher in the BEACOPP-escalated arm compared with the COPP-ABVD arm (Table 19.8).[101] The OS difference between COPP-ABVD and BEACOPP-escalated was also significant ($p < 0.002$). BEACOPP-escalated was associated with greater hematological toxicity including a higher number of platelet and red blood cell transfusions. Second malignancies including AML were reported; 9, 4, and 1 AML/MDS were reported for the BEACOPP-escalated, BEACOPP-baseline, and COPP-ABVD regimens, respectively. The total rate of secondary neoplasias was highest in the COPP/ABVD arm with 4.2% compared with 3.4% in the BEACOPP-escalated arm. One critique of this pivotal BEACOPP trial was the dose intensities of the respective regimens; the median duration of COPP-ABVD chemotherapy was 33.4 weeks as reported in an erratum (originally reported 46.3 weeks), which was 36% longer treatment duration compared to BEACOPP baseline and BEACOPP-escalated (24.4 and 24.7 weeks, respectively). The subsequent GHSG HD12 advanced-stage trial randomized 1661 patients between eight cycles of BEACOPP-escalated vs. four cycles of BEACOPP-escalated and four cycles of BEACOPP-baseline. With a median follow-up of 78 months, there have been no apparent FFTF or OS differences (Table 19.8).[179,180]

The experiences with the high efficacy but also increased toxicity of the BEACOPP-escalated principal (given in 21-day intervals) led the GHSG to consider a BEACOPP variant, in which the drug dosage and time period according to the effective dose model of Diehl *et al.*[101] would accomplish the same efficacy, but have a reduced toxicity, especially concerning the rate of AML/MDS. The result was the construction of a time intensified BEACOPP-baseline regimen given in 14-day intervals with granulocyte colony-stimulating factor (G-CSF) support for advanced Hodgkin lymphoma (BEACOPP-14). In a multicenter pilot study with 32 centers, the GHSG tested the feasibility, toxicity, and efficacy in 99 patients with stage IIB and LMM/extranodal disease (23%) or advanced-stage disease (77%).[194] At a median 34-month follow-up, the estimated FFTF was 90% and the OS was 97%. Hematotoxicity was moderate, with 75% experiencing WHO grade 3 or 4 leukopenia, 23% thrombocytopenia, and 65% anemia. Subsequently, the GHSG HD15 trial has recently completed accrual which randomized 1500 patients to eight cycles of BEACOPP-escalated vs. eight cycles BEACOPP-14 with a second randomization with or without epoetin in each arm.

Dose intensity of ABVD

One consideration with conventional ABVD is what dose intensity of ABVD is important for remission and survival. Landgren and colleagues reported that OS was significantly improved in elderly patients who received greater than 65% ABVD dose intensity.[92] Myelosuppression, especially neutropenia, is common during ABVD treatment.[100,102,146,195] Treatment strategies include either dose reduction or treatment delay, and/or use of G-CSF to maintain dose intensity, although data to support this recommendation (i.e., G-CSF with ABVD) are lacking.[196,197] Three retrospective analyses have reported that ABVD can be safely administered at very high dose intensity.[195,198,199] Furthermore, it has been shown that ABVD can be administered in full doses safely and effectively and without delay (> 99% dose intensity), and without G-CSF, irrespective of the treatment-day granulocyte count.[199] This treatment strategy needs to be tested further and confirmed in prospective multicenter trials.

Role of radiotherapy in advanced-stage Hodgkin lymphoma

A number of phase III trials investigated the role of consolidative RT after primary chemotherapy; the vast majority have shown no EFS or OS advantage.[85,95,103,142,168,200–204] The GHSG analyzed the role of low-dose (20 Gy) IFRT vs. two cycles of further chemotherapy consolidation in 288 patients in CR after initial chemotherapy with COPP-ABVD.[201] There was no significant difference in FFP or OS rates between both treatment arms. In the GHSG HD12 trial, 1661 patients were randomized to eight cycles of BEACOPP-escalated or four cycles each of BEACOPP-escalated/BEACOPP-baseline, with a second randomization for initial bulky and/or residual disease of IFRT vs. no RT.[180] Reported in abstract form, the FFTF for all patients was 86% and OS was 92% with a similar toxicity as described in the HD9 trial, after a median observation time of 4 years.[179] There is no difference among the two chemotherapy regimens or between the IFRT arm and no RT arm; however, 10% of patients in the non-RT arm received radiation according to a central panel decision (Table 19.8).

In the EORTC 20884 trial, patients with advanced-stage Hodgkin lymphoma achieving CR after six to eight cycles of MOPP-ABV hybrid were randomly assigned to receive either IFRT or no further treatment.[95,203] Those with PR after six cycles were treated with IFRT. Of 739 initial patients, 333 CR patients were randomized, and 227 patients in PR received IFRT. The 8-year EFS and OS rates were 77% and 85%, respectively, for patients without RT and 73% and 78% in the group assigned to IFRT, respectively. The 8-year EFS and OS were 76% and 84%, respectively, for patients with a PR who received IFRT. A meta-analysis showed that combined modality therapy in advanced-stage Hodgkin lymphoma prevented progression/relapse, but had no effect on OS and was associated with increased secondary malignancies.[205]

On the other hand, Johnson *et al.* analyzed results from the aforementioned ABVD regimen vs. two MDRs according to radiation received.[102] In that trial, IFRT was recommended for incomplete response or bulk disease (over 1/3 transthoracic ratio or 10 cm outside the chest) at presentation. From the end of chemotherapy (regardless of regimen), the EFS was superior for patients who received RT (5-year EFS 86% vs. 71%) as was OS (5-year OS 93% vs. 87%). FDG-PET may be a diagnostic modality that can predict advanced-stage patients who may avoid consolidative RT. As part of the recently discussed GHSG HD15 trial, FDG-PET was analyzed in 311 patients.[182] After completion of chemotherapy, patients in at least PR by CT and with at least one involved nodal site of >2.5 cm received consolidative RT if FDG-PET was positive. PET-negative (PET^-) patients received no additional RT. The FDG-PET was positive in 21% of patients and negative in 79%. The PFS for FDG-PET-negative patients was 96% compared with 86% for FDG-PET-positive patients ($p = 0.011$). Further, the negative predictive value (NPV) for PET in this analysis was 94%, after six to eight cycles of BEACOPP.

Recent/ongoing untreated advanced-stage trials

Federico *et al.* recently reported on a 307-patient phase III trial of advanced-stage (stage IIB, III, and IV) Hodgkin lymphoma which randomized patients between six cycles of ABVD vs. four escalated plus two baseline courses of BEACOPP vs. six cycles of COPPEBVCAD.[97] RT was designated for sites of previous bulky disease or for slowly or partially responding sites and 43–46% of patients on each arm received RT. CR rates were statistically similar among the three arms: 70%, 69%, and 81% for patients treated with ABVD, COPPEBV-CAD, and BEACOPP, respectively ($p = 0.130$). After a median follow-up of 41 months (range, 4–91 months), PFS was superior in BEACOPP vs. ABVD as shown in Table 19.8. The PFS advantage of BEACOPP was more apparent in patients with high IPS (3–7). The 5-year PFS of 68% for ABVD was noticeably inferior to a prior Italian trial with 5-year PFS of 85%.[100] Part of the explanation may be related to the study rules of the more recent study where patients with less than PR after the first three cycles of chemotherapy were taken off study (and typically proceeded to stem cell transplant). Johnson *et al.* presented preliminary results of a 520-patient randomized phase III trial of ABVD vs. Stanford V.[181] RT was delivered to 72% Stanford V and 53% ABVD. The overall response rate at completion of all treatment was 89% for ABVD and 90% for Stanford V. With a median 4-year follow-up, there are no apparent survival differences.

The multi-country EORTC 20012 trial continues enrollment for advanced-stage patients with IPS of 4–7 randomizing between ABVD (eight cycles) vs. eight cycles of BEACOPP (eight escalated and four baseline). Several recently activated trials are examining the role of early PET (i.e., PET-2) in advanced-stage Hodgkin lymphoma. The GHSG HD18 will randomize PET-2 patients who are negative after two cycles of BEACOPP-escalated to standard treatment with six further cycles of BEACOPP-based therapy vs. two further cycles of BEACOPP-escalated (i.e., four total cycles). FDG-PET-positive patients will have rituximab added to BEACOPP vs. continuing six cycles of BEACOPP-escalated. The United States Intergroup recently opened a phase II trial treating patients with two cycles of "full dose" ABVD,[199] as discussed before. Patients with positive FDG-PET-2 will change to six cycles of BEACOPP-escalated, while FDG-PET-2-negative patients will continue with ABVD. The United Kingdom has recently opened a phase III trial where patients with negative FDG-PET following two cycles of ABVD will have bleomycin eliminated and randomize between continuing ABVD vs. AVD. FDG-PET-2-positive patients will continue to a single arm with BEACOPP-14 therapy.

Relapsed or refractory disease

Biopsy of clinically suspected disease to pathologically prove relapsed/refractory Hodgkin lymphoma is important, as etiologies other than Hodgkin lymphoma may account for lymphadenopathy and/or tissue growth on CT and/or FDG-PET suspicious for lymphoma, including thymic hyperplasia, cysts, infections, granulomas, or benign lymph node hyperplasia.[206] In addition, the appearance of other lymphoma histologies (low-grade or aggressive NHL) or other malignancies, especially beyond 5–10 years from initial treatment, is possible. Once relapsed/refractory Hodgkin lymphoma has been pathologically proven, salvage chemotherapy should be initiated. Non-cross resistant chemotherapy regimens such as etoposide, methylprednisolone, high-dose cytarabine, and cisplatin (ESHAP), dexamethasone, high-dose cytarabine, cisplatin (DHAP), ifosfamide, carboplatin, etoposide (ICE), mitoxantrone, ifosfamide, vinorelbine, and etoposide (MINE), or dexamethasone and carmustine, etoposide, cytarabine, and melphalan (Dexa-BEAM) are associated with expected response rates of 65–85%.[146,207–209] The optimal number of chemotherapy cycles prior to HSCT is not known, although most centers advocate two to three cycles.

ASCT is standard treatment for patients with relapsed/refractory Hodgkin lymphoma. Two randomized trials were performed comparing ASCT with continued conventional chemotherapy. Schmitz *et al.* of the GHSG/European Group for Blood and Bone Marrow Transplantation conducted a randomized study of 161 patients with biopsy-proven relapsed Hodgkin disease.[209] Patients were randomized to either ASCT or continued chemotherapy. All patients initially received two cycles of Dexa-BEAM chemotherapy; patients who had achieved a CR or PR proceeded to either two more cycles of Dexa-BEAM or high-dose BEAM chemotherapy (carmustine 300 mg/m^2, etoposide 1200 mg/m^2, cytarabine 1600 mg/m^2, and melphalan 140 mg/m^2) followed by autologous stem cell infusion. The median TTF was 12 months in the Dexa-BEAM arm, but was not reached in the BEAM-transplant arm. At 3 years, 55% of transplant patients were free from treatment failure, compared with 34% in the Dexa-BEAM group ($p = 0.019$). OS at 3 years, however, was not significantly different between the two groups (65% Dexa-BEAM group vs. 71% ASCT group, $p = 0.331$). In both groups, patients treated with ASCT had a statistically significant improvement in FFS, but not OS. A 1993 trial by the BNLI randomized 40 patients with relapsed or refractory Hodgkin lymphoma to either BEAM chemotherapy (carmustine 300 mg/m^2, etoposide 800 mg/m^2, cytarabine 1600 mg/m^2, and melphalan 140 mg/m^2) followed by autologous HSCT or mini-BEAM chemotherapy (carmustine 60 mg/m^2, etoposide 300 mg/m^2, cytarabine 800 mg/m^2, melphalan 30 mg/m^2).[210] The overall response rates in the BEAM and mini-BEAM groups were 74% and 60%, respectively. At 3 years, the actuarial EFS was 53% in the BEAM group and 10% in the mini-BEAM group ($p = 0.025$).

ASCT: chemotherapy-alone conditioning

Numerous studies have investigated a variety of high-dose chemotherapy conditioning regimens with autologous HSCT. The most commonly used high-dose chemotherapy conditioning regimens are BEAM and cyclophosphamide, carmustine, and etoposide (CBV) with resultant long-term survival rates of 45–51%.[140,209,211–218] It is important to note the precise dosing of particular chemotherapy agents in each report, as different doses among regimens such as BEAM and CBV often vary from study to study. Of note, no specific chemotherapy regimen has shown definite superiority over another. Some studies have focused primarily on primary induction failure (Table 19.9), while others have combined the primary refractory patient population with those who first achieve CR but then develop relapsed disease (Table 19.10).

ASCT: radiation-based conditioning

The inclusion of radiation into the conditioning regimen with high-dose chemotherapy for relapsed and refractory patients has shown promising results with long-term DFS/EFS rates up to 68%.[146,223] The rationale for incorporating radiation into pre-transplant conditioning therapy stems from the observation that relapses often occur in nodal sites – typically in sites that were previously unirradiated – and that radiation may lower the risk of disease recurrence in these sites as compared to chemotherapy alone. Radiation protocols may involve total body irradiation (TBI)[140,213,215,219] or total lymphoid irradiation (TLI), the latter minimizing radiation exposure to dose-limiting organs such as the lungs and liver, thereby minimizing toxicity. The use of radiation as part of the initial therapy, however, may limit the use of TLI in the treatment of primary refractory or relapsed disease due to the concern over radiation-induced toxicities. It should be noted that no randomized controlled trials have been performed comparing radiation-based vs. non-radiation-containing HSCT conditioning programs.

Allogeneic HSCT

A smaller but increasing number of studies have investigated the role of allogeneic HSCT in refractory or relapsed Hodgkin lymphoma (Table 19.11). The European Group for Blood and Marrow Transplantation conducted a case-matched study of 45 patients with refractory or relapsed Hodgkin lymphoma who received a HLA-identical sibling allogeneic HSCT.[225] In the allogeneic transplant group, the 4-year actuarial probabilities of OS, PFS, relapse, and non-relapse mortality were 25%, 15%, 61%, and 48%, respectively. These same probabilities among patients who underwent ASCT were 37%, 24%, 61%, and 27%. Procedural-related mortality at four years was significantly higher in the allogeneic group – 48% compared to 27% in the autologous patients ($p = 0.041$). Twenty-five allogeneic patients developed acute graft-versus-host disease (GVHD; 55%). Additionally, 55% of patients developed chronic GVHD. The grade of acute GVHD was related to OS and relapse rates. The results suggest that an acute GVHD effect may contribute to a benefit in terms of disease relapse, but this is overshadowed by the excess mortality resulting from allogeneic transplants. Similar conclusions were drawn from a review of the transplantation experience in Hodgkin disease at the Fred Hutchinson Cancer Research Center.[237] Due to studies suggesting a prohibitive treatment-related mortality in the allogeneic setting, reduced intensity conditioning (RIC) for allogeneic HSCT has been studied with encouraging preliminary results.[212,213,233,235]

Prognosis and transplantation

Numerous studies, most retrospective, have evaluated prognostic factors for outcomes after HSCT, in particular ASCT.

Table 19.9. Autologous transplantation trials: relapsed and refractory disease[a]

Authors	No. patients (study type)	High-dose chemotherapy regimen	Outcomes
Nademanee *et al.*, 1995[219]	85, prospective	TBI/cyclophosphamide/VP-16 (26%), BCNU/ cyclophosphamide/VP-16 (74%)	Median follow-up 25 months OS 76%, 2-year DFS 58% No significant difference between regimens
Sweetenham *et al.*, 1997[217]	139, retrospective	BEAM (58%), CBV (20%), cyclophosphamide + TBI (6%), other (15%)	Median follow-up 2.75 years 5-year OS 49.4%, 5-year PFS 44.7%
Horning *et al.*, 1997[140]	119, prospective	TBI/cyclophosphamide/VP-16 (22%), BCNU/ cyclophosphamide/VP-16 (62%), CCNU/ cyclophosphamide/VP-16 (16%)	4-year OS 52%; EFS 48%; FFP 62% No difference between three regimens
Straus *et al.*, 2001[146]	65, prospective	Previously unirradiated: TLI 1800 cGy (twice daily fractions over 5 days) + cyclophosphamide and etoposide; Previously irradiated: CBV and involved field radiation	OS and EFS were 81% and 68%, respectively, in the TLI group, and 84% and 68%, respectively, in the CBV group
Sureda *et al.*, 2001[220]	494, retrospective	Cyclophosphamide + TBI, CBV, BEAM/BEAC	5-year OS 54.5%
Ferme *et al.*, 2002[208]	157, prospective	2–3 cycles of MINE + BEAM	Median follow-up 50 months 5-year survival 56%, 5-year FFP 46%
Gutierrez-Delgado *et al.*, 2003[215]	92, retrospective	TBI/cyclophosphamide/etoposide (47%), busulfan/ melphalan/thiotepa (53%)	TBI/Cy/E: OS 57%, EFS 49%, relapse 36%; Bu/Mel/T: OS 52%, EFS 42%, relapse 34%
Czyz *et al.*, 2004[214]	341, retrospective	BEAM (50%), CBV (36%), others (14%)	5-year EFS 45% 5-year OS 64%
Sureda *et al.*, 2005[221]	357, retrospective	Cyclophosphamide + TBI (7%), CBV (45%), BEAM/BEAC (31%/12%)	5-year OS 57%
Lavoie *et al.*, 2005[216]	100, retrospective	CBV (29%), CBVP (71%)	Median follow-up 11.4 years 15-year OS 54%
Engelhardt *et al.*, 2007[222]	115, retrospective	CBV (93%), cyclophosphamide/etoposide/TBI (4%), thiotepa, etoposide, cytarabine, melphalan (2%), cyclophosphamide/etoposide/cisplatin (1%)	5-year OS 58% 5-year PFS 46% TRM 16%
Evens *et al.*, 2007[223]	48, prospective	Carboplatin, cyclophosphamide, and etoposide + TLI (latter for previously unirradiated)	5-year EFS and OS for TLI/chemotherapy arm: 61% and 63%, respectively, and for chemotherapy-alone arm: 5% and 21%, respectively
Schulz *et al.*, 2008[218]	245, prospective	Intermediate risk: BEAM; poor risk: tandem transplant (CBV or BEAM followed by TBI, cytarabine, and melphalan for previously unirradiated or busulfan, cytarabine, and melphalan for previously irradiated)	5-year FFTF and OS for intermediate risk: 73% and 85%, respectively, and for poor risk: 46% and 57%, respectively

Note: [a]Minimum study size: 45 patients.
No number; BEAM: carmustine (BCNU), etoposide, cytarabine, melphalan; MINE: mitoxantrone, ifosfamide, vinorelbine, etoposide; CBV: cyclophosphamide, carmustine, etoposide; TBI: total body irradiation; TLI: total lymphoid irradiation; BEAC: carmustine, etoposide, cytarabine, cyclophosphamide; CBVP: cyclophosphamide, carmustine, etoposide, cisplatin; DFS: disease-free survival; OS: overall survival; PFS: progression-free survival; EFS: event-free survival; FFP: freedom from progression; CR: complete response; PR: partial response; TRM: treatment-related mortality; FFTF: freedom from treatment failure.

Prognostic factors in ASCT studies shown to predict survival include gender,[215] performance status,[238] bulky disease,[213] advanced stage of disease,[211,212,215] anemia,[211,238,239] and B symptoms at time of relapse;[140,146,208] the most commonly reported prognostic factors are length of initial remission (< 1 year),[146,209,211,213,239] extranodal disease at time of relapse,[140,146,213,219,240] number of regimens prior to ASCT,[212–214,219,238,240] and degree of sensitivity to salvage chemotherapy.[140,146,208,212–215,217,225,239] The GHSG developed a prognostic score based on a review of 422 patients between 1988 and 1999 with relapsed disease after standard chemotherapy, RT, or HSCT, identifying anemia, stage III/IV disease,

Table 19.10. Autologous transplantation reports: primary refractory Hodgkin lymphoma

Authors	No. patients (study type)	High-dose chemotherapy regimen	Outcomes
Reece *et al.*, 1995[224]	30, prospective	CBV ± P	Median follow-up 3.6 years PFS 42%, OS at 5 years 60%
Andre *et al.*, 1999[225]	86, case-matched	BEAM (51%), CBV (24%), TBI (2%), other (22%)	25% EFS and 35% OS (actuarial 5-yr)
Lazarus *et al.*, 1999[226]	122, retrospective	CBV (39%), other chemotherapy-only regimens (49%), TBI and chemotherapy (12%)	38% PFS and 50% OS (at 3 yrs)
Sweetenham *et al.*, 1999[227]	175, retrospective	BEAM (47%), CBV (22%), other chemotherapy-only (23%), Cy/TBI (3%), other TBI-based (5.1%)	32% PFS and 36% OS (actuarial 5-yr)
Czyz *et al.*, 2002[228]	65, retrospective	BEAM (68%), CBV (28%), other (6%)	36% PFS and 55% OS (actuarial 3-yr)
Constans *et al.*, 2003[213]	62, retrospective	CBV (40%), BEAM/BEAC (42%), other chemotherapy-only regimens (8%), Cy + TBI (10%)	15% TTF and 26% OS (actuarial 5-yr)
Schulz *et al.*, 2008[218]	77, prospective	Tandem transplant (CBV or BEAM followed by TBI, cytarabine, and melphalan for previously unirradiated or busulfan, cytarabine, and melphalan for previously irradiated)	5-year FFTF and OS: 41% and 53%

Minimum study size: 30 patients.
No.: number; BEAM: carmustine, etoposide, cytarabine, melphalan; CBV: cyclophosphamide, carmustine, etoposide; Cy: cyclophosphamide; TBI: total body irradiation; BEAC: carmustine, etoposide, cytarabine, cyclophosphamide; CBV ± P: cyclophosphamide, carmustine, etoposide ± cisplatin; OS: overall survival; PFS: progression-free survival; EFS: event-free survival; TTF: time to treatment failure; FFTF: freedom from treatment failure.

and time to relapse < 12 months as adverse prognostic factors.[239] An abnormal PET scan after salvage chemotherapy has also been shown to be a poor prognostic factor for patients proceeding to HSCT. A retrospective review of 211 patients with recurrent or refractory Hodgkin lymphoma found that functional imaging (PET or gallium scan) after salvage chemotherapy was positive in only 6/110 (5%) of patients with CR, 48/86 (56%) patients with PR, and 3/3 patients with progressive disease.[241]

Specific topics

Nodular lymphocyte predominant Hodgkin lymphoma (NLPHL)

Exclusion to the aforementioned recommendation of combined modality therapy for early-stage Hodgkin lymphoma might be nodular lymphocyte predominant Hodgkin lymphoma (NLPHL) subtype in favorable stage IA without risk factors. These patients may be treated by lymph node excision followed by a "wait and see" strategy or with 20–30 Gy IFRT alone.[242,243,244] The GHSG showed CR rates of 98% after extended-field RT, 100% after IFRT, and 95% after combined modality.[242] Furthermore, FFTF at 24 months was 100%, 92%, and 97%, respectively, while OS for all patients was 99%.

Early-stage, intermediate, and advanced-stage NLPHL has been regarded as an entity with a more indolent course, with more frequent later recurrences compared with classical Hodgkin lymphoma.[242,243] A comprehensive analysis of 394 NLPHL (total 8298 patients) showed an overall similar relapse rate to classical Hodgkin lymphoma (7.9% vs. 8.1%, respectively), but with significantly fewer "early" relapses with NLPHL (0.76% vs. 3.2%, respectively, $p = 0.02$).[245] At a median observation of 41–48 months, the FFTF for NLPHL and classical Hodgkin lymphoma were 88% and 82%, respectively ($p = 0.0093$) and OS were 96% and 92%, respectively ($p = 0.016$). Of note, a slightly increased rate of secondary NHL, typically diffuse large B-cell lymphoma, was seen with NLPHL compared with classical Hodgkin lymphoma.

The current treatment recommendation for newly diagnosed, early-stage, intermediate, and advanced-stage NLPHL is to treat according to similar regimens to classical Hodgkin lymphoma. Rituximab has shown encouraging activity as a single agent in relapsed CD20+ NLPHL with remission rates of 86–100%.[218,246,247]

An updated report from the GHSG showed that the median time to treatment progression with single-agent rituximab in relapsed/refractory NLPHL was 33 months with median OS not being reached with 63-month median follow-up.[248] Rituximab has also been combined with chemotherapy for NLPHL including rituximab combined with cyclophosphamide, doxorubicin (Adriamycin), vincristine (Oncovin), and doxorubicin (R-CHOP). Fanale and colleagues reported on their experience of outcomes of 51 NLPHL patients treated with various treatment regimens over a 10-year period.[249] Nine patients received R-CHOP with reported CR rate of 94% and EFS and OS of near

Table 19.11. Allogeneic transplantation reports in relapsed/refractory Hodgkin lymphoma

Author (year)	No. patients	Conditioning regimens	Transplant-related mortality	EFS/PFS/DFS	OS
Gajewski *et al.*, 1996[229]	100	Cyclophosphamide + TBI, cyclophosphamide + busulfan, cyclophosphamide + etoposide + lamustine, or cyclophosphamide + busulfan + etoposide	61% at 3 years	3-year DFS 15%	3-year OS 21%
Milpied *et al.*, 1996[230]	45	Allogeneic: BEAM, Bu/Cy, CBV, Chemo + TBI, other/unknown	65% at 4 years	4-year PFS 15%	4-year OS 25%
Akpek *et al.*, 2001[231]	53	Busulfan + cyclophosphamide, cyclophosphamide + TBI, or busulfan, cyclophosphamide, etoposide	At 10 years: chemotherapy-sensitive at transplant: 53%; chemotherapy-resistant: 32%	EFS at 10 years 26%	Autologous: 37% Allogeneic: 30%
Carella *et al.*, 2001[232]	17	BEAM-autologous transplant followed by fludarabine + cyclophosphamide	6% (1 death due to infection)	NR	Median follow-up 566 days: 65%
Peggs *et al.*, 2005[233]	49	Fludarabine, melphalan, alemtuzumab	4% at 100 days; 16% at 730 days	4-year PFS 32.4%	4-year OS 55.7%
Anderlini *et al.*, 2005[234]	40	Fludarabine, cyclophosphamide ± antithymocyte globulin, or fludarabine + melphalan	22% at 18 months	18-month PFS 32%	18-month OS 61%
Todisco *et al.*, 2007[235]	14	Fludarabine + cyclophosphamide MUD regimen: melphalan + alemtuzumab + fludarabine + TBI	0%	1-year PFS 36%	1-year OS 93%, 2-year OS 73%
Sureda *et al.*, 2009[236]	88	Fludarabine and melphalan	15% at 1 year, 19% at 3 years	PFS for chemotherapy-sensitive: 64% at 1 year, 40% at 3 years	OS for chemotherapy-sensitive: 80% at 1 year, 62% at 3 years

Minimum study size: 14 patients.
No.: number; BEAM: carmustine, etoposide, cytarabine, melphalan; CBV: cyclophosphamide, carmustine, etoposide; TBI: total body irradiation; Bu/Cy: busulfan/cyclophosphamide; OS: overall survival; PFS: progression-free survival; EFS: event-free survival; DFS: disease-free survival; NR: not reported.

100% for these patients. Outcomes of R-CHOP-treated NLPHL patients were significantly improved vs. all other treatment regimens. Continued clinical trial investigations incorporating rituximab into the treatment plan of NLPHL is warranted.

Acute and long-term treatment-related toxicities

In a malignancy that predominantly affects younger patients and one where the majority of patients are cured, secondary long-term toxicities are a critical consideration when choosing therapy. The most common acute side effects caused by chemotherapy for Hodgkin lymphoma include myelosuppression with associated cytopenias contributing to increased infection risk. Anemia and pulmonary toxicity can be caused by bleomycin and/or RT. The incidence of bleomycin lung toxicity in the literature is variable, though it has been reported to be up to 46% in some reports.[250,251] Risk factors for bleomycin lung toxicity include older age, cumulative bleomycin dose, renal insufficiency, pulmonary radiation, underlying lung disease, and tobacco history.[250–252] Case reports[253,254] and pre-clinical data[255,256] have suggested that G-CSF increases the incidence of bleomycin lung toxicity. A retrospective report showed a significantly increased incidence of bleomycin lung toxicity when G-CSF was used during bleomycin-containing chemotherapy for Hodgkin lymphoma (26% vs. 9% without G-CSF, $p = 0.014$) with an overall associated mortality rate of 24% (death rate 40% for patients > age 40).[257]

The most common serious long-term toxicities due to Hodgkin lymphoma therapy include: secondary cancers such as AML/MDS and solid tumors,[147–153,169] gonadal dysfunction including sterility,[258–261] hypothyroidism, typically related to

RT,[262] and cardiovascular disease including increased rates of ischemic heart disease and stroke.[147,154–159]

Many unapparent clinically important cardiovascular abnormalities are frequently encountered among Hodgkin lymphoma survivors, especially if mediastinal radiation was a component of the treatment. Adams *et al.* studied patients who had received a median of 40 Gy RT (range, 27.0–51.7 Gy) at a median age of 16.5.[154] Significant valvular defects were found in 42% of patients, while 75% had conduction defects, 57% had autonomic dysfunction, 31% persistent tachycardia, and 27% blunted hemodynamic responses to exercise. Aleman studied 1474 Hodgkin lymphoma survivors who were ≤ 40 years of age at time of treatment.[158] The risks myocardial infarction (MI) and congestive heart failure (CHF) were highly increased compared with the general population (SIRs = 3.6 and 4.9, respectively). In patients who received mediastinal radiation, the 30-year cumulative incidence of any cardiovascular disease was 35%, 13% for MI, and 20% developed valvular disorders. If given, anthracyclines significantly increased the risks of CHF and valvular disorders related to mediastinal RT. The SIR for MI was significantly elevated beginning 10 years after treatment and remained increased with longer follow-up duration. Stroke is also increased in Hodgkin lymphoma survivors. Bowers *et al.* reported that the relative risk of late-occurring stroke in Hodgkin lymphoma survivors treated with mantle irradiation was 5.63 (95% CI = 2.59–12.25) compared with their siblings.[155] The risk of cardiovascular disease, however, is not exclusively in radiation-treated patients. Swerdlow *et al.* showed that patients who received ABVD without radiation had a long-term highly increased risk of death from MI compared with the general population (SIR = 7.8; 95% CI = 1.6–22.7).[159]

The 20–25 year cumulative actuarial risk (adjusting for background incidence) of secondary cancers for Hodgkin lymphoma patients is 24–28% with the highest overall risk seen 15–20 years after treatment.[147–150,152,153] The strongest predisposing factor is radiation,[148,151,153] although some secondary cancers are seen after chemotherapy alone.[150] The most common second malignancy is breast cancer, although the rates for many other tumors including lung and gastrointestinal are also significantly increased.[148–151,153,169] Travis *et al.* showed that the cumulative risk of breast cancer in women treated for Hodgkin lymphoma is increased with increased age at time of treatment, time since diagnosis, and radiation dose. Further, the risk of secondary cancer is significant for all patient ages, and the risks have not appeared to have declined when examining the rate of second tumors from the 1960s and 1970s compared with the 1980s and 1990s (Figure 19.5).[148,151]

In terms of approximate breast cancer risks, Travis *et al.* conducted a case–control study within an international population-based cohort of 3817 female Hodgkin lymphoma survivors.[151] An example of the cumulative absolute risk of breast cancer for a woman treated at age 25 years with 20–40 Gy of RT (and no alkylator) at 10, 20, and 30 years of follow-up is 1.1%, 9.1%, and 24.6%, respectively. The comparative rates for a patient who received no RT are 0.3%, 1.9%, and 5.5%, respectively. In terms of age at time of treatment, for women treated with 20–40 Gy RT at age 20, 25, and 30 years, the cumulative absolute risk of breast cancer at 30 years of follow-up is 16.0%, 24.6%, and 34.1%, respectively. It should be noted that much of the data regarding long-term radiation-related side effects are derived from patient groups treated with older RT methods and more extensive treatment fields compared with those used today. The potential diminution of long-term toxicity, in particular second malignancies, using contemporary radiation techniques is not known.

Similar to standard frontline treatments for Hodgkin lymphoma, high-dose chemotherapy and HSCT for refractory or relapsed disease carries an increased risk of second malignancies. A retrospective analysis of French registry data found that the overall incidence of secondary malignancies among 467 autografted patients was 9%.[263] Of these, 393 patients were matched to patients who received conventional treatment. The 5-year cumulative incidence of second malignancies was 10% and 5% for the autografted and non-autografted groups, respectively, yielding a relative risk of solid tumors in the autografted group of 5.19, while the risk of AML/MDS was equal in both groups. An analysis of 1732 patients treated at the British Columbia Cancer agency found, however, no difference in second malignancy incidence between patients receiving conventional treatment and those undergoing ASCT.[216] The cumulative 15-year incidence for second malignancies among all patients was 9%. A multivariate analysis revealed that age > 35 years was the only risk variable associated with an increased risk of second malignancy. Goodman *et al.* recently showed that the relative risk of a secondary malignancy after ASCT was 6.5, while it was lower but still elevated compared with Hodgkin lymphoma patients (relative risk 2.4).[264]

Hodgkin lymphoma in the elderly

Hodgkin lymphoma in the elderly remains a disease where no standard treatment recommendations exist. Moreover, it is a population that is underrepresented in Hodgkin lymphoma prospective clinical studies and one in which survival rates are disproportionately inferior compared with younger patients. In population-based studies, the proportion of Hodgkin lymphoma patients older than 60 years ranges between 20% and 40%.[92–94] The proportion of elderly patients participating in prospective trials, however, is considerably lower.[265] With outcomes, the 5-year EFS or FFTF rates for elderly Hodgkin lymphoma patients range from 30% to 40%[96,237,266,267] with 5-year OS ranging from 40% to 55%.[95,237,266,267] This compares to 5-year EFS rates of > 70–80% and OS of > 80–90% for patients aged < 40 years.[95,96,237,267] Suboptimal staging and inadequate treatment delivery for older patients may compromise the rate of cure.[265,268] Furthermore, comorbidities may preclude the delivery of standard chemotherapy.[269,270]

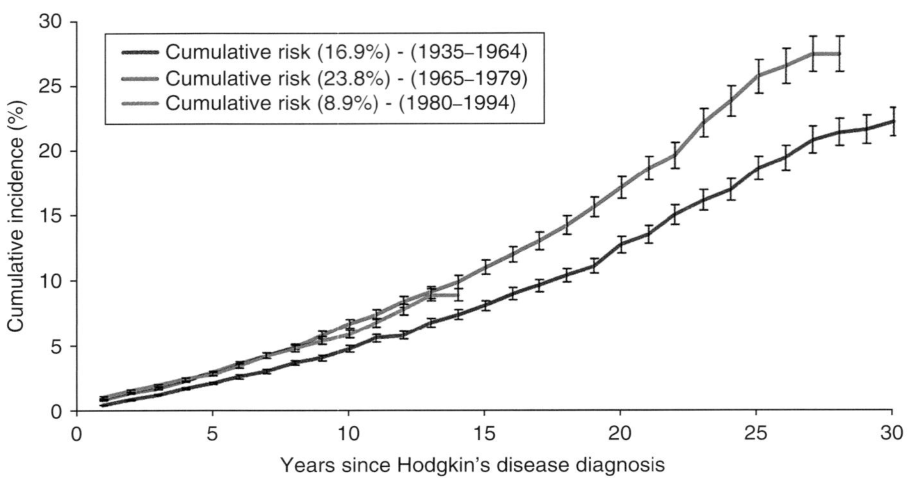

No. of patients at risk/No. person-years:

1935–1964:	(1,783/6,954)	(1,103/4,755)	(824/3,708)	(665/2,975)	(534/2,358)	(344/1,734)
1965–1979:	(8,881/39,225)	(7,036/31,546)	(5,280/18,363)	(2,196/6,333)	(577/1,100)	
1980–1994:	(8,774/28,886)	(3,187/6,565)	(91/42)			

Figure 19.5 Cumulative risk of all solid tumors among 32 591 1-year survivors of Hodgkin disease according to calendar year of diagnosis. Percentages in parentheses indicate the actuarial risk at 25 years (1935–64, 1965–79) or 14 years (1980–94). Vertical lines represent 95% CI for point estimates. From Dores GM *et al.* Second malignant neoplasms among long-term survivors of Hodgkin's disease: a population-based evaluation over 25 years. *J Clin Oncol* 2002;**20**:3484–94.[148] Reprinted with permission. © 2008 American Society of Clinical Oncology. All rights reserved.

Treatment delivery and comorbidity do not appear to completely explain the observed differences in outcome, however, implicating the biology of Hodgkin lymphoma in the elderly.[94,126,129]

Clinically, elderly Hodgkin lymphoma patients commonly present with mixed cellularity histology, EBV-positive disease, poor performance status, presence of B symptoms, absence of bulk, and with advanced stage.[91,92,96,137,267,271–275] Treatment for all stages in the elderly should be given with curative intent, although careful monitoring for treatment-related toxicity during therapy is warranted (i.e., frequent cardiac and pulmonary testing). The majority of data regarding treatment of elderly Hodgkin lymphoma patients stems from phase II and retrospective analyses (Table 19.12). The BEACOPP regimen is too toxic for patients over age 60 years.[276] ABVD can be given,[92] although bleomycin and/or doxorubicin toxicity may be prohibitive. On the randomized ABVD-based CALGB 8251 trial, the 5-year OS for patients $\geq$ age 60 years was significantly inferior compared with patients age <40 years (31% vs. 79%, respectively, $p < 0.0001$). A report by Levis *et al.* analyzed the outcome of patients ≥ 65 years who had received a registry-recommended protocol of ABVD, MOPP, or ABVD/MOPP therapy.[91] The 8-year EFS and OS were 41% and 46%, respectively, both significantly worse compared with patients < 65 years. A critical factor associated with the inferior outcomes was the 23% acute treatment-related death rate among older patients associated with ABVD-based therapy.

Support with hematopoietic growth factors should be considered, although attention should be given to the potential accentuation of bleomycin-associated lung toxicity with concurrent use of G-CSF as discussed before.[257] There are retrospective data that suggest bleomycin might not be needed to maintain efficacy of ABVD treatment, although this needs to be confirmed in a randomized study.[257,278] Less intensive regimens such as CVP/CEB (chlorambucil, vinblastine, procarbazine, prednisone/cyclophosphamide, etoposide, bleomycin) and ChlVPP (chlorambucil, vinblastine, procarbazine, prednisone) have been studied,[266,267] but they are less effective. This may be explained in part as the inclusion of anthracyclines is associated with improved outcome.[267] Of note, limited data using CHOP in elderly Hodgkin lymphoma patients appear promising.[277] International studies examining specific regimens for the elderly are ongoing.[279] Other data in elderly Hodgkin lymphoma patients exist, and have been reviewed in detail elsewhere.[217] Continued multi-center collaborations with prospective clinical trials including formal assessment of comorbidity and functional status will be critical to the successful study of Hodgkin lymphoma in the elderly.

New therapeutic options

Many biologically based strategies are currently being investigated in Hodgkin lymphoma including monoclonal antibodies and novel small molecule inhibitors (Table 19.13). Immunotherapy for Hodgkin lymphoma with monoclonal antibodies has focused primarily on CD30, as well as CD20. CD30 is a TNF receptor protein that is expressed in normal activated B and T cells, EBV-infected cells, and H-RS cells. MDX-060 (Medarex) is a fully humanized antibody to CD30 that has been shown to inhibit cell proliferation and induce apoptosis that was studied in CD30-positive lymphoma (anaplastic large cell lymphoma and classic Hodgkin lymphoma).[280] SGN-30 (Seattle Genetics) is a chimeric anti-CD30 monoclonal antibody that has been shown to increase apoptosis in Hodgkin lymphoma cell lines and sensitize these cell lines to various chemotherapeutic agents.[281] Clinical trials with these compounds thus far have

Table 19.12. Hodgkin lymphoma in the elderly: chemotherapy series[a]

Author	No. patients	Stage	Median age (years)	Treatment	Outcome
Enblad *et al.*, 1991[94]	49	54% III/IV	71	MOPP/ABVD or MOPP (71%) or ChlVPP (22%)	CR 67%, RR 43%, 5-year OS 45%
Mir *et al.*, 1993[237]	29	All advanced stage	71% 60–69	ABVD, MOPP, alternating ABVD/MOPP	5-year OS 31%
Levis *et al.*, 1994[91]	26	58% III/IV	72	ABVD-based (ABVD, MOPP-ABVD)	CR 62%, 8-year RFS 75%, EFS 41%, OS 46%
Levis *et al.*, 1996[266]	25	24% IV	72	CVP/CEB	CR 73%, 5-year RFS 47%, EFS 32%, OS 55%
Weekes *et al.*, 2002[267]	56	73% III/IV	NR	ChlVPP (n = 31), ChlVPP/ABV (n = 25)	5-year EFS and OS ChlVPP/ABV 52% and 67%, respectively, vs. 24% and 30%, respectively, ChlVPP
Macpherson *et al.*, 2002[272]	38	All advanced stage[b]	72	ODBEP	5-year DFS 49% and OS 42%
Stark *et al.*, 2002[96]	102	64% III/IV[b]	Male 69/ female 72	Heterogeneous	Median OS 26 mon and median RFS 39 mon
Enblad *et al.*, 2002[271]	31	42% III/IV	71	LVPP/OEPA	CR 67%, 5-year OS 48%
Landgren *et al.*, 2003[92]	88	69% III/IV	72	MOPP-based (n = 46), ABVD-based (n = 39), other (n = 3)	CR 49%, 5-year CSS 39%, and OS 51%
Levis *et al.*, 2004[275]	105	54% IIB–IV	71	VEPEMB	CR 76%, 5-year RFS 82%, DSS 69%, FFS 56%, and OS 64%
Ballova *et al.*, 2005[276]	68	All IIB–IV	69	COPP/ABVD vs. BEACOPP baseline	COPP/ABVD: 5-year FFTF 55%, OS 50% BEACOPP: 5-year FFTF 74%, OS 50%
Kolstad *et al.*, 2007[277]	29	62% IIB–IV	71	CHOP ± RT	CR 93%; Stage I–IIA: 3-year PFS 82%, OS 91%; Stage IIB–IV: 3-year PFS 72%, OS 67%

Note: [a]Minimum 25 patients treated.
[b]Included stage IB and IIB disease.
No.: number; FFTF: freedom from treatment failure; OS: overall survival; CR: complete remission; RT: radiation therapy; RFS: relapse-free survival; DSS: disease-specific survival; FFS: failure-free survival; PFS: progression-free survival; CSS: cause-specific survival; mon: months; EFS: event-free survival; DFS: disease-free survival; NR: not reported; CVP/CEB: chlorambucil, vinblastine, procarbazine, prednisone/cyclophosphamide, etoposide, bleomycin; ODBEP: vincristine, doxorubicin, bleomycin, etoposide, prednisone; LVPP/OEPA: chlorambucil, vinblastine, procarbazine, prednisolone/vincristine, etoposide, prednisolone, doxorubicin; VEPEMB: vincristine, cyclophosphamide, procarbazine, etoposide, mitoxantrone, and bleomycin.

shown low toxicity, although with only modest activity.[257] New-generation anti-CD30 antibodies with enhanced Fc receptor-mediated antibody activity (Medarex, MDX-1401) and with antibody–drug conjugates (Seattle Genetics, SGN-35) have been developed and are in clinical trials. SGN-35 consists of the anti-CD30 antibody chemically conjugated to the antitubulin agent, monomethyl auristatin-E (MMAE).[282]

The anti-CD20 antibody, rituximab, has been studied in classical Hodgkin lymphoma.[283] Classical Hodgkin lymphoma is not known to contain high levels of CD20 on its cell surface. However, Jones *et al.* recently documented in Hodgkin lymphoma cell lines and patient samples that there is a subpopulation of stem cells clearly related to H-RS cells which express CD20.[284] Immunoglobulin gene rearrangements were found following isolation of H-RS tumor cells from patient samples and peripheral blood mononuclear cells from Hodgkin lymphoma patients were found to express CD20 and were clonal. Further, it has been theorized that rituximab may have a role in classical Hodgkin lymphoma in part by targeting the typical large collection of surrounding non-malignant B cells which support the H-RS cells (i.e., targeting and clearing the microenvironment). Younes *et al.* treated 22 patients with recurrent nodular sclerosis Hodgkin lymphoma with six weekly doses of rituximab.[283] Response rate was 22% with median response duration of 7.8 months (range, 3.3–14.9 months). The same group has also combined rituximab with chemotherapy using rituximab with ABVD for untreated disease[285] and rituximab-gemcitabine for relapsed Hodgkin lymphoma.[286] A randomized

Table 19.13. Novel therapeutic strategies for Hodgkin lymphoma

Mechanism	Treatments
Antibody/receptor therapy	CD30, CD20, CD40, interleukin-13, TRAIL, RANKL
Radioimmunotherapy-based	Anti-CD25 and anti-CD30
Antiapoptotic molecules	Proteasome pathway inhibition, XIAP
Transcriptional pathways	HDAC inhibition, mTOR inhibition, anti-BCL2, anti-HSP-90
EBV-directed therapy	EBV-cytotoxic T-cells, LMP-2A inhibition

Notes: TRAIL: tumor necrosis factor-related apoptosis-inducing ligand; RANKL: receptor activator of nuclear factor-kappa B; XIAP: X-linked inhibitor of apoptosis proteins; HDAC: histone deacetylase; mTOR: mammalian target of rapamycin; HSP: heat shock protein; EBV: Epstein-Barr virus; LMP-2A: latent membrane protein 2A.

controlled trial would be needed to definitely prove the efficacy and safety of R-ABVD over ABVD.

Radioimmunotherapy (RIT), which incorporates radiolabeled antibodies, uses the concept of targeted antibodies, typically antiferritin and anti-CD30, to deliver radiation with yttrium-90 (^{90}Y) or iodine-131 (^{131}I) to specific tumor cells.[287] The tumor-associated protein ferritin has been used as a target.[288] ^{90}Y-labeled rabbit polyclonal antiferritin antibody has been shown to be well tolerated and have disease activity in relapsed Hodgkin lymphoma.[289] In addition, anti-CD25 monoclonal antibody has been labeled with ^{90}Y. CD25 represents an attractive target since the majority of H-RS cells, as well as many of the surrounding tumor-associated T cells, express CD25.

Small molecules to modulate intracellular pathways important for H-RS and lymphocytic and histiocytic cells are also being investigated. NF-κB, a transcription factor, has been shown to be constitutively activated in Hodgkin lymphoma and to be responsible for the pro-proliferative and antiapoptotic properties of the H-RS cells.[290] It also induces the major inhibitor molecules of apoptosis: *c-FLIP* in the extrinsic pathway of apoptosis and *XIAP* in the intrinsic pathway.[291,292] The activity of NF-κB is regulated in part by the inhibitory molecule IκBα, which in turn is inhibited by Iκ kinases (IKKs).[7,291] The reversible proteasome inhibitor, bortezomib, has been shown to be effective in H-RS cell lines with or without IκBα mutations suggesting that it has other proapoptotic properties in addition to blocking the degradation of IκBα.[293] It has been found to downregulate the antiapoptotic molecules *c-FLIP*[7] and *XIAP*,[71] leading to more apoptosis. Despite this pre-clinical activity, bortezomib has shown limited clinical activity as a single agent or in combination with dexamethasone in relapsed/refractory Hodgkin lymphoma;[294–296] but combination regimens including bortezomib to exploit potential synergistic activity should be explored. In vitro studies have shown improved apoptosis combining bortezomib with TRAIL compared with bortezomib alone.[7]

Histone deacetylase (HDAC) inhibitors are being investigated as they interfere with activation of NF-κB and mediate apoptosis through cFLIP inhibition, induction of p21, and production of reactive oxygen species.[69,297] Several HDAC inhibitors are under development for the treatment of lymphoma. The non-hydroxamate HDAC inhibitor, MGCD0103, was associated with a response rate of 46% among 28 evaluable relapsed/refractory Hodgkin lymphoma patients treated at doses ≥ 1.2 mg/kg (CR 25%). The antiapoptotic molecule XIAP is also being targeted with antisense oligonucleotides and through chemical inhibition. In addition to inhibiting the intrinsic pathway of apoptosis, XIAP also increases NF-κB via positive feedback.[291] XIAP is inhibited by second mitochondria-derived activator of caspases (Smac) when they bind in the cytosol. AEG35156 (Aegera Therapeutics) is an antisense oligonucleotide directed towards *XIAP* that has been studied in various cancer cell lines and shown to reduce XIAP levels and sensitize the cells to chemotherapeutic agents.[298] Downregulation of *XIAP* by adding small hairpin RNA (shRNA) targeting *XIAP* mRNA also achieves the same effect.[71] Trials are also investigating *m-TOR* inhibition; using everolimus (RAD001, Novartis Pharmaceuticals), Johnston *et al.* showed a 43% overall response rate (6/14) in patients with relapsed/refractory Hodgkin lymphoma.[299] Georgakis *et al.* have showed that inhibiting heat shock protein (HSP)-90 function by the small molecule 17-allylamino-17-demethoxygeldanamycin (17-AAG) in Hodgkin lymphoma results in significant apoptosis depleted AKT, decreased extracellular signal-regulated kinase (ERK) phosphorylation, and reduced cellular *FLICE*-like inhibitory levels.[300] Clinical trials targeting HSP-90 with 17-AAG in Hodgkin lymphoma are ongoing. In addition, a monoclonal antibody to interleukin-13 (TNX-650; Tanox, Inc.), a growth factor in Hodgkin lymphoma,[301] continues enrollment in a phase I trial for patients with relapsed/refractory Hodgkin lymphoma.

Other important Hodgkin lymphoma cell survival pathways have been identified in pre-clinical studies. Galectin-1 (Gal-1), a carbohydrate-binding lectin, is overexpressed in H-RS cells and contributes to the overabundance of T helper-2 (Th-2) and T regulatory (T-reg) cells in the T cell infiltrate that surrounds the H-RS cells. Gal-1 treatment of activated T-cells has been shown to favor the secretion of Th-2 cytokines and expand the FOXP3+ T-reg cells.[302] Targeting Gal-1 may be a novel way to alter the T-cell infiltrate surrounding the H-RS cells thus increasing their vulnerability to immune surveillance. The p53 gene is activated when a cell is stressed and triggers cell cycle and apoptotic regulatory pathways.[303] Murine double minute 2 (MDM2; HDM2 in humans) is an inhibitor of p53. The wildtype *p53* gene is expressed in most H-RS cells. A recently developed molecule, nutlin-3A, binds to the p53-binding site of MDM2 and stabilizes p53 to allow it to activate the apoptotic pathways. One recent study demonstrated that adding nutlin-3A to H-RS cells with the wildtype *p53* gene resulted in p53-dependent cell cycle arrest and apoptosis.[304] H-RS cells have also been found to have a large number of interleukin-4 receptors (IL-4R). In vitro studies were done showing good cytotoxicity of a permuted human IL-4 and *Pseudomonas* exotoxin (IL-4 cytotoxin). IL-4 cytotoxin was then given to mice that had Hodgkin lymphoma and resulted in a substantial doubling of the survival time of these mice as compared with the controls.[305]

Finally, EBV-targeted therapy is also being researched as a potential target for the treatment of Hodgkin lymphoma. By combining EBV transformed B cells with peripheral blood mononuclear cells, one can produce EBV-specific cytotoxic T lymphocytes that can then be given to the patient in hopes of attacking the specific EBV-infected cancer cells.[306] A 2004 study marked these infused cells and saw that they multiplied exponentially, traveled to the tumor sites, and lasted for up to 12 months. EBV viral load decreased and 5 of 14 patients achieved CR.[307] In addition to attacking EBV directly, cellular strategies directed against EBV-encoded proteins, such as LMP-2A, are also being investigated.[308]

Conclusions

Many advances have been made in the science and the treatment of Hodgkin lymphoma over the past 10–20 years. Currently more than 70–80% of all Hodgkin lymphoma patients are cured of their disease. Continued clinical and translational research is warranted in order to continue to improve the survival of Hodgkin lymphoma as well as to lessen the toxicities associated with Hodgkin lymphoma-related therapy. Ongoing and planned studies are using the principles of response-adapted (e.g., early PET) and/or risk-adapted therapy (e.g., genotypic analysis) to tailor treatments to individual patients. A multitude of new targeted compounds are being investigated in relapsed/refractory Hodgkin lymphoma. If proven efficacious and safe, these novel agents may begin to be studied in newly diagnosed patients in an attempt to decrease the amount and/or length of chemotherapy and radiation needed. In order to continue to advance the field of Hodgkin lymphoma, it is critical that international collaborative efforts continue and that oncologists offer to all Hodgkin lymphoma patients the opportunity to participate in clinical trials.

References

1. Hodgkin T. On some morbid appearances of the absorbent glands and spleen. *Medico-Chirurg Trans* 1832;**17**:68.
2. Wilks S. Cases of the enlargement of the lymphatic glands and spleen (or Hodgkin's disease) with remarks. *Guys Hosp Rep* 1865;**11**:56.
3. Greenfield WS. Specimens illustrative of the pathology of lymphadenoma and leucocythemia. *Trans Pathol Soc Lond* 1878;**29**:272.
4. Reed D. On pathological changes in Hodgkin's disease, with special reference to its relation to tuberculosis. *Johns Hopkins Hosp Rep* 1902;**10**:133.
5. Sternberg C. Uber eine eigenartige unter dem Bilde der Pseudoleukamie verlaufende Tuberculose des lymphatischen Apparates. *Ztschr Heilk* 1879;**19**:21.
6. Kanzler H, Kuppers R, Hansmann ML, *et al.* Hodgkin and Reed-Sternberg cells in Hodgkin's disease represent the outgrowth of a dominant tumor clone derived from (crippled) germinal center B cells. *J Exp Med* 1996;**184**:1495–505.
7. Kuppers R, Rajewsky K, Zhao M, *et al.* Hodgkin disease: Hodgkin and Reed-Sternberg cells picked from histological sections show clonal immunoglobulin gene rearrangements and appear to be derived from B cells at various stages of development. *Proc Natl Acad Sci U S A* 1994;**91**:10 962–6.
8. Marafioti T, Hummel M, Foss H-D, *et al.* Hodgkin and Reed-Sternberg cells represent an expansion of a single clone originating from a germinal center B-cell with functional immunoglobulin gene rearrangements but defective immunoglobulin transcription. *Blood* 2000;**95**:1443–50.
9. Swerdlow SH, Campo E, Harris NL, *et al.* (eds.) *WHO Classification of Tumours of Haematopoietic and Lymphoid Tissues*, 4th edn. Lyon, France, IARC Press, 2008.
10. DeVita VT Jr, Hubbard SM, Moxley JH, 3rd. The cure of Hodgkin's disease with drugs. *Adv Intern Med* 1983; **28**:277–302.
11. Peters M. A study of survivals in Hodgkin's disease treated radiologically. *AJR Am J Roentgenol* 1950;**63**:299.
12. DeVita VT Jr, Carbone PP. Treatment of Hodgkin's disease. *Med Ann Dist Columbia* 1967;**36**:232–34 passim.
13. http://www.seer.cancer.gov/csr/1975_2005/results_single/sect_01_table.01.pdf.
14. Katanoda K, Yako-Suketomo H. Comparison of time trends in Hodgkin and non-Hodgkin lymphoma incidence (1973–97) in East Asia, Europe and USA, from cancer incidence in five continents, Vol. IV–VIII. *Jpn J Clin Oncol* 2008;**38**:391–3.
15. Au WY, Gascoyne RD, Gallagher RE, *et al.* Hodgkin's lymphoma in Chinese migrants to British Columbia: a 25-year survey. *Ann Oncol* 2004;**15**:626–30.
16. Correa P, O'Conor GT. Epidemiologic patterns of Hodgkin's disease. *Int J Cancer* 1971;**8**:192–201.
17. Macfarlane GJ, Evstifeeva T, Boyle P, *et al.* International patterns in the occurrence of Hodgkin's disease in children and young adult males. *Int J Cancer* 1995;**61**:165–9.
18. Grufferman S, Cole P, Smith PG, *et al.* Hodgkin's disease in siblings. *N Engl J Med* 1977;**296**:248–50.
19. Lindelof B, Eklund G. Analysis of hereditary component of cancer by use of a familial index by site. *Lancet* 2001;**358**:1696–8.
20. Westergaard T, Melbye M, Pedersen JB, *et al.* Birth order, sibship size and risk of Hodgkin's disease in children and young adults: a population-based study of 31 million person-years. *Int J Cancer* 1997;**72**:977–81.
21. Goldin LR, Pfeiffer RM, Gridley G, *et al.* Familial aggregation of Hodgkin lymphoma and related tumors. *Cancer* 2004;**100**:1902–8.
22. Mack TM, Cozen W, Shibata DK, *et al.* Concordance for Hodgkin's disease in identical twins suggesting genetic

susceptibility to the young-adult form of the disease. *N Engl J Med* 1995; **332**:413–18.

23. Cozen W, Gill PS, Ingles SA, *et al.* IL-6 levels and genotype are associated with risk of young adult Hodgkin lymphoma. *Blood* 2004;**103**:3216–21.
24. Chang ET, Smedby KE, Hjalgrim H, *et al.* Family history of hematopoietic malignancy and risk of lymphoma. *J Natl Cancer Inst* 2005;**97**:1466–74.
25. Paltiel O, Schmit T, Adler B, *et al.* The incidence of lymphoma in first-degree relatives of patients with Hodgkin disease and non-Hodgkin lymphoma: results and limitations of a registry-linked study. *Cancer* 2000;**88**:2357–66.
26. Anderson LA, Pfeiffer RM, Rapkin JS, *et al.* Survival patterns among lymphoma patients with a family history of lymphoma. *J Clin Oncol* 2008;**26**:4958–65.
27. Chang ET, Zheng T, Weir EG, *et al.* Childhood social environment and Hodgkin's lymphoma: new findings from a population-based case-control study. *Cancer Epidemiol Biomarkers Prev* 2004;**13**:1361–70.
28. Gutensohn NM. Social class and age at diagnosis of Hodgkin's disease: new epidemiologic evidence for the "two-disease hypothesis". *Cancer Treat Rep* 1982;**66**:689–95.
29. Hjalgrim H, Askling J, Rostgaard K, *et al.* Characteristics of Hodgkin's lymphoma after infectious mononucleosis. *N Engl J Med* 2003;**349**:1324–32.
30. Hjalgrim H, Smedby KE, Rostgaard K, *et al.* Infectious mononucleosis, childhood social environment, and risk of Hodgkin lymphoma. *Cancer Res* 2007;**67**:2382–8.
31. Mueller N, Evans A, Harris NL, *et al.* Hodgkin's disease and Epstein-Barr virus. Altered antibody pattern before diagnosis. *N Engl J Med* 1989;**320**:689–95.
32. Hjalgrim H, Askling J, Sorensen P, *et al.* Risk of Hodgkin's disease and other cancers after infectious mononucleosis. *J Natl Cancer Inst* 2000;**92**:1522–8.
33. Staal SP, Ambinder R, Beschorner WE, *et al.* A survey of Epstein-Barr virus DNA in lymphoid tissue. Frequent detection in Hodgkin's disease. *Am J Clin Pathol* 1989;**91**:1–5.
34. Brousset P, Chittal S, Schlaifer D, *et al.* Detection of Epstein-Barr virus messenger RNA in Reed-Sternberg cells of Hodgkin's disease by in situ hybridization with biotinylated probes on specially processed modified acetone methyl benzoate xylene (ModAMeX) sections. *Blood* 1991;**77**:1781–6.
35. Brousset P, Knecht H, Rubin B, *et al.* Demonstration of Epstein-Barr virus replication in Reed-Sternberg cells of Hodgkin's disease. *Blood* 1993;**82**:872–6.
36. Glaser SL, Lin RJ, Stewart SL, *et al.* Epstein-Barr virus-associated Hodgkin's disease: epidemiologic characteristics in international data. *Int J Cancer* 1997;**70**:375–82.
37. Armstrong AA, Alexander FE, Cartwright R, *et al.* Epstein-Barr virus and Hodgkin's disease: further evidence for the three disease hypothesis. *Leukemia* 1998;**12**:1272–6.
38. Enblad G, Sandvej K, Sundstrom C, *et al.* Epstein-Barr virus distribution in Hodgkin's disease in an unselected Swedish population. *Acta Oncol* 1999;**38**:425–9.
39. Frisch M, Biggar RJ, Engels EA, *et al.* Association of cancer with AIDS-related immunosuppression in adults. *JAMA* 2001;**285**:1736–45.
40. Herida M, Mary-Krause M, Kaphan R, *et al.* Incidence of non-AIDS-defining cancers before and during the highly active antiretroviral therapy era in a cohort of human immunodeficiency virus-infected patients. *J Clin Oncol* 2003;**21**:3447–53.
41. Engels EA, Pfeiffer RM, Goedert JJ, *et al.* Trends in cancer risk among people with AIDS in the United States 1980–2002. *AIDS* 2006;**20**:1645–54.
42. Patel P, Hanson DL, Sullivan PS, *et al.* Incidence of types of cancer among HIV-infected persons compared with the general population in the United States, 1992–2003. *Ann Intern Med* 2008;**148**:728–36.
43. Grulich AE, van Leeuwen MT, Falster MO, *et al.* Incidence of cancers in people with HIV/AIDS compared with immunosuppressed transplant recipients: a meta-analysis. *Lancet* 2007;**370**:59–67.
44. Biggar RJ, Jaffe ES, Goedert JJ, *et al.* Hodgkin lymphoma and immunodeficiency in persons with HIV/AIDS. *Blood* 2006;**108**:3786–91.
45. Clifford GM, Polesel J, Rickenbach M, *et al.* Cancer risk in the Swiss HIV Cohort Study: associations with immunodeficiency, smoking, and highly active antiretroviral therapy. *J Natl Cancer Inst* 2005;**97**:425–32.
46. Clifford GM, Rickenbach M, Lise M, *et al.* Hodgkin lymphoma in the Swiss HIV Cohort Study. *Blood* 2009;**113**:5737–42.
47. Powles T, Robinson D, Stebbing J, *et al.* Highly active antiretroviral therapy and the incidence of non-AIDS-defining cancers in people with HIV infection. *J Clin Oncol* 2009;**27**:884–90.
48. Landgren O, Engels EA, Pfeiffer RM, *et al.* Autoimmunity and susceptibility to Hodgkin lymphoma: a population-based case-control study in Scandinavia. *J Natl Cancer Inst* 2006;**98**:1321–30.
49. Nieters A, Rohrmann S, Becker N, *et al.* Smoking and lymphoma risk in the European prospective investigation into cancer and nutrition. *Am J Epidemiol* 2008;**167**:1081–9.
50. Hjalgrim H, Ekstrom-Smedby K, Rostgaard K, *et al.* Cigarette smoking and risk of Hodgkin lymphoma: a population-based case-control study. *Cancer Epidemiol Biomarkers Prev* 2007;**16**:1561–6.
51. Briggs NC, Hall HI, Brann EA, *et al.* Cigarette smoking and risk of Hodgkin's disease: a population-based case-control study. *Am J Epidemiol* 2002;**156**:1011–20.
52. McCunney RJ. Hodgkin's disease, work, and the environment. A review. *J Occup Environ Med* 1999;**41**:36–46.
53. Hjalgrim H, Rasmussen S, Rostgaard K, *et al.* Familial clustering of Hodgkin lymphoma and multiple sclerosis. *J Natl Cancer Inst* 2004;**96**:780–4.
54. Nielsen NM, Rostgaard K, Rasmussen S, *et al.* Cancer risk among patients with multiple sclerosis: a population-based register study. *Int J Cancer* 2006; **118**:979–84.
55. El-Zein R, Monroy CM, Etzel CJ, *et al.* Genetic polymorphisms in DNA repair genes as modulators of Hodgkin disease risk. *Cancer* 2009;**115**:1651–9.
56. Niens M, Jarrett RF, Hepkema B, *et al.* HLA-A*02 is associated with a reduced risk and HLA-A*01 with an increased risk of developing EBV+ Hodgkin lymphoma. *Blood* 2007;**110**:3310–15.
57. Hohaus S, Massini G, D'Alo F, *et al.* Association between glutathione

S-transferase genotypes and Hodgkin's lymphoma risk and prognosis. *Clin Cancer Res* 2003;**9**:3435–40.

58. Re D, Kuppers R, Diehl V. Molecular pathogenesis of Hodgkin's lymphoma. *J Clin Oncol* 2005;**23**:6379–86.

59. Re D, Thomas RK, Behringer K, *et al.* From Hodgkin disease to Hodgkin lymphoma: biologic insights and therapeutic potential. *Blood* 2005;**105**:4553–60.

60. Schwering I, Brauninger A, Klein U, *et al.* Loss of the B-lineage-specific gene expression program in Hodgkin and Reed-Sternberg cells of Hodgkin lymphoma. *Blood* 2003;**101**:1505–12.

61. Re D, Muschen M, Ahmadi T, *et al.* Oct-2 and Bob-1 deficiency in Hodgkin and Reed Sternberg cells. *Cancer Res* 2001;**61**:2080–4.

62. Stein H, Marafioti T, Foss H-D, *et al.* Down-regulation of BOB.1/OBF.1 and Oct2 in classical Hodgkin disease but not in lymphocyte predominant Hodgkin disease correlates with immunoglobulin transcription. *Blood* 2001;**97**:496–501.

63. Kuppers R. Molecular biology of Hodgkin's lymphoma. *Adv Cancer Res* 2002;**84**:277–312.

64. Marafioti T, Hummel M, Anagnostopoulos I, *et al.* Origin of nodular lymphocyte-predominant Hodgkin's disease from a clonal expansion of highly mutated germinal-center B cells. *N Engl J Med* 1997;**337**:453–8.

65. Ohno T, Stribley JA, Wu G, *et al.* Clonality in nodular lymphocyte-predominant Hodgkin's disease. *N Engl J Med* 1997;**337**:459–65.

66. Caldwell RG, Wilson JB, Anderson SJ, *et al.* Epstein-Barr virus LMP2A drives B cell development and survival in the absence of normal B cell receptor signals. *Immunity* 1998;**9**:405–11.

67. Maggio EM, van den Berg A, de Jong D, *et al.* Low frequency of FAS mutations in Reed-Sternberg cells of Hodgkin's lymphoma. *Am J Pathol* 2003;**162**:29–35.

68. Dutton A, O'Neil JD, Milner AE, *et al.* Expression of the cellular FLICE-inhibitory protein (c-FLIP) protects Hodgkin's lymphoma cells from autonomous Fas-mediated death. *Proc Natl Acad Sci U S A* 2004;**101**:6611–16.

69. Mathas S, Lietz A, Anagnostopoulos I, *et al.* c-FLIP mediates resistance of Hodgkin/Reed-Sternberg cells to death receptor-induced apoptosis. *J Exp Med* 2004;**199**:1041–52.

70. Thomas RK, Kallenborn A, Wickenhauser C, *et al.* Constitutive expression of c-FLIP in Hodgkin and Reed-Sternberg cells. *Am J Pathol* 2002;**160**:1521–8.

71. Kashkar H, Haefs C, Shin H, *et al.* XIAP-mediated caspase inhibition in Hodgkin's lymphoma-derived B cells. *J Exp Med* 2003;**198**:341–7.

72. Muschen M, Re D, Brauninger A, *et al.* Somatic mutations of the CD95 gene in Hodgkin and Reed-Sternberg cells. *Cancer Res* 2000;**60**:5640–3.

73. Sanchez-Aguilera A, Montalban C, de la Cueva P, *et al.* Tumor microenvironment and mitotic checkpoint are key factors in the outcome of classic Hodgkin lymphoma. *Blood* 2006;**108**:662–8.

74. Gilbert R. Radiotherapy in Hodgkin's disease (malignant granulomatosis); anatomic and clinical foundations; governing principles, results. *Am J Roentgenol* 1939;**41**:198.

75. Peters M. Prophylactic treatment of adjacent areas in Hodgkin's disease. *Cancer Res* 1966;**26**:1232.

76. Austin-Seymour MM, Hoppe RT, Cox RS, *et al.* Hodgkin's disease in patients over sixty years old. *Ann Intern Med* 1984;**100**:13–18.

77. Castellino RA, Dunnick NR, Goffinet DR, *et al.* Predictive value of lymphography for sites of subdiaphragmatic disease encountered at staging laparotomy in newly diagnosed Hodgkin's disease and non-Hodgkin's lymphoma. *J Clin Oncol* 1983;**1**:532–6.

78. Mauch P, Larson D, Osteen R, *et al.* Prognostic factors for positive surgical staging in patients with Hodgkin's disease. *J Clin Oncol* 1990;**8**:257–65.

79. Rueffer U, Sieber M, Josting A, *et al.* Prognostic factors for subdiaphragmatic involvement in clinical stage I-II supradiaphragmatic Hodgkin's disease: a retrospective analysis of the GHSG. *Ann Oncol* 1999;**10**:1343–8.

80. Hernandez-Maraver D, Hernandez-Navarro F, Gomez-Leon N, *et al.* Positron emission tomography/computed tomography: diagnostic accuracy in lymphoma. *Br J Haematol* 2006;**135**:293–302.

81. Kostakoglu L, Coleman M, Leonard JP, *et al.* PET predicts prognosis after 1 cycle of chemotherapy in aggressive lymphoma and Hodgkin's disease. *J Nucl Med* 2002;**43**:1018–27.

82. Jerusalem G, Beguin Y, Fassotte MF, *et al.* Whole-body positron emission tomography using 18F-fluorodeoxyglucose for posttreatment evaluation in Hodgkin's disease and non-Hodgkin's lymphoma has higher diagnostic and prognostic value than classical computed tomography scan imaging. *Blood* 1999;**94**:429–33.

83. Cheson BD, Pfistner B, Juweid ME, *et al.* Revised response criteria for malignant lymphoma. *J Clin Oncol* 2007;**25**:579–86.

84. Doll DC, Ringenberg QS, Anderson SP, *et al.* Bone marrow biopsy in the initial staging of Hodgkin's disease. *Med Pediatr Oncol* 1989;**17**:1–5.

85. Fabian CJ, Mansfield CM, Dahlberg S, *et al.* Low-dose involved field radiation after chemotherapy in advanced Hodgkin disease: A Southwest Oncology Group randomized study. *Ann Intern Med* 1994;**120**:903–12.

86. Howell SJ, Grey M, Chang J, *et al.* The value of bone marrow examination in the staging of Hodgkin's lymphoma: a review of 955 cases seen in a regional cancer centre. *Br J Haematol* 2002; **119**:408–11.

87. Munker R, Hasenclever D, Brosteanu O, *et al.* Bone marrow involvement in Hodgkin's disease: an analysis of 135 consecutive cases. German Hodgkin's Lymphoma Study Group. *J Clin Oncol* 1995;**13**:403–9.

88. Vassilakopoulos TP, Angelopoulou MK, Constantinou N, *et al.* Development and validation of a clinical prediction rule for bone marrow involvement in patients with Hodgkin lymphoma. *Blood* 2005; **105**:1875–80.

89. Wang J, Weiss LM, Chang KL, *et al.* Diagnostic utility of bilateral bone marrow examination: significance of morphologic and ancillary technique study in malignancy. *Cancer* 2002;**94**:1522–31.

90. Lister TA, Crowther D, Sutcliffe SB, *et al.* Report of a committee convened to discuss the evaluation and staging of patients with Hodgkin's disease:

Cotswolds meeting. *J Clin Oncol* 1989;**7**:1630–6.

91. Levis A, Depaoli L, Urgesi A, *et al.* Probability of cure in elderly Hodgkin's disease patients. *Haematologica* 1994;**79**:46–54.
92. Landgren O, Algernon C, Axdorph U, *et al.* Hodgkin's lymphoma in the elderly with special reference to type and intensity of chemotherapy in relation to prognosis. *Haematologica* 2003;**88**:438–44.
93. Proctor SJ, Rueffer JU, Angus B, *et al.* Hodgkin's disease in the elderly: current status and future directions. *Ann Oncol* 2002;**13** Suppl 1:133–7.
94. Enblad G, Glimelius B, Sundstrom C. Original article: Treatment outcome in Hodgkin's disease in patients above the age of 60: a population-based study. *Ann Oncol* 1991;**2**:297–302.
95. Aleman BMP, Raemaekers JMM, Tirelli U, *et al.* Involved-field radiotherapy for advanced Hodgkin's lymphoma. *N Engl J Med* 2003;**348**:2396–406.
96. Stark GL, Wood KM, Jack F, *et al.* Hodgkin's disease in the elderly: a population-based study. *Br J Haematol* 2002;**119**:432–40.
97. Federico M, Luminari S, Iannitto E, *et al.* ABVD compared with BEACOPP compared with CEC for the initial treatment of patients with advanced Hodgkin's lymphoma: results from the HD2000 Gruppo Italiano per lo Studio dei Linfomi Trial. *J Clin Oncol* 2009;**27**:805–11.
98. Horning SJ, Hoppe RT, Breslin S, *et al.* Stanford V and radiotherapy for locally extensive and advanced Hodgkin's disease: mature results of a prospective clinical trial. *J Clin Oncol* 2002; **20**:630–7.
99. Duggan DB, Petroni GR, Johnson JL, *et al.* Randomized comparison of ABVD and MOPP/ABV hybrid for the treatment of advanced Hodgkin's disease: report of an intergroup trial. *J Clin Oncol* 2003;**21**:607–14.
100. Gobbi PG, Levis A, Chisesi T, *et al.* ABVD versus modified Stanford V versus MOPPEBVCAD with optional and limited radiotherapy in intermediate- and advanced-stage Hodgkin's lymphoma: final results of a multicenter randomized trial by the Intergruppo Italiano Linfomi. *J Clin Oncol* 2005;**23**:9198–207.
101. Diehl V, Franklin J, Pfreundschuh M, *et al.* Standard and increased-dose BEACOPP chemotherapy compared with COPP-ABVD for advanced Hodgkin's disease. *N Engl J Med* 2003;**348**:2386–95.
102. Johnson PW, Radford JA, Cullen MH, *et al.* Comparison of ABVD and alternating or hybrid multidrug regimens for the treatment of advanced Hodgkin's lymphoma: results of the United Kingdom Lymphoma Group LY09 Trial (ISRCTN97144519). *J Clin Oncol* 2005;**23**:9208–18.
103. Ferme C, Mounier N, Casasnovas O, *et al.* Long-term results and competing risk analysis of the H89 trial in patients with advanced-stage Hodgkin lymphoma: a study by the Groupe d'Etude des Lymphomes de l'Adulte (GELA). *Blood* 2006;**107**:4636–42.
104. Ertem M, Uysal Z, Yavuz G, *et al.* Immune thrombocytopenia and hemolytic anemia as a presenting manifestation of Hodgkin disease. *Pediatr Hematol Oncol* 2000;**17**:181–5.
105. Ballonoff A, Kavanagh B, Nash R, *et al.* Hodgkin lymphoma-related vanishing bile duct syndrome and idiopathic cholestasis: statistical analysis of all published cases and literature review. *Acta Oncol* 2008;**47**:962–70.
106. Meert AP, Berghmans T, Sculier JP. Hypothermia and Hodgkin's disease: case report and review of the literature. *Acta Clin Belg* 2006;**61**:252–4.
107. Audard V, Larousserie F, Grimbert P, *et al.* Minimal change nephrotic syndrome and classical Hodgkin's lymphoma: report of 21 cases and review of the literature. *Kidney Int* 2006;**69**:2251–60.
108. Gutmann B, Crivellaro C, Mitterer M, *et al.* Paraneoplastic stiff-person syndrome, heterotopic soft tissue ossification and gonarthritis in a HLA B27-positive woman preceding the diagnosis of Hodgkin's lymphoma. *Haematologica* 2006;**91**:ECR59.
109. Duhmke E, Franklin J, Pfreundschuh M, *et al.* Low-dose radiation is sufficient for the noninvolved extended-field treatment in favorable early-stage Hodgkin's disease: long-term results of a randomized trial of radiotherapy alone. *J Clin Oncol* 2001;**19**:2905–14.
110. Engert A, Schiller P, Josting A, *et al.* Involved-field radiotherapy is equally effective and less toxic compared with extended-field radiotherapy after four cycles of chemotherapy in patients with early-stage unfavorable Hodgkin's lymphoma: results of the HD8 trial of the German Hodgkin's Lymphoma Study Group. *J Clin Oncol* 2003; **21**:3601–8.
111. Noordijk EM, Carde P, Dupouy N, *et al.* Combined-modality therapy for clinical stage I or II Hodgkin's lymphoma: long-term results of the European Organisation for Research and Treatment of Cancer H7 randomized controlled trials. *J Clin Oncol* 2006;**24**:3128–35.
112. Meyer RM, Gospodarowicz MK, Connors JM, *et al.* Randomized comparison of ABVD chemotherapy with a strategy that includes radiation therapy in patients with limited-stage Hodgkin's lymphoma: National Cancer Institute of Canada Clinical Trials Group and the Eastern Cooperative Oncology Group. *J Clin Oncol* 2005;**23**:4634–42.
113. Hasenclever D, Diehl V. A prognostic score for advanced Hodgkin's disease. International Prognostic Factors Project on Advanced Hodgkin's Disease. *N Engl J Med* 1998;**339**:1506–14.
114. Klimm B, Reineke T, Haverkamp H, *et al.* Role of hematotoxicity and sex in patients with Hodgkin's lymphoma: an analysis from the German Hodgkin Study Group. *J Clin Oncol* 2005;**23**: 8003–11.
115. Friedberg JW, Fischman A, Neuberg D, *et al.* FDG-PET is superior to gallium scintigraphy in staging and more sensitive in the follow-up of patients with de novo Hodgkin lymphoma: a blinded comparison. *Leuk Lymphoma* 2004;**45**:85–92.
116. Jerusalem G, Beguin Y, Fassotte MF, *et al.* Early detection of relapse by whole-body positron emission tomography in the follow-up of patients with Hodgkin's disease. *Ann Oncol* 2003;**14**:123–30.
117. Jerusalem G, Beguin Y, Fassotte MF, *et al.* Whole-body positron emission tomography using 18F-fluorodeoxyglucose compared to standard procedures for staging patients with Hodgkin's disease. *Haematologica* 2001;**86**:266–73.
118. Stumpe KD, Urbinelli M, Steinert HC, *et al.* Whole-body positron emission tomography using fluorodeoxyglucose

for staging of lymphoma: effectiveness and comparison with computed tomography. *Eur J Nucl Med* 1998; **25**:721–8.

119. Hoekstra OS, van Lingen A, Ossenkoppele GJ, *et al.* Early response monitoring in malignant lymphoma using fluorine-18 fluorodeoxyglucose single-photon emission tomography. *Eur J Nucl Med* 1993;**20**:1214–17.

120. Torizuka T, Nakamura F, Kanno T, *et al.* Early therapy monitoring with FDG-PET in aggressive non-Hodgkin's lymphoma and Hodgkin's lymphoma. *Eur J Nucl Med Mol Imaging* 2004;**31**:22–8.

121. Zinzani PL, Tani M, Fanti S, *et al.* Early positron emission tomography (PET) restaging: a predictive final response in Hodgkin's disease patients. *Ann Oncol* 2006;**17**:1296–300.

122. Hutchings M, Loft A, Hansen M, *et al.* FDG-PET after two cycles of chemotherapy predicts treatment failure and progression-free survival in Hodgkin lymphoma. *Blood* 2006; **107**:52–9.

123. Gallamini A, Rigacci L, Merli F, *et al.* The predictive value of positron emission tomography scanning performed after two courses of standard therapy on treatment outcome in advanced stage Hodgkin's disease. *Haematologica* 2006;**91**:475–81.

124. Gallamini A, Hutchings M, Rigacci L, *et al.* Early interim 2-[18F]fluoro-2-deoxy-D-glucose positron emission tomography is prognostically superior to international prognostic score in advanced-stage Hodgkin's lymphoma: a report from a joint Italian-Danish study. *J Clin Oncol* 2007;**25**:3746–52.

125. Dann EJ, Bar-Shalom R, Tamir A, *et al.* Risk-adapted BEACOPP regimen can reduce the cumulative dose of chemotherapy for standard and high-risk Hodgkin lymphoma with no impairment of outcome. *Blood* 2007;**109**:905–9.

126. Keegan TH, Glaser SL, Clarke CA, *et al.* Epstein-Barr virus as a marker of survival after Hodgkin's lymphoma: a population-based study. *J Clin Oncol* 2005;**23**:7604–13.

127. Diepstra A, van Imhoff G, Karim-Kos H, *et al.* Latent EBV infection of Hodgkin Reed-Sternberg cells predicts adverse outcome in older adult classical Hodgkin lymphoma patients. *Seventh International Symposium on Hodgkin Lymphoma*; 2007:16a.

128. Asano N, Tamaru J, Kinoshita T, *et al.* Age-related EBV-associated B-cell lymphoproliferative disorders: comparison with EBV-positive classical Hodgkin lymphoma in elderly patients. Seventh International Symposium on Hodgkin Lymphoma; 2007:39a.

129. Gandhi MK, Tellam JT, Khanna R. Epstein-Barr virus-associated Hodgkin's lymphoma. *Br J Haematol* 2004;**125**:267–81.

130. Frisan T, Sjoberg J, Dolcetti R, *et al.* Local suppression of Epstein-Barr virus (EBV)-specific cytotoxicity in biopsies of EBV-positive Hodgkin's disease. *Blood* 1995;**86**:1493–501.

131. Kelley TW, Pohlman B, Elson P, *et al.* The ratio of FOXP3+ regulatory T cells to granzyme B+ cytotoxic T/NK cells predicts prognosis in classical Hodgkin lymphoma and is independent of bcl-2 and MAL expression. *Am J Clin Pathol* 2007;**128**:958–65.

132. Ribrag V, Koscielny S, Casasnovas O, *et al.* Pharmacogenetic study in Hodgkin lymphomas reveals the impact of UGT1A1 polymorphisms on patient prognosis. *Blood* 2009;**113**:3307–13.

133. Bonadonna G, Zucali R, Monfardini S, *et al.* Combination chemotherapy of Hodgkin's disease with adriamycin, bleomycin, vinblastine, and imidazole carboxamide versus MOPP. *Cancer* 1975;**36**:252–9.

134. Bonadonna G, Bonfante V, Viviani S, *et al.* ABVD plus subtotal nodal versus involved-field radiotherapy in early-stage Hodgkin's disease: long-term results. *J Clin Oncol* 2004;**22**:2835–41.

135. Carde P, Hagenbeek A, Hayat M, *et al.* Clinical staging versus laparotomy and combined modality with MOPP versus ABVD in early-stage Hodgkin's disease: the H6 twin randomized trials from the European Organization for Research and Treatment of Cancer Lymphoma Cooperative Group. *J Clin Oncol* 1993;**11**:2258–72.

136. Engert A, Franklin J, Eich HT, *et al.* Two cycles of doxorubicin, bleomycin, vinblastine, and dacarbazine plus extended-field radiotherapy is superior to radiotherapy alone in early favorable Hodgkin's lymphoma: final results of the GHSG HD7 trial. *J Clin Oncol* 2007;**25**:3495–502.

137. Engert A, Pleutschow H, Eich HT, *et al.* Combined modality treatment of two or four cycles of ABVD followed by involved field radiotherapy in the treatment of patients with early stage Hodgkin's lymphoma: update interim analysis of the Randomised HD10 Study of the German Hodgkin Study Group (GHSG). *Blood* 2005;**106**:2673a.

138. Ferme C, Eghbali H, Meerwaldt JH, *et al.* Chemotherapy plus involved-field radiation in early-stage Hodgkin's disease. *N Engl J Med* 2007;**357**: 1916–27.

139. Ferme C, Diviné M, Vranovsky A, *et al.* Four ABVD and involved-field radiotherapy in unfavorable supradiaphragmatic clinical stages (CS) I–II Hodgkin's lymphoma (HL): preliminary results of the EORTC-GELA H9-U Trial. *Blood* 2005; **106**:813a.

140. Horning SJ, Hoppe RT, Mason J, *et al.* Stanford-Kaiser Permanente G1 study for clinical stage I to IIA Hodgkin's disease: subtotal lymphoid irradiation versus vinblastine, methotrexate, and bleomycin chemotherapy and regional irradiation. *J Clin Oncol* 1997;**15**: 1736–44.

141. Klimm BC, Engert A, Brillant C, *et al.* Comparison of BEACOPP and ABVD chemotherapy in intermediate stage Hodgkin's lymphoma: results of the fourth interim analysis of the HD 11 trial of the GHSG. *J Clin Oncol* 2005; **23**:6507a.

142. Nachman JB, Sposto R, Herzog P, *et al.* Randomized comparison of low-dose involved-field radiotherapy and no radiotherapy for children with Hodgkin's disease who achieve a complete response to chemotherapy. *J Clin Oncol* 2002;**20**:3765–71.

143. Noordijk EM, Thomas J, Fermé C, *et al.* First results of the EORTC-GELA H9 randomized trials: the H9-F trial (comparing 3 radiation dose levels) and H9-U trial (comparing 3 chemotherapy schemes) in patients with favorable or unfavorable early stage Hodgkin's lymphoma. *J Clin Oncol* 2005;**23**:561S.

144. Press OW, LeBlanc M, Lichter AS, *et al.* Phase III randomized intergroup trial of subtotal lymphoid irradiation versus doxorubicin, vinblastine, and subtotal lymphoid irradiation for stage IA to IIA Hodgkin's disease. *J Clin Oncol* 2001;**19**:4238–44.

145. Specht L, Gray RG, Clarke MJ, Peto R. Influence of more extensive radiotherapy and adjuvant chemotherapy on long-term outcome of early-stage Hodgkin's disease: a meta-analysis of 23 randomized trials involving 3,888 patients. International Hodgkin's Disease Collaborative Group. *J Clin Oncol* 1998;**16**:830–3.

146. Straus DJ, Portlock CS, Qin J, *et al.* Results of a prospective randomized clinical trial of doxorubicin, bleomycin, vinblastine, and dacarbazine (ABVD) followed by radiation therapy (RT) versus ABVD alone for stages I, II, and IIIA nonbulky Hodgkin disease. *Blood* 2004;**104**:3483–9.

147. Aleman BM, van den Belt-Dusebout AW, Klokman WJ, *et al.* Long-term cause-specific mortality of patients treated for Hodgkin's disease. *J Clin Oncol* 2003;**21**:3431–9.

148. Dores GM, Metayer C, Curtis RE, *et al.* Second malignant neoplasms among long-term survivors of Hodgkin's disease: a population-based evaluation over 25 years. *J Clin Oncol* 2002;**20**:3484–94.

149. Metayer C, Lynch CF, Clarke EA, *et al.* Second cancers among long-term survivors of Hodgkin's disease diagnosed in childhood and adolescence. *J Clin Oncol* 2000;**18**:2435–43.

150. Swerdlow AJ, Barber JA, Hudson GV, *et al.* Risk of second malignancy after Hodgkin's disease in a collaborative British cohort: the relation to age at treatment. *J Clin Oncol* 2000;**18**:498–509.

151. Travis LB, Hill D, Dores GM, *et al.* Cumulative absolute breast cancer risk for young women treated for Hodgkin lymphoma. *J Natl Cancer Inst* 2005;**97**:1428–37.

152. Ng AK, Bernardo MVP, Weller E, *et al.* Second malignancy after Hodgkin disease treated with radiation therapy with or without chemotherapy: long-term risks and risk factors. *Blood* 2002;**100**:1989–96.

153. van Leeuwen FE, Klokman WJ, Veer MB, *et al.* Long-term risk of second malignancy in survivors of Hodgkin's disease treated during adolescence or young adulthood. *J Clin Oncol* 2000;**18**:487–97.

154. Adams MJ, Lipsitz SR, Colan SD, *et al.* Cardiovascular status in long-term survivors of Hodgkin's disease treated with chest radiotherapy. *J Clin Oncol* 2004;**22**:3139–48.

155. Bowers DC, McNeil DE, Liu Y, *et al.* Stroke as a late treatment effect of Hodgkin's disease: a report from the Childhood Cancer Survivor Study. *J Clin Oncol* 2005;**23**:6508–15.

156. Eriksson F, Gagliardi G, Liedberg A, *et al.* Long-term cardiac mortality following radiation therapy for Hodgkin's disease: analysis with the relative seriality model. *Radiother Oncol* 2000;**55**:153–62.

157. Reinders JG, Heijmen BJM, Olofsen-van Acht MJJ, *et al.* Ischemic heart disease after mantlefield irradiation for Hodgkin's disease in long-term follow-up. *Radiother Oncol* 1999;**51**:35–42.

158. Aleman BMP, van den Belt–Dusebout AW, De Bruin ML, *et al.* Late cardiotoxicity after treatment for Hodgkin lymphoma. *Blood* 2007; **109**:1878–86.

159. Swerdlow AJ, Higgins CD, Smith P, *et al.* Myocardial infarction mortality risk after treatment for Hodgkin disease: a collaborative British cohort study. *J Natl Cancer Inst* 2007; **99**:206–14.

160. Hagenbeek A, Eghbali H, Fermé C, *et al.* Three cycles of MOPP/ABV hybrid and involved-field irradiation is more effective than subtotal nodal irradiation in favorable supradiaphragmatic clinical stages I–II Hodgkin's disease: preliminary results of the EORTC-GELA H8-F randomized trial in 543 patients. *Blood* 2000; **96**:575a.

161. Eich HT, Muller RP, Engenhart-Cabillic R, *et al.* Involved-node radiotherapy in early-stage Hodgkin's lymphoma. Definition and guidelines of the German Hodgkin Study Group (GHSG). *Strahlenther Onkol* 2008;**184**:406–10.

162. Girinsky T, Specht L, Ghalibafian M, *et al.* The conundrum of Hodgkin lymphoma nodes: to be or not to be included in the involved node radiation fields. The EORTC-GELA lymphoma group guidelines. *Radiother Oncol* 2008;**88**:202–10.

163. Campbell BA, Voss N, Pickles T, *et al.* Involved-nodal radiation therapy as a component of combination therapy for limited-stage Hodgkin's lymphoma: a question of field size. *J Clin Oncol* 2008;**26**:5170–4.

164. Ferme C, Eghbali H, Hagenbeek A, *et al.* MOPP/ABV hybrid and irradiation in unfavorable supradiaphragmatic clinical stages I–II Hodgkin's disease: comparison of three treatment modalities. Preliminary results of the EORTC-GELA H8-U randomized trial in 995 patients. *Blood* 2000;**96**:576a.

165. Borchmann P, Engert A, Pluetschow A, *et al.* Dose-intensified combined modality treatment with 2 cycles of BEACOPP escalated followed by 2 cycles of ABVD and involved field radiotherapy (IF-RT) is superior to 4 cycles of ABVD and IFRT in patients with early unfavourable Hodgkin lymphoma (HL): an analysis of the German Hodgkin Study Group (GHSG) HD14 Trial. *Blood* 2008;**112**:367a.

166. Pavone V, Ricardi U, Luminari S, *et al.* ABVD plus radiotherapy versus EVE plus radiotherapy in unfavorable stage IA and IIA Hodgkin's lymphoma: results from an Intergruppo Italiano Linfomi randomized study. *Ann Oncol* 2008;**19**:763–8.

167. Canellos GP. Chemotherapy alone for early Hodgkin's lymphoma: an emerging option. *J Clin Oncol* 2005;**23**:4574–6.

168. Laskar S, Gupta T, Vimal S, *et al.* Consolidation radiation after complete remission in Hodgkin's disease following six cycles of doxorubicin, bleomycin, vinblastine, and dacarbazine chemotherapy: is there a need? *J Clin Oncol* 2004;**22**:62–8.

169. Hodgson DC, Gilbert ES, Dores GM, *et al.* Long-term solid cancer risk among 5-year survivors of Hodgkin's lymphoma. *J Clin Oncol* 2007;**25**:1489–97.

170. Bonadonna G, Valagussa P, Santoro A. Alternating non-cross-resistant combination chemotherapy or MOPP in stage IV Hodgkin's disease. A report of 8-year results. *Ann Intern Med* 1986;**104**:739–46.

171. Longo DL, Young RC, Wesley M, *et al.* Twenty years of MOPP therapy for Hodgkin's disease. *J Clin Oncol* 1986; **4**:1295–306.

172. Nicholson WM, Beard ME, Crowther D, *et al.* Combination chemotherapy in generalized Hodgkin's disease. *Br Med J* 1970;**3**:7–10.

173. Sutcliffe SB, Wrigley PF, Peto J, *et al.* MVPP chemotherapy regimen for

advanced Hodgkin's disease. *Br Med J* 1978;**1**:679–83.

174. Hancock BW. Randomised study of MOPP (mustine, Oncovin, procarbazine, prednisone) against LOPP (Leukeran substituted for mustine) in advanced Hodgkin's disease. British National Lymphoma Investigation. *Radiother Oncol* 1986;**7**:215–21.

175. McElwain TJ, Toy J, Smith E, *et al.* A combination of chlorambucil, vinblastine, procarbazine and prednisolone for treatment of Hodgkin's disease. *Br J Cancer* 1977;**36**:276–80.

176. Bakemeier RF, Anderson JR, Costello W, *et al.* BCVPP chemotherapy for advanced Hodgkin's disease: evidence for greater duration of complete remission, greater survival, and less toxicity than with a MOPP regimen. Results of the Eastern Cooperative Oncology Group study. *Ann Intern Med* 1984;**101**:447–56.

177. Santoro A, Bonadonna G, Valagussa P, *et al.* Long-term results of combined chemotherapy-radiotherapy approach in Hodgkin's disease: superiority of ABVD plus radiotherapy versus MOPP plus radiotherapy. *J Clin Oncol* 1987;**5**:27–37.

178. Canellos GP, Anderson JR, Propert KJ, *et al.* Chemotherapy of advanced Hodgkin's disease with MOPP, ABVD, or MOPP alternating with ABVD. *N Engl J Med* 1992;**327**:1478–84.

179. Diehl V, Haverkamp H, Mueller RP, *et al.* Eight cycles of BEACOPP escalated compared with 4 cycles of BEACOPP escalated followed by 4 cycles of BEACOPP baseline with or without radiotherapy in patients in advanced stage Hodgkin lymphoma (HL): Final analysis of the randomised HD12 trial of the German Hodgkin Study Group. *Blood* 2008;**112**:1558.

180. Engert A, Franklin J, Mueller RP, *et al.* HD12 Randomised Trial comparing 8 dose-escalated cycles of BEACOPP with 4 escalated and 4 baseline cycles in patients with advanced stage Hodgkin lymphoma (HL): an analysis of the German Hodgkin Lymphoma Study Group (GHSG). *Blood* 2006;**108**:99a.

181. Johnson P, Horwich A, Jack A, *et al.* Randomised comparison of the Stanford V (SV) regimen and ABVD in the treatment of advanced Hodgkin lymphoma (HL): results from a UK NCRI Lymphoma Group Study. *Blood* 2008;**112**:370a.

182. Kobe C, Dietlein M, Franklin J, *et al.* Positron emission tomography has a high negative predictive value for progression or early relapse for patients with residual disease after first-line chemotherapy in advanced-stage Hodgkin lymphoma. *Blood* 2008;**112**:3989–94.

183. Goldie JH, Coldman AJ. A mathematic model for relating the drug sensitivity of tumors to their spontaneous mutation rate. *Cancer Treat Rep* 1979; **63**:1727–33.

184. Jones SE, Haut A, Weick JK, *et al.* Comparison of adriamycin-containing chemotherapy (MOP-BAP) with MOPP-bleomycin in the management of advanced Hodgkin's disease. A Southwest Oncology Group Study. *Cancer* 1983;**51**:1339–47.

185. Viviani S, Bonadonna G, Santoro A, *et al.* Alternating versus hybrid MOPP and ABVD combinations in advanced Hodgkin's disease: ten-year results. *J Clin Oncol* 1996;**14**:1421–30.

186. Glick JH, Young ML, Harrington D, *et al.* MOPP/ABV hybrid chemotherapy for advanced Hodgkin's disease significantly improves failure-free and overall survival: the 8-year results of the intergroup trial. *J Clin Oncol* 1998; **16**:19–26.

187. Somers R, Carde P, Henry-Amar M, *et al.* A randomized study in stage IIIB and IV Hodgkin's disease comparing eight courses of MOPP versus an alteration of MOPP with ABVD: a European Organization for Research and Treatment of Cancer Lymphoma Cooperative Group and Groupe Pierre-et-Marie-Curie controlled clinical trial. *J Clin Oncol* 1994;**12**:279–87.

188. Radford JA, Rohatiner AZ, Ryder WD, *et al.* ChlVPP/EVA hybrid versus the weekly VAPEC-B regimen for previously untreated Hodgkin's disease. *J Clin Oncol* 2002;**20**:2988–94.

189. Carde P, MacKintosh FR, Rosenberg SA. A dose and time response analysis of the treatment of Hodgkin's disease with MOPP chemotherapy. *J Clin Oncol* 1983;**1**:146–53.

190. van Rijswijk RE, Haanen C, Dekker AW, *et al.* Dose intensity of MOPP chemotherapy and survival in Hodgkin's disease. *J Clin Oncol* 1989;**7**:1776–82.

191. Carella AM, Bellei M, Brice P, *et al.* High-dose therapy and autologous stem cell transplantation versus conventional therapy for patients with advanced Hodgkin's lymphoma responding to front-line therapy: long-term results. *Haematologica* 2009;**94**:146–8.

192. Federico M, Bellei M, Brice P, *et al.* High-dose therapy and autologous stem-cell transplantation versus conventional therapy for patients with advanced Hodgkin's lymphoma responding to front-line therapy. *J Clin Oncol* 2003;**21**:2320–5.

193. Arakelyan N, Berthou C, Desablens B, *et al.* Early versus late intensification for patients with high-risk Hodgkin lymphoma-3 cycles of intensive chemotherapy plus low-dose lymph node radiation therapy versus 4 cycles of combined doxorubicin, bleomycin, vinblastine, and dacarbazine plus myeloablative chemotherapy with autologous stem cell transplantation: five-year results of a randomized trial on behalf of the GOELAMS Group. *Cancer* 2008;**113**:3323–30.

194. Sieber M, Bredenfeld H, Josting A, *et al.* 14-day variant of the bleomycin, etoposide, doxorubicin, cyclophosphamide, vincristine, procarbazine, and prednisone regimen in advanced-stage Hodgkin's lymphoma: results of a pilot study of the German Hodgkin's Lymphoma Study Group. *J Clin Oncol* 2003;**21**:1734–9.

195. Chand VK, Link BK, Ritchie JM, *et al.* Neutropenia and febrile neutropenia in patients with Hodgkin's lymphoma treated with doxorubicin (Adriamycin), bleomycin, vinblastine and dacarbazine (ABVD) chemotherapy. *Leuk Lymphoma* 2006;**47**:657–63.

196. Rueda A, Sevilla I, Guma J, *et al.* Secondary prophylactic G-CSF (filgrastim) administration in chemotherapy of stage I and II Hodgkin's lymphoma with ABVD. *Leuk Lymphoma* 2001;**41**:353–8.

197. Silvestri F, Fanin R, Velisig M, *et al.* The role of granulocyte colony-stimulating factor (filgrastim) in maintaining dose intensity during conventional-dose chemotherapy with ABVD in Hodgkin's disease. *Tumori* 1994;**80**:453–8.

198. Boleti E, Mead GM. ABVD for Hodgkin's lymphoma: full-dose

chemotherapy without dose reductions or growth factors. *Ann Oncol* 2007;**18**:376–80.

199. Evens AM, Cilley J, Ortiz T, *et al.* G-CSF is not necessary to maintain over 99% dose-intensity with ABVD in the treatment of Hodgkin lymphoma: low toxicity and excellent outcomes in a 10-year analysis. *Br J Haematol* 2007;**137**:545–52.

200. Weiner MA, Leventhal B, Brecher ML, *et al.* Randomized study of intensive MOPP-ABVD with or without low-dose total-nodal radiation therapy in the treatment of stages IIB, IIIA2, IIIB, and IV Hodgkin's disease in pediatric patients: a Pediatric Oncology Group study. *J Clin Oncol* 1997;**15**:2769–79.

201. Diehl V, Loeffler M, Pfreundschuh M, *et al.* Further chemotherapy versus low-dose involved-field radiotherapy as consolidation of complete remission after six cycles of alternating chemotherapy in patients with advanced Hodgkin's disease. *Ann Oncol* 1995;**6**:901–10.

202. Raemaekers J, Burgers M, Henry-Amar M, *et al.* Patients with stage III/IV Hodgkin's disease in partial remission after MOPP/ABV chemotherapy have excellent prognosis after additional involved-field radiotherapy: interim results from the ongoing EORTC-LCG and GPMC phase III trial. The EORTC Lymphoma Cooperative Group and Groupe Pierre-et-Marie-Curie. *Ann Oncol* 1997;**8** Suppl 1:111–14.

203. Aleman BMP, Raemaekers JMM, Tomisic R, *et al.* Involved-field radiotherapy for patients in partial remission after chemotherapy for advanced Hodgkin's lymphoma. *Int J Radiat Oncol Biol Phys* 2007;**67**:19–30.

204. Johnson PW, Sydes M, Radford J, *et al.* Consolidation radiotherapy is associated with improved outcomes after chemotherapy for advanced Hodgkin lymphoma: Analysis of results from the UKLG LY09 Trial. *Blood* 2008;**112**:368a.

205. Franklin JG, Paus MD, Pluetschow A, *et al.* Chemotherapy, radiotherapy and combined modality for Hodgkin's disease, with emphasis on second cancer risk. *Cochrane Database Syst Rev* 2005;(4):CD003187.

206. Scheinpflug K, Schmitt J, Jentsch-Ullrich K, *et al.* Thymic hyperplasia following successful treatment for nodular-sclerosing Hodgkin's disease. *Leuk Lymphoma* 2003;**44**:1615–17.

207. Aparicio J, Segura A, Garcera S, *et al.* ESHAP is an active regimen for relapsing Hodgkin's disease. *Ann Oncol* 1999;**10**:593–5.

208. Ferme C, Mounier N, Divine M, *et al.* Intensive salvage therapy with high-dose chemotherapy for patients with advanced Hodgkin's disease in relapse or failure after initial chemotherapy: results of the Groupe d'Etudes des Lymphomes de l'Adulte H89 Trial. *J Clin Oncol* 2002;**20**:467–75.

209. Schmitz N, Pfistner B, Sextro M, *et al.* Aggressive conventional chemotherapy compared with high-dose chemotherapy with autologous haemopoietic stem-cell transplantation for relapsed chemosensitive Hodgkin's disease: a randomised trial. *Lancet* 2002;**359**:2065–71.

210. Linch DC, Winfield D, Goldstone AH, *et al.* Dose intensification with autologous bone-marrow transplantation in relapsed and resistant Hodgkin's disease: results of a BNLI randomised trial. *Lancet* 1993;**341**:1051–4.

211. Josting A, Rudolph C, Mapara M, *et al.* Cologne high-dose sequential chemotherapy in relapsed and refractory Hodgkin lymphoma: results of a large multicenter study of the German Hodgkin Lymphoma Study Group (GHSG). *Ann Oncol* 2005;**16**:116–23.

212. Popat U, Hosing C, Saliba RM, *et al.* Prognostic factors for disease progression after high-dose chemotherapy and autologous hematopoietic stem cell transplantation for recurrent or refractory Hodgkin's lymphoma. *Bone Marrow Transplant* 2004;**33**:1015–23.

213. Constans M, Sureda A, Terol MJ, *et al.* Autologous stem cell transplantation for primary refractory Hodgkin's disease: results and clinical variables affecting outcome. *Ann Oncol* 2003;**14**:745–51.

214. Czyz J, Dziadziuszko R, Knopinska-Postuszuy W, *et al.* Outcome and prognostic factors in advanced Hodgkin's disease treated with high-dose chemotherapy and autologous stem cell transplantation: a study of 341 patients. *Ann Oncol* 2004;**15**:1222–30.

215. Gutierrez-Delgado F, Holmberg L, Hooper H, *et al.* Autologous stem cell transplantation for Hodgkin's disease: busulfan, melphalan and thiotepa compared to a radiation-based regimen. *Bone Marrow Transplant* 2003;**32**:279–85.

216. Lavoie JC, Connors JM, Phillips GL, *et al.* High-dose chemotherapy and autologous stem cell transplantation for primary refractory or relapsed Hodgkin lymphoma: long-term outcome in the first 100 patients treated in Vancouver. *Blood* 2005;**106**:1473–8.

217. Sweetenham JW, Taghipour G, Milligan D, *et al.*, on behalf of the Lymphoma Working Party of the European Group for Blood and Marrow Transplantation. High-dose therapy and autologous stem cell rescue for patients with Hodgkin's disease in first relapse after chemotherapy: results from the EBMT. *Bone Marrow Transplant* 1997;**20**:745–52.

218. Schulz H, Rehwald U, Morschhauser F, *et al.* Rituximab in relapsed lymphocyte-predominant Hodgkin lymphoma: long-term results of a phase 2 trial by the German Hodgkin Lymphoma Study Group (GHSG). *Blood* 2008;**111**:109–11.

219. Nademanee A, O'Donnell MR, Snyder DS, *et al.* High-dose chemotherapy with or without total body irradiation followed by autologous bone marrow and/or peripheral blood stem cell transplantation for patients with relapsed and refractory Hodgkin's disease: results in 85 patients with analysis of prognostic factors. *Blood* 1995;**85**:1381–90.

220. Sureda A, Arranz R, Iriondo A, *et al.* Autologous stem-cell transplantation for Hodgkin's disease: results and prognostic factors in 494 patients from the Grupo Espanol de Linfomas/Transplante Autologo de Medula Osea Spanish Cooperative Group. *J Clin Oncol* 2001;**19**:1395–404.

221. Sureda A, Constans M, Iriondo A, *et al.* Prognostic factors affecting long-term outcome after stem cell transplantation in Hodgkin's lymphoma autografted after a first relapse. *Ann Oncol* 2005;**16**:625–33.

222. Engelhardt BG, Holland DW, Brandt SJ, *et al.* High-dose chemotherapy followed by autologous stem cell transplantation for relapsed or refractory Hodgkin lymphoma: prognostic features and outcomes. *Leuk Lymphoma* 2007;**48**:1728–35.

223. Evens AM, Altman JK, Mittal BB, *et al.* Phase I/II trial of total lymphoid irradiation and high-dose chemotherapy with autologous stem-cell transplantation for relapsed and refractory Hodgkin's lymphoma. *Ann Oncol* 2007;**18**:679–88.

224. Reece DE, Barnett MJ, Shepherd JD, *et al.* High-dose cyclophosphamide, carmustine (BCNU), and etoposide (VP16–213) with or without cisplatin (CBV +/- P) and autologous transplantation for patients with Hodgkin's disease who fail to enter a complete remission after combination chemotherapy. *Blood* 1995;**86**:451–6.

225. Andre M, Henry-Amar M, Pico JL, *et al.* Comparison of high-dose therapy and autologous stem-cell transplantation with conventional therapy for Hodgkin's disease induction failure: a case-control study. Societe Francaise de Greffe de Moelle. *J Clin Oncol* 1999;**17**:222–9.

226. Lazarus HM, Rowlings PA, Zhang MJ, *et al.* Autotransplants for Hodgkin's disease in patients never achieving remission: a report from the Autologous Blood and Marrow Transplant Registry. *J Clin Oncol* 1999;**17**:534–45.

227. Sweetenham JW, Carella AM, Taghipour G, *et al.* High-dose therapy and autologous stem-cell transplantation for adult patients with Hodgkin's disease who do not enter remission after induction: results in 175 patients reported to the European Group for Blood and Marrow Transplantation. Lymphoma Working Party. *J Clin Oncol* 1999;**17**:3101–9.

228. Czyz J, Hellmann A, Dziadziuszko R, *et al.* High-dose chemotherapy with autologous stem cell transplantation is an effective treatment of primary refractory Hodgkin's disease. Retrospective study of the Polish Lymphoma Research Group. *Bone Marrow Transplant* 2002;**30**:29–34.

229. Gajewski JL, Phillips GL, Sobocinski KA, *et al.* Bone marrow transplants from HLA-identical siblings in advanced Hodgkin's disease. *J Clin Oncol* 1996;**14**:572–8.

230. Milpied N, Fielding AK, Pearce R, *et al.* Allogeneic bone marrow transplant is not better than autologous transplant for patient with relapsed Hodgkin's disease. European Group for Blood and Bone Marrow Transplantation. *J Clin Oncol* 1996;**14**:1291–6.

231. Akpek G, Ambinder RF, Piantadosi S, *et al.* Long-term results of blood and marrow transplantation for Hodgkin's lymphoma. *J Clin Oncol* 2001; **19**:4314–21.

232. Carella AM, Beltrami G, Carella M Jr, *et al.* Immunosuppressive non-myeloablative allografting as salvage therapy in advanced Hodgkin's disease. *Haematologica* 2001;**86**:1121–3.

233. Peggs KS, Hunter A, Chopra R, *et al.* Clinical evidence of a graft-versus-Hodgkin's-lymphoma effect after reduced-intensity allogeneic transplantation. *Lancet* 2005;**365**: 1934–41.

234. Anderlini P, Saliba R, Acholonu S, *et al.* Reduced-intensity allogeneic stem cell transplantation in relapsed and refractory Hodgkin's disease: low transplant-related mortality and impact of intensity of conditioning regimen. *Bone Marrow Transplant* 2005; **35**:943–51.

235. Todisco E, Castagna L, Sarina B, *et al.* Reduced-intensity allogeneic transplantation in patients with refractory or progressive Hodgkin's disease after high-dose chemotherapy and autologous stem cell infusion. *Eur J Haematol* 2007;**78**:322–9.

236. Sureda A, Canals C, Arranz R, *et al.* Allogeneic stem cell transplantation after reduced intensity conditioning (RIC-allo) in patients with relapsed or refractory Hodgkin's lymphoma (HL). Final analysis of the HDR-Allo Protocol – a prospective clinical trial by the Grupo Español de Linfomas/ Transplante de Medula OSEA (GEL/ TAMO) and the Lymphoma Working Party (LWP) of the European Group for Blood and Marrow Transplantation (EBMT). *Blood* 2009;**114**:658a.

237. Mir R, Anderson J, Strauchen J, *et al.* Hodgkin disease in patients 60 years of age or older. Histologic and clinical features of advanced-stage disease. The Cancer and Leukemia Group B. *Cancer* 1993;**71**:1857–66.

238. Hahn T, Benekli M, Wong C, *et al.* A prognostic model for prolonged event-free survival after autologous or allogeneic blood or marrow transplantation for relapsed and refractory Hodgkin's disease. *Bone Marrow Transplant* 2005;**35**:557–66.

239. Josting A, Franklin J, May M, *et al.* New prognostic score based on treatment outcome of patients with relapsed Hodgkin's lymphoma registered in the database of the German Hodgkin's lymphoma study group. *J Clin Oncol* 2002;**20**:221–30.

240. Stiff PJ, Unger JM, Forman SJ, *et al.* The value of augmented preparative regimens combined with an autologous bone marrow transplant for the management of relapsed or refractory Hodgkin disease: a Southwest Oncology Group phase II trial. *Biol Blood Marrow Transplant* 2003;**9**:529–39.

241. Jabbour E, Hosing C, Ayers G, *et al.* Pretransplant positive positron emission tomography/gallium scans predict poor outcome in patients with recurrent/refractory Hodgkin lymphoma. *Cancer* 2007;**109**:2481–9.

242. Nogova L, Reineke T, Eich HT, *et al.* Extended field radiotherapy, combined modality treatment or involved field radiotherapy for patients with stage IA lymphocyte-predominant Hodgkin's lymphoma: a retrospective analysis from the German Hodgkin Study Group (GHSG). *Ann Oncol* 2005;**16**:1683–7.

243. Diehl V, Sextro M, Franklin J, *et al.* Clinical presentation, course, and prognostic factors in lymphocyte-predominant Hodgkin's disease and lymphocyte-rich classical Hodgkin's disease: report from the European Task Force on Lymphoma Project on Lymphocyte-Predominant Hodgkin's Disease. *J Clin Oncol* 1999;**17**:776–83.

244. Wilder RB, Schlembach PJ, Jones D, *et al.* European Organization for Research and Treatment of Cancer and Groupe d'Etude des Lymphomes de l'Adulte very favorable and favorable, lymphocyte-predominant Hodgkin disease. *Cancer* 2002;**94**:1731–8.

245. Nogova L, Reineke T, Josting A, *et al.* Lymphocyte-predominant and classical Hodgkin's lymphoma–comparison of outcomes. *Eur J Haematol Suppl* 2005; **66**:106–10.

246. Ekstrand BC, Lucas JB, Horwitz SM, *et al.* Rituximab in lymphocyte-predominant Hodgkin disease: results of a phase 2 trial. *Blood* 2003;**101**:4285–9.

247. Rehwald U, Schulz H, Reiser M, *et al.* Treatment of relapsed CD20+ Hodgkin lymphoma with the monoclonal antibody rituximab is effective and well

tolerated: results of a phase 2 trial of the German Hodgkin Lymphoma Study Group. *Blood* 2003;**101**:420–4.

248. Schulz H, Rehwald U, Morschhauser F, *et al.* Rituximab in relapsed lymphocyte-predominant Hodgkin lymphoma: long-term results of a phase-II trial by the German Hodgkin Lymphoma Study Group (GHSG). *Blood* 2008;**111**:109–11.

249. Fanale MA, Fayad L, Romaguera JE, *et al.* Experience with R-CHOP in patients with lymphocyte predominant Hodgkin lymphoma (LPHL). Seventh International Symposium on Hodgkin Lymphoma; 2007:77a.

250. Coiffier B, Lepage E, Briere J, *et al.* CHOP chemotherapy plus rituximab compared with CHOP alone in elderly patients with diffuse large-B-cell lymphoma. *N Engl J Med* 2002;**346**:235–42.

251. Sleijfer S. Bleomycin-induced pneumonitis. *Chest* 2001;**120**:617–24.

252. Azambuja E, Fleck JF, Batista RG, *et al.* Bleomycin lung toxicity: who are the patients with increased risk? *Pulm Pharmacol Ther* 2005;**18**:363–6.

253. Matthews JH. Pulmonary toxicity of ABVD chemotherapy and G-CSF in Hodgkin's disease: possible synergy. *Lancet* 1993;**342**:988.

254. Dirix LY, Schrijvers D, Druwe P, *et al.* Pulmonary toxicity and bleomycin. *Lancet* 1994;**344**:56.

255. Adach K, Suzuki M, Sugimoto T, *et al.* Granulocyte colony-stimulating factor exacerbates the acute lung injury and pulmonary fibrosis induced by intratracheal administration of bleomycin in rats. *Exp Toxicol Pathol* 2002;**53**:501–10.

256. Azoulay E, Herigault S, Levame M, *et al.* Effect of granulocyte colony-stimulating factor on bleomycin-induced acute lung injury and pulmonary fibrosis. *Crit Care Med* 2003;**31**:1442–8.

257. Martin WG, Ristow KM, Habermann TM, *et al.* Bleomycin pulmonary toxicity has a negative impact on the outcome of patients with Hodgkin's lymphoma. *J Clin Oncol* 2005;**23**: 7614–20.

258. Behringer K, Breuer K, Reineke T, *et al.* Secondary amenorrhea after Hodgkin's lymphoma is influenced by age at treatment, stage of disease, chemotherapy regimen, and the use of oral contraceptives during therapy: a report from the German Hodgkin's Lymphoma Study Group. *J Clin Oncol* 2005;**23**:7555–64.

259. Brusamolino E, Baio A, Orlandi E, *et al.* Long-term events in adult patients with clinical stage IA-IIA nonbulky Hodgkin's lymphoma treated with four cycles of doxorubicin, bleomycin, vinblastine, and dacarbazine and adjuvant radiotherapy: a single-institution 15-year follow-up. *Clin Cancer Res* 2006;**12**:6487–93.

260. Hodgson DC, Pintilie M, Gitterman L, *et al.* Fertility among female Hodgkin lymphoma survivors attempting pregnancy following ABVD chemotherapy. *Hematol Oncol* 2007;**25**:11–15.

261. Horning SJ, Rosenberg SA, Hoppe RT. Brief chemotherapy (Stanford V) and adjuvant radiotherapy for bulky or advanced Hodgkin's disease: an update. *Ann Oncol* 1996;**7** Suppl 4:105–8.

262. Illes A, Biro E, Miltenyi Z, *et al.* Hypothyroidism and thyroiditis after therapy for Hodgkin's disease. *Acta Haematol* 2003;**109**:11–17.

263. Andre M, Henry-Amar M, Blaise D, *et al.* Treatment-related deaths and second cancer risk after autologous stem-cell transplantation for Hodgkin's disease. *Blood* 1998;**92**:1933–40.

264. Goodman KA, Riedel E, Serrano V, *et al.* Long-term effects of high-dose chemotherapy and radiation for relapsed and refractory Hodgkin's lymphoma. *J Clin Oncol* 2008; **26**:5240–7.

265. Engert A, Ballova V, Haverkamp H, *et al.* Hodgkin's lymphoma in elderly patients: a comprehensive retrospective analysis from the German Hodgkin's Study Group. *J Clin Oncol* 2005;**23**:5052–60.

266. Levis A, Depaoli L, Bertini M, *et al.* Results of a low aggressivity chemotherapy regimen (CVP/CEB) in elderly Hodgkin's disease patients. *Haematologica* 1996;**81**:450–6.

267. Weekes CD, Vose JM, Lynch JC, *et al.* Hodgkin's disease in the elderly: improved treatment outcome with a doxorubicin-containing regimen. *J Clin Oncol* 2002;**20**:1087–93.

268. Erdkamp FL, Breed WP, Bosch LJ, *et al.* Hodgkin disease in the elderly. A registry-based analysis. *Cancer* 1992;**70**:830–4.

269. Janssen-Heijnen ML, van Spronsen DJ, Lemmens VE, *et al.* A population-based study of severity of comorbidity among patients with non-Hodgkin's lymphoma: prognostic impact independent of International Prognostic Index. *Br J Haematol* 2005;**129**:597–606.

270. van Spronsen DJ, Janssen-Heijnen ML, Lemmens VE, *et al.* Independent prognostic effect of co-morbidity in lymphoma patients: results of the population-based Eindhoven Cancer Registry. *Eur J Cancer* 2005;**41**:1051–7.

271. Enblad G, Gustavsson A, Sundstrom C, *et al.* Patients above sixty years of age with Hodgkin's lymphoma treated with a new strategy. *Acta Oncol* 2002;**41**:659–67.

272. Macpherson N, Klasa RJ, Gascoyne R, *et al.* Treatment of elderly Hodgkin's lymphoma patients with a novel 5-drug regimen (ODBEP): a phase II study. *Leuk Lymphoma* 2002;**43**:1395–402.

273. Feltl D, Vitek P, Zamecnik J. Hodgkin's lymphoma in the elderly: the results of 10 years of follow-up. *Leuk Lymphoma* 2006;**47**:1518–22.

274. Kim HK, Silver B, Li S, *et al.* Hodgkin's disease in elderly patients (> or = 60): clinical outcome and treatment strategies. *Int J Radiat Oncol Biol Phys* 2003;**56**:556–60.

275. Levis A, Anselmo AP, Ambrosetti A, *et al.* VEPEMB in elderly Hodgkin's lymphoma patients. Results from an Intergruppo Italiano Linfomi (IIL) study. *Ann Oncol* 2004;**15**:123–8.

276. Ballova V, Ruffer JU, Haverkamp H, *et al.* A prospectively randomized trial carried out by the German Hodgkin Study Group (GHSG) for elderly patients with advanced Hodgkin's disease comparing BEACOPP baseline and COPP-ABVD (study HD9elderly). *Ann Oncol* 2005;**16**:124–31.

277. Kolstad A, Nome O, Delabie J, *et al.* Standard CHOP-21 as first line therapy for elderly patients with Hodgkin's lymphoma. *Leuk Lymphoma* 2007;**48**:570–6.

278. Canellos GP, Duggan D, Johnson J, *et al.* How important is bleomycin in the adriamycin + bleomycin + vinblastine + dacarbazine regimen? *J Clin Oncol* 2004;**22**:1532–3.

279. Proctor SJ, White J, Jones GL. An international approach to the treatment of Hodgkin's disease in the elderly: launch of the SHIELD study programme. *Eur J Haematol Suppl* 2005;**66**:63–7.

280. Boll B, Hansen H, Heuck F, *et al.* The fully human anti-CD30 antibody 5F11 activates NF-{kappa}B and sensitizes lymphoma cells to bortezomib-induced apoptosis. *Blood* 2005;**106**:1839–42.

281. Cerveny CG, Law CL, McCormick RS, *et al.* Signaling via the anti-CD30 mAb SGN-30 sensitizes Hodgkin's disease cells to conventional chemotherapeutics. *Leukemia* 2005;**19**:1648–55.

282. Younes A, Forero-Torres A, Bartlett N, *et al.* A novel antibody-drug conjugate, SGN-35 (anti-CD30-Auristatin), induces objective responses in patients with relapsed or refractory Hodgkin lymphoma: preliminary results of a phase I tolerability study. Seventh International Symposium on Hodgkin Lymphoma; 2007:099a.

283. Younes A, Romaguera J, Hagemeister F, *et al.* A pilot study of rituximab in patients with recurrent, classic Hodgkin disease. *Cancer* 2003;**98**:310–14.

284. Jones RJ, Gocke CD, Kasamon YL, *et al.* Circulating clonotypic B cells in classic Hodgkin lymphoma. *Blood* 2009;**113** (23):5920–6.

285. Younes A, Fayad L, Goy A, *et al.* Phase II study of rituximab plus ABVD for the treatment of newly diagnosed patients with advanced stage classical Hodgkin lymphoma. Seventh International Symposium on Hodgkin Lymphoma; 2007:024a.

286. Oki Y, Pro B, Fayad LE, *et al.* Phase 2 study of gemcitabine in combination with rituximab in patients with recurrent or refractory Hodgkin lymphoma. *Cancer* 2008;**112**:831–6.

287. Klimm B, Schnell R, Diehl V, *et al.* Current treatment and immunotherapy of Hodgkin's lymphoma. *Haematologica* 2005;**90**:1680–92.

288. Vriesendorp HM, Quadri SM, Wyllie CT, *et al.* Fractionated radiolabeled antiferritin therapy for patients with recurrent Hodgkin's disease. *Clin Cancer Res* 1999;**5**:3324s–9s.

289. Decaudin D, Levy R, Lokiec F, *et al.* Radioimmunotherapy of refractory or relapsed Hodgkin's lymphoma with 90Y-labelled antiferritin antibody. *Anticancer Drugs* 2007;**18**:725–31.

290. Bargou RC, Emmerich F, Krappmann D, *et al.* Constitutive nuclear factor-kappaB-RelA activation is required for proliferation and survival of Hodgkin's disease tumor cells. *J Clin Invest* 1997;**100**:2961–9.

291. Re D, Thomas RK, Behringer K, *et al.* From Hodgkin disease to Hodgkin lymphoma: biologic insights and therapeutic potential. *Blood* 2005;**105**:4553–60.

292. Re D, Kuppers R, Diehl V. Molecular pathogenesis of Hodgkin's lymphoma. *J Clin Oncol* 2005;**23**:6379–86.

293. Zheng B, Georgakis GV, Li Y, *et al.* Induction of cell cycle arrest and apoptosis by the proteasome inhibitor PS-341 in Hodgkin disease cell lines is independent of inhibitor of nuclear factor-kappaB mutations or activation of the CD30, CD40, and RANK receptors. *Clin Cancer Res* 2004;**10**:3207–15.

294. Blum RH, Carter SK, Agre K. A clinical review of bleomycin–a new antineoplastic agent. *Cancer* 1973;**31**:903–14.

295. Younes A, Pro B, Fayad L. Experience with bortezomib for the treatment of patients with relapsed classical Hodgkin lymphoma. *Blood* 2006;**107**:1731–2.

296. Trelle S, Sezer O, Naumann R, *et al.* Bortezomib is not active in patients with relapsed Hodgkin's lymphoma: results of a prematurely closed phase II study. *Blood* 2006;**108**:2477a.

297. Rosato RR, Almenara JA, Grant S. The histone deacetylase inhibitor MS-275 promotes differentiation or apoptosis in human leukemia cells through a process regulated by generation of reactive oxygen species and induction of p21CIP1/WAF1 1. *Cancer Res* 2003;**63**:3637–45.

298. LaCasse EC, Cherton-Horvat GG, Hewitt KE, *et al.* Preclinical characterization of AEG35156/GEM 640, a second-generation antisense oligonucleotide targeting X-linked inhibitor of apoptosis. *Clin Cancer Res* 2006;**12**:5231–41.

299. Johnston PB, Ansell SM, Colgan JP, *et al.* Promising results for patients with relapsed or refractory Hodgkin lymphoma treated with the oral MTOR inhibitor everolimus (RAD001). Seventh International Symposium on Hodgkin Lymphoma; 2007:015a.

300. Georgakis GV, Li Y, Rassidakis GZ, *et al.* Inhibition of heat shock protein 90 function by 17-allylamino-17-demethoxy-geldanamycin in Hodgkin's lymphoma cells down-regulates Akt kinase, dephosphorylates extracellular signal-regulated kinase, and induces cell cycle arrest and cell death. *Clin Cancer Res* 2006;**12**:584–90.

301. Skinnider BF, Elia AJ, Gascoyne RD, *et al.* Interleukin 13 and interleukin 13 receptor are frequently expressed by Hodgkin and Reed-Sternberg cells of Hodgkin lymphoma. *Blood* 2001;**97**:250–5.

302. Juszczynski P, Ouyang J, Monti S, *et al.* The AP1-dependent secretion of galectin-1 by Reed Sternberg cells fosters immune privilege in classical Hodgkin lymphoma. *Proc Natl Acad Sci U S A* 2007;**104**:13 134–9.

303. Vogelstein B, Lane D, Levine AJ. Surfing the p53 network. *Nature* 2000;**408**:307–10.

304. Drakos E, Thomaides A, Medeiros LJ, *et al.* Inhibition of p53-murine double minute 2 interaction by nutlin-3A stabilizes p53 and induces cell cycle arrest and apoptosis in Hodgkin lymphoma. *Clin Cancer Res* 2007;**13**:3380–7.

305. Kawakami M, Kawakami K, Kioi M, *et al.* Hodgkin lymphoma therapy with interleukin-4 receptor-directed cytotoxin in an infiltrating animal model. *Blood* 2005;**105**:3707–13.

306. Bollard CM, Straathof KC, Huls MH, *et al.* The generation and characterization of LMP2-specific CTLs for use as adoptive transfer from patients with relapsed EBV-positive Hodgkin disease. *J Immunother* 2004;**27**:317–27.

307. Bollard CM, Aguilar L, Straathof KC, *et al.* Cytotoxic T lymphocyte therapy for Epstein-Barr virus+ Hodgkin's disease. *J Exp Med* 2004;**200**:1623–33.

308. Portis T, Longnecker R. Epstein-Barr virus (EBV) LMP2A mediates B-lymphocyte survival through constitutive activation of the Ras/PI3K/Akt pathway. *Oncogene* 2004;**23**:8619–28.

Chapter

20 Treatment approaches to MALT/marginal zone lymphoma

Stephanie A. Gregory and Parameswaran Venugopal

Introduction

Marginal zone lymphoma (MZL) is a distinct subtype of non-Hodgkin lymphoma that has been recognized by Revised European–American Lymphoma (REAL) and World Health Organization (WHO) classifications.[1–3] They have distinct morphologic and immunophenotypic features and a variable clinical course. This entity was traditionally designated as monocytoid B-cell lymphoma.

MZL is subdivided into three categories:

1. Extranodal MZL (EMZL) arises from mucosa-associated lymphoid tissue (MALT) identified by WHO classification as EMZL of MALT type;
2. Primary nodal MZL (PNMZL). By definition, in the WHO classification the term "nodal MZL" is used to define those cases primarily involving lymph nodes, and it excludes any case with prior or concurrent localization in an extranodal site except bone marrow, spleen, or liver; and
3. Splenic B-cell MZL (SMZL).

NMZL displays no appreciable differences in its histologic, cytologic, architectural, or phenotypic characteristics from those of EMZL. Consequently, it has been debated whether MZL with primary nodal involvement has to be considered a distinct disease or merely represents disseminated EMZL of MALT type. Therefore, the REAL classifications included MZL cases with primary lymph node involvement in a provisional category. Recently, Nathwani and colleagues identified several distinct clinical features for nodal and extranodal MZL.[4] From the clinical behavior, NMZL seems to behave more like a low-grade follicular or small lymphocytic lymphoma unlike EMZL. This suggests biologic differences between EMZL and NMZL. The WHO classification recognized NMZL as a distinct disease that must be distinguished from EMZL of MALT-type with lymph node involvement and from other small B-cell non-Hodgkin lymphomas.[2]

Extranodal marginal zone (MALT) lymphoma

Extranodal MALT lymphoma is morphologically heterogeneous: B cells including marginal zone cells, cells resembling monocytoid cells, small lymphocytes, scattered transformed cells, and often monoclonal plasma cells. The infiltrate is located in the marginal zone of reactive follicles and extends into the interfollicular region. These cells typically infiltrate the epithelium, forming lymphoepithelial lesions.

Extranodal MALT lymphoma comprises 7–8% of all non-Hodgkin lymphomas (Table 20.1) and constitutes approximately half of all primary gastric lymphomas. Geographically, higher incidence of MALT lymphomas is reported from north-east Italy, the Middle East, and the Cape region of South Africa. It predominantly occurs in adults; median age being 61 years. There is a slight female predominance (male: female 1:1.2). The post-germinal center marginal zone B cell is the postulated cell of origin. The presence of follicular center and antigen stimulation are most important for the development of marginal zone B cells. Most patients with *Helicobacter pylori* infection do not develop lymphoma. *H. pylori* is present in almost all cases of chronic gastritis that induces MALT lymphoma.[6,7] There is a 44-fold increase in risk of development of MALT lymphoma in various tissues in patients with Sjogren's syndrome. In patients with Hashimoto's the risk is threefold.

H. pylori decreases as lymphoma progresses.[8] Eradication of *H. pylori* with combination therapy causes regression of lymphoma in 75% of cases.[9] A recently published meta-analysis shows that sequential therapy (which consists of 5 days of treatment with a proton pump inhibitor and one antibiotic, usually amoxicillin, followed by a 5-day treatment with the proton pump inhibitor and two other antibiotics, usually clarithromycin and a 5-nitro-imidazole) is superior to standard triple therapy for *H. pylori* infection in patients naïve to treatment.[10] It is difficult to eradicate *H. pylori* in patients with t(11;18) and BCL10 positivity. Response of patients whose lymphoma extends beyond submucosa is also not satisfactory. Cytogenetic abnormalities are noted in many patients. The three recurrent balanced translocations seen in MALT lymphoma include: (1) t(11;18)(q21;q21) in 35%. This translocation is not observed in other lymphomas; (2) t(14;18) in 11%. The breakpoints in these cases are different from those seen in

Management of Hematologic Malignancies, ed. Susan M. O'Brien, Julie M. Vose, and Hagop M. Kantarjian. Published by Cambridge University Press.

Table 20.1. Marginal zone lymphomas as a percentage of all non-Hodgkin lymphomas

Type	Percent
MALT	7.6%
Nodal	1.8%
Splenic	< 1%

Note: Zucca *et al.*[5]

follicular lymphomas; and (3) t(1;14) (p22;q32) in < 5%, mostly in gastric and pulmonary MALT lymphomas. Trisomy 3 has been noted in 60% of cases.[11] t(11;18)(q21;q21) is believed to represent one of the most important primary events in the development of MZLs. An accurate estimation of the frequency and distribution of this abnormality among the nodal, splenic, and extranodal MZL is yet to be determined. Recent molecular genetic studies have shown that this translocation results in the fusion of the *API2* gene on chromosome 11 and a novel gene termed MALT1 on chromosome 18.

Remstein et al analyzed RNAs extracted from frozen tissue samples of 99 MZL by using reverse transcriptase-polymerase chain reaction (RT-PCR). *API2-MALT1* fusion transcripts were detected in 12 of 57 EMZL (21%) but in none of the nodal or splenic specimens. Their findings suggest that t(11;18)(q21;q21) is restricted to EMZL and that these tumors have distinct genetic etiologies in comparison with their splenic and nodal counterparts.[12]

Gastric MALT lymphomas

Diagnosis and staging

The best staging system for gastric lymphomas is still controversial.[13,14] The Blackledge staging system was recommended for general use by an international workshop in Lugano, Switzerland in 1993.[14] The TNM system using the criteria was initially developed by the American Joint Committee on Cancer (AJCC) for gastric carcinoma based on the extent of the gastric wall involvement as measured by endoscopic ultrasound. Depth of gastric wall infiltration of MALT lymphoma is reported to correlate with the risk of spread to adjacent lymph nodes.[15] Endoscopic evaluation with multiple biopsies from stomach, and upper airway examination is recommended in all cases. Computed tomography (CT) scan and other staging procedures including bone marrow examination as is currently standard practice for non-Hodgkin lymphoma are recommended. Bone marrow involvement is reported in 0–15% of cases.[16,17] Apart from morphology, immunophenotyping as well as cytogenetics should be done in the biopsy specimen. Positron emission tomography (PET) scan has recently been reported to be useful in staging of MZL.[18] *H. pylori* status should be ascertained by histology or serology.

Treatment of gastric MALT lymphoma

There are no data from controlled trails that define standard of care in patients with gastric MALT lymphoma. Published data on treatment have been mostly from retrospective studies where patients have not been adequately staged or treated uniformly. Various reports of treatment for localized MALT lymphoma with combination of surgery, radiation therapy, and chemotherapy indicate overall survival rate ranging from 80% to 90% at 5 years.[17,19–21] Localized MALT lymphoma treated with radiation therapy has excellent outcome.[22] *H. pylori* therapy alone may be sufficient as an initial therapy in patients with low-grade histology, limited-stage disease, *H. pylori* positivity, and absence of t(11;18) (Table 20.2). No difference in overall survival was noted in patients who received *H. pylori* therapy alone compared to those who received radiotherapy, chemotherapy, surgery, or combinations of these.[19] The actuarial 5-year overall survival was 82% (95% CI) in the series as a whole and at a medium follow-up at 3 years, 10 of 93 patients died all but one from a second solid tumor. A German multicenter study also confirmed that antibiotics, when use as a sole therapy, can induce long-term remission in these patients.[23] Absence of nodal involvement has been suggested as the strongest predictor for response.[24] In this study, patients without nodal involvement who were *H. pylori* positive had a complete remission (CR) rate of 79%. Chlorambucil or cyclophosphamide has been studied as a single agent to treat MALT lymphomas.[25] Patients received continuous oral doses of cyclophosphamide 100 mg/day or chlorambucil 6 mg/day for a medium duration of 18 months (8–24 months). CR rate was 75% with projected 5-year event-free survival and overall survival of 50% and 75% respectively.[25] An ongoing international study randomizes patients after initial antibiotic therapy to observation versus chlorambucil.[26] An interim analysis on the first 170 patients in this study showed that about half the patients who were treated with chlorambucil achieved histologic CR. A PCR assay showed that half the patients who had histologic response also achieved molecular CR.

Patients who do not respond to anti-*H. pylori* therapy or who are negative for *H. pylori* should receive conventional therapies for low-grade non-Hodgkin lymphoma.[27] Apart from single-agent or combination chemotherapy, anti-CD20 monoclonal antibody rituximab as a single agent has been shown to have significant clinical activity in relapsing or *H. pylori*-negative MALT lymphomas.[28] A phase II study in 35 untreated and relapsed patients with gastric and extra-gastric marginal zone/MALT lymphoma, an overall response rate of 73% with 15 CRs and 10 partial remissions[29] Median response duration was 10.5 months and with a median follow-up of 15 months, 9(26%) patients relapsed. The response was significantly higher in the chemotherapy-naïve patients with significantly longer duration of remission (22 versus 12 months).

Surgery alone has been extensively used in the past with 5-year overall survival of 91% (95% for stage I and 82% for stage II).[20] Adjuvant therapy with chemotherapy or radiotherapy

Table 20.2. Algorithm for management of marginal zone lymphomas

1. Marginal zone NHL – nodal
Use same principles as follicular lymphoma:
Localized disease:
IFRT
Advanced disease:
Observation
Single-agent or combination chemotherapy
CVP, CHOP, fludarabine-based regimens
Monoclonal antibodies
Rituximab
Radioimmunotherapy
2. Marginal zone NHL – extranodal
Gastric:
Low-grade, *H. pylori* +ve
Antimicrobial therapy
Low-grade, *H. pylori* +ve, resistant to antimicrobials
IFRT, rituximab, chemotherapy
Low-grade, *H. pylori* negative
IFRT, rituximab, chemotherapy
Intermediate or higher grade
Chemotherapy ± rituximab ± IFRT
Non-gastric:
Avoid overtreatment
Observation
Local RT
Surgery
Rituximab
Chemotherapy
3. Splenic marginal zone lymphoma
Observation
Splenectomy
Rituximab
Chemotherapy

NHL: non-Hodgkin lymphoma; IFRT: involved-field radiation therapy; CVP: cyclophosphamide, vincristine, and prednisone; CHOP: cyclophosphamide, doxorubicin, vincristine, and prednisone; RT: radiation therapy.

did not appear to contribute to the efficacy of surgery. In view of the highly effective non-surgical options available, surgery is performed less frequently for localized MALT lymphomas and, in some centers, is limited to complications like uncontrolled bleeding, obstruction, or perforation.

Monitoring of response to therapy

Apart from achieving CR, the attempt should always be made to obtain molecular remission. Patients with low grade NHL who achieve molecular remission remain without evidence of disease longer compared to those patients who have evidence of persistent disease at the molecular level. In patients with MZL either the chromosome abnormalities that are present in the pre-therapy specimen or the immunoglobulin heavy chain rearrangement can be used to monitor molecular disease.

A strict endoscopic follow-up is recommended, with multiple biopsies taken 2 months after completion of therapy and subsequently at least twice a year for 2 years. Late responses to therapy have been observed. Patients who are treated with antibiotics alone should be followed up closely for even longer, as it is unclear whether eradiation of *H. pylori* alone will cure the lymphoma. In a study of patients with MALT lymphoma who achieved CR, 32 or 86 patients relapsed at a median time of 47 (14–307) months suggesting the need for long-term monitoring in these patients.[30]

Treatment of non-gastric extranodal marginal zone lymphoma

Optimal therapy for patients with non-gastric lymphomas remains controversial. Treatment for patients with non-gastric MZLs in the International Extranodal Lymphoma Study Group (IELSG) trials usually included surgery or radiotherapy even in patients with stage IV disease. The time to progression of disease in these patients was approximately 60% at 5 years but only 18% by 10 years. However, the overall survival was 90% at 10 years. Addition of an anthracycline to a chemotherapy regimen did not improve the response rate or provide survival benefit for patients with limited disease. Similarly adjuvant chemotherapy in patients receiving radiation therapy has not been shown to improve outcome.[31] However, a low to low-intermediate International Prognostic Index (IPI) score was a significant favorable prognostic feature by multivariate analysis predicting progression-free survival, with 70% of those with 0–2 factors still free of disease at 5 years, compared with only 30% of those with 3–5 risk factors at diagnosis.[32,33]

As with the results of treatment of *H. pylori* gastric disease, anti-infective therapy has been shown to result in some responses in splenic MZL (hepatitis C), dermal MZL (*Borrelia*), and lacrimal gland MZL (*Chlamydia*).[34,35] Radiation therapy alone has been reported as effective in MALT lymphomas in the head and neck region but most patients ultimately develop relapse.[36] Chemotherapy as used in other indolent non-Hodgkin lymphoma with or without rituximab is effective. Fludarabine- and alkylator-based therapies have been shown to be very active.[37,38] Cladribine (2-chlorodeoxy adenosine; 2-CdA) has been successfully used to treat gastric as well as extra-gastric MALT lymphoma.[39]

Primary nodal marginal zone lymphoma

Primary nodal marginal zone lymphoma (PNMZL) morphologically resembles lymph nodes involved by MZL of extranodal or splenic types but without evidence of extranodal or splenic disease. It constitutes about 1.8% of all lymphoid neoplasm (see Table 20.1) and about one-third of all MZLs. Various morphologic patterns have been described, including sinusoidal, interfollicular, marginal zone (surround normal follicles), inverse follicular (surround naked follicles), and invasion of follicles and replacement of follicular center cell to produce a follicular pattern, secondary to follicular colonization. No statistically significant difference has been noted between extranodal marginal zone MALT lymphomas and NMZLs with respect to median age of onset, sex distribution, incidence of B symptoms, lactate dehydrogenase (LDH) elevation, thoracic and mesenteric lymphadenopathy, involvement of bone marrow, liver, or spleen, and IPI.[4] However, significant difference was observed between the two groups with respect to advanced disease (stage III and IV more with nodal type). MALT lymphomas tended to have larger (≥ 5 cm) masses, whereas nodal lymphomas tended to have more likelihood of initial cervical, axillary, inguinal/femoral, and para-aortic lymphadenopathy.

Treatment of primary nodal marginal zone lymphoma

As with other indolent non-Hodgkin lymphomas, observation without therapy is appropriate in patients with low tumor burden and no symptoms.

Local radiation therapy is associated with long-term disease-free intervals in limited-stage disease. In patients with high tumor burden and those with symptoms related to the lymphoma, treatment options include single-agent or combination chemotherapy, monoclonal antibodies, and combination of these agents. The common combination chemotherapy regimens include CVP (cyclophosphamide, vincristine, and prednisone), CHOP (cyclophosphamide, doxorubicin, vincristine, and prednisone), FN (fludarabine and mitoxantrane), and FND (FN plus dexamethasone). Anti-CD20 monoclonal antibody rituximab, when used as a single agent, leads to responses in half the patients with relapsed low-grade non-Hodgkin lymphoma.[40] In combination with chemotherapy, the response rates and duration of response are even higher. Radioimmunotherapy is approved for use in patients with relapsed low-grade non-Hodgkin lymphoma including MZL. The currently available radioimmunotherapy agents are ^{90}Y-ibritumomab tiuxetan (Zevalin) and ^{131}I-tositumomab (Bexxar). Both agents are murine anti-CD20 monoclonal antibodies and have higher efficacy on B-cell malignancies largely because of the cross-fire effects of radiation emitted from the radioimmunoconjugate that destroys more tumor cells than unconjugated antibodies. MZL cells express CD20 antigen more than small lymphocytic leukemia/chronic lymphatic leukemia and less than follicular lymphoma. There are no published data on the activity of radioimmunotherapy agents specifically in MZL; however, based on their activity in other CD20-positive low-grade non-Hodgkin lymphoma, there is reason to believe that this should be a very promising mode of therapy for these patients.

Stem cell transplantation

Both autologous and allogeneic stem cell transplantation (SCT) have been tried in patients with low-grade non-Hodgkin lymphoma. Although SCT can lead to durable remissions in these patients, the toxicity of the conditioning regimens is higher compared to many of the other available options like chemoimmunotherapy and radioimmunotherapy. Hence, SCT in this group of patients should be limited to investigational settings. More recent work with incorporation of monoclonal antibodies like rituximab (Rituxan) in harvest and conditioning as well as improved techniques of purging have led to promising results. If the patient is a candidate for SCT, care should be taken in sequencing of therapy of these patients to avoid potential damage to marrow stem cells from chemotherapy or radiation used in earlier therapies.

Other investigational therapies

Many investigational agents are being studied in this disease including bortezomib (Velcade) (alone or in combination with monoclonal antibodies), BCL2-antisense (oblimersen sodium [Genasense]), gallium nitrite, and other monoclonal antibodies like anti-CD22 monoclonal antibody (epratuzumab) and anti-CD52 (Campath-1H) either alone or in combination with other agents like chemotherapy.

Splenic B-cell marginal zone lymphoma

Splenic B-cell MZL (SMZL) is an indolent lymphoproliferative disease accounting for approximately 1% of all lymphomas (Table 20.1). SMZL presents with marked splenomegaly often accompanied by circulating atypical “villous lymphocytes” and hence it is also termed “splenic lymphoma with villous lymphocytes.” Functional hypersplenism with progressive pancytopenia may occur and in some cases may be the sole reason for intervention. Histologically the spleen contains nodular infiltrates involving the white and red pulp. Within the white pulp, the infiltrate has a biphasic morphology comprising of an inner zone of small lymphocytes and a peripheral (marginal) zone of larger lymphoid cells. The splenic lymph nodes and bone marrow are also usually involved by similar nodular infiltrate. Histologic differential diagnosis includes mantle cell lymphoma, follicular lymphoma, B-cell chronic lymphocytic leukemia, and benign/atypical lymphoid hyperplasia.

Treatment of splenic B-cell marginal zone lymphoma

Splenectomy is usually accompanied by resolution of symptoms as well as recovery of blood counts in patients with pancytopenia from hypersplenism. Regression of other sites of disease has been noted following splenectomy. In patients who need therapy and who are unable or unwilling for surgical procedure, chemotherapy alone or in combination with monoclonal antibody as is conventionally used in other indolent non-Hodgkin lymphoma would be the treatment of choice.

References

1. Harris NL, Jaffe ES, Stein H, *et al.* A revised European-American classification of the lymphoid neoplasms: a proposal from the International Lymphomas Study Group. *Blood* 1994;**84**:1361–92.
2. Harris NL, Jaffe ES, Diebold J, *et al.* World Health Organization classification of neoplastic diseases of the hematopoietic and lymphoid tissue: report of the Clinical Advisory Committee meeting – Airle House, Virginia, November 1997, *J Clin Oncol* 1999;**17**:3835–49.
3. Jaffe ES, Harris NL, Diebold J, Muller Hermelink HK. World Health Organization classification of neoplastic disease of the hematopoietic and lymphoid tissues. *Am J Clin Pathol* 1999;**111** Suppl 1:S8–12.
4. Nathwani BN, Anderson JR, Armitage JO, *et al.* Marginal zone B-cell lymphoma: a clinical comparison of nodal and mucosa-associated lymphoid tissue types. *J Clin Oncol* 1999;**17**:2486–92.
5. Zucca E, Bertoni F, Roggero E, *et al.* Management of rare forms of lymphoma. *Curr Opin Oncol* 1998; **10**(5):377–84.
6. Wotherspoon AC, Ortiz-Hitalgo C, Falzon MR, *et al. Helicobacter pylori* – associated gastritis and primary B-cell gastric lymphoma. *Lancet* 1991; **338**:1175–6.
7. Nakamura S, Yao T, Aoyagi K, *et al. Helicobacter pylori* and primary gastric lymphoma. A histopathologic and immunohistochemical analysis of 237 patients. *Cancer* 1997;**79**:3–11.
8. Doglioni C, Wotherspoon AC, Moschini A, *et al.* High incidence of primary gastric lymphoma in North-Eastern Italy. *Lancet* 1992;**339**:834–5.
9. Wotherspoon AC, Doglioni C, Diss TC, *et al.* Regression of primary low grade B cell gastric lymphoma of mucosa associated lymphoid tissue type after eradicating Helicobacter pylori. *Lancet* 1993;**342**:575–7.
10. Jafri NS, Hornung CA, Howden CW. Meta-analysis: sequential therapy appears superior to standard therapy for *Helicobacter pylori* infection in patients naive to treatment. *Ann Intern Med* 2008;**148**(12):1–10.
11. Wotherspoon AC, Finn TM, Isaacson PG. Trisomy 3 in low grade B cell lymphoma of mucosa-associated lymphoid tissue. *Blood* 1995;**85**:2000–4.
12. Remstein ED, James CD, Kurtin PJ. Incidence and subtype specificity of API2-MALT1 fusion translocations in extranodal, nodal and splenic marginal zone lymphomas. *Am J Pathol* 2000;**156**:1183–8.
13. De Jong D, Aleman BM, Taal BG, *et al.* Controversies and consensus in the diagnosis, work-up and treatment of gastric lymphoma: an international survey. *Ann Oncol* 1999;**10**:275–80.
14. Rohatainer A, d'Amore F, Coiffier B, *et al.* Report on a workshop convened to discuss the pathological and staging classification of gastro-intestinal tract lymphomas. *Ann Oncol* 1994;**5**:397–400.
15. Eidt S, Stolte M, Fisher R. Factors influencing lymph node infiltration in primary gastric malignant lymphomas of the mucosa-associated lymphoid tissue. *Pathol Res Pract* 1994;**190**: 1077–81.
16. Raderer M, Vorbeck F, Formanek M, *et al.* Importance of extensive staging in patients with mucosa-associated lymphoid tissue (MALT) – type lymphoma. *Br J Cancer* 2000;**83**:454–7.
17. Montalban C, Castrillo JM, Abraira V, *et al.* Gastric B-cell mucosa-associated lymphoid tissue (MALT) lymphomas: clinical-pathological study and evaluation of the prognostic factors in 143 patients. *Ann Oncol* 1995; **6**:355–62.
18. Hoffmann M, Kletter K, Becherer A, *et al.* 18-F-fluorodeoxyglucose positron emission tomography (18F-FDG-PET) for staging and follow-up of marginal zone B-cell lymphoma. *Oncology* 2003;**64**(4):336–40.
19. Pinotti G, Zucca E, Roggero E, *et al.* Clinical features, treatment and outcome in a series of 93 patients with low grade gastric MALT lymphoma. *Leuk Lymphoma* 1997;**26**:527–37.
20. Cogliatti SB, Schmid U, Schumacher U, *et al.* Primary B-cell gastric lymphoma: a clinical pathological study of 145 patients. *Gastroenterology* 1991;**101**:1159–70.
21. Schechter NR, Portlock CS, Yahalom J. Treatment of mucosa-associated lymphoid tissue lymphoma of the stomach with radiation alone. *J Clin Oncol* 1998;**16**:1916–21.
22. Tsang RW, Gospodarowicz MK, Pintilie M, *et al.* Localized mucosa-associated lymphoid tissue lymphoma treated with radiation therapy has excellent outcome. *J Clin Oncol* 2003;**21**:4157–64.
23. Neubauer A, Thiede C, Morgner A, *et al.* Cure of *Helicobacter pylori* infection and duration of remission of low-grade gastric mucosa-associated lymphoid tissue lymphoma. *J Natl Cancer Inst* 1997;**89**:1350–5.
24. Ruskone Formestraux A, Lavergne A, Aegerter PH, *et al.* Predictive factors for regression of gastric MALT lymphoma after anti-*Helicobacter pylori* treatment. *Gut* 2001;**48**:297–303.
25. Hammel P, Haioun C, Chaumette MT, *et al.* Efficacy of single-agent chemotherapy in low grade B-cell mucosa-associated lymphoid tissue lymphoma with prominent gastric expression. *J Clin Oncol* 1995;**13**:2524–9.
26. Zucca E, Roggero E, Traulle C, *et al.* Early interim report of the LY03 randomized cooperative trial of observation vs cholorambucil after anti-Helicobacter therapy in low grade gastric lymphoma. *Ann Oncol* 1999; **10** Suppl 3:25.
27. Zucca E, Carvalli F. MALT lymphomas. In: Cavalli F, Isaacson PG, Glascoyne RD, *et al. ASH Education Book.* Washington DC, American Society of Hematology. 2001; 241–58.

28. Conconi A, Thieblemont C, Martinelli G, *et al.* An international extranodal lymphoma study group phase II study of rituximab in extranodal marginal zone B-cell lymphoma (MZL). *Proc Am Soc Clin Oncol* 2001; **20**(Part 1):Abstract 1183.

29. Conconi A, Martinelli G, Thieblemont C, *et al.* Clinical activity of rituximab in extranodal marginal zone B-cell lymphoma of MALT type. *Blood* 2003;**102**:2741–5.

30. Raderer M, Streubel B, Woehrer S, *et al.* High relapse rate in patients with MALT lymphoma warrants life long follow up. *Clin Cancer Res* 2005;**11**:3349–52.

31. Aviles A, Neri N, Calva A, *et al.* Addition of a short course of chemotherapy did not improve outcome in patients with localized marginal B cell lymphoma of the orbit. *Oncology* 2006;**70**:173–6.

32. Zinzani P, Magagnoli M, Galieni P, *et al.* Nongastrointestinal low-grade mucosa associated lymphoid tissue lymphoma: analysis of 75 patients. *J Clin Oncol* 1999;**17**:1254–8.

33. Zucca E, Conconi A, Pedrinis E, *et al.* Non-gastric marginal zone B-cell lymphoma of mucosa-associated lymphoid tissue. *Blood* 2003;**101**: 2489–95.

34. Slater DN. MALT and SALT: the clue to cutaneous B-cell lymphoproliferative disease. *Br J Dermatol* 1994;**131**:557–61.

35. Musto P. Hepatitis C virus infection and B cell non-Hodgkin's lymphomas: more than a simple association. *Clin Lymphoma* 2002;**3**:150–60.

36. Wenzel C, Fiebiger W, Dieckmann K, *et al.* Extranodal marginal zone B-cell lymphoma of mucosa associated lymphoid tissue of the head and neck area: high rate of disease recurrence following local therapy. *Cancer* 2003; **97**:2236–41.

37. Zinzani PL, Stefoni V, Musuraca G, *et al.* Fludarabine-containing chemotherapy as front line treatment of nongastrointestinal mucosa-associated lymphoid tissue lymphoma. *Cancer* 2004;**100**:2190–4.

38. Thieblemont C, Berger F, Dumontet C, *et al.* Mucosa-associated lymphoid tissue lymphoma is a disseminated disease in one third of 158 patients analyzed. *Blood* 2000;**95**:802–6.

39. Jager G, Neumeister P, Brezinschek R, *et al.* Treatment of extranodal marginal zone B-cell lymphoma of mucosa-associated lymphoid tissue type with cladribine: a phase II study. *J Clin Oncol* 2002;**20**:3872–7.

40. McLaughlin P, Grillo-Lopez AJ, Link BK, *et al.* Rituximab chimeric anti-CD20 monoclonal antibody therapy for relapsed indolent lymphoma: half of patients respond to a four-dose treatment program. *J Clin Oncol* 1998;**16**(8):2825–33.

Chapter

21 Peripheral T-cell lymphomas

Matthew J. Matasar and Steven M. Horwitz

Introduction

The T-cell non-Hodgkin lymphomas are a group of uncommon malignancies that in Western countries account for 15–20% of aggressive lymphomas and between 5% and 10% of all non-Hodgkin's lymphomas (NHL).[1,2] Within the most current classification schemata, there are 21 distinct diseases that together constitute the mature T- and natural killer (NK)-cell lymphomas, diseases that range from indolent cutaneous lymphomas to aggressive malignancies that are often resistant to routine systemic therapy. Common to many of the types of T-cell lymphoma is a predilection towards extranodal disease, although sites of tropism vary among subtypes. Geographic frequencies of many subtypes, and of T-cell lymphomas as a group, are also highly variable: while only 1.5% of lymphomas are of T-cell lineage in Vancouver, Canada, 18.3% of lymphomas in Hong Kong show a T-cell phenotype. And in Asia, 47.4% of T-cell lymphomas are either NK/T-cell lymphoma, nasal type (NK/T-NT) or adult T-cell leukemia/lymphoma (ATLL), while in North America and Europe, these constitute only 7.1% and 5.3% of T-cell lymphomas, respectively.[3] These variable incidence rates may in part represent differential exposure to risk factors for T-cell lymphoma, including Epstein–Barr virus (EBV) and human T-cell leukemia virus-1 (HTLV-1). As will be explored below, the epidemiologic variety across the subtypes of T-cell lymphoma is matched by the clinical heterogeneity of these diseases, confounding investigation (or understanding) of the class of diseases as a single entity.

The most current World Health Organization (WHO) classification schema for lymphoma recognizes 20 distinct diseases under the rubric of mature T- or NK-cell lymphoma (Table 21.1).[4] These include diseases that are predominantly leukemic (T-cell prolymphocytic leukemia, T-cell large granular lymphocytic leukemia, aggressive NK-cell leukemia, and the leukemic variant of ATLL); predominantly nodal (peripheral T-cell lymphoma not otherwise specified [PTCL, NOS]), angioimmunoblastic T-cell lymphoma (AITL), both anaplastic lymphoma kinase (ALK)-positive and -negative anaplastic large cell lymphoma (ALCL), and the lymphomatous variant of ATLL); and predominantly extranodal (mycosis fungoides, Sézary syndrome, primary cutaneous CD30+ T-cell lymphoproliferative disorders, subcutaneous panniculitis-like T-cell lymphoma, extranodal NK/T-NT, enteropathy-associated T-cell lymphoma [EATL], hepatosplenic T-cell lymphoma, and the rare subtypes of primary cutaneous peripheral T-cell lymphoma). This chapter will restrict its discussion to those diseases that are nodally based or predominantly extranodal with sites other than the skin routinely involved. Others have reviewed the cutaneous T-cell lymphomas[5–13] and the predominantly leukemic lymphomas,[14–17] and these diseases will not be addressed in this chapter.

Classification

The classification of the PTCLs has seen a stepwise evolution since the 1970s, when the ability to discriminate among different lymphocyte lineages first allowed the distinction to be made. The classifications of Lukes and Collins[18] and the Kiel classification[19] were built upon the emerging understanding of immunology, but it was not until the Working Formulation was proposed in 1982 that efforts at arriving at a unified classification schema were met by any measure of success.[20] The Working Formulation, however, did not use lineage to discriminate subtypes. Subsequent revisions to classification would incorporate increasingly sophisticated understanding of biology of the malignant lymphomas. In 1994, a major revision to the classification of lymphoma was proposed, incorporating developments in morphologic, immunophenotypic, and genetic techniques, and subsequent modifications have continued to be made under the aegis of the WHO, with the original WHO classification having been published in 2000.[21] The WHO has recently published a revised classification system that further emphasizes the importance of morphology, immunophenotype, and genetics in the diagnosis of the mature T- and NK-cell lymphomas.[4]

It bears mention that the pathologic diagnosis of T-cell lymphoma can be challenging and requires significant expertise. With older systems of nomenclature, reproducibility of

Management of Hematologic Malignancies, ed. Susan M. O'Brien, Julie M. Vose, and Hagop M. Kantarjian. Published by Cambridge University Press.

Table 21.1. Mature T-cell and NK-cell neoplasms

T-cell prolymphocytic leukemia
T-cell large granular lymphocytic leukemia
Charonic lymphoproliferative disorder of NK cells
Aggressive NK-cell leukemia
Systemic EBV-positive T-cell lymphoproliferative disease of childhood
Hydroa vacciniforme-like lymphoma
Adult T-cell leukemia/lymphoma
Extranodal NK/T-cell lymphoma, nasal type
Enteropathy-associated T-cell lymphoma
Hepatosplenic T-cell lymphoma
Subcutaneous panniculitis-like T-cell lymphoma
Mycosis fungoides
Sézary syndrome
Primary cutaneous CD30-positive T-cell lymphoproliferative disorders
Lymphomatoid papulosis
Primary cutaneous anaplastic large cell lymphoma
Primary cutaneous gamma-delta T-cell lymphoma
Primary cutaneous CD8-positive aggressive epidermotropic cytotoxic T-cell lymphoma
Primary cutaneous CD4-positive aggressive epidermotropic cytotoxic T-cell lymphoma
Peripheral T-cell lymphoma, NOS
Angioimmunoblastic T-cell lymphoma
Anaplastic large cell lymphoma, ALK positive
Anaplastic large cell lymphoma, ALK negative

Note: NOS: not otherwise specified; ALK: anaplastic lymphoma kinase.
Source: From Swerdlow *et al.*[4] with permission.

diagnoses was hampered not only by difficulties inherent to the diagnostic evaluation, but also by language barriers due to differences among classification schemata. With the Working Formulation, Revised European–American Lymphoma (REAL) classification, and WHO classification, unified classification was meant to promote interobserver concordance in the diagnosis of all lymphomas. Subsequent investigations into the reproducibility of diagnosis for the PTCLs, however, have shown that difficulties persist. Experiences reported from individual referral centers have found that as many as 26% of cases referred for evaluation of a diagnosed PTCL receive a major diagnostic revision with expert hematopathology review.[22,23] The largest reported experience with expert review comes from the International Peripheral T-cell and Natural Killer/T-cell Lymphoma Study, in which 1314 cases of peripheral T- or NK/T-cell lymphomas from 22 centers worldwide underwent expert review. In this series, only 88% of cases could be confirmed as T-cell lymphomas. The remaining 12% included cases of Hodgkin lymphoma (3%), B-cell lymphomas (1.4%), diagnoses other than lymphoma (2.3%), and cases unclassifiable due to inadequate material or technical factors (3.6%).[3]

Staging

The appropriate staging of the PTCL is not substantially different from other forms of NHL, with complete physical examination, body imaging, and when relevant bone marrow biopsy. One important observation regarding staging of T-cell lymphomas is that computed tomography (CT) alone may be insufficient for determining extent of disease due to the frequent involvement of extranodal sites such as subcutaneous tissue, sinuses, and bowel. In one series of ^{18}F-fluorodeoxyglucose positron emission tomography (FDG-PET) studies in PTCL, additional sites of disease were detected in 30% of patients with FDG-PET in comparison to CT and routine physical examination.[24] Only 10% of patients were upstaged with the inclusion of FDG-PET in staging, however, as the majority of patients had stage IV disease based upon conventional staging techniques. FDG-PET may be particularly useful in the staging and subsequent management of patients with EATL, in which CT alone is often inadequate to determine extent of disease.[25] FDG-PET appears to share the limited sensitivity of CT for cutaneous disease, and careful dermatologic evaluation remains integral to the staging of T-cell lymphomas.[26] No prospective data regarding prognostic value of PET in restaging, posttreatment re-evaluation, or posttreatment surveillance are yet available.

Prognosis

The group of PTCLs collectively carries, on average, a less favorable prognosis than do B-cell lymphomas. This worse prognosis is manifest in lower response rates and complete response (CR) rates, higher rates of (and earlier) relapse, and inferior disease-specific and overall survival (OS). Prospective data guiding the management of the peripheral T-cell lymphomas are largely lacking. Historically, the peripheral T-cell lymphomas were included with the aggressive B-cell lymphomas in clinical trials, but were included in small numbers, precluding even meaningful post hoc analyses. Data from consecutive clinical trials performed by the Groupe d'Etudes des Lymphomes de l'Adulte (GELA) were analyzed retrospectively, with patients treated for T-cell lymphomas abstracted from the treatment populations.[27] The 5-year OS rate for these variably treated patients was 41%, in contrast to 53% for the patients with aggressive B-cell NHL. The difference was even more pronounced among those with higher-risk disease according to the International Prognostic Index (IPI). With this prognostic model (age, performance status, lactate dehydrogenase [LDH], extranodal sites, and stage), 5-year survival rates for patients with PTCL and two and three or more adverse risk factors were 36% and 23%, respectively. Among these high-risk groups, survival rates for patients with B-cell neoplasms were 50% greater. Furthermore, these high-risk features were disproportionately more common among those with T-cell lymphomas – in this series, 77% of patients had at least two adverse risk factors in the IPI model. Other large retrospective reports of patients with T-cell lymphomas have painted even less optimistic pictures, with one series reporting 5-year OS rates of 21% and 6% for patients with two and three or more risk factors.[28] These estimates compare unfavorably to diffuse large B-cell lymphoma (DLBCL), in which 4-year OS by risk group with modern treatment is 94% for favorable disease, 79% for intermediate-risk disease, and 54% for high-risk disease.[29]

The IPI was of course originally developed and validated in the risk stratification of patients with DLBCL.[30] And while as mentioned, the IPI does offer prognostic value in the T-cell lymphomas to some degree, the infrequency of low-risk disease alone makes it suboptimal for risk stratification in these diseases. The clinical heterogeneity of the T-cell lymphomas further complicates the application of a single model of risk to the entire class of disease. Accordingly, investigators have attempted to develop more directly applicable, and narrowly focused, prognostic models. The Italian Lymphoma Intergroup offered one such model based upon patients with peripheral T-cell lymphoma, unspecified (PTCL, NOS in the current WHO classification), largely treated with anthracycline-based chemotherapy.[31] Emerging from this retrospective analysis came the Prognostic Index for PTCL, or PIT. Advanced age (> 60 years), poor performance status (Eastern Cooperative Oncology Group [ECOG] performance status [PS] score ≥ 2), elevated LDH, and bone marrow involvement were found to be associated with worse outcomes. Unlike the IPI, distribution among risk groups was relatively even: of the five adverse risk features, 20% of cases had none, 34% had one, 26% had two, and 21% had three or four. Outcomes differed markedly across risk groups, with rates of OS at 5 years of 62.3% in the most favorable group, 52.9% for patients with one risk factor, 32.9% for those with two risk factors, and 18.3% for those with three or four risk factors.

The Italian Lymphoma Intergroup built upon this experience, incorporating findings from tissue microarrays in a second group of patients with either PTCL, NOS or AITL.[32] While multiple immunophenotypic findings were associated with inferior outcomes in univariate analysis, including expression of CD15 and expression of EBV proteins, in multivariate analysis the only finding was that the growth fraction, as measured by Ki-67, was prognostically relevant: the subset of patients whose lymphomas had Ki-67 scores of 80% or greater had lower rates of survival. The new model (PIT2) contains age > 60, ECOG PS ≥ 2, elevated LDH, and Ki-67 ≥ 80%, and was more robust in this same (non-validation) set of patients than either the IPI or original PIT (Table 21.2). Even distribution across risk groups was still not achieved, however, with 63% of patients classified as having low-risk disease (one or fewer adverse risk factors), and 25% intermediate-risk; only 12% of patients were contained in the highest-risk stratum. Nonetheless, the PIT2 represents the most robust model currently available for risk stratification of PTCL, NOS or AITL; formal models have yet to be developed for other types of PTCL, but for individual diagnoses, adverse prognostic factors will be addressed below when unique to that subtype. Appropriate risk stratification remains an important goal as efforts continue to develop and interpret clinical trials in these individually and collectively uncommon diseases.

Peripheral T-cell lymphoma, not otherwise specified

Peripheral T-cell lymphoma, not otherwise specified (PTCL, NOS) is now the preferred terminology for a collection of predominantly nodal T-cell lymphomas. Included under the rubric of PTCL, NOS are a variety of variant morphologic subtypes that had been considered distinct clinical entities in older classification schemata, such as lymphoepithelioid lymphoma (Lennert lymphoma), T-zone lymphoma, follicular T-cell lymphoma, pleomorphic T-cell lymphoma, small, medium, and large cell T-cell lymphoma, and T-immunoblastic lymphoma. While it is thought that Lennert lymphoma may follow a more indolent natural history, firm histologic criteria to distinguish among these entities were lacking, and interobserver variability for diagnosing many of these subtypes was found to lie in the range of 40–50%.[33] Furthermore, there were ultimately no reproducible data to support fundamentally different natural histories among the different morphologies.[27,28,33] Although the WHO 2008 nomenclature recognizes Lennert lymphoma, follicular T-cell lymphoma, and T-zone lymphoma as distinguishable entities, they are currently considered as variants of PTCL, NOS rather than distinct clinical entities.

Pathology

As might be expected given the nature of the diagnosis, PTCL, NOS includes a broad range of histologic entities that are better defined by what they are not, that being a specific (or specifiable) subtype of PTCL. The relative proportion of small and large cells, as well as the histologic pattern, can be heterogeneous, but does not appear to directly impact natural history or prognosis. Establishment of a malignant T-cell process by morphology and immunophenotype is required to establish the diagnosis, as is exclusion of other subtypes on similar grounds. The immunophenotype of PTCL, NOS is most frequently CD4+CD8−, with expression of CD43 and CD45RO, and variable loss of T-cell antigens, including CD3, CD5, or CD7, is seen in up to half of cases in Western series, although this is less common in Chinese patients.[33,34] Ninety percent of patients with PTCL, NOS can be shown to harbor a clonal rearrangement of the T-cell receptor (TCR). Cytogenetic abnormalities are frequently seen, with gain of material at

Table 21.2. Comparison of different prognostic models for peripheral T-cell lymphoma, not otherwise specified

Scoring system	No.	%	Relative risk of death	95% CI	p
Ann Arbor stage (n = 93)					
I	1	1	24.672	2.519 to 241.634	< 0.0001
II	19	20	0.852	0.393 to 1.848	
III	34	37	0.581	0.283 to 1.194	
IV	39	42	1		
IPI (n = 90)					
Low	24	27	0.654	0.232 to 1.847	0.1
Low-intermediate	31	34	0.785	0.304 to 2.029	
Intermediate-high	23	26	0.814	0.305 to 2.171	
High	12	13	1		
PIT group (n = 85)					
1	17	20	0.239	0.079 to 0.723	0.0043
2	27	32	0.225	0.078 to 0.647	
3	29	34	0.619	0.250 to 1.631	
4	12	14	1		
Proposed score group (n = 93)					
I	59	63	0.106	0.061 to 0.351	< 0.0001
II	23	25	0.396	0.151 to 0.967	
III	11	12	1		

Note: IPI: International Prognostic Index; PIT: Prognostic Index for PTCL, NOS.

chromosome 7q and loss of material from chromosomes 6q and 10p being the most commonly seen; over 50% of cases will demonstrate a complex karyotype.[35] *p53* gene mutations have been variably reported, and appear to confer a worse prognosis.[36,37] Ongoing work attempting to subdivide PTCL, NOS into distinct entities based upon gene expression profiling and comparative genomic hybridization may in the future allow for clinically relevant subtyping.[38]

Clinical features

PTCL, NOS represents the most common subtype of T-cell lymphoma in Western countries, accounting for between 34%[39] and 41%[33] of cases of PTCL, and approximately 6% of all NHL.[40] The median age of onset is 60 years, and a 2:1 male:female predominance is seen. Although PTCL, NOS is a predominantly nodal lymphoma, 60% of patients present with stage IV disease, and 22% with bone marrow involvement. Traditional adverse prognostic findings, including presence of B symptoms, bulky disease, impaired performance status, and extranodal dissemination are not uncommon in PTCL, NOS, resulting in a relative preponderance of high-risk patients according to the IPI.

PTCL, NOS tends to follow an aggressive clinical course, in keeping with its tendency to present with high-risk features. Despite routine use of anthracycline-based combination chemotherapy, long-term outcomes for the disease remain poor, with 5-year failure-free survival (FFS) rates of 20% and 5-year OS rates of 32%. These numbers are far lower for higher-risk disease: among that subset of patients with IPI scores of 4 or 5, estimates drop to 6% and 11%, respectively.[39]

Angioimmunoblastic T-cell lymphoma

Angioimmunoblastic T-cell lymphoma (AITL) is one of the more common peripheral T-cell lymphomas, accounting for 18% of diagnoses and approximately 5% of all NHL diagnoses in Western countries.[3] It was first described in the 1970s as a clinical syndrome of diffuse lymphadenopathy, organomegaly, anemia, and hypergammaglobulinemia. Reviews of pathology specimens noted that characteristic features in excised lymph nodes included partial effacement of the normal nodal architecture with a brisk inflammatory infiltrate of blastoid lymphocytes and dramatic vascular proliferation. These common features led to the initial names assigned to the syndrome, including angioimmunoblastic lymphadenopathy with dysproteinemia (AILD), immunoblastic lymphadenopathy, and lymphogranulomatosis X. The disease was initially felt not to represent true malignancy, but rather a hyperplastic, premalignant condition. Indeed, it was not until the availability of more sensitive immunophenotypic and molecular studies that it was demonstrated that the characteristic immunoblasts represented a monoclonal T-cell population, often with complex cytogenetic abnormalities, suggesting that the syndrome itself was in fact neoplastic in nature.

Initial investigations into the etiology of AITL suggested that any number of infectious agents may be contributing to lymphomagenesis, including fungal (*Cryptococcus*), mycobacterial (*Mycobacterium tuberculosis*), and viral.[41–44] Early work identified infection by human herpesvirus (HHV)-6 and HHV-8, although subsequent studies have failed to demonstrate that viral antigens are present in transformed lymphocytes, arguing against virally mediated oncogenesis.[45,46] Infection in patients with AITL by human immunodeficiency virus (HIV) or hepatitis C has been seen, although again no causal connection has been established. Perhaps the greatest interest has been in defining the role of EBV in development of AITL. EBV-infected lymphocytes are seen in nearly all cases of AITL; however, microdissection studies have established that it is the B-cell component of the inflammatory milieu that harbors EBV infection rather than the clonal T cells.[47,48] Typically, viral protein patterns are most consistent with latent phase infection as opposed to replicative. Patients with AITL can develop second primary lymphomas that are B cell in origin and driven by EBV infection, including diffuse large B-cell lymphoma and Burkitt's lymphoma.[49]

Pathology

The lymph node involved by AITL will classically demonstrate variable effacement of the normal underlying nodal architecture; based upon the morphologic features, investigators classify individual diagnoses into one of three patterns: in pattern I, normal nodal architecture is largely preserved intact, with hyperplastic B-cell follicles readily identified. The paracortical space will harbor the pleomorphic infiltrate and the arborizing vasculature. In pattern II, partial effacement of normal architecture is present, with only rare B-cell follicles present and with germinal center immunophenotype cells present beyond the confines of these scant follicles. The lymph node is otherwise occupied by the inflammatory and vascular proliferations characteristic of AITL. Pattern III is characterized by complete effacement of nodal architecture. Based upon limited experiences with serial biopsies, there has emerged the suggestion that the three histologic patterns represent increasingly advanced disease.[50,51]

Given the variable histologic appearance (which shares some features with a host of other conditions, both malignant and benign), and the at times minimal or absent cytologic features typically associated with lymphoid neoplasia, supportive testing with immunophenotypic and molecular studies can be helpful in confirming the diagnosis. Immunohistochemistry (IHC) can identify the diffuse CD3+ T-cell infiltrate that is predominated by CD4+CD8− cells. The immunoblasts will stain positively for B-cell markers, including CD20 and CD79a, but these B cells will not demonstrate light-chain restriction (in the absence of a coexisting EBV-associated B-NHL). A prominent follicle dendritic cell (FDC) network is present and can be highlighted with CD21 or CD23, particularly in patterns II and III. The observation based upon microdissection that the malignant T cells aberrantly coexpress the germinal center B-cell marker CD10 is felt to be rather specific for AITL. Coexpression of BCL6 and CD57 further supports the conclusion that the cell of origin of AITL is the follicular T-helper cell.[52] Cytogenetic studies will demonstrate abnormalities in as many as 90% of patients, although no abnormalities are either singularly common among cases of AITL or exclusive to AITL. However, half of patients will harbor multiple cytogenetically distinct clones, a finding that is uncommon in other lymphomas of either T-cell or B-cell origin.[53]

Table 21.3. Presenting signs and symptoms in angioimmunoblastic T-cell lymphoma

Sign/symptom	Frequency (% of patients)
B symptoms	65–85
Generalized lymphadenopathy	94–97
Nodal mass > 10 cm	17
Splenomegaly	70–73
Hepatomegaly	52–72
Rash	48–58
Ascites/effusions	23–37
Polyarthritis	18

Source: Adapted from Dogan A *et al.*[54]

Clinical features

AITL is typically a disease of the elderly, with median age of diagnosis in the seventh decade of life. Patients will typically present with a constellation of signs and symptoms (Table 21.3) including constitutional symptoms and diffuse adenopathy, and can frequently be mistakenly diagnosed with an acute infectious illness. Hepatosplenomegaly is common, and rash is present in approximately half of patients. Patients will frequently experience immune deficiency and dysregulation, and autoimmune phenomena are collectively common in patients with AITL, even if they are individually rare. Possible comorbid autoimmune diseases include Coomb's-positive hemolytic anemia, immune thrombocytopenic purpura, mixed cryoglobulinemia with associated vasculitis, autoimmune thyroid disease, and autoimmune arthritides (including rheumatoid arthritis). Common serologic abnormalities (Table 21.4) include elevation of LDH and erythrocyte sedimentation rate

Table 21.4. Laboratory abnormalities in angioimmunoblastic T-cell lymphoma

Finding	Frequency (% of patients)
Anemia	40–57
Other cytopenia(s)	20
Eosinophilia	39
Hypergammaglobulinemia	50–83
Hypogammaglobulinemia	9–27
Elevated LDH[a]	60–74
Elevated ESR[b]	45

Notes: [a]Lactate dehydrogenase.
[b]Erythrocyte sedimentation rate.
Source: Adapted from Dogan A *et al.*[54]

(ESR), cytopenias (most commonly anemia), peripheral eosinophilia, and polyclonal hypergammaglobulinemia (although hypogammaglobulinemia has also been rarely observed). Staging will typically demonstrate malignant adenopathy above and below the diaphragm in addition to lymphomatous infiltration of liver and spleen. Bone marrow biopsy may demonstrate involvement by lymphoma in approximately 60% of cases.[55]

The natural history of AITL tends to follow a moderately aggressive course, with historical median survival of between 15 months and 3 years, and 5-year survival rates of approximately one in three or less, although spontaneous remissions have been reported. Notably, the most common proximate cause of death is infectious complications, either due to systemic therapy or to the underlying immunodeficiency associated with AITL.[54] Therapy for AITL ranges from single-agent corticosteroid to multiagent anthracycline-based chemotherapy with consolidative high-dose therapy and autologous stem cell transplantation (HDT-ASCT), and will be discussed below.

Systemic anaplastic large cell lymphoma

Background

Anaplastic large cell lymphoma (ALCL) was originally described as a malignant lymphoma characterized by large, pleomorphic lymphocytes with a cohesive growth pattern and uniform expression of CD30.[56] The anaplastic lymphomas could be of B-cell, T-cell, or null (indeterminate) phenotypes, but the International Lymphoma Study Group proposed a reclassification of B-ALCL as a variant of DLBCL and grouped ALCL of T and null phenotypes as a distinct clinical entity, a recommendation that is reflected in the WHO classification.[4,57] Indeed, B-ALCL has subsequently been shown to confer a prognosis indistinct from DLBCL, whereas the natural history of ALCL (T/null) has continued to remain distinct. Although only approximately 2% of NHL in the United States, the clinical subtypes of T-ALCL are collectively second only to PTCL, NOS in frequency among T-cell lymphomas, accounting for approximately 25% of diagnosed cases. As discussed below, ALCL of T/null origin is best understood as three clinically distinct entities: ALK-positive ALCL, ALK-negative ALCL, and primary cutaneous ALCL.

Pathology

The original description of ALCL was made possible by the original description by Stein *et al.* of a novel molecule, originally named Ki-1 and subsequently CD30. CD30, a member of the tumor necrosis factor (TNF) receptor family, was noted to be expressed by a range of neoplastic processes, including the Reed–Sternberg cells of Hodgkin lymphoma as well as a subset of large cell neoplasms that had previously been classified as various diseases, ranging from seminoma to melanoma.[56,58] Subsequent immunophenotypic and genetic studies confirmed the lymphocytic lineage of these anaplastic tumors, establishing the clinical entity of ALCL. The putative cell of origin of ALCL is the CD30+ lymphoblast, present in small quantity in normal lymphoid tissues, which tends to share cytologic and immunophenotypic characteristics with the malignant lymphocytes of ALCL as well as having similar architectural distribution, largely residing in perifollicular and intrasinusoidal regions of normal lymph nodes.[59] Immunophenotypically, ALCL will frequently express mature activated T-cell markers, including CD25 and HLA-DR. Approximately 60% will express one or more T-cell antigens, including CD3, CD43, and CD45RO. One-third of cases will express neither T-cell nor B-cell markers, and will harbor neither TCR rearrangement nor immunoglobulin heavy chain (IgH) rearrangement, and are labeled as indeterminate or null lineage ALCL. Additionally, cytogenetic studies have demonstrated a unique translocation t(2;5)(p23;35) in a subset of cases, fusing the *ALK* gene from chromosome 2 with the nucleophosmin (*NPM*) gene from chromosome 5, resulting in expression of a constitutively active tyrosine kinase. Additional, less common translocations can similarly lead to overexpression of ALK, and in sum analysis, between 50% and 85% of cases of systemic ALCL demonstrate ALK expression. In addition to the dichotomy between ALK+ and ALK− ALCL, there is significant morphologic heterogeneity among cases of ALCL, with variants predominated by small cells or histiocytic infiltration reported, as well as neutrophil-rich, eosinophil-rich, sarcomatoid, and signet-cell variants; a previously described entity of Hodgkin-like ALCL has been reclassified as a variant of classical Hodgkin lymphoma based upon protein expression patterns, and this entity is not recognized in the most recent iteration of the WHO nomenclature. Lastly, while CD30+ is uniformly present in both ALK+ ALCL and ALK− ALCL, it can also be seen in a subset of cases of PTCL, NOS. Indeed, 32% of cases of PTCL, NOS may demonstrate expression of CD30 on at least a fraction of malignant lymphocytes, and in 5% of cases this will be seen in over 80% of cells.[60] Although the entity of CD30+ PTCL, NOS is difficult to distinguish reliably from ALK− ALCL, patients with this diagnosis suffer a prognosis significantly worse than ALK− ALCL, ALK+ ALCL, or PTCL, NOS not highly expressing CD30, with a 5-year FFS of 9%, and a 5-year OS of 19%.

Despite the varied morphology which ALCL can present, the clinical significance of the variant patterns remains unclear, although some feel that the small-cell variant is best considered a type of PTCL, NOS.[61] Nonetheless, independent of this morphologic variety, there exists a broad spectrum of clinical presentations of ALCL, with distinct prognoses, natural history, and optimal management strategies. ALCL can present as primary cutaneous disease, defined as disease presenting in skin without evidence of systemic involvement and without a history of an underlying lymphoproliferative disorder. Although disease can disseminate beyond the skin or regional lymph nodes in as many as 16% of patients with this diagnosis, when the disease remains limited to the skin only, it has not been shown to adversely impact OS.[62] Primary cutaneous ALCL, which is almost uniformly ALK-1 negative, lies at one end of a spectrum of CD30+ cutaneous lymphoproliferative disorders, and the discussion of these diseases is beyond the scope of this chapter.

Clinical features

This stands in contrast to systemic ALCL (hereon, ALCL), which, similar to other intermediate- or high-grade NHLs, is an aggressive but potentially curable disease. ALCL carries a bimodal age distribution, with a peak in adolescence and a second peak in late adulthood, resulting in an overall mean age of 34 years. It has long been recognized that expression of ALK confers a more favorable prognosis than does its absence, and appears to do so independently of IPI or PIT.[60] Patients with ALK-positive disease are more likely to be younger, but a similar distribution of patients across both IPI and PIT risk groups exists for both ALK-positive and ALK-negative disease. Clinical features for ALK-positive and ALK-negative disease are depicted in Table 21.5.

In the largest published series of ALCL to date, consisting of 87 cases of ALK-positive ALCL and 72 cases of ALK-negative ALCL, collected from multiple centers across North America, Europe, and Asia, the majority of patients were treated with cyclophosphamide, doxorubicin, vincristine, and prednisone (CHOP) or CHOP-like regimens regardless of ALK expression (95% of ALK-positive, and 93% of ALK-negative). Fewer than 10% of patients from each cohort received HDT/ASCR, and allogeneic stem cell transplantation was not used in consolidation of first remission. Response to anthracycline-based induction therapy was 88% and 76% for ALK-positive and ALK-negative disease, respectively, and 5-year FFS was 60% for ALK-positive, but only 36% for ALK-negative, ALCL. IPI (and PIT) contributed prognostic value; with an IPI of 3 or greater, fewer than 25% of ALK-positive, and fewer than 15% of ALK-negative, patients remained alive without recurrent disease at 5 years. Both ALK-positive and ALK-negative ALCL carried a prognosis that was superior to that associated with PTCL, NOS. Of note, despite the superior prognosis of patients with ALK-positive disease in comparison to those with ALK-negative, this may be at least in part due to a significant difference in median age for the two diseases. Although small numbers limit power to detect meaningful differences, when outcomes for the two diseases were compared within age groups, no differences were seen in OS and FFS for patients over 40 years of age. How to incorporate this observation into the management of ALK-positive ALCL remains unclear and will benefit from clinical investigation.

Management

No consensual standard of care exists for the management of the nodal PTCL (PTCL, NOS, AITL, and ALCL), either at diagnosis or for relapsed or refractory disease. The single most common therapeutic approach in newly diagnosed patients is treatment with combination anthracycline-based cytotoxic chemotherapy such as CHOP or similar regimens. While CHOP and CHOP-like regimens are commonly used for untreated PTCL, there exist no prospective data that establish this as the optimal clinical strategy. CHOP and CHOP-like regimens were defined in sequential randomized studies and the subsequent high-priority multi-regimen randomized trial as active in aggressive lymphomas, but the majority of patients in these trials were treated for DLBCL. Unfortunately, comparable work has not yet been carried out specifically for patients with nodal PTCL.

Current insights into optimal management of the newly diagnosed are largely informed, therefore, by retrospective data. One attempt at determining whether inclusion of anthracyclines in first-line therapy were as important for PTCL as it has proven to be for DLBCL emerged from the International T-cell Lymphoma Clinical/Pathological Project.[39] In contrast to aggressive B-cell disease, however, no significant difference in OS was seen in this retrospective review between patients who received anthracycline-based regimens and those receiving alternative regimens. Interpretation of these findings clearly is difficult due to the potential for confounding factors in the decision of whether or not to administer anthracycline-based therapy. Nonetheless, in part due to a lack of established regimens that are associated with outcomes superior to those achieved by CHOP or CHOP-like regimens, such treatment remains common in clinical practice. The clearest characterization of the effectiveness of CHOP in PTCL has emerged from the population-based registry maintained by the British Columbia Cancer Agency (BCCA);[63] the use of province-wide registry data allows for minimization of selection bias and captures "real-world" conditions more accurately than does extrapolation of results from clinical trials. Of the 199 patients in the BCCA report, the majority received either CHOP alone or CHOP followed by intensified consolidation. Of patients with PTCL, 64% achieved a CR to initial therapy, but 5-year OS and progression-free survival (PFS) were 35% and 29%,

Table 21.5. Clinical features of ALK-positive versus ALK-negative ALCL, systemic type

Clinical feature	ALK-pos n (%)	ALK-neg n (%)	p-value[a]	PTCL, NOS n (%)	p-value[b]
Total number of cases	87 (55)	72 (45)	-	331	-
Median age (years)	34	58	.0001	57	.30
Age < 60 years	74 (86)	42 (58)	<.0001	170 (50)	.21
Male:female	1.7:1	15:1	.74	1.9:1	.41
Stage					
I or II	30 (35)	30 (42)	.38	102 (31)	.18
III	25 (29)	15 (21)		87 (26)	
IV	31 (36)	27 (37)		145 (43)	
Elevated LDH	31 (37)	31 (46)	.28	158 (49)	.62
Performance status > 2	30 (35)	21 (30)	.56	60 (18)	.02
Nodal only disease	39 (54)	38 (49)	.52	124 (42)	.07
Extranodal sites > 1	17 (19.5)	15 (21)	.84	99 (29)	.15
Bulky disease > 10 cm	17 (21)	6 (11)	.17	19 (7)	.25
B-symptoms	52 (60)	41 (57)	.72	118 (35)	.0004
Hemoglobin < 110 g/L	17 (27)	18 (32)	.54	61 (22)	.11
Platelets < 150 × 10^9/L	6 (10)	6 (11)	.83	64 (24)	.03
IPI 0,1	40 (49)	27 (41)	.50	88 (28)	.066
2	18 (22)	13 (20)		111 (35)	
3	12 (15)	16 (24)		71 (22)	
4,5	12 (14)	10 (15)		48 (15)	
5 y FFS %	60	36	.015	20	.012
5 y OS %	70	49	.016	32	.032
5 y FFS by IPI %					
0,1	80	62		35	
2	61 p<001[c]	44 p = .0015[c]		16 p<.001[c]	
3	23	16		13	
4,5	25	13		8	
5 y OS by IPI %				13	
0,1	90	74		52	
2	68 p<001[c]	62 p<.001[c]		33 p<.001[c]	
3	23	31		16	
4,5	33	13		13	

Notes: [a]ALK-pos vs. ALK-neg.
[b]ALK-neg vs. PTCL-NOS.
[c]Comparison of IPI risk groups within specified subtype.
FFS: failure-free survival; OS: overall survival; IPI: International Prognostic Index; PS: performance status; LDH : lactate dehydrogenase.
Source: Reproduced with permission from Savage *et al.*[60]

respectively. Among patients with intermediate- or high-risk disease based upon the IPI (see below), 5-year OS was 22%. Outcomes were worse yet for patients with AITL, of whom only 13% were free from progression at 5 years. While CHOP alone may be adequate for a subset of patients with favorable risk features, the majority of patients will not enjoy durable remissions or outright cure. Indeed, for certain subtypes of extranodal T-cell lymphoma (such as hepatosplenic T-cell lymphoma and enteropathy-associated T-cell lymphoma), it appears that CHOP alone is virtually never curative.[64,65]

Unfortunately, it is easier to identify the shortcomings of CHOP as first-line therapy for PTCL than it is to demonstrate an alternative approach proven superior. Generally, attempts at improving outcomes for previously untreated patients have either intensified induction therapy or followed induction with intensified consolidative therapy. Attempts at intensifying induction therapy without consolidation have not yielded results that are demonstrably better than those with CHOP alone.[66,67] Ongoing investigations into intensified induction therapy are exploring strategies of dose-intensification (double-CHOP, dose-escalated CHOP plus etoposide [mega-CHOEP]) and drug addition (CHOP plus etoposide and gemcitabine, alemtuzumab, denileukin diftitox, or bevacizumab, to name but four such regimens).

Drawing from the experience with HDT-ASCT in poor-risk DLBCL, many have explored the potential for consolidative HDT to improve outcomes in PTCL. Individual series often suffer from retrospective methodology, limited power, and heterogeneous patient populations with multiple histologies; both selection and publication bias may further compromise the ability to interpret published case series. Two prospective studies allow for an assessment of the impact of consolidative HDT with intention-to-treat populations. The Nordic Lymphoma Group reported the results of a prospective study of CHOEP given every 14 days (CHOEP-14) and consolidative HDT-ASCT in responding patients.[68] The majority of treated patients had one of the three predominant nodal PTCLs, and patients with ALK-1-positive ALCL were excluded. The patient population was not atypical for these diseases, with a median age of 55 and with 54% classified as high-intermediate or high-risk disease based upon the IPI. Of evaluable patients, 73% (77/105) responded to CHOEP-14 and subsequently received consolidative HDT. At a median follow-up of 24 months, 67% of patients were alive. Corradini *et al.* reported results of two phase II studies in which patients were assigned to one of two treatments: multiagent high-dose sequential chemotherapy, or MACOP-B (high-dose methotrexate with leucovorin rescue, doxorubicin, cyclophosphamide, vincristine, prednisone, and bleomycin) induction followed by consolidative HDT-ASCT.[69] Among poor-risk PTCL patients, only 21% were alive 10 years after treatment, and only 18% were event free at the same time point.

The German experience with HDT-ASCT as consolidation of first-line therapy in either CR or PR for the treatment of T-cell lymphoma (predominantly PTCL, NOS and AITL) has recently been reported in abstract form.[70] In this prospective multicenter study, eligible patients received CHOP for four to six cycles, treatment with ESHAP (etoposide, methylprednisolone, cytarabine, and cisplastin) or DexaBEAM (dexamethasone, carmustine, etoposide, cytarabine, and melphalan) with stem cell mobilization, and subsequent HDT with hyperfractionated total body irradiation (TBI) and high-dose cyclophosphamide. While only 66% of newly diagnosed patients were able to proceed to HDT, the 3-year OS for the entire cohort (in an intention-to-treat analysis) was 48%, which compared favorably to their historical controls. Whereas this study did not identify prognostic factors predictive of outcome other than the PIT, the reported Spanish experience with consolidative HDT for previously untreated PTCL emphasizes the predictive power of the quality of the response to first-line therapy. Among those achieving a CR with first-line therapy and subsequently receiving consolidative therapy, 68% were alive at 5 years, and 63% were alive without evidence of new or recurrent disease. Although these numbers may be somewhat inflated by the inclusion and treatment of ALCL (regardless of ALK-1 expression), even after exclusion of more favorable ALCL patients, 5-year OS and PFS rates were 61% and 55%, respectively. The question that these and others' similar findings cannot address is whether consolidative HDT significantly alters the course of illness, or whether the "ability" to receive consolidation – or, put differently, chemotherapy-sensitive disease and good performance status – inherently confers a more favorable prognosis regardless of consolidation.

Additional experience with HDT-ASCT has been reported in the management of AITL. A retrospective review of 146 patients with AITL included patients both in first CR as well as with chemotherapy-sensitive relapsed disease, and the constituent patients received heterogeneous HDT regimens. Nonetheless, for the entire group, OS at median follow-up of 31 months was 65%; provocatively, the subset of patients transplanted in first CR enjoyed a 4-year PFS rate of 56%. Perhaps equally noteworthy is the observation that, of those patients with chemotherapy-refractory disease at HDT, only 23% were without evidence of progression at 4 years.[71] Clearly, however, none of these (or other) investigators have randomized responding patients to consolidative therapy or observation. Thus, it is difficult to offer evidence-based guidance to patients regarding the benefits of consolidative HDT. Nonetheless, the risks (at least in the selected patients reported in the literature) appear modest, as additional toxicity of HDT in this patient population is modest and reported treatment-related mortality rates are low. At the present time, in the absence of persuasive data, the decision of whether or not to embark upon consolidative HDT-ASCT for patients with poor-risk PTCL in first CR is best made on a case-by-case basis.

Relapsed/refractory disease

Historically, therapeutic decisions at time of relapse or in the management of primary refractory disease have largely borrowed from the more extensive investigational literature in the management of aggressive B-cell lymphomas. This can be seen perhaps most clearly in the application of consolidative HDT-ASCT following non-crossresistant second-line therapy, although results with this management strategy have been at best mixed. Many studies have yielded results similar to those for relapsed B-cell lymphoma, with a subset of patients experiencing long-term benefit. Of course, the published experience with this approach is limited to case series data, and thus the above concerns regarding selection and publication bias are all the more relevant here. Data reporting on consecutive-patient series reduce (but do not eliminate) such biases; one series reported the experience of 40 consecutive patients with relapsed or refractory nodal PTCL treated with the combination ifosfamide, carboplatin, and etoposide (ICE) with intent to consolidate responses with HDT-ASCT.[72] Following ICE chemotherapy, 70% of patients were deemed to be in a minimal disease state permitting consolidation, and all received planned HDT. At a median follow-up of 3 years, only 17% remained free of progression, with the majority of relapses occurring less than 6 months after HDT. Somewhat less disheartening results have been reported by the Cleveland Clinic, where 32 patients received HDT-ASCT for either PTCL, NOS or ALCL (both ALK+ and ALK−) between 1996 and 2005, the majority of which was in the relapsed setting.[73] Five-year OS and PFS were 34% and 18%, although 4 of the 5 patients (13% of cohort) with ALK+ ALCL were alive at last follow-up, potentially both identifying a subset of patients who may benefit from such therapy as well as in part explaining the difference in outcomes. Similar results have been reported by other groups, allowing for heterogeneity of treated patient populations and ranges in frequency of ALK+ ALCL across reports.[74]

Given suboptimal results of consolidative HDT in second CR, there has been interest in exploring whether a graft-versus-lymphoma effect may be achievable with allogeneic stem cell transplantation (SCT), and if so whether such treatment could provide clinical benefit as consolidative therapy for relapsed or refractory PTCL. A retrospective analysis of 77 patients receiving allogeneic SCT for PTCL of mixed histologies has been reported by Le Gouill *et al*;[75] the majority of patients had PTCL, NOS, AILT, or ALCL, the median previous lines of therapy was two (range, one to five), and 25% had progressed despite previous HDT-ASCT. Five-year OS and PFS for this cohort of patients were 57% and 53%, respectively, and treatment-related mortality was 34%. Of pretransplant characteristics, only chemoresistant disease was associated with worse event-free survival. Two patients received donor lymphocyte infusion for relapse following SCT, and both subsequently achieved durable remissions. The possible role for reduced-intensity conditioning regimens for PTCL was highlighted by a 17-patient pilot study by the Italian group.[76] Although the patients were young (median age 41 years), 15 of the 17 had relapsed disease, and half had previously received HDT-ASCT. Despite this, however, 14 of the 17 patients were alive at the median follow-up of 28 months, and 12 remained in a CR at that time point. Two-year non-relapse mortality was only 6%, while 3-year OS and PFS were 81% and 64%. In each series, several relapsing patients responded to donor lymphocyte infusions suggesting the presence of a graft-versus-lymphoma effect. While in sum, the modest literature addressing allogeneic SCT for PTCL is encouraging, the nature of the data – retrospective reviews and/or highly selected patients – does not permit adoption of allogeneic SCT as a standard of care for relapsed disease. Nonetheless, formal investigation of this strategy for patients with relapsed or refractory PTCL is warranted.

Rare subtypes

Adult T-cell leukemia/lymphoma

While epidemiologic studies in Japan during the 1970s first suggested an infectious etiology for ATLL, it was not until 1982 – after the discovery of interleukin-2 enabled researchers to culture T-cell lines in vitro – that the transforming retrovirus was first identified. The term "human T-lymphotropic virus-1," or HTLV-1, was given to this newly identified virus.

The incidence of ATLL is intimately associated with the variable geographical prevalence of HTLV-1 exposure. While ATLL is an uncommon diagnosis in those native to Western countries, accounting for $<1\%$ of lymphomas in the United States, in Japan ATLL accounts for one in four lymphomas and is six times more common than Hodgkin lymphoma.[77–79] HTLV-1 is a blood-borne pathogen with a disease latency period that can be from 10 to 40 years and can be transmitted by intravenous, sexual, breast-milk, or vertical routes. Of note, the intravenous route is limited to exposure to cellular blood products (and specifically infected T lymphocytes), due to the low-titer viremia experienced by actively infected patients. Patients exposed to HTLV-1 by the intravenous route have a greater risk of developing tropical spastic paraparesis/HTLV-1-associated myelopathy (TSP/HAM), potentially due to higher viral dose and an associated polyclonal expansion of infected cells.[80] And while the majority of the 20–30 million people worldwide believed to be infected with HTLV-1 will remain asymptomatic throughout the course of their lives, between 1% and 5% will at some time develop ATLL.[81,82]

Pathology

The diagnosis of ATLL is made based upon a combination of morphologic, immunophenotypic, and at times supporting molecular analyses in conjunction with serologic evaluation. Light microscopy will typically demonstrate infiltration of the affected organ by "flower cells," which represent activated lymphocytes with indented or lobulated nuclei. These lymphocytes are believed to be helper T cell in origin, as indicated by the predominant immunophenotype observed in ATLL: CD3+, CD4+/CD8−, CD7−, CD25+, HLA-DR+. No karyotypic abnormalities are unique to ATLL, although loss of heterozygosity of chromosome 6q has been reported in up to 50% of cases, suggesting the possibility of the presence of a relevant tumor-suppressor in the frequently deleted region. Other abnormalities can vary, and may include trisomies of chromosomes 3, 8, 9, or 21, gain of 14q32, 17p deletion, or complex cytogenetics.[83] Definitive evaluation can include demonstration of integration of HTLV-1 proviral sequences into the host genome, a technique that is far more sensitive than enzyme-linked immunosorbent assays (ELISA) for antibodies against structural components of HTLV-1, which are frequently absent (particularly from patients with predominant cutaneous manifestations of their disease, see below).[84]

Clinical features

ATLL can manifest along a broad spectrum of clinical disease, and is commonly divided into four separate categories (acute, chronic, lymphomatous, and smoldering) with non-overlapping signs and symptoms, natural histories, and responses to therapy. Acute ATLL typically manifests with constitutional symptoms, marked lymphocytosis, hepatosplenomegaly, diffuse lymphadenopathy, and cutaneous involvement. Metabolic disarray is common, most notably hypercalcemia, which will be present in approximately 70% of patients, due to the production of parathyroid hormone-related protein (PTHrp). Chronic ATLL presents without constitutional symptoms and manifests lesser degrees of lymphocytosis (typically less than 10% of circulating cells), organomegaly, and lymphadenopathy. Hypercalcemia is not a feature of chronic ATLL. Lymphomatous ATLL presents with symptoms indistinguishable from acute ATLL with the exception of an absence of hypercalcemia, but lacks a significant leukemic burden (by convention, less than 1% of circulating malignant lymphocytes). Smoldering ATLL describes the presence of a modest leukemic phase of disease in an asymptomatic individual, typically with malignant lymphocytes consisting of less than 5% of circulating cells; up to 50% of such patients will experience a spontaneous and durable remission, while the remainder will have persistent lymphocytosis. Many, although not all, such patients' diseases will subsequently progress to acute ATLL.

A significant complication of ATLL common to all subtypes is profound underlying immunodeficiency, leading to typical and atypical infections. Frequently identified pathogens include parasites (most commonly *Strongyloides stercoralis*), viruses (including cytomegalovirus [CMV]), and other organisms (such as *Candida* species and *Pneumocystis jiroveci*). Other virally mediated malignancies, including EBV-related lymphoma, akin to post-transplant lymphoproliferative disorder, and Kaposi's sarcoma, have been reported in patients with ATLL.[85,86]

Management

There exists no single standard of care for patients with ATLL, due largely to the inability of multiagent systemic cytotoxic chemotherapy to induce durable remission. General consensus recommendations on approaches to disease management have recently been published, although a lack of rigorous data from clinical trials limits the ability to offer definitive treatment recommendations.[87] Although anthracycline-based regimens (CHOP or CHOP-like regimens, including MACOP-B) can be associated with rates of complete response of up to 40%, these responses are short lived, and relapse is universal; primary refractory disease is not uncommon. Median survivals for acute, lymphomatous, and chronic types of ATLL are 8 months, 10 months, and 24 months, respectively. Treatment can be further compromised by both the immunodeficiency experienced by patients as well as the frequency of underlying organ dysfunction (particularly hepatic failure) that can limit the ability to safely administer systemic therapy. A randomized clinical trial comparing the sequenced regimen VCAP-AMP-VECP (sequentially: vincristine, cyclophosphamide, doxorubicin, and prednisone; doxorubicin, ranimustine, and prednisone; vindesine, etoposide, carboplatin, and prednisone) to CHOP given every 14 days (CHOP-14) found that the more intensified induction therapy was associated with superior rates of complete response (40% vs. 25%), but the survival benefit did not achieve statistical significance and outcomes in both arms (3-year OS of 24 and 13 months, respectively) were disappointing.[88]

Given the viral mediation of lymphomagenesis, investigators have explored the potential impact of antiviral therapy on the course of illness. Anecdotes of systemic response to treatment of CMV retinitis with foscarnet seemed a proof of principle, and ongoing work using interferon alpha (IFN-α) in combination with the antiretroviral zidovudine (AZT) has been promising. In one study that included 12 previously untreated patients, the combination yielded 7 complete responses and 4 partial responses.[89] It appears, however, that this clinical benefit is only enjoyed by patients with wild-type p53.[90] A worldwide meta-analysis of 100 patients has been reported in abstract form, documenting an overall response rate of 66%, including a 43% CR rate.[91] Patients with acute-type ATLL experienced a median survival of 12 months with this treatment, as opposed to only 9 months for those receiving chemotherapy. For those patients achieving a CR with AZT/IFN-α, however, 70% went on to live over 10 years. For patients with smoldering or chronic types of ATLL, AZT/IFN-α resulted in a 100% OS at a median follow-up of 5 years. Unfortunately, the one subtype of ATLL that AZT/IFN-α has shown the least activity in is lymphoma-type, in which it was associated with a 12-month median OS, compared to 15 months for chemotherapy. Other therapeutic agents that have been shown to have some degree of activity have included arsenic trioxide, all-*trans* retinoic acid, denileukin diftitox, alemtuzumab, and bortezomib. Although HDT-ASCT has not been shown to be of benefit for ATLL, interest in consolidative allogeneic SCT exists. Groups have reported long-term disease-free survival rates in excess of 30% in (highly selected) patients achieving a CR after allogeneic SCT.[92,93] Whether reduced-intensity or fully myeloablative preparative regimens should be preferred for the treatment of ATLL remains an open question, although only fully ablative transplants could be considered for chemotherapy-refractory disease. It is possible that incorporation of antiviral therapy or antibody-based therapy in induction and/or consolidation phases in conjunction with allogeneic SCT could further improve outcomes, and clinical trials employing such approaches are needed.

Extranodal natural killer/T-cell lymphoma, nasal type

Extranodal natural killer/T-cell (NK/T) lymphoma, nasal type (NK/T-NT) is a recently recognized diagnosis, but the first observation of destructive lesions of the face and nose was made in 1897. A series of ten patients with locally destructive central facial lesions led to the eponymous name of Stewart syndrome, but the disease was variably renamed as granuloma gangraenescens, idiopathic midline destructive disease, polymorphic reticulosis, and lethal midline granuloma. Modern pathology techniques applied retrospectively on archived biopsy material have made it clear that the majority of historical cases of the syndrome indeed represent what is now understood as NK/T-NT.[94]

NK/T-NT is rare in Western countries, although more prevalent in portions of Asia, including China, Japan, and the Koreas, and Central and South America, most notably among individuals of indigenous ancestry.[95] As with nasopharyngeal carcinoma, which shares some epidemiologic features with NK/T-NT, malignant lymphocytes can frequently be shown to be infected by EBV, and express viral proteins in patterns similar to that seen in EBV+ Hodgkin lymphoma and nasopharyngeal carcinoma.[96] It is felt that EBV is likely involved in the process of lymphomagenesis, although the literature is clouded somewhat by inclusion in some reports of historical patients with lethal midline granuloma that may not indeed have had NK/T-NT, but rather may have had other conditions that can rarely manifest similarly (such as Wegener's granulomatosis).

Pathology

Frequently, multiple biopsies will be needed before definitive pathologic diagnosis can be achieved. Morphologically, typical tumors arising in the nasal cavity will consist of a pleomorphic infiltrate, with constituent cells ranging from small mature-appearing lymphocytes to large transformed cells that can be seen invading and destroying small blood vessels. Similarly, necrosis can either be absent or extensive, which when present can further obfuscate the diagnosis. Support for the diagnosis can be derived from IHC and molecular pathology; tumor cells are characteristically positive for CD2, cytoplasmic CD3 (CD3ε), and CD45RO. CD56 is typically positive, supporting a NK cell origin, and T-cell-restricted intracellular antigen (TIA-1) is frequently expressed, suggesting a cytotoxic lymphocyte (either of NK or T lineage) as the cell of origin. As discussed, EBER positivity can be detected in many – if not all – specimens via *in situ* hybridization.[97–99] Clonal rearrangements of the TCRγδ can be detected via PCR in the majority of cases.[100]

Clinical features

NK/T-NT is most frequently diagnosed during the fifth decade of life, although it can be seen in pediatric and geriatric populations as well. A strong male preponderance has been consistently reported, with reported ratios ranging from 1.7:1 to 2.8:1. Disease most often arises in the nasal cavity, and tends to be rapidly progressive, leading to symptoms over a period of months. Common presenting symptoms include nasal obstruction, epistaxis, and facial or preorbital swelling. B symptoms are present in approximately half of patients. Laboratory analysis tends to be less informative, although the LDH can be elevated, and cytopenias would prompt greater attention to the possibility of bone marrow infiltration by the lymphoma (present in only a small minority of patients). The cervical lymph nodes are the regional nodes for the nasal cavity and paranasal sinuses, and can be demonstrated to harbor lymphoma in between 14% and 38% of individuals. Possible extranodal sites of disease beyond the nasal cavity and sinuses, either at diagnosis or relapse, include skin and central nervous system, among others.

Patients with NK/T-NT are staged according to a modified Ann Arbor system, with stage I(E) representing a single nodal or extranodal site, stage II(E) representing multiple nodal sites ipsilateral to the diaphragm or a single extranodal site with ipsilateral nodal involvement, stage III(E) involvement of lymph nodes above and below the diaphragm, with or without extranodal disease, and stage IV diffuse or disseminated disease with more than one extranodal site involved. Ann Arbor stage and the IPI score are of limited prognostic value, and fail to discriminate among risk groups as successfully for NK/T-NT as they do for other types of NHL. Other pathologic features, including expression of cytotoxic lymphocyte proteins and measures of local tumor invasion of bone or skin, appear to add prognostic value; how best to incorporate superior risk stratification into management decisions remains unclear.

Management

The optimal management of newly diagnosed NK/T-NT is unknown, and no data from randomized clinical trials are available to inform the decision. Groups have published experience with three general classes of treatment: chemotherapy only, radiation therapy only, and combined-modality therapy (CMT) programs. Chemotherapy, when given alone or within the context of CMT, has typically consisted of CHOP or CHOP-like regimens (including EPOCH [etoposide, vincristine, doxorubicin, cyclophosphamide, and prednisone], COP-BLAM-V [cyclophosphamide, vincristine, prednisolone, bleomycin, doxorubicin, and procarbazine], and ProMACE/CytaBOM [cyclophosphamide, doxorubicin, etoposide, cytarabine, bleomycin, vincristine, methotrexate, and prednisone]), although ifosfamide/etoposide-based regimens also appear to be active.[101–106] Radiation therapy (RT) doses in the literature range from 22 Gy to 65 Gy, and have been given alone, prior to chemotherapy, early in the course of CMT, or following completion of chemotherapy.

Assessing responses to different therapeutic approaches is challenging, as many patients reported were treated prior to modern immunophenotyping, and most reports do not offer important prognostic information that could help inform cross-trial comparisons. With these important caveats, some lessons emerge from the reported experiences treating NK/T-NT. Of 67 patients treated at the Queen Mary Hospital in Hong Kong, 51 patients had stage I disease, and were treated with one of a variety of chemotherapy regimens and consolidative RT to a dose of 40–50 Gy for patients achieving a CR. The reported 10-year disease-free survival was 52%, and the 10-year OS 42%.[107] The hypothesis emerging from these data that earlier RT may afford better local control, and thus better outcomes, was supported by the reported Chinese experience; among 105 patients treated with either RT or CMT, stratified, non-randomized results suggested that up-front RT was preferable to up-front chemotherapy: 83% of patients receiving up-front RT achieved a CR, as compared to only 20% of patients receiving up-front chemotherapy.[108] Among patients receiving up-front RT, there was a statistically insignificant benefit to subsequent chemotherapy (which was anthracycline-based for the majority of patients). Further experience from Sichuan University confirmed this finding, and additionally assessed dose of RT and impact on outcomes, finding that patients receiving 54 Gy or greater had significantly better DFS and OS than patients receiving 22–53 Gy.[109] Based upon this series of reports, administration of RT as the first therapy or early in the course of CMT is considered by many as the current standard of care for localized NK/T-NT lymphoma. Less of a consensus exists regarding the optimal treatment of widely disseminated disease, with many investigators electing to administer six to eight cycles of anthracycline-based chemotherapy and subsequent irradiation of sites of initially bulky disease; despite such treatment, outcomes remain poor, and such treatment is not likely to be curative. Other than transplant-based strategies, no standard of care for relapsed or refractory disease has emerged.

Given the relatively poor outcomes, even for patients with early-stage disease, and the relative chemotherapy resistance of the disease, investigation into the role for consolidative therapy, either HDT-ASCT or allogeneic SCT, would seem warranted. The literature on the role for these therapeutic modalities in NK/T-NT, unfortunately, is scarce. One report of 20 patients receiving HDT – 15 with autologous and 5 with allogeneic stem cell support – after one or two courses of systemic therapy documented some activity in poor-prognosis patients. Among the 15 patients receiving HDT-ASCT, 7 remained alive without recurrence at a median follow-up of 48 months. For the five patients receiving allogeneic transplants, there were two treatment-related mortalities and one death due to rapidly progressive disease; two patients with primary refractory disease remained alive and without evidence of recurrence at 56 and 78 months post-transplant.[110] The Japanese experience with allogeneic SCT for NK/T-NT has been reported, with 28 patients undergoing transplantation; of these, 10 remained in a CR at a median follow-up of 34 months, and no late relapses (after 10 months) were seen. Clarification of the optimal use and sequencing of these therapeutic approaches, using modern prognostic variables for stratification, is clearly needed.

Hepatosplenic T-cell lymphoma

Hepatosplenic T-cell lymphoma (HSTCL) is a rare form of PTCL, accounting for 1.4% of all T-cell lymphomas in the International T-cell NHL study.[39] Originally described in 1990 as the entity hepatosplenic $\gamma\delta$ T-cell lymphoma, the disease emerged as clinically distinct based upon unique aspects of clinical presentation, histologic pattern, and expression of clonally restricted $\gamma\delta$ T-cell receptor (TCR) by tumor cells.[111] The expression of the $\gamma\delta$ TCR has subsequently been shown not to be a prerequisite, as rare cases of otherwise clinically and pathologically stereotypical HSTCL have been reported with expression of the $\alpha\beta$ TCR.[112,113] The rarity of this disease results in the fact that the majority of our understanding of the natural history and optimal management of HSTCL is based upon small series or individual case reports. There is also significant overlap in published series, with many individual cases being reported more than once.

Pathology

Diagnosis of HSTCL is typically made based upon evaluation of splenectomy specimens or liver core-needle biopsy. Lymphomatous infiltrates in these tissues are typically made up of monomorphic, small- to medium-sized cells with pale cytoplasm. Typically, these cells demonstrate either sinusal or sinusoidal tropism, and spare the white pulp and portal triads, respectively. To date, no association with viral agents (including EBV and HHV) has been identified (despite the association with immunodeficiency). Malignant lymphocytes routinely share a specific immunophenotype: CD2+, CD3+, and $\gamma\delta$ TCR+; CD4, CD5, and CD8 are not expressed, and CD7 expression is variable. Of note, CD8 can be detected at low levels with more sensitive techniques, including flow cytometry, although immunoperoxidase stains on fresh or paraffin-embedded tissue will be negative.[114] It is not uncommon to see aberrant coexpression of NK markers, including CD56 and the NK cell immunoglobulin-like receptor CD94.[121,116] Typically, malignant lymphocytes will retain expression of TIA-1, belying their putative development from a cytotoxic T-cell precursor, although granzyme B expression is rarely retained. T-lymphoblastic lymphomas may be excluded from the pathologic differential, as HSTCL does not express terminal deoxynucleotidyl transferase (TdT).

Cytogenetic evaluations have found a recurrent abnormality of isochromosome 7q, either alone or in association with other chromosomal abnormalities, including trisomy 8. While these abnormalities are individually seen in many hematologic neoplasms, the combination of the two (while far from universally present in HSTCL) appears to be most specific for HSTCL.[65,117,118]

Clinical features

HSTCL is a disease that can occur at any age but is most often seen in teenagers or young adults, with a strong male predominance. Immunocompromised patients are overrepresented, with reports of HSTCL developing many years after solid organ transplantation. Other immune dysregulation that has antedated a diagnosis of HSTCL include Hodgkin lymphoma, acute myeloid leukemia, systemic lupus erythematosus, inflammatory bowel disease (IBD), and malarial infection.[119–121] The importance of immunosuppression as a contributor to lymphomagenesis has become particularly relevant in the light of a series of eight patients developing HSTCL following treatment with infliximab, a chimeric antibody against TNF-α approved for the treatment of IBD.[122] Although previous cases had been reported following treatment with azathioprine, and while all patients were using concomitant immunosuppressants (including azathioprine, mercaptopurine, and corticosteroids), these cases strongly suggest a significant increase in the risk of developing HSTCL in this patient population. Patients typically present with significant or dramatic hepatosplenomegaly, cytopenias, and constitutional symptoms; lymphadenopathy is modest, and may be absent. In the two largest series of HSTCL, the presenting features included splenomegaly in all but one case, and over 80% had hepatomegaly.[123,124] Spontaneous splenic rupture has been reported. The clinical course leading to diagnosis is typically aggressive, although reports exist of cases presenting far more indolently, with symptoms present for years.[65] Cytopenias are usually present, with over 85% of patients presenting with thrombocytopenia and with a majority of patients demonstrating anemia and leucopenia as well. The etiology of peripheral cytopenias is often multifactorial, with components of splenic sequestration and marrow failure due to lymphomatous infiltration frequently observed; the hemophagocytic syndrome can be present and contribute as well to both cytopenias as well as symptom burden, and autoimmune cytopenias (including immune thrombocytopenic purpura and autoimmune hemolytic anemia) can present simultaneously or precede the ultimate diagnosis of HSTCL.[125,126]

Computed tomography typically demonstrates marked hepatosplenomegaly out of proportion to adenopathy. Perhaps due in part to this pattern of distribution, FDG-PET has been of limited utility. Corresponding to liver involvement and aggressive growth rates, laboratory analyses will typically include an elevated LDH, alkaline phosphatase, and hepatic transaminases in addition to peripheral cytopenias.

Management

To date, no prospective study of optimal treatment of HSTCL, either at diagnosis or relapse, has been reported. Typically, patients will be treated with combination cytotoxic chemotherapy that is anthracycline-based (e.g., CHOP or CHOP-like regimens), albeit with disappointing results. In the two largest series, reporting on 66 patients (although at least 5 cases are reported in both series), only 6 patients survived at time of reporting. Of these, one had only achieved 3 months of follow-up, and four had received consolidative HDT (and either autologous or allogeneic SCT). Thus, conventional first-line chemotherapy alone has historically been unlikely to lead to a durable disease-free state. Primary refractory disease is common, and even for responders, duration of response or remission is typically brief. Other agents, including purine analogs and alemtuzumab, have shown activity.[124,127–129]

Given the poor prognosis for patients receiving routine multiagent chemotherapy alone, interest in consolidative therapy has emerged. In one series of six patients receiving consolidative HDT-ASCT, two patients achieved remissions of 42 and 52 months.[65] Of note, both patients received a first-line regimen that was platinum-cytarabine based, as opposed to a CHOP-like regimen, and both received consolidation immediately following induction of remission. There are no reports of durable remission with HDT-ASCT for relapsed disease. Allogeneic SCT appears to have clinical utility, with 7 of 17 patients (reported in 13 case reports) alive without relapse at times of publication, with follow-up ranging from 3 to 86 months.[130] All patients were treated following first-line induction chemotherapy; of the ten treatment failures, there were five treatment-related deaths and five relapses (all of which were within the first 18 months following SCT). More research is needed into optimization of induction therapy, conditioning regimen, and selection of cellular therapy for appropriate candidates.

Enteropathy-associated T-cell lymphoma

Enteropathy-associated T-cell lymphoma (EATL) is a rare form of peripheral T-cell lymphoma, accounting for 4.7% of all T-cell lymphomas. Originally named malignant histiocytosis of the intestine in the first reported series in 1978, 16 years after it was first hypothesized that celiac sprue could cause lymphoma and a full 133 years after Gull first suggested an association between lymphoma and steatorrhea, EATL was subsequently shown to be a lymphoproliferative disorder of the intraepithelial T lymphocyte (IEL) of the gastrointestinal tract.[131–133] EATL is intimately associated with celiac sprue and its associated enteropathy; the clinical entity of T-cell lymphoma of the intestine without associated enteropathy is even less common. A predominantly extranodal lymphoma, EATL demonstrates unique pathologic and clinical characteristics that contribute to the poor prognosis associated with the disease.

The association between EATL and celiac sprue has been well established, with investigators reporting relative risks of between 40 and 100, although the absolute risk for patients with celiac disease is low, with incidence rates of EATL estimated at 1 in 5684 person-years.[134–137] The multistage development of EATL has been reviewed by Isaacson and Du, with the process beginning with the development of celiac disease among susceptible individuals, particularly those with HLA-DQA1 and-DQB1.[138] This subsequently progresses to refractory celiac disease, and then to EATL. It is believed that in many patients, EATL arises from a progressive clonal expansion of IELs in these patients with refractory, or advanced and untreated or undiagnosed, celiac disease. Homozygosity for HLA-DQ2 in particular has been associated with increased risk of refractory celiac disease type II and subsequent development of EATL.[139] In biopsy specimens from patients with refractory celiac disease, early changes with clonal T-cell populations without overt lymphoma can frequently be identified, and "refractory sprue with clonal IELs" has become recognized as a true precursor lesion in these at-risk patients, although progression to EATL is not universal. Furthermore, this risk may be modifiable through early intervention, as will be discussed below.

Pathology

Given the predominant bowel involvement of EATL, a predominance of signs and symptoms referable to the gastrointestinal tract, the pathologic characteristics of EATL stand in relation to lymphocyte biology and bowel architecture and microenvironment. Grossly, the most typical enteroscopic findings are circumferential ulcers either restricted to the jejunum or with multiple synchronous lesions throughout the small bowel including the jejunum, with bulky luminal masses being the exception rather than the rule, and with spontaneous perforation frequently noted.[140] Microscopically, tumor histology can be variable, with a population of large or blastic lymphocytes often seen, classically with rounded nuclei and a single nucleolus, but significant pleomorphism can be observed, with malignant lymphocytes varying from small and mature to large and anaplastic.[141] Immunophenotypically, the IEL is an aberrant cytotoxic mucosal T cell that expresses CD3 cytoplasmically but has lost surface CD3, is dual CD4−/CD8−, but maintains expression of CD103, an E-cadherin ligand characteristically expressed by mucosal lymphocytes. The clonal IELs may express cytotoxic T-cell-associated proteins, including TIA-1, granzyme B, and perforin.[142,143] Anaplastic cells may coexpress CD30, and a subset of small or medium cells aberrantly can less commonly express CD56. EBV has been detected in some; of note, the proportion of EBV-positive patients was 100% among people of Mexican descent, in comparison to only 10% of European ancestry, in one series.[144] Whether this EBV+ disease truly represents EATL or more likely rather reflects bowel involvement by NK/T-NT, which can (in direct contrast with its name) present in the gastrointestinal tract, remains unclear.[145]

Molecularly, EATL will nearly universally express a clonal rearrangement of TCRβ, and will not typically undergo clonal TCRγ rearrangement.[146] Although pathognomonic cytogenetic abnormalities have not yet been defined in EATL, it is clear that recurrent genetic alterations are common. In one series of 75 cases, recurrent gains and losses of genetic material were found in 65 (87%), including gain at 5q (18%), 1q (16%), 7q (24%), and 9q (58%) and loss from chromosomes 8p and 13q (24% each) or 9p (18%).[153]

Clinical features

EATL is a disease of adulthood, with a median age of 50 years. Common symptoms at presentation include diarrhea, abdominal pain, and weight loss; B symptoms may be reported in as many as one-third of patients, although fevers and night sweats may also be precipitated by occult small bowel perforation or small bowel obstruction, each present in approximately 25% of patients at time of diagnosis. Frank abdominal masses are rare, and significant peripheral adenopathy is not typically seen. Cavitating mesenteric adenopathy has been described, although this can be either reactive or malignant in etiology. Disease, even when advanced, is typically restricted to the abdominal cavity, with extraintestinal sites of disease including lymph nodes, omentum, liver, and spleen. Laboratory abnormalities can include an elevated LDH and a microcytic anemia, due in part to iron deficiency related to malabsorption secondary to celiac disease.

Despite the strong epidemiologic association with celiac disease, EATL may be diagnosed in patients without a known history of gluten sensitivity or malabsorption. Accordingly, in patients presenting with small bowel (particularly jejeunal) lymphoma, evaluation for serologic evidence of celiac disease (e.g., antibodies to tissue transglutaminase) should be considered. Among patients with celiac disease who do not respond clinically to a gluten-free diet, a high index of suspicion for EATL must be maintained.

Following diagnosis of EATL, clinical staging routinely consists of physical examination; CT scans of the chest, abdomen, and pelvis; routine laboratory analyses; and bone marrow biopsy. The necessity of bone marrow biopsy has been called into question given the low rates of involvement reported (< 10%), but nonetheless remains a standard of care, particularly in patients for whom SCT may be a consideration. Nonetheless, with the predominant site of disease being the small bowel, significant clinical attention must be paid to evaluating the length of the bowel for multifocal disease prior to treatment planning. The contribution of FDG-PET to the staging process has been evaluated, with investigators finding that FDG-PET may be superior to CT for identification of involved regions of bowel.[148] Additionally, given the difficulty of radiographic diagnosis of EATL, it is possible that FDG-PET scanning may offer unique advantages for surveillance in patients at high risk or in post-treatment monitoring. Additional radiographic options include capsule endoscopy, which has been found to be of clinical utility in the diagnostic evaluation for EATL.[149]

Due in part to the rarity of this disease, prospective data addressing optimal management of EATL are lacking. Most patients are either diagnosed at time of, or subsequently will undergo, small bowel resection; unfortunately, complete surgical resection, even when disease is limited to the small bowel (CSIE), is not considered curative. Treatments that have been reported have most often been anthracycline-based multiagent chemotherapeutic regimens, including CHOP, VAMP (vincristine, doxorubicin, high-dose methotrexate, and prednisolone), and PEACE-BOM (prednisolone, etoposide, doxorubicin, cyclophosphamide, bleomycin, vincristine, and high-dose methotrexate). Systemic therapy alone infrequently leads to durable remissions; in a single-institution series of 31 patients, the 1-year and 5-year failure-free survival rates were 19.4% and 3.2%, respectively, and OS was poor (1-year OS was 38.7%, 5-year OS 19.7%, and median OS was 7.5 months). These poor outcomes may in part be due to the underlying physiologic compromise often seen at diagnosis of EATL, with surgical emergencies and significant malnutrition often complicating both diagnostic evaluation and subsequent therapy; as many as 50% of patients historically have been unable to complete a full course of planned systemic therapy due to these and other factors. In a multicenter prospective, non-randomized study of intestinal NHL of all types, 28 patients with EATL were treated with CHOP every 21 days; these patients experienced a 2-year OS of only 28%.[150] Others have reported treatment with alemtuzumab as a single agent or in combination with low-dose gemcitabine, HyperCVAD (cyclophosphamide, vincristine, infusional doxorubicin, and dexamethasone alternating with high-dose methotrexate and cytarabine), ProMACE-CytaBOM, and CHOEP (cyclophosphamide, doxorubicin, etoposide, vincristine, and prednisone).[151,152]

The inadequacy of available first-line therapy for EATL has prompted consideration of further intensification of induction therapy and attempts to offer consolidation therapy to responding patients. Published reports of either standard (CHOP or CHOP-like) or intensified induction chemotherapy with consolidative HDT-ASCT have included small numbers of patients, but one series of six patients treated with ifosfamide, etoposide, and epirubicin, then with high-dose methotrexate, and subsequently consolidated with HDT-ASCT reported complete responses in four patients lasting up to 4 years at last follow-up.[153] As the patient with refractory celiac disease with atypical IELs is known to be at high risk of subsequent progression to EATL, treatment of patients in this phase of disease has been proposed as one possible way to improve outcomes. Seven such patients received HDT-ASCT without prior induction chemotherapy in one published report receiving fludarabine and melphalan conditioning following granulocyte colony-stimulating factor (G-CSF) mobilization.[154] At a median follow-up of 15 months, there was one death attributed to progressive neuroceliac disease. All three of the patients with follow-up beyond 12 months demonstrated partial responses as measured by flow cytometric analysis of the IEL population at repeat duodenal biopsy. The feasibility and utility of allogeneic SCT in treatment of EATL is unknown, with reports limited to individual cases.

Future directions

The combination of unfortunately poor outcomes with current therapy, a lack of consensus standard-of-care for relapsed or refractory disease in particular, and a relative dearth of compounds approved for (and effective in) the treatment of T-cell lymphomas has made these diseases increasingly popular foci of clinical investigation. Significant promise can be found both in the use of agents approved by the United States Food and Drug Administration (FDA) for the treatment of other malignancies as well as investigation agents that have shown some evidence of activity against peripheral T-cell lymphomas.

Many agents currently available in the treatment of other diseases – including cutaneous T-cell lymphoma – have been evaluated in patients with relapsed disease, including denileukin diftitox, alemtuzumab, and gemcitabine. Use of the diphtheria/interleukin-2 fusion protein, denileukin diftitox, was associated with a 48% response rate when given as a single agent to patients with relapsed PTCL, and treated patients experienced a median PFS of 6 months.[155] Alemtuzumab, a monoclonal antibody against the surface glycoprotein CD52, has also demonstrated single-agent activity in relapsed PTCL, with an overall response rate of 60% and with manageable toxicity, including a rate of reactivation of CMV of 10%.[156] Based in part on such results, on the non-overlapping toxicity of monoclonal antibody-based immunotherapy and cytotoxic chemotherapy, and on the profound success of the combination of CHOP and rituximab, investigators are pursuing whether inclusion of alemtuzumab in first-line anthracycline-based therapy may improve outcomes. In a study by the Gruppo Italiano Terapie Innovative nei Linfomie (GITIL), CHOP plus subcutaneous alemtuzumab for previously untreated PTCL (predominantly PTCL, NOS) was associated with a CR rate of 71%, although the median duration of response was only 11 months and significant infectious sequelae (including CMV reactivation and Jacob–Creutzfeldt viral reactivation, among others) were reported.[157] Others continue to investigate the application of alemtuzumab as consolidative therapy following anthracycline-based treatment.[158] As for cytotoxic therapies, gemcitabine – a pyrimidine analog with structural similarities to cytarabine with activity in multiple solid tumors – has shown promise in both Hodgkin lymphoma and NHLs. An initial report of ten patients with relapsed or refractory T-cell lymphomas reported an overall response rate of 60%,[159] and subsequent investigations have used gemcitabine in combination with other FDA-approved or novel agents. The combination of gemcitabine, cisplatin, and methylprednisolone was associated with a 69% overall response rate and a 19% CR rate in relapsed or refractory disease, with a suggestion that EATL and AITL in particular may be sensitive to this combination. Investigations into incorporation of gemcitabine into anthracycline-based regimens for previously untreated disease are ongoing.[160]

In addition to evaluation of currently available agents, active investigation worldwide is ongoing into the identification and development of novel agents in the treatment of PTCL. Two agents that have shown particular promise are pralatrexate and depsipeptide. Pralatrexate is a novel antifolate that was designed for higher affinity for reduced folate carrier type I and increased polyglutamation, resulting in increased internalization of the drug in tumor tissues and more prolonged intracellular retention once internalized. Promising activity was reported in early clinical trials treating patients with relapsed or refractory disease, with a 45% overall response rate and a 40% CR rate – the highest CR rate with single-agent therapy in this patient population reported to date.[161] Depsipeptide is an inhibitor of histone deacetylase (HDAC) that was initially found to have activity in cutaneous T-cell lymphoma and was subsequently shown to have activity in PTCL. In a National Cancer Institute-sponsored multicenter phase II study, depsipeptide was associated with a 30% response rate in relapsed or refractory PTCL.[162] Both agents are undergoing formal investigation with international registration trials, and would be, if approved, the first agent(s) specifically indicated for non-cutaneous PTCL. Numerous other drugs are the subjects of earlier-phase investigation and may hold promise, including monoclonal antibodies other than alemtuzumab (including antibodies against CD4, CD2, and CD30, among others); other agents in the class of HDAC inhibitors; purine analogs, including clofarabine and nelarabine; and proteosome inhibitors such as bortezomib.

With an increasing interest in T-cell lymphomas and so many new agents with at least anecdotal activity, the problem of the lack of effective therapies to offer patients with PTCL is being replaced by new issues such as efficient evaluation of new therapies for these uncommon and heterogeneous lymphomas. Fortunately, physicians and patients are becoming aware of the unique challenges of PTCL and increasingly understand that the only way to make progress is to move beyond the anecdotes and participate in well-designed prospective trials. Whether utilizing new upfront combination regimens, HDT-ASCT, or novel drugs for the still too common relapsed patients, it is only through these well-designed trials that we can move forward in an understandable way. These trials will allow us to identify the most active of the new agents and/or combinations of therapies, and ultimately move beyond CHOP as the primary therapy for patients with PTCL.

References

1. Ascani S, Zinzani P, Gherlinzoni F, *et al.* Peripheral T-cell lymphomas. Clinicopathologic study of 168 cases diagnosed according to the REAL classification. *Ann Oncol* 1997; **8**(6):583–92.
2. Anderson J, Armitage J, Weisenburger D. Epidemiology of the non-Hodgkin's lymphomas: distributions of the major subtypes differ by geographic locations. *Ann Oncol* 1998;**9**(7):717–20.
3. Vose J, Armitage J, Weisenberger D. International T-Cell Lymphoma Project. International peripheral T-cell and natural killer/T-cell lymphoma study: pathology findings and clinical outcomes. *J Clin Oncol* 2008;**26** (25):4124–30.
4. Swerdlow SH, Campo E, Harris NL, *et al.* (eds.) *WHO Classification of Tumours of Haematopoietic and Lymphoid Tissues*, 4th edn. Lyon, France, IARC Press, 2008.
5. Willemze R, Jansen PM, Cerroni L, *et al.* Subcutaneous panniculitis-like T-cell lymphoma: definition, classification, and prognostic factors: an EORTC Cutaneous Lymphoma Group Study of 83 cases. *Blood* 2008;**111** (2):838–45.
6. Querfeld C, Kuzel TM, Guitart J, *et al.* Primary cutaneous CD30+ lymphoproliferative disorders: new insights into biology and therapy. *Oncology (Williston Park)* 2007;**21** (6):689–96.
7. Olsen E, Vonderheid E, Pimpinelli N, *et al.* Revisions to the staging and classification of mycosis fungoides and Sezary syndrome: a proposal of the International Society for Cutaneous Lymphomas (ISCL) and the cutaneous lymphoma task force of the European Organization of Research and Treatment of Cancer (EORTC). *Blood* 2007;**110**(6):1713–22.
8. Kim YH, Willemze R, Pimpinelli N, *et al.* TNM classification system for primary cutaneous lymphomas other than mycosis fungoides and Sezary syndrome: a proposal of the International Society for Cutaneous Lymphomas (ISCL) and the Cutaneous Lymphoma Task Force of the European Organization of Research and Treatment of Cancer (EORTC). *Blood* 2007;**110**(2):479–84.
9. Willemze R, Jaffe ES, Burg G, *et al.* WHO-EORTC classification for cutaneous lymphomas. *Blood* 2005;**105** (10):3768–85.
10. Querfeld C, Rosen ST, Guitart J, *et al.* The spectrum of cutaneous T-cell lymphomas: new insights into biology and therapy. *Curr Opin Hematol* 2005;**12**(4):273–8.
11. Querfeld C, Guitart J, Kuzel TM, *et al.* Primary cutaneous lymphomas: a review with current treatment options. *Blood Rev* 2003;**17**(3):131–42.
12. Liu HL, Hoppe RT, Kohler S, *et al.* CD30+ cutaneous lymphoproliferative disorders: the Stanford experience in lymphomatoid papulosis and primary cutaneous anaplastic large cell lymphoma. *J Am Acad Dermatol* 2003;**49**(6):1049–58.
13. Foss F. Overview of cutaneous T-cell lymphoma: prognostic factors and novel therapeutic approaches. *Leuk Lymphoma* 2003;**44** Suppl 3:S55–61.
14. Osuji N, Matutes E, Catovsky D, *et al.* Histopathology of the spleen in T-cell large granular lymphocyte leukemia and T-cell prolymphocytic leukemia: a comparative review. *Am J Surg Pathol* 2005;**29**(7):935–41.
15. Sokol L, Loughran T Jr. Large granular lymphocyte leukemia. *Oncologist* 2006;**11**(3):263–73.
16. Suzuki R, Suzumiya J, Nakamura S, *et al.* Aggressive natural killer-cell leukemia revisited: large granular lymphocyte leukemia of cytotoxic NK cells. *Leukemia* 2004;**18**(4): 763–70.
17. Ryder J, Wang X, Bao L, *et al.* Aggressive natural killer cell leukemia: report of a Chinese series and review of

the literature. *Int J Hematol* 2007;**85**(1):18–25.

18. Lukes R, Collins R. Lukes-Collins classification and its significance. *Cancer Treat Rep* 1977;**61**(6):971–9.
19. Lennert K, Mohri N, Stein H, *et al.* The histopathology of malignant lymphoma. *Br J Haematol* 1975;**31**:193–203.
20. The Non-Hodgkin's Lymphoma Pathologic Classification Project. National Cancer Institute sponsored study of classifications of non-Hodgkin's lymphomas: summary and description of a working formulation for clinical usage. *Cancer* 1982;**49**:2112–35.
21. Harris NL, Jaffe ES, Diebold J, *et al.* The World Health Organization classification of hematological malignancies report of the Clinical Advisory Committee Meeting, Airlie House, Virginia, November 1997. *Mod Pathol* 2000;**13**(2):193–207.
22. Kukreti V, Patterson B, Callum J. Pathology the gold standard: a retrospective analysis of discordant "second-opinion" lymphoma pathology and its impact on patient care. *Blood* 2006;**108**:348.
23. Matasar M, Shi W, Silberstein J, *et al.* Expert second opinion pathology review of lymphoma in the era of the World Health Organization classification. *Blood* 2007;**110**(11):3317.
24. Horwitz S, Foss F, Goldfarb S. FDG-PET scans as an additional staging study for T-cell lymphomas: high rates of positivity do not result in frequent changes in stage. *Blood* 2006;**108**(11):2399.
25. Hadithi M, Mallant M, Oudejans J, *et al.* 18F-FDG PET versus CT for the detection of enteropathy-associated T-cell lymphoma in refractory celiac disease. *J Nucl Med* 2006;**47**(10):1622–7.
26. Kako S, Izutsu K, Ota Y, *et al.* FDG-PET in T-cell and NK-cell neoplasms. *Ann Oncol* 2007;**18**(10):1685–90.
27. Gisselbrecht C, Gaulard P, Lepage E, *et al.* Prognostic significance of T-cell phenotype in aggressive non-Hodgkin's lymphomas. Groupe d'Etudes des Lymphomes de l'Adulte (GELA). *Blood* 1998;**92**(1):76–82.
28. Lopez-Guillermo A, Cid J, Salar A, *et al.* Peripheral T-cell lymphomas: initial features, natural history, and prognostic factors in a series of 174 patients diagnosed according to the REAL Classification. *Ann Oncol* 1998;**9**(8):849–55.
29. Sehn LH, Berry B, Chhanabhai M, *et al.* The revised International Prognostic Index (R-IPI) is a better predictor of outcome than the standard IPI for patients with diffuse large B-cell lymphoma treated with R-CHOP. *Blood* 2007;**109**(5):1857–61.
30. Shipp M, Harrington D, Anderson T. A predictive model for aggressive NHL: the international non-Hodgkin's lymphoma prognostic factors project. *N Engl J Med* 1993;**329**:987.
31. Gallamini A, Stelitano C, Calvi R, *et al.* Peripheral T-cell lymphoma unspecified (PTCL-U): a new prognostic model from a retrospective multicentric clinical study. *Blood* 2004;**103**(7):2474–9.
32. Went P, Agostinelli C, Gallamini A, *et al.* Marker expression in peripheral T-cell lymphoma: a proposed clinical-pathologic prognostic score. *J Clin Oncol* 2006;**24**(16):2472–9.
33. Rudiger T, Weisenburger D, Anderson J, *et al.* Peripheral T-cell lymphoma (excluding anaplastic large-cell lymphoma): results from the Non-Hodgkin's Lymphoma Classification Project. *Ann Oncol* 2002;**13**(1):140–9.
34. Au WY, Ma SY, Chim CS, *et al.* Clinicopathologic features and treatment outcome of mature T-cell and natural killer-cell lymphomas diagnosed according to the World Health Organization classification scheme: a single center experience of 10 years. *Ann Oncol* 2005;**16**(2):206–14.
35. Nelson M, Horsman DE, Weisenburger DD, *et al.* Cytogenetic abnormalities and clinical correlations in peripheral T-cell lymphoma. *Br J Haematol* 2008;**141**(4):461–9.
36. Pescarmona E, Pignoloni P, Puopolo M, *et al.* p53 over-expression identifies a subset of nodal peripheral T-cell lymphomas with a distinctive biological profile and poor clinical outcome. *J Pathol* 2001;**195**(3):361–6.
37. Moller M, Gerdes A, Skjodt K, *et al.* Disrupted p53 function as predictor of treatment failure and poor prognosis in B- and T-cell non-Hodgkin's lymphoma 1. *Clin Cancer Res* 1999;**5**(5):1085–91.
38. Ballester B, Ramuz O, Gisselbrecht C, *et al.* Gene expression profiling identifies molecular subgroups among nodal peripheral T-cell lymphomas. *Oncogene* 2005;**25**(10):1560–70.
39. Vose J. International Peripheral T-Cell Lymphoma (PTCL) Clinical and Pathologic Review Project: poor outcome by prognostic indices and lack of efficacy with anthracyclines. *Blood* 2005;**106**:811a.
40. Armitage JO, Weisenburger DD. New approach to classifying non-Hodgkin's lymphomas: clinical features of the major histologic subtypes. Non-Hodgkin's Lymphoma Classification Project. *J Clin Oncol* 1998;**16**(8):2780–95.
41. Matz L, Papadimitriou J, Carroll J, *et al.* Angioimmunoblastic lymphadenopathy with dysproteinemia. *Cancer* 1977;**40**(5):2152–60.
42. Rho R, Laddis T, McQuain C, *et al.* Miliary tuberculosis in a patient with Epstein-Barr virus-associated angioimmunoblastic lymphadenopathy. *Ann Hematol* 1996;**72**(5):333–5.
43. Shamoto M, Suchi T. Intracytoplasmic type A virus-like particles in angioimmunoblastic lymphadenopathy. *Cancer* 1979;**44**(5):1641–3.
44. Sallah S, Gagnon G. Angioimmunoblastic lymphadenopathy with dysproteinemia: emphasis on pathogenesis and treatment. *Acta Haematol* 1998;**99**:57–64.
45. Luppi M, Marasca R, Barozzi P, *et al.* Frequent detection of human herpesvirus-6 sequences by polymerase chain reaction in paraffin-embedded lymph nodes from patients with angioimmunoblastic lymphadenopathy and angioimmunoblastic lymphadenopathy-like lymphoma. *Leuk Res* 1993;**17**(11):1003–11.
46. Luppi M, Barozzi P, Garber R, *et al.* Expression of human herpesvirus-6 antigens in benign and malignant lymphoproliferative diseases. *Am J Pathol* 1998;**153**(11):815–23.
47. Weiss L, Jaffe E, Liu X, *et al.* Detection and localization of Epstein-Barr viral genomes in angioimmunoblastic lymphadenopathy and angioimmunoblastic lymphadenopathy-like lymphoma. *Blood* 1992;**79**(7):1789–95.
48. Brauninger A, Spieker T, Willenbrock K, *et al.* Survival and clonal expansion

of mutating "forbidden" (immunoglobulin receptor-deficient) Epstein-Barr virus-infected B cells in angioimmunoblastic T cell lymphoma. *J Exp Med* 2001;**194**(7):927–40.

49. Zettl A, Lee S, Rüdiger T, *et al.* Epstein-Barr virus-associated B-cell lymphoproliferative disorders in angioimmunoblastic T-cell lymphoma and peripheral T-cell lymphoma, unspecified. *Am J Clin Pathol* 2002; **117**(3):368–79.
50. Attygalle A, Al-Jehani R, Diss T, *et al.* Neoplastic T cells in angioimmunoblastic T-cell lymphoma express CD10. *Blood* 2002;**99**(2): 627–33.
51. Attygalle A, Kyriakou C, Dupuis J, *et al.* Histologic evolution of angioimmunoblastic T-cell lymphoma in consecutive biopsies: clinical correlation and insights into natural history and disease progression. *Am J Surg Pathol* 2007;**31**(7):1077–88.
52. de Leval L, Rickman D, Thielen C, *et al.* The gene expression profile of nodal peripheral T-cell lymphoma demonstrates a molecular link between angioimmunoblastic T-cell lymphoma (AITL) and follicular helper T (TFH) cells. *Blood* 2007;**109**(11): 4952–63.
53. Smith J, Hodges E, Quin C, *et al.* Frequent T and B cell oligoclones in histologically and immunophenotypically characterized angioimmunoblastic lymphadenopathy. *Am J Pathol* 2000;**156**(2):661–9.
54. Dogan A, Attygalle A, Kyriakou C. Angioimmunoblastic T-cell lymphoma. *Br J Haematol* 2003;**121**(5):681–91.
55. Ghani A, Krause J. Bone marrow biopsy findings in angioimmunoblastic lymphadenopathy. *Br J Haematol* 1985;**61**(2):203–13.
56. Stein H, Mason D, Gerdes J, *et al.* The expression of the Hodgkin's disease associated antigen Ki-1 in reactive and neoplastic lymphoid tissue: evidence that Reed-Sternberg cells and histiocytic malignancies are derived from activated lymphoid cells. *Blood* 1985;**66**(4): 848–58.
57. Weisenburger D, Anderson J, Diebold J, *et al.* Systemic anaplastic large-cell lymphoma: results from the non-Hodgkin lymphoma classification project. *Am J Hematol* 2001; **67**(3):172–8.
58. Falini B, Pileri S, Stein H, *et al.* Variable expression of leucocyte-common (CD45) antigen in CD30 (Ki1)-positive anaplastic large-cell lymphoma: implications for the differential diagnosis between lymphoid and nonlymphoid malignancies. *Hum Pathol* 1990;**21**(6):624–9.
59. Stein H, Gerdes J, Schwab U, *et al.* Identification of Hodgkin and Sternberg-Reed cells as a unique cell type derived from a newly-detected small-cell population. *Int J Cancer* 1982;**30**(4):445–59.
60. Savage KJ, Harris NL, Vose JM, *et al.* ALK-negative anaplastic large-cell lymphoma (ALCL) is clinically and immunophenotypically different from both ALK-positive ALCL and peripheral T-cell lymphoma, not otherwise specified: report from the International Peripheral T-Cell Lymphoma Project. *Blood* 2008; **111**(12):5496–504.
61. Hodges K, Collins R, Greer J, *et al.* Transformation of the small cell variant Ki-1+ lymphoma to anaplastic large cell lymphoma: pathologic and clinical features. *Am J Surg Pathol* 1999; **23**(1):49–58.
62. Bekkenk MW, Geelen FA, van Voorst Vader PC, *et al.* Primary and secondary cutaneous CD30(+) lymphoproliferative disorders: a report from the Dutch Cutaneous Lymphoma Group on the long-term follow-up data of 219 patients and guidelines for diagnosis and treatment. *Blood* 2000; **95**(12):3653–61.
63. Savage KJ, Chhanabhai M, Gascoyne RD, *et al.* Characterization of peripheral T-cell lymphomas in a single North American institution by the WHO classification. *Ann Oncol* 2004; **15**(10):1467–75.
64. Gale J, Simmonds P, Mead G, *et al.* Enteropathy-type intestinal T-cell lymphoma: clinical features and treatment of 31 patients in a single center. *J Clin Oncol* 2000;**18**(4):795.
65. Belhadj K, Reyes F, Farcet JP, *et al.* Hepatosplenic gammadelta T-cell lymphoma is a rare clinicopathologic entity with poor outcome: report on a series of 21 patients. *Blood* 2003;**102** (13):4261–9.
66. Gressin R, Peoch M, Deconinck E. The VIP-ABVD regimen is not superior to the CHOP 21 for the treatment of non epidermotropic peripheral T cell lymphoma. Final results of the LTP95 protocol of the GOELAMS. *Blood* 2006;**108**:697a.
67. Liang R, Loke S, Chan A. The prognostic factors for peripheral T-cell lymphomas. *Hematol Oncol* 1992; **10**(3–4):135–40.
68. d'Amore F, Lauritzsen G, Jantunen E, *et al.* 15. Clinical Results in Lymphoma II: 071 high-dose therapy (HDT) and autologous stem cell transplant as first line treatment in peripheral t-cell lymphomas. *Ann Oncol* 2005; **16**(suppl 5):v56.
69. Corradini P, Tarella C, Zallio F, *et al.* Long-term follow-up of patients with peripheral T-cell lymphomas treated up-front with high-dose chemotherapy followed by autologous stem cell transplantation. *Leukemia* 2006; **20**(9):1533–8.
70. Reimer P, Rudiger T, Einsele H, *et al.* Autologous stem cell transplantation as first-line therapy in peripheral T cell lymphomas: results of a prospective multicenter study. *J Clin Oncol* 2009; **27**(1):106–13.
71. Kyriakou C, Canals C, Goldstone A, *et al.* High-dose therapy and autologous stem-cell transplantation in angioimmunoblastic lymphoma: complete remission at transplantation is the major determinant of Outcome-Lymphoma Working Party of the European Group for Blood and Marrow Transplantation. *J Clin Oncol* 2008;**26**(2):218–24.
72. Horwitz S, Moskowitz C, Kewalramani T, *et al.* Second-line therapy with ICE followed by high dose therapy and autologous stem cell transplantation for relapsed/refractory peripheral T-cell lymphomas: minimal benefit when analyzed by intent to treat. *Blood* 2005;**106**(11):2679.
73. Smith SD, Bolwell BJ, Rybicki LA, *et al.* Autologous hematopoietic stem cell transplantation in peripheral T-cell lymphoma using a uniform high-dose regimen. *Bone Marrow Transplant* 2007;**40**(3):239–43.
74. Song KW, Mollee P, Keating A, *et al.* Autologous stem cell transplant for relapsed and refractory peripheral T-cell lymphoma: variable outcome according to pathological subtype. *Br J Haematol* 2003;**120**(6): 978–85.

75. Le Gouill S, Milpied N, Buzyn A, *et al.* Graft-versus-lymphoma effect for aggressive T-cell lymphomas in adults: a study by the Societe Francaise de Greffe de Moelle et de Therapie Cellulaire. *J Clin Oncol* 2008;**26** (14):2264–71.

76. Corradini P, Dodero A, Zallio F, *et al.* Graft-versus-lymphoma effect in relapsed peripheral T-cell non-Hodgkin's lymphomas after reduced-intensity conditioning followed by allogeneic transplantation of hematopoietic cells. *J Clin Oncol* 2004;**22**(11):2172–6.

77. Proietti F, Carneiro-Proietti A, Catalan-Soares B, *et al.* Global epidemiology of HTLV-I infection and associated diseases. *Oncogene* 2005;**24**(39): 6058–68.

78. Arisawa K, Soda M, Endo S, *et al.* Evaluation of adult T-cell leukemia/ lymphoma incidence and its impact on non-Hodgkin lymphoma incidence in southwestern Japan. *Int J Cancer* 2000;**85**(3):319–24.

79. Nicot C. Current views in HTLV-I-associated adult T-cell leukemia/ lymphoma. *Am J Hematol* 2005;**78** (3):232–9.

80. Yamano Y, Nagai M, Brennan M, *et al.* Correlation of human T-cell lymphotropic virus type 1 (HTLV-1) mRNA with proviral DNA load, virus-specific CD8+ T cells, and disease severity in HTLV-1-associated myelopathy (HAM/TSP). *Blood* 2002; **99**(1):88–94.

81. Murphy E, Hanchard B, Figueroa J, *et al.* Modelling the risk of adult T-cell leukemia/lymphoma in persons infected with human T-lymphotropic virus type I. *Int J Cancer* 1989; **43**(2):250–3.

82. Cleghorn F, Manns A, Falk R, *et al.* Effect of human T-lymphotropic virus type I infection on non-Hodgkin's lymphoma incidence. *J Natl Cancer Inst* 1995;**87**:1009–14.

83. Itoyama T, Chaganti R, Yamada Y, *et al.* Cytogenetic analysis and clinical significance in adult T-cell leukemia/ lymphoma: a study of 50 cases from the human T-cell leukemia virus type-1 endemic area, Nagasaki. *Blood* 2001; **97**(11):3612–20.

84. Takemoto S, Matsuoka M, Yamaguchi K, *et al.* A novel diagnostic method of adult T-cell leukemia: monoclonal integration of human T-cell lymphotropic virus type I provirus DNA detected by inverse polymerase chain reaction. *Blood* 1994;**84**(9): 3080–5.

85. Greenberg S, Jaffe E, Ehrlich G, *et al.* Kaposi's sarcoma in human T-cell leukemia virus type I-associated adult T-cell leukemia. *Blood* 1990;**76**(5): 971–6.

86. Tobinai K, Ohtsu T, Hayashi M, *et al.* Epstein-Barr virus (EBV) genome carrying monoclonal B-cell lymphoma in a patient with adult T-cell leukemia-lymphoma. *Leuk Res* 1991;**15**(9): 837–46.

87. Tsukasaki K, Hermine O, Bazarbachi A, *et al.* Definition, prognostic factors, treatment, and response criteria of adult T-cell leukemia-lymphoma: a proposal from an international consensus meeting. *J Clin Oncol* 2009;**27**(3): 453–9.

88. Tsukasaki K, Utsunomiya A, Fukuda H, *et al.* VCAP-AMP-VECP compared with biweekly CHOP for adult T-cell leukemia-lymphoma: Japan Clinical Oncology Group Study JCOG9801. *J Clin Oncol* 2007;**25**(34):5458–64.

89. Hermine O, Allard I, Levy V, *et al.* A prospective phase II clinical trial with the use of zidovudine and interferon-alpha in the acute and lymphoma forms of adult T-cell leukemia/lymphoma. *Hematol J* 2002;**3**(6):276–82.

90. Datta A, Bellon M, Sinha-Datta U, *et al.* Persistent inhibition of telomerase reprograms adult T-cell leukemia to p53-dependent senescence. *Blood* 2006;**108**(3):1021–9.

91. Bazarbachi A, Panelatti G, Ramos J, *et al.* A worldwide meta-analysis on the use of zidovudine and interferon-alpha for the treatment of adult T-cell leukemia/lymphoma. *Blood* 2007; **110**(11):2049.

92. Utsunomiya A, Miyazaki Y, Takatsuka Y, *et al.* Improved outcome of adult T cell leukemia/lymphoma with allogeneic hematopoietic stem cell transplantation. *Bone Marrow Transplant* 2001;**27**(1):15–20.

93. Kami M, Hamaki T, Miyakoshi S, *et al.* Allogeneic haematopoietic stem cell transplantation for the treatment of adult T-cell leukaemia/lymphoma. *Br J Haematol* 2003;**120**(2):304–9.

94. Jaffe E, Chan J, Su I, *et al.* Report of the Workshop on Nasal and Related Extranodal Angiocentric T/Natural Killer Cell Lymphomas. Definitions, differential diagnosis, and epidemiology. *Am J Surg Pathol* 1996; **20**(1):103–11.

95. Aozasa K, Takakuwa T, Hongyo T, *et al.* Nasal NK/T-cell lymphoma: epidemiology and pathogenesis. *Int J Hematol* 2008;**87**(2):110–17.

96. Chiang A, Tao Q, Srivastava G, *et al.* Nasal NK- and T-cell lymphomas share the same type of Epstein-Barr virus latency as nasopharyngeal carcinoma and Hodgkin's disease. *Int J Cancer* 1996;**68**(3):285–90.

97. Tao Q, Ho F, Loke S, *et al.* Epstein-Barr virus is localized in the tumour cells of nasal lymphomas of NK, T or B cell type. *Int J Cancer* 1995;**60**(3):315–20.

98. Chiang A, Chan A, Srivastava G, *et al.* Nasal T/natural killer (NK)-cell lymphomas are derived from Epstein-Barr virus-infected cytotoxic lymphocytes of both NK- and T-cell lineage. *Int J Cancer* 1997;**73**(3):332–8.

99. Van Gorp J, Weiping L, Jacobse K, *et al.* Epstein-Barr virus in nasal T-cell lymphomas (polymorphic reticulosis/ midline malignant reticulosis) in western China. *J Pathol* 1994; **173**(2):81–7.

100. Oyoshi MK, Nagata H, Kimura N, *et al.* Preferential expansion of V gamma 9-J gamma P/V delta 2-J delta 3 gammadelta T cells in nasal T-cell lymphoma and chronic active Epstein-Barr virus infection. *Am J Pathol* 2003;**162**(5):1629–38.

101. Kim W, Song S, Ahn Y, *et al.* CHOP followed by involved field radiation: is it optimal for localized nasal natural killer/T-cell lymphoma? *Ann Oncol* 2001;**12**(3):349–52.

102. Lee J, Kim W, Park Y, *et al.* Nasal-type NK/T cell lymphoma: clinical features and treatment outcome. *Br J Cancer* 2005;**92**:1226–30.

103. Lee J, Park Y, Kim W, *et al.* Extranodal nasal type NK/T-cell lymphoma: elucidating clinical prognostic factors for risk-based stratification of therapy. *Eur J Cancer* 2005;**41** (10):1402–8.

104. Kim T, Park Y, Lee S, *et al.* Local tumor invasiveness is more predictive of survival than International Prognostic Index in stage IE/IIE extranodal NK/T-cell lymphoma, nasal type. *Blood* 2005;**106**(12):3785–90.

105. Liang R. Diagnosis and management of primary nasal lymphoma of T-cell or NK-cell origin. *Clin Lymphoma Myeloma* 2000;**1**(1):33–7.

106. Lee K, Yun T, Kim D, *et al.* First-line ifosfamide, methotrexate, etoposide and prednisolone chemotherapy +/− radiotherapy is active in stage I/II extranodal NK/T-cell lymphoma. *Leuk Lymphoma* 2006;**47**(7):1274–82.

107. Chim C-S, Ma S-Y, Au W-Y, *et al.* Primary nasal natural killer cell lymphoma: long-term treatment outcome and relationship with the International Prognostic Index. *Blood* 2004;**103**(1):216–21.

108. Li Y, Yao B, Jin J, *et al.* Radiotherapy as primary treatment for stage IE and IIE nasal natural killer/T-cell lymphoma. *J Clin Oncol* 2006;**24**(1):181–9.

109. Peng YL, Huang HQ, Lin XB, *et al.* Clinical outcomes of patients with peripheral T-cell lymphoma (PTCL) treated by EPOCH regimen. *Ai Zheng* 2004;**23**(8):943–6.

110. Suzuki R, Suzumiya J, Nakamura S, *et al.* Hematopoietic stem cell transplantation for natural killer-cell lineage neoplasms. *Bone Marrow Transplant* 2006;**37**(4):425–31.

111. Cooke C, Krenacs L, Stetler-Stevenson M, *et al.* Hepatosplenic T-cell lymphoma: a distinct clinicopathologic entity of cytotoxic gamma delta T-cell origin. *Blood* 1996;**88**(11): 4265–74.

112. Suarez F, Wlodarska I, Rigal-Huguet F, *et al.* Hepatosplenic alpha beta T-cell lymphoma: an unusual case with clinical, histologic, and cytogenetic features of gammadelta hepatosplenic T-cell lymphoma. *Am J Surg Pathol* 2000;**24**(7):1027–32.

113. Macon W, Levy N, Kurtin P, *et al.* Hepatosplenic [alpha][beta] T-cell lymphomas: a report of 14 cases and comparison with hepatosplenic [gamma][delta] T-cell lymphomas. *Am J Surg Pathol* 2001;**25**(3):285–96.

114. Ahmad E, Kingma D, Jaffe E, *et al.* Flow cytometric immunophenotypic profiles of mature gamma delta T-cell malignancies involving peripheral blood and bone marrow. *Cytometry B Clin Cytom* 2005;**67**(1):6–12

115. Wong K, Chan J, Matutes E, *et al.* A distinctive aggressive lymphoma type. *Am J Surg Pathol* 1995;**19**(6): 718–26.

116. Chan J, Sin V, Wong K, *et al.* Nonnasal lymphoma expressing the natural killer cell marker CD56: a clinicopathologic study of 49 cases of an uncommon aggressive neoplasm. *Blood* 1997;**89** (12):4501–13.

117. Jonveaux P, Daniel MT, Martel V, *et al.* Isochromosome 7q and trisomy 8 are consistent primary, non-random chromosomal abnormalities associated with hepatosplenic T gamma/delta lymphoma. *Leukemia* 1996;**10**(9): 1453–5.

118. Coventry S. Consistency of isochromosome 7q and trisomy 8 in hepatosplenic gammadelta T-cell lymphoma: detection by fluorescence in situ hybridization of a splenic touch-preparation from a pediatric patient. *Pediatr Dev Pathol* 1999;**2** (5):478–83.

119. Santos E, Raez L, Salvatierra J, *et al.* Primary hepatic non-Hodgkin's lymphomas: case report and review of the literature. *Am J Gastroenterol* 2003;**98**(12):2789–93.

120. Hassan R, Franco S, Stefanoff C, *et al.* Hepatosplenic T-cell lymphoma following seven malaria infections. *Pathol Int* 2006;**56**(11):668–73.

121. Shale M, Kanfer E, Panaccione R, *et al.* Hepatosplenic T cell lymphoma in inflammatory bowel disease. *Gut* 2008;**57**(12):1639–41.

122. Mackey A, Green L, Liang L, *et al.* Hepatosplenic T cell lymphoma associated with infliximab use in young patients treated for inflammatory bowel disease. *J Pediatr Gastroenterol Nutr* 2007;**44**(2):265–7.

123. Weidmann E. Hepatosplenic T cell lymphoma. A review on 45 cases since the first report describing the disease as a distinct lymphoma entity in 1990. *Leukemia* 2000;**14**(6):991–7.

124. Grigg A. 2'-Deoxycoformycin for hepatosplenic gammadelta T-cell lymphoma. *Leuk Lymphoma* 2001;**42** (4):797.

125. Allory Y, Challine D, Haioun C, *et al.* Bone marrow involvement in lymphomas with hemophagocytic syndrome at presentation: a clinicopathologic study of 11 patients in a Western institution. *Am J Surg Pathol* 2001;**25**(7):865–74.

126. Chin M, Mugishima H, Takamura M, *et al.* Hemophagocytic syndrome and hepatosplenic gammadelta T-cell lymphoma with isochromosome 7q and 8 trisomy. *J Pediatr Hematol Oncol* 2004;**26**(6):375–8.

127. Iannitto E, Barbera V, Quintini G, *et al.* Hepatosplenic gammadelta T-cell lymphoma: complete response induced by treatment with pentostatin. *Br J Haematol* 2002;**117**(4):995–6.

128. Aribi A, Kantarjian H, O'Brien S, *et al.* Combination therapy with alemtuzumab and pentostatin is effective and has acceptable toxicity in patients with T-lymphoid neoplasms. *J Clin Oncol* 2007;**25**(18 Suppl):7037.

129. Jaeger G, Bauer F, Brezinschek R, *et al.* Hepatosplenic gammadelta T-cell lymphoma successfully treated with a combination of alemtuzumab and cladribine. *Ann Oncol* 2008; **19**(5):1025–6.

130. Konuma T, Ooi J, Takahashi S, *et al.* Allogeneic stem cell transplantation for hepatosplenic gammadelta T-cell lymphoma. *Leuk Lymphoma* 2007; **43**(3):630–2.

131. Gull W. Fatty stools from disease of the mesenteric glands. *Guy's Hosp Rep* 1855;**1**:369–72.

132. Isaacson P, Wright D. Intestinal lymphoma associated with malabsorption. *Lancet* 1978;**1** (8055):67–70.

133. Isaacson PG, O'Connor NT, Spencer J, *et al.* Malignant histiocytosis of the intestine: a T-cell lymphoma. *Lancet* 1985;**2**(8457):688–91.

134. Holmes G, Prior P, Lane M, *et al.* Malignancy in coeliac disease–effect of a gluten free diet. *Gut* 1989;**30**(3):333–8.

135. Trier J. Celiac sprue. *N Engl J Med* 1991;**325**(24):1709–19.

136. Leonard J, Tucker W, Fry J, *et al.* Increased incidence of malignancy in dermatitis herpetiformis. *Br Med J (Clin Res Ed)* 1983;**286**(6358):16–18.

137. Catassi C, Fabiani E, Corrao G, *et al.* Risk of non-Hodgkin lymphoma in celiac disease. *Am Med Assoc* 2002; **287**(11):1413–19.

138. Isaacson P, Du M. Gastrointestinal lymphoma: where morphology meets molecular biology. *J Pathol* 2005; **205**(2):255–74.

139. Al-Toma A, Goerres M, Meijer J, *et al.* Human leukocyte antigen–DQ2 homozygosity and the development of refractory celiac disease and enteropathy-associated T-cell

lymphoma. *Clin Gastroenterol Hepatol* 2006;**4**(3):315–19.

140. Gale J, Simmonds P, Mead G, *et al.* Enteropathy-type T-cell lymphoma: clinical features and treatment of 31 patients in a single institution. *J Clin Oncol* 2000;**18**:795–803.

141. Cellier C, Delabesse E, Helmer C, *et al.* Refractory sprue, coeliac disease, and enteropathy-associated T-cell lymphoma. *Lancet* 2000;**356** (9225):203–8.

142. Russell G, Nagler-Anderson C, Anderson P, *et al.* Cytotoxic potential of intraepithelial lymphocytes (IELs). Presence of TIA-1, the cytolytic granule-associated protein, in human IELs in normal and diseased intestine. *Am J Pathol* 1993;**143**(2):350–4.

143. De Bruin P, Connolly C, Oudejans J, *et al.* Enteropathy-associated T-cell lymphomas have a cytotoxic T-cell phenotype. *Histopathology* 1997; **31**(4):313–17.

144. Quintanilla-Martinez L, Lome-Maldonado C, Ott G, *et al.* Primary non-Hodgkin's lymphoma of the intestine: high prevalence of Epstein-Barr virus in Mexican lymphomas as compared with European cases. *Blood* 1997;**89**(2):644–51.

145. Ko Y, Ree H, Kim W, *et al.* Clinicopathologic and genotypic study of extranodal nasal-type natural killer/ T-cell lymphoma and natural killer precursor lymphoma among Koreans. *Cancer* 2000; **89**(10):2106–16.

146. Daum S, Weiss D, Hummel M, *et al.* Frequency of clonal intraepithelial T lymphocyte proliferations in enteropathy-type intestinal T cell lymphoma, coeliac disease, and refractory sprue. *Gut* 2001; **49**(6):804–12.

147. Zettl A, Ott G, Makulik A, *et al.* Chromosomal gains at 9q characterize enteropathy-type T-cell lymphoma. *Am J Pathol* 2002;**161**(5):1635–45.

148. Hoffmann M, Vogelsang H, Kletter K, *et al.* 18F-fluoro-deoxy-glucose positron emission tomography (18F-FDG-PET) for assessment of enteropathy-type T cell lymphoma. *Gut* 2003;**52**(3):347–51.

149. Culliford A, Daly J, Diamond B, *et al.* The value of wireless capsule endoscopy in patients with complicated celiac disease. *Gastrointest Endosc* 2005;**62**(1): 55–61.

150. Daum S, Ullrich R, Heise W, *et al.* Intestinal non-Hodgkin's lymphoma: a multicenter prospective clinical study from the German Study Group on Intestinal non-Hodgkin's Lymphoma. *J Clin Oncol* 2003;**21**(14): 2740–6.

151. Enblad G, Hagberg H, Erlanson M, *et al.* A pilot study of alemtuzumab (anti-CD52 monoclonal antibody) therapy for patients with relapsed or chemotherapy-refractory peripheral T-cell lymphomas. *Blood* 2004; **103**(8):2920–4.

152. Soldini D, Mora O, Cavalli F, *et al.* Efficacy of alemtuzumab and gemcitabine in a patient with enteropathy-type T-cell lymphoma. *Br J Haematol* 2008; **142**(3):484–6.

153. Bishton M, Haynes A. Combination chemotherapy followed by autologous stem cell transplant for enteropathy-associated T cell lymphoma. *Br J Haematol* 2007;**136**(1): 111–13.

154. Al-toma A, Visser O, van Roessel H, *et al.* Autologous hematopoietic stem cell transplantation in refractory celiac disease with aberrant T cells. *Blood* 2007;**109**(5):2243–9.

155. Dang N, Pro B, Hagemeister F, *et al.* Phase II trial of denileukin diftitox for relapsed/refractory T-cell non-Hodgkin lymphoma. *Br J Haematol* 2007; **136**(3):439–47.

156. Zinzani PL, Alinari L, Tani M, *et al.* Preliminary observations of a phase II study of reduced-dose alemtuzumab treatment in patients with pretreated T-cell lymphoma. *Haematologica* 2005; **90**(5):702–3.

157. Gallamini A, Zaja F, Patti C, *et al.* Alemtuzumab (Campath-1H) and CHOP chemotherapy as first-line treatment of peripheral T-cell lymphoma: results of a GITIL (Gruppo Italiano Terapie Innovative nei Linfomi) prospective multicenter trial. *Blood* 2007;**110**(7):2316–23.

158. Trumper L, Hohloch K, Kloess M, *et al.* CHOP/CHOEP-14 followed by consolidation with alemtuzumab in untreated aggressive T-cell lymphomas (DSHNHL 2003–1): feasibility and toxicity of a phase II trial of the German High Grade Non-Hodgkin's Lymphoma Group DSHNHL. *J Clin Oncol* 2006;**24** (18 Suppl):7538.

159. Sallah S, Wan JY, Nguyen NP. Treatment of refractory T-cell malignancies using gemcitabine. *Br J Haematol* 2001;**113**(1):185–7.

160. Kim JG, Sohn SK, Chae YS, *et al.* CHOP plus etoposide and gemcitabine (CHOP-EG) as front-line chemotherapy for patients with peripheral T cell lymphomas. *Cancer Chemother Pharmacol* 2006;**58**(1):35–9.

161. O'Connor O, Hamlin P, Gerecitano J. Pralatrexate (PDX) produces durable complete remissions in patients with chemotherapy resistant precursor and peripheral T-cell lymphomas: results of the MSKCC phase I/II experience. *Blood* 2006;**108**:122a.

162. Piekarz R, Wright J, Frye R, *et al.* Final results of a phase 2 NCI multicenter study of romidepsin in patients with relapsed peripheral T-cell lymphoma (PTCL). *Blood* 2009;**114**(22):1657.

Chapter 22

Mycosis fungoides and Sézary syndrome

Christiane Querfeld and Steven T. Rosen

Introduction

Cutaneous T-cell lymphomas (CTCL) represent a clinically and biologically heterogeneous group of non-Hodgkin lymphomas with clonal proliferation of malignant T lymphocytes homing into the skin according to the new revised World Health Organization and European Organization for Research and Treatment of Cancer (WHO–EORTC) consensus classification for cutaneous lymphomas.[1] Mycosis fungoides (MF) and the aggressive and leukemic variant Sézary syndrome (SS), collectively referred to as CTCL, are the most common and best studied entities. CTCL include other entities such as lymphomatoid papulosis (LyP) and primary cutaneous anaplastic large T-cell lymphoma (ALCL), which belong to the CD30+ lymphoproliferative disorders and other rare diseases with distinct clinical features (Table 22.1).

MF disease is characterized by a chronic, slowly progressing course.[2] The clinical manifestations typically include erythematous patches, evolving into plaques and/or tumors (Figure 22.1a–c). Patients usually present with a prolonged history of a skin rash in sun-protected areas such as lower abdomen, upper thighs, buttocks, and breasts in women. Patients with cutaneous patch/plaque disease have an excellent prognosis and a normal life expectancy compared with age-matched individuals. However, 20% of patients progress into more aggressive and advanced disease with either cutaneous or extracutaneous tumor manifestations. Three major variants have been recognized in the new WHO–EORTC classification including granulomatous slack skin, clinically characterized by the development of erythematous lax skin folds and histologically by a granulomatous T-cell infiltrate and loss of elastic fibers, folliculotropic MF, characterized by involvement of hair follicles with or without mucin deposition often leading to alopecia, and pagetoid reticulosis (Woringer–Kolopp disease), presenting as a slowly enlarging, solitary psoriasiform patch with intraepidermal involvement of atypical (pagetoid) T cells expressing a CD4−CD8+ phenotype.

SS is an aggressive variant of CTCL with a leukemic component. SS represents approximately 3–5% of newly diagnosed patients with CTCL.[1,3] It is characterized by circulating, atypical, malignant T lymphocytes with cerebriform nuclei (Sézary cells), the presence of erythroderma, and often lymphadenopathy. Severe pruritus, ectropion, alopecia, dystrophic nails, and palmoplantar keratoderma with fissures are common associated features (Figure 22.2). Patients with MF may develop erythroderma, leading to a disorder termed erythrodermic MF. In contrast to patients with SS, there is low if any blood involvement.[3]

Epidemiology

Cutaneous lymphomas are a group of rare diseases that represent 3.9% of all non-Hodgkin lymphoma. MF represents the most common type of CTCL comprising 50% of all cutaneous lymphomas. The incidence of CTCL has risen consistently since 1973 with an overall annual age-adjusted incidence of 6.4 cases per million population.[4,5] Incidence was higher among males and blacks and increases with age. A substantial geographic variation in incidence is seen in the United States based on 13 cancer registries (SEER-13). Data suggest an interesting association with higher physician density and higher socioeconomic status. Patients with MF and SS are at significantly increased risk of developing a second primary lymphoma, in particular Hodgkin lymphoma.[6]

Etiology

Several groups have proposed microbiologic, environmental, and occupational factors in the etiology of CTCL, but none have yet been verified. It has been suggested that the condition results from persistent antigen stimulation with an increased risk for the development of CTCL in patients exposed to chemicals or pesticides; however, recent studies on the subject produced controversial results.[7,8] Unlike adult T-cell leukemia/lymphoma (ATLL), which is etiologically associated with human T-lymphocyte virus 1 (HTLV-1), most patients with CTCL are serologically negative for HTLV-1.[9] Other investigators have found serologic evidence for Epstein–Barr virus (EBV) and cytomegalovirus (CMV), but evidence is scarce.[10,11]

Management of Hematologic Malignancies, ed. Susan M. O'Brien, Julie M. Vose, and Hagop M. Kantarjian. Published by Cambridge University Press.

Table 22.1. The new WHO–EORTC consensus classification for primary cutaneous lymphomas with relative frequency and 5-year survival

WHO–EORTC	Frequency (%)	5-year survival (%)
Cutaneous T-cell and NK-cell lymphoma		
Indolent		
Mycosis fungoides	44	88
• Follicular MF	4	80
• Pagetoid reticulosis	<1	100
• Granulomatous slack skin	<1	100
CD30+ lymphoprolif. diseases		
• Anaplastic large cell lymphoma	8	95
• Lymphomatoid papulosis	12	100
Subcutaneous panniculitis-like T-cell lymphoma	1	82
CD4+ small/medium pleomorphic T-cell lymphoma	2	72
Aggressive		
Sézary syndrome	3	24
Cutaneous peripheral T-cell lymphoma, unspecified	2	16
• Cutaneous aggressive CD8+ T-cell lymphoma	<1	18
• Cutaneous γ/δ T-cell lymphoma	<1	–
Cutaneous NK/T-cell lymphoma, nasal type	<1	–
Cutaneous B-cell lymphoma		
Indolent		
Follicle center cell lymphoma	11	95
Marginal zone lymphoma	7	99
Intermediate clinical behavior		
Large B-cell lymphoma of the leg	4	55
Cutaneous diffuse large B-cell lymphoma, other	<1	50
Intravascular large B-cell lymphoma	<1	65

Source: Produced from Willemze *et al.*[1]

Immunosuppression and/or immunosuppressive therapy might be a risk factor for the development of CTCL, as documented in patients following organ transplant or treatment of Hodgkin lymphoma, and in human immunodeficiency virus (HIV)-positive patients.[12–14]

Molecular and biologic characteristics

The pathogenesis of MF/SS is characterized by an altered immune biology and the accumulation of cytogenetic abnormalities during disease progression.[15] Immunophenotyping studies revealed that the neoplastic T cells in MF/SS typically bear a CD4+ T-helper/memory antigenic profile with frequent loss of the CD7 and/or CD26 antigen in advanced stages.[16] Absence of CD26 expression on atypical circulating CD4+ T cells is a highly sensitive marker for diagnosis and therapeutic monitoring of patients with SS.[16] The malignant cells show clonal rearrangements for the gene that encodes the T-cell receptor (TCR).[17] Persistent activation of the neoplastic T cells is demonstrated by the constitutive phosphorylation of intracellular signaling protein Stat3.[18] These cells may express the activation markers CD45RO and the interleukin 2 (IL-2) alpha receptor (CD25).[19]

Microarray studies have been performed to reveal unique gene expression patterns of CTCL. Several genes involved in the pathogenesis of CTCL have been identified. Expression profiles showed upregulation of genes involved in the tumor necrosis factor (TNF)-signaling pathway and decreased expression of tumor suppressor genes such as transforming growth factor beta (TGF-β) receptor II while *EPHA4* and *TWIST* were overexpressed.[20,21] Aberrant expression of *STAT4*, *GATA3*, T-plastin, CD1D, TRAIL, CDO1, and DNM3 were also found and may serve as potential targets for novel treatment strategies.[22,23] Patients with large cell transformation show chromosomal clonal evolution with changes in ploidy levels and structural aberrations.[24] Evidence of epigenetic silencing of hypermethylation of individual genes or gene-specific promoters and microsatellite instability is associated with tumor progression in advanced stages of CTCL.[25,26]

The skin-homing mechanism of malignant T cells is not completely elucidated, but may be partially explained by their expression of specific chemokine receptors and adhesion molecules. Data have shown that skin homing T cells isolated from patients with MF/SS express cutaneous lymphocyte antigen (CLA), chemokine receptor (CCR)-4, and CCR-10, which bind to their corresponding skin-derived ligands on endothelial cells, keratinocytes, and/or Langerhans cells, thereby facilitating migration into the dermis and epidermis.[27] The CXCR4 chemokine receptor might also have a role in skin homing of Sézary cells. Furthermore, loss of CD26 has been shown to enhance migration of cell lines derived from patients with SS.[28]

The clinical course is accompanied by dysregulated synthesis of Th-1/Th-2 cytokines. The skewed ratio of T-helper cell type 1 (Th-1) and type 2 (Th-2) has been hypothesized to be critical for disease progression.[29] In advanced stages there is a dominant Th-2 cytokine profile leading to an impaired cell-mediated immune response. The number of reactive cytotoxic CD8+ T cells and dendritic cells, which are characteristic in early patch stage cutaneous lesions, tend to decrease with increase of neoplastic CD4+ T cells and correlate with disease progression.[30,31] Disease progression has also been

(a)

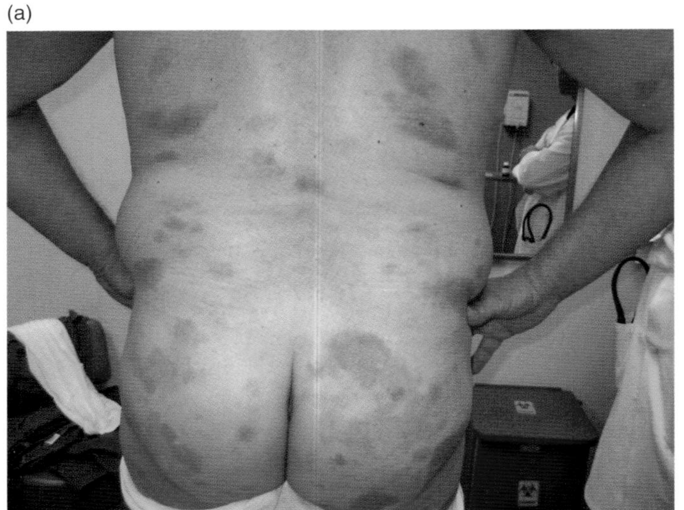

(b)

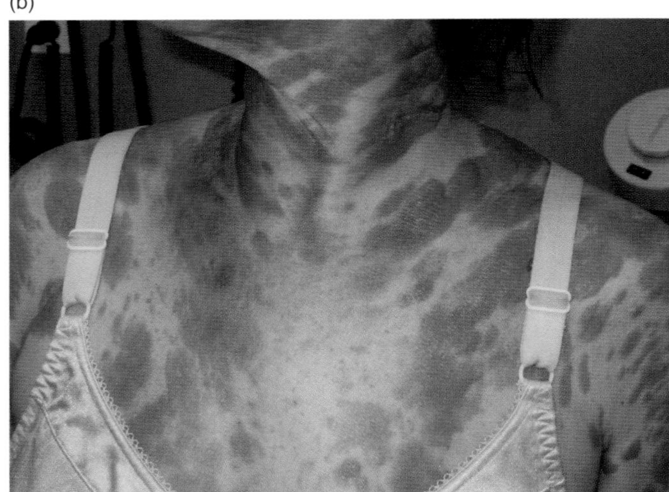

(c)

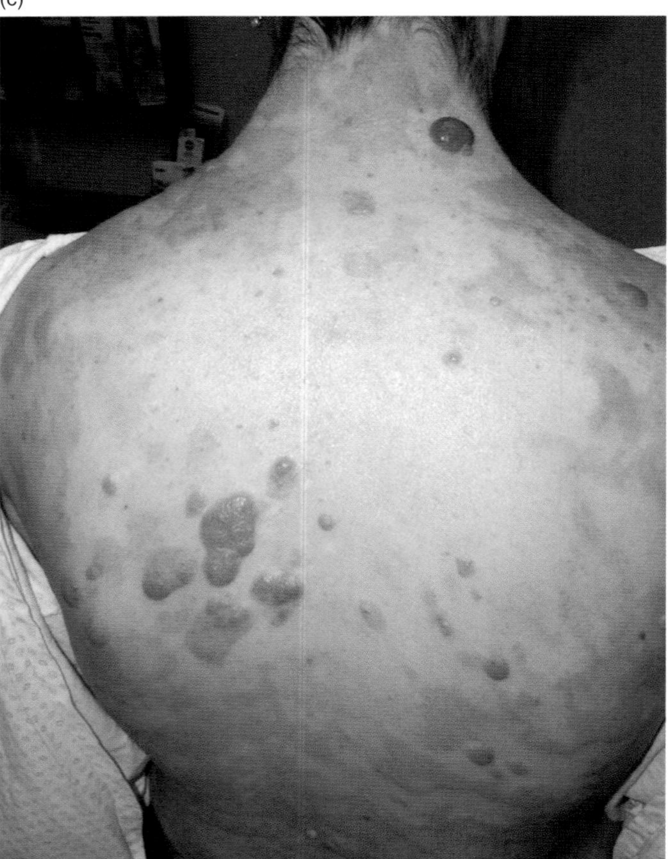

Figure 22.1 Clinical presentation of patients with mycosis fungoides, patch (a), plaque (b), and tumor stage (c).

associated with a substantial reduction in the normal T-cell receptor repertoire. In addition, recent data suggest that MF/SS may be associated with alterations in regulatory T cells (Tregs) that contribute to the immune suppression seen with these disorders.

Clinical manifestation

Early stages of MF can typically present with patches. The early patch stage may resemble eczema, psoriasis, secondary syphilis, atopic dermatitis, or "pre-mycotic" parapsoriasis. Diagnosis is often delayed or missed in early-stage patients pretreated

(a)

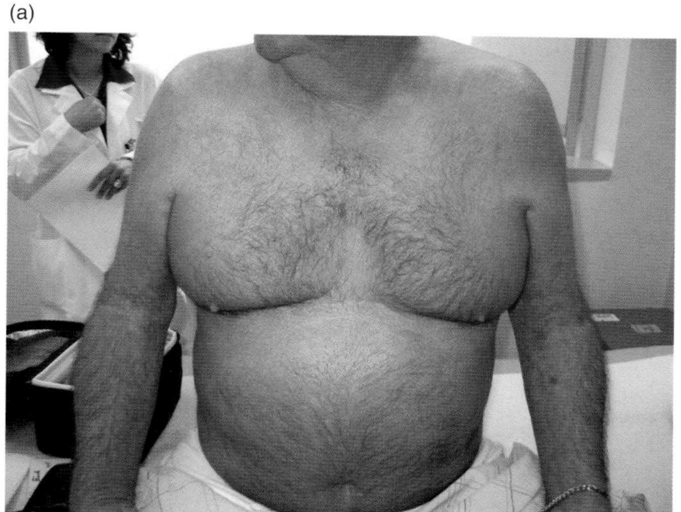

(b)

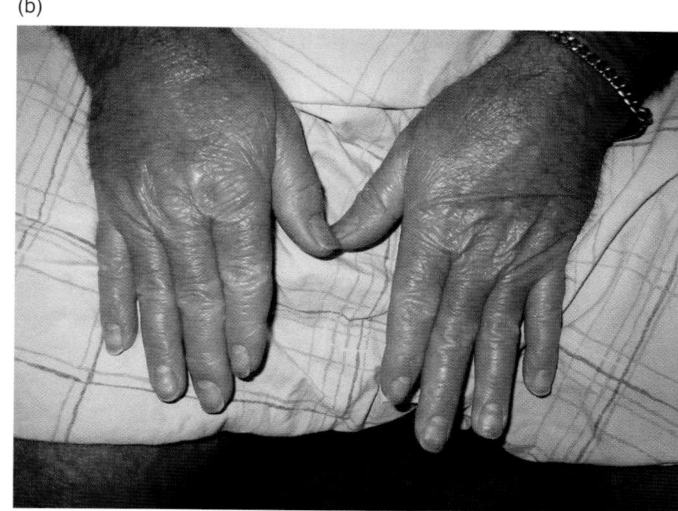

Figure 22.2 Patient with Sézary syndrome with generalized exfoliative erythroderma (a) and palmar keratoderma (b).

with topical corticosteroids. Most patients have multiple biopsies before being diagnosed. The interval between the onset of skin lesions to the definitive diagnosis ranges from 4 to 10 years, with a mean of 6 years. To further complicate diagnosis, observations about invisible MF cases with recalcitrant pruritus have been reported and documented MF variants mimicking a plethora of benign disorders. With progressive invasion and infiltration of the skin by the malignant T cells patches evolve into plaques and/or tumors. In advanced stages of MF the patients show a combination of patches, plaques, and nodular/tumor lesions or diffuse erythroderma.

Patients with SS mostly present with severe disabling pruritus. The skin appearance may vary from mild erythema to generalized exfoliative erythroderma with keratoderma and fissures on palms and soles. Other problems include electrolyte imbalance, hypothermia, hair loss, and eye changes (ectropion). Lymphadenopathy is often but not always present. Diagnosis may be missed in the elderly whose symptoms of dry skin and pruritus are attributed to advanced age. Cutaneous drug reactions, infectious conditions, generalized seborrheic dermatitis, psoriasis, and chronic photosensitivity reactions may resemble erythrodermic MF.

Diagnosis

Several histologic features are useful in establishing a diagnosis of MF/SS.[32] In most cases, it consists of an upper-dermal band-like lymphocytic infiltrate with atypical lymphocytes with cerebriform nuclei, variable findings of inflammatory cells, and epidermal involvement with solitary cells or clusters of malignant lymphocytes (Pautrier's microabscesses). Tumor lesions express more diffuse and deep infiltrates with diminished epidermotropism. A large cell phenotype is not an uncommon feature in tumor stage MF. Biopsies from erythrodermic MF or SS often lack epidermotropism or Pautrier's microabscesses and may show a mild perivascular or superficial dermal infiltrate of atypical lymphocytes and minimal exocytosis of these cells into the epidermis. As MF has numerous variants histopathology may also show involvement of hair follicles and other skin adnexae, granulomatous changes, or vascular and subcutaneous tissue infiltration.

Immunophenotyping by immunohistochemistry on skin biopsies or flow cytometry on skin and blood samples has an important role in the evaluation of CTCL. Studies have demonstrated an increased CD4/CD8 ratio, loss of subset markers such as CD26 and CD7, and aberrant expression or loss of pan-T-cell markers such as CD2, CD3, and CD5 in many affected patients.[16]

In its earliest stages, MF is often diagnosed as dermatitis and a definitive diagnosis may be difficult to establish, therefore the presence of a dominant T-cell clone is an important diagnostic criterion. Clonal rearrangements can be detected both by Southern blotting or by using the polymerase chain reaction (PCR) single-strand conformational polymorphism analysis, which is the most sensitive technique to detect clonality.[33,34] These molecular studies represent an important adjuvant procedure, in association with histopathology and immunophenotyping, to support the clinical diagnosis.

All patients with MF/SS should initially be seen and co-managed by a multidisciplinary cutaneous lymphoma team consisting of members from dermatology and oncology with the support of other health professionals such as radiation oncologists, pathologists, and clinical psychologists. Routine evaluation should include complete physical examination, complete blood count with differential and peripheral blood smear for Sézary cell count, chemistry panel with lactate dehydrogenase (LDH), skin biopsy for histology, immunophenotyping, and gene rearrangement studies, and lymph node biopsies in cases with enlarged nodes at presentation to establish the diagnosis and staging. Baseline and serial photographs of the skin are of great value. Serologic tests for HIV and HTLV-1 should be considered in certain patients. Diagnosis in early stages of MF has been improved due to advances in T-cell receptor (TCR) gene rearrangement analyses with increased sensitivity and specificity.[17,35] Imaging studies should be reserved for patients with clinical and laboratory findings suggestive of systemic disease or prominent lymphadenopathy. Bone marrow biopsy is a consideration in advanced-stage disease. Histopathologic and molecular results should be correlated with clinical findings and patients classified according to the WHO–EORTC consensus classification.

Staging and prognosis

Accurate staging of patients with MF/SS is essential both for its prognostic value and for treatment decisions. In contrast to the staging system that is traditionally used for other lymphomas, the widely used and recommended staging system for CTCL relies on the TNMB (tumor, node, metastasis, blood) classification adopted by Bunn and Lamberg in 1979[36] that has been revised to include blood stage (Tables 22.2 and 22.3). It considers the extent of skin involvement (T), presence of lymph node (N) and visceral disease (M), and detection of Sézary cells in the peripheral blood (B).

Patients with stage IA disease (T1, N0, M0) have limited patch/plaque disease with less than 10% of body surface area involvement. Patients are usually asymptomatic and may remain at this stage for years. As patches and plaques involve more than 10% of the body surface area, patients are classified as stage IB disease (T2, N0, M0). Stage IIA disease (T1–2, N1, M0) includes the skin findings of stage IA or IB disease with the additional presence of lymphadenopathy. Stage IIB (T3, N0/1, M0) is associated with the development of skin tumors, which may arise de novo or in preexisting patches or plaques with or without associated lymphadenopathy. Patients with erythroderma have stage III disease (IIIA: T4, N0, M0; IIIB: T4, N1, M0). Involvement of nodes by tumor cells (LN3, LN4) without visceral involvement is classified as stage IVA (T1–4, NP1, M0), and with visceral and/or bone marrow involvement classified as stage IVB (T1–4, N0–NP1, M1). The International Society for Lymphoma (ISCL) has recommended definitions based on the degree of blood involvement for subsets of erythrodermic CTCL (E-CTCL) to address the differences among E-CTCL.[3] B1-rating would be defined as Sézary cell count of less than 1000 cells/m^3 or less than 20% Sézary cells on peripheral smear. B2-rating would be more than 1000 cells/m^3 or greater than 20% Sézary cells on peripheral smear.

Histologic classification of lymph node (LN) involvement is also used as prognostic value and for treatment decisions in patients diagnosed with MF/SS.[38] It was found that the LN class correlates with disease progression and survival.[38,39] Moreover, detection of a monoclonal T-cell population within nodes is associated with an inferior survival and outcome regardless of the LN class.[40] LN1-rating defines reactive changes, LN2 and LN3 nodes describe small or large clusters

Table 22.2. Revised TNMB classification for patients with mycosis fungoides and Sézary syndrome

T (skin)	
T1	Limited patch/plaque (< 10% of BSA)
T2	Generalized patch/plaque (> 10% of BSA)
T3	Tumors
T4	Generalized erythroderma
N (nodes)	
N0	No clinically abnormal peripheral lymph nodes
N1	Clinically abnormal peripheral lymph nodes
NP0	Biopsy performed, not CTCL
NP1	Biopsy performed, CTCL
LN0	Uninvolved
LN1	Reactive lymph node
LN2	Dermatopathic node, small clusters of convoluted cells (< 6 cells per cluster)
LN3[a]	Dermatopathic node, large clusters of convoluted cells (> 6 cells per cluster)
LN4[a]	Lymph node effacement
M (viscera)	
M0	No visceral metastasis
M1	Visceral metastasis
B (blood)	
B0	Atypical circulating cells not present (< 5%)
B1	Atypical circulating cells present (> 5%)

Note: [a]Pathologically involved lymph nodes.
TNMB: tumor, node, metastasis, blood; BSA: body surface area.
Source: Olsen *et al.*[37]

Table 22.3. Stage classification for patients with mycosis fungoides and Sézary syndrome

Stage	T	N	NP	M
IA	1	0	0	0
IB	2	0	0	0
IIA	1/2	1	0	0
IIB	3	0/1	0	0
III	4	0/1	0	0
IVA	1–4	0/1	1	0
IVB	1–4	0/1	0/1	1

Source: Olsen *et al.*[37]

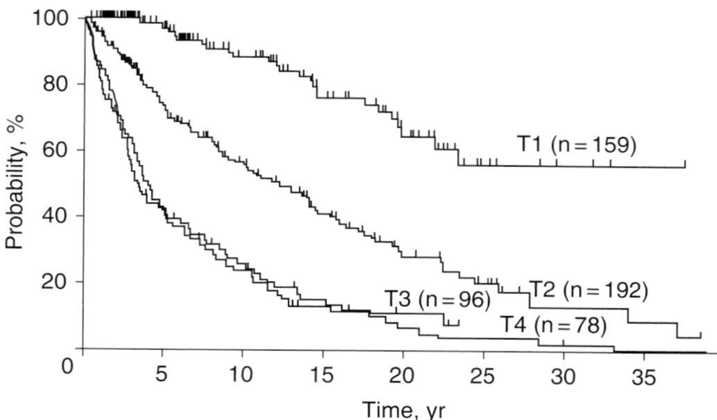

Figure 22.3 An update of the Stanford experience shows the actuarial overall survival of 525 patients with mycosis fungoides and Sézary syndrome according to their T-classification at diagnosis (T1–T4).[41] The risk for disease progression correlates with the severity of the initial skin presentation.

of atypical cells in paracortical T-cell regions, while LN4 nodes define frank effacement.

The Stanford experience with MF/SS demonstrates the impact of stage on overall survival (Figure 22.3). The risk for disease progression correlates with the severity of the initial skin presentation.

Prognostic markers

The most important predictive factors for survival remain the T classification, extracutaneous manifestation, and patient age.[41] In addition, several independent adverse prognostic factors have been identified including large cell transformation, follicular mucinosis, thickness of tumor infiltrate, and increased LDH and β_2-microglobulin.[42,43] Patients with large circulating Sézary cells were also found to have a worse prognosis. A high Sézary cell count, loss of T-cell subset markers such as CD5 and CD7, and chromosomal abnormalities in T cells are also independently associated with a poor outcome.[44] The existence of a blood clonal T-cell population, detected by PCR, was of poor predictive survival value independent of the T stage and lymph node involvement.[45] The increased number of cytotoxic CD8+ T lymphocytes in the dermal infiltrate, as well as the density of epidermal Langerhans cells greater than 90 cells/mm^2 is associated with a better prognosis.[30,46]

Treatment options

The development of treatment strategies for patients with CTCL is influenced by the extent of disease (TNMB stage) and its impact on the patient's quality of life. Prolonged complete remissions have been obtained in patients with limited disease, though it is not clear that the disease has been cured. A trial randomizing patients to sequential topical and subsequent single-agent chemotherapy versus an intervention with multiagent chemotherapies combined with electron beam radiation failed to show a survival benefit.[47]

Early stage (IA to IIA) MF has a favorable prognosis. The disease is mostly limited to the upper dermis and epidermis, which makes skin-directed therapies appealing. Current topical therapies include corticosteroids, nitrogen mustard (mechlorethamine), carmustine (1,3-bis(2-chloroethyl)-I-nitrosourea, BCNU), bexarotene, phototherapy with psoralens and ultraviolet light A (PUVA), UVB or narrowband (NB)-UVB, and total skin electron beam therapy (TSEBT).[48] Refractory patients in early stages benefit from combination therapies such as PUVA or NB-UVB with low-dose systemic bexarotene or interferon alpha (IFN-α). Treatment goals in advanced stages of MF/SS should be to reduce tumor burden, to relieve symptoms, to delay disease progression, and to preserve quality of life. In particular, SS is known to be refractory to most therapies and historically no treatment has been demonstrated to modify significantly the natural course of this disease. Current approaches focus upon biologic agents and reconstitution of the immune function using interferons, IL-12, extracorporeal photopheresis (ECP), oral bexarotene, monoclonal antibodies, recombinant toxins, and combinations of the aforementioned for disease control. Single or localized skin tumors are ideally treated with spot-radiation. Mono- or polychemotherapies are best reserved for patients with rapidly progressing disease that needs immediate palliation. High-dose chemotherapy followed by allogeneic stem cell transplantation (SCT) might be an option for younger patients with advanced disease refractory to multiple regimens. A representative treatment algorithm amended from the EORTC therapeutic recommendations is presented in Figure 22.4.

Topical treatments

Phototherapy

Phototherapy is one of the traditional treatment modalities in CTCL. Of the available phototherapies PUVA therapy has been widely used with established benefit in early-stage MF for more than 25 years. It involves treatment with orally administered 8-methoxypsoralen (8-MOP [UVADEX]) that sensitizes the skin to UVA irradiation. The initial UVA dosage is approximately 0.5 J/cm^2 and will be increased per treatment as tolerated or up to the minimal erythema dose. Patients are required to use proper eye protection for 12–24 hours after a PUVA treatment to prevent the formation of cataracts. PUVA has been successfully utilized since 1976 in the treatment of early-stage MF, but was also found to moderately affect skin lesions of patients with advanced MF/SS.[49] Therapy is typically given three times a week until complete remission (CR) is achieved. Additional maintenance therapy can be administered while gradually reducing PUVA to once every 4–6 weeks, to maintain longer remission times. Several studies confirmed high remission rates in early stages of MF with reported CR in up to 71.4% of patients.[50,51] PUVA has also been successfully applied in the treatment of hypopigmented MF.[52] Although being effective in clearing superficial lesions, PUVA has its limitations in clearing deeply infiltrated lesions. Still,

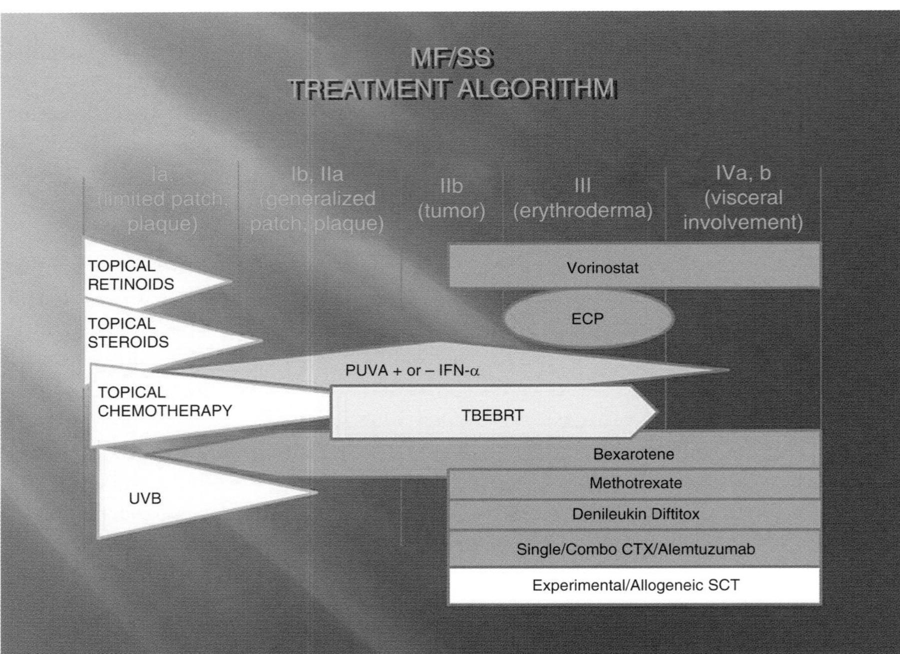

Figure 22.4 Treatment algorithm for mycosis fungoides/Sézary syndrome according to Zic and Pinter-Brown. CTX, chemotherapy; TBEBRT, total body external beam radiation therapy.

the Scandinavian Mycosis Fungoides Study Group reported an overall response rate of 82% with CR in 8 (47%) and partial remission (PR) in 6 of 17 (35%) patients with cutaneous tumor stage. Most of these patients, however, had concomitant therapy with topical nitrogen mustard or systemic chemotherapy. Long-term remissions of more than 8 years have been reported in patients with early-stage MF.[53] Disease-free survival rates for stage IA at 5 and 10 years were 56% and 30%, respectively and for stage IB/IIA 74% and 50%. The most common reported acute side effects were erythema, pruritus, and nausea, which were usually mild at presentation and generally manageable with dose adjustments of UVA or 8-MOP or dose interruptions. Long-term exposure was associated with an increased risk for developing chronic photodamage and non-melanoma skin cancer in about one-third of patients. Two multicenter, dose-randomized evaluations of oral low-dose bexarotene (75 mg or 150 mg daily for 24 weeks) and PUVA in patients with stage IB–IIA CTCL are ongoing in the USA and Europe. Preliminary results have shown a similar response rate as PUVA monotherapy, but the results were achieved with lower cumulative Joules (J. Guitart, personal communication, 2008). Folliculotropic MF is often less responsive to PUVA. Combined treatment with low-dose bexarotene or IFN-α may be considered in such cases.

The efficacy of broadband UVB is more limited to patch stage, while PUVA is also effective in clearing plaques. The effects of UVB phototherapy were retrospectively evaluated in 37 patients with MF limited to patch/plaque disease.[54] Seventy-one percent achieved CR with a median duration of 22 months. Eighty-three percent of patients with disease limited to patches achieved remission, whereas none of the patients with plaque disease achieved remission. NB-UVB is considered to be less carcinogenic and may offer an alternative treatment option in early-stage MF, but randomized clinical trials are needed to confirm its efficacy and long-term remission rates. In three small retrospective analyses patients with clinical stage IA/IB and parapsoriasis and treated with NB-UVB showed CR rates between 54.2% and 83%.[55,56] However, remission times were short and a maintenance schedule has been difficult to establish. Patients with darker skin may still not respond as well as light-skinned patients.[56]

Corticosteroids

Topical corticosteroids are easy to apply and frequently prescribed for patients with limited patches (stage IA). In an investigational trial, 79 patients were treated daily with topical class I–III corticosteroids.[57] Thirty-two (63%) of stage T1 patients and seven (25%) of stage T2 patients achieved complete clearing. Thirteen patients (40%) with stage T1 and two patients (29%) with stage T2 relapsed; however, the median observation time was only 9 months. Reported side effects were minor skin irritation in two patients, reversible skin atrophy in one patient, and reversible depression of serum cortisol levels in ten patients. A more recent clinical observation from the same treatment center reported similar efficacy in about 100 patients with T1 and 50 patients with T2 stage when treated with a topical class I corticosteroid (clobetasol 0.05% ointment) as first-line treatment.[58] Treatment was applied twice daily and generally well tolerated with no signs of adrenal insufficiency detected.

Nitrogen mustard

Nitrogen mustard (mechlorethamine) is a classic alkylating agent. The topical formulation has been widely used as a first-line treatment of early-stage MF since 1959. It may be applied locally or to the entire skin once daily. Nitrogen mustard-induced DNA damage has been the primary mechanism responsible for its systemic anticancer effects, but the mechanism of action of the topical formulation remains elusive. It does not appear to act through its alkylating properties, but rather induces cell-mediated antitumor responses via delayed hypersensitivity reactions.[59,60]

Many investigators have demonstrated the efficacy of topical nitrogen mustard at a concentration of 0.1–0.2% in an aqueous or ointment base (Aquaphor) with reported CR in up to 72% of early-stage MF patients and occasional long-term remissions of more than 8 years.[61] Updates on 203 patients with MF (clinical stage I–III) treated with topical nitrogen mustard demonstrated its efficacy with reported CR rates of 76–80% for patients with stage IA, and 35–68% for those with stage IB disease.[62] Skin clearance may require 6 months or longer and is followed by maintenance therapy; however, there is no evidence that prolonged maintenance is beneficial. Only 11% of patients maintain CR after 10 years. The most common side effect was irritant contact dermatitis and hypersensitivity reaction. No secondary malignancies related to therapy were reported. New formulations that are better tolerated are currently under investigation.

Carmustine

Another type of topical chemotherapy that has been employed for MF is the nitrosourea alkylating agent BCNU. Like nitrogen mustard it interferes with DNA synthesis through alkylation. Topical BCNU can be used daily in either solution or ointment form.[63] Five milliliters of a 0.2% BCNU alcoholic stock solution will be diluted in 60 mL of water and applied to the total skin once daily. Clearance rates in 44 (86%) of 51 T1 and 18 (47%) of 38 T2 patients appear to be similar to those with nitrogen mustard.[64] Patients almost always develop erythema at site of application. Although irritant and/or allergic reactions occur less frequently, the cutaneous toxicity may be greater with the development of progressing teleangiectasias and reported bone marrow suppression from systemic absorption. Mild leukopenia occurred in 3.7% of patients. At Northwestern we have abandoned the use of this compound because of its skin toxicity.

Retinoids

Bexarotene 1% gel (Targretin) was approved by the US Food and Drug Administration (FDA) for early-stage MF in 2000 and has become an important addition to skin-directed therapies in limited disease, but it is extremely expensive and causes frequent skin irritation, which makes it unlikely that bexarotene gel would be used in patients with more than 10% of skin involvement.[62] Bexarotene gel is applied slightly to patches or plaques and is most effective and best tolerated when used twice daily. Topical bexarotene has been evaluated in a dose-escalating trial with concentrations ranging from 0.1% to 1.0%.[65] Median treatment duration with bexarotene gel was 10.5 months. The CR rate was 21% with a 63% overall response rate and a 75% response rate in treatment-naïve patients. The median duration of remission was 24 months. A multinational phase III study of patients with refractory and/or persistent early-stage MF, treated with 1% bexarotene gel in a dose frequency escalating fashion, demonstrated an overall response rate of 44% with CR in 8%.[66] The median duration was less favorable at 7 months. A pilot study with 0.1% tazarotene gel, a widely used retinoic acid receptor (RAR)-selective retinoid for psoriasis, was conducted in 20 patients with early-stage MF.[67] Daily application for 6 months resulted in similar responses compared to bexarotene gel and may be an alternative approach to topical bexarotene.

Radiation

Patients with localized tumors (stage IIB) respond very well to localized orthovoltage radiation. Granulomatous slack skin may also benefit from radiation, although experiences are very limited.[1] TSEBT may be used in patients with more disseminated cutaneous disease. It is a treatment in which ionizing radiation is administered to the entire skin surface penetrating to the dermis. The standard total dose is 36 Gy delivered with electrons of at least 4 MeV energy and fractionated over 8–10 weeks. Reported CR rates range from 40% to 98% among patients with T1 and T2 stage; however, relapse rates are high.[68,69] These results were confirmed by a recent update on 57 patients with T1/T2 stage.[70] Twenty-one patients (87.5%) with T1 and 28 patients with T2 (84.5%) achieved CR. The median duration of remission was 26 months. Long-term analysis revealed that 75% T1 patients and 25% with T2 were disease-free after 5 years. Nearly all patients developed skin-related side effects including erythema, teleangiectasia, xerosis, nail dystrophy, and/or reversible alopecia. An increased risk of non-melanoma skin cancer was not observed. TSEBT may be repeated for palliative effects, although at reduced doses. Adjuvant therapy including PUVA, ECP, and IFN-α may improve the duration of response. Improvement in disease-free survival, but not in overall survival, has been reported in T1/T2 patients treated with adjuvant PUVA therapy.[71]

Systemic treatments

Interferon

IFN-α is one of the most effective single agents in the treatment of CTCL. The available subtypes IFN-α2a (Roferon A) and IFN-α2b (Intron A) do not differ in their activity and have shown a wide range of biologic effects, including antiviral, antiproliferative, and immunomodulatory. The exact mechanism with which they exert their antitumor effects remains unknown. Th-1 cytokines support cytotoxic T-cell-mediated immunity and it has been speculated that IFN-α maintains or enhances a Th-1-cell population balance for an effective cell-mediated response to malignant T lymphocytes. IFN-α was first reported in 1986 by Bunn *et al.* for the treatment of advanced and heavily pretreated MF/SS with an overall response rate of 45%.[72] Subsequent reported overall response rates ranged from 29% to 74% of patients with median durations from 4 to 42 months.[73–75] Higher response rates were seen in early-stage MF patients.

IFN-α is generally given as long-term therapy, although the optimal dose and duration in CTCL has not been established. Various dosages and treatment schedules have been used. The initial trials used very high doses, but significant toxicities in nearly all patients have defined the limits of its clinical application. Therapy should be initiated at low doses between 1 and 3 million units (MU) three times weekly with gradual escalation to 9–12 MU daily or as tolerated. The combination therapy IFN-α and PUVA, first reported by Kuzel *et al.* in 1995, resulted in very high response rates and showed superiority to other combinations with retinoids or ECP.[76] Thirty-nine patients with advanced disease (IB–IVB) were treated with IFN-α2a (12 MU 3 × weekly) and PUVA (3 × weekly) with an overall response rate of 92% and CR in 62% of patients. The median duration was 28 months. The development of neutralizing antibodies has been associated with IFN-α therapy with variable impact on response rates. The IFN-α/PUVA combination has been shown to inhibit the development of neutralizing antibodies.[77] Side effects are based on dosage and schedule and can be divided into acute and chronic. Initially, almost all patients develop temporary flu-like symptoms. Chronic side effects can be anorexia, fatigue, depression, alopecia, cytopenia, and impaired liver function. Pegylated IFN-α, with the advantage of once weekly injection, is more convenient to administer than standard IFN-α, and has demonstrated similar if not improved efficacy and tolerability in other malignancies. A pilot study is currently being performed to investigate its effects in patients with CTCL.

Retinoids/rexinoids

Retinoids are vitamin A derivatives that have important effects on cell growth, terminal differentiation, and apoptosis and have been used to treat CTCL since the early 1980s with reported benefits in several small studies.[62] Response rates ranged from 44% to 67% with CR rates from 21% to 35% and median response duration around 8 months. Common effects consisted of skin and mucous membrane dryness. Bexarotene, a new retinoid X receptor (RXR)-selective retinoid, was approved in 1999 for the treatment of relapsed/refractory CTCL at early and advanced stages. In vitro studies have shown that bexarotene treatment induces apoptosis in CTCL cell lines and tumor regression in animal models, although its precise mechanisms are unknown.[78] The approval of bexarotene capsules was based on two multicenter open-label phase II–III clinical trials in 152 patients with early and advanced stages of CTCL who had failed or were refractory to two or more standard therapies.[79,80] In the early-stage trial, 58 patients randomized to doses of 6.5, 300, or 650-mg/m^2 daily achieved response rates (defined as a greater than 50% improvement in skin lesions) of 20%, 54%, and 67%, respectively.[79] Median time to response was 8 weeks. In the advanced-stage trial with 94 patients, response rates of 45% and 55% have been observed with daily doses of 300 or 650 mg/m^2, respectively, and an overall response rate of 48%.[80] However, only 6% (6/94) of patients achieved a CR. Median duration of response was short at 10 months. A significantly higher clinical response to oral bexarotene was achieved in patients by controlling dose-limiting hypertriglyceridemia with two concomitantly administered lipid-lowering agents compared to those taking one or no lipid-lowering agents. Retrospectively collected comparison data suggest that there may be little difference in efficacy between the RXR-selective retinoid bexarotene and the RAR-specific retinoid all-*trans* retinoic acid (ATRA). The bexarotene-treated group had an overall response rate of 21% compared to the ATRA-treated group with 12%.[81] Compared to previously published data, bexarotene achieved significantly lower response rates possibly related to differences in response criteria and patient inclusion criteria.

Bexarotene has been combined with other therapies such as PUVA, IFN-α, IFN-γ, and extracorporal photopheresis (ECP) in patients with advanced disease or refractory to prior treatments.[82] Bexarotene induces upregulation of the high-affinity IL-2 receptor on T cells in vitro and provided the rationale for combining bexarotene with IL-2 fusion protein (denileukin diftitox, Ontak) to enhance susceptibility of malignant cells.[83] In a phase I study using this combination approach in 14 patients with MF, 57% (8) of patients achieved a response, with CR in 4 patients (28%).[84]

The most common significant side effects experienced in both early- and advanced-stage trials were hypertriglyceridemia, hypercholesterolemia, central hypothyroidism, and leukopenia requiring additional treatment with lipid-lowering agents such as statins, 3-hydroxy-3-methyl-glutaryl-CoA (HMG-CoA) reductase inhibitors, or fenofibrates, and thyroid hormone replacement.[79,80] The concomitant use of gemfibrozil (Gemcor) is contraindicated as it increases plasma concentration of bexarotene and triglyceride levels, possibly related to cytochrome P450 3A4 isoenzyme inhibition. Oral bexarotene can be considered as first-line treatment for patients with stage IB and higher as a single agent or at reduced dose in combination with PUVA with serum lipids and thyroid parameters carefully monitored. The combined regimen may not increase response rates, but has the advantage of decreased dose requirements for both PUVA and bexarotene.

Extracorporeal photopheresis

Extracorporeal photopheresis (ECP) was approved in 1988 by the FDA for the palliative treatment of patients with CTCL. It also has been effective in the treatment of graft-versus-host disease (GVHD) and autoimmune diseases. Circulating mononuclear cells are separated by a leukapheresis-based method, mixed with 8-MOP, exposed to UVA light (1–2 J/cm^2) that activates the 8-MOP causing cross-linking of DNA, and reinfused to the patient. One suggested mechanism of action is induction of apoptosis in circulating malignant T lymphocytes with subsequent release of tumor antigens leading to a systemic antitumor response against the malignant T-cell clone. Quite recently, immunomodulatory effects via the induction of antigen-specific regulatory T cells have been suggested.[85] Still, the relative importance of these findings for the treatment of CTCL is not clear. Treatment is empirically given on two consecutive days every 14–28 days. It usually takes several months to see an improvement and is especially of benefit for both erythrodermic MF and SS with circulating neoplastic T cells. In 1987 Edelson *et al.* reported on preliminary results of the first multicenter trial for ECP in CTCL with a PR or CR in 27 of 37 patients (73%).[86] Of the responding patients 24 had exfoliative erythroderma. Mean time to response was 22 weeks. Subsequently performed studies on ECP have shown various degrees of overall response rates ranging from 31% to 73% of patients when used as monotherapy.[87] ECP has not been found to be as effective in patients with cutaneous patch, plaque, or tumor stages (IA to IIB).[88] Optimal candidates for ECP are patients with SS with less than 2 years of disease onset, modest tumor burden and circulating neoplastic cells, and almost normal counts of circulating CD8+ T cells and natural killer (NK) cells. Prolonged response rates have been reported when combined with IFN-α, bexarotene, granulocyte colony-stimulating factor (G-CSF), or TESBT.[87,89,90] Fludarabine with subsequent treatment with ECP seemed to increase the response rate, although no survival benefit was seen.[91] In this non-randomized trial, overall response rate was 63.2% versus 29.5% in patients with fludarabine monotherapy. There have been few adverse events related to ECP treatment including catheter-related infection and hypotension caused by volume shifts.

Alemtuzumab

Monoclonal antibodies (mAb) can mediate antitumor effects through three major mechanisms including intrinsic cytotoxic activity, antibody-dependent cellular cytotoxicity (ADCC), and activation of complement-dependent cytolysis. Alemtuzumab (Campath) is a humanized IgG_1 mAb that targets the CD52 antigen abundantly expressed on normal and malignant B and T cells, but not on hematopoietic stem cells. It is FDA-approved for the treatment of chronic lymphoid leukemia (CLL). An update on alemtuzumab reported more than 50% response rates with 32% CR in two studies conducted with heavily pretreated relapsed/refractory MF/SS patients.[92] Results were most promising in patients with SS. Median response duration was 12 months. The compound, however, can be associated with significant hematologic toxicities and infectious complications consisting of reactivation of CMV, herpes zoster, miliary tuberculosis, and pulmonary aspergillosis. In particular, this can be a problem when used in heavily pretreated patients. Cytopenias and prolonged immunosuppression require prophylactic antibiotic, antiviral, and antifungal treatment, and potential support with G-CSF. One group observed adverse cardiac events such as congestive heart failure, arrhythmia, and left ventricular dysfunction associated with alemtuzumab therapy. The availability of a subcutaneous preparation has been of great value for patients with SS with a favorable toxicity profile.

Denileukin diftitox

Denileukin diftitox (Ontak) is a recombinant fusion protein that contains the portion of IL-2 that interacts with the IL-2R, coupled to a component of diphtheria toxin. After binding to the IL-2R on neoplastic T cells it is internalized and induces apoptosis. The IL-2R consists of three subunits, the α-chain (CD25), β-chain (CD122), and γ-chain (CD132). Denileukin diftitox targets preferentially the intermediate-(β/γ-chain) and high-affinity IL-2R (α/β/γ-chain) on malignant T lymphocytes. The degree of CD25 expression is highly variable and dependent on the tissue site. Current anti-CD25 antibodies only recognize one component of the receptor and therefore can be inaccurate in predicting response although investigators have recently found evidence that the baseline level of CD25 expression on skin biopsies in CTCL patients correlated with their clinical response to denileukin diftitox.[93] Denileukin diftitox has been approved by the FDA in 1999 for the treatment of patients with CTCL refractory to standard treatment options. In general, response rates in patients with relapsed and refractory MF/SS range from 30% to 37%.[19] Adverse effects include acute infusion-related events such as fever, rash, chills, dyspnea, and hypotension, and later effects such as myalgias, elevated serum transaminases, and vascular leak syndrome (VLS). The incidence of acute infusion-related events and VLS was significantly decreased with premedication of 8 mg dexamethasone, in addition to a significantly improved overall response rate of 57% (8 of 14 patients). In vitro, bexarotene is known to upregulate the expression of the high-affinity form of IL-2R in malignant T cells enhancing their susceptibility to denileukin diftitox, which prompted a phase II study with bexarotene combined with denileukin diftitox using escalating doses of bexarotene up to 300 mg/m^2. An overall response rate of 57% was seen in mostly relapsed and refractory MF/SS patients with manageable toxicities.[84] However, all patients had been premedicated with dexamethasone.

Histone deacetylase inhibitors

The degree of histone acetylation correlates with open chromatin, which allows various transcription factors access to the promoters of target genes. These genes are silenced by histone deacetylases, which remove acetyl groups from histones, which form complexes with DNA (nucleosome). HDAC inhibitors may restore the expression of tumor suppressor and/or cell cycle regulatory genes by increasing the acetylation of histones. Vorinostat (suberoylanilide hydroxamic acid or SAHA), romidepsin (depsipeptide, FK228), and LBH589 are potent class I and II HDAC inhibitors and have shown in vitro and in vivo cytotoxic activity against CTCL and various hematologic malignancies and solid tumors.[94–96]

Vorinostat (Zolinza) is an oral inhibitor of histone acetylase and histone deacetylase regulatory enzymes and was approved in 2006 by the FDA for the treatment of patients with CTCL with stage IB and higher who had progressive, persistent, or recurrent disease following two systemic therapies. The recommended vorinostat dose is 400 mg orally once daily with food. Phase I trials supporting approval were conducted at academic centers in the USA and Canada that enrolled 74 patients with CTCL with stage IB and higher who had failed two systemic therapies, one of which must have been bexarotene.[97] The overall response rate was modest with PR seen in 22 of 74 patients (29.7%) with only one complete responder observed. All patients received vorinostat at a dose of 400 mg once daily which could be reduced for toxicity to 300 mg orally daily or 300 mg orally five days a week. Median duration of response was 168 days and median time to progression was 202 days.

A phase II trial assessed several dosing regimens. When given to 33 heavily pretreated CTCL patients, vorinostat produced an overall response rate of 24.2% (8 patients).[98] Intermittent dosing was less effective than sustained dosing at 400 mg/day. The 300 mg twice-daily regimen had higher toxicity with no additional clinical benefit over the 400 mg once-daily regimen. No CR was observed.

Intriguingly, this study showed that nearly half of the patients with CTCL also experienced significant pruritus relief with vorinostat therapy and, hence, a marked improvement in their quality of life. The most common serious toxicities (grade 3 and 4) were thrombocytopenia, anemia, dehydration, vomiting, hypotension, infection, sepsis, pulmonary embolism, and deep venous thrombosis. These toxicities were reversible upon discontinuation of the drug.

The mechanism of action of vorinostat in CTCL has not been fully elucidated. Laboratory investigations have demonstrated that vorinostat causes apoptosis in CTCL lines and in malignant T cells of patients with CTCL.[94] Furthermore, skin biopsies of CTCL patients at baseline and during treatment showed decreased vessel density, a decreased number of dermal lymphocytes, and changes in p-STAT3 localization after treatment.[98] It is conceivable that vorinostat has pleiotropic effects affecting multiple pathways in CTCL and thus may provide an advantage for advanced and/or refractory stages with inactivation of several tumor suppressor genes involved in DNA repair, cell cycle, and apoptosis signaling pathways.[99]

Romidepsin is an HDAC inhibitor that is in phase II trials for MF/SS after demonstrating activity in phase I studies. As a single agent, it has achieved a reported overall and durable response rate of 36% in patients with CTCL.[100,101] In combination with denileukin diftitox, romidepsin has shown increased expression of the IL-2 receptor and cumulative toxicity. LBH589 is another HDAC inhibitor currently in phase II/III clinical development in patients with CTCL. LBH589 has inhibited cell proliferation and induced apoptosis in preclinical models and exhibited efficacy in advanced-stage patients in phase I studies.[96] Other HDAC inhibitors such as LAQ824 and PXD101 (belinostat) are also under investigation.

Single-agent chemotherapy

Oral chlorambucil, methotrexate, or etoposide have all been used as single-agent chemotherapy with similar efficacy producing complete responses of 25–35% in patients with advanced stages IIB–IVB with a median response duration of 3–22 months. Among single-agent chemotherapies, pegylated doxorubicin (Doxil) and the nucleoside analogs pentostatin (deoxycoformycin, Nipent) and gemcitabine (2′, 2′-difluorodeoxycytidine, Gemzar) are reported to be particularly effective.

Pegylated doxorubicin

The pegylated liposomal encapsulated anthracycline doxorubicin was developed to decrease the risk of cardiotoxicity experienced with conventional doxorubicin while preserving the antitumor efficacy. Anthracyclines work by deforming the DNA structure of tumor cells and terminating their biologic function. Pegylated doxorubicin was empirically tested in MF/SS patients and showed an overall response rate of 80% with CR in six of ten patients (60%).[102] More recent published multicenter data of pegylated doxorubicin in 34 patients with recurrent or recalcitrant CTCL revealed a response rate of 88.2%.[103] Twenty-seven patients (79.4%) achieved CR with a median duration of 12 months ranging from 9.5 to 44 months. The drug is usually well tolerated and not associated with alopecia.

Nucleoside analogs

The pyrimidine nucleoside analog gemcitabine is metabolized intracellularly to its active metabolites gemcitabine diphosphate and triphosphate with the latter incorporated into DNA resulting in inhibition of DNA synthesis and induction of apoptosis. Gemcitabine has shown clinical activity in patients with advanced CTCL with a low toxicity profile.[104,105] It was investigated at two centers in a phase II trial at a dosage of 1200 mg/m^2 (using traditional 3-weekly dosing every 28 days over 30 minutes) in 44 patients with clinical stage IIB–IV MF/SS.[104] Twelve percent of patients achieved CR and 26% of patients achieved PR, with a median duration of 15 months and 10 months, respectively. Gemcitabine at a similar dose schedule achieved higher response rates in 32 patients with untreated MF, peripheral T-cell lymphoma (unclassified), and SS.[105] The overall response rate was 75% with CR in 22% and PR in 53% of patients. The reported median duration was 10 months.

Pentostatin is an FDA-approved purine analog for hairy cell leukemia that inhibits adenosine deaminase. Adenosine deaminase deficiency, an inherited disorder that has been found in patients with severe combined immunodeficiency characterized by a deficiency of both B and T cells, provided the rationale to use pentostatin in clinical trials for CTCL and other non-Hodgkin lymphoma. The efficacy and toxicity of pentostatin was evaluated in several non-randomized trials for patients with T-cell malignancies. Only a limited number of CTCL patients (3 to 18 patients) were included. The reported median response rate was 41% (range 33–67%) with CR in 6% (4) of patients.[107] Various dosing regimens were applied ranging from 4 mg/m^2 per week or biweekly, 5 mg/m^2 $\times$ 3 days every 28 days, or at 35- to 71-day intervals. More recently, the MD Anderson experience in 32 MF/SS patients with stage IIB–IV was presented. Patients were treated with 5 mg/m^2 $\times$ 3 days every 3 weeks with an overall response rate of 31% and 2/32 CR.[106] Durations were usually short ranging from 1.3 to 16+ months. Reported common side effects of pentostatin were myelosuppression, infection, gastrointestinal, and elevated liver function tests.

Fludarabine (9-β-D-arabinosyl-2-fluoroadenine) and cladribine (2-chlorodeoxyadenosine, 2-CdA, Leustatin) are halogenated purine analogs that are resistant to degradation by adenosine deaminase. Both are metabolized to their triphosphate forms, which lead to the inhibition of ribonucleotide reductase, DNA polymerases, and DNA repair. Experience with fludarabine as monotherapy is limited. Results of a multicenter study with 31 patients with advanced disease showed a modest response rate of 19% with CR in 3% of patients.[108] Fludarabine is associated with significant and long-lasting myelosuppression. Two studies with 2-CdA in refractory advanced-stage disease conducted by Kuzel *et al.* and Saven *et al.* showed an overall response rate in 28% and 47% of patients with CR in 14% and 20% of patients with short duration.[109,110] The most significant toxicities encountered were prolonged myelosuppression and infectious complications.

Two non-randomized studies have evaluated IFN-α combined with fludarabine or pentostatin. Response rates have not shown to be superior to single-agent or IFN-α therapy.[111] As aforementioned, fludarabine with sequential ECP has increased response rates, but did not affect overall survival.[91]

Temozolomide

Temozolomide, an oral analog of dacarbazine (DTIC) that is used for metastasized melanoma, exerts its main cytotoxic effects by the alkylation of DNA. It has shown activity in a small number of patients with relapsed MF and SS.[112] Temozolomide is currently being evaluated in a phase II trial for patients with refractory advanced stages of MF/SS.[113] Patients with MF/SS have been shown to have low levels of DNA repair enzyme O^6 alkylguanine DNA alkyltransferase (AGT) and may be particularly sensitive to this alkylator.[114] Preliminary data have been reported with a more than 50% decrease in tumor burden in 5 of 19 evaluable patients with MF/SS (26%) with a median duration of 4 months. Twelve of 16 patients tested did not express AGT. Patients with AGT expression did not respond to treatment.

Multiagent chemotherapy

There were no randomized trials comparing combined regimens with single-agent regimens. However, combination approaches with anthracycline-based therapies have been shown to achieve higher response rates, although a prolonged relapse-free or overall survival has not been seen. A retrospective study on 81 patients with primary cutaneous lymphomas (46 primary cutaneous B-cell lymphomas and 35 CTCL) treated with cyclophosphamide, vincristine, and prednisone (COP) or cyclophosphamide, doxorubicin, vincristine, and prednisone (CHOP) regimens reported an overall response rate of 40% in CTCL patients with CR in 23% of patients. The median response duration was 5.7 months and median survival was 19 months.[115] A phase II trial with the etoposide, vincristine, doxorubicin, cyclophosphamide, and oral prednisolone (EPOCH) regimen in 15 patients with refractory CTCL resulted in an overall response rate of 80%.[116] Twenty-seven percent (4) of patients achieved a CR, and 53% (8) of patients achieved a PR with a median duration of 8 months and overall survival of 13.5 months. Significant hematologic toxicity occurred in eight patients (53%). A more recently published combination approach with ESHAP (etoposide, cisplatin, high-dose cytarabine, prednisolone) showed no advantage in patients with advanced CTCL compared to previously reported results. ESHAP resulted in a CR in 2 patients of 11 treated, with short duration of PR in 7 patients, while severe toxicity was observed in 90% of patients, especially myelosuppression and infectious complications.

Stem cell transplantation

The concept of high-dose combined chemotherapy followed by autologous SCT (ASCT) or peripheral blood stem cell support has curative potential in various non-Hodgkin lymphomas, but experience in CTCL is limited. ASCT has yielded disappointing results. Despite reported effective responses with CR in most patients treated, relapses are frequent and may occur rapidly.[117,118] Allogeneic transplants are known to achieve much more durable CR, most likely due to an immune-mediated graft-versus-lymphoma (GVL) effect. Response durations as far as 6 years post-transplant have been reported suggesting that it may be a curative option.[119] It does, however, carry a higher risk of treatment-related mortality including life-threatening infections and GVHD. Reduced-intensity non-myeloablative (mini) allogeneic SCT potentially offers a GVL effect with lesser toxicities related to the conditioning regimen. A recent series of three young patients with advanced, refractory CTCL, who underwent non-myeloablative allogeneic transplantation, demonstrated only brief periods of disease remission, despite the evidence of GVL effects, indicating that there was insufficient GVL effect to control the disease.[120] Allogeneic SCT should be a consideration in younger patients with aggressive and advanced disease resistant to standard treatment options as a potentially curative option.

Investigational treatments

Monoclonal antibodies

Therapeutic effects of a chimeric (mouse/human) anti-CD4 antibody had been observed as an active agent in MF/SS as early as in 1991. Zanolimumab is a fully human anti-CD4 ($IgG_1\kappa$) mAb that targets the CD4 receptor expressed on T-helper/memory cells. The major mechanism of action for zanolimumab is believed to be through antibody-dependent cellular cytotoxicity. In vivo analyses have indicated that zanolimumab depletes the activated CD4+ $CD45RO^+$ T-cell memory subset. The efficacy and safety of zanolimumab in patients with refractory CTCL has been assessed in two multicenter, open-label phase II trials.[121] Forty-seven patients with treatment refractory CTCL (38 patients with MF, 9 with SS) were included. Patients received 17 weekly infusions of zanolimumab (early-stage patients, 280 or 560 mg; advanced-stage patients, 280 or 980 mg). A clinical response according to the Composite Assessment of Index Lesion Disease Activity Score and Physician's Global Assessment was reported in 13 patients with early and advanced MF and 2 patients with SS. A higher response rate of 56% with a median duration of 81 weeks was achieved with greater doses in early and advanced stages. In general, treatment was well-tolerated with no dose-related toxicities. The most frequently reported adverse events included low-grade infections and eczematous dermatitis similar to erythroderma and seborrhea seen in patients with advanced HIV. A pivotal phase III study is ongoing.

Cytokines

Immunomodulatory cytokines are thought to enhance cytotoxic cell-mediated activity. Human recombinant IL-2 (rIL-2) has raised interest because of its ability to induce regression in a minority of patients with CTCL. Recent results of a phase II study with subcutaneous rIL-2-based therapy could not reproduce similar efficacy compared to previous reports.[122] Overall response rate of 18% and median response duration of 3 months suggest that subcutaneously administered rIL-2 is largely ineffective as therapy in patients with relapsed and refractory CTCL. Treatment with IL-12 achieved higher response rates of 43% in 23 patients.[123] An increased level of CD8+ and/or TIA-1+ T cells in regressing cutaneous lesions suggested induction of a cytotoxic-T-cell antitumor response.

Immunomodulatory agents

Host immune function appears to play an integral role in mediating responses in MF. Toll-like receptor (TLR) agonists such as imiquimod (Aldara) and CpG-7909 enhance immune responses via activation of TLR-7, 8, and/or 9. CpG-7909 (CpG oligonucleotide) is a TLR-9 agonist known to induce Th-1-induced immune responses via dendritic cell activation. Preliminary results demonstrate that the cytotoxic CD8+ T-cell population increased within tumor infiltrates after systemic administration.[124] Due to the small number of patients, results are inconclusive without frank evidence of efficacy. Lenalidomide (CC-5013, Revlimid), an oral immunomodulatory thalidomide analog, is currently being used in clinical trials to treat various hematologic malignancies and solid tumors. The immunomodulatory properties such as T-cell co-stimulation with induction of Th-1 cytokine production and cytotoxic activity along with antiangiogenic, antiproliferative, and proapoptotic properties provided the rationale to use this agent in patients with MF/SS. Preliminary data from an ongoing phase II trial have shown efficacy in heavily pretreated patients with advanced MF/SS with mild toxicities.[125]

Proteosome inhibitors

The proteosome inhibitor bortezomib has been approved by the FDA for the treatment of multiple myeloma and mantle cell lymphoma. A phase II trial of bortezomib has demonstrated activity in previously treated patients with CTCL.[126] Patients received a traditional dose of 1.3 mg/m^2 intravenously on days 1, 4, 8, and 11, every 21 days for a total of six cycles. The ten patients with MF had an overall response rate of 70% (one CR and six PR). The CR has exceeded 12 months and three of the PRs remained in remission at 14, 4, and 7 months at the time of the report. The most common side effect included grade 3 neutropenia, thrombocytopenia, and sensory neuropathy.

Survival and outcome

The prognosis of patients with MF is excellent in early stages with a low mortality risk. Patients with early stage (IA–IIA) MF should be treated with skin-targeted modalities to achieve CR. In most instances therapies are not curative and recurrences of disease occur frequently; however, the long-term survival is not affected by relapse status. At later stages, patients have a decreased survival, with most deaths caused by infections due to the impaired immune system. Stage-dependent therapies are thought to decrease the risk of further disease progression and transformation into aggressive large-cell lymphoma. In the past, most investigational and standard treatment strategies have focused on physical measures for the primary end point of efficacy. CTCL is a disease with visible manifestations commonly accompanied by pruritus, burning sensations, and pain with a significant detriment to patients' quality of life.[127]

Patients with clinical stage IB have a higher chance (20%) of disease progression compared to patients with clinical stage IA disease (10%). Patients with advanced-stage (IIB–IVB) MF/SS have a significantly decreased survival. Data published in the literature show a 5-year survival of 40% for stage IIB and 25% for stage III. Treatment goals should be disease palliation, improvement of survival, and improvement of quality of life. No regimen has been proven to prolong survival in advanced stages; therefore, immunomodulatory regimens should be used initially to reduce the need for cytotoxic therapies with more damaging side effects. Treatment-associated toxicities can be pronounced particularly in elderly patients with comorbid medical conditions, poor performance status, and/or severe skin disease or in patients whose life expectancy is short.

Dose adjustments in those patients are often required to preserve quality of life as treatment is always regarded to be palliative and greater disease elimination does not outweigh the increased risk for toxicities.

The development of new biologic therapies, chemotherapies, and combinations thereof and the participation in national and international studies offers patients with CTCL various treatment options.

References

1. Willemze R, Jaffe ES, Burg C, *et al.* WHO-EORTC classification for cutaneous lymphomas. *Blood* 2005;**105**(10):3768–85.
2. Querfeld C, Guitart J, Kuzel TM, *et al.* Primary cutaneous lymphomas: a review with current treatment options. *Blood Rev* 2003;**17**(3):131–42.
3. Vonderheid EC, Bernengo MG, Burg G, *et al.* Update on erythrodermic cutaneous T-cell lymphoma: report of the International Society for Cutaneous Lymphomas. *J Am Acad Dermatol* 2002;**46**(1):95–106.
4. Criscione VD, Weinstock MA. Incidence of cutaneous T-cell lymphoma in the United States, 1973–2002. *Arch Dermatol* 2007;**143**(7):854–9.
5. Weinstock MA, Gardstein B. Twenty-year trends in the reported incidence of mycosis fungoides and associated mortality. *Am J Public Health* 1999; **89**(8):1240–4.
6. Huang KP, Weinstock MA, Clarke CA, *et al.* Second lymphomas and other malignant neoplasms in patients with mycosis fungoides and Sezary syndrome: evidence from population-based and clinical cohorts. *Arch Dermatol* 2007;**143**(1):45–50.
7. Koh HK, Charif M, Weinstock MA. Epidemiology and clinical manifestations of cutaneous T-cell lymphoma. *Hematol Oncol Clin North Am* 1995;**9**(5):943–60.
8. Morales-Suarez-Varela MM, Olsen J, Johansen P, *et al.* Occupational exposures and mycosis fungoides. A European multicentre case-control study (Europe). *Cancer Causes Control* 2005;**16**(10):1253–9.
9. Wood GS, Schaffer JM, Boni R, *et al.* No evidence of HTLV-I proviral integration in lymphoproliferative disorders associated with cutaneous T-cell lymphoma. *Am J Pathol* 1997;**150** (2):667–73.
10. Herne KL, Talpur R, Breuer-McHam J, *et al.* Cytomegalovirus seropositivity is significantly associated with mycosis fungoides and Sezary syndrome. *Blood* 2003;**101**(6):2132–6.
11. Gupta RK, Ramble J, Tong CY, *et al.* Cytomegalovirus seroprevalence is not higher in patients with mycosis fungoides/Sezary syndrome. *Blood* 2006;**107**(3):1241–2.
12. Ravat FE, Spittle MF, Russell-Jones R. Primary cutaneous T-cell lymphoma occurring after organ transplantation. *J Am Acad Dermatol* 2006;**54**(4): 668–75.
13. Kaufman D, Gordon LI, Variakojis D, *et al.* Successfully treated Hodgkin's disease followed by mycosis fungoides: case report and review of the literature. *Cutis* 1987;**39**(4):291–6.
14. Wilkins K, Turner R, Dolev JC, *et al.* Cutaneous malignancy and human immunodeficiency virus disease. *J Am Acad Dermatol* 2006;**54**(2):189–206; quiz 207–10.
15. Whittaker S. Biological insights into the pathogenesis of cutaneous T-cell lymphomas (CTCL). *Semin Oncol* 2006;**33**(1 Suppl 3):S3–6.
16. Sokolowska-Wojdylo M, Wenzel J, Gaffal E, *et al.* Absence of CD26 expression on skin-homing CLA+ CD4+ T lymphocytes in peripheral blood is a highly sensitive marker for early diagnosis and therapeutic monitoring of patients with Sezary syndrome. *Clin Exp Dermatol* 2005;**30** (6):702–6.
17. Wood GS, Tung RM, Haeffrer AC, *et al.* Detection of clonal T-cell receptor gamma gene rearrangements in early mycosis fungoides/Sezary syndrome by polymerase chain reaction and denaturing gradient gel electrophoresis (PCR/DGGE). *J Invest Dermatol* 1994;**103**(1):34–41.
18. Eriksen KW, Kaltoft K, Mikkelsen G, *et al.* Constitutive STAT3-activation in Sezary syndrome: tyrphostin AG490 inhibits STAT3-activation, interleukin-2 receptor expression and growth of leukemic Sezary cells. *Leukemia* 2001;**15** (5):787–93.
19. Saleh MN, LeMaistre CF, Kuzel TM, *et al.* Antitumor activity of DAB389IL-2 fusion toxin in mycosis fungoides. *J Am Acad Dermatol* 1998;**39**(1):63–73.
20. Tracey L, Villuendas R, Dotor AM, *et al.* Mycosis fungoides shows concurrent deregulation of multiple genes involved in the TNF signaling pathway: an expression profile study. *Blood* 2003;**102**(3):1042–50.
21. van Doorn R, Dijkman R, Vermeer MH, *et al.* Aberrant expression of the tyrosine kinase receptor EphA4 and the transcription factor twist in Sezary syndrome identified by gene expression analysis. *Cancer Res* 2004;**64**(16):5578–86.
22. Booken N, Gratchev A, Utikal J, *et al.* Sezary syndrome is a unique cutaneous T-cell lymphoma as identified by an expanded gene signature including diagnostic marker molecules CDO1 and DNM3. *Leukemia* 2008;**22**(2):393–9.
23. Karenko L, Hahtola S, Ranki A. Molecular cytogenetics in the study of cutaneous T-cell lymphomas (CTCL). *Cytogenet Genome Res* 2007; **118**(2–4):353–61.
24. Prochazkova M, Chevret E, Beylot-Barry M, *et al.* Large cell transformation of mycosis fungoides: tetraploidization within skin tumor large cells. *Cancer Genet Cytogenet* 2005;**163**(1):1–6.
25. van Doorn R, Zoutman WH, Dijkman R, *et al.* Epigenetic profiling of cutaneous T-cell lymphoma: promoter hypermethylation of multiple tumor suppressor genes including BCL7a, PTPRG, and p73. *J Clin Oncol* 2005;**23** (17):3886–96.
26. Rubben A, Kempf W, Kadin ME, *et al.* Multilineage progression of genetically unstable tumor subclones in cutaneous T-cell lymphoma. *Exp Dermatol* 2004;**13**(8):472–83.
27. Kupper TS, Fuhlbrigge RC. Immune surveillance in the skin: mechanisms and clinical consequences. *Nat Rev Immunol* 2004;**4**(3):211–22.
28. Narducci MG, Scala E, Bresin A, *et al.* Skin homing of Sezary cells involves SDF-1-CXCR4 signaling and down-regulation of CD26/ dipeptidylpeptidase IV. *Blood* 2006;**107** (3):1108–15.
29. Vowels BR, Lessin SR, Cassin M, *et al.* Th-2 cytokine mRNA expression in

skin in cutaneous T-cell lymphoma. *J Invest Dermatol* 1994;**103**(5):669–73.

30. Goteri G, Filosa A, Mannello B, *et al.* Density of neoplastic lymphoid infiltrate, CD8+ T cells, and CD1a+ dendritic cells in mycosis fungoides. *J Clin Pathol* 2003;**56**(6):453–8.
31. Lee BN, Duvic M, Tang CK, *et al.* Dysregulated synthesis of intracellular type 1 and type 2 cytokines by T cells of patients with cutaneous T-cell lymphoma. *Clin Diagn Lab Immunol* 1999;**6**(1):79–84.
32. Guitart J, Kennedy J, Ronan S, *et al.* Histologic criteria for the diagnosis of mycosis fungoides: proposal for a grading system to standardize pathology reporting. *J Cutan Pathol* 2001;**28**(4):174–83.
33. Costa C, Gallardo F, Pujol RM, *et al.* Comparative analysis of TCR-gamma gene rearrangements by Genescan and polyacrylamide gel-electrophoresis in cutaneous T-cell lymphoma. *Acta Derm Venereol* 2004;**84**(1):6–11.
34. Costa C, Gallardo F, Bellosillo B, *et al.* Analysis of T-cell receptor gamma gene rearrangements by PCR-Genescan and PCR-polyacrylamide gel electrophoresis in early-stage mycosis fungoides/large-plaque parapsoriasis. *Dermatology* 2003;**207**(4):418–19.
35. Murphy M, Signoretti S, Kadin ME, *et al.* Detection of TCR-gamma gene rearrangements in early mycosis fungoides by non-radioactive PCR-SSCP. *J Cutan Pathol* 2000;**27**(5):228–34.
36. Bunn PA Jr, Lamberg SI. Report of the Committee on Staging and Classification of Cutaneous T-Cell Lymphomas. *Cancer Treat Rep* 1979;**63**(4):725–8.
37. Olsen E, Vonderheid E, Pimpinelli N, *et al.* Revisions to the staging and classification of mycosis fungoides and Sézary syndrome: a proposal of the International Society for Cutaneous Lymphomas (ISCL) and the Cutaneous Lymphoma Task Force of the European Organization of Research and Treatment of Cancer (EORTC). *Blood* 2007;**110**:1713–22.
38. Sausville EA, Eddy JL, Makuch RW, *et al.* Histopathologic staging at initial diagnosis of mycosis fungoides and the Sezary syndrome. Definition of three distinctive prognostic groups. *Ann Intern Med* 1988;**109**(5):372–82.
39. Sausville EA, Warsham GF, Matthews MJ, *et al.* Histologic assessment of lymph nodes in mycosis fungoides/Sezary syndrome (cutaneous T-cell lymphoma): clinical correlations and prognostic import of a new classification system. *Hum Pathol* 1985;**16**(11):1098–109.
40. Kern DE, Kidd PG, Moe R, *et al.* Analysis of T-cell receptor gene rearrangement in lymph nodes of patients with mycosis fungoides. Prognostic implications. *Arch Dermatol* 1998;**134**(2):158–64.
41. Kim YH, Liu HL, Mraz-Gernhard S, *et al.* Long-term outcome of 525 patients with mycosis fungoides and Sezary syndrome: clinical prognostic factors and risk for disease progression. *Arch Dermatol* 2003;**139**(7):857–66.
42. Diamandidou E, Colome M, Fayad L, *et al.* Prognostic factor analysis in mycosis fungoides/Sezary syndrome. *J Am Acad Dermatol* 1999; **40**(6 Pt 1):914–24.
43. Diamandidou E, Colome-Grimmer M, Fayad L, *et al.* Transformation of mycosis fungoides/Sezary syndrome: clinical characteristics and prognosis. *Blood* 1998;**92**(4):1150–9.
44. Scarisbrick JJ, Whittaker S, Evans AV, *et al.* Prognostic significance of tumor burden in the blood of patients with erythrodermic primary cutaneous T-cell lymphoma. *Blood* 2001; **97**(3):624–30.
45. Grange F, Hedelin G, Joly P, *et al.* Prognostic factors in primary cutaneous lymphomas other than mycosis fungoides and the Sezary syndrome. The French Study Group on Cutaneous Lymphomas. *Blood* 1999;**93**(11):3637–42.
46. Meissner K, Michaelis K, Rehpenning W, *et al.* Epidermal Langerhans' cell densities influence survival in mycosis fungoides and Sezary syndrome. *Cancer* 1990;**65**(9):2069–73.
47. Kaye FJ, Bunn PA Jr, Steinberg SM, *et al.* A randomized trial comparing combination electron-beam radiation and chemotherapy with topical therapy in the initial treatment of mycosis fungoides. *N Engl J Med* 1989;**321**(26):1784–90.
48. Querfeld C, Rosen ST, Kuzel TM. Cutaneous T-cell lymphoma (Mycosis fungoides and Sézary's syndrome). In: Rakel RE, Bape ET, eds. *Conn's Current Therapy*, 58th edn., Section 13: Diseases of the skin. Philadelphia, USA, Saunders Elsevier. 2006; 955–62.
49. Gilchrest BA, Parrish JA, Tanenbaum L, *et al.* Oral methoxsalen photochemotherapy of mycosis fungoides. *Cancer* 1976;**38**(2):683–9.
50. Honigsmann H, Brenner W, Rauschmeier W, *et al.* Photochemotherapy for cutaneous T cell lymphoma. A follow-up study. *J Am Acad Dermatol* 1984;**10**(2 Pt 1):238–45.
51. Herrmann JJ, Roenigk HH Jr, Hurria A, *et al.* Treatment of mycosis fungoides with photochemotherapy (PUVA): long-term follow-up. *J Am Acad Dermatol* 1995;**33**(2 Pt 1):234–42.
52. Akaraphanth R, Douglass MC, Lim HW. Hypopigmented mycosis fungoides: treatment and a 6(1/2)-year follow-up of 9 patients. *J Am Acad Dermatol* 2000;**42**(1 Pt 1):33–9.
53. Querfeld C, Rosen ST, Kuzel TM, *et al.* Long-term follow-up of patients with early-stage cutaneous T-cell lymphoma who achieved complete remission with psoralen plus UV-A monotherapy. *Arch Dermatol* 2005;**141**(3):305–11.
54. Ramsay DL, Lish KM, Yalowitz CB, *et al.* Ultraviolet-B phototherapy for early-stage cutaneous T-cell lymphoma. *Arch Dermatol* 1992;**128**(7):931–3.
55. Gambichler T, Breuckmann F, Bom S, *et al.* Narrowband UVB phototherapy in skin conditions beyond psoriasis. *J Am Acad Dermatol* 2005;**52**(4):660–70.
56. Gathers RC, Scherschun L, Malick F, *et al.* Narrowband UVB phototherapy for early-stage mycosis fungoides. *J Am Acad Dermatol* 2002;**47**(2):191–7.
57. Zackheim HS, Kashani-Sabet M, Amin S. Topical corticosteroids for mycosis fungoides. Experience in 79 patients. *Arch Dermatol* 1998;**134**(8):949–54.
58. Zackheim HS. Treatment of patch-stage mycosis fungoides with topical corticosteroids. *Dermatol Ther* 2003;**16**(4):283–7.
59. Klein E, Rosner D, Holtermann OA, *et al.* Nonspecific antigen reactions. *Natl Cancer Inst Monogr* 1976;**44**:87–97.
60. Vonderheid EC, Ekbote SK, Kerrigan K, *et al.* The prognostic significance of delayed hypersensitivity to dinitrochlorobenzene and mechlorethamine hydrochloride in cutaneous T cell lymphoma. *J Invest Dermatol* 1998;**110**(6):946–50.
61. Vonderheid EC, Tan ET, Kantor AF, *et al.* Long-term efficacy, curative potential, and carcinogenicity of topical mechlorethamine chemotherapy in cutaneous T cell lymphoma. *J Am Acad Dermatol* 1989;**20**(3):416–28.

62. Querfeld C, Nagelli LV, Rosen ST, *et al.* Bexarotene in the treatment of cutaneous T-cell lymphoma. *Expert Opin Pharmacother* 2006;7(7):907–15.

63. Zackheim HS. Topical carmustine (BCNU) in the treatment of mycosis fungoides. *Dermatol Ther* 2003;**16** (4):299–302.

64. Zackheim HS, Epstein EH Jr, Crain WR. Topical carmustine (BCNU) for cutaneous T cell lymphoma: a 15-year experience in 143 patients. *J Am Acad Dermatol* 1990;**22**(5 Pt 1):802–10.

65. Breneman D, Duvic M, Kuzel T, *et al.* Phase 1 and 2 trial of bexarotene gel for skin-directed treatment of patients with cutaneous T-cell lymphoma. *Arch Dermatol* 2002;**138**(3):325–32.

66. Heald P, Mehlmaller M, Martin AG, *et al.* Topical bexarotene therapy for patients with refractory or persistent early-stage cutaneous T-cell lymphoma: results of the phase III clinical trial. *J Am Acad Dermatol* 2003;**49**(5):801–15.

67. Apisarnthanarax N, Talpur R, Ward S, *et al.* Tazarotene 0.1% gel for refractory mycosis fungoides lesions: an open-label pilot study. *J Am Acad Dermatol* 2004;**50**(4):600–7.

68. Hoppe RT, Cox RS, Fuks Z, *et al.* Electron-beam therapy for mycosis fungoides: the Stanford University experience. *Cancer Treat Rep* 1979;**63** (4):691–700.

69. Jones GW, Hoppe RT, Glatstein E. Electron beam treatment for cutaneous T-cell lymphoma. *Hematol Oncol Clin North Am* 1995;**9**(5):1057–76.

70. Ysebaert L, Truc G, Dalac S, *et al.* Ultimate results of radiation therapy for T1-T2 mycosis fungoides (including reirradiation). *Int J Radiat Oncol Biol Phys* 2004;**58**(4):1128–34.

71. Quiros PA, Jones GW, Kacinski BM, *et al.* Total skin electron beam therapy followed by adjuvant psoralen/ultraviolet-A light in the management of patients with T1 and T2 cutaneous T-cell lymphoma (mycosis fungoides). *Int J Radiat Oncol Biol Phys* 1997;**38**(5):1027–35.

72. Bunn PA, Ihde DC, Foon KA. The role of recombinant interferon-alfa-Za in the therapy of cutaneous T-cell lymphomas. *Cancer* 1986;**57**:1689–95.

73. Vonderheid EC, Thompson R, Smiles KA, *et al.* Recombinant interferon alfa-2b in plaque-phase mycosis fungoides. Intralesional and low-dose intramuscular therapy. *Arch Dermatol* 1987;**123**(6):757–63.

74. Kohn EC, Steiss RG, Sausville EA, *et al.* Phase II trial of intermittent high-dose recombinant interferon alfa-2a in mycosis fungoides and the Sezary syndrome. *J Clin Oncol* 1990;**8**(1):155–60.

75. Olsen EA, Bunn PA. Interferon in the treatment of cutaneous T-cell lymphoma. *Hematol Oncol Clin North Am* 1995;**9** (5):1089–107.

76. Kuzel TM, Roenigk HH Jr, Samuelson E, *et al.* Effectiveness of interferon alfa-2a combined with phototherapy for mycosis fungoides and the Sezary syndrome. *J Clin Oncol* 1995;**13**(1):257–63.

77. Kuzel TM, Roenigk HH Jr, Samuelson E, *et al.* Suppression of anti-interferon alpha-2a antibody formation in patients with mycosis fungoides by exposure to long-wave UV radiation in the A range and methoxsalen ingestion. *J Natl Cancer Inst* 1992;**84**(2):119–21.

78. Zhang C, Hazarika P, Ni X, *et al.* Induction of apoptosis by bexarotene in cutaneous T-cell lymphoma cells: relevance to mechanism of therapeutic action. *Clin Cancer Res* 2002;**8**(5):1234–40.

79. Duvic M, Martin AG, Kim Y, *et al.* Phase 2 and 3 clinical trial of oral bexarotene (Targretin capsules) for the treatment of refractory or persistent early-stage cutaneous T-cell lymphoma. *Arch Dermatol* 2001;**137**(5):581–93.

80. Duvic M, Hymes K, Heald P, *et al.* Bexarotene is effective and safe for treatment of refractory advanced-stage cutaneous T-cell lymphoma: multinational phase II-III trial results. *J Clin Oncol* 2001;**19**(9):2456–71.

81. Querfeld C, Rosen ST, Guitart J, *et al.* Comparison of selective retinoic acid receptor- and retinoic X receptor-mediated efficacy, tolerance, and survival in cutaneous t-cell lymphoma. *J Am Acad Dermatol* 2004;**51**(1):25–32.

82. Talpur R, Ward S, Aspisarnthanarax N, *et al.* Optimizing bexarotene therapy for cutaneous T-cell lymphoma. *J Am Acad Dermatol* 2002;**47**(5):672–84.

83. Gorgun G, Foss F. Immunomodulatory effects of RXR rexinoids: modulation of high-affinity IL-2R expression enhances susceptibility to denileukin diftitox. *Blood* 2002;**100**(4):1399–403.

84. Foss F, Demierre MF, DiVenuti G. A phase-1 trial of bexarotene and denileukin diftitox in patients with relapsed or refractory cutaneous T-cell lymphoma. *Blood* 2005;**106**(2):454–7.

85. Maeda A, Schwarz A, Kernebeck K, *et al.* Intravenous infusion of syngeneic apoptotic cells by photopheresis induces antigen-specific regulatory T cells. *J Immunol* 2005;**174**(10):5968–76.

86. Edelson R, Berger C, Gasparro F, *et al.* Treatment of cutaneous T-cell lymphoma by extracorporeal photochemotherapy. Preliminary results. *N Engl J Med* 1987;**316**(6):297–303.

87. Zic JA. The treatment of cutaneous T-cell lymphoma with photopheresis. *Dermatol Ther* 2003;**16**(4):337–46.

88. Child FJ, Mitchell TJ, Whittaker SJ, *et al.* A randomized cross-over study to compare PUVA and extracorporeal photopheresis in the treatment of plaque stage (T2) mycosis fungoides. *Clin Exp Dermatol* 2004;**29**(3):231–6.

89. Wilson LD, Jones GW, Kim D, *et al.* Experience with total skin electron beam therapy in combination with extracorporeal photopheresis in the management of patients with erythrodermic (T4) mycosis fungoides. *J Am Acad Dermatol* 2000;**43**(1 Pt 1):54–60.

90. Suchin KR, Cucthiara AJ, Gottleib SL, *et al.* Treatment of cutaneous T-cell lymphoma with combined immunomodulatory therapy: a 14-year experience at a single institution. *Arch Dermatol* 2002;**138**(8):1054–60.

91. Quaglino P, Fierro MT, Rossotto GL, *et al.* Treatment of advanced mycosis fungoides/Sezary syndrome with fludarabine and potential adjunctive benefit to subsequent extracorporeal photochemotherapy. *Br J Dermatol* 2004;**150**(2):327–36.

92. Dearden CE, Matutes E, Catovsky D. Alemtuzumab in T-cell malignancies. *Med Oncol* 2002;**19** Suppl:S27–32.

93. Talpur R, Jones DM, Alencar AJ, *et al.* CD25 expression is correlated with histological grade and response to denileukin diftitox in cutaneous T-cell lymphoma. *J Invest Dermatol* 2006;**126** (3):575–83.

94. Zhang C, Richon V, Ni X, *et al.* Selective induction of apoptosis by histone deacetylase inhibitor SAHA in cutaneous T-cell lymphoma cells: relevance to mechanism of therapeutic action. *J Invest Dermatol* 2005;**125**(5):1045–52.

95. Piekarz RL, Robey RW, Zhan Z, *et al.* T-cell lymphoma as a model for the use of histone deacetylase inhibitors in cancer therapy: impact of depsipeptide on molecular markers, therapeutic targets, and mechanisms of resistance. *Blood* 2004;**103**(12):4636–43.

96. Prince HM, George DJ, Johnstone R, *et al.* LBH589, a novel histone deacetylase

inhibitor (HDACi), treatment of patients with cutaneous T-cell lymphoma (CTCL). Changes in skin gene expression profiles related to clinical response following therapy. *J Clin Oncol* (2006 ASCO Annual Meeting Proceedings Part I) 2006;**24**(185):Abstract 7501.

97. Olsen E, Kim Y, Kuzel T, *et al.* Vorinostat (suberoylanilide hydroxamic acid, SAHA) is clinically active in advanced cutaneous T-cell lymphoma (CTCL): results of a phase IIB trial. *J Clin Oncol* (2006 ASCO Annual Meeting Proceedings Part I) 2006;**24**(185):Abstract 7500.

98. Duvic M, Talpur R, Nix, *et al.* Phase 2 trial of oral vorinostat (suberoylanilide hydroxamic acid, SAHA) for refractory cutaneous T-cell lymphoma (CTCL). *Blood* 2007;**109**(1):31–9.

99. Querfeld CR, Rosen ST. Epigenetic modulation of gene transcription: a new therapeutic modality in CTCL? *Am J Hematol Oncol* 2007;**6**(5 Suppl 7):23–5.

100. Sandor V, Bakke S, Robey RW, *et al.* Phase I trial of the histone deacetylase inhibitor, depsipeptide (FR901228, NSC 630176), in patients with refractory neoplasms. *Clin Cancer Res* 2002;**8**(3):718–28.

101. Piekarz RL, Robey R, Sandor V, *et al.* Inhibitor of histone deacetylation, depsipeptide (FR901228), in the treatment of peripheral and cutaneous T-cell lymphoma: a case report. *Blood* 2001;**98**(9):2865–8.

102. Wollina U, Graefe T, Kaatz M. Pegylated doxorubicin for primary cutaneous T cell lymphoma: a report on ten patients with follow-up. *Ann N Y Acad Sci* 2001;**941**:214–16.

103. Wollina U, Dummer R, Brockmeyer NH, *et al.* Multicenter study of pegylated liposomal doxorubicin in patients with cutaneous T-cell lymphoma. *Cancer* 2003;**98**(5):993–1001.

104. Zinzani PL, Baliva G, Magagnoli M, *et al.* Gemcitabine treatment in pretreated cutaneous T-cell lymphoma: experience in 44 patients. *J Clin Oncol* 2000;**18**(13):2603–6.

105. Marchi E, Alinari L, Tani M, *et al.* Gemcitabine as frontline treatment for cutaneous T-cell lymphoma: phase II study of 32 patients. *Cancer* 2005;**104**(11):2437–41.

106. Tsimberidou AM, Giles F, Duvic M, *et al.* Phase II study of pentostatin in advanced T-cell lymphoid malignancies: update of an M.D. Anderson Cancer Center Series. *Cancer* 2004;**100**(2):342–9.

107. Bunn PA Jr, Hoffman S J, Norris D, *et al.* Systemic therapy of cutaneous T-cell lymphomas (mycosis fungoides and the Sezary syndrome). *Ann Intern Med* 1994;**121**(8):592–602.

108. Von Hoff DD, Dohlberg S, Hartstock R J, *et al.* Activity of fludarabine monophosphate in patients with advanced mycosis fungoides: a Southwest Oncology Group study. *J Natl Cancer Inst* 1990;**82**(16):1353–5.

109. Kuzel TM, Hurria A, Samuelson E, *et al.* Phase II trial of 2-chlorodeoxyadenosine for the treatment of cutaneous T-cell lymphoma. *Blood* 1996;**87**(3):906–11.

110. Saven A, Carrera C J, Carson DA, *et al.* 2-Chlorodeoxyadenosine: an active agent in the treatment of cutaneous T-cell lymphoma. *Blood* 1992;**80**(3):587–92.

111. Foss FM, Ihde DC, Breneman DL, *et al.* Phase II study of pentostatin and intermittent high-dose recombinant interferon alfa-2a in advanced mycosis fungoides/Sezary syndrome. *J Clin Oncol* 1992;**10**(12):1907–13.

112. Tani M, Fina M, Alinari L, *et al.* Phase II trial of temozolomide in patients with pretreated cutaneous T-cell lymphoma. *Haematologica* 2005;**90**(9):1283–4.

113. Rosen ST, Guitart J, Martone B, *et al.* Phase II trial of temozolomide for treatment of mycosis fungoides/Sézary syndrome (MF/SS). *Proc Am Soc Clin Oncol* 2002;**21**:140.

114. Dolan ME, McRae BL, Ferries-Rowe E, *et al.* O6-alkylguanine-DNA alkyltransferase in cutaneous T-cell lymphoma: implications for treatment with alkylating agents. *Clin Cancer Res* 1999;**5**(8):2059–64.

115. Fierro MT, Quaglino P, Savoia P, *et al.* Systemic polychemotherapy in the treatment of primary cutaneous lymphomas: a clinical follow-up study of 81 patients treated with COP or CHOP. *Leuk Lymphoma* 1998;**31**(5–6):583–8.

116. Akpek G, Keh HK, Bogen S, *et al.* Chemotherapy with etoposide, vincristine, doxorubicin, bolus cyclophosphamide, and oral prednisone in patients with refractory cutaneous T-cell lymphoma. *Cancer* 1999;**86**(7):1368–76.

117. Bigler RD, Crilley P, Micaily B, *et al.* Autologous bone marrow transplantation for advanced stage mycosis fungoides. *Bone Marrow Transplant* 1991;**7**(2):133–7.

118. Russell-Jones R, Child F, Olavaria E, *et al.* Autologous peripheral blood stem cell transplantation in tumor-stage mycosis fungoides: predictors of disease-free survival. *Ann N Y Acad Sci* 2001;**941**:147–54.

119. Oyama Y, Guitart J, Kuzel TM, *et al.* High-dose therapy and bone marrow transplantation in cutaneous T-cell lymphoma. *Hematol Oncol Clin North Am* 2003;**17**(6):1475–83, xi.

120. Herbert KE, Spencer A, Gigg A, *et al.* Graft-versus-lymphoma effect in refractory cutaneous T-cell lymphoma after reduced-intensity HLA-matched sibling allogeneic stem cell transplantation. *Bone Marrow Transplant* 2004;**34**(6):521–5.

121. Kim YH, Duvic M, Obitz E, *et al.* Clinical efficacy of zanolimumab (HuMax-CD4): two phase 2 studies in refractory cutaneous T-cell lymphoma. *Blood* 2007;**109**(11):4655–62.

122. Querfeld C, Rosen ST, Guitart J, *et al.* Phase II trial of subcutaneous injections of human recombinant interleukin-2 for the treatment of mycosis fungoides and Sezary syndrome. *J Am Acad Dermatol* 2007;**56**(4):580–3.

123. Rook AH, Zaki MH, Wysocka M, *et al.* The role for interleukin-12 therapy of cutaneous T cell lymphoma. *Ann N Y Acad Sci* 2001;**941**:177–84.

124. Wysocka M, Benoit BM, Newton S, *et al.* Enhancement of the host immune responses in cutaneous T-cell lymphoma by CpG oligodeoxynucleotides and IL-15. *Blood* 2004;**104**(13):4142–9.

125. Querfeld C, Kuzel TM, Guitart J, *et al.* Preliminary results of a phase II study of CC-5013 (Lenalidomide, Revlimid™) in patients with cutaneous T-cell lymphoma. *Blood* 2005;**106**(11):936a–7a.

126. Zinzani PL, Musuraca G, Tani M, *et al.* Phase II trial of proteasome inhibitor bortezomib in patients with relapsed or refractory cutaneous T-cell lymphoma. *J Clin Oncol* 2007;**25**(27):4293–7.

127. Demierre MF, Tien A, Miller D. Health-related quality-of-life assessment in patients with cutaneous T-cell lymphoma. *Arch Dermatol* 2005;**141**(3):325–30.

Chapter 23

Central nervous system lymphoma

Elizabeth R. Gerstner and Tracy T. Batchelor

Introduction

Central nervous system (CNS) lymphoma may be isolated to the brain or leptomeninges in the absence of systemic disease (primary CNS lymphoma) or may occur as a neurologic complication of systemic lymphoma (secondary CNS lymphoma), usually in the form of leptomeningeal dissemination.

Primary CNS lymphoma

Primary central nervous system lymphoma (PCNSL) is an uncommon variant of extranodal non-Hodgkin lymphoma (NHL) that can affect multiple parts of the neuraxis including the eyes, brain, leptomeninges, or spinal cord. PCNSL accounts for approximately 3% of all the primary CNS tumors diagnosed each year in the United States and approximately 2–3% of all cases of NHL diagnosed each year. The incidence of PCNSL has increased over the past three decades, largely because of the human immunodeficiency virus (HIV) pandemic, but recent data suggest that the incidence has stabilized or is decreasing.[1] Acquired or congenital immunodeficiency is the only established risk factor for PCNSL.

Since PCNSL is a rare malignancy, it has been challenging to study, which partially explains why it has been difficult to establish an effective standard of care for this type of lymphoma. In PCNSL, remission may be achieved for a few years but the tumor relapses in most cases. This chapter will focus on non-HIV-related CNS lymphoma since HIV-associated lymphomas are covered elsewhere.

Pathology and biology

Approximately 90% of non-HIV-associated PCNSL cases are diffuse large B-cell type with the remaining 10% consisting of poorly characterized low-grade lymphomas, Burkitt lymphomas, or T-cell lymphomas.[2] Less is known about these latter, rare forms of PCNSL. Low-grade lymphomas are typically B cell as well and are analogous to systemic low-grade lymphomas. Prognosis is more favorable for low-grade CNS lymphoma.[3] T-cell lymphomas are pathologically heterogeneous and most appear to arise subcortically leading to a greater incidence of seizures in these patients.[4] A single patient has been reported with natural killer/T-cell CNS lymphoma.[5] Burkitt lymphoma with or without Epstein–Barr virus (EBV) infection and neurolymphomatosis are very rare variants of CNS lymphoma.

The more common diffuse large B-cell type of PCNSL is angiocentric and composed of immunoblasts or centroblasts that cluster around small cerebral vessels (Figure 23.1). Reactive T-cell infiltrates can also be present in varying degrees, sometimes making it difficult for a pathologist to discriminate between PCNSL and a reactive process. The presence of T-cell infiltrates is associated with a better prognosis for PCNSL patients.[6] PCNSL likely arises from late germinal center or post-germinal center extraneural lymphoid cells and may localize to the CNS because of a poorly understood neurotropism.[7]

Few systematic studies of the molecular pathology of PCNSL have been performed largely due to the lack of adequate tumor specimens for research purposes. The vast majority of PCNSL patients are diagnosed by stereotactic needle biopsy so that most of the tissue specimen is consumed by the diagnostic evaluation. Nevertheless, sharing of tissue specimens across multiple institutions has led to some preliminary observations highlighting the unique biologic properties of PCNSL as compared to systemic NHL. Immunophenotyping demonstrated that the majority of PCNSLs express BCL6, a germinal center marker, and MUM-1, a marker of activated B cells. Gene expression studies have demonstrated three gene "signatures" associated with PCNSL analogous to the signatures identified in systemic diffuse large B-cell lymphomas: germinal center B-cell (GCB), activated B-cell (ABC), and type 3 large B-cell lymphoma.[8] Brain lymphoma is distinguished from nodal large B-cell lymphoma by expression of regulators of the unfolded protein response (UPR) signaling pathway, by the oncogenes *c-MYC* and *Pim-1*, and by distinct regulators of apoptosis. Interleukin-4 (IL-4), a B-cell growth factor, is expressed by both tumor vessels and tumor cells in PCNSL but not in normal brain endothelia. Several IL-4-associated genes are highly

Management of Hematologic Malignancies, ed. Susan M. O'Brien, Julie M. Vose, and Hagop M. Kantarjian. Published by Cambridge University Press.

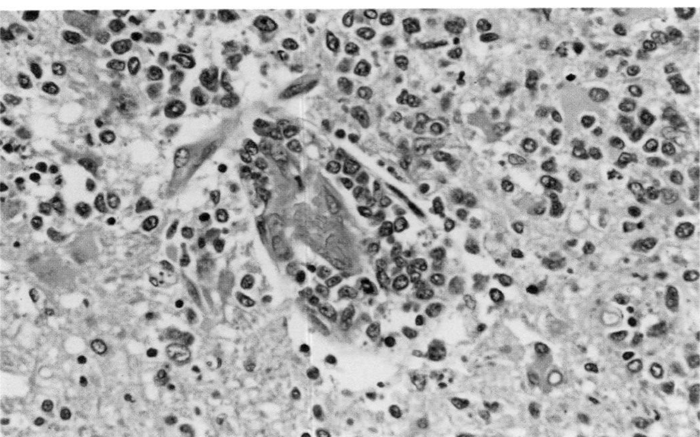

Figure 23.1 Microscopic section from a tumor specimen in a patient with PCNSL. The tumor cells are pleomorphic with large nuclei and a coarse chromatin pattern. Tumor cells are clustered around a cerebral blood vessel in a pattern typical for PCNSL. (Hematoxylin and eosin stain.)

expressed in PCNSL including X-box binding protein 1 (XBP-1), a regulator of the UPR. The expression of UPR-related genes is important for cell survival under stressful conditions such as hypoxia so activation of this pathway may promote tumor cell survival as well. There is also expression of STAT6, a mediator of IL-4 signaling, by tumor cells and tumor endothelia in PCNSL. High expression levels of STAT6 are associated with short survival in PCNSL patients treated with high-dose methotrexate.[8] In addition, extracellular matrix genes, particularly those involved in cell adhesion, were found to be upregulated.[9]

Clinical features

As in most CNS disorders, the presentation of PCNSL tends to reflect the location of the tumor. A single brain mass is observed in 70% of patients at the time of diagnosis.[10,11] In 248 immunocompetent patients diagnosed with PCNSL, 43% had neuropsychiatric signs, 33% had symptoms or signs of increased intracranial pressure, 14% had seizures, and 4% had ocular symptoms.[10] Seizures tend to be less common than with other types of brain tumors probably because the disease involves predominantly subcortical white matter rather than epileptogenic gray matter. Typically, patients do not present with B symptoms such as fever, weight loss, or night sweats.

Primary intraocular lymphoma (PIOL) of the retina, vitreous, and optic nerve without other CNS or systemic involvement is a rare subtype of PCNSL. In addition, 10–20% of patients with PCNSL are found to have concurrent ocular involvement. Patients with ocular lymphoma often complain of non-specific symptoms like floaters and blurred vision. As many as 80% of patients with PIOL have bilateral disease and approximately 56–80% of patients eventually develop leptomeningeal or brain parenchymal disease.[12–15] However, in the largest published series of PIOL cases aggressive treatments including whole brain radiation or systemic chemotherapy did not improve progression-free survival (PFS) or overall survival (OS) over ocular-focused treatment alone.[14]

Diagnostic evaluation

The International PCNSL Collaborative Group (IPCG) has established guidelines for the diagnostic evaluation of a patient with suspected PCNSL (Table 23.1).[16] These guidelines are important for establishing the extent of disease for PCNSL patients and for confirming that disease is limited to the CNS. Contrast-enhanced MRI (contrast-enhanced CT if MRI is not obtainable), lumbar puncture if not contraindicated, complete ophthalmologic examination, CT of the chest/abdomen/pelvis, and bone marrow biopsy should be done in all newly diagnosed patients. The cerebrospinal fluid (CSF) specimen should be analyzed for cell count, protein, glucose, cytology, flow cytometry, and immunoglobulin heavy chain (*IGH*) gene rearrangement. IGH gene rearrangement has been reported to have a specificity of 97% but a sensitivity of only 54% for detecting the presence of B-cell clonality.[17] Blood tests for HIV, complete blood count, basic metabolic panel, and lactate dehydrogenase (LDH) level are also recommended. Testicular examination should be performed in all male patients and testicular ultrasound should be considered. The role of body positron emission tomography (PET) imaging has not been defined but may offer another important tool to screen for the possibility of asymptomatic systemic lymphoma.

The search for occult systemic lymphoma has become increasingly important as disease may not be restricted to the nervous system in a subpopulation of patients with CNS lymphoma. In a study of 24 "primary" CNS lymphoma patients, Jahnke *et al.* used polymerase chain reaction (PCR) for analysis of clonally rearranged IGH genes. Identical dominant PCR products were identified in the bone marrow aspirates, blood samples, and tumor biopsy specimens in 2/24 patients. In one of these patients, follow-up IGH PCR 24 months after diagnosis yielded a persistent monoclonal blood product despite a complete response in the CNS. In addition, an oligoclonal pattern of IGH rearrangement was identified in the tumor biopsy specimen, bone marrow aspirate, and peripheral blood from an additional two patients.[18] These studies suggest that a subset of patients with "primary" CNS lymphoma actually harbor occult systemic lymphoma. Prospective, long-term follow-up studies will be necessary to further elucidate the frequency and importance of subclinical systemic disease in CNS lymphoma patients and whether the presence of these monoclonal cell populations increases the risk of systemic relapse.

Neuroimaging

Contrast-enhanced cranial MRI is the imaging modality of choice in evaluating a patient for the diagnosis of PCNSL (Figure 23.2). If MRI is not possible or is contraindicated, a contrast-enhanced cranial CT scan is recommended. PCNSL tends to enhance homogeneously on both MRI and CT, is

Table 23.1. International Primary CNS Lymphoma Collaborative Group (IPCG) guidelines for baseline evaluation for clinical trials

Pathology	Clinical	Laboratory	Imaging
Centralized review of pathology	Complete medical and neurologic examination	HIV serology	Contrast-enhanced cranial MRI[a]
Immunophenotyping	Dilated eye examination including slit lamp evaluation	Serum LDH level	CT of chest, abdomen, and pelvis
	Record prognostic factors (age, performance status)	CSF cytology, flow cytometry, IGH PCR	Bone marrow biopsy with aspirate
	Serial evaluation of cognitive function[b]	24-hour urine collection for creatinine clearance[c]	Testicular ultrasound in elderly males

Note: [a]Contrast-enhanced cranial CT should be obtained in patients who have a contraindication for MRI or who cannot tolerate MRI.
[b]Mini-mental status examination is used commonly although improved instruments are being developed.
[c]For patients who will receive high-dose methotrexate.
Source: Adapted from Abrey *et al.*[16]

iso- or hyperintense on T2 images, and may be bright on diffusion-weighted images. In immunocompetent patients, lesions are solitary in 65% of cases and are located in the hemisphere (38%), thalamus/basal ganglia (16%), corpus callosum (14%), periventricular region (12%), and cerebellum (9%).[20] Isolated spinal cord involvement is rare and observed in $< 1\%$ of cases so spinal imaging is only needed if warranted based on clinical suspicion or to screen for leptomeningeal involvement if lumbar puncture cannot be performed.

Prognostic markers

The identification of prognostic markers in PCNSL enables physicians to discuss prognosis with individual patients and may eventually allow the application of risk-adjusted therapeutic strategies. In addition, knowledge of important prognostic markers is critical for the design and analysis of clinical trials.

In one review, the International Extranodal Lymphoma Study Group (IELSG) identified age older than 60, Eastern Cooperative Oncology Group (ECOG) performance status greater than 1, elevated serum LDH level, high CSF protein concentration, and involvement of deep regions of the brain as independent predictors of worse prognosis.[21] The 2-year survival rates were 80%, 48%, and 15% in patients with 0–1 factors, 2–3 factors, and 4–5 factors, respectively.

In another study, investigators divided patients with PCNSL into three groups: those < 50 years of age, those ≥ 50 years of age with a Karnofsky performance status (KPS) ≥ 70, and those ≥ 50 years of age with a KPS < 70.[22] Based on these divisions, significant differences in OS and failure-free survival were observed. As these variables are easily obtained in virtually all subjects (patients often do not have all the IELSG prognostic markers at diagnosis), this model may prove useful in future clinical trials for risk stratification.

The search for biomarkers of prognosis for patients with PCNSL is an active area of investigation. BCL6, a tumor suppressor gene expressed in 22–100% of patients,[23–25] has been associated with improved prognosis. Both PFS (20.5 months vs. 10.1 months)[26] and OS (101 months vs. 14.7 months)[23,27] are longer in PCNSL patients with BCL6 expression. These findings are consistent with the observation that BCL6 expression is a favorable prognostic marker in patients with systemic NHL.[25,28,29] As noted above, expression of STAT6 was associated with shorter survival in PCNSL patients.

Treatment

As with systemic forms of NHL, the available treatment options for PCNSL include corticosteroids, chemotherapy, and radiation. Resection of PCNSL is not a viable treatment option except in the atypical patient experiencing acute brain herniation due to increased intracranial pressure. The relative rarity of PCNSL makes studying the disease difficult so the optimal treatment is still debated. The IPCG has recommended guidelines for assessing response to treatment in an attempt to standardize the study of the disease and allow comparison across individual phase II trials (Table 23.2).[16] The "IPCG criteria" should be adopted in prospective clinical trials for this rare disease.

Corticosteroids

Corticosteroids alone produce tumor regression on neuroimaging studies in 40% of patients likely through direct tumor cell lysis and reduction of tumor-associated edema.[30] Moreover, initial radiographic response to corticosteroids in newly diagnosed PCNSL patients is a significant favorable prognostic marker with survival of 117 months in responders versus 5.5 months in non-responders.[31] However, despite this initial response to corticosteroids, patients typically relapse quickly and require alternate treatment strategies. Moreover, corticosteroids should be withheld if possible prior to a diagnostic biopsy since these drugs may cause significant tumor lysis leading to diagnostic inaccuracy at the time of microscopic analysis.

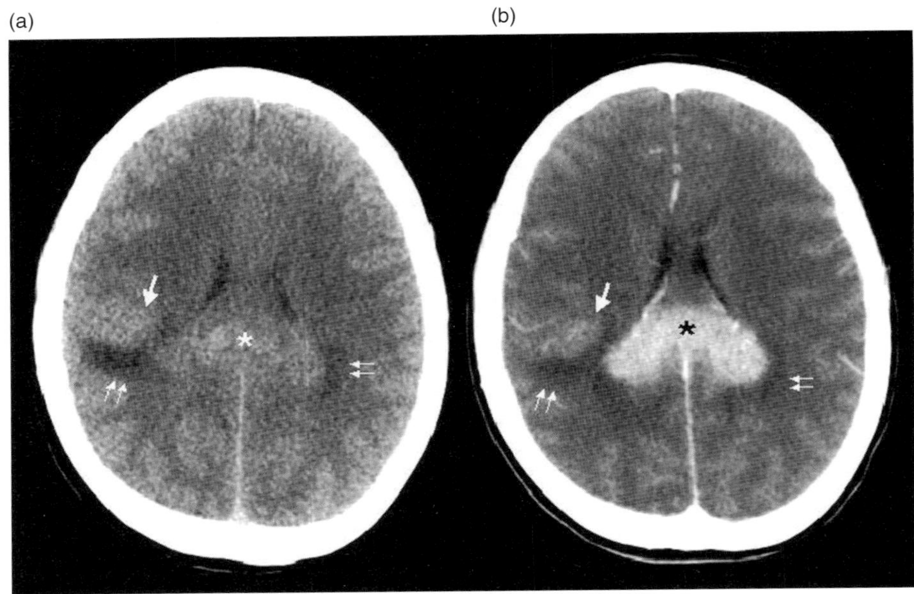

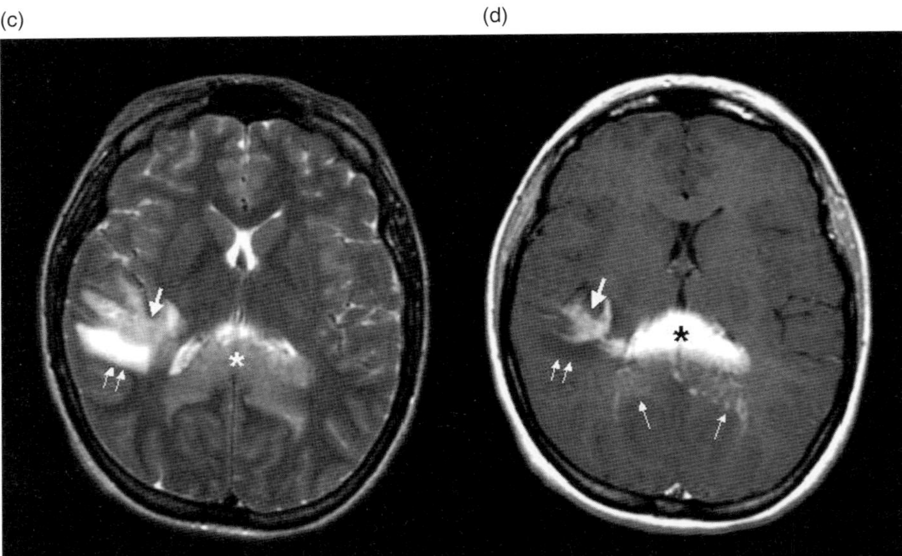

Figure 23.2 Axial CT images in a patient with PCNSL (a and b). The first CT image without contrast (a) shows an infiltrative mass that expands the splenium of the corpus callosum (*asterisk*) and spreads into the right parietal lobe (*single arrow*), which is isodense with respect to gray matter. After administration of contrast (b), the masses enhance homogeneously. Mild low attenuation edema surrounds the lesions (*double arrows*). Reprinted with permission from Batchelor *et al. N Engl J Med* 2005; **352**:185–94.[19] Figures 23.2 (c) and (d) show axial MR images of the same patient in (a) and (b). An axial T2-weighted MR image (c) shows that the splenial (*asterisk*) and right parietal (*single thick arrow*) lesions are isointense with respect to gray matter. Right parietal edema is T2-hyperintense (*double arrows*). An axial T1-weighted MR image after contrast (d) shows that the lesions enhance intensely. Linear enhancing structures emanating from the corpus callosum indicate tumor spread through the Virchow–Robin perivascular spaces in a pattern characteristic for PCNSL (*single thin arrows*). Adjacent edema is T1-hypointense (*double arrows*). Permission from *NEJM*.

Surgery

Attempts at gross total resection have been unsuccessful in improving survival in patients with PCNSL mostly because of the infiltrative nature of the tumor.[32] In addition, PCNSL is a multifocal cancer involving the leptomeninges, the eyes, or the deep regions of the brain making total tumor resection impossible. Median survival following surgery alone is only 1–4 months.[33] Consequently, once the diagnosis is achieved with stereotactic biopsy, surgery has little role in the management of PCNSL.

Radiation

Whole brain radiation therapy (WBRT) was historically the modality of choice to treat PCNSL given the multifocal and infiltrative nature of the tumor. However, WBRT alone is inadequate therapy in PCNSL patients with CSF dissemination of their tumor. Initial radiographic response to WBRT is achieved in 90% of PCNSL patients but relapse usually occurs within a few months.[34] In studies of patients receiving WBRT alone, the median OS varied from 13 to 18 months and 5-year OS was 18–35%.[35,36] A radiation dose–response relationship exists for PCNSL as dose reduction from 45 Gy to 30 Gy might increase the risk of relapse.[37] Considering the significant neurotoxicity associated with WBRT, especially in persons over the age of 60, hyperfractionated WBRT (in addition to chemotherapy) has been proposed as a method to reduce radiation-associated toxicity to the brain. Unfortunately, this approach does not eliminate neurotoxicity but does delay the onset of neurotoxicity.[38] Consequently, while WBRT is effective for the initial control of disease, it produces delayed neurotoxicity,

Table 23.2. International Primary CNS Lymphoma Collaborative Group (IPCG) guidelines for response assessment for clinical trials

Response	Brain imaging	Corticosteroid dose	Eye exam	CSF cytology
CR	No enhancing disease	None	Normal	Negative
CRu	No enhancing disease	Any	Normal	Negative
	Minimal enhancing disease	Any	Minor RPE abnormality	Negative
PR	50% decrease in enhancement	NA	Minor RPE abnormality or normal	Negative
	No enhancing disease	NA	Decrease in vitreous cells or retinal infiltrate	Persistent or suspicious
PD	25% increase in enhancement	NA	Recurrent or new disease	Recurrent or positive
	Any new site of disease			
SD	All scenarios not covered by responses above			

Notes: CR: complete response; CRu: unconfirmed complete response; PR: partial response; PD: progressive disease; RPE: retinal pigment; SD: stable disease; NA: not available.
Source: Adapted from Abrey *et al.*[16]

especially in those older than 60, causing cognitive deficits and diminishing quality of life. For this reason, WBRT is often deferred in patients > 60 with newly diagnosed PCNSL.

Combined modality therapy

Considering the disappointing outcomes with surgery or radiation alone, chemotherapy was added to WBRT in an attempt to improve survival. Numerous studies with various chemotherapy drugs have been reported in PCNSL and there is no compelling evidence for the superiority of any one regimen (Table 23.3). Typical agents used to treat systemic NHL (ex. cyclophosphamide, doxorubicin, vincristine as components of CHOP) are associated with limited blood–brain barrier (BBB) penetration so have limited efficacy in PCNSL. Methotrexate (MTX), a folate antagonist that interferes with DNA synthesis, is the most effective agent for PCNSL but has limited penetration into the CNS because of its high degree of ionization at physiologic pH. Using microdialysis catheters, investigators measured the penetration of 12 g/m^2 of IV methotrexate into brain tumor tissue.[54] The ratio of brain extracellular fluid MTX to plasma MTX was only 0.13. This low penetration is an important reason that high-dose MTX (HD-MTX, $\geq$ 3.5 g/m^2) is necessary to achieve cytotoxic intratumoral concentrations. In addition to dose, infusion duration appears to be important; a 3-hour infusion of 100 mg/kg of MTX resulted in greater tumor shrinkage than a 6-hour infusion.[55]

Combination regimens involving MTX and WBRT are associated with a radiographic response in > 50% of patients and a 2-year survival of 43–73%.[30] In a retrospective study, Shenkier *et al.* reviewed the response to three different treatment strategies over 13 years: WBRT with or without CHOP (cyclophosphamide, doxorubicin, vincristine, and prednisone); combined modality treatment with MTX (1 g/m^2) and WBRT; or HD-MTX (8 g/m^2) alone. Only age > 60, elevated LDH, and omission of MTX were associated with a worse outcome – otherwise OS was similar across the different strategies.[56]

Because of this demonstrated efficacy, MTX forms the backbone of most combined modality regimens and most are associated with similar survival rates, but it is the toxicity that varies among the different regimens. There is no consensus on which specific combination is superior. One commonly used combination regimen involving MTX, vincristine, procarbazine, cytarabine, and WBRT was associated with an overall response rate (ORR) of 91%, a PFS of 24 months, and an OS of 36.9 months.[41] Toxicity was notable for 8 patient deaths and 12 cases of clinically significant neurotoxicity in the 98 patients studied. A subsequent study administered a lower dose of post-chemotherapy WBRT (23.4 Gy) to patients who achieved a complete response (CR) to chemotherapy and full-dose WBRT (45 Gy) to those who did not.[45] Overall 2-year survival was estimated to be 67% and no treatment-related neurotoxicity was observed. In a multicenter trial using MTX, teniposide, carmustine, methylprednisolone, intrathecal (IT) MTX, IT cytarabine, and WBRT an ORR of 81% and median OS of 46 months was observed, but 10% of patients died from treatment-related complications.[42] Toxicity was deemed excessive when MTX (3.5 g/m^2) was combined with IDHAP (idarubicin, dexamethasone, cytarabine [cytosine arabinoside; Ara-C], cisplatin) and bromodeoxyuridine, an agent to enhance the lytic effects of WBRT.[57] While the ORR reported in these studies is encouraging, the high frequency of treatment-related toxicity is a significant concern.

A common finding in these trials is that patients who respond to initial chemotherapy have improved outcomes. In a review of 55 consecutive PCNSL patients treated at a single center, patients who could not tolerate MTX had a median survival of 46 days while those < 60 years old who achieved a CR with MTX-based treatment had a median survival of

Table 23.3. Selected treatment studies

	Chemotherapy regimen	n	IT chemo	WBRT	CR	PR	OS (mo)	PFS (mo)
Chemotherapy with RT								
Abrey *et al.*, 2000[39]	MTX (3.5 g/m^2), procarbazine, vincristine, cytarabine	52	MTX	45 Gy	87% (45/52)	8% (4/52)	60	NA
Ferreri *et al.*, 2001[40]	MTX (3 g/m^2), procarbazine, vincristine	13	None	36–45 Gy	77%[a] (10/13)	15%[a] (2/13)	2-yr survival 80%	25+
DeAngelis *et al.*, 2002[41]	MTX (2.5 g/m^2), procarbazine, vincristine, dexamethasone, cytarabine	102	MTX	45 Gy	58%[a] (29/50)	36%[a] (18/50)	36.9	24
Poortsmans *et al.*, 2003[42]	MTX (3 g/m^2), teniposide, carmustine	52	Cytarabine, MTX	30 Gy with 10 Gy boost	69% (36/52)	12% (6/52)	46	NA
Omuro *et al.*, 2005[43]	MTX (1 g/m^2), thiotepa, procarbazine	17	MTX	41.4 Gy with 14.4 Gy boost	76% (13/17)	12% (2/17)	18	32
Gavrilovic *et al.*, 2006[39,44b]	MTX (3.5 g/m^2), procarbazine, vincristine, cytarabine	57	MTX	45 Gy in those < 60 yo	56% (27/48)	33% (16/48)	51	129
Shah *et al.*, 2007[45]	MTX (3.5 g/m^2), rituximab, procarbazine, vincristine, cytarabine	30	None	23.4 Gy if CR, 45 Gy if not CR	77% (23/30)	NA	2-yr survival 67%	40[c]
Yamanaka *et al.*, 2007[46]	MTX (1 g/m^2), rituximab, pirarubicin, procarbazine, prednisone	11	None	Deferred if > 60 yo, 20 Gy given for CR after chemo	55%[a] (6/11)	36%[a] (4/11)	NA (54 +/− 40% at 2 yrs)	NA
Chemotherapy without RT								
Pels *et al.*, 2003[47]	MTX (5 g/m^2), vincristine, ifosfamide, dexamethasone, cyclophosphamide, cytarabine, vindesine	65	Prednisolone, MTX, cytarabine	None	61% (37/61)	10% (6/65)	50	21
Hoang-Xuan *et al.*, 2003[48]	MTX (1 g/m^2), lomustine, procarbazine, methylprednisolone	50	Cytarabine, MTX	None	42% (21/50)	6% (3/50)	14.3	10.6
Gerstner *et al.*, 2008[49,50b]	MTX (8 g/m^2)	25	None	None	48% (12/25)	NA	55.4	12.8
Intra-arterial chemotherapy								
McAllister *et al.*, 2000[51]	IA MTX after BBBD with mannitol, IV cyclophosphamide, etoposide	74	None	None	65% (48/74)	19% (14/74)	40.7	NA
Doolittle *et al.*, 2000[52]	IA MTX (5 g total dose), cyclophosphamide, etoposide after BBBD mannitol	53	None	None	75% (40/53)	15% (8/53)	NA	NA
Sonoda *et al.*, 2007[53]	IA ACNU	63	None	36–50 Gy	75% (43/57)	25% (14/57)	39	26

Note: [a]Prior to RT – post-RT results not available.
[b]This study is an update of a previous study.
[c]Estimated.
RT: radiation therapy; MTX: methotrexate; IT: intrathecal; IA: intra-arterial; IV: intravenous; BBBD: blood–brain barrier disruption; ACNU: nimustine; NA: not available.

56 months. However, 40% of the patients did not complete chemotherapy because of toxicity or disease progression.[58]

Chemotherapy alone

The combined modality protocols enumerated above are often associated with delayed neurotoxicity, particularly in those patients older than 60 years who received WBRT. Because of this high frequency of neurotoxicity, there has been interest in studies of chemotherapy alone, reserving WBRT for patients who relapse.

In a phase II, multicenter study of 25 patients using IV MTX ($8\,g/m^2$), the outcomes included a CR proportion of 52%, PFS of 12.8 months, OS of 55.4 months and median disease-specific survival of 73.2+ months.[49,50] These results suggest that up to 25% of patients with PCNSL may be cured with MTX alone. In a study of ten elderly patients with PCNSL treated with MTX alone ($8\,g/m^2$ followed by $3.5\,g/m^2$) the ORR was 90% with a median OS of 36 months.[59] In addition, toxicity was acceptable, demonstrating that MTX can be both safe and effective in an elderly patient population if used without adjuvant radiation. MTX combined with temozolomide may also be beneficial in elderly patients.[60]

Methotrexate-based, multiagent chemotherapy regimens without WBRT have received considerable attention. A regimen consisting of MTX, lomustine (CCNU), procarbazine, methylprednisolone, IT MTX, and IT cytarabine in patients > 60 was associated with a median OS of 14.3 months and a decreased risk of neurotoxicity.[48] Another multiagent regimen consisting of MTX, cytarabine, vincristine, ifosfamide, cyclophosphamide, and IT MTX/cytarabine/prednisolone was studied in a phase II trial of 65 patients and was associated with a 71% ORR and a median OS of 50 months. Despite these promising results 6 patients died from treatment-related complications and 12 patients experienced Ommaya reservoir infections.[47]

Blood–brain barrier disruption (BBBD) is a strategy aimed at circumventing the BBB in order to deliver higher concentrations of chemotherapeutic agents to the CNS. Doolittle *et al.* reported complete radiographic responses in 40/53 patients with PCNSL treated with intra-arterial (IA) MTX, IV cyclophosphamide, and etoposide following BBBD with IA mannitol.[51] Moreover, long-term follow-up of the patients treated with IA MTX demonstrated maintenance of cognitive function.[53] However, BBBD is technically complex and should only be performed in centers with expertise and experience in the technique.

Intrathecal chemotherapy

A controversial issue in the management of PCNSL is the role of IT chemotherapy. Historical comparisons have determined that there appears to be no difference in OS when IT MTX is added to regimens that already include high doses of IV MTX.[61] By giving IV MTX in lieu of IT chemotherapy, the risk of Ommaya placement, IT-related chemical meningitis, and infection can be avoided. As mentioned above, the IV dose must be high enough, though, and administered over a rapid enough time interval for MTX to penetrate into the CSF and tumor. However, patients with concurrent brain and leptomeningeal lymphoma will often require IT chemotherapy.

High-dose chemotherapy with stem cell rescue

Initial studies of autologous stem cell transplantation (ASCT) for patients with newly diagnosed PCNSL have yielded mixed results (Table 23.4). Brevet *et al.* achieved an initial CR in 6/6 patients following completion of induction (4 patients) and ASCT (remaining 2 patients); two died from relapse after 9 and 23 months while the other four remained disease-free at a median follow up of 41.5 months.[62] In a study of induction chemotherapy (MTX $3.5\,g/m^2$ for five cycles and cytarabine $3\,g/m^2$ for two cycles) followed by BEAM (carmustine,

Table 23.4. Studies of high-dose chemotherapy and ASCT in newly diagnosed PCNSL

	No. of pts entered into study	No. of pts who underwent ASCT	No. of pts with PR/CR following ASCT	OS
Brevet *et al.*[62]	6	6	6	35.5 months
Abrey *et al.*[63]	28	14	10	3-year survival: 60%
Cheng *et al.*[64]	7	7	6	NA[a]
Illerhaus *et al.*[65]	30	23	21	5-year survival: 87%
Montemurro *et al.*[66]	23	16	13	2-year survival: 61%[b]
Illerhaus *et al.*[67]	13	11	11	3-year survival: 76.9%

Notes: [a]5 patients still relapse free at end of study at 5, 8, 24, 36, and 42 months.
[b]Estimated.
pts: patients; ASCT: autologous stem cell transplantation, OS: overall survival; PR: partial response; CR: complete response; NA: not available.

etoposide, cytarabine, melphalan) and ASCT in 28 patients with newly diagnosed PCNSL, 14 achieved at least a partial response to induction chemotherapy and then received BEAM and ASCT. Among these 14 transplanted patients, 8 progressed at a median of 2.3 months following ASCT.[63] In a multicenter study of 30 newly diagnosed PCNSL patients under the age of 65, Illerhaus *et al.* reported on the subset of 23 patients who received high-dose chemotherapy plus ASCT followed by hyperfractionated WBRT.[65] All 21 patients who were assessed after WBRT had achieved CR. After a median follow-up of 63 months the 5-year OS was 87% in those who received ASCT and 69% for all 30 patients initially enrolled into the study. ASCT may be effective in patients with poor prognostic features as well.[64] Neurotoxicity was low in patients < 60 years old in these studies but aggressive induction chemotherapy seems to be necessary. It is likely that high-dose chemotherapy and ASCT will assume an increasingly important role in younger patients with PCNSL in the newly diagnosed or relapsed setting.

Salvage therapy

Despite aggressive treatment, the majority of patients with PCNSL progress or relapse and require salvage therapy. The best management of relapsed or refractory PCNSL has yet to be determined and has only been studied in small patient series. In general, the prognosis for patients with relapsed or progressive PCNSL is poor with a median survival of approximately 4 months.[68] For patients who initially experienced a CR to a chemotherapy regimen that included MTX, retreatment with MTX alone may be effective. Twenty-two patients who previously responded to MTX were treated at relapse with MTX ($8\,g/m^2$); the ORR was 91% and the median OS was 61.9 months.[69]

Temozolomide, an alkylating agent with good CSF penetration, was associated with a 26% radiographic response proportion in 23 patients previously treated with MTX-containing chemotherapy with or without WBRT.[70] Rituximab, a monoclonal antibody to CD20, has been added to temozolomide in two studies of relapsed or progressive PCNSL, yielding a median survival of 8 and 14 months.[71,72] Intraventricular rituximab (10–25 mg) was determined to be feasible in a phase I study of patients with relapsed or refractory lymphomatous meningitis (LM) but further testing is needed.[73] An unexpected observation in this study was a radiographic response of brain parenchymal lymphoma in one case and two patients with intraocular lymphoma who experienced disease resolution and/or clinical improvement in vision.

Topotecan, a topoisomerase I inhibitor, was administered to 27 patients with relapsed or refractory PCNSL. The ORR was 33% with 9 patients achieving a CR or partial response, and the OS was 8.4 months.[74] However, 8 of 12 patients still alive at 6 months exhibited symptoms of neurotoxicity. Other chemotherapy regimens studied have included etoposide (VP-16), ifosfamide, and cytarabine (cytosine arabinoside [Ara-C]) (VIA) and procarbazine, lomustine (CCNU), and vincristine (PCV).[75,76] Using VIA, the 12-month OS was 41% and with PCV, it was 57%. These results are summarized in Table 23.5.

Table 23.5. Selected salvage therapy trials in PCNSL

Treatment	n	Pts with PR/CR	OS (months)
WBRT[77]	27	20	10.9
WBRT[78]	48	38	16
MTX[69]	22	20	61.9
HDT/ASCT[79]	22	16	63.7% at 36 months
PCV[76]	7	6	>16
TMZ[70]	23	6	3.5
TMZ + rituximab[72]	15	8	14
TMZ + rituximab[71]	7	7	8
Topotecan[74]	27	9	8.4
VIA[75]	16	6	41% at 12 months
Stereotactic radiosurgery[80]	9 with 17 tumors	13/17 tumors	58% at 12 months

Notes: Pts: patients; HDT: high-dose chemotherapy; ASCT: autologous stem cell transplantation; PCV: procarbazine, lomustine, vincristine; TMZ: temozolomide; VIA: etoposide, ifosfamide, cytarabine; OS: overall survival; PR: partial response; CR: complete response; MTX: methotrexate; WBRT: whole brain radiation therapy.

In a study of 20 refractory or relapsed PCNSL and ocular lymphoma patients using thiotepa, busulfan, and cyclophosphamide as induction chemotherapy followed by ASCT, there was an 80% CR proportion (16/20) and a 3-year probability of survival of 63.7%.[79] Although this study included a highly selected salvage patient population, these results are encouraging and should be confirmed in other studies of this approach in relapsed or refractory PCNSL patients.

Radiation as a salvage therapy has also been explored. Following WBRT, 74–79% of patients with relapsed or refractory PCNSL can achieve a radiographic response.[77,78] Median survival after radiation treatment is 10.9–16 months, with those less than 60 years old faring better. Stereotactic radiosurgery (SRS) was studied in nine patients as salvage therapy for relapse and was given with chemotherapy in seven of the nine patients.[80] Patients had a 1-year survival of 58% and a 1-year intracranial relapse-free rate of 22% suggesting that perhaps SRS may palliate local symptoms but does not affect distant spread.

Neurotoxicity

Neurotoxicity is a well-known, delayed consequence of treatment of PCNSL with chemoradiation (WBRT + chemotherapy) or WBRT alone. It is more common in patients older

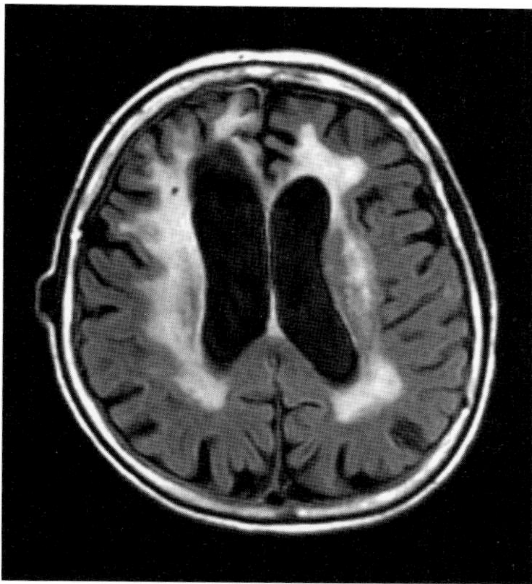

Figure 23.3 Neurotoxicity. Cranial FLAIR MR images from a 67-year-old patient with PCNSL 1 year after achieving a CR to WBRT. The patient developed memory failure, gait ataxia, and incontinence in the post-radiation setting. There is increased signal throughout the cerebral white matter, cortical atrophy, and ventricular enlargement.

than 60 and may present as a subcortical dementia with gait ataxia and incontinence. MRI typically reveals periventricular white matter abnormalities, cortical atrophy, and ventricular enlargement (Figure 23.3). These changes typically appear 6–12 months following WBRT but it is important to note that radiographic changes do not always correlate with clinical symptoms. Pathologic studies have demonstrated demyelination, neuronal loss, gliosis, and rarefaction of the white matter.[81] Large vessel atherosclerosis has been observed as well, implicating vascular injury and resultant tissue ischemia as one possible mechanism for neurotoxicity. Although the pathophysiology of treatment-related neurotoxicity is multifactorial, toxicity to neural progenitor cells is likely to play a pivotal role.[82]

Studies examining neurotoxicity have several methodologic limitations including lack of baseline evaluations, different definitions of cognitive impairment, and small numbers.[83] In one study of PCNSL patients, the 5-year cumulative incidence of neurotoxicity was 24% and the use of WBRT was the only significant predictor of development of neurotoxicity on multivariate analysis.[84] This is in contrast to chemotherapy alone in which less decline in cognitive function is observed despite evidence of white matter changes on MRI.[83,85,86] Attention, executive function, memory (particularly verbal), and psychomotor speed are the cognitive domains typically affected. Unfortunately, there is no effective treatment for neurotoxicity, and patients often die from complications of neurotoxicity without evidence of recurrent lymphoma. In order to better assess these changes, the IPCG has proposed a battery of cognitive and quality-of-life tests to be included in all prospective PCNSL trials.[83]

Secondary CNS lymphoma

CNS dissemination of NHL is much more common than in Hodgkin lymphoma. More than 60% of secondary lymphoma cases involve the leptomeninges while isolated brain parenchymal lesions are rare.[87] Specific groups of patients with NHL who are at higher risk of CNS dissemination have been identified. Extranodal lymphoma such as testicular lymphoma has a higher predisposition to involve the CNS than other forms of NHL. Burkitt lymphoma also has a high risk of CNS dissemination. The role of prophylactic IT chemotherapy for these high-risk cases remains controversial but is recommended by some authorities.[88]

Lymphoma cells may reach the leptomeninges by direct extension from local metastases, by hematologic dissemination, or by perineural tracking along cranial or peripheral nerves. Once cancer cells gain access to the CSF, they can disseminate throughout CSF pathways by bulk flow. Tumor cells typically settle in the basal cisterns, posterior fossa, and cauda equina because of slower CSF flow in these areas. These deposits may then become sources for continuous shedding of malignant cells into the CSF.

Diagnosis

Patients with LM can present with signs of obstructed CSF flow, multifocal neurologic signs, or altered mental status. CSF obstruction occurs when tumor cells block flow or reabsorption of CSF leading to signs and symptoms of increased intracranial pressure and communicating hydrocephalus. The clinical hallmark of LM is multifocal neurologic signs and symptoms along the neuraxis. Any new occurrence of focal numbness/weakness, headache, back/radicular pain, or incontinence in a patient with lymphoma should prompt consideration of LM. Following a history and physical examination searching for the multifocal signs and symptoms mentioned above, contrast-enhanced MRI or CT should be done. Imaging should focus on the suspected source of the symptoms but scanning the brain and entire spine often identifies asymptomatic lesions, and brain imaging is recommended prior to diagnostic lumbar puncture. Radiographic findings suggestive of LM include enhancement of the leptomeninges or communicating hydrocephalus and is observed in 43–52% of patients. However, leptomeningeal enhancement is non-specific and can also be seen in patients with infection, inflammation, trauma, or following lumbar puncture. CSF examination is the most informative investigation to confirm LM with a sensitivity of 67–93%. CSF studies that should be obtained are similar to the diagnostic evaluation in patients with PCNSL – cell count, protein, glucose, cytology, flow cytometry, and IGH gene rearrangement. The lumbar puncture may need to be repeated since the yield of CSF cytology increases from 50% to 85% from the first lumbar puncture to the third. Rarely, a biopsy is necessary if MRI and CSF examination are non-diagnostic.

Treatment

Unfortunately, the prognosis for patients with LM or parenchymal disease is poor with a survival of less than 5 months if the patient presents with relapsed disease. Consequently, treatment is often palliative although some patients do respond and have a sustained survival with therapy, especially those < 60 or those who receive MTX-based chemotherapy.[87] Radiation has a limited role in LM with minimal impact on OS unless there is bulky disease that chemotherapy cannot penetrate. Intrathecal chemotherapy by Ommaya reservoir with MTX, thiotepa, or cytarabine has traditionally been the mainstay of treatment. The liposomal formulation of cytarabine extends the half-life of the drug from 3 hours to 141 hours allowing for treatment every 2 weeks versus twice a week with MTX, thiotepa, or non-liposomal cytarabine. In one small study, liposomal cytarabine had an improved cytologic response rate when compared with standard cytarabine.[89] As mentioned above, intraventricular rituximab is currently under evaluation as a potential treatment for LM in NHL patients.[73] Systemic chemotherapies that incorporate IV MTX therapy may result in cytologic responses.[90,91] MTX-based chemotherapy and/or WBRT are typically used in patients with brain parenchymal relapses. Myeloablative therapies with SCT have been studied in small trials and show some promise with CR rates ranging from 23% to 61%.[92,93]

CNS post-transplant lymphoproliferative disorder

Post-transplant lymphoproliferative disorder (PTLD) of the CNS (CNS-PTLD) arises in the setting of immunosuppression and is similar to PCNSL in that it is typically an aggressive, angiocentric B-cell tumor. More often than not, the tumor is associated with EBV infection. CNS-PTLD occurs in < 7% of transplant patients and can develop months to years following transplant.[94] Neuroimaging typically reveals multifocal, heterogeneously enhancing brain masses with extensive tumor-associated edema. Treatment consists of reduced immunosuppression, radiation, chemotherapy, antivirals, or rituximab.[95] Survival is poor in patients who do not respond to reduction of immunosuppression or are older than 40 years old. Some patients with isolated CNS involvement may respond to rituximab, radiation, or MTX-based chemotherapy.[95,96]

Conclusions

PCNSL is a distinct and rare type of NHL. Evaluation requires proper assessment of the brain, eyes, CSF, and body in order to confirm that the tumor is restricted to the CNS. The rarity of PCNSL and the difficulty in obtaining tissue for molecular studies has limited development of effective treatments. As a result, there is no consensus on the optimal management strategy for patients with PCNSL. It appears reasonable, particularly in those patients older than 60 years, to withhold WBRT until relapse in order to avoid neurotoxicity. MTX is clearly the backbone of chemotherapy for PCNSL but it is unclear which drugs should be added to MTX to improve survival and whether or not low-dose radiation with chemotherapy can avoid delayed neurotoxicity.

Secondary CNS lymphoma, typically NHL, most often presents with leptomeningeal dissemination but brain parenchymal disease can occur as well. Diagnostic evaluation consists of history, physical examination, contrast-enhanced cranial and spine MRI, and CSF examination. Treatment is primarily palliative but therapeutic benefit may be achieved with IT chemotherapy or with systemic chemotherapy regimens that include MTX or ASCT.

References

1. Kadan-Lottick N, Sklusarek M, Gurney J. Decreasing incidence rates of primary central nervous system lymphoma. *Cancer* 2002;**95**:193–202.
2. Miller DC, Hochberg FH, Harris NL, *et al.* Pathology with clinical correlations of primary central nervous system non-Hodgkin's lymphoma. The Massachusetts General Hospital experience 1958–1989. *Cancer* 1994;**74**:1383–97.
3. Jahnke K, Korfel A, Komm J, *et al.* International study on low-grade primary central nervous system lymphoma. *Ann Neurol* 2006; **59**:755–62.
4. Shenkier T, Blay JY, O'Neill BP, *et al.* Primary CNS lymphoma of T-cell origin: a descriptive analysis from the international primary CNS lymphoma collaborative group. *J Clin Oncol* 2005;**23**:2233–9.
5. Kaluza V, Rao DS, Said JW, *et al.* Primary extranodal nasal-type natural killer/T-cell lymphoma of the brain: a case report. *Hum Pathol* 2006; **37**:769–72.
6. Ponzoni M, Berger F, Chassagne-Clement C, *et al.* Reactive perivascular T-cell infiltrate predicts survival in primary central nervous system B-cell lymphomas. *Br J Haematol* 2007;**138**:316–23.
7. Camilleri-Broët S, Crinière E, Broët P, *et al.* A uniform activated B-cell-like immunophenotype might explain the poor prognosis of primary central nervous system lymphomas: analysis of 83 cases. *Blood* 2006;**107**:190–6.
8. Rubenstein J, Fridlyand J, Shen A, *et al.* Gene expression and angiotropism in primary CNS lymphoma. *Blood* 2006;**107**:3716–23.
9. Tun HW, Personett D, Baskerville KA, *et al.* Pathway analysis of primary central nervous system lymphoma. *Blood* 2008;**111**:3200–10.
10. Bataille B, Delwail V, Menet E, *et al.* Primary intracerebral malignant lymphoma: report of 248 cases. *J Neurosurg* 2000;**92**:261–6.
11. Newell M, Hoy J, Cooper S, *et al.* Human immunodeficiency virus-related primary central nervous system lymphoma: factors influencing survival in 111 patients. *Cancer* 2004;**100**:2627–34.

12. Batchelor TT, Kolak G, Ciordia R, *et al.* High-dose methotrexate for intraocular lymphoma. *Clin Cancer Res* 2003;**9**:711–15.

13. Akpek EK, Ahmed I, Hochberg FH, *et al.* Intraocular-central nervous system lymphoma: clinical features, diagnosis, and outcomes. *Ophthalmology* 1999;**106**:1805–10.

14. Grimm SA, Pulido JS, Jahnke K, *et al.* Primary intraocular lymphoma: an International Primary Central Nervous System Lymphoma Collaborative Group Report. *Ann Oncol* 2007;**18**:1851–5.

15. Char DH, Ljung BM, Miller T, *et al.* Primary intraocular lymphoma (ocular reticulum cell sarcoma) diagnosis and management. *Ophthalmology* 1988;**95**:625–30.

16. Abrey L, Batchelor T, Ferreri A, *et al.* Report of an international workshop to standardize baseline evaluation and response criteria for primary CNS lymphoma. *J Clin Oncol* 2005;**23**: 5034–43.

17. Ekstein D, Ben-Yehuda D, Slyusarevsky E, *et al.* CSF analysis of IgH gene rearrangement in CNS lymphoma: relationship to the disease course. *J Neurol Sci* 2006;**247**:39–46.

18. Jahnke K, Hummel M, Korfel A, *et al.* Detection of subclinical systemic disease in primary CNS lymphoma by polymerase chain reaction of the rearranged immunoglobulin heavy-chain genes. *J Clin Oncol* 2006;**24**:4754–7.

19. Batchelor TT, Buchbinder BR, Harris NL. Case records of the Massachusetts General Hospital. Weekly clinicopathological exercises. Case 1-2005. A 35-year-old woman with difficulty walking, headache, and nausea. *N Engl J Med* 2005; **352**(2): 185–94.

20. Kuker W, Nagele T, Korfel A, *et al.* Primary central nervous system lymphomas (PCNSL): MRI features at presentation in 100 patients. *J Neurooncol* 2005;**72**:169–77.

21. Ferreri A, Blay J, Reni M, *et al.* Prognostic scoring system for primary CNS lymphomas: the International Extranodal Lymphoma Study Group experience. *J Clin Oncol* 2003;**21**: 266–72.

22. Abrey LE, Ben-Porat L, Panageas KS, *et al.* Primary central nervous system lymphoma: the Memorial Sloan-Kettering Cancer Center prognostic model. *J Clin Oncol* 2006; **24**:5711–15.

23. Braaten K, Betensky R, de Leval L, *et al.* BCL-6 expression predicts improved survival in patients with primary central nervous system lymphoma. *Clin Cancer Res* 2003;**9**:1063–9.

24. Larocca LM, Capello D, Rinelli A, *et al.* The molecular and phenotypic profile of primary central nervous system lymphoma identifies distinct categories of the disease and is consistent with histogenetic derivation from germinal center-related B cells. *Blood* 1998;**92**:1011–19.

25. Takeshita M, Iwashita A, Kurihara K, *et al.* Histologic and immunohistologic findings and prognosis of 40 cases of gastric large B-cell lymphoma. *Am J Surg Pathol* 2000;**24**:1641–69.

26. Levy O, DeAngelis LM, Filippa DA, *et al.* Bcl-6 predicts improved prognosis in primary central nervous system lymphoma. *Cancer* 2007;**112**:151–6.

27. Lin C, Kuo K, Chuang S, *et al.* Comparison of the expression and prognostic significance of differentiation markers between diffuse large B-cell lymphoma of the central nervous system origin and peripheral nodal origin. *Clin Cancer Res* 2006;**12**:1152–6.

28. Rosenwald A, Wright G, Chan W. Lymphoma/Leukemia Molecular Profiling Project. The use of molecular profiling to predict survival after chemotherapy for diffuse large-B-cell lymphoma. *N Engl J Med* 2002;**346**:1937–47.

29. Lossos I, Jones C, Warnke R, *et al.* Expression of a single gene, BCL-6, strongly predicts survival in patients with diffuse large B-cell lymphoma. *Blood* 2001;**98**:945–51.

30. Ferreri A, Abrey L, Blay J, *et al.* Summary statement on primary central nervous system lymphomas from the Eighth International Conference on Malignant Lymphoma, Lugano, Switzerland, June 12 to 15, 2002. *J Clin Oncol* 2003;**21**:2407–14.

31. Mathew BS, Carson K, Grossman SA. Initial response to glucocorticoids *Cancer* 2006;**106**:383–7.

32. Bellinzona M, Roser F, Ostertag H, *et al.* Surgical removal of primary central nervous system lymphomas (PCNSL) presenting as space occupying lesions: a series of 33 cases. *Eur J Surg Oncol* 2005;**31**:100–5.

33. Batchelor T, Loeffler J. Primary CNS lymphoma. *J Clin Oncol* 2006; **24**:1281–8.

34. Nelson D, Martz K, Bonner H, *et al.* Non-Hodgkin's lymphoma of the brain: can high dose, large volume radiation therapy improve survival? Report on a prospective trial by the Radiation Therapy Oncology Group (RTOG): RTOG 8315. *Int J Radiat Oncol Biol Phys* 1992;**23**:9–17.

35. Shibamoto Y, Ogino H, Hasegawa M, *et al.* Results of radiation monotherapy for primary central nervous system lymphoma in the 1990s. *Int J Radiat Oncol Biol Phys* 2005;**62**:809–13.

36. Ishikawa H, Hasegawa M, Tamaki Y, *et al.* Comparable outcomes of radiation therapy without high-dose methotrexate for patients with primary central nervous system lymphoma. *Jpn J Clin Oncol* 2003;**33**:443–9.

37. Bessell E, Lopez-Guillermo A, Villa S, *et al.* Importance of radiotherapy in the outcome of patients with primary CNS lymphoma: an analysis of the CHOD/BVAM regimen followed by two different radiotherapy treatments. *J Clin Oncol* 2002;**20**:231–6.

38. Fisher B, Seiferheld W, Schultz C, *et al.* Secondary analysis of Radiation Therapy Oncology Group study (RTOG) 9310: an intergroup phase II combined modality treatment of primary central nervous system lymphoma. *J Neurooncol* 2005;**74**: 201–5.

39. Abrey LE, Yahalom J, DeAngelis LM. Treatment for primary CNS lymphoma: the next step. *J Clin Oncol* 2000;**18**:3144–50.

40. Ferreri AJ, Reni M, Dell'Oro S, *et al.* Combined treatment with high-dose methotrexate, vincristine and procarbazine, without intrathecal chemotherapy, followed by consolidation radiotherapy for primary central nervous system lymphoma in immunocompetent patients. *Oncology* 2001;**60**:134–40.

41. DeAngelis L, Seiferheld W, Schold S, *et al.* Combination chemotherapy and radiotherapy for primary central nervous system lymphoma: Radiation Therapy Oncology Group Study 93–10. *J Clin Oncol* 2002;**20**:4643–8.

42. Poortmans P, Kluin-Nelemans H, Haaxma-Reiche H, *et al.* High-dose methotrexate-based chemotherapy followed by consolidating radiotherapy in non-AIDS-related primary central nervous system lymphoma: European Organization for Research and Treatment of Cancer Lymphoma Group Phase II Trial 20962. *J Clin Oncol* 2003;**21**:4483–8.

43. Omuro A, DeAngelis L, Yahalom J, *et al.* Chemoradiotherapy for primary CNS lymphoma: an intent-to-treat analysis with complete follow-up. *Neurology* 2005;**64**:69–74.

44. Gavrilovic IT, Hormigo A, Yahalom J, *et al.* Long-term follow-up of high-dose methotrexate-based therapy with and without whole brain irradiation for newly diagnosed primary CNS lymphoma. *J Clin Oncol* 2006; **24**:4570–4.

45. Shah G, Yahalom J, Correa D, *et al.* Combined immunochemotherapy with reduced whole-brain radiotherapy for newly diagnosed primary CNS lymphoma. *J Clin Oncol* 2007; **25**:4730–5.

46. Yamanaka R, Homma J, Sano M, *et al.* Immuno-chemotherapy with a combination of rituximab, methotrexate, pirarubicin and procarbazine for patients with primary CNS lymphoma – a preliminary report. *Leuk Lymphoma* 2007;**48**:1019–22.

47. Pels H, Schmidt-Wolf IG, Glasmacher A, *et al.* Primary central nervous system lymphoma: results of a pilot and phase II study of systemic and intraventricular chemotherapy with deferred radiotherapy. *J Clin Oncol* 2003;**21**:4489–95.

48. Hoang-Xuan K, Taillandier L, Chinot O, *et al.* Chemotherapy alone as initial treatment for primary CNS lymphoma in patients older than 60 years: a multicenter phase II study (26952) of the European Organization for Research and Treatment of Cancer Brain Tumor Group. *J Clin Oncol* 2003;**21**:2726–31.

49. Batchelor T, Carson K, O'Neill A, *et al.* Treatment of primary CNS lymphoma with methotrexate and deferred radiation therapy: a report of the NABTT 96–07. *J Clin Oncol* 2003;**21**:1044–9.

50. Gerstner ER, Carson K, Grossman S, *et al.* Long-term outcome in PCNSL patients treated with high-dose methotrexate and deferred radiation. *Neurology* 2008;**70**:401–2.

51. McAllister LD, Doolittle ND, Guastadisegni PE, *et al.* Cognitive outcomes and long-term follow-up results after enhanced chemotherapy delivery for primary central nervous system lymphoma. *Neurosurgery* 2000;**46**:51–60.

52. Doolittle N, Miner M, Hall W, *et al.* Safety and efficacy of a multicenter study using intraarterial chemotherapy in conjunction with osmotic opening of the blood-brain barrier for the treatment of patients with malignant brain tumors. *Cancer* 2000;**88**:637–47.

53. Sonoda Y, Matsumoto K, Kakuto Y, *et al.* Primary CNS lymphoma treated with combined intra-arterial ACNU and radiotherapy. *Acta Neurochir (Wien)* 2007;**149**:1183–9.

54. Olson J, Blakeley J, Grossman S, *et al.* Differences in the distribution of methotrexate into high grade gliomas following intravenous administration as monitored by microdialysis, are associated with blood-brain-barrier integrity. *J Clin Oncol* (2006 ASCO Annual Meeting Proceedings Part I) 2006;**24**(185): Abstract 1548.

55. Hiraga S, Arita N, Ohnishi T, *et al.* Rapid infusion of high-dose methotrexate resulting in enhanced penetration into cerebrospinal fluid and intensified tumor response in primary central nervous system lymphomas. *J Neurosurg* 1999; **91**:221–30.

56. Shenkier TN, Voss N, Chhanabhai M, *et al.* The treatment of primary central nervous system lymphoma in 122 immunocompetent patients: a population-based study of successively treated cohorts from the British Colombia Cancer Agency. *Cancer* 2005;**103**:1008–17.

57. Dabaja BS, McLaughlin P, Ha CS, *et al.* Primary central nervous system lymphoma: phase I evaluation of infusional bromodeoxyuridine with whole brain accelerated fractionation radiation therapy after chemotherapy. *Cancer* 2003;**98**:1021–8.

58. Hodson D, Bowles K, Cooke L, *et al.* Primary central nervous system lymphoma: a single-centre experience of 55 unselected cases. *Clin Oncol (R Coll Radiol)* 2005;**17**:185–91.

59. Rubenstein JL, Kim J, Ozawa T, *et al.* Anti-VEGF antibody treatment of glioblastoma prolongs survival but results in increased vascular cooption. *Neoplasia* 2000;**2**:306–14.

60. Omuro A, Taillandier L, Chinot O, *et al.* Temozolomide and methotrexate for primary central nervous system lymphoma in the elderly. *J Neurooncol* 2007;**85**:207–11.

61. Khan R, Shi W, Thaler H, *et al.* Is intrathecal methotrexate necessary in the treatment of primary CNS lymphoma? *J Neurooncol* 2002; **58**:175–8.

62. Brevet M, Garidi R, Gruson B, *et al.* First-line autologous stem cell transplantation in primary CNS lymphoma. *Eur J Haematol* 2005;**75**:288–92.

63. Abrey L, Moskowitz C, Mason W, *et al.* Intensive methotrexate and cytarabine followed by high-dose chemotherapy with autologous stem-cell rescue in patients with newly diagnosed primary CNS lymphoma: an intent-to-treat analysis. *J Clin Oncol* 2003;**21**:4151–6.

64. Cheng T, Forsyth P, Chaudhry A, *et al.* High-dose thiotepa, busulfan, cyclophosphamide and ASCT without whole-brain radiotherapy for poor prognosis primary CNS lymphoma. *Bone Marrow Transplant* 2003; **31**:679–85.

65. Illerhaus G, Marks R, Ihorst G, *et al.* High-dose chemotherapy with autologous stem-cell transplantation and hyperfractionated radiotherapy as first-line treatment of primary CNS lymphoma. *J Clin Oncol* 2006; **24**:3865–70.

66. Montemurro M, Kiefer T, Schüler F, *et al.* Primary central nervous system lymphoma treated with high-dose methotrexate, high-dose busulfan/ thiotepa, autologous stem-cell transplantation and response-adapted whole-brain radiotherapy: results of the multicenter Ostdeutsche Studiengruppe Hamato-Onkologie OSHO-53 phase II study. *Ann Oncol* 2007;**18**:665–71.

67. Illerhaus G, Müller F, Feuerhake F, *et al.* High-dose chemotherapy and autologous stem-cell transplantation without consolidating radiotherapy as first-line treatment for primary lymphoma of the central nervous system. *Haematologica* 2008; **93**:147–8.

68. Jahnke K, Thiel E, Martus P, *et al.* Relapse of primary central nervous system lymphoma: clinical features, outcome and prognostic factors. *J Neurooncol* 2006;**80**:159–65.

69. Plotkin S, Betensky R, Hochberg F, *et al.* Treatment of relapsed central nervous system lymphoma with high-dose methotrexate. *Clin Cancer Res* 2004;**10**:5643–6.

70. Reni M, Mason W, Zaja F, *et al.* Salvage chemotherapy with temozolomide in primary CNS lymphomas: preliminary results of a phase II trial. *Eur J Cancer* 2004;**40**:162–8.

71. Wong ET, Tishler R, Barron L, *et al.* Immunochemotherapy with rituximab and temozolomide for central nervous system lymphomas. *Cancer* 2004;**101**:139–45.

72. Enting R, Demopoulos A, DeAngelis L, *et al.* Salvage therapy for primary CNS lymphoma with a combination of rituximab and temozolomide. *Neurology* 2004;**63**:901–3.

73. Rubenstein JL, Fridlyand J, Abrey L, *et al.* Phase I study of intraventricular administration of rituximab in patients with recurrent CNS and intraocular lymphoma. *J Clin Oncol* 2007; **25**:1350–6.

74. Fischer L, Thiel E, Klasen H, *et al.* Prospective trial on topotecan salvage therapy in primary CNS lymphoma. *Ann Oncol* 2006;**17**:1141–5.

75. Arellano-Rodrigo E, Lopez-Guillermo A, Bessell EM, *et al.* Salvage treatment with etoposide (VP-16), ifosfamide and cytarabine (Ara-C) for patients with recurrent primary central nervous system lymphoma. *Eur J Haematol* 2003;**70**:219–24.

76. Herrlinger U, Brugger W, Bamberg M. PCV salvage chemotherapy for recurrent primary CNS lymphoma. *Neurology* 2000;**54**:1707–8.

77. Nguyen P, Chakravarti A, Finkelstein D, *et al.* Results of whole-brain radiation as salvage of methotrexate failure for immunocompetent patients with primary CNS lymphoma. *J Clin Oncol* 2005;**23**:1507–13.

78. Hottinger AF, DeAngelis LM, Yahalom J, *et al.* Salvage whole brain radiotherapy for recurrent or refractory primary CNS lymphoma. *Neurology* 2007;**69**:1178–82.

79. Soussain C, Suzan F, Hoang-Xuan K, *et al.* Results of intensive chemotherapy followed by hematopoietic stem-cell rescue in 22 patients with refractory or recurrent primary CNS lymphoma or intraocular lymphoma. *J Clin Oncol* 2001;**19**:742–9.

80. Sakamoto M, Oya N, Mizowaki T, *et al.* Initial experiences of palliative stereotactic radiosurgery for recurrent brain lymphomas. *J Neurooncol* 2006; 77:53–8.

81. Lai RA, Lauren E, Rosenblum MK, *et al.* Treatment-induced leukoencephalopathy in primary CNS lymphoma: a clinical and autopsy study. *Neurology* 2004;**62**:451–6.

82. Monje M, Mizumatsu S, Fike J, *et al.* Irradiation induces neural precursor cell dysfunction. *Nat Med* 2002; **8**:955–62.

83. Correa D, Maron L, Harder H, *et al.* Cognitive functions in primary central nervous system lymphoma: literature review and assessment guidelines. *Ann Oncol* 2007;**18**:1145–51.

84. Omuro A, Ben-Porat L, Panageas K, *et al.* Delayed neurotoxicity in primary central nervous system lymphoma. *Arch Neurol* 2005;**62**:1595–600.

85. Correa D, Anderson N, Glass A, *et al.* Cognitive functions in primary central nervous system lymphoma patients treated with chemotherapy and stem cell transplantation: preliminary findings. *Clin Adv Hematol Oncol* 2003;**1**:490.

86. Fliessbach K, Helmstaedter C, Urbach H, *et al.* Neuropsychological outcome after chemotherapy for primary CNS lymphoma: a prospective study. *Neurology* 2005;**64**:1184–8.

87. Doolittle ND, Abrey LE, Shenkier TN, *et al.* Brain parenchyma involvement as isolated central nervous system (CNS) relapse of systemic non-Hodgkin lymphoma: an International Primary CNS Lymphoma Collaborative Group report. *Blood* 2008;**111**:1085–93.

88. Hollender A, Kvaloy S, Nome O, *et al.* Central nervous system involvement following diagnosis of non-Hodgkin's lymphoma: a risk model. *Ann Oncol* 2002;**13**:1099–107.

89. Glantz MJ, Jaeckle KA, Chamberlain MC, *et al.* A randomized controlled trial comparing intrathecal sustained-release cytarabine (DepoCyt) to intrathecal methotrexate in patients with neoplastic meningitis from solid tumors. *Clin Cancer Res* 1999;**5**:3394–402.

90. Bokstein F, Lossos A, Lossos IS, *et al.* Central nervous system relapse of systemic non-Hodgkin's lymphoma: results of treatment based on high-dose methotrexate combination chemotherapy. *Leuk Lymphoma* 2002;**43**:587–93.

91. Glantz MJ, Cole BF, Recht L, *et al.* High-dose intravenous methotrexate for patients with nonleukemic leptomeningeal cancer: is intrathecal chemotherapy necessary? *J Clin Oncol* 1998;**16**:1561–7.

92. Gleissner B, Chamberlain M. Treatment of CNS dissemination in systemic lymphoma. *J Neurooncol* 2007; **84**:107–17.

93. Kasamon YL, Jones RJ, Piantadosi S, *et al.* High-dose therapy and blood or marrow transplantation for non-Hodgkin lymphoma with central nervous system involvement. *Biol Blood Marrow Transplant* 2005; **11**:93–100.

94. Castellano-Sanchez AA, Li S, Qian J, *et al.* Primary central nervous system posttransplant lymphoproliferative disorders. *Am J Clin Pathol* 2004;**121**:246–53.

95. Schiff D, O'Neill B, Plotkin S, *et al.* Isolated central nervous system post-transplant lymphoproliferative disorder (CNS-PTLD): The International Primary CNS Lymphoma Collaborative Group experience. *Proceedings of the Seventh Congress of the European Association for Neuro-Oncology* 2006; Abstract 022.

96. Buell JF, Gross TG, Hanaway MJ, *et al.* Posttransplant lymphoproliferative disorder: significance of central nervous system involvement. *Transplant Proc* 2005;**37**:954–5.

Chapter 24

HIV-related lymphomas

Caroline M. Behler and Lawrence D. Kaplan

Epidemiology/etiology

Ever since the beginning of the HIV/AIDS pandemic, it has been recognized that in addition to the increased risk of opportunistic and other infections, the incidence of malignancy is much greater in people with HIV/AIDS (PWHA) than that of the general population. This risk is likely a direct result of the immune dysfunction from chronic HIV infection, though concomitant viral infections including Epstein–Barr virus (EBV), human herpesvirus 8 (HHV-8), and human papilloma virus (HPV) also play a role. While the incidence of cancers is increased both for PWHA and immunosuppressed organ transplant patients, the risk of non-Hodgkin (NHL) and Hodgkin (HL) lymphomas appears to be significantly greater in the setting of HIV/AIDS compared to the transplant population.[1,2]

This risk of NHL is 25- to 200-fold increased in PWHA compared to those without HIV,[3–6] and risk appears to increase with duration of HIV infection[3,7] as well as with lower CD4 counts.[8,9] The risk of HL, while not considered an AIDS-defining illness (ADI) by the Centers for Disease Control, is increased by about 5- to 15-fold in PWHA;[4–6,10–12] however, its incidence is decreased with lower CD4 counts.[13] Since the widespread introduction of highly active antiretroviral therapy (HAART) in the mid-1990s, the incidence of ADIs and mortality among PWHA has decreased dramatically[14] and many studies have reported an increase in the proportion of ADIs attributable to HIV-related lymphomas (HRL).[15–18] The most recent epidemiologic data demonstrate a clear decrease in the risk of NHL associated with HAART,[9,19–22] with sharp decline in the hazard ratio for NHL incidence within the first 5 months after initiation of HAART.[22] The incidence of HL, however, appears to have risen since the institution of HAART,[13,23,24] with a higher risk in patients using HAART[24] and in those with higher CD4 counts.[13] In the SMART (Strategies for Management of Antiretroviral Therapy) study, in which patients with a CD4 count greater than 350 cells/μL were randomized to either receive continuous antiretroviral therapy (viral suppression, VS arm) or no antiretroviral therapy unless CD4 count fell to less than 250 cells/μL (drug conservation, DC arm), the rates of both Kaposi's sarcoma (KS) and lymphoma were increased in patients who had interrupted antiretroviral therapy. While the difference in lymphoma incidence (1.1/1000 person-years in the DC arm versus 0.3/1000 person-years in the VS arm) did not reach statistical significance, and neither CD4 count nor viral load predicted development of malignancy, the numbers were small.[25]

The widespread use of HAART also appears to have changed the distribution of lymphoma subtypes. Data from the San Diego County cancer and AIDS registry showed that, while the incidence of all grades of lymphoma decreased from pre- to post-HAART era, the proportion of HRL attributable to intermediate-grade lymphoma (primarily diffuse large B-cell lymphoma [DLBCL]) increased from 33% to 49% and the proportion of high-grade lymphoma (primarily high-grade immunoblastic DLBCL) decreased from 38% to 19%. The proportion of Burkitt lymphoma (BL) increased from 4% to 9%. Primary CNS lymphoma (PCNSL) decreased from 28% to 17%.[21] A different study from Los Angeles County showed a lower prevalence of small non-cleaved lymphoma (BL) but a higher prevalence of DLBCL in the HAART era. While the median CD4 count at HRL diagnosis had declined, median survival remained unchanged.[26] Among patients with HL, the annual incidence of mixed cellularity HL is higher than that of nodular sclerosing and lymphocyte-depleted HL. The incidence of all HL subtypes declines with lower CD4 counts, an effect that is more pronounced in nodular sclerosing. Thus, mixed cellularity is more prevalent than other subtypes of HL in PWHA.[13] HIV-related lymphomas have been categorized by the World Health Organization (WHO) into three main categories: those arising in immunocompetent patients, those arising specifically in HIV-positive patients, and those occurring in other immunodeficiency states (Table 24.1).[27]

Prognosis

Prior to the introduction of HAART, outcomes of therapy for HRL were poor, due to poor tolerance of therapy from

Management of Hematologic Malignancies, ed. Susan M. O'Brien, Julie M. Vose, and Hagop M. Kantarjian. Published by Cambridge University Press.

Table 24.1. WHO classification of lymphoid neoplasms

I. Lymphoma also occurring in immunocompetent patients
(a) Burkitt and Burkitt-like lymphoma
(b) Diffuse large B-cell lymphoma
(i) Centroblastic
(ii) Immunoblastic (including primary CNS lymphoma)
(c) Extranodal marginal zone lymphoma of mucosa-associated lymphoid tissue type (MALT lymphoma) (rare)
(d) Peripheral T-cell lymphoma (rare)
(e) Classical Hodgkin lymphoma
II. Lymphoma occurring more specifically in HIV-positive patients
(a) Primary effusion lymphoma
(b) Plasmablastic lymphoma of the oral cavity
III. Lymphoma also occurring in other immunodeficiency states
(a) Polymorphic B-cell lymphoma (PTLD-like) (rare)

Note: PTLD: post-transplant lymphoproliferative disorder.
Source: Adapted from Raphael *et al.*[27]

impaired bone marrow reserve related to advanced HIV infection and involvement with lymphoma, and advanced immune dysfunction with infectious complications. Complete remission (CR) was achieved in 30–60% and median overall survival (OS) was only 5–8 months.[28–31] Poor prognostic factors included patient/HIV-related factors such as a history of AIDS, CD4 count < 100 cells/μL, Karnofsky performance status (KPS) of less than 70%, injection drug use and age of 35 years or older, and disease factors such as advanced stage (III or IV) and elevated lactate dehydrogenase (LDH) level.[30,32–34] Several studies have suggested that the International Prognostic Index (IPI) developed for aggressive NHL in 1993[35] is also applicable to patients with HIV-related NHL (HIV-NHL) both in the pre-HAART[34,36] and HAART[37] eras. Since the introduction of HAART in the mid-1990s, prognosis has improved remarkably, and response rates and survival now approach those of HIV-negative patients with lymphoma.[38–41] Outcomes of patients with HIV-related HL (HIV-HL) appear to be most significantly impacted by successful therapy for HIV.[42–44] One study demonstrated that the mortality rate at 3 years for patients with HIV-HL who did not receive HAART was 5.6 times that of those who did. Two-year OS was significantly improved in those who received HAART (74% versus 30%, $p < 0.001$) and HAART-responders had overwhelmingly better survival compared to those without response (88% versus 19%, $p = 0.0002$).[44]

While CD4 count < 100 cells/μL is clearly associated with worse outcomes in HRL,[37,45,46] and HAART use is associated with improved prognosis in HRL,[47] many studies examining prognostic factors for HRL since the introduction of HAART have shown that HIV-specific factors (prior AIDS diagnosis, CD4 count) are not associated with outcomes by multivariate analysis.[39,48] On the other hand, both lower IPI score[39,48] and histologic subtype (DLBCL versus BL or T-cell NHL)[48,49] are independently associated with both response rate and survival, and lack of CR achievement is associated with significantly worse survival.[39,48,49] Prognosis for patients with HIV-related Burkitt and Burkitt-like lymphoma (HIV-BL) appears to be worse than for HIV-negative patients with BL/BLL, though this can largely be attributed to the use of the same chemotherapy regimens as for HIV-related DLBCL (HIV-DLBCL) rather than the more effective shorter-course, intensive regimens designed for BL.[49,50]

Diagnosis and staging

As in lymphoma occurring in HIV-negative individuals, excisional biopsy of a lymph node or other involved site is preferable to establish an accurate diagnosis, although a generous core biopsy may be adequate. Fine needle aspiration with flow cytometry should only be used if this is impossible. In certain cases, evaluation of cytogenetics or fluorescence *in situ* hybridization (FISH) can be useful, for example, in distinguishing DLBCL from BLL (by evaluating for lack or presence of *c-MYC* rearrangement). Physical examination should include evaluation of all nodal sites.

Use of antiretrovirals with chemotherapy

Because of its clear impact on HIV-specific survival and improved tolerance of and outcomes from chemotherapy, HAART has become an integral part of therapy for HRL. Not only does effective HAART therapy lead to improved immune function and fewer infectious complications, but it may improve lymphoma control independently of these effects.

However, chemotherapy can lead to depletion of predominantly T- but also B-lymphocyte and natural killer cells even in immunocompetent patients.[51,52] The decline of the CD4+ T-cell subset may be more pronounced than that of CD8+ T-cells and take months to a year to recover, as illustrated by a study in patients treated for breast cancer.[53] Significant changes in T-, B-, and natural killer cell subsets but no change in HIV viral load were observed in patients treated with chemotherapy and HAART for HRL. Median CD4 count fell from a pretreatment level of 138 to 77 cells/μL after 3 months, then increased back to 139 cells/μL at 1 month and 187 cells/μL at 3 months after completion of chemotherapy; however, the percentage of CD4+ T cells did not change significantly during the study period. B lymphocytes also fell significantly with chemotherapy and took longer to recover, but returned to pretreatment levels by 3 months after completion of therapy.[54]

A different study comparing HAART therapy (stavudine, lamivudine, and indinavir) with either reduced-dose CHOP (cyclophosphamide, doxorubicin, vincristine, prednisone) or full-dose CHOP with granulocyte colony-stimulating factor (G-CSF) for patients with HIV-NHL, 49% of whom had received prior three-drug antiretroviral therapy, showed a significant increase in median CD4 count during the study.[55] Individual effects can vary considerably; it is safest to assume CD4 count will decline with chemotherapy, and to use opportunistic infection (OI) prophylaxis accordingly.

Antiretrovirals can interfere with cytotoxic drug metabolism, and the HAART regimen and/or chemotherapy dosage may need adjustment. While zidovudine (AZT) may have antineoplastic activity and has been studied in combination with methotrexate for HRL,[56] its use during chemotherapy is in most cases not recommended due to myelosuppressive effects. Non-nucleoside reverse transcriptase inhibitors (NNRTIs) and protease inhibitors (PIs) can inhibit drug metabolism through the cytochrome P450 and CYP3A4 pathways.[57,58] A study investigating efficacy, toxicity, and pharmacokinetics of HAART with chemotherapy for HIV-NHL showed a significant 1.5-fold decrease in cyclophosphamide clearance, but no difference in doxorubicin clearance and no excess hematologic toxicity in comparison to historical controls.[55] A prospective analysis of patients with HIV-NHL treated with CDE (infusional cyclophosphamide, doxorubicin, and etoposide) showed a significantly lower median day 10 neutrophil count in patients treated with PIs compared to the non-PI group (0.2 versus 0.7×10^6/L, $p = 0.012$), and a higher rate of grade 3/4 infections requiring hospitalization (48% versus 25%, $p = 0.0025$) but no difference in disease-free survival (DFS), relapse-free survival (RFS), or OS.[59] While HAART has been associated with improved prognosis in HIV-HL,[38–44] patients with advanced HIV and/or bone marrow involvement may have less tolerance for standard HL regimens, and pharmacokinetic interactions resulting in severe neutropenia have been reported with Stanford V (doxorubicin, vinblastine, mechlorethamine, etoposide, vincristine, bleomycin, prednisone)[60] and ABVD (doxorubicin, bleomycin, vinblastine, dacarbazine).[61] In the latter report, severe neutropenia with fever followed three courses of ABVD despite dose-reduction of vinblastine and increased G-CSF dosing. Metabolism of vinblastine occurs predominantly by the cytochrome P450 3A4 isoenzyme, which is inhibited by ritonavir. Once lopinavir-ritonavir were interrupted 48 hours before and after chemotherapy, neutropenia resolved, even with resumption of full-dose vinblastine. Future studies of HRL treatment with HAART and chemotherapy should include careful pharmacokinetic and pharmacodynamic monitoring, and the concept of temporary interruption of PI-boosted antiretroviral therapy should be studied prospectively before any formal recommendations can be made. Until more prospective data are available to support the interruption of HAART therapy during chemotherapy, HAART should not be held; chemotherapy doses should be modified as necessary based on toxicity.

Even in the HAART era, CD4 counts less than 100 or 50 cells/μL have been shown to predict lower rates of CR.[45,46,62] Patients presenting with extremely low CD4 counts are typically those without a prior known HIV diagnosis or who have not received routine HIV care. With continued improvement in HIV screening, this situation will hopefully become much less common. Treatment of HRL should begin as soon as the staging workup is complete; it is not advisable to postpone treatment of HRL until HIV parameters improve on HAART. For patients with a new diagnosis of HIV, it is advisable to initiate HAART after the first course of chemotherapy is administered.

Aggressive B-cell non-Hodgkin lymphoma

Clinical features

DLBCL, the most common subtype of HRL, accounts for about 60–80% of subjects enrolled in clinical trials for aggressive HRL. As in HIV-negative DLBCL, HIV-DLBCL can present variably, but most commonly presents with advanced disease. Sixty percent to 80% present with stage III/IV disease with bone marrow involvement in approximately 15–25%, and 40–70% with elevated LDH. Thirty percent to 70% have an IPI of 2 or greater. Median CD4 count at presentation is usually about 130 cells/μL, and about 30% have CD4 count < 200 cells/μL.[45,60,63–65]

Pathology

The morphologic and immunophenotypic features of HIV-DLBCL are identical to those of HIV-negative DLBCL; however, the immunoblastic variant occurs with higher frequency, up to 50% of HIV-DLBCL, especially in advanced HIV.[66] Figure 24.1 shows the characteristic morphology of centroblastic DLBCL, with a predominance of centroblasts with vesicular chromatin, prominent nucleoli, and abundant cytoplasm. Immunoblastic DLBCL shares features of centroblastic and plasmablastic lymphoma, and probably represents a stage between the two along the spectrum from lymphoid to plasmacytoid differentiation. Immunophenotyping shows DLBCL to be positive for pan-B-cell markers such as CD19, CD20, and

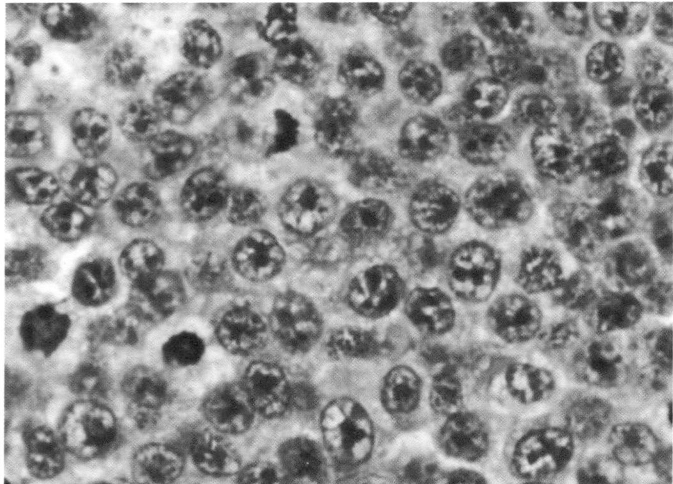

Figure 24.1 Diffuse large B-cell lymphoma. Hematoxylin and eosin (H&E) stain of lymph node biopsy shows a predominance of centroblasts with abundant cytoplasm, vesicular chromatin, and prominent nucleoli (original magnification × 1000). Courtesy of Patrick Treseler, MD, Department of Pathology, University of California, San Francisco.

CD22; centroblastic DLBCL tends to be CD10 and BCL6 positive (consistent with germinal center differentiation) while immunoblastic DLBCL tends to be negative for these markers. On the contrary, immunoblastic DLBCL (post-germinal center) is usually positive for the plasma cell markers CD138 and MUM1.[66,67] EBV expression has been shown in about 30–50% of DLBCL,[68,69] and evidence of EBV infection has been shown to correlate with the immunoblastic phenotype.[67,70,71] Incidence of immunoblastic lymphoma is increased about 1.5-fold in PWHA with KS even when adjusted for gender, age, HIV risk group, calendar year, and CD4 count.[72] While HHV-8 has been associated with some cases of plasmablastic lymphoma,[73–76] it has not been established whether HHV-8 infection plays a role in immunoblastic DLBCL. DLBCL with plasmablastic differentiation has been associated with TP53 deletion in 85% of cases analyzed by FISH.[77] (Table 24.2.)

Treatment

Chemotherapy trials

Due to poor outcomes earlier in the HIV/AIDS pandemic, investigators hypothesized that reduced-intensity chemotherapy regimens might improve treatment outcomes. A randomized trial of standard-dose m-BACOD (methotrexate, bleomycin, doxorubicin, cyclophosphamide, vincristine, and dexamethasone) with granulocyte–macrophage-colony stimulating factor (GM-CSF) versus low-dose m-BACOD with GM-CSF as indicated showed that while the low-dose arm were more likely to die from recurrent HRL, the standard-dose arm had increased mortality from infectious complications, resulting in similarly poor median survival (35 versus 31 weeks in the standard-dose and low-dose arms, respectively) in this group treated before the HAART era.[29] The French–Italian cooperative group began a trial in 1993 randomizing 485 patients to one of two high-, intermediate-, or low-intensity chemotherapy regimens based on HIV risk score, determined by performance status, prior AIDS, and CD4 counts below 100 cells/μL. After 1996 the protocol was modified to include HAART therapy. Good-risk patients received ACVBP (doxorubicin, cyclophosphamide, vindesine, bleomycin, and prednisolone) or CHOP, intermediate-risk patients received CHOP or low-dose CHOP, and poor-risk patients received low-dose CHOP or VS (vincristine, steroid). While 5-year OS dropped from about 50% in the good-risk to 24% in the intermediate-risk group and 3–11% in the poor-risk group, similar OS rates were seen within each risk group regardless of chemotherapy randomization. However, as the study was not powered to detect differences within risk groups, this result should be interpreted with caution. Multivariate analysis did show an impact on OS according to HAART therapy, HIV score, and IPI score in this pre- and post-HAART era group.[64] As the majority of patients in this study were treated in the pre-HAART era, it is not clear if the results are generalizable to the current population of patients with HRL. CHOP has also been investigated with the substitution of liposomal doxorubicin for standard doxorubicin in escalating doses of 50–80 mg/m^2. CR rate was 75% and median duration of response 15.6 months.[79] A comparison of modified CHOP (m-CHOP) to full-dose CHOP combined with G-CSF showed lower CR rate (30% versus 40%) and more grade 3/4 neutropenia (25% versus 12%) in the m-CHOP arm,[55] supporting dose intensity with G-CSF support in patients treated for HRL.

Given preclinical data suggesting possible superiority of infusional over bolus administration of chemotherapy and clinical evidence showing high efficacy of infusional regimens,[80] several groups have investigated the use of infusional chemotherapy regimens for HRL. Investigators at the National Cancer Institute reported favorable results with the EPOCH regimen, which combines dose-adjusted etoposide, doxorubicin, and vincristine, given as a 96-hour infusion, with cyclophosphamide and prednisone. Seventy-four percent of the 39 patients treated achieved CR, DFS was 92%, and OS was 60% with 53 months median follow-up. Notably, the majority of patients had a high- or high-intermediate risk IPI score, and 41% had a CD4 count of 100 cells/μL or fewer. Despite the relatively poor-risk group, severe neutropenia occurred in 30% of cycles, febrile neutropenia in 13%, and no deaths occurred during treatment.[46] It is noteworthy that patients with CD4 $< 100/\mu L$ had OS of only 16%.

Another infusional regimen, CDE, resulted in a 45% CR rate, and 2-year OS and FFS rates of 43% and 36%, respectively, in 55 patients treated in both the pre- and post-HAART era. Grade 4 neutropenia occurred in 75% of patients treated, but while treatment-related mortality was 10% in the pre-HAART patients, none died during treatment in the post-HAART group.[81] A summary of the major trials of chemotherapy for HIV-related aggressive NHL is shown in Table 24.3.

ChemoImmunotherapy

The use of rituximab, a humanized anti-CD20 antibody, in the treatment of CD20+ lymphomas has become nearly ubiquitous since the initial report of improved OS in elderly patients with CD20+ lymphoma treated with rituximab and CHOP compared to CHOP alone.[83] Several clinical trials have been conducted to explore the use of rituximab in HRL, as summarized in Table 24.4.

A pooled analysis of 74 patients receiving rituximab with CDE (R-CDE) from three phase II trials showed a CR rate of 70% and 2-year OS of 64%,[84] an apparent improvement over previously reported results of CDE alone.[81] However, the rate of infectious complications was significant, with 14% opportunistic infections and 23% non-opportunistic infections attributed to therapy, and 8% infection-related death.

A randomized trial performed by the AMC (Academisch Medisch Centum Universiteit van Amsterdam) comparing rituximab with CHOP (R-CHOP) to CHOP for patients with aggressive B-cell HRL showed no statistically significant difference in CR/CRu (CR, unspecified) (58% and 47%, $p = 0.147$)

Table 24.2. HIV-associated B-cell NHL

Pathology	CD4 count	Clinical features	Morphology	Immunophenotype	EBV	HHV-8	Genetics
Diffuse large B-cell lymphoma	Low > high	Aggressive, often advanced stage, extranodal involvement common	Diffuse infiltrate replacing normal lymph node architecture, large cells with large nuclei, prominent nucleoli, vesicular chromatin centroblastic: irregular nuclear contour; 2–4 nucleoli close to nuclear membrane; scant cytoplasm; may have interspersed immunoblasts (up to 90%) immunoblastic: > 90% immunoblasts; round to oval nuclei; large, centrally located nucleoli; more abundant, basophilic cytoplasm	(+) CD19, 20, 22, 79a; some (+) CD5 or 10, *BCL6*; (–) CD138, *MUM1*	Centroblastic: 30–40% Immunoblastic: 80–90%	No	*BCL2* (t(14;18)) 20–30%, *BCL6* 30%
Primary central nervous system lymphoma	CD4 < 100	Aggressive, localized to CNS	Usually immunoblastic DLBCL	(+) CD19, 20, 22, 79a; some (+) CD5 or 10, *BCL6*; (–) CD138, *MUM1*	> 90%	No	
Burkitt lymphoma	High > low	Highly aggressive, extranodal site involvement very common, high risk for CNS involvement, bulky disease	Classical: intermediate-size cells, deeply basophilic cytoplasm with prominent vacuoles, frequent mitoses and apoptoses with interspersed macrophages ("starry-sky" appearance) Atypical/Burkitt-like: intermediate-size cells, more pleiomorphism in nuclear and cellular size and shape, fewer/more prominent nucleoli	(+) CD19, 20, 22, CD10, *BCL6*; (–) CD5, 23, surface IgM	Burkitt (classical) 30% Burkitt-like: 30–50% Plasmacytoid Burkitt: 50–70%	No	100% *C-MYC* (8q24) translocation: t(8;14), t(2;8), t(8;22)
Plasmablastic lymphoma	Low	Classically involves oral cavity but also nodal and other extranodal sites, aggressive	Intermediate-large cells; round to oval, eccentric nuclei; prominent nucleoli; basophilic cytoplasm with paranuclear hof, frequent "starry-sky" pattern	(+) CD138, VS38c, CD38, EMA, *MUM1*, clg; (–) CD20, CD45; weak-variable CD 79a, (–) *BCL6*	> 50%	No	p53 deletion in 75%
Primary effusion lymphoma	CD4 < 100	< 5% HIV	Large cells with large, irregular nuclei, prominent nucleoli, abundant basophilic cytoplasm, may have cytoplasmic vacuoles	(+) EMA, CD71, CD38, *MUM1*, CD138; (–) CD19, CD20, CD79a, slg; occasionally (+)	100%	100%	Trisomy 12, trisomy 7 1q21-q25 aberrations, *BCL6* mutations

Note: EMA: epithelial membrane antigen; clg: cytoplasmic immunoglobulin; slg: surface immunoglobulin.

Sources: Grogg *et al.*,[66] Carbone *et al.*,[67] MacMahon *et al.*,[68] Jaffe *et al.*,[69] Simonitsch-Klupp *et al.*,[77] Gaidano *et al.*[78]

Table 24.3. Chemotherapy for HIV-related aggressive NHL

Reference	n	DLBCL/ BL (%)	Stage III/ IV (%)	aaIPI ≥2 (%)	Median CD4 (cells/μL)	CD4 count (cells/μL)	Regimen	CR, PR (%)	Survival
Kaplan *et al.*[29]	198	62/26	65	NR	100–107	79% < 200	m-BACOD	52, 26	7-mo median OS
							reduced m-BACOD	41, 28	8-mo median OS
Sparano *et al.*[82]	14	64/36	64	NR	87	55% < 100	CDE	71, 21	17-mo median OS
Ratner *et al.*[55]	65	52/28	60	NR	138	NR	m-CHOP (n = 40) CHOP + G-CSF (n = 25)	30, 30 48, 9	NR NR
Little *et al.*[46]	39	78/18	67	59	198	41% < 100	EPOCH	74, 13	60% (53-mo median follow-up)
Levine *et al.*[79]	24	79/8	67		112	54% < 100	CHOP[a]	75, 13	58% at 1 year
Sparano *et al.*[81]	98	78/22	76	67	160	37% < 100	CDE	45, 12	13-mo median OS
Mounier *et al.*[64]	485	54/20	62	47	129	39% < 200	ACVBP (good risk) CHOP (good risk) CHOP (int risk) Ld-CHOP (int risk) Ld-CHOP (poor risk) VS (poor risk)	61, 16 51, 15 49, 9 32, 16 20, 12 5, 15	51% est. 5-yr OS 47% 28% 24% 11% 3%

Notes: [a]With liposomal doxorubicin.
[aa]IPI: age-adjusted International Prognostic Index; NR: not recorded; Ld: low dose.

or median OS (139 and 110 weeks) in the two arms. Inferior lymphoma control in the CHOP arm appeared to be offset by the increase in infection-related mortality in the R-CHOP arm, which was most pronounced in patients with CD4 count < 50 cells/μL, with 60% of such deaths occurring in this subgroup.[45] In contrast, a subsequent phase II trial of R-CHOP in 61 patients with good- or intermediate-risk HRL showed 77% CR/CRu and 75% estimated 2-year overall survival. Twenty-five percent of patients had neutropenic fever, there were two occurrences of sepsis and one opportunistic infection, and the only death occurred in a patient with infection and progressive lymphoma.[65] Only four patients had CD4 counts < 50 cells/μL in this study. Another phase II study of R-CHOP included 20% patients with poor-risk IPI scores, and demonstrated 69% CR, 56% 3-year OS; IPI score and response to HAART were predictive of response and survival. However, infection-related death occurred in 9% of patients.[85]

The AMC 034 randomized phase II trial compared EPOCH given with concurrent rituximab (R-EPOCH) to EPOCH followed by sequential weekly rituximab (EPOCH-R) for 6 weeks for HRL. Toxicity was similar between the two arms (15–16% grade 3/4 febrile neutropenia, 7–10% death), but CR/CRu rate was 69% in the concurrent arm and 53% in the sequential arm. Multivariate analysis including treatment arm (concurrent versus sequential rituximab administration), CD4 count < 100 cells/μL, elevated LDH, performance status, and antiretroviral therapy showed that concurrent administration of rituximab was significantly associated with achievement of CR/CRu.[86] In addition to *Pneumocystis carinii* pneumonia prophylaxis, all patients in this trial received quinolone neutropenic prophylaxis. A randomized phase III trial comparing R-EPOCH and R-CHOP in HIV-negative patients with intermediate-grade lymphoma is currently underway through the Cancer and Leukemia Group B (CALGB) cooperative group.

Some of the differences in outcomes among these trials of chemotherapy with rituximab may have been due to patient selection; however, HIV-infected individuals appear to be at an increased risk of infectious complications, especially those with

Table 24.4. Immunochemotherapy for HIV-related aggressive NHL

Reference	n	DLBCL/BL (%)	Stage III/IV (%)	IPI ≥ 2 (%)	Median CD4 (cells/μL)	CD4 count (cells/μL)	Regimen	CR, PR (%)	Survival
Spina *et al.*[84]	74	65/28	70	58	161	NR	R-CDE	70, 5	64% 2-yr OS
Kaplan *et al.*[45]	150	80/9	79	47	133	67% < 200	R-CHOP	58, 8	32-mo median OS
							CHOP	47, 8	25-mo median OS
Boue *et al.*[65]	61	69/26	42	29	172	20% < 100	R-CHOP	77, 10	75% 2-yr OS
Ribera *et al.*[85]	81	100/0	70	68	158	NR	R-CHOP	69, 9	56% 3-yr OS
Levine *et al.*[86]	51	69/25	84%	69	181	31% < 100	R-EPOCH[a]	69, 14	80% 1-yr OS
	55	78/15	75	64	194	31% < 100	EPOCH-R[b]	53, 22	78% 1-yr OS

Notes: [a]Rituximab administration with each cycle of EPOCH.
[b]Rituximab weekly × 6 after completion of EPOCH chemotherapy.

severe AIDS. Hypogammaglobulinemia after the use of rituximab has also been reported in the setting of other immunosuppressive treatments,[87] after autologous stem cell transplantation,[88,89] and in a patient with HIV-related DLBCL treated with R-CHOP.[90] Prolonged neutropenia is an uncommon but well-documented complication of rituximab that has been described in both immunocompetent and post-autologous transplant patients,[91–93] and CD4 lymphopenia has been shown to be an independent risk factor for febrile neutropenia and death in patients receiving cytotoxic chemotherapy for cancer.[94] Although concern about increased infectious complications with the use of rituximab in HRL remains, its use is still strongly encouraged. Caution is advised in those with severe immunosuppression, and antibiotic prophylaxis against bacterial and *Pneumocystis carinii* infections is strongly recommended regardless of CD4 count.

Burkitt and Burkitt-like lymphoma

Clinical features

BL and a morphologic variant, BLL, comprises the second most common HRL after DLBCL, and accounts for approximately 30–40% of all HIV-NHL.[69,95] Commonly presenting with rapidly progressive symptoms and extranodal disease, involvement of the gastrointestinal tract, bone marrow, liver, and spleen are relatively common. Meningeal involvement is also relatively common, up to approximately 10–20% in most published reports,[49,95–99] requiring both assessment of cerebrospinal fluid (CSF) and intrathecal prophylaxis in all patients presenting with BL/BLL. One series reported a similar proportion of BL patients with stage IV disease among HIV-positive and -negative patients (74% and 66%, respectively).[95]

Pathologic features

Classical BL features monomorphic, medium-size lymphoid cells with interspersed apoptotic figures and histiocytes, imparting a "starry-sky" pattern on low-power light microscopy (Figure 24.2a). Nuclei are round and uniform with several small nucleoli, and cytoplasm is intensely basophilic with numerous vacuoles (Figure 24.2b). Immunophenotyping reveals surface expression of CD20 and CD10, and proliferative rate is typically very high. The hallmark finding is the translocation t(8;14) or a variant resulting in rearrangement of *c-MYC*. BLL shares all of these features but has more cellular pleiomorphism, with interspersed larger cells and cells with abundant cytoplasm, and nuclei with more prominent nucleoli.[69,100] A plasmacytoid variant of BL has also been described specifically in association with AIDS, with eccentric nuclei and abundant, immunoglobulin-containing cytoplasm.[66] Evidence of EBV expression is present in 30% of classical BL, 30–50% of BLL, and 50–70% of BL with plasmacytoid differentiation.[66,69] (Table 24.2.)

Treatment

Since the introduction of HAART, the difference in survival between HIV-DLBCL and HIV-BL has increased significantly due to improvements in survival of HIV-DLBCL and increased intensity of chemotherapy for HIV-BL, which was previously inadequate.[49,50] For example, R-CDE resulted in lower CR rates (52% versus 77%, $p = 0.05$) and higher risk of death (hazard ratio [HR] = 2.24; 95% confidence intervals [CI] = 1.01–4.97) for patients with HIV-BL compared to HIV-DLBCL.[50]

A retrospective analysis of outcomes in HIV-BL compared to HIV-negative BL patients showed a significantly lower

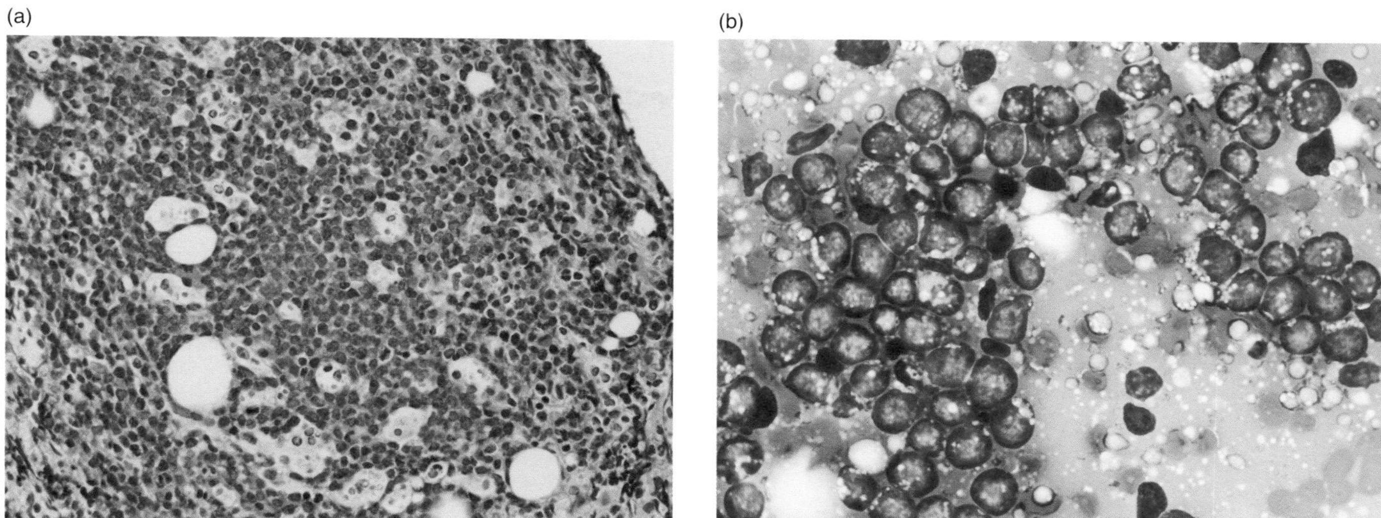

Figure 24.2 Burkitt lymphoma: (a) A × 500 view of a bone marrow core biopsy from a patient with HIV-BL, showing a dense population of monomorphic, medium-size lymphoid cells with interspersed apoptotic figures and histiocytes, imparting a "starry-sky" pattern. (b) A × 1000 view of the touch prep, showing round and uniform nuclei, and basophilic cytoplasm with numerous vacuoles. Courtesy of Mark Lu, MD, PhD, Department of Pathology, San Francisco Veterans Affairs Medical Center.

Table 24.5. Chemotherapy for HIV-related Burkitt or Burkitt-like NHL

Reference	n	Stage IV (%)	Median CD4 (cells/μL)	CD4 count (cells/μL)	Regimen	CR (%)	2-year OS (%)
Cortes *et al.*[96]	13	31	77	38% < 100	HyperCVAD	92	52% 2-yr OS
Astrow *et al.*[101]	23	83 III/IV	240		McMaster	39	49% OS at 4.5 months med follow-up
	21	81 III/IV	140		Conventional[a]	38	
Wang *et al.*[98]	8	88	149		CODOX-M/IVAC	63	60% 2-yr EFS
	14	33			other	67	60% 2-yr EFS
Oriol *et al.*[97]	14	57 III/IV	420	21% < 200	PETHEMA LAL3/97	77	51% 2-yr OS
Hoffmann *et al.*[99]	20	55	254		GMALL	75	55% 2-yr OS
	31	64			CHOP	40	34% 2-yr OS
Galicier *et al.*[102]	63	100	239		LMB86	70	47% 2-yr OS

Note: [a]CHOP, CDE, COMP, ProMACE-CytaBOM
COMP: cyclophosphamide, vincristine, methotrexate, prednisone; ProMACE-CytaBOM: cyclophosphamide, doxorubicin, etoposide, cytarabine, bleomycin, vincristine, methotrexate, and prednisone; EFS: event-free survival.

response to therapy for HIV-BL (CR 40% versus 65%, p = 0.03), which most likely reflected the less intensive chemotherapy regimens used in the HIV-BL group (CHOP or modified CHOP-like) compared to the HIV-negative BL group. There was no difference in CR rate among PWHA who had AIDS prior to the diagnosis of BL compared to those without a prior AIDS diagnosis. Median OS was also significantly shorter for those with HIV-BL (7 months versus median not reached in HIV-negative BL, p = 0.0001).[95]

The use of short-course, intensive chemotherapy regimens for BL in immunocompetent individuals has shown promising results for patients with HIV-BL (Table 24.5). HyperCVAD alternating with high-dose methotrexate and cytarabine resulted in 92% CR lasting a median of 31 months and 12 months median OS; best outcomes were in those who received HAART concurrently. The protocol was amended in the last year of accrual to include rituximab; however, it was not reported how many patients actually received this.[96] A non-randomized comparison of outcomes with CODOX-M/IVAC (cyclophosphamide, doxorubicin, vincristine, methotrexate/ifosfamide, etoposide, cytarabine) versus less-intensive regimens in HIV-BL has shown similar efficacy with 63–67% CR and 60% 2-year event-free survival (EFS) regardless of type of therapy. However, among high-risk patients (both

HIV-negative and -positive patients), CR and EFS rates were substantially better after CODOX-M/IVAC, without a significant difference in myelosuppression and infectious complications.[98] However, given further clinical experience with this regimen, excessive myelosuppression has been seen with high-dose methotrexate given on day 10 of CODOX-M in patients with HIV-BL, especially those with bone marrow involvement or baseline cytopenias. For this reason, the AMC phase II trial of R-CODOX-M/IVAC in HIV-associated BL and atypical BL has moved the methotrexate from day 10 to day 15 and reduced the dose from 5520 to 3000 mg/m^2. Additionally, this trial investigates the use of rituximab with each cycle, infusional rather than bolus ifosfamide and etoposide, and vincristine dose capped at 2 mg/m^2. Patients with BL treated with the PETHEMA-LAL3/97 regimen had similar outcomes regardless of HIV status. CR rates were not significantly different, 71% in HIV-BL and 77% in HIV-negative BL cases, and the estimated 2-year OS was 51% for the group as a whole.[97] Another study, however, showed similarly poor outcomes in HIV-BL patients treated with either high-intensity (the McMaster protocol, which involves two month-long induction regimens) or less intensive chemotherapy, with 39% CR and only 36% long-term lymphoma-free survival. Of the 23 patients treated with the McMaster regimen, 100% had grade 4 hematologic toxicity and 30% of patients died during treatment; however, all of the nine patients achieving CR were cured. Seventy-five percent of stage I patients were alive and in CR with only 4.5 months median follow-up, half of whom received conventional chemotherapy.[101] Given excessive treatment-related toxicity and mortality, the McMaster approach cannot be recommended for treatment of HIV-BL.

A retrospective study of the GMALL (German Multicenter Study Group for Adult ALL) protocol versus CHOP-like chemotherapy for patients with HIV-BL/BLL showed that the GMALL protocol resulted in a significantly higher rate of CR (75% versus 40%, $p = 0.02$) and a non-significant difference in 2-year OS (55% versus 34%, $p = 0.17$), though the study may not have had enough statistical power to detect an OS difference. Of note, 65% of GMALL patients and only 32% of the CHOP patients received HAART after the diagnosis of BL/BLL and a higher proportion of the GMALL patients had a CD4 count > 200 cells/μL (78% versus 43% in the CHOP group, $p = 0.03$). Thirteen of 20 patients treated with the GMALL protocol suffered from infectious complications (neutropenic fever, sepsis, aspergillosis), but none of these were fatal and 9 of these 13 patients were able to receive at least four cycles.[99]

One prospective study of therapy for HIV-BL was conducted by Galicier and colleagues, who examined the effects of the LMB86 regimen in 63 patients with HIV infection and stage IV BL. CR was achieved in 70%, almost all patients experienced grade 4 bone marrow toxicity, and seven patients died as a result of treatment. Two-year OS was 47% and DFS 68%.[102]

Given the poor outcomes of HIV-BL treated with CHOP or similar regimens, all patients with adequate organ function and performance status should be treated with intensive, shorter-course therapy designed for highly aggressive lymphoma with a high growth fraction, such as CODOX-M/IVAC, HyperCVAD, GMALL, or LMB86. It is not yet clear if the addition of rituximab improves outcomes in HIV-BL; however, its use should be considered in patients with CD4 count > 50 cells/μL.

Plasmablastic lymphoma

Clinical features

While plasmablastic lymphoma (PBL) has been described in HIV-negative individuals, it appears to be more common in those who are immunosuppressed due to solid organ transplant,[103,104] or receiving immunosuppressive treatment for other diseases.[105,106] In PWHA, PBL classically occurs in the oral cavity but also with extra-oral involvement in a substantial number of cases.[76,107–109] A review of all PBL case reports and case series showed that 66% of cases were oral, 34% were extra-oral, including those with skin, gastrointestinal tract, lymph node, and bone marrow involvement. Seventy-nine percent of these cases were in PWHA, and an additional 10% had immunosuppression from other causes. In PWHA median CD4 count at presentation was 120 cells/μL.[76] Another review of HIV-associated PBL showed that median age was 38 years, 49% presented with stage I and 34% with stage IV disease, and 65% of cases presented in the oral cavity.[75] Compared to patients with DLBCL (either centroblastic or immunoblastic), patients with PBL tend to present with more extranodal disease, B symptoms, and a higher IPI.[77]

Pathologic features

PBL is distinguished from DLBCL by its morphologic and immunophenotypic plasmacytoid differentiation. Histology usually shows a diffuse infiltrate of large lymphoid cells with central or eccentric round to oval nuclei, prominent nucleolus or nucleoli, abundant basophilic cytoplasm, and often apoptotic and mitotic figures indicative of a high proliferative rate (Figure 24.3).[76,77,110,111] PBL typically lacks expression of B- and T-cell markers such as CD20 and PAX5 and does not express BCL6, but usually shows expression of CD79a, the plasma cell markers CD138 and VS38c, epithelial membrane antigen (EMA), MUM-1, and immunoglobulin light chains[73,75,76,78,110–114] (Table 24.2). PBL can be distinguished from immunoblastic DLBCL by lack of CD20 expression and greater morphologic plasmacytoid differentiation, and from multiple myeloma by large cell/plasmablastic appearance, as well as the lack of other findings consistent with multiple myeloma (lytic bone lesions, paraprotein, renal failure, and hypercalcemia).

As with other types of HIV-related lymphoma, many investigators have sought evidence for EBV and HHV-8 infection in PBL. According to a review of published PBL cases, EBV is present in about 75% of cases tested[75,76] and 17% are positive for HHV-8.[76] While one group of investigators failed to find

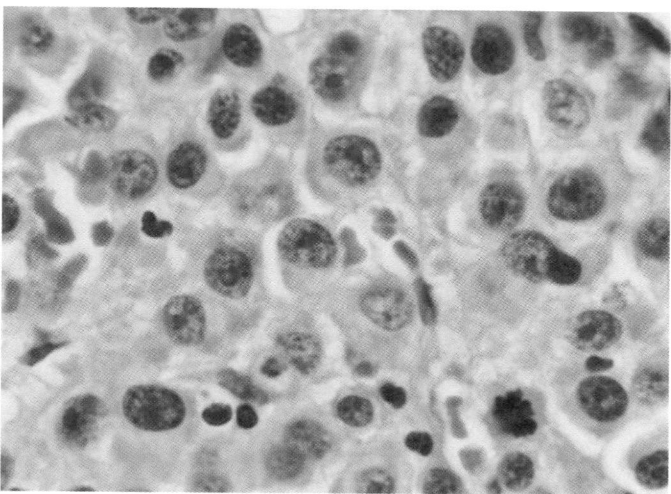

Figure 24.3 Plasmablastic lymphoma: H&E stain of lymph node biopsy shows a diffuse infiltrate of large lymphoid cells with central and eccentric round to oval nuclei, prominent nucleoli, and abundant eosinophilic-basophilic cytoplasm. A high proliferative rate is evident, with both apoptotic and mitotic figures present (original magnification × 1000). Courtesy of Patrick Treseler, MD, Department of Pathology, University of California, San Francisco.

evidence of HHV-8 by both immunohistochemistry and DNA-based polymerase chain reaction (PCR) in nine cases of oral cavity PBL,[111] HHV-8 expression has been demonstrated in many cases of PBL by reverse transcriptase-PCR (RT-PCR),[73,74,110] and also in non-oral cavity PBL.[115]

Treatment and prognosis

While there are case reports of HIV-positive PBL (HIV-PBL) patients treated effectively with HAART alone,[116–118] the standard approach has been to use a CHOP-like regimen with or without radiation therapy. There are no prospective data on response rates to any one therapeutic strategy. CHOP is the most commonly used chemotherapy regimen, used in 30% of reported cases, followed by EPOCH or CODOX-M/IVAC in 25%, and radiation therapy alone or in combination has been used in 29%.[75] Among cases that reported response to therapy, 66% achieved a CR to initial therapy but 29% had progressive disease, and 25% eventually relapsed.[75]

PBL tends to be more resistant to standard chemotherapy than DLBCL: one study reported 47% CR for PBL, 73% for centroblastic DLBCL, and 57% for immunoblastic DLBCL, though these differences were not statistically significant.[77] Survival also appears to be shorter, with a median OS of 14 months for PBL, versus estimated 5-year survival of 56% and 57% for centroblastic and immunoblastic DLBCL, respectively ($p < 0.002$), a difference that was particularly apparent in the low and low-intermediate IPI risk groups.[77]

While responses to therapy are poor, survival with PBL may be improving: reported median survival used to be 5.5 months earlier in the AIDS epidemic,[110] but more recently approaches 14–15 months.[75,77] A case series published in 2004 described six patients with HIV-PBL treated with either CHOP or CODOX-M/IVAC and one of whom received therapy for a synchronous diagnosis of anal squamous cell carcinoma. Five of six were in CR with a median follow-up of 22 months, and the other patient died of progressive disease after refusing therapy.[113] Given the biologic similarity between PBL and plasma cells, agents active in multiple myeloma, such as thalidomide, lenalidomide, or bortezomib, may also be effective for PBL either alone or in combination with chemotherapy; however, this approach remains investigational.

Primary effusion lymphoma

Clinical features

In 1989, Knowles and colleagues reported a case of a highly aggressive form of lymphoma presenting as malignant pleural effusions that lacked B- and T-cell lineage-specific antigens but did express antigens associated with B- and T-cell activation, showed evidence of antigen receptor gene rearrangement, and was positive for EBV-DNA by Southern blot analysis.[119] Subsequently other investigators described body cavity-based lymphoma, later named primary effusion lymphoma (PEL), which manifests as malignant pleural effusions, pericardial effusions, and/or ascites, without predominant lymph node involvement or extranodal masses.[119–121] PEL comprises $< 5\%$ of all HIV-associated NHL,[66,119,122] and occurs only rarely in HIV-negative individuals. It presents primarily as a malignant effusion(s) with minimal associated nodal or extranodal involvement; BL or DLBCL with a significant amount of nodal or solid extranodal involvement also presenting with malignant effusion(s) is not considered PEL. A "solid variant" of PEL has been described involving the gastrointestinal tract, skin, and lymph nodes that has similar immunophenotypic features and is also associated with HHV-8,[66,123] though these cases may actually represent PBL. The majority of reported PEL cases are homosexual males with median age in the mid-30s to mid-40s[124–126] with CD4 count < 200 cells/μL,[124,126] and often with poor performance status.[125]

Pathologic features

Morphologic features of PEL bridge those of immunoblastic, plasmablastic, and anaplastic large cell lymphoma. The cells are large, with large, round, irregular nuclei, prominent nucleoli, and abundant basophilic cytoplasm that may have prominent vacuoles. PEL with more plasmacytoid differentiation may have a perinuclear hof. Increased mitotic and apoptotic activity is often described (Figure 24.4).[66,69,127–129] Immunophenotyping typically reveals lymphoid and plasmacytoid markers such as CD30, CD45, EMA, CD71, MUM1, CD38, and CD138. B-cell antigens such as CD19, CD20, CD79a, and surface or cytoplasmic immunoglobulins are commonly absent.[66,69,119,124,128] One report of four PEL cases described two with T-cell phenotype and two with null phenotype, but all expressing CD30, and variable CD138 and EMA[129]

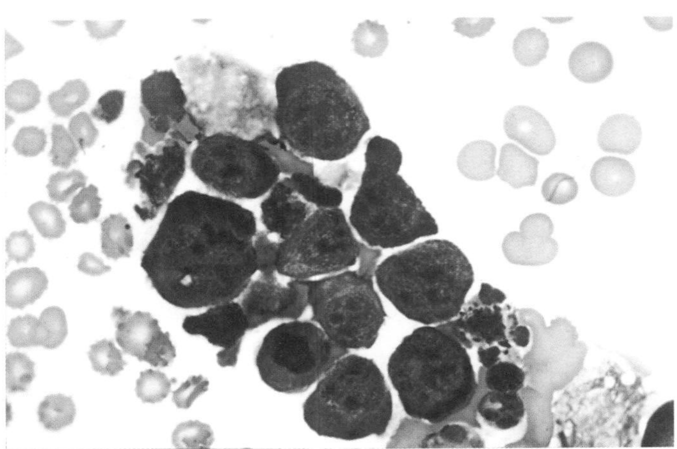

Figure 24.4 Primary Effusion Lymphoma: PEL cells are large, with large, round, irregular nuclei, prominent nucleoli, and abundant basophilic cytoplasm. Some of the cells exhibit plasmacytoid differentiation, with a perinuclear hof (original magnification × 1000). Courtesy of Patrick Treseler, MD, University of California, Department of Pathology, San Francisco.

(Table 24.2). Gene expression profiling (GEP) has been shown to distinguish PEL as a separate subtype from other AIDS- and non-AIDS-related NHL when compared to both cell lines and primary human lymphoma cells. The PEL GEP is similar to that of EBV-positive immunoblasts and plasma cells, and distinct from that of germinal center or memory B cells. This suggests that PEL may be more closely related to PBL than other AIDS-related lymphoma subtypes, a finding that is consistent with the PEL immunophenotype.[130] GEP has also been shown to differentiate PEL from other lymphomatous effusions (BL presenting as primary lymphomatous effusions), as well as EBV-positive and EBV-negative PEL.[131]

After the discovery of a novel herpesvirus in association with KS (KS-associated herpesvirus, KSHV, or HHV-8),[132] this same virus was also found to be present almost universally in PEL.[111,122,124,125,128,129,133] EBV infection is present in the majority of cases.[124,125,128,130,131,133]

Treatment and prognosis

While PEL is an aggressive lymphoma with an associated median OS of approximately 6 months or less,[122,124–126,128] there are a few reports of spontaneous regression with HAART alone.[125,126,128] Most patients treated with chemotherapy receive CHOP or a modified, CHOP-like regimen. Simonelli and colleagues compared outcomes of 11 patients with PEL with 11 patients with oral cavity PBL, 76 patients with immunoblastic DLBCL, and 75 patients with centroblastic DLBCL. PEL patients presented with worse performance score and when treated with CHOP-like therapy had a CR rate of 42% and a significantly worse 2-year OS compared with patients with centroblastic DLBCL (33% versus 53%, respectively, $p = 0.0002$).[125]

Boulanger and colleagues examined 28 cases of HIV-positive patients with PEL, including one who achieved CR with HAART alone. Five patients were treated with interferon alpha, three of whom also received cidofovir. Twelve received intensive chemotherapy, either ACVBP (doxorubicin, cyclophosphamide, vindesine, bleomycin, and prednisone) or a CHOP-like regimen (cyclophosphamide, doxorubicin, prednisone, and either vincristine or etoposide) with high-dose methotrexate (2.5–3 g/m^2), and the rest received an anthracycline and/or cyclophosphamide-based regimen, some of these with methotrexate. In this series, 50% achieved CR, and with 3.8 years median follow-up, 32% of patients were alive. Of the patients that died, 14 had progressive lymphoma, 4 died of infection and/or chemotherapy toxicity, and 1 died of disseminated visceral KS. Multivariate analysis showed that only performance status greater than 2, based on the Eastern Cooperative Oncology Group (ECOG) scale (HR = 5.84; 95% CI = 1.76–19.33), and absence of HAART before PEL diagnosis (HR = 3.26; 95% CI = 1.14–9.34) were associated with shorter survival.[126]

A randomized, controlled, crossover trial of valganciclovir in 26 men (16 HIV-positive and 10 HIV-negative) with HHV-8 infection showed a reduction in HHV-8 replication with valganciclovir,[134] but it is not known if this will be a useful treatment modality in HHV-8-associated malignancies as no significant association between HHV-8 viral load and response to therapy has been demonstrated.[135]

One group showed that nuclear factor-kappa B (NF-κB) was constitutively activated in both cell lines and patient samples of HHV-8-associated lymphoma. Inhibition of NF-κB in PEL cells resulted in downregulation of interleukin 6 (IL-6) and a significant increase in apoptosis, only when IκB was stabilized.[136] These data suggest that NF-κB inhibition may be a useful treatment for PEL. Proteasome inhibitors act at least in part by inhibition of NF-κB through decreased degradation of IκB; however, their activity against PEL has not yet been demonstrated.

Primary central nervous system lymphoma

Epidemiology

Although the relative risk of PCNSL in the pre-HAART era was reportedly 3600 times that in the general population[137] the risk has dramatically declined since the introduction of HAART, with a 0.42 relative risk (99% CI = 0.26–0.40) of PCNSL compared to the pre-HAART era.[138] According to Surveillance, Epidemiology, and End Results (SEER) data, PCNSL incidence declined sharply after 1995 in people between ages 20 and 59 years, with no change in age-adjusted incidence for those 60 years and older.[139] Incidence of HIV-PCNSL in the HAART era is now approximately 1 case per 1000 person-years.[138,140]

Clinical features

During the early AIDS epidemic, PCNSL was the second most common cerebral mass-lesion in PWHA after toxoplasmosis.[141] PCNSL tends to occur only in patients with advanced AIDS, with CD4 count at presentation usually < 50 cells/μL.[8,140,142] Patients can present with altered mental status, lethargy, seizure, ataxia, and/or focal neurologic symptoms. Approximately half of patients with PCNSL have an isolated brain lesion and half present with two or more lesions.[142,143] The majority of PCNSL cases are not associated with systemic lymphoma; however, ocular involvement can occur. Staging workup should include magnetic resonance imaging (MRI) of the brain with gadolinium, lumbar puncture, and ophthalmologic exam. Positron emission tomography (PET) and/or computed tomography (CT) scans of the neck, chest, abdomen, and pelvis and bone marrow biopsy are relatively low-yield tests, and MRI of the spine with gadolinium should be performed if signs or symptoms warrant it or if there is evidence of leptomeningeal disease on initial workup.[144]

Pathology

Most cases of PCNSL are high-grade or immunoblastic DLBCL,[100,142] and more than 95% PCNSL are associated with latent EBV infection (Table 24.2). The EBV genome is present in most PCNSL tissue samples tested by FISH. While standard cytology examination of the CSF often does not reveal malignant cells, the EBV genome can be detected by PCR in most cases. This was first reported in 1993 by Cinque and colleagues, who performed nested PCR using probes for EBNA-1 (EBV-nuclear antigen-1) on CSF samples taken within 180 days of death from 85 patients with HIV and CNS disorders at necropsy. Sixteen of 16 PCNSL tissue specimens tested expressed EBER (EBV-encoded nuclear RNA transcripts) by FISH, and all 17 patients with PCNSL had evidence of EBV in their CSF by PCR, as opposed to only 1 of 68 patients without PCNSL.[145]

Diagnosis

Radiographic imaging (CT and MRI) usually reveals a well-circumscribed, enhancing focal brain lesion (or lesions). On MRI, lesions are iso-intense to gray matter on T2-weighted images, often with surrounding edema.[146] PCNSL involves the periventricular white matter, frontal lobes, basal ganglia, corpus callosum, and thalamus; cerebellum and brainstem involvement are less common.[142,146] Nuclear medicine modalities can also be useful for distinguishing PCNSL from non-malignant brain lesions, including single photon emission computed tomography (SPECT)[147] and PET.[148–150] Because PCNSL are highly proliferative and metabolically active tumors, they tend to show markedly increased SPECT or PET uptake compared to background tissue, even though the metabolic activity of the brain is already quite high. This effect can be rapidly attenuated, however, in patients that have started taking CNS-penetrating corticosteroids such as dexamethasone, which may lead to a false-negative result.[151]

Because the radiographic appearance of PCNSL can be similar to that of cerebral abscess from *Toxoplasma gondii*, patients with a positive serum *T. gondii* IgG not receiving appropriate prophylaxis may warrant a trial of therapy with pyrimethamine plus sulfadiazine (or clindamycin in those who cannot tolerate sulfadiazine); however, a very large or life-threatening lesion may require immediate biopsy.

CSF should be examined for protein, glucose, cell count, differential, cytology, and EBV PCR. While CSF examination is often benign in PCNSL, several studies have indicated that CSF EBV PCR may be useful diagnostically. A prospective study of 122 PWHA with focal brain lesions in 1994–6 showed a sensitivity and specificity for CSF EBV PCR of 80% and 100%, respectively, and a positive predictive value (PPV) and negative predictive value (NPV) of 100% and 90%, respectively.[152] PPV of CSF EBV PCR performed on 26 patients with clinical CNS disease diagnosed between 1998 and 2002 was only 29%. Only two patients had PCNSL, for which both had a positive PCR test. Five patients with non-malignant disease had a false-positive PCR, yielding a specificity of only 33%. The different test characteristics in the second study are most likely due to the fact that subjects were not selected on the basis of characteristic radiologic findings, as well as reduced overall incidence of PCNSL in the post-HAART era, both leading to a lower prevalence of PCNSL in this population. A subsequent study of 55 patients with similar entry criteria found positive CSF EBV PCR in both patients with PCNSL as well as in the 18 patients with other diagnoses. Using a cutoff of 10 000 copies/mL, specificity was improved to 96% and PPV to 66%;[153] however, this approach has not been validated prospectively. Caution should also be exercised in using this test to rule out PCNSL in patients on ganciclovir, as diagnostic yield in patients with PCNSL may be reduced.[154]

While tissue biopsy remains the gold standard in diagnosis of PCNSL, in patients for whom the morbidity of brain biopsy would be too high, the combination of clinical, radiographic, and CSF findings, including PCR for EBV, can yield the correct diagnosis in the majority of cases. For example, Antinori and colleagues investigated the combination of SPECT and CSF EBV PCR for distinction of PCNSL and non-malignant neurologic disorders among 31 patients with HIV and focal brain lesions. The combination (SPECT) uptake and EBV PCR had 100% sensitivity, 89% specificity, 87% PPV, and 100% NPV.[147] Future studies of the combination of PET/CT and other novel imaging modalities with CSF analysis, including EBV PCR, gene expression profiling, and proteomic analysis may eliminate the need for brain biopsy in the future.

Treatment and prognosis

As with other HRL, outcomes in HIV-related PCNSL have improved significantly in the HAART era. Increased OS has been associated with the use of HAART after diagnosis,[142,155] effectiveness of HAART therapy (decrease in viral load by $\geq 0.5 \log_{10}$ mL and increase in CD4 count by 50 cells/μL or more),[155] and with receipt of radiation therapy (RT).[142,155] These results can be difficult to interpret as the numbers of subjects tend to be small, studies are not randomized, and patients who receive cranial radiation are also more likely to receive HAART and have a higher performance status. A retrospective study of 111 patients with HIV-PCNSL showed median OS of 50 days, but 92 days for those who received RT and 38 days for those who did not. Completion of ≥ 30 Gray (Gy) RT was associated with improved OS as a continuous variable, indicative of a dose–response effect, but failure to complete RT was also associated with an ECOG performance status ≥ 3 and age > 40 years.[142] While RT can result in 50–75% clinical or radiographic response, treatment is rarely curative and progression usually occurs within weeks to months.[144,156]

High-dose methotrexate has been shown to be an effective treatment for PCNSL in HIV-negative individuals,[157–159] and outcomes appear to be favorable in PWHA as well. One study reported on ten patients with HIV-PCNSL, all of whom received methotrexate 3 g/m^2. Eight patients also received thiotepa and procarbazine, and all received intrathecal or intraventricular methotrexate followed by whole brain RT. Of seven assessable patients (excluding one early death), 57% had CR after chemotherapy, 86% at the end of treatment. Median OS was 3.5 months for the entire cohort, and 7 months for eight patients who completed therapy.[157] Jacomet and colleagues enrolled 15 patients with HIV-PCNSL in a pilot study, 10 with confirmed histologic diagnosis (group 1) and 15 with diagnosis based on characteristic radiographic findings (group 2) who did not respond to therapy for toxoplasmosis. Subjects were treated with methotrexate 3 g/m^2 every 14 days for up to six cycles; achieving CR in seven subjects, but in only three of the ten with histologic confirmation. Median survival was 290 days overall, 73 days for group 1 and 383 days for group 2.[160] Subjects with newly diagnosed PCNSL should be initiated on HAART immediately, and treated with curative intent with high-dose methotrexate on a bi-weekly basis until two cycles beyond CR or eight cycles. Because of the poor outcomes of cranial radiotherapy, including its late toxicity, radiation should be reserved for those who are refractory or relapse after chemotherapy, or who cannot tolerate chemotherapy.

Overall outcome of therapy for PCNSL in the setting of HIV infection remains suboptimal and efforts should be made to encourage clinical trial participation.

Leptomeningeal lymphoma

Risk factors

CNS involvement of systemic HRL occurs in up to 17–23% of cases, 3–14% at diagnosis.[161–165] Risk factors for CNS involvement include Burkitt histology, bone marrow involvement, involvement of more than one extranodal site, increased serum LDH, paranasal sinus or paraspinal involvement, CD4 count < 100 cells/μL, and EBV infection of the primary tumor.[161–163,166] The risk of CNS involvement at diagnosis and of CNS relapse appears to have decreased in the HAART era. A retrospective analysis of 131 patients with HRL diagnosed between 1986 and 2006 showed that HAART was associated with a decreased risk of leptomeningeal involvement of HRL, with leptomeningeal involvement in 14% of subjects not on HAART and none of the subjects on HAART.[163]

Diagnosis

In patients who have signs or symptoms or are otherwise at high risk to have leptomeningeal involvement of lymphoma, standard tests include CSF examination for cell count and differential, protein, glucose, and cytologic examination, and MRI of the brain with gadolinium. However, routine workup can often miss true leptomeningeal disease in a substantial number of cases. A series comparing the results of standard CSF cytology to CSF flow cytometry examined CSF of 51 patients with a new diagnosis of lymphoma considered to be at high risk of CNS involvement (diagnosis of AIDS-related lymphoma, BL, or DLBCL with ≥ 2 extranodal sites, and elevated LDH or bone marrow involvement), 25% of who were HIV positive. Nine patients with relapsed DLBCL who did not meet these criteria, but were clinically suspected to have CNS disease, had CSF examination as well. Eleven (22%) newly diagnosed and three (33%) relapsed patients were found to have CNS involvement by positive flow cytometry; only one in each group would have been detected by CSF cytology alone. There were no cases with positive CSF cytology that were not also positive by flow cytometry.[166] A subsequent series looked at CSF cytology and flow cytometry in 42 patients considered to be at high risk for CNS relapse by elevated LDH plus at least two extranodal sites, bone marrow involvement, or diagnosis of BL; HIV status was not mentioned. Eleven had evidence of leptomeningeal lymphoma by flow cytometry, only four of who would have been diagnosed by cytologic examination alone. Three of the four cases with positive cytology had neurologic symptoms.[167] CSF PCR for EBV has been shown to be positive in most cases of leptomeningeal HRL, with sensitivity and specificity of 90% and 100% respectively, PPV 100%, and NPV 98%; however, in that particular study the diagnosis of leptomeningeal lymphoma was made by standard means: neurologic symptoms, imaging, and/or CSF cytology. Of seven patients who did not initially have leptomeningeal involvement but subsequently developed CNS relapse, only one had initially positive CSF EBV PCR at diagnosis of lymphoma and the other six were only PCR positive at diagnosis of relapse.[164] Thus, this approach is not useful for predicting who may be high risk for CNS relapse at the initial lymphoma diagnosis.

In patients with a relatively high risk of occult leptomeningeal disease (more than one extranodal site of lymphoma, high-grade histology, paranasal or paraspinous involvement, and/or bone marrow involvement with elevated LDH but no neurologic symptoms), CSF should be sent for cytology, cell count, differential, protein, and glucose. Flow cytometry and PCR for EBV should be evaluated if the initial workup is negative and there is a clinical suspicion of leptomeningeal disease. Symptomatic patients are likely to have positive cytology, and in this subset flow cytometry may not be required.

Prophylaxis and treatment

No prospective, randomized trial has demonstrated a proven benefit of prophylactic therapy to prevent CNS recurrence for patients with HRL; however, prophylaxis should be considered in high-risk patients. Desai and colleagues treated 62 patients with CDE, five of who had lymphomatous meningitis at diagnosis and were treated with whole brain RT (30 Gy) and intrathecal (IT) chemotherapy (methotrexate and/or cytarabine). Thirty-one subjects were assigned to receive prophylactic IT chemotherapy due to lymphomatous bone marrow involvement and/or high-grade histology. Three refused IT therapy, and one of these had parenchymal brain recurrence. Of the 28 who received IT chemotherapy, three had CNS recurrence, two in the leptomeninges and one parenchymal. Of the 26 subjects who did not meet criteria for IT prophylaxis, none had leptomeningeal recurrence, but one had a parenchymal relapse. Three of the four CNS recurrences occurred in the setting of systemic recurrence or progression.[165] Thus, the available data do not clearly support the practice of administering IT prophylaxis to all patients with HIV-NHL. As IT therapy does not penetrate the brain parenchyma deeply, it may not provide prophylaxis against parenchymal recurrence. Patients with a high risk for leptomeningeal involvment include those with disease involving the paranasal sinuses, epidural space, testis, and >2 extranodal sites with elevated LDH. These patients should undergo IT prophylaxis. However, there is no standard approach for this. In the AMC and at University of California, San Francisco (UCSF) we generally administer four doses (weekly during the first cycle of chemotherapy) of IT cytarabine or methotrexate. BL/BLL have a very high risk of leptomeningeal involvement at diagnosis and/or recurrence, and should all receive IT prophylaxis in addition to intravenous chemotherapy that penetrates the CSF.

Hodgkin lymphoma

Clinical features

HIV infection clearly increases the risk of HL, and unlike HIV-NHL the risk may be increased in patients with preserved CD4 counts compared to those with severe immune deficiency.[13] PWHA with HL are more likely to present with advanced-stage disease, B symptoms, and extranodal disease than their HIV-negative counterparts.[168–171] Early on in the HIV/AIDS epidemic, survival with HL was poor; however, since the widespread use of HAART survival has improved significantly, and now approaches that of HIV-negative individuals with HL.[42,43]

While all subtypes can occur in PWHA, the proportion of mixed cellularity and lymphocyte-depleted subtypes appears to be greater than in the HIV-negative population, especially in those with more advanced HIV/AIDS,[13,44,168–170,172] although in one study mixed cellularity and nodular sclerosis occurred at a similar rate, both making up 60% of the cases in that series.[172]

Pathologic features

The Reed–Sternberg (RS) cell in HIV-HL has similar features as in HL occurring in HIV-negative patients, with expression of CD15 and CD30, a small subset expressing CD20, and negative for CD45. EBER and latent membrane protein-1 (LMP-1) expression is also extremely common, indicating a greater role of EBV infection in HIV-HL.[172,173] While one study showed that the inflammatory background cell composite of HIV-HL was characterized by a predominance of CD8-positive T lymphocytes over CD4-positive T lymphocytes,[172] it has also been shown to have a decreased number of activated cytotoxic cells expressing granzyme B and intratumoral activated cytotoxic T-lymphocytes.[174]

Treatment

Prior to HAART, toxicity of chemotherapy and prednisone for patients with HIV-HL was a considerable concern for treating physicians. However, a less intensive regimen, EBV (epirubicin, bleomycin, and vinblastine) combined with AZT yielded only 53% CR and 55% 2-year DFS rates.[175] EBVP (epirubicin, bleomycin, vinblastine, and prednisone) given with both AZT or dideoxinosyne (ddI) with G-CSF support led to 74% CR, 3-year OS and DFS of 32% and 53%, respectively.[176]

The regimen with the most published experience in HIV-HL is ABVD. The AIDS Clinical Trial Group (ACTG) reported that ABVD with G-CSF support but no HAART led to 43% CR, median OS of 18 months, and DFS 13 months.[177] A subsequent case series of eight patients with HIV-HL treated with ABVD (two with HAART) described 100% CR, median CR duration of 43 months (range 22–90 months), and 44 months median OS with no relapses reported.[178] A retrospective study reported by the GESIDA (Groupo de Estudia de SIDA) and GELCAB (Grup per l'Estudi dels Limfomes de Catalunya i Balears) groups from Spain reported 87% CR with ABVD and HAART, with 82% of patients completing all planned cycles of therapy, 76% 5-year OS, and 71% EFS; HAART response was significantly associated with both OS and EFS. However, 6 of 62 patients died during induction, two due to sepsis and three due to HL- and HIV-related events.[179]

Spina and colleagues postulated that concurrent HAART in combination with Stanford V (doxorubicin, vinblastine, meclorethamine, etoposide, vincristine, bleomycin, prednisone), a short-term, intensive regimen incorporating RT for high-risk patients, might yield higher response rates and better survival. Sixty-nine percent of patients were able to complete the full planned treatment, and 81% achieved CR. Estimated OS and DFS were 51% and 68%, respectively. Results were dramatically different among patients with International Prognostic Score (IPS) <2 compared to those with IPS >2, with freedom from progression (FFP) of 84% and 41% and OS of 76% and 33%, respectively, suggesting that higher-risk patients may require more intensive therapy.[60] In a small series of 12 patients treated with BEACOPP (bleomycin, etoposide, doxorubicin, cyclophosphamide, vincristine, procarbazine, and prednisone) without concurrent HAART, CR was 100% but grade 3/4 neutropenia occurred in 75% of patients, and 25% died during the study period.[180]

As in HIV-NHL, there are many active regimens in HIV-HL but no randomized controlled trials, as demonstrated by a recent Cochrane review.[181] However, the data to date confirm that patients with HIV-HL should be treated aggressively up front, as for their HIV-negative counterparts, and dose adjustments made based on toxicity, especially for those taking ritonavir, and those with extensive bone marrow involvement and/or advanced HIV/AIDS.

T-cell lymphoma

Epidemiology

While not considered an AIDS-defining malignancy, the risk for T-cell NHL (T-NHL) does appear to be increased in PWHA. This is a more recent finding in the literature, which may be in part due to improved diagnostic techniques since the early AIDS epidemic. By linking AIDS and cancer registry data from 1978 to 1996, Biggar *et al.* found that, of 120 114 NHL cases, 9% of NHL occurred in PWHA, and 36% (3804) were reported to have non-specific histologies. In the early 1980s, 8% of all NHL cases had immunophenotypic data, but in the 1990s this proportion increased to 29%. Of the non-specific AIDS-NHL cases, 11% (402) had immunophenotypic data, and of these 11% (45) had T-cell markers. One percent (96 cases) of HIV-NHL of all AIDS-linked NHLs were classified specifically as having T-cell histology, and of the 51% with immunophenotypic data, 94% confirmed T-cell phenotype.[5] In this study, the relative risk of T-NHL within the first 4–27 months of AIDS onset was 15.0 (95% CI = 10.0–21.7), compared to the risk in HIV-negative patients, a risk increase that was seen across all subtypes identified. A report describing HRL cases in Peru surprisingly found 27% of cases to be T-NHL.[182]

Clinical features

Case reports describe a high proportion of stage IV disease with extranodal involvement, including skin, bone marrow, liver, lung, nasal cavity, gastrointestinal tract, and peritoneal cavity.[171,183,184] One report showed a statistically significantly higher proportion of bone marrow (45% vs. 15%, $p = 0.019$) and skin (36% vs. 2%, $p < 0.001$) in T- compared to B-NHL, respectively; while there were trends to a higher rate of pleural and bone involvement, these were not statistically significant. CD4 count at diagnosis is typically below 200 cells/μL, and the majority of cases reported were not on HAART at diagnosis of T-NHL. A large proportion present with stage IV disease (44–90%) and B symptoms (38–82%).[182,185]

Pathologic features

Most T-NHL subtypes have been reported to occur in PWHA. In the study by Biggar and colleagues, 13 had mycosis fungoides (MF), 36 peripheral T-cell lymphoma (PTCL), 13 cutaneous, 11 adult T-cell leukemia/lymphoma (ATLL), and 1 angiocentric.[5] There have been many case reports and case series demonstrating the heterogeneity of HIV-related T-NHL (HIV-T-NHL), though PTCL and anaplastic large cell lymphoma (ALCL) appear to be the most common subtypes. Immunophenotyping usually shows expression of CD45, lack of B-cell markers such as CD19, 20, and 22, and presence of T-cell markers (CD3, 4, 8), natural killer cell markers (CD56, CD57), or, in some cases of ALCL, a null phenotype (no T- or B-cell markers) but expression of CD30.[185] A series of three peripheral T-cell lymphoma, not otherwise specified (PTCL, NOS) cases described a cytotoxic phenotype (positive for CD3, CD8, TIA-1, and granzyme B) with clonal rearrangement of the T-cell receptor-γ (TCR-γ).[186] Evidence of clonal EBV expression can be found in about half to three-quarters of ALCL cases.[183,184,187]

Treatment and prognosis

There have been no prospective clinical trials to address the optimal therapy for HIV-T-NHL. Looking at results reported in case series, CHOP or CHOP-like regimens are commonly used, with mixed results. Of eight patients from the University of Southern California AIDS-Lymphoma registry treated with CHOP, three of three patients with ALCL achieved CR and lived 3.6–54.6+ months. Outcomes of CHOP in PTCL, NOS were poor, with four achieving PR and one PD. Four patients with relapse were salvaged with ESHAP (etoposide, methylprednisolone, cytarabine, cisplatin), and one PTCL, NOS patient was alive and in CR at 81.3 months follow-up. The overall median survival for T-NHL was 10.6 months, and 6.6 months for B-NHL ($p = 0.013$).[185] The Peruvian study described the treatment of eight patients alive at diagnosis of T-NHL. Two were treated with HAART without chemotherapy, and one achieved CR (also received corticosteroids); the other who was treated with surgery had "non-progressive lymphoma." There was no significant difference in survival between T- and B-NHL, and the only predictors of death by multivariate analysis were stage IV disease and lack of CD4 count availability.[182]

Multicentric Castleman's disease

Epidemiology

Castleman's disease comprises two distinct diseases, unicentric and multicentric; in HIV infection the most common presentation is as multicentric Castleman's disease (MCD). MCD may present in isolation (primary MCD) or in the setting of other diseases, such as HIV, plasma-cell dyscrasias, and other lymphomas (secondary MCD). It is associated with low CD4 count (mean CD4 156 cells/μL in one analysis) and with KS and KSHV-associated NHL.[188,189]

Clinical features

MCD presents with generalized lymphadenopathy, constitutional symptoms such as fever and weight loss, varying degrees of hepatomegaly, respiratory symptoms, and edema, as well as anemia or pancytopenia.[187] Laboratory examination often reveals polyclonal hypergammaglobulinemia, hypoalbuminemia, elevated levels of IL-6, IL-10, and C-reactive protein, and a measurable KSHV-viral load.[188,190–192]

Pathologic features

MCD is typically not a clonal disorder, with pathology revealing hyperplastic germinal centers, germinal center angiosclerosis, expansion of plasma cells in interfollicular regions, and dilatation of the sinuses.[193,194] KSHV is present in all HIV-associated MCD and most cases of HIV-negative MCD.[195,196] B-cells in MCD are notable for high levels of viral IL-6 production, which may play a role in vascular endothelial growth factor secretion and B-cell proliferation.[192,196] Cases of MCD with scattered medium to large plasmablastic cells associated with HIV-infection have been described as a "plasmablastic variant." While the cells containing KSHV have plasmablastic or immunoblastic features, are often IgM-lambda-restricted, and sometimes found in clusters or sheets,[189,196–198] these are usually found to be polyclonal.[199] However, aggressive lymphoma may arise out of MCD: in a prospective cohort study in which 60 patients with HIV and MCD were followed for a median of 20 months, 14 developed NHL (all KSHV and/or EBV-associated), suggesting a 15-fold increased incidence of NHL in patients with HIV-MCD.[189] Large cell lymphoma arising from KSHV-associated MCD is almost always positive for KSHV.[196]

Treatment and prognosis

An important component of therapy for HIV-associated MCD is treatment of the underlying HIV infection with HAART. Some HIV-associated MCD cases have been reported to regress with HAART therapy alone.[200] While cytotoxic chemotherapy with drugs such as etoposide, vinblastine, and liposomal doxorubicin can be effective, most of the published clinical experience has been with rituximab monotherapy. One prospective study enrolled five patients with HIV-associated MCD for treatment with four weekly infusions of rituximab. CR was achieved in three patients, who remained free of any evidence of disease with a follow-up of 4–14 months; the other two patients died shortly after receiving rituximab without any evidence of response. Both of these patients were very ill with severe autoimmune manifestations at the time of treatment.[201] A phase II trial of rituximab treatment for 21 patients with HIV-associated MCD reported remission of symptoms in 20 patients, and 14 had a radiologic response. Two-year DFS was 79%, OS 95%,[202] an improvement over the median survival of 14 months prior to the availability of rituximab.[188] Rituximab has also been evaluated prospectively for maintenance therapy in patients who have responded to, but cannot be discontinued from, chemotherapy. Twenty-four patients with a median time on chemotherapy were enrolled, and treated with four weekly doses of rituximab. Ninety-two percent had sustained remission of therapy at day 60, and four relapsed before day 365. Rituximab was well tolerated, though of 12 patients with KS, 8 experienced an exacerbation of KS.[203] Case reports describe the successful use of rituximab in combination with cytotoxic chemotherapy for MCD, including CVP (cyclophosphamide, vincristine, prednisone),[204] CHOP, and liposomal doxorubicin,[205] as well as with thalidomide.[206]

Antiviral therapy has had limited success in MCD, with sustained clinical improvement in one of three patients given 21 days of daily ganciclovir,[207] and five of five patients progressing during weekly cidofovir for 3 weeks followed by every other week.[208]

Splenectomy resulted in improvement of fevers and cytopenias in a retrospective analysis of ten patients with MCD; eight were alive with 41 months median follow-up, though six of those subsequently received chemotherapy for KS (four) and progressive MCD (two).[209] While there are no published comparisons of rituximab to rituximab in combination with other therapies, or cytotoxic chemotherapy alone, rituximab is the recommended first-line therapy. However, choice of therapy should be guided by clinical judgement, including the extent of disease and the patient's organ function and performance status.

Stem cell transplantation

High-dose chemotherapy followed by autologous stem cell transplantation (ASCT) should be strongly considered for all patients with relapsed or refractory HRL. ASCT has been shown to be the optimal therapy for HIV-negative patients with relapsed or refractory lymphoma.[210,211] Patients with HIV infection do not appear to experience an increase in toxicity and infectious complications compared to HIV-negative patients, and clinical outcomes appear to be similar (Table 24.6). Patients selected to undergo ASCT for relapsed/refractory HRL in general must have adequate control of HIV (stable or undetectable viral load, CD4 count greater than 50 cells/μL) and no active opportunistic infections.[218] While CR or chemosensitivity is also a requirement for ASCT, there are not many published data on salvage regimens for HRL. One study reported a 53% overall response rate for patients with relapsed/refractory HRL treated with high-dose cytarabine and cisplatin regimens (ESHAP or DHAP [dexamethasone, cytarabine, cisplatin]).[219]

The first major prospective ASCT series to be reported included 20 patients with relapsed or refractory HRL (18 NHL

Table 24.6. Autologous stem cell transplant for HIV-related lymphoma

Reference	Prep	n	Transplanted	CR	Engraftment		TRM	Follow-up (mo)	OS
					ANC > 0.5	Plt > 20K			
Re *et al.*[212]	BEAM	20	65%	8/16	10 d	13 d	0	12	55% 9 mo
Gabarre *et al.*[213]	various	14	100%	10/14	12 d	11 d	0	32	50% 9 mo
Krishnan *et al.*[214]	CBV	20	100%	17/20	11 d	10 d	5%	32	85% 32 mo
Serrano *et al.*[215]	BEAM	14	79%	8/14	16 d	20 d	3 prior to txplt	30	71% 21 mo
Balsalobre *et al.*[216]	various	44			11 d	14 d		36	60% 36 mo
Spitzer *et al.*[217]	Bu-Cy	27	74%	10/19	11 d	13 d	4%	6	74% 6 mo

Note: BEAM: etoposide, cytarabine, and melphalan; CBV: cyclophosphamide, carmustine (BCNU), and etoposide; Bu-Cy: busulfan and cyclophosphamide; txplt: transplant; TRM: transplant-related mortality.

and 2 HL). Patients younger than 55 years with bulky or extranodal disease and who had not received prior radiation (n = 3) were treated with fractionated total body irradiation (TBI) with etoposide and cyclophosphamide. All others (n = 17) received CBV (cylophosphamide, carmustine [BCNU], etoposide) without TBI. All patients were on HAART and median CD4 count was 175 cells/μL; 11 had to discontinue HAART due to mucositis and gastrointestinal toxicity. Febrile neutropenia occurred in eight patients, gram-positive bacteremia in five and grade 3/4 hepatotoxicity, engraftment syndrome in two, and BCNU-induced pneumonitis in one. One patient died of treatment-related toxicity and two patients died of disease relapse within 4 months after transplant. With 32 months median follow-up, OS and PFS were 85% and 81%, respectively. CD4 counts returned to pretransplant levels by the first year after transplant, and 76% had undetectable viral loads.[214] Eleven patients with relapsed or refractory HRL (seven NHL and four HL) treated with BEAM or BEAC (carmustine [BCNU], etoposide, cytarabine, plus melphalan or cyclophosphamide, respectively) had a median time to neutrophil engraftment of 16 days, and no treatment-related mortality. With a median follow-up of 30 months after ASCT, EFS is 65%.[215] Re and colleagues reported another prospective study of BEAM-ASCT for relapsed or refractory HRL with concurrent HAART. Ten of 16 enrolled patients were able to undergo transplant. Median time to engraftment was 10 days, and there were no treatment-related deaths. Eight of nine assessable patients achieved CR relapse; six were alive and in CR at a median of 8 months after transplant.[212]

The AIDS Malignancy Consortium (AMC) studied a dose-reduced busulfan and cyclophosphamide regimen for ASCT in 27 patients with HRL. All patients received a HAART regimen that excluded ritonavir and zidovudine, and all received a single dose of intrathecal cytarabine prior to conditioning. Of 20 patients transplanted, median time to neutrophil recovery was 11 days. One treatment-related death occurred due to veno-occlusive disease with multiorgan failure. CR rate at day 100 after ASCT was 53%.[217]

A retrospective review by the European Group for Blood and Marrow Transplantation (EBMT) analyzed outcomes of 44 patients with HIV-NHL undergoing autotransplant. Twenty-two patients were in CR at the time of transplant, and 18 were in PR or chemosensitive relapse. Most patients received BEAM or a similar preparative regimen, and more than 90% received HAART though this had to be discontinued in nine patients. Neutrophil engraftment occurred at a median of 8 days, and platelets reached 20 000/μL by a median of 14 days. Three patients died of bacterial infection, one from an HIV-related complication, five from complications of ASCT (including one myelodysplasia), and 11 died from progressive NHL. OS was 60% at a median follow-up of 36 months.[216]

No studies have prospectively compared the results of ASCT among different subtypes of HRL; however, a retrospective analysis suggested that patients with PBL do poorly after ASCT, in comparison to patients with centroblastic or immunoblastic DLBCL. All three of the PBL patients who underwent ASCT in this series relapsed within 6 months and died of progressive lymphoma; seven of the ten patients with centroblastic DLBCL were still alive and in CR with a median of 51 months follow-up.[77] One case report described a favorable outcome of ASCT for PBL.[173]

There are a variety of conditioning regimens that appear to be safe and effective for relapsed or refractory HRL; some of the differences in reported outcomes may be due to variability in patient selection. The studies to date support the use of ASCT for patients with relapsed or refractory HRL with adequate organ function, HIV control, and with chemosensitive disease. Future studies will need to address optimal selection of patients for ASCT (tumor histology, HIV parameters), type of HAART and timing with regard to the preparative regimen and engraftment, and duration and type of post-transplant antibiotic, antifungal, and antiviral prophylaxis.

References

1. Grulich AE, van Leeuwen MT, Falster MO, *et al.* Incidence of cancers in people with HIV/AIDS compared with immunosuppressed transplant recipients: a meta-analysis. *Lancet* 2007;**370**(9581):59–67.
2. Serraino D, Piselli P, Busnach G, *et al.* Risk of cancer following immunosuppression in organ transplant recipients and in HIV-positive individuals in southern Europe. *Eur J Cancer* 2007;**43**(14):2117–23.
3. Rabkin CS, Hilgartner MW, Hedberg KW, *et al.* Incidence of lymphomas and other cancers in HIV-infected and HIV-uninfected patients with hemophilia. *JAMA* 1992;**267**(8):1090–4.
4. Goedert JJ, Cote TR, Virgo P, *et al.* Spectrum of AIDS-associated malignant disorders. *Lancet* 1998; **351**(9119):1833–9.
5. Biggar RJ, Kirby KA, Atkinson J, *et al.* Cancer risk in elderly persons with HIV/AIDS. *J Acquir Immune Defic Syndr* 2004;**36**(3):861–8.
6. Serraino D, Boschini A, Carrieri P, *et al.* Cancer risk among men with, or at risk of, HIV infection in southern Europe. *AIDS* 2000;**14**(5):553–9.
7. Munoz A, Schrager LK, Bacellar H, *et al.* Trends in the incidence of outcomes defining acquired immunodeficiency syndrome (AIDS) in the Multicenter AIDS Cohort Study: 1985–1991. *Am J Epidemiol* 1993;**137**(4):423–38.
8. Pluda JM, Venzon DJ, Tosato G, *et al.* Parameters affecting the development of non-Hodgkin's lymphoma in patients with severe human immunodeficiency virus infection receiving antiretroviral therapy. *J Clin Oncol* 1993;**11**(6):1099–107.
9. Kirk O, Pedersen C, Cozzi-Lepri A, *et al.* Non-Hodgkin lymphoma in HIV-infected patients in the era of highly active antiretroviral therapy. *Blood* 2001;**98**(12):3406–12.
10. Hessol NA, Katz MH, Liu JY, *et al.* Increased incidence of Hodgkin disease in homosexual men with HIV infection. *Ann Intern Med* 1992;**117**(4):309–11.
11. Frisch M, Biggar RJ, Engels EA, *et al.* Association of cancer with AIDS-related immunosuppression in adults. *JAMA* 2001;**285**(13):1736–45.
12. Grulich AE, Li Y, McDonald A, *et al.* Rates of non-AIDS-defining cancers in people with HIV infection before and after AIDS diagnosis. *AIDS* 2002;**16**(8):1155–61.
13. Biggar RJ, Jaffe ES, Goedert JJ, *et al.* Hodgkin lymphoma and immunodeficiency in persons with HIV/AIDS. *Blood* 2006;**108**(12):3786–91.
14. Palella FJ Jr, Delaney KM, Moorman AC, *et al.* Declining morbidity and mortality among patients with advanced human immunodeficiency virus infection. HIV Outpatient Study Investigators. *N Engl J Med* 1998;**338**(13):853–60.
15. Mocroft A, Katlama C, Johnson AM, *et al.* AIDS across Europe, 1994–98: the EuroSIDA study. *Lancet* 2000;**356**(9226):291–6.
16. Matthews GV, Bower M, Mandalia S, *et al.* Changes in acquired immunodeficiency syndrome-related lymphoma since the introduction of highly active antiretroviral therapy. *Blood* 2000;**96**(8):2730–4.
17. Dore GJ, Li Y, McDonald A, *et al.* Impact of highly active antiretroviral therapy on individual AIDS-defining illness incidence and survival in Australia. *J Acquir Immune Defic Syndr* 2002;**29**(4):388–95.
18. Gates AE, Kaplan LD. Biology and management of AIDS-associated non-Hodgkin's lymphoma. *Hematol Oncol Clin North Am* 2003;**17**(3):821–41.
19. Besson C, Goubar A, Gabarre J, *et al.* Changes in AIDS-related lymphoma since the era of highly active antiretroviral therapy. *Blood* 2001; **98**(8):2339–44.
20. Bonnet F, Balestre E, Thiebaut R, *et al.* Factors associated with the occurrence of AIDS-related non-Hodgkin lymphoma in the era of highly active antiretroviral therapy: Aquitaine Cohort, France. *Clin Infect Dis* 2006; **42**(3):411–17.
21. Diamond C, Taylor TH, Aboumrad T, *et al.* Changes in acquired immunodeficiency syndrome-related non-Hodgkin lymphoma in the era of highly active antiretroviral therapy: incidence, presentation, treatment, and survival. *Cancer* 2006;**106**(1):128–35.
22. Polesel J, Clifford GM, Rickenbach M, *et al.* Non-Hodgkin lymphoma incidence in the Swiss HIV Cohort Study before and after highly active antiretroviral therapy. *AIDS* 2008; **22**(2):301–6.
23. Engels EA, Pfeiffer RM, Goedert JJ, *et al.* Trends in cancer risk among people with AIDS in the United States 1980–2002. *AIDS* 2006;**20**(12):1645–54.
24. Clifford GM, Polesel J, Rickenbach M, *et al.* Cancer risk in the Swiss HIV Cohort Study: associations with immunodeficiency, smoking, and highly active antiretroviral therapy. *J Natl Cancer Inst* 2005;**97**(6):425–32.
25. Silverberg MJ, Neuhaus J, Bower M, *et al.* Risk of cancers during interrupted antiretroviral therapy in the SMART study. *AIDS* 2007;**21**(14):1957–63.
26. Levine AM, Seneviratne L, Espina BM, *et al.* Evolving characteristics of AIDS-related lymphoma. *Blood* 2000;**96**(13): 4084–90.
27. Raphael M, Borisch B, Jaffe ES. Immunodeficiency associated lymphoproliferative disorders. In: Jaffe ES, Harris NL, Stein H, *et al.*, eds. *World Health Organization Classification of Tumours: Pathology and Genetics of Tumours of Haematopoietic and Lymphoid Tissues.* Lyon, France, IRC Press. 2001; 255–71.
28. Kaplan LD, Abrams DI, Feigal E, *et al.* AIDS-associated non-Hodgkin's lymphoma in San Francisco. *JAMA* 1989;**261**(5):719–24.
29. Kaplan LD, Straus DJ, Testa MA, *et al.* Low-dose compared with standard-dose m-BACOD chemotherapy for non-Hodgkin's lymphoma associated with human immunodeficiency virus infection. National Institute of Allergy and Infectious Diseases AIDS Clinical Trials Group. *N Engl J Med* 1997;**336**(23):1641–8.
30. Levine AM, Sullivan-Halley J, Pike MC, *et al.* Human immunodeficiency virus-related lymphoma. Prognostic factors predictive of survival. *Cancer* 1991;**68**(11):2466–72.
31. Gisselbrecht C, Oksenhendler E, Tirelli U, *et al.* Human immunodeficiency virus-related lymphoma treatment with intensive combination chemotherapy. French-Italian Cooperative Group. *Am J Med* 1993;**95**(2):188–96.
32. Vaccher E, Tirelli U, Spina M, *et al.* Age and serum lactate dehydrogenase level are independent prognostic factors in human immunodeficiency virus-related non-Hodgkin's lymphomas: a single-institute study of 96 patients. *J Clin Oncol* 1996;**14**(8):2217–23.
33. Straus DJ, Huang J, Testa MA, *et al.* Prognostic factors in the treatment of

human immunodeficiency virus-associated non-Hodgkin's lymphoma: analysis of AIDS Clinical Trials Group protocol 142–low-dose versus standard-dose m-BACOD plus granulocyte-macrophage colony-stimulating factor. National Institute of Allergy and Infectious Diseases. *J Clin Oncol* 1998;**16**(11):3601–6.

34. Rossi G, Donisi A, Casari S, *et al.* The International Prognostic Index can be used as a guide to treatment decisions regarding patients with human immunodeficiency virus-related systemic non-Hodgkin lymphoma. *Cancer* 1999;**86**(11):2391–7.

35. The International Non-Hodgkin's Lymphoma Prognostic Factors Project. A predictive model for aggressive non-Hodgkin's lymphoma. *N Engl J Med* 1993;**329**(14):987–94.

36. Navarro JT, Ribera JM, Oriol A, *et al.* International prognostic index is the best prognostic factor for survival in patients with AIDS-related non-Hodgkin's lymphoma treated with CHOP. A multivariate study of 46 patients. *Haematologica* 1998;**83**(6): 508–13.

37. Bower M, Gazzard B, Mandalia S, *et al.* A prognostic index for systemic AIDS-related non-Hodgkin lymphoma treated in the era of highly active antiretroviral therapy. *Ann Intern Med* 2005;**143** (4):265–73.

38. Vaccher E, Spina M, Talamini R, *et al.* Improvement of systemic human immunodeficiency virus-related non-Hodgkin lymphoma outcome in the era of highly active antiretroviral therapy. *Clin Infect Dis* 2003;**37**(11):1556–64.

39. Lim ST, Karim R, Tulpule A, *et al.* Prognostic factors in HIV-related diffuse large-cell lymphoma: before versus after highly active antiretroviral therapy. *J Clin Oncol* 2005;**23**(33):8477–82.

40. Navarro JT, Lloveras N, Ribera JM, *et al.* The prognosis of HIV-infected patients with diffuse large B-cell lymphoma treated with chemotherapy and highly active antiretroviral therapy is similar to that of HIV-negative patients receiving chemotherapy. *Haematologica* 2005;**90**(5):704–6.

41. Tam HK, Zhang ZF, Jacobson LP, *et al.* Effect of highly active antiretroviral therapy on survival among HIV-infected men with Kaposi sarcoma or non-Hodgkin lymphoma. *Int J Cancer* 2002;**98**(6):916–22.

42. Ribera JM, Navarro JT, Oriol A, *et al.* Prognostic impact of highly active antiretroviral therapy in HIV-related Hodgkin's disease. *AIDS* 2002;**16** (14):1973–6.

43. Gerard L, Galicier L, Boulanger E, *et al.* Improved survival in HIV-related Hodgkin's lymphoma since the introduction of highly active antiretroviral therapy. *AIDS* 2003; **17**(1):81–7.

44. Hentrich M, Maretta L, Chow KU, *et al.* Highly active antiretroviral therapy (HAART) improves survival in HIV-associated Hodgkin's disease: results of a multicenter study. *Ann Oncol* 2006; **17**(6):914–19.

45. Kaplan LD, Lee JY, Ambinder RF, *et al.* Rituximab does not improve clinical outcome in a randomized phase 3 trial of CHOP with or without rituximab in patients with HIV-associated non-Hodgkin lymphoma: AIDS-Malignancies Consortium Trial 010. *Blood* 2005;**106**(5):1538–43.

46. Little RF, Pittaluga S, Grant N, *et al.* Highly effective treatment of acquired immunodeficiency syndrome-related lymphoma with dose-adjusted EPOCH: impact of antiretroviral therapy suspension and tumor biology. *Blood* 2003;**101**(12):4653–9.

47. Lascaux AS, Hemery F, Goujard C, *et al.* Beneficial effect of highly active antiretroviral therapy on the prognosis of AIDS-related systemic non-Hodgkin lymphomas. *AIDS Res Hum Retroviruses* 2005;**21**(3):214–20.

48. Miralles P, Berenguer J, Ribera JM, *et al.* Prognosis of AIDS-related systemic non-Hodgkin lymphoma treated with chemotherapy and highly active antiretroviral therapy depends exclusively on tumor-related factors. *J Acquir Immune Defic Syndr* 2007; **44**(2):167–73.

49. Lim ST, Karim R, Nathwani BN, *et al.* AIDS-related Burkitt's lymphoma versus diffuse large-cell lymphoma in the pre-highly active antiretroviral therapy (HAART) and HAART eras: significant differences in survival with standard chemotherapy. *J Clin Oncol* 2005;**23**(19):4430–8.

50. Spina M, Simonelli C, Talamini R, *et al.* Patients with HIV with Burkitt's lymphoma have a worse outcome than those with diffuse large-cell lymphoma also in the highly active antiretroviral therapy era. *J Clin Oncol* 2005;**23** (31):8132–3; author reply 8133–4.

51. Mackall CL, Fleisher TA, Brown MR, *et al.* Lymphocyte depletion during treatment with intensive chemotherapy for cancer. *Blood* 1994;**84**(7):2221–8.

52. Cheson BD. Infectious and immunosuppressive complications of purine analog therapy. *J Clin Oncol* 1995;**13**(9):2431–48.

53. Hakim FT, Cepeda R, Kaimei S, *et al.* Constraints on CD4 recovery postchemotherapy in adults: thymic insufficiency and apoptotic decline of expanded peripheral CD4 cells. *Blood* 1997;**90**(9):3789–98.

54. Powles T, Imami N, Nelson M, *et al.* Effects of combination chemotherapy and highly active antiretroviral therapy on immune parameters in HIV-1 associated lymphoma. *AIDS* 2002; **16**(4):531–6.

55. Ratner L, Lee J, Tang S, *et al.* Chemotherapy for human immunodeficiency virus-associated non-Hodgkin's lymphoma in combination with highly active antiretroviral therapy. *J Clin Oncol* 2001;**19**(8):2171–8.

56. Tosi P, Gherlinzoni F, Visani G, *et al.* AZT plus methotrexate in HIV-related non-Hodgkin's lymphomas. *Leuk Lymphoma* 1998;**30**(1–2):175–9.

57. Smith PF, DiCenzo R, Morse GD. Clinical pharmacokinetics of non-nucleoside reverse transcriptase inhibitors. *Clin Pharmacokinet* 2001; **40**(12):893–905.

58. Chiba M, Nishime JA, Lin JH. Potent and selective inactivation of human liver microsomal cytochrome P-450 isoforms by L-754,394, an investigational human immune deficiency virus protease inhibitor. *J Pharmacol Exp Ther* 1995; **275**(3):1527–34.

59. Bower M, McCall-Peat N, Ryan N, *et al.* Protease inhibitors potentiate chemotherapy-induced neutropenia. *Blood* 2004;**104**(9):2943–6.

60. Spina M, Gabarre J, Rossi G, *et al.* Stanford V regimen and concomitant HAART in 59 patients with Hodgkin disease and HIV infection. *Blood* 2002;**100**(6):1984–8.

61. Makinson A, Martelli N, Peyriere H, *et al.* Profound neutropenia resulting

from interaction between antiretroviral therapy and vinblastine in a patient with HIV-associated Hodgkin's disease. *Eur J Haematol* 2007;**78**(4):358–60.

62. Moore DA, Benepal T, Portsmouth S, *et al.* Etiology and natural history of neutropenia in human immunodeficiency virus disease: a prospective study. *Clin Infect Dis* 2001;**32**(3):469–75.

63. Seneviratne L, Espina BM, Nathwani BN, *et al.* Clinical, immunologic, and pathologic correlates of bone marrow involvement in 291 patients with acquired immunodeficiency syndrome-related lymphoma. *Blood* 2001; **98**(8):2358–63.

64. Mounier N, Spina M, Gabarre J, *et al.* AIDS-related non-Hodgkin lymphoma: final analysis of 485 patients treated with risk-adapted intensive chemotherapy. *Blood* 2006;**107**(10):3832–40.

65. Boue F, Gabarre J, Gisselbrecht C, *et al.* Phase II trial of CHOP plus rituximab in patients with HIV-associated non-Hodgkin's lymphoma. *J Clin Oncol* 2006;**24**(25):4123–8.

66. Grogg KL, Miller RF, Dogan A. HIV infection and lymphoma. *J Clin Pathol* 2007;**60**(12):1365–72.

67. Carbone A, Gaidano G, Gloghini A, *et al.* Differential expression of BCL-6, CD138/syndecan-1, and Epstein-Barr virus-encoded latent membrane protein-1 identifies distinct histogenetic subsets of acquired immunodeficiency syndrome-related non-Hodgkin's lymphomas. *Blood* 1998;**91**(3):747–55.

68. MacMahon EM, Glass JD, Hayward SD, *et al.* Epstein-Barr virus in AIDS-related primary central nervous system lymphoma. *Lancet* 1991;**338** (8773):969–73.

69. Jaffe ES, Harris NL, Stein H, *et al.* *World Health Organization Classification of Tumours: Pathology and Genetics of Tumours of Haematopoietic and Lymphoid Tissues.* Lyon; Oxford: IARC Press; Oxford University Press (distributor); 2001.

70. Raphael MM, Audouin J, Lamine M, *et al.* Immunophenotypic and genotypic analysis of acquired immunodeficiency syndrome-related non-Hodgkin's lymphomas. Correlation with histologic features in 36 cases. French Study Group of Pathology for HIV-Associated Tumors. *Am J Clin Pathol* 1994; **101**(6):773–82.

71. Hamilton-Dutoit SJ, Rea D, Raphael M, *et al.* Epstein-Barr virus-latent gene expression and tumor cell phenotype in acquired immunodeficiency syndrome-related non-Hodgkin's lymphoma. Correlation of lymphoma phenotype with three distinct patterns of viral latency. *Am J Pathol* 1993;**143**(4): 1072–85.

72. Engels EA, Rosenberg PS, Frisch M, *et al.* Cancers associated with Kaposi's sarcoma (KS) in AIDS: a link between KS herpesvirus and immunoblastic lymphoma. *Br J Cancer* 2001;**85**(9): 1298–303.

73. Cioc AM, Allen C, Kalmar JR, *et al.* Oral plasmablastic lymphomas in AIDS patients are associated with human herpesvirus 8. *Am J Surg Pathol* 2004; **28**(1):41–6.

74. Deloose ST, Smit LA, Pals FT, *et al.* High incidence of Kaposi sarcoma-associated herpesvirus infection in HIV-related solid immunoblastic/ plasmablastic diffuse large B-cell lymphoma. *Leukemia* 2005;**19**(5):851–5.

75. Castillo J, Pantanowitz L, Dezube BJ. HIV-associated plasmablastic lymphoma: lessons learned from 112 published cases. *Am J Hematol* 2008; **83**(10):804–9.

76. Riedel DJ, Gonzalez-Cuyar LF, Zhao XF, *et al.* Plasmablastic lymphoma of the oral cavity: a rapidly progressive lymphoma associated with HIV infection. *Lancet Infect Dis* 2008;**8**(4):261–7.

77. Simonitsch-Klupp I, Hauser I, Ott G, *et al.* Diffuse large B-cell lymphomas with plasmablastic/plasmacytoid features are associated with TP53 deletions and poor clinical outcome. *Leukemia* 2004;**18**(1):146–55.

78. Gaidano G, Cerri M, Capello D, *et al.* Molecular histogenesis of plasmablastic lymphoma of the oral cavity. *Br J Haematol* 2002;**119**(3):622–8.

79. Levine AM, Tulpule A, Espina B, *et al.* Liposome-encapsulated doxorubicin in combination with standard agents (cyclophosphamide, vincristine, prednisone) in patients with newly diagnosed AIDS-related non-Hodgkin's lymphoma: results of therapy and correlates of response. *J Clin Oncol* 2004;**22**(13):2662–70.

80. Wilson WH, Grossbard ML, Pittaluga S, *et al.* Dose-adjusted EPOCH chemotherapy for untreated large B-cell lymphomas: a pharmacodynamic approach with high efficacy. *Blood* 2002;**99**(8):2685–93.

81. Sparano JA, Lee S, Chen MG, *et al.* Phase II trial of infusional cyclophosphamide, doxorubicin, and etoposide in patients with HIV-associated non-Hodgkin's lymphoma: an Eastern Cooperative Oncology Group Trial (E1494). *J Clin Oncol* 2004;**22**(8):1491–500.

82. Sparano JA, Wiernik PH, Strack M, *et al.* Infusional cyclophosphamide, doxorubicin, and etoposide in human immunodeficiency virus- and human T-cell leukemia virus type I-related non-Hodgkin's lymphoma: a highly active regimen. *Blood* 1993;**81**(10): 2810–15.

83. Coiffier B, Lepage E, Briere J, *et al.* CHOP chemotherapy plus rituximab compared with CHOP alone in elderly patients with diffuse large-B-cell lymphoma. *N Engl J Med* 2002; **346**(4):235–42.

84. Spina M, Jaeger U, Sparano JA, *et al.* Rituximab plus infusional cyclophosphamide, doxorubicin, and etoposide in HIV-associated non-Hodgkin lymphoma: pooled results from 3 phase 2 trials. *Blood* 2005; **105**(5):1891–7.

85. Ribera JM, Oriol A, Morgades M, *et al.* Safety and efficacy of cyclophosphamide, adriamycin, vincristine, prednisone and rituximab in patients with human immunodeficiency virus-associated diffuse large B-cell lymphoma: results of a phase II trial. *Br J Haematol* 2008; **140**(4):411–19.

86. Levine AM, Lee J, Kaplan L, *et al.* Efficacy and toxicity of concurrent rituximab plus infusional EPOCH in HIV-associated lymphoma: AIDS Malignancy Consortium Trial 034. *J Clin Oncol* 2008;**26**:Abstract 8527.

87. Cabanillas F, Liboy I, Pavia O, *et al.* High incidence of non-neutropenic infections induced by rituximab plus fludarabine and associated with hypogammaglobulinemia: a frequently unrecognized and easily treatable complication. *Ann Oncol* 2006; **17**(9):1424–7.

88. Nishio M, Fujimoto K, Yamamoto S, *et al.* Hypogammaglobulinemia with a selective delayed recovery in memory B cells and an impaired isotype expression after rituximab administration as an adjuvant to

autologous stem cell transplantation for non-Hodgkin lymphoma. *Eur J Haematol* 2006;**77**(3):226–32.

89. Shortt J, Spencer A. Adjuvant rituximab causes prolonged hypogammaglobulinaemia following autologous stem cell transplant for non-Hodgkin's lymphoma. *Bone Marrow Transplant* 2006;**38**(6):433–6.

90. Miles SA, McGratten M. Persistent panhypogammaglobulinemia after CHOP-rituximab for HIV-related lymphoma. *J Clin Oncol* 2005; **23**(1):247–8.

91. Chaiwatanatorn K, Lee N, Grigg A, *et al.* Delayed-onset neutropenia associated with rituximab therapy. *Br J Haematol* 2003;**121**(6):913–18.

92. Cairoli R, Grillo G, Tedeschi A, *et al.* High incidence of neutropenia in patients treated with rituximab after autologous stem cell transplantation. *Haematologica* 2004;**89**(3):361–3.

93. Cattaneo C, Spedini P, Casari S, *et al.* Delayed-onset peripheral blood cytopenia after rituximab: frequency and risk factor assessment in a consecutive series of 77 treatments. *Leuk Lymphoma* 2006;**47**(6):1013–17.

94. Borg C, Ray-Coquard I, Philip I, *et al.* CD4 lymphopenia as a risk factor for febrile neutropenia and early death after cytotoxic chemotherapy in adult patients with cancer. *Cancer* 2004; **101**(11):2675–80.

95. Spina M, Tirelli U, Zagonel V, *et al.* Burkitt's lymphoma in adults with and without human immunodeficiency virus infection: a single-institution clinicopathologic study of 75 patients. *Cancer* 1998;**82**(4):766–74.

96. Cortes J, Thomas D, Rios A, *et al.* Hyperfractionated cyclophosphamide, vincristine, doxorubicin, and dexamethasone and highly active antiretroviral therapy for patients with acquired immunodeficiency syndrome-related Burkitt lymphoma/leukemia. *Cancer* 2002;**94**(5):1492–9.

97. Oriol A, Ribera JM, Esteve J, *et al.* Lack of influence of human immunodeficiency virus infection status in the response to therapy and survival of adult patients with mature B-cell lymphoma or leukemia. Results of the PETHEMA-LAL3/97 study. *Haematologica* 2003;**88**(4):445–53.

98. Wang ES, Straus DJ, Teruya-Feldstein J, *et al.* Intensive chemotherapy with cyclophosphamide, doxorubicin, high-dose methotrexate/ifosfamide, etoposide, and high-dose cytarabine (CODOX-M/IVAC) for human immunodeficiency virus-associated Burkitt lymphoma. *Cancer* 2003; **98**(6):1196–205.

99. Hoffmann C, Wolf E, Wyen C, *et al.* AIDS-associated Burkitt or Burkitt-like lymphoma: short intensive polychemotherapy is feasible and effective. *Leuk Lymphoma* 2006; **47**(9):1872–80.

100. Carbone A. AIDS-related non-Hodgkin's lymphomas: from pathology and molecular pathogenesis to treatment. *Hum Pathol* 2002; **33**(4):392–404.

101. Astrow AB, Tarabay G, Salerno VE, *et al.* Long-term survival in patients with human immunodeficiency virus-associated small non-cleaved cell lymphoma: the role for short course intensive chemotherapy. *Hematol Oncol* 2003;**21**(3):131–40.

102. Galicier L, Fieschi C, Borie R, *et al.* Intensive chemotherapy regimen (LMB86) for St Jude stage IV AIDS-related Burkitt lymphoma/leukemia: a prospective study. *Blood* 2007; **110**(8):2846–54.

103. Nicol I, Boye T, Carsuzaa F, *et al.* Post-transplant plasmablastic lymphoma of the skin. *Br J Dermatol* 2003;**149**(4):889–91.

104. Borenstein J, Pezzella F, Gatter KC. Plasmablastic lymphomas may occur as post-transplant lymphoproliferative disorders. *Histopathology* 2007; **51**(6):774–7.

105. Robak T, Urbanska-Rys H, Strzelecka B, *et al.* Plasmablastic lymphoma in a patient with chronic lymphocytic leukemia heavily pretreated with cladribine (2-CdA): an unusual variant of Richter's syndrome. *Eur J Haematol* 2001;**67**(5–6):322–7.

106. Redmond M, Quinn J, Murphy P, *et al.* Plasmablastic lymphoma presenting as a paravertebral mass in a patient with Crohn's disease after immunosuppressive therapy. *J Clin Pathol* 2007;**60**(1):80–1.

107. Sharma R, Abdou S, Plymyer MR, *et al.* Disseminated plasmablastic lymphoma. *J Am Coll Surg* 2004;**199**(4):654–5.

108. Hausermann P, Khanna N, Buess M, *et al.* Cutaneous plasmablastic lymphoma in an HIV-positive male: an unrecognized cutaneous manifestation. *Dermatology* 2004; **208**(3):287–90.

109. Jambusaria A, Shafer D, Wu H, *et al.* Cutaneous plasmablastic lymphoma. *J Am Acad Dermatol* 2008;**58**(4):676–8.

110. Delecluse HJ, Anagnostopoulos I, Dallenbach F, *et al.* Plasmablastic lymphomas of the oral cavity: a new entity associated with the human immunodeficiency virus infection. *Blood* 1997;**89**(4):1413–20.

111. Carbone A, Gaidano G, Gloghini A, *et al.* BCL-6 protein expression in AIDS-related non-Hodgkin's lymphomas: inverse relationship with Epstein-Barr virus-encoded latent membrane protein-1 expression. *Am J Pathol* 1997;**150**(1):155–65.

112. Flaitz CM, Nichols CM, Walling DM, *et al.* Plasmablastic lymphoma: an HIV-associated entity with primary oral manifestations. *Oral Oncol* 2002; **38**(1):96–102.

113. Teruya-Feldstein J, Chiao E, Filippa DA, *et al.* CD20-negative large-cell lymphoma with plasmablastic features: a clinically heterogenous spectrum in both HIV-positive and -negative patients. *Ann Oncol* 2004;**15**(11):1673–9.

114. Folk GS, Abbondanzo SL, Childers EL, *et al.* Plasmablastic lymphoma: a clinicopathologic correlation. *Ann Diagn Pathol* 2006;**10**(1):8–12.

115. Zanetto U, Martin CA, Sapia S, *et al.* Re: Cioc AM, Allen C, Kalmar J, *et al.* Oral plasmablastic lymphomas in AIDS patients are associated with human herpesvirus 8. *Am J Surg Pathol* 2004;**25**:41–46. *Am J Surg Pathol* 2004;**28**(11):1537–8; author reply 1538.

116. Nasta SD, Carrum GM, Shahab I, *et al.* Regression of a plasmablastic lymphoma in a patient with HIV on highly active antiretroviral therapy. *Leuk Lymphoma* 2002;**43**(2):423–6.

117. Lester R, Li C, Phillips P, *et al.* Improved outcome of human immunodeficiency virus-associated plasmablastic lymphoma of the oral cavity in the era of highly active antiretroviral therapy: a report of two cases. *Leuk Lymphoma* 2004; **45**(9):1881–5.

118. Nuovo GJ. Re: Cioc AM, Allen C, Kalmar J, *et al.* Oral plasmablastic lymphomas in AIDS patients are associated with human herpesvirus 8.

Am J Surg Pathol 2004;**25**:41–46. *Am J Surg Pathol* 2004;**28**(9):1252–3.

119. Knowles DM, Inghirami G, Ubriaco A, *et al.* Molecular genetic analysis of three AIDS-associated neoplasms of uncertain lineage demonstrates their B-cell derivation and the possible pathogenetic role of the Epstein-Barr virus. *Blood* 1989;**73**(3):792–9.
120. Green I, Espiritu E, Ladanyi M, *et al.* Primary lymphomatous effusions in AIDS: a morphological, immunophenotypic, and molecular study. *Mod Pathol* 1995;**8**(1):39–45.
121. Walts AE, Shintaku IP, Said JW. Diagnosis of malignant lymphoma in effusions from patients with AIDS by gene rearrangement. *Am J Clin Pathol* 1990;**94**(2):170–5.
122. Carbone A, Tirelli U, Gloghini A, *et al.* Herpesvirus-like DNA sequences selectively cluster with body cavity-based lymphomas throughout the spectrum of AIDS-related lymphomatous effusions. *Eur J Cancer* 1996;**32A**(3):555–6.
123. Chadburn A, Hyjek E, Mathew S, *et al.* KSHV-positive solid lymphomas represent an extra-cavitary variant of primary effusion lymphoma. *Am J Surg Pathol* 2004;**28**(11):1401–16.
124. Komanduri KV, Luce JA, McGrath MS, *et al.* The natural history and molecular heterogeneity of HIV-associated primary malignant lymphomatous effusions. *J Acquir Immune Defic Syndr Hum Retrovirol* 1996;**13**(3):215–26.
125. Simonelli C, Spina M, Cinelli R, *et al.* Clinical features and outcome of primary effusion lymphoma in HIV-infected patients: a single-institution study. *J Clin Oncol* 2003;**21**(21):3948–54.
126. Boulanger E, Gerard L, Gabarre J, *et al.* Prognostic factors and outcome of human herpesvirus 8-associated primary effusion lymphoma in patients with AIDS. *J Clin Oncol* 2005;**23** (19):4372–80.
127. Ansari MQ, Dawson DB, Nador R, *et al.* Primary body cavity-based AIDS-related lymphomas. *Am J Clin Pathol* 1996;**105**(2):221–9.
128. Nador RG, Cesarman E, Chadburn A, *et al.* Primary effusion lymphoma: a distinct clinicopathologic entity associated with the Kaposi's sarcoma-associated herpes virus. *Blood* 1996;**88**(2):645–56.
129. Brimo F, Michel RP, Khetani K, *et al.* Primary effusion lymphoma: a series of 4 cases and review of the literature with emphasis on cytomorphologic and immunocytochemical differential diagnosis. *Cancer* 2007;**111**(4):224–33.
130. Klein U, Gloghini A, Gaidano G, *et al.* Gene expression profile analysis of AIDS-related primary effusion lymphoma (PEL) suggests a plasmablastic derivation and identifies PEL-specific transcripts. *Blood* 2003;**101**(10):4115–21.
131. Fan W, Bubman D, Chadburn A, *et al.* Distinct subsets of primary effusion lymphoma can be identified based on their cellular gene expression profile and viral association. *J Virol* 2005; **79**(2):1244–51.
132. Chang Y, Cesarman E, Pessin MS, *et al.* Identification of herpesvirus-like DNA sequences in AIDS-associated Kaposi's sarcoma. *Science* 1994;**266**(5192):1865–9.
133. Cesarman E, Chang Y, Moore PS, *et al.* Kaposi's sarcoma-associated herpesvirus-like DNA sequences in AIDS-related body-cavity-based lymphomas. *N Engl J Med* 1995; **332**(18):1186–91.
134. Casper C, Krantz EM, Corey L, *et al.* Valganciclovir for suppression of human herpesvirus-8 replication: a randomized, double-blind, placebo-controlled, crossover trial. *J Infect Dis* 2008;**198**(1):23–30.
135. Simonelli C, Tedeschi R, Gloghini A, *et al.* Characterization of immunologic and virological parameters in HIV-infected patients with primary effusion lymphoma during antiblastic therapy and highly active antiretroviral therapy. *Clin Infect Dis* 2005;**40**(7):1022–7.
136. Keller SA, Hernandez-Hopkins D, Vider J, *et al.* NF-κB is essential for the progression of KSHV- and EBV-infected lymphomas in vivo. *Blood* 2006;**107**(8):3295–302.
137. Cote TR, Manns A, Hardy CR, *et al.* Epidemiology of brain lymphoma among people with or without acquired immunodeficiency syndrome. AIDS/Cancer Study Group. *J Natl Cancer Inst* 1996;**88**(10):675–9.
138. International Collaboration on HIV and Cancer. Highly active antiretroviral therapy and incidence of cancer in human immunodeficiency virus-infected adults. *J Natl Cancer Inst* 2000;**92**(22):1823–30.
139. Kadan-Lottick NS, Skluzacek MC, Gurney JG. Decreasing incidence rates of primary central nervous system lymphoma. *Cancer* 2002;**95**(1):193–202.
140. Bower M, Powles T, Nelson M, *et al.* Highly active antiretroviral therapy and human immunodeficiency virus-associated primary cerebral lymphoma. *J Natl Cancer Inst* 2006;**98**(15):1088–91.
141. Gray F, Gherardi R, Scaravilli F. The neuropathology of the acquired immune deficiency syndrome (AIDS). A review. *Brain* 1988;**111**(Pt 2):245–66.
142. Newell ME, Hoy JF, Cooper SG, *et al.* Human immunodeficiency virus-related primary central nervous system lymphoma: factors influencing survival in 111 patients. *Cancer* 2004;**100**(12): 2627–36.
143. Raez LE, Patel P, Feun L, *et al.* Natural history and prognostic factors for survival in patients with acquired immune deficiency syndrome (AIDS)-related primary central nervous system lymphoma (PCNSL). *Crit Rev Oncog* 1998;**9**(3–4):199–208.
144. Kasamon YL, Ambinder RF. AIDS-related primary central nervous system lymphoma. *Hematol Oncol Clin North Am* 2005;**19**(4):665–87, vi–vii.
145. Cinque P, Brytting M, Vago L, *et al.* Epstein-Barr virus DNA in cerebrospinal fluid from patients with AIDS-related primary lymphoma of the central nervous system. *Lancet* 1993;**342**(8868):398–401.
146. Thurnher MM, Thurnher SA, Schindler E. CNS involvement in AIDS: spectrum of CT and MR findings. *Eur Radiol* 1997;**7**(7):1091–7.
147. Antinori A, De Rossi G, Ammassari A, *et al.* Value of combined approach with thallium-201 single-photon emission computed tomography and Epstein-Barr virus DNA polymerase chain reaction in CSF for the diagnosis of AIDS-related primary CNS lymphoma. *J Clin Oncol* 1999;**17**(2):554–60.
148. Hoffman JM, Waskin HA, Schifter T, *et al.* FDG-PET in differentiating lymphoma from nonmalignant central nervous system lesions in patients with AIDS. *J Nucl Med* 1993;**34**(4):567–75.
149. Pierce MA, Johnson MD, Maciunas RJ, *et al.* Evaluating contrast-enhancing brain lesions in patients with AIDS by using positron emission tomography. *Ann Intern Med* 1995;**123**(8):594–8.
150. Heald AE, Hoffman JM, Bartlett JA, *et al.* Differentiation of central nervous

system lesions in AIDS patients using positron emission tomography (PET). *Int J STD AIDS* 1996;**7**(5):337–46.

151. Roelcke U, Leenders KL. Positron emission tomography in patients with primary CNS lymphomas. *J Neurooncol* 1999;**43**(3):231–6.

152. Cingolani A, De Luca A, Larocca LM, *et al.* Minimally invasive diagnosis of acquired immunodeficiency syndrome-related primary central nervous system lymphoma. *J Natl Cancer Inst* 1998; **90**(5):364–9.

153. Corcoran C, Rebe K, van der Plas H, *et al.* The predictive value of cerebrospinal fluid Epstein-Barr viral load as a marker of primary central nervous system lymphoma in HIV-infected persons. *J Clin Virol* 2008; **42**(4):433–6.

154. Bossolasco S, Falk KI, Ponzoni M, *et al.* Ganciclovir is associated with low or undetectable Epstein-Barr virus DNA load in cerebrospinal fluid of patients with HIV-related primary central nervous system lymphoma. *Clin Infect Dis* 2006;**42**(4):e21–5.

155. Skiest DJ, Crosby C. Survival is prolonged by highly active antiretroviral therapy in AIDS patients with primary central nervous system lymphoma. *AIDS* 2003;**17**(12):1787–93.

156. Chamberlain MC, Kormanik PA. AIDS-related central nervous system lymphomas. *J Neurooncol* 1999; **43**(3):269–76.

157. Ferreri AJ, Reni M, Pasini F, *et al.* A multicenter study of treatment of primary CNS lymphoma. *Neurology* 2002;**58**(10):1513–20.

158. Ferreri AJ, Reni M, Villa E. Therapeutic management of primary central nervous system lymphoma: lessons from prospective trials. *Ann Oncol* 2000;**11**(8):927–37.

159. Batchelor T, Carson K, O'Neill A, *et al.* Treatment of primary CNS lymphoma with methotrexate and deferred radiotherapy: a report of NABTT 96-07. *J Clin Oncol* 2003;**21**(6):1044–9.

160. Jacomet C, Girard PM, Lebrette MG, *et al.* Intravenous methotrexate for primary central nervous system non-Hodgkin's lymphoma in AIDS. *AIDS* 1997;**11**(14):1725–30.

161. Sarker D, Thirlwell C, Nelson M, *et al.* Leptomeningeal disease in AIDS-related non-Hodgkin's lymphoma. *AIDS* 2003;**17**(6):861–5.

162. Hill QA, Owen RG. CNS prophylaxis in lymphoma: who to target and what therapy to use. *Blood Rev* 2006; **20**(6):319–32.

163. Navarro JT, Vall-Llovera F, Mate JL, *et al.* Decrease in the frequency of meningeal involvement in AIDS-related systemic lymphoma in patients receiving HAART. *Haematologica* 2008;**93**(1):149–50.

164. Cingolani A, Gastaldi R, Fassone L, *et al.* Epstein-Barr virus infection is predictive of CNS involvement in systemic AIDS-related non-Hodgkin's lymphomas. *J Clin Oncol* 2000;**18** (19):3325–30.

165. Desai J, Mitnick RJ, Henry DH, *et al.* Patterns of central nervous system recurrence in patients with systemic human immunodeficiency virus-associated non-hodgkin lymphoma. *Cancer* 1999;**86**(9):1840–7.

166. Hegde U, Filie A, Little RF, *et al.* High incidence of occult leptomeningeal disease detected by flow cytometry in newly diagnosed aggressive B-cell lymphomas at risk for central nervous system involvement: the role of flow cytometry versus cytology. *Blood* 2005;**105**(2):496–502.

167. Di Noto R, Scalia G, Abate G, *et al.* Critical role of multidimensional flow cytometry in detecting occult leptomeningeal disease in newly diagnosed aggressive B-cell lymphomas. *Leuk Res* 2008;**32**(8):1196–9.

168. Gold JE, Altarac D, Ree HJ, *et al.* HIV-associated Hodgkin disease: a clinical study of 18 cases and review of the literature. *Am J Hematol* 1991; **36**(2):93–9.

169. Errante D, Zagonel V, Vaccher E, *et al.* Hodgkin's disease in patients with HIV infection and in the general population: comparison of clinicopathological features and survival. *Ann Oncol* 1994; **5** (Suppl 2):37–40.

170. Andrieu JM, Roithmann S, Tourani JM, *et al.* Hodgkin's disease during HIV1 infection: the French registry experience. French Registry of HIV-associated Tumors. *Ann Oncol* 1993; **4**(8):635–41.

171. Tirelli U, Errante D, Dolcetti R, *et al.* Hodgkin's disease and human immunodeficiency virus infection: clinicopathologic and virologic features of 114 patients from the Italian Cooperative Group on AIDS and Tumors. *J Clin Oncol* 1995;**13**(7):1758–67.

172. Thompson LD, Fisher SI, Chu WS, *et al.* HIV-associated Hodgkin lymphoma: a clinicopathologic and immunophenotypic study of 45 cases. *Am J Clin Pathol* 2004;**121**(5):727–38.

173. Dawson MA, Schwarer AP, McLean C, *et al.* AIDS-related plasmablastic lymphoma of the oral cavity associated with an IGH/MYC translocation–treatment with autologous stem-cell transplantation in a patient with severe haemophilia-A. *Haematologica* 2007; **92**(1):e11–12.

174. Bosch Princep R, Lejeune M, Salvado Usach MT, *et al.* Decreased number of granzyme B+ activated CD8+ cytotoxic T lymphocytes in the inflammatory background of HIV-associated Hodgkin's lymphoma. *Ann Hematol* 2005;**84**(10):661–6.

175. Errante D, Tirelli U, Gastaldi R, *et al.* Combined antineoplastic and antiretroviral therapy for patients with Hodgkin's disease and human immunodeficiency virus infection. A prospective study of 17 patients. The Italian Cooperative Group on AIDS and Tumors (GICAT). *Cancer* 1994;**73**(2):437–44.

176. Errante D, Gabarre J, Ridolfo AL, *et al.* Hodgkin's disease in 35 patients with HIV infection: an experience with epirubicin, bleomycin, vinblastine and prednisone chemotherapy in combination with antiretroviral therapy and primary use of G-CSF. *Ann Oncol* 1999;**10**(2):189–95.

177. Levine AM, Li P, Cheung T, *et al.* Chemotherapy consisting of doxorubicin, bleomycin, vinblastine, and dacarbazine with granulocyte-colony-stimulating factor in HIV-infected patients with newly diagnosed Hodgkin's disease: a prospective, multi-institutional AIDS clinical trials group study (ACTG 149). *J Acquir Immune Defic Syndr* 2000;**24**(5):444–50.

178. Gastaldi R, Martino P, Gentile G, *et al.* Hodgkin's disease in HIV-infected patients: report of eight cases usefully treated with doxorubicin, bleomycin, vinblastine and dacarbazine (ABVD) plus granulocyte colony-stimulating factor. *Ann Oncol* 2002;**13**(7):1158–60.

179. Xicoy B, Ribera JM, Miralles P, *et al.* Results of treatment with doxorubicin,

bleomycin, vinblastine and dacarbazine and highly active antiretroviral therapy in advanced stage, human immunodeficiency virus-related Hodgkin's lymphoma. *Haematologica* 2007;**92**(2):191–8.

180. Hartmann P, Rehwald U, Salzberger B, *et al.* BEACOPP therapeutic regimen for patients with Hodgkin's disease and HIV infection. *Ann Oncol* 2003; **14**(10):1562–9.

181. Marti-Carvajal AJ, Cardona AF, Rodriguez ML. Interventions for treating AIDS-associated Hodgkin's lymphoma in treatment-naive adults. *Cochrane Database Syst Rev* 2007;Issue 2: CD006149. DOI: 10.1002/14651858. CD006149.pub2.

182. Collins JA, Hernandez AV, Hidalgo JA, *et al.* High proportion of T-cell systemic non-Hodgkin lymphoma in HIV-infected patients in Lima, Peru. *J Acquired Immune Defic Syndr* 2005;**40**(5):558–64.

183. Chadburn A, Cesarman E, Jagirdar J, *et al.* CD30 (Ki-1) positive anaplastic large cell lymphomas in individuals infected with the human immunodeficiency virus. *Cancer* 1993;**72**(10):3078–90.

184. Nosari A, Cantoni S, Oreste P, *et al.* Anaplastic large cell (CD30/Ki-1+) lymphoma in HIV+ patients: clinical and pathological findings in a group of ten patients. *Br J Haematol* 1996; **95**(3):508–12.

185. Arzoo KK, Bu X, Espina BM, *et al.* T-cell lymphoma in HIV-infected patients. *J Acquir Immune Defic Syndr* 2004; **36**(5):1020–7.

186. Ruco LP, Di Napoli A, Pilozzi E, *et al.* Peripheral T cell lymphoma with cytotoxic phenotype: an emerging disease in HIV-infected patients? *AIDS Res Hum Retroviruses* 2004; **20**(2):129–33.

187. Carbone A, Gloghini A, Volpe R, *et al.* High frequency of Epstein-Barr virus latent membrane protein-1 expression in acquired immunodeficiency syndrome-related Ki-1 (CD30)-positive anaplastic large-cell lymphomas. Italian Cooperative Group on AIDS and Tumors. *Am J Clin Pathol* 1994; **101**(6):768–72.

188. Oksenhendler E, Duarte M, Soulier J, *et al.* Multicentric Castleman's disease in HIV infection: a clinical and pathological study of 20 patients. *AIDS* 1996;**10**(1):61–7.

189. Oksenhendler E, Boulanger E, Galicier L, *et al.* High incidence of Kaposi sarcoma-associated herpesvirus-related non-Hodgkin lymphoma in patients with HIV infection and multicentric Castleman disease. *Blood* 2002;**99** (7):2331–6.

190. Oksenhendler E, Carcelain G, Aoki Y, *et al.* High levels of human herpesvirus 8 viral load, human interleukin-6, interleukin-10, and C reactive protein correlate with exacerbation of multicentric Castleman disease in HIV-infected patients. *Blood* 2000; **96**(6):2069–73.

191. Aoki Y, Yarchoan R, Wyvill K, *et al.* Detection of viral interleukin-6 in Kaposi sarcoma-associated herpesvirus-linked disorders. *Blood* 2001;**97**(7): 2173–6.

192. Aoki Y, Tosato G, Fonville TW, *et al.* Serum viral interleukin-6 in AIDS-related multicentric Castleman disease. *Blood* 2001;**97**(8):2526–7.

193. Baloon G, Cesarman E. *Castleman's Disease.* Hamilton, ON, BC Decker, 2006.

194. Navarro WH, Kaplan LD. AIDS-related lymphoproliferative disease. *Blood* 2006;**107**(1):13–20.

195. Casper C. The aetiology and management of Castleman disease at 50 years: translating pathophysiology to patient care. *Br J Haematol* 2005; **129**(1):3–17.

196. Carbone A, Cesarman E, Spina M, *et al.* HIV-associated lymphomas and gamma-herpesviruses. *Blood* 2009; **113**(6):1213–24.

197. Dupin N, Diss TL, Kellam P, *et al.* HHV-8 is associated with a plasmablastic variant of Castleman disease that is linked to HHV-8-positive plasmablastic lymphoma. *Blood* 2000;**95**(4):1406–12.

198. Amin HM, Medeiros LJ, Manning JT, *et al.* Dissolution of the lymphoid follicle is a feature of the HHV8+ variant of plasma cell Castleman's disease. *Am J Surg Pathol* 2003; **27**(1):91–100.

199. Du MQ, Liu H, Diss TC, *et al.* Kaposi sarcoma-associated herpesvirus infects monotypic (IgM lambda) but polyclonal naive B cells in Castleman disease and associated lymphoproliferative disorders. *Blood* 2001;**97**(7):2130–6.

200. Lanzafame M, Carretta G, Trevenzoli M, *et al.* Successful treatment of Castleman's disease with HAART in two HIV-infected patients. *J Infect* 2000;**40**(1):90–1.

201. Marcelin AG, Aaron L, Mateus C, *et al.* Rituximab therapy for HIV-associated Castleman disease. *Blood* 2003;**102** (8):2786–8.

202. Bower M, Powles T, Williams S, *et al.* Brief communication: rituximab in HIV-associated multicentric Castleman disease. *Ann Intern Med* 2007;**147**(12):836–9.

203. Gerard L, Berezne A, Galicier L, *et al.* Prospective study of rituximab in chemotherapy-dependent human immunodeficiency virus associated multicentric Castleman's disease: ANRS 117 CastlemaB Trial. *J Clin Oncol* 2007;**25**(22):3350–6.

204. Fragasso A, Mannarella C, Ciancio A, *et al.* Complete remission and virologic response to combined chemoimmunotherapy (R-CVP) followed by rituximab maintenance in HIV-negative, HHV-8 positive patient with multicentric Castleman disease. *Leuk Lymphoma* 2008;**49**(11):2224–6.

205. Bestawros A, Michel R, Seguin C, *et al.* Multicentric Castleman's disease treated with combination chemotherapy and rituximab in four HIV-positive men: a case series. *Am J Hematol* 2008;**83**(6):508–11.

206. Stary G, Kohrgruber N, Herneth AM, *et al.* Complete regression of HIV-associated multicentric Castleman disease treated with rituximab and thalidomide. *AIDS* 2008;**22**(10):1232–4.

207. Casper C, Nichols WG, Huang ML, *et al.* Remission of HHV-8 and HIV-associated multicentric Castleman disease with ganciclovir treatment. *Blood* 2004;**103**(5):1632–4.

208. Berezne A, Agbalika F, Oksenhendler E. Failure of cidofovir in HIV-associated multicentric Castleman disease. *Blood* 2004;**103**(11):4368–9; author reply 4369.

209. Coty PC, Astrow AB, Gallinson D. Splenectomy is an effective treatment for HIV-associated multicentric Castleman's disease. *Blood* 2003; **102**:Abstract 3899.

210. Philip T, Guglielmi C, Hagenbeek A, *et al.* Autologous bone marrow transplantation as compared with salvage chemotherapy in relapses of chemotherapy-sensitive non-Hodgkin's lymphoma. *N Engl J Med* 1995;**333** (23):1540–5.

211. Nademanee A, Molina A, Dagis A, *et al.* Autologous stem-cell transplantation for poor-risk and relapsed intermediate- and high-grade non-Hodgkin's lymphoma. *Clin Lymphoma* 2000;**1**(1):46–54.

212. Re A, Cattaneo C, Michieli M, *et al.* High-dose therapy and autologous peripheral-blood stem-cell transplantation as salvage treatment for HIV-associated lymphoma in patients receiving highly active antiretroviral therapy. *J Clin Oncol* 2003;**21**(23):4423–7.

213. Gabarre J, Marcelin AG, Azar N, *et al.* High-dose therapy plus autologous hematopoietic stem cell transplantation for human immunodeficiency virus (HIV)-related lymphoma: results and impact on HIV disease. *Haematologica* 2004;**89**(9):1100–8.

214. Krishnan A, Molina A, Zaia J, *et al.* Durable remissions with autologous stem cell transplantation for high-risk HIV-associated lymphomas. *Blood* 2005;**105**(2):874–8.

215. Serrano D, Carrion R, Balsalobre P, *et al.* HIV-associated lymphoma successfully treated with peripheral blood stem cell transplantation. *Exp Hematol* 2005;**33**(4):487–94.

216. Balsalobre BN, Serrano D, Re A, *et al.* Autologous stem cell transplantation (ASCT) in HIV associated lymphoma (HIV-Ly) patients: The EBMT Lymphoma Working Party (EBMT-LWP) experience. *Blood* 2006;**108**:Abstract 3042.

217. Spitzer TR, Ambinder RF, Lee JY, *et al.* Dose-reduced busulfan, cyclophosphamide, and autologous stem cell transplantation for human immunodeficiency virus-associated lymphoma: AIDS Malignancy Consortium study 020. *Biol Blood Marrow Transplant* 2008;**14**(1):59–66.

218. Wagner-Johnston ND, Ambinder RF. Blood and marrow transplant for lymphoma patients with HIV/AIDS. *Curr Opin Oncol* 2008;**20**(2):201–5.

219. Bi J, Espina BM, Tulpule A, *et al.* High-dose cytosine-arabinoside and cisplatin regimens as salvage therapy for refractory or relapsed AIDS-related non-Hodgkin's lymphoma. *J Acquir Immune Defic Syndr* 2001;**28**(5):416–21.

Chapter 25

Lymphoblastic lymphoma

Anuj Mahindra and John W. Sweetenham

Introduction

Lymphoblastic lymphoma (LBL) is a rare disease which accounts for approximately 2% of all non-Hodgkin lymphomas (NHLs).[1] Most commonly it is of T-cell immunophenotype with about 20% being B cell. LBL is morphologically and immunophenotypically identical to acute lymphoblastic leukemia (ALL). The World Health Organization (WHO) classification of lymphoid neoplasms unifies these entities as precursor T-cell and B-cell lymphoblastic leukemia/lymphoma. In the clinical literature, treatment approaches to LBL and ALL have been parallel but have developed separately. In view of the rarity of LBL and the variable (and arbitrary) clinical distinction between LBL and ALL, reported results have been variable and the optimal treatment approaches remain uncertain.

Clinical presentation

In adults, it is usually diagnosed in males (2:1 ratio), with a peak incidence in the second decade of life. T-cell lymphoblastic lymphoma (T-LBL) typically presents as symptomatic supradiaphragmatic adenopathy. Cough, shortness of breath, and B symptoms are common. A large anterior mediastinal mass can result in respiratory distress and accompanying pleural and pericardial effusions can lead to tracheal obstruction or cardiac tamponade. Bone marrow involvement at presentation is seen in approximately 50% of the patients. Central nervous system (CNS) involvement is variable ranging from 0% to 26% at presentation in different studies[2–11] and is typically leptomeningeal rather than parenchymal. Hence cytologic evaluation of spinal fluid is recommended in all patients at the time of diagnosis. Primary intra-abdominal adenopathy at presentation is unusual.

B-cell lymphoblastic lymphomas behave differently, frequently involve extranodal sites such as skin, and are not characterized by male predominance or mediastinal mass. An aggressive B-cell variant is characterized by a high incidence of osteolytic bone lesions.

Diagnostic evaluation includes:

- Complete blood count, chemistry profile, and lactate dehydrogenase (LDH)
- CT of the chest, abdomen, and pelvis
- Bone marrow aspiration and biopsy including testing for T-cell receptor (TCR) gene rearrangements – bone marrow evaluation if positive is sufficient for diagnosis
- Lumbar puncture with cytology
- Mediastinal biopsy, if no other easily accessible site of disease
- MR imaging of the spine or head in case of suspected epidural or leptomeningeal disease.

The Ann Arbor staging system is commonly used for staging. Most patients present with stage III or IV disease and B symptoms. Although the St. Jude staging system is also used for this disease, reports in the adult literature do not show this system to have more prognostic value.

Pathologic features and pathogenesis

Lymphoblastic lymphoma is characterized by a diffuse growth pattern composed of medium-to-large lymphoblasts with round or convoluted nuclei with very fine chromatin, inconspicuous nucleoli, distinct nuclear membranes, and a scant rim of basophilic cytoplasm (Figure 25.1). Tingible body macrophages may at times give a "starry-sky" pattern. Terminal deoxynucleotidyl transferase (TdT) positivity is seen in 96% of lymphoblastic lymphoma cases unlike other B- and T-cell NHL, which are typically TdT negative. In addition, T-cell markers CD7, CD5, CD2, and cytoplasmic CD3 characterize T-LBL. The B-cell types express the pan-B-cell markers such as CD19 and CD79a in addition to TdT.

Morphologically, T-cell ALL (T-ALL) and T-LBL are indistinguishable and both are characterized by expression of cell surface antigens that correspond to stages of normal T-cell ontogeny. The similar morphologic, immunophenotypic, and genotypic features of T-ALL and T-LBL have led to the belief that they represent different presentations of a single disease

Management of Hematologic Malignancies, ed. Susan M. O'Brien, Julie M. Vose, and Hagop M. Kantarjian. Published by Cambridge University Press.

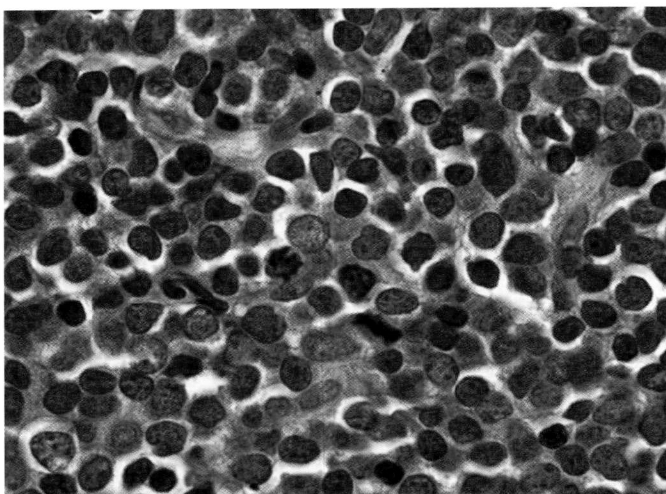

Figure 25.1 Lymphoblastic lymphoma. Courtesy of Eric Hsi, MD, Cleveland Clinic, Cleveland.

entity. Gene expression profiling, however, reveals intrinsic differences between the two entities.[12] In this study, the gene expression profiles of T-ALL and T-LBL samples obtained from Children's Oncology Group (COG) tumor banks were analyzed using DNA arrays. Prediction analysis of microarrays identified a subset of genes, which accurately classified all 19 T-ALL and T-LBL samples with an overall misclassification error rate of 0. Immunohistochemical validation of protein expression of selected genes identified by microarray analysis confirmed overexpression of *MLL-1* in T-LBL tumor cells compared to T-ALL and CD47 in T-ALL tumor cells when compared to T-LBL. This implies an underlying difference in the biology of the two entities.

Treatment

Pediatric LBL was treated with radiotherapy alone before 1970, and the 5-year survival rate was only 10%, with frequent leukemic transformations in the later course of the disease: adult survivors beyond 2 years were rare. Initial success with conventional NHL chemotherapy protocols (CHOP [cyclophosphamide, doxorubicin {hydroxydaunomycin}, vincristine {Oncovin}, and prednisone] and the similar COMP [cyclophosphamide, vincristine {Oncovin}, methotrexate, and prednisone], BACOP [bleomycin, doxorubicin {Adriamycin}, cyclophosphamide, vincristine {Oncovin}, and prednisone], and m-BACOD [methotrexate, bleomycin, doxorubicin {Adriamycin}, cyclophosphamide, vincristine {Oncovin}, and dexamethasone] protocols) was also limited to a complete remission (CR) rate of 53–71% and a disease-free survival (DFS) rate of 23–53%.[9,13–17] The outcomes in studies using some of the standard "CHOP"-like induction regimens are summarized in Table 25.1.

With the addition of an anthracycline, usually daunorubicin or doxorubicin, to the backbone ALL therapy of vincristine, prednisone, and, often, L-asparaginase, CR rates of 72–92% have been achieved in adults.[18] Given the high CR rate in ALL patients observed with these four-drug induction regimens, it has been difficult to consistently demonstrate improvement in overall CR rates with the addition of other drugs, including cyclophosphamide or cytarabine, except in T-lineage ALL, where they seem to improve CR, DFS, and overall survival rates.[18] Consistent with these findings, improvements in long-term outcome were achieved with ALL-type regimens for T-LBL, and in multiple series, CR rates of 55–100% and DFS rates of 45–65% have been reported.[2,10,11,17,19–22] The outcomes in studies using some of the intensive ALL-like induction regimens are summarized in Table 25.2.

Among the intensive ALL-like induction regimens mentioned in Table 25.2, considering the DFS and overall survival, the HyperCVAD regimen has been one of the more widely adopted regimens. Thomas *et al.*[2] reported the outcome of 33 adult LBL patients treated at MD Anderson Cancer Center with intensive chemotherapy using the HyperCVAD regimen (fractionated cyclophosphamide, vincristine, doxorubicin [Adriamycin], and dexamethasone) or the modified HyperCVAD regimen used for ALL. Modifications included the addition of a postinduction high-dose anthracycline and cytarabine course consisting of liposomal daunorubicin 150 mg/m^2 intravenously over 12 hours on days 1 and 2 with cytarabine 1.5 g/m^2 by continuous infusion over 24 hours daily on days 1 and 2 (i.e., nine instead of eight induction-consolidation courses were given). Prednisone (200 mg) was given orally daily for 5 days. Maintenance therapy consisted of mercaptopurine, methotrexate, monthly vincristine, and prednisone (POMP) for 24 months. During maintenance two intensification courses were administered during months 9 and 12 consisting of etoposide and L-asparaginase. At diagnosis, 80% of patients had a T-cell immunophenotype, 70% had stage III or IV disease, 70% had mediastinal involvement, and 9% had CNS disease. Overall, 91% of patients achieved CR, and the estimated 3-year overall survival rate with standard HyperCVAD was 83%, with a progression-free survival rate of 77%. Modification of the HyperCVAD regimen with anthracycline intensification did not improve outcome. This suggests that early consolidation with high-dose methotrexate and cytarabine may be beneficial for long-term progression-free survival.

There was no induction mortality reported with the HyperCVAD regimen. Grades 3–4 infections were observed in 24% of patients during induction and 56% of patients during consolidation. While the results of the HyperCVAD regimen reflect an improvement compared to earlier regimens, the intensity of the regimen leads to appreciable toxicity and further clinical trials are needed to delineate dose intensity, timing of mediastinal radiation, and duration of maintenance therapy.

An earlier study by the German Multicenter Study Group[11] reported the outcome of 45 adult patients with T-LBL (age range 15–61 years) treated with two protocols designed for adult ALL. The study included an eight-drug standard

Table 25.1. Outcomes with "standard" induction regimens

	Regimen	n	DFS	OS
Anderson *et al.*[17]	COMP	40 (pediatric)	34% (5 yr)	45% (5 yr)
Colgan *et al.*[13]	CHOP-like	39	49% (6 yr)	51% (6 yr)
Jost *et al.*[14]	MACOP-B + ASCT	20	31% (3 yr)	48% (3 yr)
Kaiser *et al.*[15]	CHOP-like	29	38% (3 yr)	41% (3 yr)
Le Gouill *et al.*[9]	ACVBP-like	92	22% (3 yr)	32% (3 yr)
van Imhoff *et al.*[16]	CHOP-like	15	40% (5-yr EFS)	46% (5 yr)

Notes: COMP: cyclophosphamide, vincristine, methotrexate, prednisone; CHOP: cyclophosphamide, doxorubicin, vincristine, prednisone; MACOP-B: methotrexate with leucovorin rescue, doxorubicin, cyclophosphamide, vincristine, prednisone, and bleomycin; ASCT: autologous stem cell transplantation; ACVBP: doxorubicin, cyclophosphamide, vindesine, bleomycin, and prednisone; DFS: disease-free survival; EFS: event-free survival; OS: overall survival.

Table 25.2. Outcomes with "intensive" induction regimens

	Regimen	n	DFS	OS
Anderson *et al.*[17]	LSA_2L_2	124 (pediatric)	64% (5 yr)	67% (5 yr)
Coleman *et al.*[23]	ALL-type	44	56% (3-yr FFS)	56% (3 yr)
Slater *et al.*[19]	ALL-type	51	NA	45% (5 yr)
Bernasconi *et al.*[22]	LBL-type	31	45% (3-yr RFS)	59% (3 yr)
Morel *et al.*[10]	ALL-type	80	46% (30 mo)	51% (30 mo)
Hoelzer *et al.*[11]	LBL-type	5	62% (7 yr)	51% (7 yr)
Thomas *et al.*[2]	HyperCVAD	33	66% (3 yr)	70% (3 yr)
Jabbour *et al.*[7]	LMT-98	27	44% (5-yr FFP)	63% (5 yr)
Song *et al.*[8]	Hybrid ALL/NHL	34	68% (4-yr FFS)	72% (4 yr)

Notes: HyperCVAD: hyperfractionated cyclophosphamide, vincristine, doxorubicin, and dexamethasone alternating with high-dose methotrexate and cytarabine; DFS: disease-free survival; FFP: freedom from progression; OS; overall survival; NA: not available.

induction administered over 8 weeks including prophylactic cranial (24 Gy) and mediastinal irradiation (24 Gy) followed by consolidation and reinduction therapy. Seventy-three percent of the patients had stage III/IV disease and 91% showed a mediastinal tumor. CR was achieved in 42 patients (93%), partial remission (PR) in 2 patients (4%), and 1 patient died during induction. Fifteen patients (36%) relapsed within 12 months with 47% of relapses occurring in the mediastinum despite mediastinal irradiation. The estimates for overall survival, continuous CR, and DFS at 7 years are 51%, 65%, and 62%, respectively. The high incidence of mediastinal relapse in this study argues for appropriate dose consolidation mediastinal irradiation. The 7-year estimates indicate the need for improved consolidation and maintenance treatments.

A potential treatment algorithm for the initial treatment of lymphoblastic lymphoma is outlined in Figure 25.2.

Management of CNS disease

Involvement of the CNS at presentation occurs in 7–20% of patients with LBL. The CNS is a frequent site of relapse in the absence of CNS prophylaxis.[2]

In the series of Coleman *et al.*[23] early administration of intrathecal methotrexate and the addition of prophylactic cranial irradiation reduced the incidence of CNS relapse from 29% to 3% when compared with historical controls treated on an earlier, less intensive regimen, but there was no significant improvement in survival. Taken as a whole, CNS relapse rates range from 3% to 42% in studies using intrathecal chemotherapy prophylaxis alone, from 3% to 15% in studies using a combination of cranial radiation and intrathecal therapy, and from 42% to 100% in studies not incorporating any CNS-directed therapy (usually with NHL programs).[24] The Pediatric Oncology Group study[25] found that the CNS relapse rate was similar whether prophylaxis was intrathecal therapy alone or was cranial radiation and intrathecal therapy. Many programs have eliminated irradiation because of concerns about the long-term neurologic sequelae.[24] Despite prophylactic intrathecal prophylaxis with or without radiation therapy, leptomeningeal relapses still occur in some patients, thus suggesting that the intensity of systemic chemotherapy (e.g., high-dose methotrexate) may have a role in the reduction of CNS recurrence.

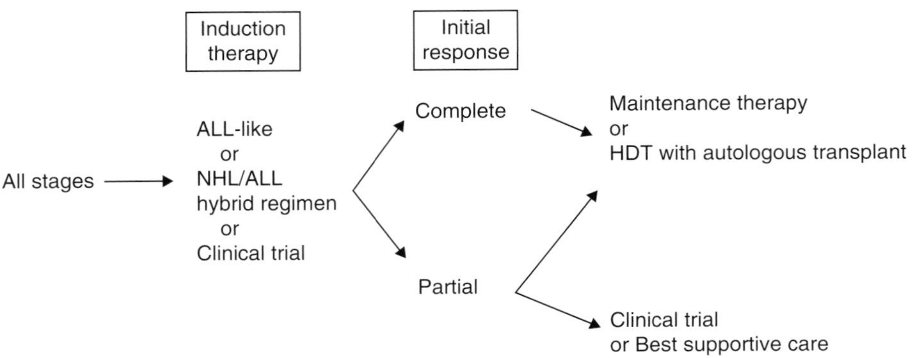

Figure 25.2 Treatment algorithm for initial therapy of lymphoblastic lymphoma. HDT: high-dose therapy.

Mediastinal radiation

Since the mediastinum is a common site of presentation and patients may present with bulky disease, adjuvant mediastinal radiation has been investigated. Since radiation therapy has not been shown to improve survival in the pediatric population and has long-term consequences including risk of secondary malignancies and cardiac toxicity, radiation is not considered standard treatment. However, in adults, the mediastinum is a frequent site of recurrence and hence the role of mediastinal radiation remains debatable.

MD Anderson retrospectively reviewed their data on 47 adult patients with LBL to investigate the role of mediastinal radiation therapy in patients who achieve a CR to chemotherapy.[26] None of the 19 patients who received mediastinal radiation experienced mediastinal recurrence, whereas 8 of 24 patients who did not get radiation had mediastinal relapse. Patients who received local radiation therapy had significantly better local disease control; a 5-year actuarial local control of 100% compared with a rate of 67% in patients who did not receive local radiation therapy ($p = 0.01$). This did not translate into an improved overall freedom-from-progression rate or overall survival rate. A major confounding factor was that 16 of 19 patients who received mediastinal radiation therapy had HyperCVAD, while most of the patients without radiation (18 of 24) had other forms of chemotherapy. Larger studies are needed to define the role of local radiation therapy for local disease control.

Stem cell transplantation

While intensive chemotherapy regimens, based on ALL protocols, have improved outcomes, considering the high relapse rates, stem cell transplantation (SCT), both autologous and allogeneic, has been used as consolidation in first remission in LBL patients (Table 25.3).

A recent retrospective study from British Columbia reported the outcome in 34 adults with T-LBL diagnosed and treated from July 1987 to March 2005.[8] Treatment, before planned SCT, consisted of a NHL/acute lymphoblastic leukemia hybrid chemotherapy protocol (28 patients) or a standard NHL chemotherapy regimen (6 patients). Median follow-up of

Table 25.3. Stem cell transplantation in first remission

	Regimen	n	DFS	OS
Jost *et al.*[14]	MACOP-B + auto SCT	20	31% (3 yr)	48% (3 yr)
Sweetenham *et al.*[27]	Various induction regimens + auto SCT	105	63% (6 yr)	64% (6 yr)
Bouabdallah *et al.*[20]	ALL-type + auto or allo SCT	62	8% (5-yr EFS)	60% (5 yr)
Song *et al.*[8]	Hybrid ALL/NHL + auto or allo SCT	34	8% (4-yr EFS)	72% (4 yr)

the 23 surviving patients was 51 months (range 13–142 months). Twenty-nine proceeded to SCT (4 allogeneic, 25 autologous). For all 34 patients, 4-year overall survival and event-free survival were 72% and 68%, respectively. For patients proceeding to SCT, the 4-year overall survival and event-free survival were 79% and 73%, respectively. All patients who received allografts are alive without disease at 38–141 months since diagnosis. For patients who received autografts, the 4-year event-free survival is 69%.

The European Group for Blood and Marrow Transplantation (EBMT) reported outcomes of 214 patients who underwent autologous transplantation after chemotherapy, including conventional lymphoma chemotherapy or ALL-like regimens.[5] Of 105 patients undergoing transplantation in first complete remission (CR1), long-term overall survival was 63% as compared with only 31% in those undergoing transplantation after initial disease progression. The Dutch–Belgian Hemato-Oncology Cooperative Group subsequently reported a phase II study in which 15 patients with LBL underwent two courses of high-dose induction chemotherapy followed by autologous transplantation;[17] 13 of 15 patients responded to initial chemotherapy and completed the entire treatment protocol. At 5 years, the estimated overall survival was 46% and event-free survival was 40%, suggesting that early transplantation might improve outcomes.

The EBMT and the United Kingdom Lymphoma Group conducted a randomized controlled trial in which of the 98 patients eligible for randomization, 65 were randomized, 31 to autologous SCT (ASCT) and 34 to conventional chemotherapy.[27] Main reasons for failure to randomize included patient refusal, early progression or death on induction therapy, excessive toxicity of induction regimen, and elective allogeneic SCT. With a median follow-up of 37 months, the actuarial 3-year relapse-free survival rate was 24% for the chemotherapy arm and 55% for the ASCT arm (hazard ratio = 0.55 in favor of the ASCT arm; $p = 0.065$). A difference in overall survival at three years was not detected (56% vs. 45%; $p = 0.71$). Potential reasons for lack of difference in overall survival included insufficient power given the small number of randomized patients. Slow accrual led to the early termination of the trial. A post hoc power calculation indicated that a different conclusion would have been unlikely.

The International Bone Marrow Transplant Registry (IBMTR) and the Autologous Blood and Marrow Transplant Registry (ABMTR) reported the outcomes of 128 patients who underwent autologous and 76 patients who underwent HLA-identical sibling SCT from 1989 to 1998.[4] The median age of autologous transplant patients was 31 years (range, 2–67 years) and 27 years (range, 5–53 years) for those who received HLA-identical sibling SCTs. Patients receiving autologous transplants were older, more likely to receive peripheral blood stem cells, more likely to receive transplants before 1994, and less likely to receive a total body irradiation (TBI)-containing conditioning regimen than allogeneic transplant recipients. The 5-year adjusted probabilities of survival were 39% (95% CI = 29–49%) after allogeneic transplantation and 44% (95% CI = 36–52%) after autologous transplantation; $p = 0.47$. Advanced disease status and poor performance status at transplantation were predictive of higher mortality. The 5-year cumulative incidences of transplant-related mortality (TRM) were 25% (95% CI = 16–36%) after allogeneic transplantation and 5% (95% CI = 2–10%) after autologous transplantation; $p < 0.001$. The 5-year cumulative incidences of relapse were 34% (95% CI = 23–45%) after allogeneic transplantation and 56% (95% CI = 45–65%) after autologous transplantation; $p = 0.004$.

The EBMT reported a registry matched study of allogeneic SCT for lymphoma.[3] The report included 314 patients with lymphoblastic lymphoma. Bone marrow involvement was detected in 52% and CNS involvement in 12% of the patients. Median progression-free survival after allogeneic transplantation was 7.6 months and median overall survival was 1 year. The actuarial progression-free survival at 4 years was 38% and overall survival was 42%. The actuarial procedure-related mortality at 4 years was 33%.

The above data indicate that, as has been seen in other hematologic malignancies, allogeneic transplant leads to a lower relapse rate but the increased TRM leads to an inferior overall survival compared to autologous transplantation. We do not recommend allogeneic transplantation outside the context of a clinical trial.

The improved outcome in patients receiving intensive induction[2] at diagnosis compared to patients receiving a non-intensive induction like CHOP followed by autologous transplantation[14] indicates the importance of the induction regimen in this disease. In the setting of intensive induction, the role of autologous transplant for consolidation in CR1 remains unclear. A potential treatment algorithm for treatment at the time of diagnosis is outlined in Figure 25.2.

Prognosis

Clinically, CNS disease or bone marrow involvement at presentation have been reported as adverse prognostic factors.[2,8] However, no clinically reproducible risk factors have been identified. This may be a reflection of the small sample size in the various studies.

A recent study looking at a retrospective evaluation of 41 cytoplasmic CD3+ T-LBL by assessing stage of maturation arrest based on TCR immunogenotyping and immunohistochemistry allowed the identification of three subcategories: 11 immature IM0/D-LBL showed no TCR or only incomplete *TCRD* DJ rearrangement and corresponded to cytoplasmic CD3+ precursors of uncertain lineage. Sixteen mature TCRDdel-LBL showed biallelic *TCRD* deletion and both *TCRG* and *TCRB* rearrangement, consistent with TCRαβ lineage restriction. Fourteen intermediate LBL (Int-LBL) showed complete *TCRD* VDJ and *TCRG* VJ rearrangement, with *TCRB* VDJ rearrangement in the majority. All Int-LBL expressed *HOX11/TLX1* or *HOXA9* transcripts and a proportion of the latter were associated with *CALM-AF10* or *NUP214-ABL* fusion transcripts. IM0/D-LBL were restricted to adults with extrathymic disease and bone marrow involvement, whereas Int-LBL and TCRDdel-LBL were found in children and adults with predominantly thymic disease. In adults, the Int-LBL subgroup was associated with a significantly superior clinical outcome. This subgroup can be identified either by TCR immunogenotyping or *HOXA9/TLX1* transcript quantification.[6]

Future directions

There is evidence for a pro-oncogenic role for Notch-transduced signals in the development of T-ALL in mice and humans. A recent study attempted to characterize the downstream pathways that transmit pro-oncogenic signals.[28] To identify these pathways, protein microarrays were used to profile the phosphorylation state of 108 epitopes on 82 distinct signaling proteins in a panel of 13 T-cell leukemia cell lines treated with a gamma-secretase inhibitor (GSI) to inhibit Notch signals. The microarray screen detected GSI-induced hypophosphorylation of multiple signaling proteins in the mTOR pathway. Withdrawal of Notch signals prevented stimulation of the mTOR pathway by mitogenic factors. The findings collectively suggest that the mTOR pathway is positively regulated by Notch in T-ALL cells. Simultaneous blockade of the mTOR and Notch pathway with small-molecule inhibitors resulted in synergistic suppression of T-ALL growth.

Another promising area is the development of drugs that preferentially target T cells. In a recent study, nelarabine was administered to 26 patients with T-ALL and 13 with T-LBL on an alternate day schedule (days 1, 3, and 5) at 1.5 g/m^2 per day.[29] Cycles were repeated every 22 days. CR was 31% (95% CI = 17%–48%). Overall response rate was 41% (95% CI = 26%–58%). Principal toxicity was grade 3 or 4 neutropenia and thrombocytopenia, occurring in 37% and 26% of patients, respectively. The promising activity merits further study in the first-line setting.

The optimal management strategy for lymphoblastic lymphoma remains unclear. Promising and comparable results, as discussed above, have been reported with intensive ALL-like chemotherapy regimens alone and with NHL/ALL hybrid regimens followed by consolidation with ASCT in first remission. A better understanding of the biology of the disease and the signaling pathways involved should lead to improved therapeutic options in the future.

References

1. Anonymous. A clinical evaluation of the International Lymphoma Study Group classification of non-Hodgkin's lymphoma. The Non-Hodgkin's Lymphoma Classification Project. *Blood* 1997;**89**:3909–18.
2. Thomas DA, O'Brien S, Cortes J, *et al.* Outcome with the hyper-CVAD regimens in lymphoblastic lymphoma. *Blood* 2004;**104**:1624–30.
3. Peniket AJ, Ruiz de Elvira MC, Taghipour G, *et al.* An EBMT registry matched study of allogeneic stem cell transplants for lymphoma: allogeneic transplantation is associated with a lower relapse rate but a higher procedure-related mortality rate than autologous transplantation. *Bone Marrow Transplant* 2003;**31**:667–78.
4. Levine JE, Harris RE, Loberiza FR Jr, *et al.* A comparison of allogeneic and autologous bone marrow transplantation for lymphoblastic lymphoma. *Blood* 2003;**101**: 2476–82.
5. Sweetenham JW, Liberti G, Pearce R, *et al.* High-dose therapy and autologous bone marrow transplantation for adult patients with lymphoblastic lymphoma: results of the European Group for Bone Marrow Transplantation. *J Clin Oncol* 1994;**12**:1358–65.
6. Baleydier F, Decouvelaere AV, Bergeron J, *et al.* T cell receptor genotyping and HOXA/TLX1 expression define three T lymphoblastic lymphoma subsets which might affect clinical outcome. *Clin Cancer Res* 2008;**14**: 692–700.
7. Jabbour E, Koscielny S, Sebban C, *et al.* High survival rate with the LMT-89 regimen in lymphoblastic lymphoma (LL), but not in T-cell acute lymphoblastic leukemia (T-ALL). *Leukemia* 2006;**20**:814–19.
8. Song KW, Barnett MJ, Gascoyne RD, *et al.* Primary therapy for adults with T-cell lymphoblastic lymphoma with hematopoietic stem-cell transplantation results in favorable outcomes. *Ann Oncol* 2007;**18**:535–40.
9. Le Gouill S, Lepretre S, Briere J, *et al.* Adult lymphoblastic lymphoma: a retrospective analysis of 92 patients under 61 years included in the LNH87/ 93 trials. *Leukemia* 2003;**17**:2220–4.
10. Morel P, Lepage E, Brice P, *et al.* Prognosis and treatment of lymphoblastic lymphoma in adults: a report on 80 patients. *J Clin Oncol* 1992;**10**:1078–85.
11. Hoelzer D, Gokbuget N, Digel W, *et al.* Outcome of adult patients with T-lymphoblastic lymphoma treated according to protocols for acute lymphoblastic leukemia. *Blood* 2002; **99**:4379–85.
12. Raetz EA, Perkins SL, Bhojwani D, *et al.* Gene expression profiling reveals intrinsic differences between T-cell acute lymphoblastic leukemia and T-cell lymphoblastic lymphoma. *Pediatr Blood Cancer* 2006;**47**:130–40.
13. Colgan JP, Andersen J, Habermann TM, *et al.* Long-term follow-up of a CHOP-based regimen with maintenance therapy and central nervous system prophylaxis in lymphoblastic non-Hodgkin's lymphoma. *Leuk Lymphoma* 1994;**15**:291–6.
14. Jost LM, Jacky E, Dommann-Scherrer C, *et al.* Short-term weekly chemotherapy followed by high-dose therapy with autologous bone marrow transplantation for lymphoblastic and Burkitt's lymphomas in adult patients. *Ann Oncol* 1995;**6**:445–51.
15. Kaiser U, Uebelacker I, Havemann K. Non-Hodgkin's lymphoma protocols in the treatment of patients with Burkitt's lymphoma and lymphoblastic lymphoma: a report on 58 patients. *Leuk Lymphoma* 1999;**36**:101–8.
16. van Imhoff GW, van der Holt B, MacKenzie MA, *et al.* Short intensive sequential therapy followed by autologous stem cell transplantation in adult Burkitt, Burkitt-like and lymphoblastic lymphoma. *Leukemia* 2005;**19**:945–52.
17. Anderson JR, Wilson JF, Jenkin DT, *et al.* Childhood non-Hodgkin's lymphoma. The results of a randomized therapeutic trial comparing a 4-drug regimen (COMP) with a 10-drug regimen (LSA2-L2). *N Engl J Med* 1983;**308**:559–65.
18. Larson RA, Dodge RK, Burns CP, *et al.* A five-drug remission induction regimen with intensive consolidation for adults with acute lymphoblastic leukemia: cancer and leukemia group B study 8811. *Blood* 1995;**85**:2025–37.
19. Slater DE, Mertelsmann R, Koziner B, *et al.* Lymphoblastic lymphoma in adults. *J Clin Oncol* 1986;**4**:57–67.
20. Bouabdallah R, Xerri L, Bardou VJ, *et al.* Role of induction chemotherapy and bone marrow transplantation in adult lymphoblastic lymphoma: a report on 62 patients from a single center. *Ann Oncol* 1998;**9**:619–25.
21. Zinzani PL, Bendandi M, Visani G, *et al.* Adult lymphoblastic lymphoma: clinical features and prognostic factors in 53 patients. *Leuk Lymphoma* 1996;**23**:577–82.
22. Bernasconi C, Brusamolino E, Lazzarino M, *et al.* Lymphoblastic lymphoma in adult patients: clinicopathological features and response to intensive multiagent chemotherapy analogous to that used in acute lymphoblastic leukemia. *Ann Oncol* 1990;**1**:141–6.
23. Coleman CN, Picozzi VJ Jr, Cox RS, *et al.* Treatment of lymphoblastic lymphoma in adults. *J Clin Oncol* 1986;**4**:1628–37.

24. Thomas DA, Kantarjian HM. Lymphoblastic lymphoma. *Hematol Oncol Clin North Am* 2001;**15**:51–95, vi.

25. Hvizdala EV, Berard C, Callihan T, *et al.* Lymphoblastic lymphoma in children–a randomized trial comparing LSA2-L2 with the A-COP+ therapeutic regimen: a Pediatric Oncology Group Study. *J Clin Oncol* 1988;**6**:26–33.

26. Dabaja BS, Ha CS, Thomas DA, *et al.* The role of local radiation therapy for mediastinal disease in adults with T-cell lymphoblastic lymphoma. *Cancer* 2002;**94**:2738–44.

27. Sweetenham JW, Santini G, Qian W, *et al.* High-dose therapy and autologous stem-cell transplantation versus conventional-dose consolidation/ maintenance therapy as postremission therapy for adult patients with lymphoblastic lymphoma: results of a randomized trial of the European Group for Blood and Marrow Transplantation and the United Kingdom Lymphoma Group. *J Clin Oncol* 2001;**19**:2927–36.

28. Chan SM, Weng AP, Tibshirani R, *et al.* Notch signals positively regulate activity of the mTOR pathway in T-cell acute lymphoblastic leukemia. *Blood* 2007;**110**:278–86.

29. DeAngelo DJ, Yu D, Johnson JL, *et al.* Nelarabine induces complete remissions in adults with relapsed or refractory T-lineage acute lymphoblastic leukemia or lymphoblastic lymphoma: Cancer and Leukemia Group B study 19801. *Blood* 2007;**109**: 5136–42.

Chapter

26 Burkitt lymphoma

Julie M. Vose

Introduction

Burkitt lymphoma (BL) is an uncommon B-cell lymphoma characterized by high proliferation rate and cytogenetic changes related to c-Myc proto-oncogene overexpression. It encompasses a heterogeneous group of highly aggressive B-cell lymphoma. It is seen frequently in children and young adults in the endemic areas. As the result of the world epidemic of AIDS, the number of adult BL cases has increased significantly in the last few decades. In the United States, BL has an incidence of 1200 patients per year.

This lymphoma was first described by Denis Burkitt in 1958 in children in Africa.[1] This type of endemic BL was described in children with jaw tumors with eventual spread to extranodal sites, particularly the bone marrow and leptomeninges. In the USA, BL is more commonly diagnosed in adult patients over age 40 years. According to the Surveillence, Epidemiology and End Results (SEER) registry, 59% of the BL cases in the USA are in patients over the age of 40 years.

The challenge of correctly identifying the BL in an individual patient becomes particularly critical as BL is rapidly fatal if not treated rapidly and appropriately with brief intensive chemotherapy. Initiation of the correct treatment early has yielded excellent results; however, when patients with BL were treated with regimens for diffuse large B-cell lymphoma (DLBCL), the long-term outcomes were inferior.[2–4] On the other hand, the intensive therapy is not the favored choice for DLBCL, since it is associated with higher toxicity. Therefore, the need for more advanced modalities to establish the accurate diagnosis is crucial to avoid under-treatment or over-treatment of the patients.

Historical background

BL was first described by Dr. Denis Burkitt, an Irish surgeon who was working for the Colonial Medical Service in Uganda. He noted a high incidence of rapid-growing tumor affecting the jaws of African children in the endemic areas of malaria. At that time, Dr. Burkitt described the tumor as a form of sarcoma.[5] Three years later, the tumor was recognized histologically as a malignant lymphoma by Burkitt and O'Connor when they studied a series of cases that involved extranodal sites in African children that shared the geographical distribution, histologic features, and high incidence of jaw involvement.[6,7]

BL accounts for over half of all childhood cancers in endemic areas and 40–50% of childhood non-Hodgkin lymphomas (NHLs) in non-endemic areas (America and Western Europe).[8] In contrast, it is a rare lymphoma in adults, except in HIV-positive patients; it constitutes 1–2% of all non-HIV adult lymphomas in Western Europe and the USA.[9]

The World Health Organization (WHO) classified BL on the basis of geographical distribution and clinical presentation into three subtypes; endemic, sporadic, and immunodeficiency-associated BL. These subtypes share the same morphologic and immunohistologic features. The endemic variant is the prototype and the most common form; it describes cases that have been observed in children in equatorial Africa and Papua New Guinea with a pattern of geographical distribution corresponding with endemic malaria falciparum. The highest risk of BL is seen between 10 degrees north and south of the equator;[10] it has a tendency to occur in low, warm, and humid lands.[11] It is also an important disease in areas such as the Middle East, North Africa, and parts of South America. It is characterized by high incidence of jaw and other facial bones involvement. Central nervous system (CNS) and bone marrow (BM) involvement in children have been reported in 12% and 22% of cases, respectively.[12] Nearly all of endemic cases are associated with Epstein–Barr Virus (EBV) infection.

In contrast, the sporadic form describes cases that occur outside the endemic distribution of the disease; it is seen in industrialized nations such as in North America and Europe. It accounts for a minor percentage of adult lymphoma; it peaks in the second and third decades. It is a highly aggressive disease with high propensity to invade BM and CNS; they are involved in 30–38% and 13–17% of cases, respectively.[13]

Management of Hematologic Malignancies, ed. Susan M. O'Brien, Julie M. Vose, and Hagop M. Kantarjian. Published by Cambridge University Press.

Lymph nodes are noted to be involved more often in adults than in children. Whereas the jaw is the most common affected site in the endemic form, it is infrequently involved in sporadic Burkitt.[14] The abdomen is the most common site in sporadic cases, particularly terminal ileum, cecum, and intra-abdominal lymph nodes; however, it occurs in other sites like ovaries, kidneys, pancreas, liver, omentum, Waldeyer's ring, and breast;[15] breast involvement is observed almost exclusively in girls at the onset of puberty and in lactating women.[16] Malignant pleural effusion and ascites were reported with BL.[9] One-third of patients have B symptoms at presentation (unexplained fever higher than 38°C [100.4°F] in the prior month, unexplained weight loss greater than 10% in the past 6 months, and recurrent drenching night sweats in the prior month). Patients with abdominal disease usually present with abdominal mass or pain, bowel obstruction symptoms, gastrointestinal bleeding, or syndrome mimicking an acute appendicitis.

The third group is immunodeficiency-associated BL which is seen in HIV-positive patients, to a lesser extent in post-transplant recipients,[17] and in some individuals with congenital immunodeficiency.[18] BL is much more seen in HIV-positive individuals; it occurs over a thousand times more often in HIV-positive individuals than in the general population in the sporadic areas.[19] Now, it accounts for 30–40% of all HIV-associated NHLs.[20] It is a recent expanding variant that was sharply escalated by the wide spread of HIV and it has become one of the most devastating complications of AIDS in industrialized countries. Compared to other AIDS-associated NHLs, BL occurs in younger patients with higher CD4 count. Since the prevalence of highly active antiretroviral therapy (HAART) in 1996, the prognosis of HIV-associated NHL has improved significantly with the standard chemotherapy protocols, except for Burkitt, which continues to carry an unsatisfied prognosis with the current chemotherapy. It is usually presented clinically in more aggressive course, the majority of the patients diagnosed with stage III and IV disease as well as wide dissemination and BM involvement.[21] Relapse with CNS involvement tends to occur early in the course of the disease.[22] Post-transplant BL was observed to occur after a relatively long interval after the transplant, with a mean of 4.5 years.[17]

Pathology and biology

Histologically, classic BL is characterized by a diffuse pattern of uniform round to ovoid medium-sized cells (12 μm) with round nuclei that contain coarse chromatin and multiple nucleoli with a high nuclear-to-cytoplasmic ratio. It has a moderately abundant basophilic cytoplasm that contains numerous lipid vacuoles. The hallmark of BL histologically is the presence of starry-sky appearance seen under low-power microscope; it is created by numerous macrophages containing ingested apoptotic tumor cells as a consequence of rapid proliferation and high rate of apoptosis (Figure 26.1). The rate of cell division is extremely high as reflected by the presence of a large number of mitotic figures and high fraction of actively growing cells demonstrated by Ki-67 which is nearly 100% in BL. The classic form is seen in almost all endemic cases and in most pediatric sporadic cases.

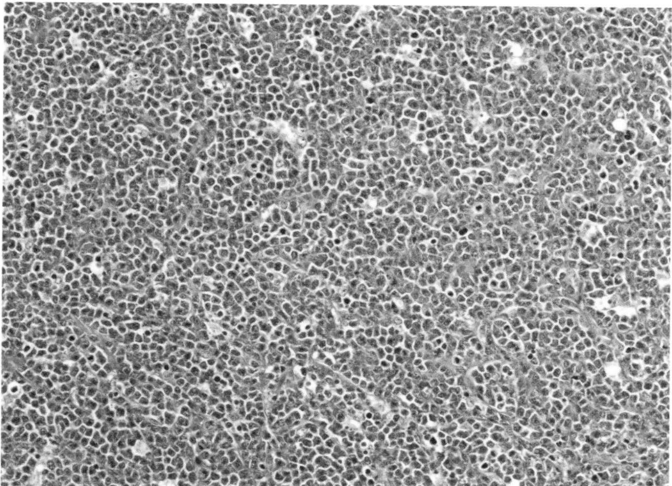

Figure 26.1 Hematoxylin and eosin (H&E) stain of Burkitt lymphoma with the "starry-sky" appearance.

The WHO classification identified Burkitt lymphoma and leukemia as a single entity of peripheral B-cell lymphoma with two related morphologic variants in addition to the classical form; BL with plasmacytoid differentiation and atypical BL/Burkitt-like lymphoma (BLL). Those variants share the genetic and immunophenotypic criteria, but they have atypical morphologic features.

There are many distinctions between BL and DLBCL (Table 26.1). However, BLL has morphologic features intermediate between BL and DLBCL. It is differentiated by larger nuclear size, greater shape pleomorphism, fewer numbers of more prominent nucleoli, and the presence of some admixed large centroblasts; it is seen frequently in sporadic adult cases. The revised European–American lymphoma classification gave BLL a provisional status.[23] It had been a confusing entity for clinicians where they found themselves reluctant to choose between treating the disease as BL or as DLBCL, which has a significant impact on the outcome based on the precise diagnosis. Later on, the Southwest Oncology Group reported that BLL is an entity of high-grade lymphoma much closer to BL than DLBCL, and it can be differentiated based on phenotypical and molecular features; a higher proliferation index (PI) average has been noted in BLL cases compared to DLBCL.[24]

The WHO classification resolved the dilemma by recognizing BLL as a morphologic variant of BL that requires intensive therapy. BLL was defined as lymphoma with morphologic features intermediate between BL and DLBCL with high Ki-67 fraction of the neoplastic cells, at least 99%. Cases with a high proliferation fraction or with t(8;14) and typical morphologic features of DLBCL, and cases that are morphologically

Table 26.1. Differences between Burkitt lymphoma and DLBCL

	Burkitt lymphoma	DLBCL
Epidemiology	1–2% of NHL	30% of NHL
Morphology	Starry-sky appearance	Large cells
Immunophenotype	CD10+, CD19+, CD20+, CD22+, CD79a+, CD5−, monotypic sIg+, TdT	CD19+, CD20+, CD22+, CD45+, CD79a+, PAX5+, monotypic sIg±, CD5±, CD10±
Ki-67	100%	53%
Genetics	c-Myc+, BCL6+, BCL2 neg	BCL2 (30% +), BCL6 (30% +), c-Myc (10% +)
Treatment	R-CODOX-M/IVAC or R-HyperCVAD or R-EPOCH	R-CHOP

Notes: R-CODOX-M/IVAC: rituximab plus cyclophosphamide, vincristine, doxorubicin, high-dose methotrexate, and intrathecal therapy alternating with ifosfamide, etoposide, high-dose cytarabine, and intrathecal therapy; R-CHOP: cyclophosphamide, doxorubicin, vincristine, and prednisone; R-Hyper CVAD: rituximab plus hyperfractionated cyclophosphamide, vincristine, doxorubicin, and dexamethosone; R-EPOCH: etoposide, prednisone, vincristine, cyclophosphamide, and doxorubicin with rituximab and intrathecal methotrexate; TdT: terminal deoxyribonucleotide transferase; sIg: surface immunoglobulin.

intermediate between BL and DLBCL with lower proliferation fraction, should be considered DLBCL rather than BLL.[24,25]

BL with plasmacytoid differentiation variant is reported frequently in HIV-associated cases. It is distinguished by nuclear pleomorphism, frequent single nucleolus, abundant eccentric basophilic cytoplasm, and evidence of monotypic intracytoplasmic immunoglobulins; in contrast to the uniform appearance of the classic form, section reveals more heterogeneity in BL with plasmacytoid differentiation.

BL cell markers are compatible with germinal center origin based on data from sequence analysis of the somatic mutated immunoglobulin heavy chain variable-region genes and frequent expression of B-cell surface markers on the cells;[26] in addition, some cases of endemic BL show evidence of ongoing somatic hypermutation which supports the germinal center origin as somatic hypermutation is apparently confined to germinal center B cells.[27]

Immunophenotyping features

BL cells are derived from mature B-cell lineage and typically express monotypic surface IgM, CD19, CD20, CD22, CD10, BCL6, and CD79a, and are negative for CD5, CD23, nuclear terminal deoxyribonucleotide transferase (TdT), and BCL2.[9] Lack of the surface immunoglobulins was reported in few cases of Burkitt.[28] The presence of CD10 and BCL6 expression in BL cells supports the germinal center origin of Burkitt cells.[29]

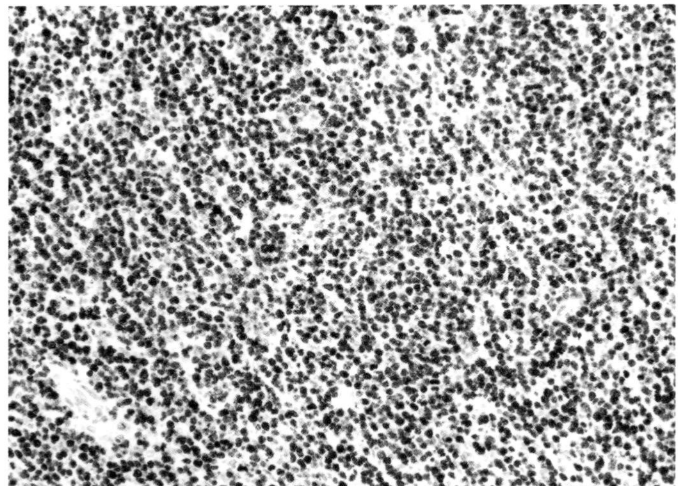

Figure 26.2 Ki-67 stain of Burkitt lymphoma with 100% staining.

A remarkable feature of BL is high growth fraction demonstrated by extremely high Ki-67 PI that reaches 100%[9] (Figure 26.2). BL in leukemic phase usually express mature immunophenotypes that distinguish blast cells from classic precursor B-cell ALL.[30]

BLL demonstrates more phenotypical diversity; it exhibits a lower proliferation rate as measured by Ki-67 compared with the classic form and more frequent expression of BCL2.[31] On the other hand, some cases of DLBCL were found to exhibit overlapping immunophenotypes with BL with high proliferation rate,[32] which means distinguishing BLL from DLBCL is not always feasible based on immunophenotypic characteristics alone. Expression of CD21 is seen in EBV-positive cases since it is an EBV-viral receptor.[33] Therefore, it presents in the vast majority of endemic cases which correlated with high incidence of EBV infection in this variant.

Molecular genetics

c-MYC encodes a transcription factor. It normally has an influence on the cell cycle regulation, cellular differentiation, and apoptosis.[34] Dysregulation of the gene is the key element in BL pathogenesis at the cellular level. Translocation of c-Myc oncogene is universal in BL; it juxtaposes the c-Myc oncogene location at 8q24 and one of the three immunoglobin loci on chromosome 2, 14, or 22. The commonest translocation is (8;14), which is observed in 80% of the cases; it occurs between c-Myc oncogene and Ig heavy chain gene (*IGH*). Fifteen percent of BL cases have t(2;8), where the translocation occurs between c-Myc and Kappa light chain gene, and the remaining 5% have (8;22) translocation between c-Myc and Lambda light chain gene.[35] In addition, one-third of the BL cases also have alterations at the p53 gene at 17p. The detection of translocations is not always feasible by performing routine cytogenetics; using fluorescence *in situ* hybridization (FISH) or long-segment polymerase chain reaction increases the chance of identifying the translocations.[28]

The position of breakpoint in relation to c-Myc gene at chromosome 8 and *IGH* at chromosome 14 is not constant and it was reported to be variable in individuals with BL. Studies found a correlation between the site of breakpoint at the chromosomes and the geographical distribution of BL. In the endemic form, the breakpoint on chromosome 8 tends to occur upstream of the c-Myc gene, while the breakpoint in the *IGH* locus is usually located within the joining segment. In sporadic and HIV-associated cases, the translocation breakpoint falls often within the c-Myc gene on chromosome 8 and in the *IGH* switch region in chromosome 14.[34] This may suggest a presence of diverse pathogenesis for the different variants of BL which may reflect the clinical variability between endemic and sporadic subtypes.

Making BL diagnosis more challenging, c-Myc was found to be overexpressed in a percentage of DLBCL cases; it is estimated that 5–15% of DLBCL harbor the c-Myc rearrangement.[36] It is also seen infrequently in other malignancies such as mantle cell lymphoma, follicular lymphoma, and multiple myeloma; translocation in these tumors is usually a secondary event in contrast to BL cases that have a de novo translocation. However, some cases of BLL were found missing the c-Myc translocation.[37,38]

The presence of both (8;14)(q24;q32) and (14;18)(q32;q21) translocations in malignancy cells at the same time is referred to as the dual hit or translocation; it was found that tumors harboring this combination have more aggressive disease, present in more advanced stages, and have worse prognosis.[39] The t(14;18) causes overexpression of BCL2, and it is seen frequently in follicular lymphoma and to a lesser extent in DLBCL. It mediates cell survival prolongation through apoptosis inhibition, and when this mutation is present in alliance with c-Myc overexpression, cell proliferation is enhanced,[40] and a synergic effect is created on the growth speed of tumor and the resistance for chemotherapy. Dual translocation has been reported in BL cases, especially BLL,[41] as well as DLBCL;[42] however, it occurs in transforming follicular lymphoma as well. Patients with dual transformation usually have a worse outcome compared to simple translocation. More complex cases with triple translocations in BL were reported,[43] and it was also linked to poor prognosis. Management approach in such complex translocation cases is not well defined yet; however, intensive therapy remains the standard of care, and the role of stem cell transplantation (SCT) in patients with these translocations is not yet established.

Gene profile studies

Differentiating BL from DLBCL can be extremely difficult in some cases, yet the distinction has important therapeutic implications; using molecular technology has imparted new insights in the accurate diagnosis. Genetic signature was introduced in the past few years to compare the gene expression based on the differential expression of thousands of genes, creating a global picture of cell activity. Recent studies conducted by Dave *et al.*[37] and Hummel *et al.*[38] reported a more reliable approach in subclassification of mature aggressive B-cell lymphoma by gene expression profiling using DNA microarrays. They found that 17%[37] and 34%[38] of cases identified to have the Burkitt gene expression profile had previously been called DLBCL or unclassifiable high-grade lymphoma. On the contrary, 0.5–4% of the cases that had been called BL or BLL lacked the genetic signature of BL, which implies that these cases could represent DLBCL or other high-grade lymphoma rather than BL. Both studies demonstrated the superiority of using gene signature in BL diagnosis over WHO criteria. The results showed preferred prognosis for patients without the molecular signature of BL, but the retrospective design of the studies couldn't allow addressing of the accurate correlation between diagnosis and chemotherapy response.

Clinical evaluation

Most adult patients with BL in the USA present with a large abdominal mass or less commonly rapidly enlarging neck or groin nodes. The patients often have "B" symptoms and evidence for tumor lysis syndrome. BM involvement is present approximately 70% of the time and leptomeningeal disease is present about 40% of the time. Extranodal involvement can occur in a number of different locations including bone, testes, ovaries, liver, or gastrointestinal tract. After the diagnosis has been made by a biopsy, the patient needs to be staged as quickly as possible with computed tomographic (CT) imaging of the chest, abdomen, or pelvis, BM biopsy, and lumbar puncture. Routine lab tests for blood counts, renal and liver tests, and electrolyte evaluation should also be done in a timely manner. There is not a lot of published information on ^{18}F-fluorodeoxyglucose positron emission tomography (FDG-PET) in BL; however, it may be helpful in picking up other extranodal disease such as occult bone disease. The patients are at very high risk for tumor lysis syndrome and should be monitored very closely once the diagnosis is made and treatment is initiated for organ damage due to this complication.

Treatment of Burkitt lymphoma

Prior to the initiation of treatment, the patients must be given aggressive bicarbonate hydration, and allopurinol or rasburicase to prevent tumor lysis syndrome. The initial trials of BL treatment by using standard protocols had failed to obtain acceptable outcomes; when BL was treated with conventional NHL or acute lymphoblastic leukemia (ALL) regimens, complete response (CR) rate ranged between 30% and 70% with cure rate between 0% and 30%,[2–4] which can be attributed to the fact that viable cells in Burkitt are able to recover fast and reenter the cell cycle with rapid growth rate between the chemotherapy cycles. The introduction of intensive chemotherapy given over a relatively short interval provided an ideal strategy for this obstacle; however, adult patients do not tolerate these intensive regimens as well as pediatric patients.

Table 26.2. Treatment results for Burkitt lymphoma

Study	Regimen	No.	Median age (range)	CR%	DFS%	EFS%	OS%
Bernstein *et al.* (83)	Stanford	18	25 (15–75)	78	71.3 at 1 y	N/A	66.8 at 2 y
Lopez *et al.* (107)	MD Anderson 81-01 and 84-30	44	32 (17–72)	80	60 at 5 y	N/A	52 at 5 y
McMaster *et al.* (108)	Vanderbilt	20	44.5 (21–69)	85	60 at 5 y	N/A	N/A
Hoelzer *et al.* (81)	B-NHL83	24	33 (15–38)	63	50 at 8 y	N/A	49 at 8 y
	B-NHL86	35	36 (18–65)	74	71 at 4 y		51 at 4 y
Soussain *et al.* (82)	LMP 84 and 86	65	26 (17–65)	89	N/A	71 at 3 y	74 at 3 y
Divine *et al.* (83)	LMB 81, 84, 86, and 89	51	33	83	N/A	61 at 2 y	66 at 2 y
Divine *et al.* (84)	LMB	72	33 (18–76)	72		65 at 2 y	70 at 2 y
McGrath *et al.* (80)	CODOX-M/IVAC	41	24			92	
Adde *et al.* (85)	CODOX-M/IVAC	26	25 (18–59)	92.3	N/A	84 at 1 y	N/A

Most of the adult BL regimens have largely been adopted from pediatric protocols.[44–46] Although intensive chemotherapy improved the outcome markedly in pediatric BL, increased age was an independent factor associated with inferior outcome in most trials. The German Multicenter Study Group for Adult ALL (GMALL) developed two protocols for adult BL derived from the pediatric Berlin, Frankfurt, Munster (BFM) regimen; these protocols are B-NHL 83 and B-NHL 86.[46] Those studies reported 4- to 8-year overall survival (OS) around 50%, which was a significant improvement compared to earlier dismal outcome. Toxicities were high with these protocols, including hematologic and neurologic toxicities; 40% of patients could not complete the entire assigned regimen.

After the success that the lymphoma malignant B-cell (LMB) protocol achieved in pediatrics, a retrospective review of 65 HIV-negative patients was done to evaluate its efficacy in the adult population. The study included patients that were diagnosed with small non-cleaved cell lymphoma (SNCL) or ALL L3; the majority of the patients had advanced disease. Age ranged between 17 and 65. They were treated with LMB 84 and 86. CR was 89% and 3-year OS was 74%. Three-year OS was 100% among patients with stage I and II compared to 57% among patients with stage IV or ALL L3. The LMB protocol involves cytoreduction phase with COP regimen which includes low-dose cyclophosphamide, vincristine, and prednisone, followed by two induction cycles with COPADM that includes high dose of methotrexate, cyclophosphamide, vincristine, doxorubicin, and prednisone; then one to two consolidation cycles that contain cytarabine, and one to four maintenance cycles.[47]

To support the previous results, a prospective trial of LMB in adults was performed on 51 patients with median age of 33. A CR of 83% was achieved, with 2-year event-free survival (EFS) and OS of 61% and 66%, respectively. The multivariate analysis showed poor survival rate associated with the presence extranodal involvement and failing to respond to cytoreductive therapy.[48] Subsequently, a more recent prospective study of the LMB protocol on 72 adult patients with BL was published in 2005. The study reported CR of 72% and 2-year EFS and OS of 65% and 70%, respectively. Worse outcome was associated with increased lactate dehydrogenase and increased age; analysis showed 2-year OS of 84% in patients < 33 years compared to 60% in patients > 33 years.[49] The major reported adverse effect in LMB studies was myelosuppression.[47–49] Although the LMB protocol has proved its efficacy in adults, survival rate didn't reach the pediatric rate.

The CODOX-M/IVAC protocol has gained the interest of many oncologists due to the excellent curable potential it has attained. It consists of alternating therapy between cyclophosphamide, vincristine, doxorubicin, high-dose methotrexate, and intrathecal therapy and ifosfamide, etoposide, high-dose cytarabine, and intrathecal therapy (Table 26.2).

The alternating regimen with IVAC was developed by McGrath. He conducted a trial of four cycles of CODOX/IVAC on 41 patients, including children and adults, with SNCL. The study reported 2-year EFS of 92% with identical survival outcomes obtained in children and adult groups. The study reported similar prognosis for adults and children when they were treated with CODOX/IVAC, but young adults were enrolled in the study with median age of 24. The reported therapy toxicities were mucositis and neurotoxicity.[45]

Two years later, Adde, who was a partner in the previous study, reported updated results of four cycles of alternating CODOX-M/IVAC protocol in advanced B-cell lymphomas. The regimen was given to 66 high-risk patients, including children and young adults; 55 patients had BL/BLL and 11 patients had DLBCL. The EFS was 85% at 1 year and beyond, and Adde reported that significant improvement in survival rate is achieved by adding alternating therapy to the previous CODOX-M regimen. The study confirmed the prior results seen in children and young adults with a median age of 25.[50]

To confirm the value of CODOX-M/IVAC protocol in adults, the United Kingdom Lymphoma Group conducted an international, prospective phase II study with some

Table 26.3. Treatment results for Burkitt lymphoma

Study	Regimen	No.	Median age (range)	CR%	DFS%	EFS%	OS%
Bernstein *et al.*[44]	Stanford	18	25 (15–75)	78	71.3 at 1 yr	NA	66.8 at 2 yrs
McMaster *et al.*[56]	Vanderbilt	20	44.5 (21–69)	85	60 at 5 yrs	NA	NA
Hoelzer *et al.*[46]	B-NHL83	24	33 (15–38)	63	50 at 8 yrs	NA	49 at 8 yrs
	B-NHL86	35	36 (18–65)	74	71 at 4 yrs		51 at 4 yrs
Soussain *et al.*[47]	LMB 84 and 86	65	26 (17–65)	89	NA	71 at 3 yrs	74 at 3 yrs
Divine *et al.*[48]	LMB 81, 84, 86, and 89	51	33	83	NA	61 at 2 yrs	66 at 2 yrs
Divine *et al.*[49]	LMB	72	33 (18–76)	72	NA	65 at 2 yrs	70 at 2 yrs
McGrath *et al.*[45]	CODOX-M/IVAC	41	24			92	
Adde *et al.*[50]	CODOX-M/IVAC	26	25 (18–59)	92.3	NA	84 at 1 yr	NA
Mead *et al.*[51]	CODOX-M/IVAC	52	35 (16–60)	75	NA	64.6 at 2 yrs	72.8 at 2 yrs
Thomas *et al.*[53]	HyperCVAD	26	58 (17–79)	81	61 at 3 yrs	NA	49 at 3 yrs
Thomas *et al.*[54]	R-HyperCVAD	31	46 (17–77) 29% > 60	86	88 at 3 yrs	80 at 3 yrs	88 at 3 yrs
Kujawski *et al.*[57]	High-dose CHOP, mid-cycle MTX	11	51 (33–71)	91		73 at 22 mo	82 at 22 mo

Notes: MTX: methotrexate; NA: not available.

modification in the original protocol of CODOX/IVAC on 52 HIV-negative patients with age ranging between 16 and 60 with median age of 35. Eighty percent of the cases were considered high risk by International Prognostic Index-based criteria. Low-risk patients received three cycles of modified CODOX-M, while the high-risk group was given four cycles of alternating modified CODOX-M and IVAC. Two-year OS and EFS for all patients were 73% and 65%, respectively. In the low-risk group 2-year OS and EFS were 82% and 83%, respectively, versus 70% and 60% for 2-year OS and EFS, respectively, in high-risk patients. The study revealed a trend of worsening EFS in older age and advanced disease.[51] Reported side effects were myelosuppression and mucositis. Close outcome was obtained from a small prospective study using the modified McGrath regimen performed by the Dana Farber Cancer Institute. The 2-year EFS was 64% in the entire study, with 100% in the low-risk group versus 60% in the high-risk group; toxicity was less in this modified regimen compared to McGrath's original protocol.[52]

The MD Anderson Cancer Center developed the HyperCVAD protocol which has been used exclusively in adult BL. The regimen includes hyperfractionated cyclophosphamide, vincristine, doxorubicin, dexamethasone, and CNS prophylaxis. The trial was performed on 28 adult patients with median age of 58. The CR was 81% and the 3-year OS was 49%. The study was performed in relatively elderly patients compared to the previously mentioned studies as 46% of patients were older than 60.[53]

Since Burkitt cells strongly express CD20 on the surface and as rituximab is a monoclonal antibody against CD20, the advent of rituximab to the preexisting regimens was investigated in anticipation of improving adults' survival without adverse impact on toxicity. A trial by Thomas *et al.* revealed very promising results in elderly treatment. The study examined the addition of rituximab to HyperCVAD protocol in 31 patients; the median age was 46 and 29% of the patients engaged in the study were older than 60 years. The CR was 86%, and the 3-year OS, EFS, and disease-free survival (DFS) were 89%, 80%, and 88%, respectively. In patients older than 60 years, 3-year OS was 89%. Survival enhancement without therapy toxicity worsening was noted in the study, which represents an evolutionary achievement in the unfavorable elderly age group. In comparison to HyperCVAD regimen in adults, HyperCVAD plus rituximab yielded similar CR; on the other hand, a superior outcome in regard of 3-year OS, EFS, and DFS was achieved. Presence of CNS disease was not a prognostic factor in this study.[54] The most recent National Comprehensive Cancer Network (NCCN) guidelines in BL treatment considered CHOP (cyclophosphamide, doxorubicin, vincristine, and prednisone) as an inadequate regimen for BL. However, it recommended using CODOX-M or HyperCVAD for low-risk patients, and CODOX-M/IVAC ± rituximab or HyperCVAD alternating with methotrexate + cytarabine ± R for HR patients, and SCT has to be considered for patients with relapsed disease.[55] The results with these regimens are outlined in Table 26.3.

The role of autologous or allogeneic bone marrow transplant is still controversial. Although some studies reported that intensive therapy followed by SCT may improve the survival,[55,58] it has not been proved yet as consolidation therapy, especially after the introduction of chemoimmunotherapy that has achieved excellent outcomes and if the significant procedure-related mortality risk is considered. In a study investigating the efficacy of autologous SCT in adults with BL/BLL, a superior OS was obtained from treating relapsed chemosensitive disease. Compared to conventional regimens, the 3-year OS was 72% after the first CR, 37% in relapsed chemosensitive disease, and 7% in relapsed chemoresistant BL.[59] In a more recent study performed on chemoradiotherapy and stem cell transplant as primary therapy in sporadic BL, 3-year EFS was 50%.[58] The potential benefit of graft-versus-lymphoma by using allogeneic transplant did not affect the relapse rate and OS based on the current existing data.[60] The place of autologous and allogeneic stem cell transplants in BL remains uncertain.

CNS prophylaxis is one of the main keys in BL treatment, since the CNS is a common site for relapse in the absence of such treatment; relapse had occurred in 30–50% of patients with BL prior to the introduction of intensive chemotherapy with CNS prophylaxis. However, it can be skipped in patients with completely resected disease in the absence of CNS involvement with the intention to limit therapy toxicity. CNS prophylaxis and therapy have been used as intrathecal and systemic therapy in Burkitt protocols; intrathecal methotrexate with or without cytarabine and hydrocortisone has been popular in the current regimens.

Special situations

HIV-positive Burkitt lymphoma

Studies have demonstrated a worse prognosis of Burkitt in HIV-positive patients compared to HIV-negative patients. The immunocompromised state of the HIV-positive patients had precluded the use of intensive chemotherapy in the past; however, the introduction of HAART in HIV management supported the immune system and created more capability to mount the opportunistic infections during the course of therapy, which has allowed the application of more intense therapy. Recent successful clinical trials using different intensive regimens were reported, which count as one of the major advances in HIV-associated BL treatment.[61] In contrast to the encouraging results that rituximab has provided in HIV-negative adult BL, the role of rituximab in HIV-positive BL remains controversial as trials revealed increased serious infection in the rituximab group.[62,63] A low CD4 count and poor performance status predicted for inferior survival. More recently, dose-adjusted R-EPOCH (etoposide, prednisone, vincristine, cyclophosphamide, doxorubicin, with rituximab and intrathecal methotrexate) has had very good outcomes but with short follow-up so far.[64]

Burkitt lymphoma in the elderly

According to the SEER database, approximately 30% of BL patients are over the age of 60 years. Patients in this age group have a very difficult time tolerating the intense high-dose regimens such as the McGrath regimen or the Hyper-CVAD regimens. Although R-CHOP is not a very good alternative, the use of R-EPOCH may be a good alternative in this age group.

Conclusions

Dramatic advances continue to be made in the diagnosis and treatment of BL. A rapid and accurate diagnosis is needed to provide the optimal therapy. Therefore, more clear criteria should be made for diagnosis, and new identification modalities such as gene expression profile need to be involved in the uncertain cases. Treatment of adult BL has improved remarkably in the last few years by introducing very intensive "pediatric" or "acute leukemia" protocols. Delay in therapy can have tragic results, but with rapid diagnosis and with the prompt initiation of an appropriate treatment regimen the majority of adults will be cured.

References

1. Coakley D. Denis Burkitt and his contribution to haematology/oncology. *Br J Haematol* 2006;**135**:17–25.
2. McGrath IT, Janus C, Edwards BK, *et al.* An effective therapy for both undifferentiated (including Burkitt's) lymphomas and lymphoblastic lymphomas in children and young adults. *Blood* 1984;**63**:1102–11.
3. Bernasconi C, Brusamolino E, Pagnucco G, *et al.* Burkitt's lymphoma/leukemia: a clinicopathologic study on 24 adult patients. *Leukemia* 1991;**5** (Suppl 1):90–4.
4. Kantarjian HM, Walters RS, Keating MJ, *et al.* Results of the vincristine, doxorubicin, and dexamethasone regimen in adults with standard- and high-risk acute lymphocytic leukemia. *J Clin Oncol* 1990;**8**:994–1004.
5. Burkitt DP. Sarcoma involving jaws in African children. *Br J Surg* 1958; **46**:218–23.
6. Burkitt D, O'Conor GT. Malignant lymphoma in African children; I, clinical syndrome. *Cancer* 1961; **14**:258–69.
7. O'Conor GT. Malignant lymphoma in African children. II. A pathological entity. *Cancer* 1961;**14**:270–83.
8. Wilson JF, Jenkin RD, Anderson JR, *et al.* Studies on the pathology of non-Hodgkin's lymphoma of childhood. I. The role of routine histopathology as a prognostic factor. A report from the Children's Cancer Study Group. *Cancer* 1984;**53**:1695–704.
9. Diebold J, Jaffe E, Raphael M, *et al.* Burkitt lymphoma. In: Jaffe E, Harris N, Stein H, *et al.*, eds. *World Health Organization Classification of Tumours: Pathology and Genetics of Tumors of Hematopoietic and Lymphoid Tissues.* Lyon, France, IARC Press. 2001; 181–4.
10. Cardy A, Sharp L, Little J. Burkitt's lymphoma: a review of the epidemiology. *Kuwait Med J* 2001; **33**(4):293–306.
11. Makata AM, Toriyama K, Kamidigo NO, *et al.* The pattern of pediatric solid malignant tumors in Western Kenya, East Africa, 1979–1994: an analysis based on histopathologic study. *Am J Trop Med Hyg* 1996;**54**:343–7.

12. Cairo MS, Sposto R, Perkins SL, *et al.* Burkitt's and Burkitt-like lymphoma in children and adolescents: a review of the Children's Cancer Group experience. *Br J Haematol* 2003;**120**:660–70.
13. Blum KA, Lozanski G, Byrd JC. Adult Burkitt leukemia and lymphoma. *Blood* 2004;**104**:3009–20.
14. Sariban E, Donahue A, McGrath IT. Jaw involvement in American Burkitt's lymphoma. *Cancer* 1984;**53**:141–6.
15. McGrath IT, Sariban E. Clinical features of Burkitt's in the USA. *IARC Sci Publ* 1985;**1**:119–27.
16. Hugh JC, Jackson FI, Hanson J, *et al.* Primary breast lymphoma. An immunohistologic study of 20 new cases. *Cancer* 1990;**66**:2602–11.
17. Gong JZ, Stenzel TT, Bennett ER, *et al.* Burkitt lymphoma arising in organ transplant recipients: a clinicopathologic study of five cases. *Am J Surg Pathol* 2003;**27**:818–27.
18. Ferry JA. Burkitt's lymphoma: clinicopathologic features and differential diagnosis. *Oncologist* 2006;**11**:375–83.
19. Knowles DM. Etiology and pathogenesis of AIDS-related non-Hodgkin's lymphoma. *Hematol Oncol Clin North Am* 2003;**17**:785–820.
20. Gabarre J, Raphael M, Lepage E, *et al.* Human immunodeficiency virus-related lymphoma: relation between clinical features and histological subtypes. *Am J Med* 2001;**11**:704–11.
21. Sandler AS, Kaplan LD. Diagnosis and management of systemic non-Hodgkin's lymphoma in HIV. *Hematol Oncol Clin North Am* 1996;**10**:1111–24.
22. Ostronoff M, Soussain C, Zambon E, *et al.* Burkitt's lymphoma in adults: a retrospective study of 46 cases. *Nouv Rev Fr Hematol* 1992;**34**:389–97.
23. Harris NL, Jaffe ES, Stein H, *et al.* A revised European-American classification of lymphoid neoplasms: a proposal from the International Lymphoma Study Group. *Blood* 1994; **84**:1361–92.
24. Braziel RM, Arber DA, Slovak ML, *et al.* The Burkitt-like lymphomas: a Southwest Oncology Group study delineating phenotypic, genotypic, and clinical features. *Blood* 2001; **97**:3713–20.
25. Harris N, Jaffe E, Diebold J, *et al.* World Health Organization classification of neoplastic diseases of the hematopoietic and lymphoid tissues: report of the Clinical Advisory Committee meeting-Airlie House, Virginia, November 1997. *J Clin Oncol* 1999;**17**:3835–49.
26. Jain R, Roncella S, Hashimoto S, *et al.* A potential role for antigen selection in the clonal evolution of Burkitt's lymphoma. *J Immunol* 1994;**153**:45–52.
27. Chapman CJ, Wright D, Stevenson FK. Insight into Burkitt's lymphoma from immunoglobulin variable region gene analysis. *Leuk Lymphoma* 1998; **30**:257–67.
28. Burmeister T, Schwartz S, Horst HA, *et al.* Molecular heterogeneity of sporadic adult Burkitt-type leukemia/lymphoma as revealed by PCR and cytogenetics: correlation with morphology, immunology and clinical features. *Leukemia* 2005;**19**:1391–8.
29. Falini B, Fizzotti M, Pileri S, *et al.* Bcl-6 protein expression in normal and neoplastic lymphoid tissues. *Ann Oncol* 1997;**8** (Suppl 2):101–4.
30. Van der Burg M, Barendregt BH, van Wering ER, *et al.* The presence of somatic mutations in immunoglobulin genes of B cell acute lymphoblastic leukemia (ALL L3) supports assignment as Burkitt's leukemia-lymphoma rather than B-lineage ALL. *Leukemia* 2001;**15**:1141–3.
31. Macpherson N, Lesack D, Klasa R, *et al.* Small noncleaved, non-Burkitt's (Burkitt-like) lymphoma: cytogenetics predict outcome and reflect clinical presentation. *J Clin Oncol* 1999; **17**:1558–67.
32. Haralambieva E, Boerma EJ, van Imhoff GW, *et al.* Clinical, immunophenotypic, and genetic analysis of adult lymphomas with morphologic features of Burkitt lymphoma. *Am J Surg Pathol* 2005;**29**:1086–94.
33. McGrath IT, Freeman CB, Bizzo P, *et al.* Characterization of lymphoma-derived cell lines: comparison of cell lines positive and negative for Epstein-Barr virus nuclear antigen. II. Surface markers. *J Natl Cancer Inst* 1980; **64**:477–83.
34. Hecht J, Aster J. Molecular biology of Burkitt's lymphoma. *J Clin Oncol* 2000;**18**:3703–21.
35. Pelicci PG, Knowles DM 2nd, McGrath I, *et al.* Chromosomal breakpoints and structural alterations of the c-myc locus differ in endemic and sporadic forms of Burkitt lymphoma. *Proc Natl Acad Sci U S A* 1986;**83**:2984–8.
36. McClure RF, Remstein ED, Macon WR, *et al.* Adult B-cell lymphomas with Burkitt-like morphology are phenotypically and genotypically heterogeneous with aggressive clinical behavior. *Am J Surg Pathol* 2005;**29**:1652–60.
37. Dave SS, Fu K, Wright GW, *et al.* Molecular diagnosis of Burkitt's lymphoma. *N Engl J Med* 2006; **354**:2431–42.
38. Hummel M, Bentink S, Berger H, *et al.* A biologic definition of Burkitt's lymphoma from transcriptional and genomic profiling. *N Engl J Med* 2006;**354**:2419–30.
39. Johnson NA, Savage KJ, Ludkovski O, *et al.* Lymphomas with concurrent BCL2 and MYC translocations: the critical factors associated with survival. *Blood* 2009;**114**:2273–9.
40. Hockenbery D, Nunez G, Milliman C, *et al.* Bcl-2 is an inner mitochondrial membrane protein that blocks programmed cell death. *Nature* 1990;**348**:334–6.
41. Thangavelu M, Olopade O, Beckman E, *et al.* Clinical, morphologic, cytogenetic characteristics of patients with lymphoid malignancies characterized by both t(14;18)(q32;q21) and t(8;14)(q24;q32) or t(8;22)(q24;q11). *Genes Chromosomes Cancer* 1990;**2**:147–58.
42. Le Gouill S, Talmant P, Touzeau C, *et al.* The clinical presentation and prognosis of diffuse large B-cell lymphoma with t(14;18) and 8q24/c-MYC rearrangement. *Haematologica* 2007;**92**(10):1335–42.
43. Zimonjic DB, Keck-Waggoner C, Popescu NC. Novel genomic imbalances and chromosome translocations involving c-myc gene in Burkitt's lymphoma. *Leukemia* 2001;**15**:1582–8.
44. Bernstein JI, Coleman CN, Strickler JG, *et al.* Combined modality therapy for adults with small noncleaved cell lymphoma (Burkitt's and non-Burkitt's types). *J Clin Oncol* 1986;**4**:847–58.
45. McGrath I, Adde M, Shad A, *et al.* Adults and children with small non-cleaved cell lymphoma have a similar excellent outcome when treated with the same chemotherapy regimen. *J Clin Oncol* 1996;**14**:925–34.
46. Hoelzer D, Ludwig WD, Thiel E, *et al.* Improved outcome in adult B-cell acute

lymphoblastic leukemia. *Blood* 1996; **87**:495–508.

47. Soussain C, Patte C, Ostronoff M, *et al.* Small noncleaved cell lymphoma and leukemia in adults. A retrospective study of 65 adults treated with the LMB pediatric protocols. *Blood* 1995; **85**:664–74.
48. Divine M, Cassasus P, Koscielny S, *et al.* Adult Burkitt lymphoma. A prospective multicenter trial with the LMB protocol. *Proc Am Soc Clin Oncol*, 2000;**19**:Abstract 80.
49. Divine M, Casassus P, Koscielny S, *et al.* Burkitt lymphoma in adults: a prospective study of 72 patients treated with an adapted pediatric LMB protocol. *Ann Oncol* 2005;**16**:1928–35.
50. Adde M, Shad A, Venzon D, *et al.* Additional chemotherapy agents improve treatment outcome for children and adults with advanced B-cell lymphomas. *Semin Oncol* 1998;**25**:33–9; discussion 45–8.
51. Mead GM, Sydes MR, Walewski J, *et al.* An international evaluation of CODOX-M and CODOX-M alternating with IVAC in adult Burkitt's lymphoma: results of United Kingdom Lymphoma Group LY06 study. *Ann Oncol* 2002;**13**:1264–74.
52. LaCasce A, Howard O, Li S, *et al.* Modified McGrath regimens for adults with Burkitt and Burkitt-like lymphomas: preserved efficacy with decreased toxicity. *Leuk Lymphoma* 2004;**45**:761–7.
53. Thomas D, Cortes J, O'Brien S, *et al.* Hyper-CVAD program in Burkitt's type adult acute lymphoblastic leukemia. *J Clin Oncol* 1999;**17**:2461–70.
54. Thomas DA, Faderl S, O'Brien S, *et al.* Chemoimmunotherapy with hyper-CVAD plus rituximab for the treatment of adult Burkitt and Burkitt-type lymphoma or acute lymphoblastic leukemia. *Cancer* 2006;**106**:1569–80.
55. Nademanee A, Molina A, O'Donnell MR, *et al.* Results of high-dose therapy and autologous bone marrow/stem cell transplantation during remission in poor-risk intermediate and high-grade lymphoma: international index high and high-intermediate risk group. *Blood* 1997;**90**:3844–52.
56. McMaster ML, Johnson DH, Greer JP, *et al.* A brief-duration combination chemotherapy for elderly patients with poor-prognosis non-Hodgkin's lymphoma. *Cancer* 1991;**67**:1487–92.
57. Kujawski LA, Longo WL, Williams EC, *et al.* A 5-drug regimen maximizing the dose of cyclophosphamide is effective therapy for adult Burkitt or Burkitt-like lymphomas. *Cancer Invest* 2007;**25**:87–93.
58. Song KW, Barnett MJ, Gascoyne RD, *et al.* Haematopoietic stem cell transplantation as primary therapy of sporadic adult Burkitt lymphoma. *Br J Haematol* 2006;**133**(6):634–7.
59. Sweetenham J, Pearce R, Taghipour G, *et al.* Adult Burkitt's and Burkitt-like non-Hodgkin's lymphoma–outcome for patients treated with high-dose therapy and autologous stem-cell transplantation in the first remission or at relapse: results from the European Group for Blood and Marrow Transplantation. *J Clin Oncol* 1996; **14**:2465–72.
60. Grigg AP, Seymour JF. Graft versus Burkitt's lymphoma effect after allogeneic marrow transplantation. *Leuk Lymphoma* 2002;**43**:889–92.
61. Cortes J, Thomas D, Rios A, *et al.* Hyperfractionated cyclophosphamide, vincristine, doxorubicin, and dexamethasone and highly active antiretroviral therapy for patients with acquired immunodeficiency syndrome-related Burkitt lymphoma/leukemia. *Cancer* 2002;**94**:1492–9.
62. Boue F, Gabarre J, Gisselbrecht C, *et al.* Phase II trial of CHOP plus rituximab in patients with HIV-associated non-Hodgkin's lymphoma. *J Clin Oncol* 2006;**24**:4123–8.
63. Kaplan LD, Lee JY, Ambinder RF, *et al.* Rituximab does not improve clinical outcome in a randomized phase 3 trial of CHOP with or without rituximab in patients with HIV-associated non-Hodgkin lymphoma: AIDS-Malignancies Consortium Trial 010. *Blood* 2005;**106**:1538–43.
64. Dunleavy K, Little RF, Pittaluga S, *et al.* A prospective study of dose-adjusted EPOCH with rituximab in adults with newly diagnosed Burkitt lymphoma: a regimen with high efficacy and low toxicity. *Blood* 2008;**112**:3606a.

Index

ABVD regimen in Hodgkin lymphoma 380–382
  dose intensity 383

acute lymphoblastic leukemia (ALL) 18–19, 43–61
  adolescents and young adults 57–58
  Burkitt-type 18–19
  CD20 antigen 47
  chemotherapy
    induction 48
    intrathecal 55
    regimens 48, 49
  clinical features 44
  CNS prophylaxis 50–51
  CNS relapse rate 50–51
  consolidation therapy 48–50
  cranial irradiation 50
    mature B-cell disease 55
  cytogenetics 44–46
  differential diagnosis 46–47
  environmental factors 44
  epidemiology/etiology 43–44
  HOX gene family 19
  HyperCVAD regimen 53–55
  hyperdiploidy 45
  hypodiploidy 45
  IKZF1 gene abnormalities 18
  IL3-IGH translocation 19
  immunophenotyping 44
  incidence 43
  induction chemotherapy 48
  inherited syndromes 43–44
  intrathecal chemotherapy 55
  laboratory features 44
  leukocyte count 47
  mAb targeting 60
  maintenance therapy 50
  mature B-cell 52–55
    CNS involvement 55
  microRNAs 46
  minimal residual disease 47–48
  molecular genetics 46
  morphology 44
  mTOR pathway 491
    targeting 60
  myeloid antigen coexpression 47
  neutropenia management 58–59
  Notch signaling 491
    inhibition 60
  NOTCH1 gene mutations 19, 46, 60
  older adults 58
  pathology 44–46
  patient age 47
  pediatric 43–44
  Philadelphia-positive 18, 45, 54–57
    older adults 58
  ploidy groups 18
  precursor 19
  precursor B-cell 45–47, 60–61
  prognostic factors 47
  relapse 59
  risk factors 43–44
  salvage regimens 59
  stem cell transplantation 51–53, 56
    relapsed disease 59
  supportive care 58–59
  targeted therapies 60–61
  T-cell 60–61
    lymphoblastic lymphoma differential diagnosis 487–488
    Notch signaling 491
  therapy-related 43
  translocations 18, 19, 45–46
  treatment 48–53
  tumor lysis syndrome 53, 59

acute myeloid leukemia (AML) 16–18
  11q23 abnormalities 17
  antibody-directed chemotherapy 28–29
  CEBPA gene mutation 18
  classification 141–143
  consolidation treatment 29
  core binding factor abnormalities 16–17
  cytogenetic risk classification 34
  del(5q) abnormalities 17
  del(7q) abnormalities 17
  FLT3 gene mutations 17
  fludarabine-based induction combinations 29
  gene mutations 35–36
  gene overexpression 35–36
  growth factors 27
  immunologic approaches 31–34
  induction chemotherapy 26–27
    complete disease remission 26–27
    response definition 26–27
  management 26–38
  minimal residual disease 35–36
  MLL gene abnormalities 17
  molecular information 35–36
  molecular targets 38
  monosomy 5 17
  monosomy 7 17
  novel agents 36–37
  NPM1 gene mutation 17–18
  Pgp overexpression 27–28
  prognostic factors 32, 34–35
    validated 34–35
  remission rates 26–27
  resistance modulation 27–28
  retinoic acid receptor alpha abnormalities 17
  stem cell transplantation 28–31, 36
    relapse risk 30–31
    second remission 31
  treatment outcomes 29
  trisomy 8 17
  WT1 gene 18

acute promyelocytic leukemia (APL) 131–137
  all-*trans* retinoic acid treatment 29, 132–135
  arsenic trioxide therapy 133, 135–136
    rescue therapy 136–137
    simultaneous chemotherapy 135
  CD33 134
  9-cis-RA 132
  clinical signs 131
  consolidation therapy 135
  cytarabine 135–136
  FLT3 receptor 134
  gemtuzumab ozogamicin therapy 134
  immunophenotype 134
  induction therapy 134–135
  maintenance therapy 136
  PML gene structure 131–132
  PML protein 131–132
  PML-RARα 132–133
  RARα 132
    variant translocations 133
  stem cell transplantation 136–137
  supportive measures 134–135
  t(15;17) molecular architecture 131
  treatment 134
    relapsed disease 136–137

acute promyelocytic leukemia differentiation syndrome (APL-DS) 135

adolescents and young adults, ALL treatment 57–58

adult T-cell leukemia/lymphoma (ATLL) 240, 419–421
  acute 420
  antiviral therapy 420
  chemotherapy 420
  CHOP regimen 420
  chronic 420
  clinical features 420
  diagnosis 419–420
  epidemiology 419
  HIV-related 476
  HTLV-1 exposure 419–420
  immunodeficiency 420
  infections 420
  interferon 420
  management 420–421
  pathology 419–420
  smoldering 420
  stem cell transplantation 420–421
  survival 420
  zidovudine 420

aggressive B-cell non-Hodgkin lymphoma *see* diffuse large B-cell lymphoma (DLBCL), HIV-related

alemtuzumab
CLL 87–88
fludarabine-refractory patients 91
salvage therapy 90
CMV reactivation 88
follicular lymphoma 351–352
mantle cell lymphoma 323
mycosis fungoides/Sézary syndrome 441

alkylating agents
CLL 85–86
myelodysplastic syndrome risk 103
therapy-related ALL 43
Waldenstrom's macroglobulinemia treatment 215

all-*trans* retinoic acid (ATRA)
AML management 29
APL management 29, 132–135

amyloidosis, systemic 184–190
AL 155, 185
bortezomib 189–190
chemotherapy
high-dose with stem cell transplantation 186
standard 188–189
classification 185
diagnosis 184–186
diagnostic criteria 156
immune modulatory derivatives 189
immunoglobulin light chain 155, 184–190
lenalidomide 189
localized 190
monoclonal protein screening 184–185
novel therapies 189–190
number of organs involved 190
organ involvement 187
outcome prediction 190
primary 155
prognostic factors in treatment decisions 190
proteosome inhibitors 189
Schnitzler's syndrome progression 200
staging 186
thalidomide 189
treatment 185–190
algorithm 188–190
response 187
troponin T 190
Waldenstrom's macroglobulinemia 211–212

anaplastic large cell lymphoma 240–242, 415–419
ALK gene 241, 415
CD30 415–416
chemotherapy 416–418
relapsed/refractory disease 419
CHOP regimen 416–418
clinical features 416, 417
histology 241
HIV-related 476
management 416–418
morphologic variants 416
pathology 415–416
primary cutaneous 242, 416, 432
relapsed/refractory disease 418–419
stem cell transplantation 419
translocations 415

anaplastic lymphoma kinase *(ALK)* gene
anaplastic large cell lymphoma 241, 415
T-cell non-Hodgkin lymphoma 268

anemia
cold agglutinin hemolytic anemia 211
multiple myeloma 173
Waldenstrom's macroglobulinemia 211, 212
see also refractory anemia

angiogenesis, multiple myeloma 160

angiogenesis inhibitors, mantle cell lymphoma 325

angioimmunoblastic T-cell lymphoma (AITL) 242, 412, 413–415
autoimmune disease association 414
clinical features 414–415
EBV association 414
etiology 414
laboratory abnormalities 415
natural history 415
pathology 414
treatment 415

anthracyclines
ALL treatment 48
diffuse large B-cell lymphoma 290–291
induction chemotherapy for AML 26

antibody-directed chemotherapy
AML management 28–29
anti-CD33 antibodies 28

anti-CD20 antibodies
cryoglobulinemia 196
follicular lymphoma 354
Hodgkin lymphoma 391–392
mantle cell lymphoma 322–323
see also rituximab

anti-CD22 antibodies
follicular lymphoma 352–353
radioimmunoconjugates/immunotoxins 353
mantle cell lymphoma 323

anti-CD25 antibodies, Hodgkin lymphoma 392

anti-CD30 antibodies, Hodgkin lymphoma 390–391

anti-CD33 antibodies, antibody-directed chemotherapy 28

anti-CD52 antibodies, mantle cell lymphoma 323

anti-CD80 antibodies, follicular lymphoma 353

anti-idiotype vaccines, mantle cell lymphoma 323

antilymphocyte globulins, myelodysplastic syndromes 109–110

antisense oligonucleotides, mantle cell lymphoma 325–326

antithymocyte globulins, myelodysplastic syndromes 109–110

antiviral therapy
adult T-cell leukemia/lymphoma 420
HIV-related multicentric Castleman's disease 477

AP12 gene, lymphoma 265

AP23573 mTOR inhibitor, mantle cell lymphoma 325

AP24534 multikinase inhibitor 74

apoptosis
Hodgkin lymphoma 371
targeting in mantle cell lymphoma 325–326

arsenic trioxide
acute promyelocytic leukemia 133, 135–136
rescue therapy 136–137
simultaneous chemotherapy 135
myelodysplastic syndromes 111

L-asparaginase
ALL treatment 48, 50
adolescents and young adults 57
older adults 58
see also PEG-asparaginase

aspirin, polycythemia vera 148

ataxia–telangiectasia, ALL risk 43

ATM gene, mantle cell lymphoma 311–312

atomic bomb survivors, ALL risk 44

autoantibodies, IgM 210

autoimmune diseases
angioimmunoblastic T-cell lymphoma association 414
Hodgkin lymphoma association 370

azacitidine
chronic myelomonocytic leukemia therapy 111
myelodysplastic syndromes 110

B cells, hairy cell association 117

B-cell lymphoma
molecular aberrations 260
rituximab monotherapy 346–347
somatic hypermutations 268
see also non-Hodgkin lymphoma, B-cell

B-cell neoplasms, mature 231–238
lymphoid leukemias 239

B-cell prolymphocytic leukemia 121

BCL2, antisense oligonucleotides in mantle cell lymphoma 325–326

BCL2 family inhibitors
follicular lymphoma 358
mantle cell lymphoma 326

BCL2 family targeted therapies, CLL 91

BCL2 gene 263–264
diffuse large B-cell lymphoma 290
mantle cell lymphoma 311–312
PCR analysis 261

BCL6 gene
diffuse large B-cell lymphoma 290
FISH analysis 264
lymphoma 264–265
primary central nervous system lymphoma 451

Bcr-Abl oncoprotein
CML 68–69
imatinib resistance 71

BEACOPP regimen, Hodgkin lymphoma 381, 383

bendamustine
CLL 86
mantle cell lymphoma 320

bevacizumab, mantle cell lymphoma 325

bexarotene, mycosis fungoides/ Sézary syndrome 439, 440
Bing–Neel syndrome 212
BL-22 recombinant immunotoxin, hairy cell leukemia 125
bleomycin toxicity 388
blood–brain barrier disruption, primary CNS lymphoma 455
Bloom's syndrome, ALL risk 43
B-lymphoblastic leukemia/ lymphoma (B-ALL/LBL) 231
bone marrow
  Burkitt lymphoma 44, 497
  hairy cell leukemia 118
  Hodgkin lymphoma 372
  lymphoblastic lymphoma 491
  Waldenstrom's macroglobulinemia 208, 213
bortezomib
  amyloidosis treatment 189–190
  follicular lymphoma 358
  Hodgkin lymphoma 392
  mantle cell lymphoma 324
  multiple myeloma 168–169, 171
    side effects 174
  mycosis fungoides/Sézary syndrome 444
  Waldenstrom's macroglobulinemia 217–218
bosutinib, CML therapy 73–74
Burkitt-like lymphoma 234–235, 266, 468–470
  ALL 18–19
  chemotherapy 468–470
  classification 495–496
  clinical features 468
  EBV 468
  pathologic features 468
  treatment 468–470
Burkitt leukemia 234
Burkitt lymphoma 234–235, 494–500
  biology 495–496
  bone marrow involvement 44, 497
  cell markers 496
  chemotherapy 468–470, 497–500
  classification 494–496
  clinical evaluation 497
  clinical features 468
    c-MYC gene 265–266
  c-Myc gene 496–497
  CNS lymphoma 449, 457
  CNS prophylaxis 500
  DLBCL differential diagnosis 495, 496
  EBV 468
  elderly patients 500
  endemic 494
  epidemiology 494–495
  extranodal disease 497
  gene profile studies 497
  histology 495, 496
  HIV-related 466, 468–470, 495, 500
    histology 469
  IGH gene 265–266
  imaging 497
  immunodeficiency associated 495
  immunophenotyping 496
  molecular genetics 496–497
  pathologic features 468, 495–496
  with plasmacytoid differentiation variant 496
  sporadic 494–495
  stem cell transplantation 499–500
  translocations 265–266, 497
  treatment 468–470, 497–500
  tumor lysis syndrome prevention 497
calcium supplementation, multiple myeloma 172
cardiovascular disease, nodular lymphocyte predominant Hodgkin lymphoma 389
carfilzomib (PR171), mantle cell lymphoma 325
carmustine, mycosis fungoides/ Sézary syndrome 439
Castleman's disease *see* multicentric Castleman's disease
CCAAT/enhancer binding protein alpha (CEBPA), AML 18
CCND1 proto-oncogene, lymphoma 265
CD11c, hairy cell leukemia 120–121, 125
CD20 antigen, ALL 47, 55, 60
CD20-directed antibodies, Waldenstrom's macroglobulinemia 216
CD22 antigen, ALL 60
CD25, hairy cell leukemia 120–121, 125
CD30, anaplastic large cell lymphoma 415–416
CD33, acute promyelocytic leukemia 134
CD95 mutations, Hodgkin lymphoma 371
CD103, hairy cell leukemia 120–121, 125
CEBPA gene mutation, AML 18
celiac disease, enteropathy-type T-cell lymphoma association 423–425
central nervous system lymphoma 449–458
  clinical features 450
  clinical trials evaluation 451, 453
  dissemination 457
  secondary 457–458
    chemotherapy 458
    diagnosis 457
    treatment 458
  see also primary central nervous system lymphoma
central nervous system post-transplant lymphoproliferative disorder 458
c-FLIP, Hodgkin lymphoma 371, 392
chlorambucil, Waldenstrom's macroglobulinemia treatment 215
CHOP (cyclophosphamide, doxorubicin, vincristine, prednisone) therapy 217
  adult T-cell leukemia/ lymphoma 420
  anaplastic large cell lymphoma 416–418
  diffuse large B-cell lymphoma 290–291
    advanced disease 291–292
    treatment improvement 293
  follicular lymphoma 341
    rituximab combination 354
  mantle cell lymphoma 317, 318
  Waldenstrom's macroglobulinemia 217
chromosomal abnormalities
  CLL 82
  imatinib resistance 71
chromosomal translocations
  detection methods for lymphomas 258–260
  leukemia 1
chromosome 6 deletions, Waldenstrom's macroglobulinemia 207
chromosome 14 breakpoints 264
chronic eosinophilic leukemia not otherwise specified (CEL-NOS) 141
chronic lymphocytic leukemia (CLL) 19–20, 81–93
  alemtuzumab therapy 87–88
    consolidation therapy 88
    fludarabine-refractory patients 91
    salvage therapy 90
  alkylating agent therapy 85–86
  BCL2 family targeted therapies 91
  bendamustine therapy 86
  chromosomal abnormalities 82
  cladribine therapy 86
    salvage therapy 89
  classification 84
  cyclophosphamide therapy 84
  diagnosis 81, 82
    scoring system 82
  differential diagnosis 82
  FISH analysis 82
  fludarabine therapy 84, 86
    salvage therapy 89
  fludarabine-refractory patients 90–91
  IGHV gene 268
  IgV_H genes 83–84
  mantle cell lymphoma differentiation 269
  oblimersen sodium 91
  pentostatin 87
    salvage therapy 89
  prognosis 81–84
  prognostic factors 84
  purine analogs 86–87, 90–91
  rituximab therapy 84, 87
    fludarabine-refractory patients 91
    induction and consolidation therapy 87
    induction therapy 87
    salvage therapy 89–90
  staging 81, 83
  stem cell transplantation 91–93
  treatment
    first-line 85
    fludarabine-refractory patients 90–91
    indications 84–85
    response assessment 84–85
    response criteria 85
    salvage therapy 88–90
  ZAP-70 expression 84
chronic lymphocytic leukemia/ small lymphocytic lymphoma (CLL/SLL) 238
  prognostic markers 238
chronic lymphoproliferative diseases 19–20
chronic myeloid leukemia (CML) 20, 68–76, 141
  accelerated phase 68–69
  Bcr-Abl oncoprotein 68–69
  blastic phase 68–69

chronic myeloid leukemia (CML) (*cont.*)
  bosutinib therapy 73–74
  chronic phase 68–69
  dasatinib therapy 72–73, 75–76
  diagnosis 69, 145
  differential diagnosis 69–70
  epidemiology 68
  etiology 68
  FISH analysis 69
  imatinib therapy 70–72, 75, 76
    dose escalation 71–72
    interferon combination 75
    resistance 71, 75
    response optimization 70–71
  incidence 68
  interferon therapy 75
  manifestations 69
  multikinase inhibitors 74
  nilotinib therapy 73, 75–76
  non-tyrosine kinase inhibitors 74–75
  omacetaxine therapy 74–75
  pathogenesis 68–69
  Philadelphia chromosome 68–69
  response assessment 71
  RT-PCR 69
  signs/symptoms 69
  staging 69
  stem cell transplantation 70
  translocations 69
  treatment 70–76
    combination 75
    decision-making 76
    resistance prevention 75–76
    response assessment 71
  trisomy 8 69
  tyrosine kinase inhibitors 70–72, 75
    second-generation 72–76

chronic myelomonocytic leukemia (CMML) 105–107
  hypomethylating agents 110–111

chronic myeloproliferative diseases
  CML 20
  non-CML 20–21

chronic myeloproliferative neoplasia (MPN) 20

chronic neutrophilia leukemia 141

cigarette smoking
  ALL risk 44
  Hodgkin lymphoma association 371

9-cis-retinoic acid, acute promyelocytic leukemia 132

cKIT mutations, AML 36

cladribine
  CLL 86
    fludarabine-refractory patients 90–91
    salvage therapy 89
  hairy cell leukemia 123–125
    retreatment 125
  infections 124
  Waldenstrom's macroglobulinemia treatment 215–217

clofarabine
  AML management 37
  Ara-C combination 37
  myelodysplastic syndromes 111
  relapsed ALL 59

clonality detection methods, lymphomas 258–260

clorezatine, AML management 37

CMC-544 immunoconjugate, follicular lymphoma 353

c-Myc gene, Burkitt lymphoma 496–497

cold agglutinin hemolytic anemia 211

comparative genomic hybridization (CGH), lymphoma 262

computed tomography (CT)
  Burkitt lymphoma 497
  hepatosplenic T-cell lymphoma 423
  lymphoma 277–278
  peripheral T-cell lymphoma 411
  primary central nervous system lymphoma 452
    HIV-related 473

connective tissue disease, cryoglobulinemia 194–195

core binding factor (CBF) abnormalities in AML 16–17

corticosteroids
  ALL treatment
    adolescents and young adults 57
    mature B-cell 53
  amyloidosis treatment 188–189
  multiple myeloma 171
  mycosis fungoides/Sézary syndrome 438
  primary central nervous system lymphoma 451

cranial irradiation, ALL treatment 50

cryoglobulinemia 194–196
  anti-CD20 therapy 196
  HCV association 196
  IgM 210
  interferon 196
  laboratory studies 195
  pathology 195
  plasma exchange/plasmapheresis 196
  rituximab therapy 196
  signs/symptoms 195
  splenectomy for hypersplenism 196
  treatment 196
  Waldenstrom's macroglobulinemia 210, 211

cutaneous anaplastic large cell lymphoma (C-ALCL) 242, 416, 432

cutaneous CD30-positive T-cell lymphoproliferative disorders 242

cutaneous T-cell lymphomas 432
  $p16^{INK4a}$ tumor suppressor gene 269
  pathogenesis 433
  see also anaplastic large cell lymphoma, primary cutaneous; lymphomatoid papulosis; mycosis fungoides; Sézary syndrome

CVP (cyclophosphamide, vincristine, and prednisone), follicular lymphoma 355

cyclin D1
  lymphoma 265
  mantle cell lymphoma 309, 312
    cyclin D1-negative 311
    overexpression 310–311

cyclophosphamide
  ALL treatment 48–50
    adolescents and young adults 57
    mature B-cell 53
    older adults 58
  CLL 84
  multiple myeloma 171
  POEMS syndrome treatment 193
  Waldenstrom's macroglobulinemia treatment 216–217

ciclosporin, AML management 27–28

cytarabine (cytosine arabinoside [Ara-C]
  acute promyelocytic leukemia 135–136
  ALL treatment 48–50
    adolescents and young adults 57
  clofarabine combination 37
  consolidation chemotherapy for AML 29
  induction chemotherapy for AML 26
  secondary central nervous system lymphoma 458

cytomegalovirus (CMV) reactivation with alemtuzumab 88

darbepoetin, myelodysplastic syndrome treatment 108–109

dasatinib, CML 72–73, 75–76

daunorubicin
  ALL treatment 48
    adolescents and young adults 57
    older adults 58
  induction chemotherapy for AML 26

DCC-2036 multikinase inhibitor 74

death receptor pathway, targeting in follicular lymphoma 353–354

decitabine, myelodysplastic syndromes 110–111

del(5q) abnormalities, AML 17

del(7q) abnormalities, AML 17

dendritic cells, follicular lymphoma 339

denileukin diftitox, mycosis fungoides/Sézary syndrome 441

depsipeptide, peripheral T-cell lymphoma 426

dexamethasone, ALL treatment 48–50

dickkopf 1 (DDK1), multiple myeloma 163–164

diffuse large B-cell lymphoma (DLBCL) 231–235
  activated B-cell-like 266–267
  anatomic site-specific 234
  anthracyclines 290–291
  arising in HHV-8-associated MCD 233
  BCL2 gene 263–264, 290
  BCL6 gene 290
  Burkitt lymphoma differential diagnosis 495–496
  CHOP therapy 290–291
    advanced disease 291–292
    treatment improvement 293
  chronic inflammation-association 233–234

clinical presentation 286–287
CNS recurrence 295–296
diagnosis 286–287
EBV-associated
immunodeficiency 233
non-immunodeficient 233–234
of the elderly 233–234
etoposide prophylaxis 296
gene expression profiling 288–290
gene expression subgroups 266–267
germinal center B-cell-like 266–267
HHV-8 associated 233
high-dose chemotherapy with stem cell transplantation 294–295
histology 464
HIV-related 464–468
chemoimmunotherapy 465–468
chemotherapy 465, 467
clinical features 464
infusional chemotherapy 465
pathology 464–465
rituximab 465–468
treatment 465–468
viral infections 465
immunohistochemistry 290
initial therapy
advanced disease 291–292
localized disease 290–291
International Prognostic Index 288, 290
lymph nodes 287
minimal residual disease
adjuvant strategies 299
reduction 293–294
not otherwise specified 231–235
primary refractory 295
prognosis 288–290
recurrence in CNS 295–296
relapsed 296–301
allogeneic stem cell transplantation 299–300
non-transplant eligible patients 300
rituximab 291
advanced disease 291–292
CNS recurrence 295–296
induction therapy 294
treatment improvement 293
staging 287–288
stem cell transplantation 294–295
adjuvant strategies for minimal residual disease 299
allogeneic 299–300
autologous 296–299
conditioning regimens 298
non-myeloablative 300
patient outcome 297
reduced-intensity transplants 300
relapsed disease 296–299
residual disease detection 297
salvage regimens 298
subgroups 267, 286, 289
treatment 286–301
high-dose chemotherapy with stem cell transplantation 294–295
infusional administration 293
minimal residual disease reduction 293–294
primary refractory 295
relapsed disease 296–301
stem cell transplantation for relapsed disease 296–299

DNA microarray technology, lymphoma 262

Down syndrome *see* trisomy 21

doxorubicin
ALL treatment 48–50
adolescents and young adults 57
pegylated 442

eltrombopag, myelodysplastic syndromes 109

enteropathy-type T-cell lymphoma 243, 423–425
celiac disease association 423–425
chemotherapy 425
chromosomal alterations 268
clinical features 424
cytogenetics 424
intraepithelial T lymphocytes 423–424
management 424–425
pathology 424
staging 424

environmental factors, ALL risk 44

epigenetic therapy, myelodysplastic syndromes 110–111

EPOCH regimen, mantle cell lymphoma 317–318

epratuzumab
ALL treatment 60
follicular lymphoma 352–353
mantle cell lymphoma 323

Epstein–Barr virus (EBV)
angioimmunoblastic T-cell lymphoma 414
Burkitt lymphoma 468
HIV-related diffuse large B-cell lymphoma 465
HIV-related Hodgkin lymphoma 475
HIV-related lymphomas 462
HIV-related primary CNS lymphoma 473
HIV-related T-cell lymphoma 476
Hodgkin lymphoma 375
association 369–370
therapy targeting 393
large B-cell lymphomas 233
plasmablastic lymphoma 470–471
primary effusion lymphoma 472
systemic EBV-positive T-cell LPD of childhood 244

erythropoietin, myelodysplastic syndrome treatment 108–109

essential thrombocythemia 141, 144
clinical manifestations 145–146
diagnosis 145
epidemiology 145
hydroxyurea 148
JAK2 mutations 147–148
laboratory features 146–147
megakaryocytes 144
pregnancy 149–150
prognosis 147
risk stratification 148
treatment 148
WHO classification 143

European Organization for Research and Treatment of Cancer (EORTC), cutaneous lymphoma classification 246–247

everolimus, mantle cell lymphoma 325

extracorporeal photopheresis, mycosis fungoides/Sézary syndrome 440–441

extranodal natural killer T-cell lymphoma, nasal type 421–423
chemotherapy 421–422
clinical features 421
epidemiology 421
management 421–422
pathology 421
radiation therapy 421–422
staging 421
stem cell transplantation with high-dose chemotherapy 422

extraosseous plasmacytoma 237–238

ezatiostat, myelodysplastic syndromes 111

Fanconi's anemia, ALL risk 43

farnesyl transferase inhibition, AML management 37

^{18}F-fluorodeoxyglucose/positron emission tomography (FDG-PET)
Burkitt lymphoma 497
hepatosplenic T-cell lymphoma 423
Hodgkin lymphoma 372
outcome prediction 374–375
lymphoma
indications 280
response assessment 280
restaging 279
staging 278–279
during treatment 279
multiple myeloma 164
peripheral T-cell lymphoma 411

FGFR1 abnormalities, MPN 21

filgrastim, neutropenia 108–109

FIP1L1-PDGFRA fusion, MPN 21

flavopiridol
ALL treatment 60–61
mantle cell lymphoma 327

FLT3 gene mutations, AML 17, 34–36

FLT3 inhibitors, AML management 34, 38

FLT3 receptor, acute promyelocytic leukemia 134

fludarabine
AML management 29
CLL 84, 86
salvage therapy 89
follicular lymphoma 354–355
mantle cell lymphoma 319–320
monoclonal gammopathy of undetermined significance with peripheral neuropathy 198
mycosis fungoides/Sézary syndrome 443
rituximab combination 354–355
Waldenstrom's macroglobulinemia 215–217

fluorescence *in situ* hybridization (FISH)
CLL 82
CML 69
lymphomas 260–261, 264, 266
multicolor for lymphoma 262

fms-related tyrosine kinase 3 (FLT3) *see* FLT3 *entries*

follicular lymphoma
alemtuzumab 351–352
algorithm for approach to patients 345
anti-CD20 antibodies 354
anti-CD22 antibodies 352–353

follicular lymphoma (*cont.*)
radioimmunoconjugates/ immunotoxins 353
anti-CD80 antibodies 353
BCL2 family inhibitors 358
biology 338–339
bortezomib 358
chemotherapy timing 343–344
CHOP therapy 341
rituximab combination 354
CMC-544 immunoconjugate 353
CVP regimen 355
death receptor pathway targeting 353–354
dendritic cells 339
dual model 339
epratuzumab 352–353
FLIPI 339–340
fludarabine, rituximab combination 354–355
galiximab 353
gene expression signatures 340–341
gene profiling data extrapolation 341–342
gene profiling microarrays 341
IL-2 therapy 344
immunohistochemical biomarkers 341–342
interferon 344
chemotherapy and rituximab combination 355–356
karyotype abnormalities 338
lexatumumab 353–354
MALT lymphoma distinction 270
mapatumumab 353–354
nodal marginal zone lymphoma distinction 269
ofatumumab 354
oligonucleotide microarrays 341
pathogenesis 338–339
prognosis 338–339
prognostic factors 339–342
radioimmunotherapy 356–357
risk stratification 339–342
rituximab 344–347
chemotherapy combination 350, 354–356
extended schedules 347–351
maintenance therapy 347–351
maintenance therapy following chemoimmunotherapy 349–351
maintenance therapy following chemotherapy 349
RNAse A 353
small molecules 358–359
SNPs 341
stem cell transplantation with high-dose chemotherapy 357–358
survival prediction 340–341
T cells 339
translocations 338
treatment 342–359
biologic agents 344
chemotherapy 342–344
chemotherapy combination with rituximab 350, 354–356
chemotherapy novel agents 358–359
goals 359
monoclonal antibodies 344–357
monoclonal antibody radioimmunotherapy 356–357
proteasome inhibitors 358
timing of initiation 342–344
watchful waiting 343

Follicular Lymphoma International Prognostic Index (FLIPI) 339, 340

follicular lymphoma/leukemia 20, 235–236
BCL2 gene 263–264
$p16^{INK4a}$ tumor suppressor gene 269

fractures, multiple myeloma 172

free light chain (FLC) assay 155–158

French–American–British (FAB) classification
ALL 44
APL 131
myelodysplastic syndromes 105–106

galectin-1, Hodgkin lymphoma 392

galiximab, follicular lymphoma 353

gamma-secretase inhibitor (GSI) 491

gemcitabine, mycosis fungoides/ Sézary syndrome 442

gemtuzumab ozogamicin (GO)
acute promyelocytic leukemia 134
AML management 28, 36–37

gene amplifications/deletions in leukemia 14

gene expression
changes in leukemia 14–16
profiling in lymphoma 262

gene mutations, leukemia 1

granulocyte colony-stimulating factor (G-CSF)
ALL treatment 48, 58–59
AML treatment 27, 29

granulocyte–macrophage colony-stimulating factor (GM-CSF)
ALL treatment 58–59
AML treatment 27
neutropenia 108–109

growth factors
AML 27
hematopoietic, myelodysplastic syndromes 108–109

hairy B-cell lymphoproliferative disorder 117

hairy cell leukemia 116–126
acid phosphatase staining 120
biology 116–117
BL-22 recombinant immunotoxin therapy 125
blood lakes 119
blood studies 118
bone marrow 118
cladribine therapy 123–125
retreatment 125
clinical features 117–118
cytochemistry 119
cytopenia 125
diagnosis and treatment strategy 125
differential diagnosis 121
electron microscopy 119–120
epidemiology/etiology 116
familial 116
histology 119
immunophenotype 120–121
interferon therapy 122
retreatment 125
laboratory features 118–121
liver 119
lymph nodes 119
minimal residual disease 125
monocytopenia association 116
pancytopenia 118
pathology 117–121
pentostatin therapy 123
retreatment 125
presenting features 118
purine nucleoside analogs 122–124
rituximab salvage therapy 125
salvage therapies 124–125
spleen 118–119
splenectomy 121–122
treatment 121–126
failure 124

hairy cell leukemia-variant 121

hairy cells 116, 119
B-cell association 117
immunoglobulins 117
ontogeny 116–117
p53 mutations 117

heat-shock protein 90, Hodgkin lymphoma 392

heavy chain diseases 237

Helicobacter pylori in MALT lymphoma 404–405
treatment 405

hepatitis C virus, cryoglobulinemia association 196

hepatosplenic T-cell lymphoma 243, 422–423
chemotherapy 423
clinical features 423
cytogenetics 422–423
imaging 423
immunosuppression 423
management 423
pathology 422–423
stem cell therapy with high-dose chemotherapy 423

highly active antiretroviral therapy (HAART)
HIV-related lymphoma association 462
chemotherapy use 463–464
prognosis 462–463
HIV-related multicentric Castleman's disease 477
HIV-related primary central nervous system lymphoma 473–474
Hodgkin lymphoma 370
non-Hodgkin lymphoma association 462

histone deacetylases (HDAC)
Hodgkin lymphoma 392
mantle cell lymphoma 326

histone deacetylase (HDAC) inhibitors, mycosis fungoides/Sézary syndrome 441–442

HIV infection
Hodgkin lymphoma association 370
large B-cell lymphomas associated with EBV 233
primary central nervous system lymphoma 449

HIV-related lymphomas 462–478
antiretrovirals use with chemotherapy 463–464
chemotherapy
with stem cell transplantation 477–478
use with antiretrovirals 463–464
diagnosis 463
diffuse large B-cell lymphoma 464–468
epidemiology/etiology 462
HAART association 462

chemotherapy use 463–464
prognosis 462–463
Hodgkin lymphoma 475–476
leptomeningeal lymphoma 474–475
multicentric Castleman's disease 477
plasmablastic lymphoma 466, 470–471
primary central nervous system lymphoma 466, 472–474
primary effusion lymphoma 466, 471–472
prognosis 462–463
relapsed/refractory 477–478
staging 463
stem cell transplantation 477–478
T-cell lymphoma 476
viral infections 462
see also Burkitt-like lymphoma; Burkitt lymphoma

HLA class II expression, Hodgkin lymphoma 375

Hodgkin and Reed–Sternberg (H-RS) cells 371
HIV-related Hodgkin lymphoma 475
IL-4 receptors 393

Hodgkin lymphoma 244–245, 367–393
ABVD regimen 380–382
advanced stage 374
IPS 374
radiation therapy 383–384
treatment 380–387
trials 384
anti-CD20 antibodies 391–392
anti-CD25 antibodies 392
anti-CD30 antibodies 390–391
apoptotic pathways 371
autoimmune factors 370–371
BEACOPP regimen 381, 383
biology 371
bone marrow involvement 372
bortezomib 392
CD95 mutations 371
cell morphology 245
c-FLIP 371, 392
cigarette smoking 371
classical 244–245, 371
lymphocyte-depleted 244–245
lymphocyte-rich 244
mixed cellularity 244
nodular sclerosis 244
classification 373
clinical presentation 373
clonal B cells 371
cumulative risk 390
early stage 374, 378
chemotherapy alone 378–380
favorable 375–377
treatment 375–380
unfavorable 377–378
EBV association 369–370, 375
therapy targeting 393
elderly 389–390
clinical presentation 390
treatment 390, 391
epidemiology 367–371
etiology 369–371
extranodal disease 373
FDG-PET 372
outcome prediction 374–375
galectin-1 392
genetic factors 369, 371
HAART treatment 370
histone deacetylases 392
HIV infection association 370
HIV-related 475–476
chemotherapy 475–476
clinical features 475
EBV 475
pathologic features 475
treatment 475–476
HLA class II expression 375
hsp-90 inhibition 392
hybrid regimens 380–382
IKKs 371, 392
incidence 367–371
infections 369–370
intermediate stage 379
MOPP regimen 380–382
dose intensity 383
NF-κB 371, 392
nodular lymphocyte predominant 244–245, 371, 387–389
bleomycin toxicity 388
cardiovascular disease 389
rituximab therapy 387–388
secondary cancers after treatment 388–389
stages 387
toxicity of treatment 388–389
treatment 387–389
p16^{INK4a} tumor suppressor gene 269
p53 mutations 392–393
prevalence 367–371
prognosis 374–375
radiotherapy 383–384
relapsed/refractory disease 384–387
rituximab 391–392
staging 371–373
stem cell transplantation
allogeneic 385, 388
autologous 385, 386, 387
chemotherapy-alone conditioning 385
prognosis 385–387
radiation-based conditioning 385
transcription 371
treatment 375–387
advanced stage 380–387
biological therapies 390–391
chemotherapy 375–383
chemotherapy dose intensity 383
chemotherapy trials 384
early stage 375–380
intermediate stage 377–379
new therapeutic options 390–393
radioimmunotherapy 392
radiotherapy 377–378
risk factor groups 374
small molecules 392
Tregs 375
XIAP antiapoptotic molecule 392

HOX gene family, ALL 19

human herpesvirus 8 (HHV8)
diffuse large B-cell lymphoma 233
HIV-related diffuse large B-cell lymphoma 465
HIV-related lymphomas 462
plasmablastic lymphoma 470–471
primary effusion lymphoma 472

human papilloma virus (HPV), HIV-related lymphomas 462

human T-cell lymphotropic virus (HTLV) 419–420

hydroa vacciniforme-like lymphoma 244

hydroxyurea
essential thrombocythemia 148
polycythemia vera 148
primary myelofibrosis 149

hypercalcemia, multiple myeloma 172

HyperCVAD regimen, mantle cell lymphoma 318–319

hyperviscosity syndrome
IgM 208–210
multiple myeloma 173
Waldenstrom's macroglobulinemia 208–210, 212–213

hypomethylating agents, myelodysplastic syndromes 110–111

ibritumomab tiuxetan, mantle cell lymphoma 323–324

idarubicin, induction chemotherapy for AML 26

idiopathic thrombocytopenic purpura (ITP), Hodgkin lymphoma association 370

IG gene, rearrangements
lymphoid malignancy clonal marker 257–258
in lymphoma 257, 261

IGH gene
Burkitt lymphoma 265–266
PCR analysis of gene locus 259

IgH translocations
monoclonal gammopathy of undetermined significance 158
plasma cell leukemia 175
smoldering multiple myeloma 161

IGHV gene, B-cell lymphoma 268

IgM, Waldenstrom's macroglobulinemia 208–212

IgM-related neuropathy, Waldenstrom's macroglobulinemia 210

IgV$_H$ genes, CLL 83–84

Iκ kinases (IKKs), Hodgkin lymphoma 371, 392

IKZF1 gene abnormalities, ALL 18

IL3-IGH translocation, ALL 19

imatinib
CML treatment 70–72, 75, 76
cytogenetic response 70–71
dose escalation 71–72
interferon combination 75
Philadelphia-positive ALL 55–58
resistance 71, 75

IMiDs, side effects in multiple myeloma 173–174

immune modulation therapy
mycosis fungoides/Sézary syndrome 444
myelodysplastic syndromes 109–110

immunodeficiency
adult T-cell leukemia/lymphoma 420
hepatosplenic T-cell lymphoma 423
mycosis fungoides 433–434
Sézary syndrome 433–434

immunodeficiency-associated lymphoproliferative disease 246

immunoglobulin M (IgM)
autoantibody activity 210

immunoglobulin M (IgM) (*cont.*)
cold agglutinin hemolytic anemia 211
cryoglobulinemia 210
hyperviscosity syndrome 208–210
tissue deposition 211–212
Waldenstrom's macroglobulinemia 208–212
physicochemical/ immunologic properties 209
treatment response 220–221

immunoglobulins (Ig)
hairy cells 117
monoclonal 155–158
quantitative studies 155

immunologic approaches, AML management 31–34

immunoproliferative small intestinal disease (IPSID) 237

infections
adult T-cell leukemia/ lymphoma 420
cladribine 124
cryoglobulinemia 194–195
Hodgkin lymphoma 369–370
multiple myeloma 173
pentostatin 123

INNO-406, ALL treatment 60

interferon therapy
adult T-cell leukemia/ lymphoma 420
cryoglobulinemia treatment 196
follicular lymphoma 344
chemotherapy and rituximab combination 355–356
hairy cell leukemia 122
retreatment 125
hairy cells 122
imatinib combination 75
multiple myeloma maintenance therapy 171
mycosis fungoides/Sézary syndrome 439–440
with PUVA 439–440

interleukin 2 (IL-2)
AML management 31–34
follicular lymphoma 344
mycosis fungoides/Sézary syndrome 444

interleukin 3 (IL-3), multiple myeloma 163–164

interleukin 4 (IL-4) receptors, H-RS cells 393

interleukin 7 (IL-7), multiple myeloma 163–164

interleukin 12 (IL-12), mycosis fungoides/Sézary syndrome 444

International Prognostic Index (IPI)
diffuse large B-cell lymphoma 288, 290
follicular, mantle cell lymphoma 313–314
follicular lymphoma 339
Hodgkin lymphoma 374
peripheral T-cell lymphoma 411–412

International Prognostic Scoring System (IPPS), myelodysplastic syndromes 106

International Working Group response criteria, myelodysplastic syndromes 109

intraepithelial T lymphocytes (IELs), enteropathy-type T-cell lymphoma 423, 424

intravascular large B-cell lymphoma (IVLBCL) 234

ionizing radiation
ALL risk 44
CML risk 68
myelodysplastic syndrome risk 103

iron chelation therapy, myelodysplastic syndromes 108

ITK gene, peripheral T-cell lymphoma, not otherwise specified 268

JAK2 mutations
MPN 20–21
myeloproliferative neoplasms 144, 147–148
polycythemia vera 147
primary myelofibrosis 148
refractory anemia with ringed sideroblasts and thrombocytosis 107

Kaposi's sarcoma, HIV-related multicentric Castleman's disease association 476–477

Kaposi's sarcoma-associated herpes virus (KSHV), HIV-related multicentric Castleman's disease 476–477

Ki-67 proliferation index
mantle cell lymphoma 314–317
peripheral T-cell lymphoma 412

lactate dehydrogenase (LDH), mycosis fungoides/Sézary syndrome 435, 437

large B-cell lymphoma 234
ALK-positive 234
see also diffuse large B-cell lymphoma (DLBCL)

lenalidomide
amyloidosis treatment 189
mantle cell lymphoma 325
multiple myeloma 172
mycosis fungoides/Sézary syndrome 444
myelodysplastic syndromes 110
primary myelofibrosis 149
side effects in multiple myeloma 173–174
Waldenstrom's macroglobulinemia 218–219

lenalidomide-dexamethasone, multiple myeloma 168

leptomeningeal lymphoma, HIV-related 474–475
CSF examination 474–475
diagnosis 474–475
intrathecal chemotherapy 475
prophylaxis 475
risk factors 474
treatment 475

leukemia
chromosomal translocations 1
gene amplifications 14, 16
gene deletion 14, 16
gene expression changes 14–16
gene mutations 1, 15
methylation 16
molecular pathology 1–21
translocations 2

leukemoid reactions, CML differential diagnosis 69

lexatumumab, follicular lymphoma 353–354

liver disease
cryoglobulinemia 194–195
hairy cell leukemia 119

lymphoblastic lymphoma 487–492
B-cell 487
bone marrow disease prognosis 491
chemotherapy 488–489
CNS disease 489
intrathecal 489
clinical presentation 487
CNS disease
management 489
prognosis 491
cranial radiation 489
diagnosis 487
intensive induction regimens 489
mediastinal radiation 490
nelarabine 492
pathology/pathogenesis 487–488
prognosis 489, 491
radiation/therapy
cranial 489
mediastinal 490
relapse 489
staging 487
stem cell transplantation 490–491
T-cell 487–488
treatment 488–489
algorithm 490

lymphoid leukemias, mature B-cell neoplasms 238

lymphomas
AP12 gene 265
BCL6 gene 264–265
CCND1 proto-oncogene 265
chromosomal translocation detection methods 258–260
classification 289
clonality detection methods 258–260
comparative genomic hybridization 262
CT scans 277–278
cyclin D1 265
cytogenetic analysis 258–260
diagnostic algorithm 258
DNA microarray technology 262
dual translocation 266
FDG-PET
indications 280
response assessment 280
restaging 279
staging 278–279
during treatment 279
FISH analysis 260–261, 264, 266
gene expression profiling 262
IG gene rearrangements 257
PCR analysis 261
International Harmonization Project 279–280
IWG guidelines 277–278
IWG response criteria 279–280
leukemic component 235
mature B-cell neoplasms 231–238
molecular diagnostics limitations 270
molecular pathology 270
morphologic patterns 232
multicolor FISH 262
occult systemic 450
p16^{INK4a} tumor suppressor gene 269

p53 mutations 268–269
PCR analysis 261–262
PET/CT imaging 278–279
precursor lymphoid neoplasms 231
response criteria 279–283
clinical trials 281
revised 280–283
Southern blot analysis 260
staging 277–279, 289
TCR gene rearrangements 257
PCR analysis 261
testicular 457
TP53 gene 268–269
translocations 264, 266
treatment 277–278
WHO classification 228–247, 410
see also named lymphomas

lymphomatoid granulomatosis 233–234

lymphomatoid papulosis 242, 432

lymphoplasmacytic lymphoma 207–221, 237
see also Waldenstrom's macroglobulinemia (WM)

lymphoproliferative disease
cryoglobulinemia 194–195
immunodeficiency-associated 246

M protein 155–158
monoclonal gammopathy of undetermined significance 158
with peripheral neuropathy 197

magnetic resonance imaging (MRI), primary CNS lymphoma 450–452, 457
HIV-related 473

mantle cell lymphoma 236, 308–327
alemtuzumab 323
angiogenesis inhibitors 325
anti-CD20 antibodies 322–323
anti-CD22 antibodies 323
anti-CD52 antibodies 323
antisense oligonucleotides 325–326
AP23573 therapy 325
apoptosis targeting 325–326
ATM gene 311–312
BCL2 family inhibitors 326
BCL2 gene 311–312
bendamustine 320
bevacizumab 325
biologic agents 324–325
bortezomib 324
carfilzomib (PR171) 325
cell of origin 309–310
CHOP therapy 317–318
chromosome translocations 310
clinical presentation 312–313
CLL differentiation 269
cyclin D1 309, 312
overexpression 310–311
cyclin D1-negative 311
cytologic variants 310
diagnosis 308–309
epidemiology 308
EPOCH regimen 317–318
epratuzumab 323
everolimus 325
extrinsic pathway targeting 326
flavopiridol 327
fludarabine 319–320
follicular IPI 313–314
gastrointestinal tract involvement 314
genomic defects 311–313
graft-versus-tumor effect 323
high-dose therapy with stem cell transplantation 320
histone deacetylases 326
HyperCVAD regimen 318–319
ibritumomab tiuxetan 323–324
idiotype vaccine 323
initial oncogenic event 310
Ki-67 proliferation index 314–317
lenalidomide 325
lymphoma prognostic index 315
microRNAs 315–316
monoclonal antibodies 322–323
mTOR inhibitors 325
NF-κB stabilizers 327
novel cytotoxics 320
NPI-0052 325
nucleoside analogs 319–320
p16^{INK4a} tumor suppressor gene 269
p53 311–312
pathogenesis 309–310, 313
pathology 308–309
pixantrone 320
PKC inhibitors 327
PRAD1 gene 310
prognostic factors 313–316
proliferation gene expression signature 316
proteasome inhibitors 324–325
radioimmunotherapy 320, 323–324
rituximab 320–322
secondary genomic alterations 311–312
SNPs 315–316
somatic mutations 309–310
stem cell transplantation 320–321
allogeneic 323
subtypes 309
survival pathway dysregulation 312–313
TBI 320
temsirolimus 325
thalidomide 325
tositumomab 323–324
translocations 309
treatment 316–327
chemotherapy 317–320, 322
immune-based therapy 322–323
VGEF-trap 325
Wnt signaling pathway 311–312

mapatumumab, follicular lymphoma 353–354

marginal zone lymphoma 404–408
extranodal 404–406
non-gastric 406
management algorithm 406
nodal 236–237
follicular lymphoma distinction 269
primary nodal 404, 407
radioimmunotherapy 407
radiotherapy 407
stem cell transplantation 407
treatment 407
splenic 121, 404, 407–408
see also mucosa-associated lymphoid tissue (MALT) lymphoma

mastocytosis, systemic 141

megakaryocytes, essential thrombocythemia 144

melphalan
amyloidosis treatment 186, 188–189
POEMS syndrome treatment 193

6-mercaptopurine, ALL treatment 48–50
adolescents and young adults 57

methotrexate
ALL treatment 48–50
adolescents and young adults 57
intrathecal 50
CNS lymphoblastic lymphoma 489
HIV-related primary central nervous system lymphoma 474
primary central nervous system lymphoma 453–456
secondary central nervous system lymphoma 458

methylation, leukemia 16

microRNAs 14–16
ALL 46
mantle cell lymphoma 315–316

Miller–Fisher syndrome 210

mitoxantrone
ALL treatment 48–50
induction chemotherapy for AML 26

MK-0457 multikinase inhibitor 74

MLL gene abnormalities in AML 17

monoclonal B-cell lymphocytosis 19
diagnosis 83

monoclonal gammopathy of undetermined significance (MGUS) 155, 158–161
clinical features 160
cytogenetic changes 158
diagnostic criteria 156
differential diagnosis 160
epidemiology 158
IgH translocations 158
M protein 158
management 161
pathogenesis 158
with peripheral neuropathy 198
peripheral neuropathy-associated 196–198
clinical features 197
fludarabine 198
IVIG therapy 198
M protein 197
pathogenesis 196–197
plasma exchange 197
rituximab 198
treatment 197–198
prognosis 160–161
progression risk to multiple myeloma 158, 160, 162
risk stratification 162
serum free light chain ratio 160–161

monoclonal proteins
laboratory testing 155–158
screening in amyloidosis 184–185

monocytoid B lymphocyte 117

monocytopenia, hairy cell leukemia association 116

monosomy 5, AML 17

monosomy 7, AML 17

MOPP (mechlorethamine, vincristine, procarbazine, and prednisone), Hodgkin lymphoma 380–382
dose intensity 383

motor neuron disease, Waldenstrom's macroglobulinemia 210

MPL mutations
MPN 21
myeloproliferative neoplasms 144

mTOR pathway
ALL 60, 491
inhibitors 325

mucosa-associated lymphoid tissue (MALT) lymphoma 236–237
extranodal marginal zone lymphoma 236, 404–406
follicular lymphoma distinction 270
gastric 405–406
chemotherapy 405
diagnosis 405
response to therapy 406
rituximab 405
staging 405
surgical management 405–406
treatment 405–406
Helicobacter pylori 404–405
treatment 405
t(11;18) translocation 265

multicentric Castleman's disease 233
HIV-related 477
antiviral therapy 477
chemotherapy 477
clinical features 477
epidemiology 476–477
HAART 477
Kaposi's sarcoma association 476–477
pathologic features 477
prognosis 477
rituximab 477
splenectomy 477
treatment 477

multikinase inhibitors, CML 74

multiple myeloma (MM) 155, 162–174
anemia 173
angiogenesis 160
bone disease identification 163
bone lesion pathogenesis 163–164
bone marrow studies 163
bortezomib 171
side effects 174
clinical features 162
complications 172–173
constipation risk with treatment 174
corticosteroids 171
cyclophosphamide 171
diagnosis 162–164
diagnostic criteria 156
differential diagnosis 164
epidemiology 162
FDG-PET 164
hypercalcemia 172
hyperviscosity syndrome 173
hypothyroidism risk with treatment 174
IgM 174
infections 173
initial therapy
patients eligible for stem cell therapy 165–169
patients ineligible for stem cell therapy 169
interferon maintenance therapy 171
laboratory studies 162–163
lenalidomide 172
side effects 173–174
management 165–172
high-risk disease 170
investigational 444
maintenance therapy 171
newly diagnosed disease 166
relapsed disease 171–172
monoclonal gammopathy of undetermined significance differential diagnosis 160
myelosuppression risk with treatment 174
novel agent side effects 173–174
pamidronate maintenance therapy 171
pathogenesis 158–160
peripheral neuropathy risk with treatment 174
prognosis 162, 164–165
progression from monoclonal gammopathy of undetermined significance 158, 160, 162
renal insufficiency 173, 174
response criteria 167
risk stratification 165
serum protein electrophoresis 159
side effects with novel agents 173–174
skeletal lesions 163, 172
skin rash risk with treatment 173–174
smoldering 161–162
clinical features 161
diagnostic criteria 156
differential diagnosis 161
IgH translocation 161
M proteins 161
management 161–162
prognosis 161
progression to symptomatic disease 161
risk stratification 161
staging 164
stem cell transplantation 165, 169–170
allogeneic 170
autologous 169–170
tandem autologous 170
teratogenicity risk of treatment 173
thalidomide 171
maintenance therapy 171
side effects 173–174
venous thromboembolism risk 173

c-MYC oncogene
Burkitt lymphoma 265–266
overexpression in ALL 53

mycosis fungoides 243, 432–445
alemtuzumab 441
bexarotene 439–440
biologic characteristics 433–434
bortezomib 444
carmustine 439
chemotherapy
multiagent 443
single agent 442–443
classification 432–433, 436
clinical signs 432, 434–435
corticosteroids 438
denileukin diftitox 441
diagnosis 435–436
epidemiology 432
etiology 432–433
extracorporeal photopheresis 440–441
fludarabine 443
gemcitabine 442
histone deacetylase inhibitors 441–442
HIV-related 476
IL-2 444
IL-12 444
immunodeficiency 433–434
immunomodulatory agents 444
immunophenotyping 435
interferon 439–440
lactate dehydrogenase 435, 437
lenalidomide 444
management 435–436
molecular characteristics 433–434
monoclonal antibodies 441
investigational 444
nitrogen mustard 439
$p16^{INK4a}$ tumor suppressor gene 269
pathogenesis 433
pegylated doxorubicin 442
pentostatin 442–443
phototherapy 437–438
prognosis 444–445
prognostic markers 437
proteosome inhibitors 444
radiation therapy 439
retinoids 439, 440
romidepsin 442
staging 436–437
stem cell transplantation 443
survival 437
T helper cell dysregulation 433–434
temozolomide 443
treatment 437–444
algorithm 438
systemic 439–443
topical 437–439
vorinostat 442
zanolimumab 444

myelodysplastic syndromes 103–112
antilymphocyte globulins 109–110
antithymocyte globulins 109–110
arsenic trioxide therapy 111
azacitidine therapy 110
classification 105–107, 141–143
clinical features 103–104
clofarabine therapy 111
CML differential diagnosis 69
cytogenetic abnormalities 104–105
darbepoietin therapy 108–109
decitabine therapy 110–111
eltrombopag therapy 109
epidemiology/etiology 103
epigenetic therapy 110–111
erythropoietin therapy 108–109
ezatiostat therapy 111
hematopoietic growth factors 108–109
high-intensity therapy 111–112
hypocellular 107
hypomethylating agent therapy 110–111
immune modulation therapy 109–110
International Prognostic Scoring System 106
International Working Group response criteria 109
investigational therapies 111
iron chelation therapy 108
karyotype 105
laboratory features 103–104
lenalidomide therapy 110
low-intensity therapy 108–109
morphologic criteria of dysplasia 104
with myelofibrosis 107
neutropenia 108–109
obatoclax therapy 111
pathogenesis 104–105
risk factors 103
romiplostim therapy 109
stem cell transplantation 112
supportive therapy 108–109
survival 105
thrombocytopenia 109

treatment 107–112
algorithm 107
tyrosine kinase inhibitors 111

myelofibrosis *see* primary myelofibrosis

myeloid neoplasms, WHO classification 142

myeloproliferative neoplasms 107, 141–150
chronic
chronic myeloproliferative neoplasia 20
CML 20
non-CML 20–21
classification 141–143
clinical manifestations 145–146
CML differential diagnosis 69
cytogenetics 144
diagnosis 144–145
epidemiology 145
historical perspective 141
JAK2 mutations 144, 147–148
laboratory features 146–147
molecular pathogenesis 144
morphology 141–143
MPL mutations 144
pregnancy management 149–150
prognosis 147
TET2 mutations 144
treatment 148–150
unclassifiable 141

narrowband ultraviolet light B (NB-UVB), mycosis fungoides/Sézary syndrome 438

natural killer (NK)-cell leukemias
aggressive 240
mature 238–240

natural killer (NK)-cell neoplasms 242–244

natural killer T-cell lymphoma, nasal type *see* extranodal natural killer T-cell lymphoma, nasal type

necrobiotic xanthogranuloma 199
clinical signs 199
disease course 199
pathogenesis 199
treatment 199

nelarabine
lymphoblastic lymphoma 492
relapsed ALL treatment 59

neutropenia
management in ALL 58–59
myelodysplastic syndromes 108–109

nilotinib
CML 73, 75–76
Philadelphia-positive ALL 57

nitrogen mustard, mycosis fungoides/Sézary syndrome 439

non-Hodgkin lymphoma (NHL)
B-cell
cells of high-grade/low-grade 233
molecular genetics 263–266
epidemiology 308
HAART association 462
T-cell
ALK gene 268
molecular genetics 268
NPM1 gene mutation 268
see also named lymphomas

non-tyrosine kinase inhibitors, CML treatment 74–75

Notch signaling, T-ALL 491

NOTCH1 gene mutations
ALL 19, 46, 60
T-ALL 231

Notch1 inhibition, ALL 60

NPI-0052 proteasome inhibitor, mantle cell lymphoma 325

nuclear factor-κB (NF-κB)
Hodgkin lymphoma 371, 392
inhibition in primary effusion lymphoma 472

nuclear factor-κB (NF-κB) stabilizers, mantle cell lymphoma 327

nucleophosmin *(NPM1)* gene mutation
AML 17–18, 35–36
T-cell non-Hodgkin lymphoma 268

nucleoside analogs
mantle cell lymphoma 319–320
mycosis fungoides/Sézary syndrome 442
Waldenstrom's macroglobulinemia treatment 215–216

obatoclax, myelodysplastic syndromes 111

oblimersen sodium, CLL 91

ofatumumab, follicular lymphoma 354

older adults
ALL treatment 58
myelodysplastic syndrome risk 103

oligonucleotide microarrays, follicular lymphoma 341

omacetaxine, CML therapy 74–75

osteonecrosis of the jaw, multiple myeloma 172

osteoprotegerin, multiple myeloma 163–164

p16^{INK4a} tumor suppressor gene, lymphoma 269

p53 mutations
hairy cells 117
Hodgkin lymphoma 392–393
lymphoma 268–269
mantle cell lymphoma 311–312

pamidronate, multiple myeloma maintenance therapy 171

PDGFRB rearrangement 21

PEG-asparaginase, ALL treatment 59–60

pentostatin
CLL 87
salvage therapy 89
hairy cell leukemia 123
retreatment 125
infections 123
mycosis fungoides/Sézary syndrome 442–443

peripheral neuropathy
cryoglobulinemia 195
monoclonal gammopathy of undetermined significance-associated 196–198

peripheral T-cell lymphoma 410–426
chemotherapy 425
classification 410–411
diagnosis 410–411
HIV-related 476
imaging 411
IPI 411–412
Ki-67 proliferation index 412
management 425–426
not otherwise specified 268, 412
clinical features 413
pathology 412–413
novel agents 426
PIT 412
prognosis 411–413
staging 411

P-glycoprotein (Pgp) overexpression in AML 27–28

PHA-739538 multikinase inhibitor 74

Philadelphia chromosome
ALL 18, 45, 54–57
older adults 58
CML 20, 68–69

phlebotomy, polycythemia vera 148

phototherapy with psoralens and ultraviolet light (PUVA), mycosis fungoides/Sézary syndrome 437–438
with interferon 439–440

pixantrone, mantle cell lymphoma 320

plasma cell dyscrasias 155–175
diagnostic criteria 156

plasma cell leukemia 174–175
cytogenetics 175
definition 174–175
epidemiology 175
IgH translocation 175
prognosis 175
stem cell therapy 175
treatment 175

plasma cell myeloma 237–238

plasmablastic lymphoma 233, 466, 470–471
chemotherapy 471
clinical features 470
histology 471
pathologic features 470–471
prognosis 471
treatment 471
viral infections 470–471

PML gene 131–132

PML protein, acute promyelocytic leukemia 131–132

PML-RARα, acute promyelocytic leukemia 132–133

POEMS syndrome 156, 190–193
bone lesions 192
cyclophosphamide 193
diagnostic criteria 191
high-dose chemotherapy with stem cell transplantation 193
melphalan 193
pathogenesis 190
pathology 191–193
physical limitations 193
symptoms/signs 191
treatment 193
response 194
Waldenstrom's macroglobulinemia 210

polycythemia vera 141, 144
aspirin therapy 148
clinical manifestations 145–146
diagnosis 144–145
epidemiology 145
hydroxyurea 148
JAK2 mutations 147
laboratory features 146–147
phlebotomy 148
pregnancy 149–150
prognosis 147

polycythemia vera (*cont.*)
  risk stratification 148
  secondary 146
  treatment 148
  WHO classification 143
polymerase chain reaction (PCR), lymphomas 261–262
pomalidomide, primary myelofibrosis 149
positron emission tomography (PET)
  HIV-related primary central nervous system lymphoma 473
  see also ^{18}FDG positron emission tomography (FDG-PET)
positron emission tomography/computed tomography (PET/CT), lymphoma 278–279
post-transplant lymphoproliferative disorder of the central nervous system 458
power lines, high-voltage, ALL risk 44
PR171 (carfilzomib), mantle cell lymphoma 325
PRAD1 gene, mantle cell lymphoma 310
pralatrexate, peripheral T-cell lymphoma 426
prednisone, ALL treatment in older adults 58
pregnancy, myeloproliferative neoplasms 149–150
primary central nervous system lymphoma 449–457
  BCL6 tumor suppressor gene 451
  biology 449–450
  blood–brain barrier disruption 455
  chemotherapy 453–456
  combined modality therapy 453–455
  corticosteroids 451
  cytogenetics 449
  diagnosis 450–451
  high-dose chemotherapy with stem cell transplantation 455–456
  histology 450
  HIV-related 449, 466, 472–474
    chemotherapy 474
    clinical features 472–473
    CSF examination 473
    diagnosis 473
    EBV 473
    epidemiology 472
    HAART 473–474
    methotrexate 474
    neuroimaging 473
    pathology 473
    prognosis 473–474
    radiation therapy 473–474
    treatment 473–474
  immunophenotyping 449
  intrathecal chemotherapy 455
  methotrexate 453–456
  neuroimaging 450–452
    HIV-related 473
  neurotoxicity of treatment 456–457
  pathology 449–450
  primary intraocular lymphoma 450
  prognostic markers 451
  radiotherapy 452–453, 456
    in combined modality therapy 453–455
  rituximab 456
  salvage therapy 456
  stem cell transplantation 455–456
  surgery 452
  temozolomide 456
  topotecan 456
  treatment 451–457
primary effusion lymphoma 233, 466
  antiviral treatment 472
  chemotherapy 472
  clinical features 471
  gene expression profiling 472
  histology 472
  HIV-related 471–472
  NF-κB inhibition 472
  pathologic features 471–472
  prognosis 472
  proteasome inhibitors 472
  treatment 472
  viral infections 472
primary intraocular lymphoma (PIOL) 450
primary mediastinal large B-cell lymphoma (PMBL) 234, 266–267
  consolidative radiation 301
  pathology 301
  prognosis 301
  treatment 300–301
primary myelofibrosis 141, 144, 149
  clinical manifestations 146
  epidemiology 145
  hydroxyurea therapy 149
  JAK2 mutations 148
  laboratory features 147
  lenalidomide therapy 149
  pomalidomide therapy 149
  prognosis 147
  stem cell transplantation 148–149
  treatment 148–149
  WHO classification 143
primary T-cell lymphoma 242
  HIV-related 476
  not otherwise specified 242
Prognostic Index for PTCL, peripheral T-cell lymphoma 412
proteasome inhibitors
  follicular lymphoma 358
  mantle cell lymphoma 324–325
  primary effusion lymphoma 472
  resistance 324
  Waldenstrom's macroglobulinemia 217–218
protein kinase C (PKC) inhibitors, mantle cell lymphoma 327
proteosome inhibitors, mycosis fungoides/Sézary syndrome 444
PSC-833, AML management 27–28
purine nucleoside analogs
  CLL 86–87, 90–91
  hairy cell leukemia 122–124
    retreatment 125
5q-syndrome 105
radiation therapy
  HIV-related primary central nervous system lymphoma 473–474
  Hodgkin lymphoma 383–384
  mycosis fungoides/Sézary syndrome 439
  myelodysplastic syndrome risk 103
  primary central nervous system lymphoma 452–453, 456
radioimmunotherapy
  follicular lymphoma 356–357
  Hodgkin lymphoma 392
  mantle cell lymphoma 320, 323–324
  primary nodal marginal zone lymphoma 407
radiologists, CML risk 68
RANKL (receptor activator of nuclear factor-κB ligand), multiple myeloma 163–164
rapamycin, ALL treatment 60
RARα, acute promyelocytic leukemia 132
  variant translocations 133
Reed–Sternberg cells *see* Hodgkin and Reed–Sternberg (H-RS) cells
refractory anemia 105–106
  with excess of blasts (RAEB) 105–106
  with excess of blasts in transformation (RAEB-t) 105–106
  with ringed sideroblasts (RARS) 105–106
  with ringed sideroblasts and thrombocytosis (RARS-T) 107
renal insufficiency
  cryoglobulinemia 195
  multiple myeloma 173–174
resistance modulation, AML 27–28
retinoic acid receptor alpha (RARA) abnormalities in AML 17
retinoids, mycosis fungoides/Sézary syndrome 439, 440
reverse transcriptase-polymerase chain reaction (RT-PCR), CML 69
rheumatoid arthritis, Hodgkin lymphoma association 370
rituximab
  ALL treatment 55, 60
  B-cell lymphoma monotherapy 346–347
  CLL 84, 87
    fludarabine-refractory patients 91
    salvage therapy 89–90
  cryoglobulinemia 196
  diffuse large B-cell lymphoma 291
    advanced disease 291–292
    CNS recurrence 295–296
    induction therapy 294
    treatment improvement 293
  follicular lymphoma 344–347
    chemotherapy combination 354–356
    extended schedules 347–351
    maintenance therapy 347–351
    maintenance therapy following chemoimmunotherapy 349–351
    maintenance therapy following chemotherapy 349

gastric MALT lymphoma 405
hairy cell leukemia salvage therapy 125
HIV-related diffuse large B-cell lymphoma 465–468
HIV-related multicentric Castleman's disease 477
Hodgkin lymphoma 391–392
HyperCVAD regimen combination 318
mantle cell lymphoma 320–322
monoclonal gammopathy of undetermined significance with peripheral neuropathy 198
nodular lymphocyte predominant Hodgkin lymphoma 387–388
primary central nervous system lymphoma 456
resistance 351
Waldenstrom's macroglobulinemia treatment 216–217

RNAse A, follicular lymphoma 353

romidepsin, mycosis fungoides/Sézary syndrome 442

romiplostim, myelodysplastic syndromes 109

sarcoidosis, Hodgkin lymphoma association 370

Schnitzler's syndrome 199–200
diagnosis 200
disease progression 200
laboratory findings 199–200
pathophysiology 199
treatment 200

scleromyxedema 198–199
clinical signs 198
diagnosis 198
pathogenesis 198
pathology 198
treatment 198–199

gamma-secretase inhibitor (GSI) 491

serum free light chain assay 155–158
monoclonal gammopathy of undetermined significance 160–161

serum immunofixation (IF) 155

serum protein electrophoresis (SPEP) 155
multiple myeloma 159

Sézary syndrome 243–244, 432–445
alemtuzumab 441
bexarotene 439–440
biologic characteristics 433–434
bortezomib 444
carmustine 439
chemotherapy
multiagent 443
single-agent 442–443
classification 432–433, 436
clinical signs 432, 434–435
corticosteroids 438
denileukin diftitox 441
diagnosis 435–436
epidemiology 432
etiology 432–433
extracorporeal photopheresis 440–441
fludarabine 443
gemcitabine 442
histone deacetylase inhibitors 441–442
IL-2 444
IL-12 444
immunodeficiency 433–434
immunomodulatory agents 444
immunophenotyping 435
interferon 439–440
lactate dehydrogenase 435, 437
lenalidomide 444
management 435–436
molecular characteristics 433–434
monoclonal antibodies 441
investigational 444
nitrogen mustard 439
p16^{INK4a} tumor suppressor gene 269
pathogenesis 433
pegylated doxorubicin 442
pentostatin 442–443
phototherapy 437–438
prognosis 444–445
prognostic markers 437
proteosome inhibitors 444
radiation therapy 439
retinoids 439–440
romidepsin 442
staging 436–437
stem cell transplantation 443
survival 437
T helper cell dysregulation 433–434
temozolomide 443
treatment 437–444
algorithm 438
investigational 444
systemic 439–443
topical 437–439
vorinostat 442
zanolimumab 444

single nucleotide polymorphisms (SNPs)
follicular lymphoma 341
mantle cell lymphoma 315–316

single photon emission computed tomography (SPECT), HIV-related primary CNS lymphoma 473

SKI-606, ALL treatment 60

small lymphocytic lymphoma (SLL) 81

smoldering myeloma (SMM) 155

solitary plasmacytoma 155
of bone 237–238
diagnostic criteria 156

Southern blot analysis, lymphomas 260

spinal cord compression, multiple myeloma 172

spleen, hairy cell leukemia 118–119

splenectomy
cryoglobulinemia 196
HIV-related multicentric Castleman's disease 477

splenic lymphoma with villous lymphocytes (SLVL) 121

splenic marginal zone lymphoma 236–237

stem cell transplantation
acute promyelocytic leukemia 136–137
adult T-cell leukemia/lymphoma 420–421
ALL treatment 51–53, 56
relapsed disease 59
allogeneic
anaplastic large cell lymphoma 419
Burkitt lymphoma 499–500
CLL 91–93
diffuse large B-cell lymphoma 299–300
follicular lymphoma 358
Hodgkin lymphoma 385, 388
lymphoblastic lymphoma 491
mantle cell lymphoma 323
AML management 28–31, 36
relapse risk 30–31
second remission 31
amyloidosis 186
anaplastic large cell lymphoma 419
autologous
adult T-cell leukemia/lymphoma 420–421
Burkitt lymphoma 499–500
CLL 91
diffuse large B-cell lymphoma 296–299
follicular lymphoma 357–358
lymphoblastic lymphoma 490–491
Burkitt lymphoma 499–500
CLL 91–93
CML 70
diffuse large B-cell lymphoma
with high-dose chemotherapy 294–295
relapsed disease 296–299
extranodal natural killer T-cell lymphoma, nasal type 422
follicular lymphoma 357–358
hepatosplenic T-cell lymphoma 423
with high-dose chemotherapy
amyloidosis 186
diffuse large B-cell lymphoma 294–295
extranodal natural killer T-cell lymphoma, nasal type 422
follicular lymphoma 357–358
hepatosplenic T-cell lymphoma 423
HIV-related lymphomas 477–478
mantle cell lymphoma 320–321
POEMS syndrome 193
primary central nervous system lymphoma 455–456
TBI in conditioning regimen 320, 323–324
HIV-related lymphomas 477–478
Hodgkin lymphoma
allogeneic 385, 388
autologous 385–387
chemotherapy-alone conditioning 385
prognosis 385–387
radiation-based conditioning 385
lymphoblastic lymphoma 490–491
mantle cell lymphoma 321
with high-dose therapy 320
multiple myeloma 165, 169–170
mycosis fungoides/Sézary syndrome 443
myelodysplastic syndromes 112
non-myeloablative 92–93, 300
plasma cell leukemia 175
POEMS syndrome 193
primary central nervous system lymphoma 455–456
primary myelofibrosis 148–149

stem cell transplantation (*cont.*)
primary nodal marginal zone lymphoma 407
reduced intensity transplants 300
relapse risk in AML 30–31
Waldenstrom's macroglobulinemia 219–220
subcutaneous panniculitis-like T-cell lymphoma 243
SYK gene, peripheral T-cell lymphoma, not otherwise specified 268
systemic amyloidosis *see* amyloidosis, systemic
systemic anaplastic large cell lymphoma 240–242, 415–419
systemic EBV-positive T-cell LPD of childhood 244
systemic mastocytosis 141
T-cell/histiocyte-rich large B-cell lymphoma (THRLBCL) 234
T cells, follicular lymphoma 339
tartrate-resistant acid phosphatase (TRAP), hairy cell leukemia 119, 120
T-bet transcription factor, hairy cell leukemia 120
T-cell large granular lymphocytic leukemia (T-LGLL) 238–239
T-cell leukemias, mature 238–240
T-cell lymphomas
CNS lymphoma 449
HIV-related 476
chemotherapy 476
clinical features 476
EBV 476
epidemiology 476
pathologic features 476
prognosis 476
treatment 476
molecular aberrations 260
primary 242
HIV-related 476
not otherwise specified 242
see also cutaneous T-cell lymphomas; hepatosplenic T-cell lymphoma; peripheral T-cell lymphoma
T-cell neoplasms
extranodal mature 242–244
nodal mature 242
T-cell non-Hodgkin lymphoma, molecular genetics 268
T-cell prolymphocytic leukemia 239–240
T-cell regulatory cells (Tregs), Hodgkin lymphoma 375
TCR gene rearrangements
lymphoid malignancy clonal marker 257–258
lymphoma 257
PCR analysis 261
temozolomide
mycosis fungoides/Sézary syndrome 443
primary central nervous system lymphoma 456
temsirolimus, mantle cell lymphoma 325
TET2 mutations, myeloproliferative neoplasms 144
thalidomide
amyloidosis treatment 189
mantle cell lymphoma 325
multiple myeloma 171
maintenance therapy 171
side effects 173–174
smoldering multiple myeloma 161–162
Waldenstrom's macroglobulinemia 218–219
thalidomide-dexamethasone, multiple myeloma 167–168, 171
6-thioguanine, ALL treatment 57
thrombocytopenia, myelodysplastic syndromes 109
tipifarnib, AML management 37
T-lymphoblastic leukemia/ lymphoma (T-ALL/LBL) 231
topoisomerase II inhibitors
myelodysplastic syndrome risk 103
therapy-related ALL 43
topotecan, primary central nervous system lymphoma 456
tositumomab, mantle cell lymphoma 323–324
total body irradiation (TBI), mantle cell lymphoma 320
TP53 gene, lymphoma 268–269
trisomy 8
AML 17
CML 69
trisomy 21, ALL risk 43
troponin T, amyloidosis 190
tumor lysis syndrome
ALL 53, 59
Burkitt lymphoma 497
tyrosine kinase inhibitors
AML management 36
CML 70–72, 75
second-generation 72–74
myelodysplastic syndromes 111
Philadelphia-positive ALL 55–57
second-generation 72–76
ubiquitin–proteasome pathway 358
urine immunofixation (IF) 155
urine protein electrophoresis (UPEP) 155
valganciclovir, primary effusion lymphoma 472
vertebroplasty, multiple myeloma 172
VGEF-trap, mantle cell lymphoma 325
vincristine
ALL treatment 48–50
adolescents and young adults 57
older adults 58
sphingosomal preparation 59
vitamin D deficiency, multiple myeloma 172
vorinostat, mycosis fungoides/ Sézary syndrome 442
Waldenstrom's macroglobulinemia (WM) 155, 207–221
alkylator therapy 215
autoantibody activity 210
biochemical investigations 212
bone marrow
biochemistry 213
microenvironment 208
bortezomib therapy 217–218
CD20-directed antibody therapy 216
chromosome 6 deletions 207
cladribine 217
clinical features 208–209
clonal cells 207–208
cold agglutinin hemolytic anemia 211
cryoglobulinemia 210–211
cyclophosphamide therapy 216–217
cytogenetics 207
diagnostic criteria 156
epidemiology 207
etiology 207
fludarabine 217
genetic factors 207
hematologic abnormalities 212
hyperviscosity syndrome 208–210, 212–213
IgM 212
physicochemical/ immunologic properties 209
tissue deposition 211–212
treatment response 220–221
IgM multiple myeloma differential diagnosis 174
IgM-mediated morbidity 208–212
IgM-related neuropathy 210
imaging 213
laboratory investigations 208–209, 212–213
lenalidomide 218–219
lymph node biopsy 213
neoplastic cell infiltration 212
nucleoside analog therapy 215–216
pathogenesis 207
prognosis 213
prognostic scoring systems 214
proteasome inhibitor therapy 217–218
rituximab therapy 216–217
Schnitzler's syndrome progression 200
serum viscosity 212–213
stem cell transplantation 219–220
thalidomide therapy 218–219
treatment 213–221
combination 216–217
frontline 214–217
high-dose with stem cell transplantation 219–220
response criteria 220–221
salvage therapy 217–219
Wilms tumor, AML 18
Wnt signaling pathway, mantle cell lymphoma 311–312
World Health Organization (WHO)
ALL classification 44
Burkitt lymphoma classification 494–496
CLL classification 81
essential thrombocythemia classification 143
follicular lymphoma classification 235–236
lymphoid neoplasm classification 463, 487
lymphoma classification 228–247, 410, 463, 487
clinical features 229
clinical implications 229
entities 229–246

essential elements 228–229
genetic aberrations 228
immunophenotype 228
morphology 228
myelodysplastic syndrome classification 106
myeloid neoplasms classification 142
myeloproliferative neoplasms classification 141–143
polycythemia vera classification 143
primary myelofibrosis classification 143

World Health Organization – European Organization for Research and Treatment of Cancer (WHO–EORTC), cutaneous lymphoma classification 246–247

WT1 gene, AML 18

XIAP antiapoptotic molecule, Hodgkin lymphoma 392

XL228 multikinase inhibitor 74

zanolimumab, mycosis fungoides/Sézary syndrome 444

ZAP-70 expression, CLL 84

zidovudine, adult T-cell leukemia/lymphoma 420

Zosquidar, AML management 27–28